Textbook of Equine Veterinary Nursing

Textbook of Equine Veterinary Nursing

Edited by Rosina Lillywhite and Marie Rippingale

WILEY Blackwell

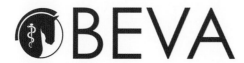

The contents of this book have been approved by The British Equine Veterinary Association (BEVA)

This edition first published 2025
© 2025 John Wiley & Sons Ltd

Registered Offices
John Wiley & Sons, Inc., 111 River Street, Hoboken, NJ 07030, USA
John Wiley & Sons Ltd, New Era House, 8 Oldlands Way, Bognor Regis, West Sussex, PO22 9NQ, UK

For details of our global editorial offices, customer services, and more information about Wiley products visit us at www.wiley.com.

Wiley also publishes its books in a variety of electronic formats and by print-on-demand. Some content that appears in standard print versions of this book may not be available in other formats.

Library of Congress Cataloging-in-Publication Data applied for:

Paperback ISBN: 9781119861942

Cover Design: Wiley
Cover Images: Courtesy of Dr Franci Boyer, Marie Rippingale, and Sarah Baillie

Set in 9.5/12.5pt STIXTwoText by Straive, Pondicherry, India

Printed in Singapore
M120246_041224

Contents

List of Contributors

Tamsyn Amos
Priestwood Physiotherapy
Sitterlow Farm
Parwich
Ashbourne
UK

Sarah Baillie
Equine Veterinary Medical Center
Doha
Qatar

Alison Bennell
Philip Leverhulme Equine Hospital
University of Liverpool
Wirral
UK

Lyndsey Bett
Glasgow Equine Hospital and Practice
University of Glasgow
Weipers Centre
Glasgow
UK

Jane Devaney
Philip Leverhulme Equine Hospital
University of Liverpool
Wirral
UK

Dominique Doyle
The Donkey Sanctuary
Sidmouth
Devon
UK

Natalie Karla Fisk
Rossdales Equine Hospital & Diagnostic Centre
Newmarket
Suffolk
UK

Victoria Gregory
Glasgow Equine Hospital and Practice
University of Glasgow
Weipers Centre
Glasgow
UK

Lisa Harrison
Rossdales Equine Hospital & Diagnostic Centre
Newmarket
Suffolk
UK

Rosie Heath
Mickleham
Dorking
Surrey
UK

Kassie Hill
Cliffe Equine Vets
Harbens Farm
East Sussex
England
UK

Susan L. Holt
University of Bristol
Bristol
UK

George Hunt
E C Straiton & Partners LTD
The Veterinary Hospital
Penkridge
Stafford
UK

Lynn Irving
Village Vet
Milton
England
UK

Kate Lambert
Pool House Equine Hospital
Crown Inn Farm
Lichfield
UK

Nicola Rose
Ash Vale
Guildford
Surrey
UK

Kate Loomes
Rainbow Equine Hospital
Rainbow Farm
Malton
North Yorkshire
UK

Lucy Middlecote
Linnaeus Veterinary Limited
Solihull
West Midlands
UK

Bonny Millar
Equicomms
CVS House
Norfolk
UK

Victoria Milne
Lantra Awards
Stoneleigh Park
Coventry
UK

Louise Pailor
Wright and Morten Equine Clinic
Somerford Park Clinic

Somerford
England
UK

Judith Parry
Bottle Green Training Ltd
Derby
UK

Sophie Pearson
Bottle Green Training Ltd
Derby
UK

Phillippa Pritchard
Liphook Equine Hospital
Liphook
Hampshire
UK

Marie Rippingale
Bottle Green Training Ltd
Derby
UK

Rosina Lillywhite
VetPartners Nursing School
Greenforde Business Park
Petersfield
UK

Chloe Skewes
The Donkey Sanctuary
Sidmouth
Devon
UK

Nicola Smith
Lantra Awards
Coventry
England
UK

Cassie Woods
Lower House Equine Clinic
Plas Cerrig Lane
Llanymynech
Oswestry
Shropshire
Llanymynech
UK

Foreword

During the past 20 years, there has been tremendous progress in the teaching and training of equine veterinary nurses (EVNs) in the United Kingdom. There are now several well-established colleges across the country that offer a range of excellent courses through which qualification can be achieved. I am constantly impressed by the dedication, enthusiasm, rigour and thoroughness with which both trainees and teachers carry out EVN training, and it is a privilege to write a foreword to this new *Textbook of Equine Veterinary Nursing*.

Creating a supportive and collaborative environment in which knowledge is gained, transferred and disseminated is essential for professional development. I consider myself extremely fortunate to have worked in Peter Rossdales' practice for the past 27 years, where the culture and ethos encourages talented individuals to better themselves. My surgical mentor, colleague and former business partner, Professor Tim Greet, undoubtedly deserves huge credit for his work in championing the cause of the skilled, dedicated modern EVNs. Together with my colleagues, as a practice, we remain hugely invested in our equine veterinary nursing team, and in the veterinary nursing profession at large. This of course has paid great dividends whereby EVNs are undoubtedly the foundation on which the delivery of first-class patient care in our hospital depends. It has been, and continues to be, a real delight to see trainee nurses joining our team, flourish and become highly skilled individuals who often develop specialist areas of expertise and niche interests.

One of my frustrations has been that EVN careers did not have sufficient longevity. Too many good nurses became lost, professionally unsatisfied or disillusioned. I am pleased that modern flexible working and better prospects of pay and career progression have allowed many valuable individuals to be retained within nursing teams and to exert influence within leadership roles.

In 2025, there is an unprecedented recruitment and retention problem for veterinary surgeons within our profession. In my view, it is essential that veterinary nurses are considered an important part of the solution for this. Now is an ideal time for the modern equine nursing profession to step up and seize opportunities for sustained long-term career progress. There must of course be appropriate recognition and remuneration for the level of skill and responsibility. This is very much parallel to our National Health Service, where nurses and nurse practitioners are now recognised as an incredibly important resource upon which our human health care infrastructure depends.

I believe that EVNs and their supporting bodies should look forward optimistically to the future and be encouraged to embrace the opportunities which allow equine veterinary nursing to reach another level of excellence. This will of course require changes in the Veterinary Surgeons Act and in particular Schedule 3. I believe this matter is under current and continued review by the Royal College of Veterinary Surgeons, and I sincerely hope this is seen as an opportunity rather than a threat.

For all that I have mentioned about the importance of teaching, training, learning and collaboration, it is also important to have consolidated reference to the current wealth of information in one place. For this reason, I am delighted that this fantastic brand new textbook has been produced. I have no doubt that it will become the 'Gold Standard' of reference for current and future generations of veterinary nurses.

I wholeheartedly congratulate the authors and editors for the dedication and attention to detail which has gone into putting together this comprehensive textbook. As our knowledge continues to advance, and as the equine nursing profession continues to evolve, let us hope that this book will become the first of many editions in the years to come.

Richard Payne
Specialist in Equine Surgery
Clinical Director, Rossdales Equine Hospital

Preface

A lot has changed in the world of equine veterinary nursing since the first equine nursing qualification was launched over 20 years ago. These changes inspired us to write a new textbook for equine veterinary nurses. This book has taken into consideration the significant changes to the different equine nursing syllabi and the changing tide within equine nursing. This was designed to be a book written by equine nurses for equine nurses.

Equine veterinary nursing is a field that demands dedication, knowledge and a deep understanding of equine anatomy and physiology, behaviour and veterinary care. As the bond between humans and horses strengthens, the importance of skilled and compassionate equine nursing professionals is becoming increasingly evident.

This comprehensive textbook is designed to serve as an indispensable guide for students, practising equine veterinary nurses and anyone who has a passion for gold standard equine veterinary care. Whether you are just starting your journey into equine veterinary nursing or are an experienced professional seeking to expand your knowledge and skills, this book will be a reliable source of information and guidance.

This book has been designed to provide readers with a well-rounded understanding of equine health, welfare and nursing care to ensure that the highest standards of veterinary care and animal welfare are delivered in practice. To achieve this, the textbook is organised into thematic sections that will lead the reader carefully through the various aspects of equine veterinary nursing care. We hope the layout will suit learners with a diverse range of learning styles, as chapters contain a wealth of knowledge based on the most up-to-date resources and practical tips from experts in the field. Illustrations, photographs and charts support the content to enhance readers' understanding.

We express our gratitude to the countless equine nursing professionals and veterinarians whose dedication and passion have contributed to the development of this textbook and to our families for their support during this process.

We hope it will be a valuable resource in the journey towards becoming an exceptional equine veterinary nurse.

Marie Rippingale – acknowledgements: I extend particular thanks to Dr. Francis Boyer for his endless tolerance and support, and for contributing so many fantastic photographs that were used as figures in this textbook. Thanks also to my horses, Harry and Boris, and my donkeys, Billy and Tilly, for being such fantastic models for those photographs. I also extend my appreciation to Nicole-Kingsley-Smith (owner of Boris) and my parents, Raymond and Margaret Rippingale, for all their help and unwavering support throughout this journey. A special thanks has to go to Petal, my little springer spaniel and constant companion, who has been present by my side throughout every meeting, writing and editing session for this manuscript.

Rosina Lillywhite – acknowledgements: I extend my heartfelt gratitude to my husband, Carl Lillywhite, for his unwavering support throughout the writing journey. This endeavour would have been far more daunting without his steadfast encouragement. In addition, I express my deepest appreciation to my two incredible children: Olivia and Jacob. Their enthusiasm for my work in equine nursing and their eagerness to learn about ways to aid equids have been a constant source of inspiration and joy.

Our hope is that this book not only equips you with the skills and knowledge you need but also nurtures a deep appreciation for the remarkable work equine veterinary practice offers. We invite you to embark on this educational journey with enthusiasm and dedication, as equine veterinary nursing is not just a profession but a calling that requires a heartfelt commitment to the well-being of the equine patients in our care.

May this textbook be your guide, reference and inspiration as you explore the multifaceted world of Equine Veterinary Nursing.

Rosina Lillywhite and Marie Rippingale

About the Companion Website

This book is accompanied by a companion website:

www.wiley.com/go/equineveterinarynursing

This website includes:

- Images used in the text as Chapter wise PPTs
- MCQs

1

Operational Requirements in Equine Practice

Rosina Lillywhite

VetPartners Nursing School, Petersfield, United Kingdom

Glossary

Hazard A hazard is a dangerous phenomenon, substance, human activity or condition. It may cause loss of life, injury or other health impacts and property damage [1].

Risk Risk is the possibility of something bad happening. Risk involves uncertainty about the effects/implications of an activity concerning something that humans value, often focusing on negative, undesirable consequences [1].

Risk assessment A risk assessment is simply a careful examination of what could cause harm to people to enable precautions to be taken to prevent injury and ill health [1].

1.1 Aims of Health and Safety

Effective health and safety within a veterinary practice aims to ensure the well-being and safety of all individuals involved, including staff, clients and animals. The specific aims can be summarised as follows:

- Reduction of risks: Effective health and safety practices aim to identify, assess and minimise risks within the veterinary practice. This involves conducting thorough risk assessments to identify potential hazards, such as dangerous equipment, hazardous substances or unsafe working conditions. The risks can be significantly reduced or eliminated by implementing appropriate controls and safety measures, such as providing personal protective equipment (PPE), establishing safe work procedures and maintaining a clean and organised environment.

- Utilising assessments, controls and quality improvement: Health and safety assessments are crucial to identify hazards and assess risks within the veterinary practice. Regular inspections and evaluations of the premises, equipment and procedures are conducted to ensure compliance with relevant health and safety regulations. Controls, such as engineering controls like ventilation systems and administrative controls like training programs, are implemented to prevent or minimise risks. Additionally, continuous quality improvement processes are established to monitor and enhance health and safety practices within the veterinary practice.

- Identification of animals: It is essential to accurately identify animals within a veterinary practice to ensure proper care and minimise potential risks. This involves maintaining thorough records that include the animal's identity, such as name, species, breed, age and any relevant medical history. Additionally, information regarding the animal's temperament and behaviour is essential for staff to handle and interact with the animals safely and appropriately. Each patient should have an identity tag attached to their mane and additional tags attached to any equipment that clients leave at the practice. Details on the tag include the name of the patient, the name of the client, the procedure to be performed and the date the patient was admitted.

Effective health and safety measures within a veterinary practice consider clients' and staff's specific needs and vulnerabilities. Some individuals may be at special risk due to various factors, such as:

- Asthma: Steps should be taken to minimise exposure to allergens or irritants that could trigger asthma attacks. This may involve proper ventilation, regular cleaning and avoiding known allergens.

Textbook of Equine Veterinary Nursing, First Edition. Edited by Rosina Lillywhite and Marie Rippingale.
© 2025 John Wiley & Sons Ltd. Published 2025 by John Wiley & Sons Ltd.
Companion website: www.wiley.com/go/equineveterinarynursing

- Visual or hearing impediments: Adequate measures should be in place to ensure effective communication with individuals who have visual or hearing impairments. This may include using visual aids, written instructions or providing sign language interpreters.
- Impaired literacy: Clear and easily understandable communication materials should be provided to accommodate individuals with impaired literacy. This could involve using visual aids, simple language and providing necessary assistance.
- Pregnancy: Pregnant staff members should be provided with appropriate information and support to ensure their safety and the well-being of the developing foetus. This may involve modifying work tasks or providing additional protective measures.
- Age: Special consideration should be given to younger and older individuals regarding their physical capabilities and vulnerabilities. Adjustments may be necessary to accommodate their specific needs and ensure their safety (adjustments may include ensuring the elderly can sit if required and the young are not left unattended on a yard).
- Disabilities: Individuals with disabilities should be provided with reasonable accommodations to ensure their safety and ability to perform their job responsibilities effectively. This may include modifying workstations, providing assistive devices or offering additional support as needed.

By considering the specific needs and risks associated with these individuals, veterinary practices can create a safe and inclusive environment that promotes the well-being of all staff and clients.

1.2 Health and Safety Legislation

In the United Kingdom, health and safety legislation is governed by various acts and regulations that aim to protect worker's and the general public's health, safety and welfare. The primary legislation that forms the foundation of health and safety regulations in the United Kingdom is the Health and Safety at Work Act 1974 (HSWA) and other health and safety legislation in the United Kingdom include [2]:

Health and Safety at Work Act 1974 (HSWA)

This is a primary piece of legislation in the United Kingdom that sets out the legal framework for workplace health and safety. It applies to all employers, employees, self-employed individuals and anyone who controls workplaces and the health and safety of others. Some key aspects of the HSWA are as follows [2]:

- General duties [2]: The HSWA places general duties on employers, employees, self-employed individuals and others to ensure the health, safety and welfare of individuals at work. These duties include:
  - Employers: Have a duty to provide a safe working environment, including safe equipment, proper training and competent supervision. Employers must also ensure the health and safety of others who may be affected by the work activities, such as visitors or the public.
  - Employees: Have a duty to take reasonable care of their own health and safety, as well as that of others who may be affected by their actions at work. They should follow the provided training, use safety equipment properly and report any hazards or concerns to their employer.
  - Self-employed individuals: They are responsible for ensuring their health and safety and that of others affected by their work activities. They must safely conduct their work and comply with relevant regulations.
- Risk assessment: The HSWA requires employers to conduct risk assessments to identify hazards in the workplace and evaluate the associated risks. Risk assessments should be reviewed regularly and updated as necessary. The aim is to identify suitable control measures to eliminate or minimise risks to health and safety.
- Consultation and information: The HSWA emphasises the importance of consultation and communication between employers and employees regarding health and safety matters. Employers must consult with safety representatives or employee representatives on health and safety issues, and employees should be provided with relevant information and training.
- Enforcement and inspections: The Health and Safety Executive (HSE) is the regulatory body responsible for enforcing health and safety laws in Great Britain. The Act grants the HSE powers to inspect workplaces, investigate accidents, issue improvement or prohibition notices if necessary and prosecute those who fail to comply with the legislation.
- Offences and penalties: The HSWA establishes various offences and penalties for non-compliance with health and safety duties. Serious breaches of the HSWA can result in fines, imprisonment or both. The Act also provides for the liability of company directors, managers and other individuals who have consented to or connived in an offence.
- Application to other workplaces: The HSWA applies to a wide range of workplaces, including offices, factories,

construction sites, mines, offshore installations and other premises where people work. It also covers activities that may affect the health and safety of individuals, such as construction work, maintenance and use of equipment.

- The HSWA 1974 is a broad and comprehensive piece of legislation that sets the foundation for health and safety management in the United Kingdom. It establishes the general duties and responsibilities of employers, employees and others and provides a legal framework for promoting a safe and healthy working environment.

Management of Health and Safety at Work Regulations 1999

The Management of Health and Safety at Work Regulations 1999 (MHSWR) is pivotal in ensuring workers' health, safety and welfare in the United Kingdom. These regulations, introduced under the HSWA, provide a comprehensive framework for managing workplace risks and fostering a safety culture. The key provisions of the MHSWR highlight their significance in safeguarding workplace well-being [3].

Risk Assessment
Central to the MHSWR is the requirement for employers to systematically assess workplace risks. Risk assessment involves identifying hazards, evaluating their potential harm and implementing suitable mitigation control measures. This process is critical for creating a safe working environment and preventing accidents, injuries and occupational illnesses [4].

Competent Personnel
Under the MHSWR, employers are obligated to appoint competent individuals to assist with health and safety management. These competent persons possess the necessary knowledge, skills and experience to provide expert guidance on risk assessment, control measures and compliance with relevant regulations. Their involvement ensures that health and safety considerations are prioritised and effectively addressed [3].

Health Surveillance
The regulations recognise the importance of monitoring workers' health in certain high-risk occupations. Employers must implement health surveillance measures to assess and monitor the impact of work-related hazards on employees' well-being. This may involve regular medical examinations, assessments and monitoring of specific health indicators to detect early signs of work-related illnesses and take appropriate preventive measures [3].

Information, Instruction and Training
Effective communication and education form the cornerstone of the MHSWR. Employers are required to provide employees with comprehensive information, instruction and training to ensure they have the necessary knowledge and skills to carry out their work safely. This includes informing workers about potential hazards, safe working practices, emergency procedures and correctly using PPE.

Cooperation and Collaboration
The MHSWR emphasises the importance of cooperation and collaboration between employers, employees and safety representatives. Employers should consult with workers and their representatives on health and safety matters, providing them opportunities to contribute their expertise, report concerns and participate in decision-making processes. This collaborative approach fosters shared responsibility for workplace safety.

Record Keeping
Accurate record keeping is an essential aspect of the MHSWR. Employers must maintain records of risk assessments, training, accidents, incidents and any measures taken to control workplace risks. These records serve as valuable resources for monitoring compliance, identifying trends, evaluating the effectiveness of control measures, and facilitating continuous improvement in health and safety performance.

Workplace (Health, Safety and Welfare) Regulations 1992

These regulations aim to ensure the health, safety and welfare of individuals in workplaces. These regulations provide guidance on various aspects of the working environment to create safe and healthy conditions for employees. Some key provisions of the Workplace Regulations are as follows [3]:

Workplace Conditions
The regulations outline specific requirements for workplace conditions, including ventilation, temperature, lighting, cleanliness and space. Employers are obligated to provide adequate ventilation to maintain a suitable working environment and prevent discomfort due to a lack of fresh air. They must also ensure that the workplace temperature is reasonable and comfortable, considering factors such as the nature of the work being carried out. Adequate lighting is essential to prevent accidents and facilitate safe working conditions. Additionally, employers are responsible for maintaining cleanliness and providing sufficient space to ensure the welfare and well-being of employees.

Sanitary Facilities

The Workplace Regulations emphasise the provision of adequate sanitary facilities. Employers must provide clean and functional toilets, washbasins and other necessary facilities for personal hygiene. These facilities should be conveniently located and maintained in good working order to ensure the health and welfare of employees.

Drinking Water

The regulations require employers to provide suitable drinking water for employees. The water should be easily accessible, clean and free from any potential contamination that may pose a risk to health. Employers must ensure the water supply is regularly checked and maintained to meet appropriate standards.

Rest and Break Areas

Employers are encouraged to provide rest and break areas to allow employees to take regular breaks and rest periods during the workday. These areas should be clean, comfortable and adequately equipped to enable employees to relax and take their breaks in a suitable environment.

Traffic Routes and Passageways

The Workplace Regulations address the need for safe traffic routes and passageways within workplaces. Employers must ensure that pedestrian routes are clearly marked, free from obstructions and designed to prevent accidents and injuries. Adequate measures should be in place to separate pedestrians from vehicles and to ensure the safe movement of vehicles within the workplace.

Safety in Maintenance and Repair

The regulations highlight the importance of maintaining a safe environment during maintenance and repair work. Employers must take measures to prevent potential hazards arising from maintenance activities, such as ensuring the safe use of equipment, providing appropriate training and implementing suitable control measures to safeguard the well-being of employees involved in such work.

Compliance and Enforcement

The Workplace Regulations are enforced by the HSE in Great Britain and the Health and Safety Executive for Northern Ireland (HSENI) in Northern Ireland. These bodies may conduct inspections and investigations to ensure compliance with the regulations. Non-compliance with the Workplace Regulations can lead to enforcement action, including fines or prosecution.

The Workplace (Health, Safety and Welfare) Regulations 1992 provide a comprehensive framework for maintaining safe and healthy working conditions. They place specific obligations on employers to ensure appropriate workplace conditions, sanitary facilities, drinking water, rest areas and safe traffic routes. Compliance with these regulations helps protect employees' well-being and welfare and creates a conducive environment for productivity and overall workplace satisfaction.

Control of Substances Hazardous to Health (COSHH) Regulations 2002

COSHH is a set of regulations in the United Kingdom that aim to protect workers from the risks associated with exposure to hazardous substances. These regulations place responsibilities on employers to control and manage hazardous substances in the workplace. Some key aspects of the COSHH Regulations are as follows.

Hazardous Substances

The COSHH Regulations define hazardous substances as any substances that have the potential to cause harm to health. This includes substances classified as toxic, harmful, corrosive, irritant or sensitising, as well as carcinogenic, mutagenic or harmful to reproduction. The regulations apply to a wide range of substances, including chemicals, dusts, fumes, gases and biological agents.

Risk Assessment

Employers must conduct a thorough risk assessment for all hazardous substances in the workplace. The assessment involves identifying and evaluating the risks associated with the substances, considering factors such as exposure routes, the nature of the work and the potential health effects. The aim is to implement suitable control measures to eliminate or minimise the risks.

Control Measures

Based on the risk assessment, employers must implement control measures to prevent or adequately control exposure to hazardous substances. Control measures may include substituting hazardous substances with less harmful alternatives, using engineering controls such as ventilation or enclosure systems, implementing safe work practices, providing PPE and ensuring proper storage, handling and disposal of hazardous substances.

Monitoring and Health Surveillance

The COSHH Regulations emphasise the importance of monitoring and health surveillance to assess and manage the health risks associated with hazardous substances. Employers may be required to monitor the levels of hazardous substances in the workplace atmosphere and regularly review exposure measurements. Health surveillance involves monitoring the health of employees who are exposed to hazardous substances to detect early signs of any adverse health effects and take appropriate preventive measures.

Information, Instruction and Training

Employers have a duty to provide employees with comprehensive information, instruction and training regarding the hazardous substances they may encounter in their work. This includes providing details about the potential risks, control measures in place, safe working practices and emergency procedures. Training should also cover the proper use, maintenance and limitations of any PPE provided.

Storage, Handling and Disposal

The COSHH Regulations set out requirements for the safe storage, handling and disposal of hazardous substances. Employers must ensure that hazardous substances are stored in appropriate containers, clearly labelled and stored in designated areas to prevent accidental exposure. Proper handling procedures, including the use of suitable equipment and precautions, should be followed. Disposal of hazardous substances must be carried out in accordance with relevant regulations and guidelines.

Record Keeping and HSE Notifications

Employers are required to maintain records of risk assessments, monitoring results, health surveillance and training provided to employees. These records serve as evidence of compliance and support the ongoing management of hazardous substances in the workplace. In some instances, employers may need to notify the HSE about the use of particularly hazardous substances.

Compliance with the COSHH Regulations is essential for protecting the health and safety of workers who may be exposed to hazardous substances. Employers can effectively manage the risks associated with hazardous substances and create safer working environments by conducting risk assessments, implementing control measures, providing information and training and monitoring exposure levels.

In January 2010, new regulations came into force regarding the classification, labelling and packaging of substances and mixtures (The European Regulation [EC] No. 1272/2008 on classification, labelling and packaging of substances and mixtures – the CLP Regulation) [5]. These regulations changed the symbols used for hazards and replaced the black printing on orange-yellow rectangles that have been used to date; now, nine hazard pictograms with black symbols on a white background with red-rimmed rhombuses are used to provide warnings. Table 1.1 shows the old symbols compared to the new ones

and explains their meaning. From June 2015, using the new symbols for all hazardous materials became mandatory.

Personal Protective Equipment at Work Regulations 1992

This sets the regulations in the United Kingdom that aim to ensure the proper selection, use and maintenance of PPE in the workplace. These regulations place responsibilities on employers to provide suitable PPE to protect their employees from workplace hazards. Some key aspects of the PPE at Work Regulations are as follows.

Risk Assessment

Employers are required to conduct a thorough risk assessment to identify hazards and assess the need for PPE. The risk assessment should consider the nature of the work, potential hazards and the effectiveness of other control measures. If hazards cannot be adequately controlled by other means, employers must provide appropriate PPE to mitigate the risks.

Selection of PPE

The regulations emphasise the importance of selecting suitable PPE that effectively protects against the identified risks. Employers should consider factors such as the nature of the hazards, the tasks being performed, ergonomic considerations and employees' individual requirements. PPE should be of the correct size, fit and durability to ensure its effectiveness.

Providing and Maintaining PPE

Employers are responsible for providing PPE to employees free of charge. The PPE should be suitable for the identified risks and in good working condition. Employers must ensure that PPE is properly maintained, inspected, worn and replaced when necessary. Regular checks and maintenance should be conducted to ensure that PPE remains effective and does not pose any additional risks to the wearer.

Instruction, Training and Information

Employers must provide employees with proper instruction, training and information on the use, storage, maintenance and limitations of the provided PPE. Employees should be aware of how to correctly wear and adjust PPE and understand the importance of using it as directed. Instruction and training should also cover the potential risks associated with not using PPE or using it incorrectly.

Table 1.1 COSHH symbols used for hazard identification [2].

Old pictogram and classification	New pictogram and classification	Precautions
Corrosive	Corrosive	This symbolises a corrosive material that causes serious skin burns and eye damage; eye damage may be permanent and may corrode metals • Wear suitable PPE • Keep away from metals • Avoid contact with skin and eyes • Wear a mask or respirator if using sprays to avoid inhalation
Dangerous to the environment	Hazardous to the environment, a hazard to the aquatic environment	Toxic and has a damaging effect on both land and aquatic environments • Should not be released into the environment • Should not be used near water sources • Containers should be disposed of appropriately
Flammable	Flammable	Flammable when exposed to sources such as heat. Some sources may emit flammable gases if contacted by water. Substances include Flammable gases, flammable liquids, flammable solids, flammable aerosols and organic peroxides • Wear suitable PPE • Keep substances away from ignition sources • Use locked flame retardant storage • Keep away from sunlight
Toxic	Acute toxicity (severe)	Material that will cause severe toxicity even in a small amount. The effects seen may be life-threatening • Wear suitable PPE • Do not ingest • Do not allow contact with skin or mucous membranes • Dispose of safely
Explosive	Explosive	The substance may explode if exposed to an ignition source. Sources may include heat, shock and friction • Wear PPE • Avoid sources of ignition • Store in suitable storage facilities • Dispose of safely
Oxidising	Oxidising	Materials can burn even without oxygen and may intensify fires with combustible materials • Use only as directed • Wear PPE • Store in an airtight container and away from children • Keep away from ignition sources • Dispose of safely

Table 1.1 (Continued)

Old pictogram and classification	New pictogram and classification	Precautions
Hazard	Health hazard/hazardous to the ozone layer	A substance that may cause irritation or less severe toxicity. It may also damage the ozone layer if realised • Wear PPE • Avoid contact with eye and skin • Do not inhale • Avoid releasing into the environment • Care when disposing
	Serious health hazard	With short- or long-term exposure, the substance may pose a severe risk to health • Wear PPE • Avoid contact with skin and eyes • Wear a mask or respirator • Store in a cool, dry environment • Store away from children and animals
	Gas under pressure	Contains a pressurised gas; if realised, gas may be cold or flammable • Store in a secure gas cabinet • Use wall fastenings to prevent falling • Keep away from direct sunlight • Keep away from sources of ignition

Source: Rosina Lillywhite.

Employee Responsibilities

Employees are responsible for using PPE as instructed and reporting any defects or issues with their PPE to their employer. They should also take care of the provided PPE and ensure its proper storage and maintenance when not in use.

Compatibility and Comfort

Employers should consider the compatibility and comfort of the PPE when selecting and providing it to employees. PPE should not cause additional risks or discomfort that could hinder the ability of employees to perform their work safely and effectively. Adequate consideration should be given to the PPE's ergonomics, weight, fit and breathability.

Review and Evaluation

Employers should regularly review and evaluate the effectiveness of the provided PPE through ongoing risk assessments, employee feedback and incident reporting.

If changes in work processes, hazards or technology occur, the suitability and effectiveness of the PPE should be reassessed and necessary adjustments should be made.

Compliance with the Personal Protective Equipment at Work Regulations 1992 ensures that employees are adequately protected from workplace hazards by providing, using and maintaining suitable PPE. By conducting risk assessments, selecting appropriate PPE, providing proper instruction and training, and regularly reviewing the effectiveness of the PPE, employers can create safer working environments and prevent injuries or illnesses caused by workplace hazards.

Reporting of Injuries, Diseases and Dangerous Occurrences Regulations 2013 (RIDDOR)

RIDDOR is a set of regulations in the United Kingdom that requires employers, self-employed individuals and individuals in control of work premises to report certain types of workplace incidents. RIDDOR ensures that significant workplace incidents, injuries, diseases and dangerous occurrences are reported to the appropriate regulatory authorities. The key aspects of the Reporting of Injuries, Diseases and Dangerous Occurrences Regulations 2013 are as follows:

Reportable Injuries

Employers are required to report specified workplace injuries that result in death, major injuries or certain types of accidents. Under the Reporting of Injuries, Diseases and Dangerous Occurrences Regulations (RIDDOR) 2013, there is a list of specific reportable injuries. These injuries include:

- Fractures other than to fingers, thumbs and toes.
- Amputations.
- Dislocations of the shoulder, hip, knee or spine.
- Loss of sight, either temporary or permanent.
- Chemical or hot metal burn to the eye or any penetrating injury to the eye.
- Injury resulting from an electric shock or electrical burn leading to unconsciousness or requiring resuscitation or admittance to a hospital for more than 24 hours.
- Any burn injury (including scalding) requiring admittance to a hospital for more than 24 hours.
- Scalping requiring hospital treatment.
- Unconsciousness caused by asphyxia or exposure to harmful substances or biological agents.
- Acute illness resulting from exposure to a substance or biological agent.
- Acute illness requiring medical treatment where there is reason to believe it resulted from exposure to a biological agent or its toxins or infected material.
- Injuries requiring the person injured to be admitted to a hospital for more than 24 hours for treatment.

It is important to note that this is a general overview of the specific reportable injuries. The full and definitive list of reportable injuries can be found in Schedule 1 of RIDDOR 2013. This list provides more detailed descriptions and additional specific injuries that fall within the scope of RIDDOR.

Occupational Diseases

Certain work-related diseases are reportable under RIDDOR. The specific work-related diseases that require reporting under RIDDOR include:

- Carpal Tunnel Syndrome: This is a condition that affects the hand and wrist, causing numbness, tingling and weakness due to compression of the median nerve.
- Hand-Arm Vibration Syndrome (HAVS): HAVS is a condition caused by prolonged exposure to vibrating tools or machinery, resulting in symptoms such as numbness, tingling and reduced dexterity in the hands and fingers.
- Occupational dermatitis: This refers to skin inflammation or irritation caused by exposure to hazardous substances in the workplace, such as chemicals, irritants or allergens.
- Occupational asthma: Occupational asthma is a type of asthma triggered by exposure to substances present in the workplace, such as dust, chemicals or fumes.
- Occupational cancer: This includes certain types of cancer that are linked to specific workplace exposures, such as lung cancer due to exposure to asbestos or bladder cancer due to exposure to certain chemicals (aromatic amines, such as benzidine and beta-naphthylamine).
- Occupational silicosis: Silicosis is a lung disease caused by inhalation of silica dust, commonly found in industries such as mining, construction and sandblasting.
- Occupational noise-induced hearing loss: This refers to hearing loss or damage caused by exposure to excessive noise levels in the workplace over an extended period.

It is important to note that these are examples of work-related diseases that require reporting under RIDDOR. The regulations cover a wide range of occupational diseases, and the specific requirements for reporting may vary depending on the circumstances and severity of the disease. For a comprehensive list and detailed guidance, it is recommended to refer to RIDDOR 2013 and accompanying guidance provided by the HSE.

Dangerous Occurrences

RIDDOR requires reporting dangerous occurrences that happen in connection with work activities. Dangerous occurrences refer to near misses or incidents that have the potential to cause significant harm or serious accidents. Examples of dangerous occurrences include the collapse of lifting equipment, explosion or fire, accidental release of a hazardous substance and incidents involving the failure of machinery or equipment.

Specified Injuries to Members of the Public

In addition to reporting injuries and dangerous occurrences to employees, RIDDOR also requires reporting of specified injuries to members of the public who are affected by work-related activities. This includes incidents occurring on or off work premises that result in death or certain types of injuries to members of the public.

Investigating and Learning From Incidents

RIDDOR promotes the importance of investigating and learning from incidents to prevent future occurrences. Employers should conduct thorough investigations to identify the root causes of incidents and implement necessary measures to prevent similar incidents from happening again.

Reporting under RIDDOR involves notifying the appropriate regulatory authorities about certain workplace incidents, injuries, diseases and dangerous occurrences. Some key points regarding reporting under RIDDOR are as follows:

Who Is Responsible for Reporting

Employers, self-employed individuals and individuals in control of work premises have a legal obligation to report incidents under RIDDOR. This includes companies, organisations and individuals responsible for the management and supervision of work activities.

Reporting Timeframes

Incidents falling within the scope of RIDDOR must be reported within specified timeframes. The timeframes vary depending on the type of incident:

- Fatal accidents: Must be reported immediately or as soon as practicable.
- Major injuries: Must be reported within 10 days of the incident.
- Occupational diseases: Must be reported as soon as they are diagnosed, and work-relatedness is suspected.
- Dangerous occurrences: Must be reported immediately or within 10 days of the incident, depending on the specific occurrence.

How to Report

Reports can be made through various channels, including:

- Online reporting: The HSE provides an online reporting system for submitting incident reports.
- Telephone reporting: Incidents can be reported by calling the HSE Incident Contact Centre.

Additional Responsibilities

In addition to reporting incidents, employers have other responsibilities under RIDDOR, such as conducting investigations into incidents, maintaining records of incidents and cooperating with regulatory authorities during investigations.

It is important to consult the official guidance the HSE provides for detailed instructions, specific reporting requirements and any updates or changes to the reporting process under RIDDOR.

Compliance with RIDDOR is essential for ensuring that significant workplace incidents, injuries, diseases and dangerous occurrences are properly reported and investigated.

By promptly reporting incidents and learning from them, employers and regulatory authorities can work together to improve workplace safety, prevent accidents and protect the health and well-being of employees and the public.

The Manual Handling Operations Regulations 1992 (MHOR)

This set of regulations in the United Kingdom aims to protect workers from the risks associated with manual handling activities. Manual handling refers to the lifting, lowering, carrying, pushing or pulling of loads by hand or bodily force. The regulations provide guidance and requirements for employers to assess, control and minimise the risks associated with manual handling. Some key aspects of the MHORs 1992 are as follows:

Risk Assessment

Employers are required to conduct a thorough risk assessment of manual handling tasks in the workplace. The assessment should identify potential hazards, evaluate the risks involved and determine appropriate control measures to reduce the risk of injury. The assessment should take into account factors such as the nature of the task, the characteristics of the load, the working environment and the capabilities of the individuals involved.

Avoidance and Reduction of Risk

The regulations prioritise the avoidance of manual handling activities where reasonably practicable. Employers are encouraged to implement measures to eliminate or reduce the need for manual handling, such as using mechanical aids or redesigning work processes. If manual handling is necessary, employers must take steps to minimise the risk to employees' health and safety.

Training and Instruction

Employers are responsible for providing training and instruction to employees involved in manual handling tasks. This includes educating employees on safe manual handling techniques, correct posture, proper lifting and carrying methods and appropriate handling aids and equipment. Training should also cover recognising potential hazards and reporting any concerns or incidents related to manual handling.

Physical Capability and Fitness

Employers should consider employees' physical capabilities and fitness when assigning manual handling tasks. It is important to match the task to the individual's capabilities, ensuring that the load can be handled safely without risk of injury. Reasonable adjustments should be made for individuals with specific needs or physical limitations.

Review and Evaluation

Employers are encouraged to regularly review and evaluate manual handling tasks, control measures and the effectiveness of training and instruction. This includes monitoring for any changes in work processes, load characteristics or employees' physical capabilities. If necessary, adjustments should be made to control measures to ensure ongoing safety.

Employee Consultation and Involvement

Employees should be consulted and involved in assessing and controlling manual handling risks. Employee input can provide valuable insights into the practicalities of the tasks, potential hazards and the effectiveness of control measures. Consultation can also help identify areas for improvement and promote a culture of health and safety within the workplace.

The MHOR sets out the maximum weight limit permissible to handle at work. Figure 1.1 shows what these limits are in relation to both men and women; these limits differ depending on how close the weight is to the body.

By complying with the MHOR 1992, employers can effectively identify and manage the risks associated with manual handling activities. Through risk assessments, control measures, training and regular review, employers can create safer working environments, reduce the likelihood of manual handling injuries and protect the health and well-being of their employees.

The Lifting Operations and Lifting Equipment Regulations 1998 (LOLER)

LOLER is a set of United Kingdom regulations that aim to ensure the safe use of lifting equipment in the workplace. The following is only a general overview of LOLER; it is important to consult the specific regulations and seek professional advice to ensure compliance in the context of equine veterinary practice. Some key points are as follows [6]:

Scope of LOLER

LOLER applies to any lifting equipment used at work, including hoists, cranes, lifts and other devices used for lifting or lowering loads. It covers both mobile and fixed lifting equipment.

Duties and Responsibilities [6]

The regulations impose certain duties and responsibilities on employers, employees and those in control of lifting equipment. Some key responsibilities include:

- Ensuring that lifting equipment is safe, properly maintained and suitable for the intended use.

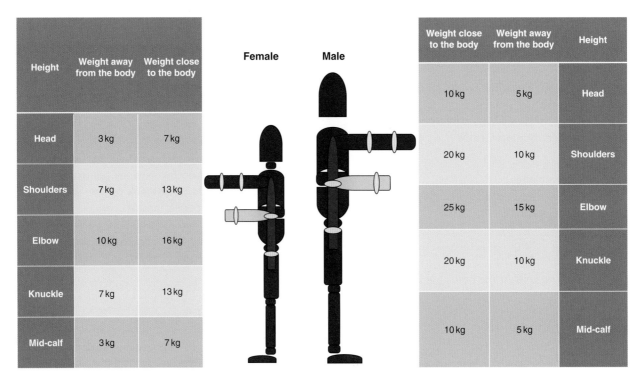

Height	Weight away from the body	Weight close to the body
Head	3 kg	7 kg
Shoulders	7 kg	13 kg
Elbow	10 kg	16 kg
Knuckle	7 kg	13 kg
Mid-calf	3 kg	7 kg

Weight close to the body	Weight away from the body	Height
10 kg	5 kg	Head
20 kg	10 kg	Shoulders
25 kg	15 kg	Elbow
20 kg	10 kg	Knuckle
10 kg	5 kg	Mid-calf

Figure 1.1 Manual handling guidelines for maximum weight limits at work. *Source:* Rosina Lillywhite.

- Providing adequate training, instruction and supervision for employees involved in lifting operations.
- Conducting thorough examinations and inspections of lifting equipment by competent persons at specified intervals.

Thorough Examination

LOLER requires that lifting equipment undergoes a thorough examination by a competent person (this should be someone who is trained and qualified in the inspection of lifting equipment) at regular intervals. The examination should ensure that the equipment is safe to use, properly maintained and complies with relevant safety standards. Hoist and lifting equipment in equine practice should be inspected every 6–12 months depending on the equipment and usage.

External Trained Inspector Duties [6]

- Ensuring that the hoist is suitable for the intended purpose and has the appropriate lifting capacity.
- Regularly inspecting the hoist for any signs of wear, damage or malfunctions.
- Providing adequate training for personnel involved in hoisting operations, including safe handling of animals and correct use of the hoist.
- Consulting with specialist veterinary equipment suppliers or professionals for specific guidance on the use and maintenance of hoists in equine veterinary practice.

It is crucial to review the full text of LOLER and seek guidance from regulatory authorities, professional bodies or health and safety consultants to ensure compliance with the specific requirements of LOLER and any additional regulations or guidelines applicable to equine veterinary practice.

The Waste (England and Wales) Regulations 2011

Waste disposal is regulated in the United Kingdom to ensure proper management and environmental protection. Several regulations govern waste disposal, with the key legislation being the Environmental Protection Act 1990 and the Waste (England and Wales) Regulations 2011. Important aspects of the waste disposal regulations include:

Duty of Care

The duty of care applies to anyone who produces, carries, keeps, treats or disposes of waste. It requires individuals and organisations to take all reasonable measures to prevent waste's escape or illegal disposal. This includes ensuring proper storage, transportation, and disposal of waste and keeping records and providing information when transferring waste to others.

Waste Hierarchy

The waste hierarchy is a key principle in waste management. It emphasises the need to prevent waste generation, promote reuse, recycle and recover energy from waste before resorting to disposal. The regulations encourage individuals and organisations to follow this hierarchy and make efforts to minimise waste generation and maximise resource recovery.

Waste Classification

Waste is classified based on its properties and potential environmental and health impacts. The regulations define different categories of waste, including hazardous waste, non-hazardous waste and inert waste. Proper classification is important as it determines the appropriate handling, storage and disposal methods for different types of waste.

Waste Carriers and Brokers

Individuals or businesses involved in the transportation of waste are required to register as waste carriers or brokers with the appropriate regulatory authority. This helps to ensure that waste is transported by authorised and responsible parties, minimising the risk of illegal dumping or mishandling.

Waste Management Licenses and Permits

Certain waste management activities like operating waste treatment facilities or landfills may require specific permits or licenses. These permits ensure that waste management activities are carried out in compliance with environmental standards and regulations.

Duty to Separate and Segregate Waste

The regulations encourage the segregation of waste at the source to facilitate recycling and proper disposal. Businesses and individuals are encouraged to separate different types of waste, such as recyclables, organic waste and hazardous waste, to enable effective waste management and resource recovery.

Landfill Regulations

The Landfill Directive, implemented through the Waste (England and Wales) Regulations 2011, sets standards and requirements for landfill operations. It aims to minimise the environmental impacts of landfilling, such as soil, water and air pollution. The regulations impose restrictions on the types of waste that can be landfilled and require compliance with specific operational and monitoring requirements.

Compliance with waste disposal regulations is essential to protect the environment and human health, and promote sustainable waste management practices. Individuals and organisations need to understand their responsibilities, follow proper waste management procedures and work towards minimising waste generation and maximising recycling and resource recovery.

The Hazardous Waste Regulations 2005

The Hazardous Waste Regulations 2005 are a set of regulations in the United Kingdom that specifically address the management, classification and disposal of hazardous waste. These regulations aim to protect human health and the environment by ensuring that hazardous waste is handled, stored, transported and disposed of safely and responsibly. Here are key aspects of the Hazardous Waste Regulations 2005.

Definition of Hazardous Waste
The regulations provide a definition of hazardous waste based on its properties, as determined by the European Waste Catalogue (EWC) codes. Hazardous waste is classified based on its potential to cause harm to human health or the environment due to its toxic, corrosive, infectious, explosive or other hazardous properties.

Duty of Care
The Hazardous Waste Regulations impose a duty of care on waste producers, carriers and handlers to ensure that hazardous waste is managed appropriately. This includes preventing the escape or harm of hazardous waste, maintaining proper documentation and ensuring that waste is transferred to authorised carriers or facilities.

Classification and Labelling
Hazardous waste must be properly classified and labelled to indicate its hazardous properties. The regulations require waste producers to accurately determine the EWC codes and hazardous properties of the waste they produce. This classification is crucial for ensuring the waste is handled and disposed of correctly.

Storage and Packaging
Hazardous waste must be stored in suitable containers or storage facilities to prevent leaks, spills or any escape that may harm human health or the environment. Proper packaging, labelling and segregation of hazardous waste are necessary to avoid cross-contamination and to ensure safe handling.

Transfer and Documentation
Proper documentation must be maintained when hazardous waste is transferred from the waste producer to a carrier or waste management facility. Waste transfer notes should include information about the waste's origin, classification, quantity and destination and the parties involved in the transfer.

Treatment and Disposal
Hazardous waste should undergo appropriate treatment to reduce its hazardous properties or render it safe for disposal. Treatment may include physical, chemical or biological processes. Hazardous waste must be disposed of at authorised facilities that have the necessary permits and comply with environmental regulations.

Penalties and Enforcement
Non-compliance with the Hazardous Waste Regulations can result in penalties, fines or legal action. Environmental regulatory authorities, such as the Environment Agency in England or the Scottish Environment Protection Agency in Scotland, have powers to monitor, inspect and enforce compliance with the regulations.

Waste producers, carriers and handlers must familiarise themselves with the requirements and obligations outlined in the Hazardous Waste Regulations 2005. They should consult the official guidance provided by the environmental regulatory authorities for detailed information on waste classification, storage, transportation and disposal procedures to ensure compliance with the regulations and promote the safe management of hazardous waste.

Exact waste disposal requirements are set out by individual waste collection companies. Table 1.2 shows the general types of waste produced and the correct disposal method.

The Health and Safety (Display Screen Equipment) Regulations 1992

The Health and Safety (Display Screen Equipment) Regulations 1992, often referred to as the DSE Regulations, are a set of guidelines and regulations aimed at safeguarding the health and well-being of employees who use DSE regularly during their work. The regulations were introduced in the United Kingdom and are part of broader efforts to address potential health risks associated with using computers, laptops, tablets and other display screen devices in the workplace [6].

Key provisions of the Health and Safety Display Screen Regulations 1992:

Table 1.2 Types of waste and correct disposal methods.

Types of waste	Description	Bin/bag type
Hazardous waste		
Infectious	Infectious waste bags, also known as clinical waste bags or biohazard bags, are used to collect and store waste contaminated with potentially infectious materials. These bags are made of robust and leak-proof material and are often colour-coded following industry standards, such as using orange bags for infectious waste (waste that contains potentially harmful microorganisms that can infect hospital patients, staff and the general public). They may have biohazard symbols or markings to indicate their contents	
Cytotoxic and cytostatic	Cytotoxic and cytostatic waste should be segregated from other types of healthcare waste to prevent cross-contamination. Use dedicated containers that are clearly labelled and distinguishable from general waste bins. Colour-coded bins, such as purple-lidded yellow bins, may be used to indicate their specific purpose	
Sharps	Sharps containers are designed to collect used needles, syringes, lancets and other sharps items. These puncture-resistant containers have a secure lid to prevent accidental injuries and contamination. They are typically colour-coded, often with a bright yellow bottom with an orange lid sharps with an orange lid contain infectious sharps	
Non-hazardous waste		
Offensive	Offensive waste is non-infectious waste, which is unpleasant and may cause offence to those coming into contact with it. It includes: • Outer dressings and protective clothing, e.g. masks, gowns and gloves that are not contaminated with body fluids • Hygiene waste and sanitary protection, e.g. nappies and incontinence pads • Autoclaved laboratory waste Offensive waste should only be placed in a yellow and black striped 'Tiger' bag	
Pharmaceutical	The blue waste stream is used for waste medicinal products that are not cytotoxic or cytostatic Blue-stream pharmaceutical waste bins must be sent for incineration at a suitably authorised facility. Blue-lidded containers are for any waste containing non-hazardous medicinal drugs that are expired, unused, contaminated, damaged, denatured or no longer needed	

(Continued)

Table 1.2 (Continued)

Types of waste	Description	Bin/bag type
Sharps	Sharps containers are designed to collect used needles, syringes, lancets and other sharps items. These puncture-resistant containers have a secure lid to prevent accidental injuries and contamination. They are typically colour-coded, often with a bright yellow bottom with a yellow lid. Sharps with a yellow lid contain non-infectious sharps	
	Animal byproducts	
Cadavers	The disposal of equine cadavers (deceased horses) is an essential aspect of equine management to ensure proper biosecurity, environmental protection and public health. Incineration: Incineration involves the controlled burning of the cadaver in a specialised facility. This method effectively destroys the remains, reducing the risk of disease transmission. Incineration can be carried out on-site or at dedicated facilities. Burial: Burial involves burying the equine cadaver in a designated burial site that complies with local regulations. The burial site should be located away from water sources, ensuring minimal environmental impact. Depth and site requirements may vary and local authorities should be consulted	
Body parts	Disposal of anatomical waste materials that are potentially infectious or biohazardous use of red-lidded containers to indicate that the waste inside is anatomical in nature and requires special handling and disposal procedures	
	Domestic waste	
Non-recycling	General waste disposal bins may be used to collect non-hazardous or non-infectious waste generated in healthcare settings, such as packaging materials, food waste or non-contaminated items. These bins are typically designed for easy waste disposal and are often colour-coded for different waste streams, following standard waste management practices	
Recycling	The disposal of recycling refers to the proper management and handling of recyclable materials to ensure they are processed and reused in an environmentally sustainable manner. Recycling helps conserve resources, reduce waste and minimise environmental impact	

Source: Rosina Lillywhite.

- Scope of application: The regulations apply to all employers whose employees habitually use DSE as a significant part of their work duties for continuous or extended periods. It covers a wide range of job roles, from office workers using computers to control room operators and data entry personnel.
- Risk assessments: Employers must conduct a thorough assessment of the health and safety risks associated with using DSE in the workplace. This assessment includes identifying potential hazards and evaluating factors such as workstation layout, equipment, lighting and the work environment.
- Ergonomic workstations: Employers must ensure that DSE workstations are ergonomically designed to promote comfort and minimise the risk of health problems. This includes providing adjustable chairs, properly positioned screens, adjustable keyboards and adequate lighting.
- Breaks and rest periods: Employees who regularly use DSE are entitled to adequate breaks or changes in work tasks to minimise the potential strain on their eyes, muscles and overall well-being. These breaks should be given at appropriate intervals, and the work should not be continuously demanding.
- Eye tests: Employers are required to provide free eye tests to employees who use DSE regularly. If the eye test indicates that specific glasses or corrective lenses are needed solely for DSE use, the employer must provide them at no cost to the employee.
- Training and information: Employers are responsible for providing adequate training and information to employees on how to set up their workstations correctly, adjust their posture and minimise health risks associated with DSE use.
- New employees and job changes: Employers must ensure that new employees who will be using DSE as part of their job role receive proper training and information before commencing work. Similarly, employees who change their workstations or job tasks must be provided with appropriate training and information.
- Health surveillance: Employers should offer health surveillance to employees who are at particular risk due to their work with DSE.

Employers must comply with the DSE regulations to protect their employees from potential health risks associated with prolonged DSE use. Failure to adhere to these regulations can result in legal consequences and potential harm to the well-being of the workforce. By creating ergonomic work environments, providing adequate training and conducting risk assessments, employers can foster a healthier and more productive workplace for DSE users [6].

Legionella Testing

Legionella is a type of bacteria that can cause a severe form of pneumonia known as Legionnaires' disease. The bacteria are commonly found in freshwater environments, such as lakes and streams, but they can also thrive in man-made water systems, including cooling towers, hot tubs, water tanks and plumbing systems. The bacteria *Legionella pneumophila* is responsible for the majority of Legionnaires' disease cases. It is transmitted to humans primarily through the inhalation of contaminated water droplets or aerosols. It is important to note that Legionella is not transmitted from person to person, meaning it is not contagious.

Consequences of contracting Legionnaires' disease:

- Legionnaires' disease: This is the severe form of infection caused by the Legionella bacteria. Symptoms typically appear within 2–10 days after exposure and may include high fever, chills, cough, muscle aches, headaches and difficulty breathing. In severe cases, patients may develop pneumonia, which can be life-threatening, especially for those with weakened immune systems or underlying health conditions.
- Pontiac fever: This is a milder and more common form of Legionella infection. It is a flu-like illness with symptoms such as fever, headache, muscle aches and fatigue. Unlike Legionnaires' disease, Pontiac fever does not affect the lungs and is usually not life-threatening. Symptoms typically appear within 24–48 hours after exposure and may last for several days.
- Long-term effects: Survivors of Legionnaires' disease may experience lingering health issues, such as fatigue, neurological symptoms and respiratory problems. In some cases, the recovery period can be prolonged, and individuals may require ongoing medical care and support.
- Outbreaks and public health concerns: Legionnaires' disease outbreaks can occur when a source of Legionella contamination affects multiple people in a specific area or facility. These outbreaks can lead to significant public health concerns, investigations and measures to control and prevent further transmission.

In the United Kingdom, the requirements for Legionella testing and control are outlined in the Health and Safety Executive's Approved Code of Practice and Guidance document known as 'Legionnaires' disease: The control of Legionella bacteria in water systems (ACOP L8). Here are the key requirements for Legionella testing in the United Kingdom [7]:

Risk assessment: Employers or those in control of premises are required to conduct a suitable and sufficient risk assessment of the water systems within their premises.

The risk assessment should identify and assess the risk of exposure to Legionella bacteria and should be reviewed regularly or whenever there is a significant change in the water system [7].

Competent person: A competent person or an appointed competent contractor should perform the risk assessment and manage and control Legionella risks. This person should have the necessary knowledge, skills and expertise to effectively assess and manage Legionella risks [7].

Control measures: The risk assessment should identify appropriate control measures to manage and minimise the risk of Legionella contamination. Control measures may include temperature monitoring, water treatment, regular cleaning and disinfection and maintenance of water systems [7].

Monitoring and testing: Routine monitoring and testing for Legionella should be conducted as part of the overall control measures. This includes regular water sampling and testing for the presence of Legionella bacteria. The frequency and extent of testing should be based on the risk assessment and should be determined by a competent person.

Documentation: Employers or duty holders are required to maintain up-to-date records of the risk assessment, control measures implemented and the results of monitoring and testing. These records should be readily available for inspection by enforcing authorities. It is important to note that the frequency and extent of Legionella testing may vary depending on the risk assessment findings. Higher-risk systems may require more frequent testing, while lower-risk systems may have less regular testing. The ACOP L8 guides the recommended frequencies for different types of systems [7].

Additionally, it is important to follow the guidelines provided by the United Kingdom HSE, local authorities and other relevant regulatory bodies to ensure compliance with specific requirements and any updates or changes to regulations. For detailed and up-to-date information, it is recommended to refer to the ACOP L8 and consult with qualified professionals or specialists in Legionella risk assessment and control [7].

Asbestos Testing

Asbestos testing requirements in the United Kingdom for workplace testing are governed by the Control of Asbestos Regulations 2012. These regulations aim to protect workers and others from the risks associated with exposure to asbestos in the workplace. Asbestos is a hazardous material known to cause serious health issues, including lung diseases and various cancers [8].

The key requirements for asbestos testing in the United Kingdom workplace are as follows [8]:

- Asbestos Management Survey: Employers are legally responsible for identifying and managing asbestos-containing materials (ACMs) in their workplaces. An asbestos management survey is the initial step to identify the presence, location and condition of any ACMs. This survey assesses the risk of exposure and helps develop a management plan to prevent the release of asbestos fibres into the air.
- Refurbishment and Demolition Survey: Before any refurbishment or demolition work occurs, a survey must be carried out. This survey is more intrusive than the management survey and involves thorough inspection and sampling of suspected ACMs to determine their presence and condition.
- Asbestos sampling and analysis: Sampling of suspected ACMs must be done by trained and competent personnel. An accredited laboratory then analyses the samples to confirm the presence and type of asbestos fibres.
- Risk assessment and management plan: Based on the survey findings and asbestos analysis, a risk assessment should be conducted to evaluate the potential risks of asbestos exposure to workers and others in the vicinity. A management plan should be put in place to mitigate these risks and ensure the safe handling, removal or encapsulation of ACMs.
- Asbestos register: Employers must keep an up-to-date asbestos register, which includes information about the location, condition and type of asbestos-containing materials in the workplace. This register should be readily accessible to all employees and relevant contractors.
- Training and information: Employers must provide adequate asbestos awareness training to employees who may encounter ACMs during their work. Training should cover the risks associated with asbestos exposure, safe work practices and procedures to follow in case of accidental disturbance.
- Licensed contractors: Only licensed contractors are allowed to undertake the work for higher-risk asbestos removal work. Licensing ensures contractors have the expertise, equipment and procedures to safely handle asbestos.
- Health surveillance: Employers should provide appropriate health surveillance to workers who are likely to be exposed to asbestos fibres, as required by the regulations.

Compliance with these asbestos testing and management requirements is crucial to protect workers' health and ensure legal compliance in the United Kingdom workplace. Employers should take asbestos-related risks seriously and take appropriate measures to prevent exposure to this hazardous material [8].

1.3 Risk Assessments

A risk assessment is a systematic process of identifying, analysing and evaluating potential risks or hazards that could impact a project, process or organisation. It involves assessing these risks' likelihood and potential impact and developing strategies to mitigate or manage them effectively. A risk assessment aims to proactively identify and understand potential risks to make informed decisions and take appropriate actions to minimise their negative consequences. It helps organisations prioritise their resources, allocate budgets and implement controls to reduce the likelihood and impact of risks. Risk assessments can be conducted in various contexts, such as business projects, health and safety management, information security, environmental impact studies and financial planning. The process typically involves the following steps [8]:

- Risk identification: Identifying and documenting potential risks affecting the project or organisation.
- Risk analysis: Assessing the likelihood and impact of each identified risk, considering factors such as probability, severity, frequency and vulnerability.
- Risk evaluation: Prioritising risks based on their significance and determining which risks require immediate attention and mitigation efforts.
- Risk treatment: Develop strategies and action plans to mitigate, avoid, transfer or accept the identified risks.

Risk monitoring and review: Continuously monitoring and reviewing the effectiveness of risk management strategies and controls and adjusting them as needed. A well-executed risk assessment helps organisations anticipate and prepare for potential risks, reduces the likelihood of costly surprises, improves decision-making and enhances overall resilience [8].

Writing a detailed risk assessment involves documenting the risk assessment process's findings, analysis and recommendations. The following is a step-by-step guide on how to write a comprehensive risk assessment report [8].

Introduction

- Provide an overview of the purpose and objectives of the risk assessment.
- State the scope and boundaries of the assessment (e.g. specific project, department or organisation). Include a brief description of the methodology used for the assessment [8].

Executive Summary

- Summarise the key findings, high-priority risks and major recommendations.
- Highlight the overall risk profile and any critical areas of concern.
- Keep the summary concise and focused on the most significant aspects.

Methodology

- Describe the approach and methods used to conduct the risk assessment.
- Explain the data sources, tools, techniques and stakeholders involved.
- Provide any limitations or constraints encountered during the assessment.

Risk Identification

- Present a comprehensive list of identified risks organised by relevant categories.
- Include a brief description of each risk, highlighting its potential impact and likelihood.
- Assign unique identifiers or codes to facilitate reference throughout the report [8].

Risk Analysis

- Assess and analyse each identified risk in detail.
- Evaluate the likelihood or probability of occurrence for each risk.
- Evaluate each risk's potential impact or consequences on the organisation, project or process.
- Use a consistent rating scale or methodology to quantify and compare risks.
- Present the risk analysis results in a structured and easy-to-understand format, such as tables or charts.

Risk Evaluation

- Evaluate the risks based on their analysis results.
- Consider additional factors such as legal and regulatory requirements, stakeholder concerns and risk tolerance levels.
- Prioritise the risks based on their severity and significance.
- Highlight any risks that require immediate attention or urgent mitigation measures.

Risk Treatment

- Provide recommendations for managing and mitigating the identified risks.
- Propose specific risk treatment strategies for each high-priority risk.
- Clearly outline the actions, controls or measures that need to be implemented.
- Describe any contingency plans or alternative approaches for risk management.

Risk Monitoring and Review

- Outline the process for ongoing monitoring and review of the risks and risk management measures.
- Define key performance indicators or metrics to track the effectiveness of risk controls.
- Specify the frequency and responsibilities for monitoring and reporting on risk status.

Conclusion

- Summarise the main findings and conclusions of the risk assessment.
- Emphasise the importance of proactive risk management and the need for ongoing vigilance.
- Consider highlighting any areas of uncertainty or areas requiring further investigation.

Appendices

- Include any supporting documentation, data or detailed analysis that may be relevant but too extensive for the main report.
- Attach any supplementary information, references or resources used during the risk assessment.

To maintain clarity, concise language should be used and the information should be presented logically and in an organised fashion. The report should be tailored to the intended audience: senior management, project stakeholders or regulatory bodies [8].

Table 1.3 shows an example of a detailed risk assessment for trips and slips in veterinary practice; this should be utilised alongside Figure 1.2, which is the grading matrix for the risk assessment; this should be used to combine the severity and likelihood scores to give the overall risk score.

1.4 Fire Safety

The Regulatory Reform (Fire Safety) Order 2005 primarily governs United Kingdom fire safety requirements and legislation. This legislation places responsibilities on both employers and employees to ensure the safety of individuals in the workplace. Some key points to consider are as follows [9]:

- **Responsible person:** The employer or the person in control of the premises is designated as the 'Responsible Person' under the legislation. This could be the employer, business owner, occupier or managing agent.
- **Fire risk assessment:** The Responsible Person must carry out a fire risk assessment of the premises to identify potential hazards, evaluate the level of risk and implement appropriate fire safety measures. The assessment should be regularly reviewed and updated as necessary.
- **Fire safety measures:** Based on the fire risk assessment findings, the Responsible Person must implement suitable fire safety measures. This includes providing appropriate firefighting equipment, maintaining fire detection and alarm systems, establishing emergency evacuation procedures and ensuring the availability of escape routes.
- **Training and information:** Employers must provide adequate fire safety training to employees, including instruction on the correct use of firefighting equipment and evacuation procedures. Information about the risks identified in the fire risk assessment should also be communicated to employees.
- **Fire drills and evacuation plans:** Employers should conduct regular fire drills to familiarise employees with evacuation procedures and ensure effective responses in the event of a fire. The evacuation plan should be clearly displayed, indicating escape routes, assembly points and any specific roles or responsibilities.
- **Maintenance and testing:** It is essential to regularly maintain and test fire safety equipment, such as fire extinguishers, fire alarms, emergency lighting and sprinkler systems. Records of maintenance activities and tests should be kept.
- **Cooperation and coordination:** In multi-occupancy buildings, collaboration and coordination among employers or responsible persons are crucial to ensure fire safety. They should communicate and cooperate to address shared fire safety issues, evacuation plans and emergency response procedures.

Non-compliance with fire safety legislation can result in penalties, including fines or imprisonment. Employers and

Table 1.3 Risk assessment for slips and trips in veterinary practice.

Slips, trips and falls

Activity	Hazard description	Personnel at risk	Existing controls in place	Risk rating Likelihood	Severity	Risk Level	Additional control measures required	New risk rating Likelihood	Severity	Risk Level
Accessing and exiting the building. Moving around the practice outside.	Slip or fall on ice or mud outside, causing bruises, cuts, sprains, and strains. Potential for dislocation or break of the limb in extreme cases.	All employees, students and visitors	Suitable footwear to be worn at all times; Grit to be applied to icy patches in the car park etc.; Mud to be cleared around the edge of the building; Ensure suitable lighting is provided and report any issues; Clear snow before applying grit	2	3	6	Mark off any known high-risk areas in extreme conditions	1	3	3
Accessing and exiting the building. Moving around the practice outside.	Trips or falls on uneven ground in the car park.	All employees, students and visitors	Notify the maintenance team if an area is posing a continued risk; Wear suitable footwear at all times; Plan a safe route to avoid uneven ground where possible; Provide suitable lighting in external areas	2	3	6		2	3	6
Moving around within the building	Trips or falls over items left in walkways equipment, stock, post, empty boxes, rubbish etc.	All employees, students and visitors	Ensure all walkways remain tidy at all times, stock, post etc. to be stored away properly, not on the floor or out of the way; All employees responsible for ensuring this happens; Remove empty boxes and rubbish to designated areas; Report any damaged flooring	2	2	4		2	2	4

(Continued)

Table 1.3 (Continued)

Slips, trips and falls

Activity	Hazard		Existing controls in place	Risk rating			Additional control measures required	New risk rating		
	Hazard description	Personnel at risk		Likelihood	Severity	Risk Level		Likelihood	Severity	Risk Level
Moving around within the building	Trip over open desk drawers, filing cabinet drawers	All employees, students and visitors	Do not leave desk draws or filing cabinet drawers open. Shut if a risk is identified.	1	3	3		1	3	3
Moving around within the building	Trip over electrical cables, extension leads, mats	All employees, students and visitors	Ensure computer cables and all electrical cables are correctly tidied away, and avoid crossing walkways. If unavoidable to cross a walkway, use suitable covers. Ensure static mats are of suitable wait and replace if edges curl	2	2	4		2	2	4
Moving around within the building	Slip-on wet floor could lead to a bad sprain or possibly even breakage of limb.	All employees, students and visitors	Ensure all spillages are promptly wiped up Ensure plenty of products to clean up spillage Use wet floor signs until dry Ensure mud/door mats in entry points to dry wet shoes	2	2	4		2	2	4
General Precautions	Slips, trips, falls	All employees, students and visitors	All employees are to be responsible for the tidiness and cleanliness of the offices and to report any concerns to the practice principles.			0		0	0	0

Source: Rosina Lillywhite.

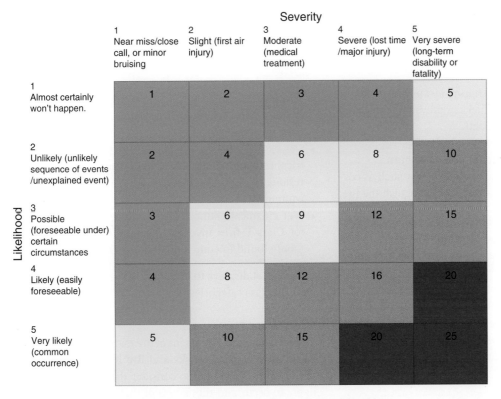

Figure 1.2 Risk grading matrix for a risk assessment. *Source:* Rosina Lillywhite.

employees must familiarise themselves with their specific obligations under the Regulatory Reform (Fire Safety) Order 2005 and seek guidance from fire safety professionals or local fire authorities if needed [9].

The Fire Triangle

The fire triangle, also known as the combustion triangle, is a simple model used to understand the three essential elements required for a fire to occur and sustain itself (Figure 1.3). These elements are heat, fuel and oxygen. Without any one of these components, a fire cannot start or continue to burn. The fire triangle is a fundamental concept in fire safety and firefighting.

- Heat: Is the first element of the fire triangle. It is the energy that raises the temperature of the fuel to its ignition point. The ignition point is the temperature at which the fuel starts to undergo a chemical reaction with oxygen, releasing heat and light, resulting in combustion. Heat can be generated from various sources, such as open flames, electrical sparks, hot surfaces, friction or chemical reactions.
- Fuel: Is the second element of the fire triangle. It refers to any material that can burn and sustain combustion. Common examples of fuel include wood, paper, cloth, gasoline, natural gas, oil and plastics. Different fuels have different ignition points and burn at varying rates. The

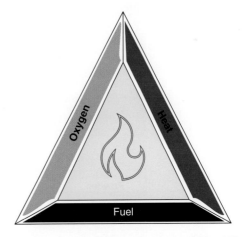

Figure 1.3 The fire triangle. *Source:* Rosina Lillywhite.

type and amount of fuel present in a fire can significantly influence its intensity and spread.
- Oxygen: Is the third element of the fire triangle. It is essential for the combustion process, as it acts as an oxidiser, enabling the fuel to burn. When the fuel's molecules combine with oxygen, they undergo a rapid chemical reaction called oxidation, producing heat, light and combustion byproducts such as smoke and gases. The presence of oxygen in the air (typically around 21% in ambient air) allows fires to spread and sustain themselves.

The interaction of these three elements is what sustains a fire. Removing any one of the elements can extinguish the fire. Fire safety measures often focus on controlling one or more aspects of the fire triangle. For instance:

- Cooling: Reducing the temperature by applying water or other cooling agents to the fuel can prevent the material from reaching its ignition point.
- Starvation: Removing or reducing the fuel supply can deprive the fire of the material needed to burn.
- Smothering: Cutting off the oxygen supply, such as covering the fire with a fire blanket, can extinguish the fire.

Understanding the fire triangle helps individuals and firefighters assess fire risks, develop fire safety plans and implement effective firefighting strategies to control and extinguish fires safely.

Fire Extinguishers

In the United Kingdom, fire extinguishers play a crucial role in fire safety and are an essential part of the fire protection measures in various premises [9].

Types of Fire Extinguishers

Different types of fire extinguishers are available, each designed to tackle specific types of fires. The most common types in the United Kingdom are [9]:

- Water extinguishers (red label): Suitable for Class A fires involving solid materials like wood, paper or fabric.
- Foam extinguishers (cream label): Effective on Class A and B fires involving flammable liquids such as petrol, oil or paints.
- Powder extinguishers (blue label): Suitable for Class A, B and C fires, which include flammable gases like propane or butane.
- CO_2 extinguishers (black label): Designed for use on electrical fires and flammable liquids. They do not leave any residue, making them suitable for areas with sensitive equipment.
- Wet chemical extinguishers (yellow label): Specifically for Class F fires involving cooking oils and fats, commonly found in commercial kitchens.

Figure 1.4 displays the available fire extinguishers in the relevant class categories.

Selection and Placement

The selection and placement of fire extinguishers should be based on the specific risks and fire hazards present in a premises. It is essential to consider the type of fire that is likely to occur and the nature of the materials in the surrounding environment. The number and location of fire extinguishers should comply with British Standard BS 5306, which provides guidelines for fire extinguisher

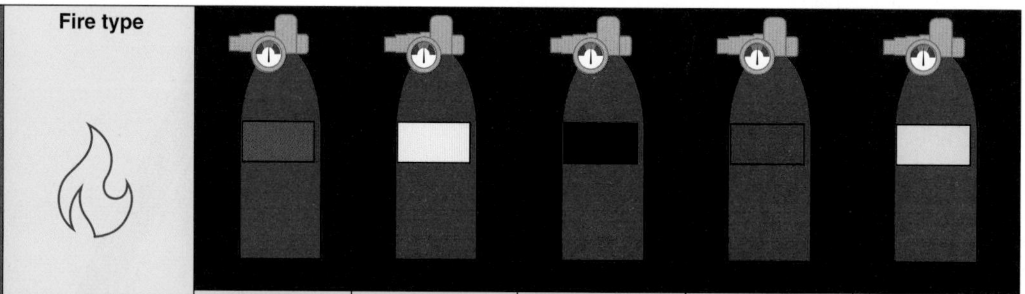

Classification	Fire type	Powder	Foam	CO²	Water	Wet Chemical
Class A	Solids (e.g. wood, plastic, paper)	✓	✓	✗	✓	✗
Class B	Flammable Liquids (e.g. solvents, paints, fuels)	✓	✓	✓	✗	✗
Class C	Gases (e.g. butane, propane, LPG)	✓	✗	✗	✗	✗
Class D	Metals (e.g. lithium, magnesium)	✓	✗	✗	✗	✗
Electrical	Equipment (e.g. computers, servers, TVs)	✓	✗	✓	✗	✗
Class F	Cooking Oils (e.g. cooking fats, oilve oil)	✗	✗	✗	✗	✓

Figure 1.4 Fire extinguishers and relevant class categories. *Source:* Rosina Lillywhite.

provision. Generally, fire extinguishers should be easily accessible, prominently located and positioned along escape routes and near potential fire hazards [9].

Maintenance and Inspection

Fire extinguishers in the United Kingdom must undergo regular maintenance and inspection to ensure they are in proper working condition. The maintenance should be carried out by a competent person who is trained in fire extinguisher servicing. The maintenance frequency and requirements are outlined in British Standard BS 5306 Part 3. This involves routine visual checks, periodic servicing and pressure testing at specified intervals. Records of maintenance activities should be kept, including dates, details of servicing and any repairs or replacements [9].

Training and Proper Use

Employees and occupants of premises should receive proper training on fire safety, including instruction on how to use fire extinguishers effectively and safely. Training should cover the identification of fire types, selecting the appropriate extinguisher and the correct techniques for operation. It is important to note that while fire extinguishers can be a valuable tool in tackling small fires, their use should be limited to situations where it is safe to do so. In case of larger or spreading fires, the immediate priority should be an evacuation and notifying the fire services. It is advisable to consult with fire safety professionals or local fire authorities for specific guidance on fire extinguishers and their requirements based on individual premises and local regulations [9].

Fire Notices

In the United Kingdom, several types of fire notices may be required in a workplace to ensure fire safety information is communicated effectively. The specific requirements can vary based on the nature of the premises and the applicable regulations. Some common types of fire notices are as follows [9]:

- Fire action notice: This notice provides instructions to building occupants on what actions to take in the event of a fire. It typically includes guidance on raising the alarm, calling emergency services, evacuation procedures, assembly points and any specific roles or responsibilities individuals may have during an emergency.
- Fire exit signs: These signs are used to indicate the location of emergency exits and escape routes. They are designed to be highly visible and should comply with relevant safety standards. Fire exit signs often feature a pictogram of a running person or an arrow indicating the direction of the exit.

- Fire equipment signs: These signs identify the location and type of fire safety equipment in the premises. They may include signs for fire extinguishers, fire blankets, fire alarms, emergency lighting or other firefighting equipment. The signs typically consist of symbols or images representing the specific equipment.
- Fire assembly point signs: These signs indicate the designated assembly point or points where occupants should gather after evacuating the building. The signs are usually placed in outdoor areas away from the building and should be clearly visible to ensure a safe and organised assembly during emergencies.
- Fire safety information signage: These signs provide general fire safety information and awareness. They may include signs indicating fire escape routes, fire assembly point locations, general fire safety reminders or instructions on reporting fire hazards.

It is important to consult the specific region's applicable fire safety regulations and standards to determine the specific requirements for fire notices in individual workplaces. Additionally, engaging with fire safety professionals or local fire authorities can provide valuable guidance and ensure compliance with relevant regulations [9].

1.5 Personal Protective Equipment (PPE)

In veterinary practice, various types of PPE are used to ensure the safety of veterinary staff when handling hazardous substances or performing procedures that may pose a risk of exposure. Infomration regarding some common types of PPE found in veterinary practice, their uses and when they are required is presented below [4]:

- Gloves: Disposable gloves, typically made of latex, nitrile or vinyl, protect the hands from contact with chemicals, bodily fluids, pathogens and other potentially harmful substances. Gloves are required when handling medications, cleaning contaminated areas, performing procedures involving bodily fluids or tissues and during surgery.
- Face masks protect the respiratory system, including surgical masks or respirators (such as N95). They are particularly important when there is a risk of airborne transmission of infectious diseases or when working in environments with dust, fumes or strong odours. Face masks should be worn during procedures that generate aerosols, such as dental surgery, or when working with animals suspected or confirmed to have respiratory infections.

- Protective eyewear: Safety glasses, goggles or face shields are worn to protect the eyes from potential splashes, sprays or debris that could cause injury or contamination. They are necessary when handling hazardous substances, performing surgeries, dental procedures.
- Protective clothing: Veterinary staff often wear protective clothing, such as lab coats or gowns, to protect their skin and clothing from contamination. These garments act as a barrier against chemicals, bodily fluids or other substances encountered during procedures. Protective clothing should be worn when handling hazardous substances, during surgery or when there is a risk of contamination during patient care. Protective clothing can also be worn in the form of non-disposable gloves when handling horses to protect the handler from burns or injury if the horse pulls away suddenly. A riding helmet of an appropriate standard should also be worn when handling equine patients.
- Respiratory protection: Respiratory protection, such as respirators or masks with specific filters, may be required in certain situations where there is a risk of airborne hazards or exposure to harmful gases, fumes or chemicals. This includes working with hazardous chemicals, performing procedures generating aerosols or working in environments with poor ventilation.
- Footwear: Sturdy, closed-toe shoes or boots should be worn to protect the feet from accidental spills, falls or sharp objects. Proper footwear is important in any veterinary setting to reduce the risk of injuries.

The use of PPE in veterinary practice is dictated by the specific hazards present and the procedures being performed. It is important to assess the risks associated with each task and ensure that appropriate PPE is provided and worn by all personnel involved. Regular training and reinforcement of PPE use are essential to promote a safe working environment and minimise the risk of exposure to hazards [4].

Radiation PPE is used in veterinary practice when working with or around sources of ionising radiation. Different types of PPE commonly used for radiation protection are as follows [4, 10]:

- Lead aprons: Lead aprons are worn to protect the body from scattered radiation during diagnostic imaging procedures such as X-rays or fluoroscopy. These aprons are made of lead or lead-equivalent materials and provide shielding to the torso, abdomen and reproductive organs.
- Thyroid shields/collars: Thyroid shields or collars are leaded shields that are worn around the neck and thyroid area during radiation procedures. They protect the thyroid gland from direct or scattered radiation.

- Lead gloves: Lead gloves are used to protect the hands and fingers when handling or working near radiation sources. They provide shielding against direct contact with radioactive materials or X-ray equipment.
- Lead glasses: Lead glasses, also known as radiation safety glasses, are designed to protect the eyes from radiation exposure. They have leaded lenses to reduce the penetration of X-rays or other forms of ionising radiation.
- Radiation monitoring devices: In addition to PPE, personnel working with radiation may use radiation monitoring devices such as dosimeters or film badges. These devices measure and track the amount of radiation to which an individual has been exposed, helping to ensure that exposure levels remain within safe limits.

It is important to note that radiation PPE should be accompanied by adherence to proper radiation safety protocols and practices. Veterinary staff working with radiation should receive appropriate training on radiation safety, including the correct use and maintenance of PPE, handling and storage of radiation sources and the principles of radiation protection. Furthermore, regulatory requirements and guidelines regarding radiation safety may vary between countries or regions. Following local authorities' specific regulations and recommendations is crucial, and consulting with a radiation safety officer or expert to ensure compliance with all necessary precautions (see Chapter 7 for further information).

1.6 Accident Reporting

The accident report process in a veterinary practice typically involves documenting any incidents or accidents that occur within the facility. This process is important for maintaining a safe working environment, ensuring proper treatment of animals and managing liability concerns. While specific practices may vary, here is a general outline of the accident report process in a veterinary practice [11]:

- Immediate response: When an accident or incident occurs, the veterinary staff should provide immediate care to injured animals or individuals. They should also assess the situation to ensure the safety of everyone present.
- Notify supervisor: The staff members involved in the incident should inform their immediate supervisor or manager about what happened. Depending on the practice's protocols, this can be done verbally or through a designated reporting system.
- Document details: The person responsible for filing the accident report should gather all relevant information about the incident. This includes the incident's date,

time and location, names of individuals involved, description of what happened and any relevant details or observations.

- Collect witness statements: If there were witnesses to the accident, their statements should be collected as well. These statements can provide additional perspectives and help establish an accurate account of the incident.
- Report completion: The staff member responsible for the accident report should complete the necessary forms or documents using the gathered information. This may include a standardised accident report form provided by the practice or specific software or digital systems used for reporting.
- Review and investigation: The supervisor or manager should review the completed accident report and may conduct an investigation if necessary. The purpose is to understand the causes of the accident, identify any underlying issues and take appropriate measures to prevent similar incidents in the future.
- Corrective actions: Based on the findings of the review and investigation, the veterinary practice should implement any necessary corrective actions. This may involve additional training, modifications to protocols or procedures or making changes to the physical environment to enhance safety.
- Communication and follow-up: The supervisor or manager should communicate the findings and any implemented corrective actions to the individuals involved in the accident and other relevant staff members. Regular follow-up may be required to monitor progress and ensure that the necessary changes are effective.
- Recordkeeping: All accident reports, witness statements, investigation findings and related documentation should be appropriately filed and maintained as part of the practice's recordkeeping system. If required, this information may be used for future reference, insurance purposes or legal matters.

It is important to note that specific protocols and requirements may vary between veterinary practices, so it is advisable to consult individual practice's policies and procedures for precise instructions on the preferred accident reporting process [11].

Figure 1.5 shows an example of an accident report form that could be used in practice.

1.7 Maintaining Equipment in Practice

Maintaining practice equipment in a veterinary practice is essential for providing high-quality care to animals and ensuring the smooth functioning of the facility. Some key points to consider for the maintenance of practice equipment are as follows [12]:

- Regular inspections: Perform routine inspections of all equipment to identify any signs of wear, damage or malfunction. This includes diagnostic machines, surgical instruments, anaesthesia equipment, dental tools and imaging devices. Check for loose or broken parts, frayed cables, leaks and any other issues affecting the equipment's performance.
- Create a maintenance schedule: Establish a maintenance schedule for different types of equipment. This schedule should outline the frequency of inspections, cleaning, calibration and servicing based on the manufacturer's recommendations. Develop a system to keep track of maintenance tasks and ensure they are completed on time.
- Cleaning and disinfection: Clean and disinfect equipment regularly to prevent the spread of infections. Follow the manufacturer's instructions for cleaning and using appropriate disinfectants. Pay special attention to items that come in contact with animals or biological samples, such as examination tables, surgical instruments and laboratory equipment [13].
- Calibration and calibration logs: Calibration is crucial for accurate readings and measurements from diagnostic equipment. Establish a calibration schedule and maintain a log of all calibration activities. Some equipment may require professional calibration, so ensure arrangements with qualified technicians or service providers are made.
- Repairs and replacements: Promptly address any equipment malfunctions or damages. Train staff members to identify problems and report them to the appropriate authority. Depending on the severity of the issue, repairs or replacement of equipment may be necessary. Keep spare parts, if available, for quick repairs.
- Staff training: Train the veterinary staff on equipment use, cleaning and maintenance. Ensure they understand the importance of regular maintenance and encourage them to report any concerns or issues promptly. The knowledgeable staff can contribute to identifying problems early and preventing further damage.
- Documentation: Maintain detailed records of all equipment maintenance activities, including inspections, cleaning, repairs and calibration. Documenting these tasks helps track the equipment's history, identify recurring issues and demonstrate compliance during audits or inspections.
- Collaborate with suppliers: Maintain contact with equipment suppliers or manufacturers to stay updated on maintenance recommendations, software updates and any recalls or safety notices. They can provide valuable

ACCIDENT INVESTIGATION REPORT			
Company Name		Unit/Contract:	
Incident location			
Date of incident		Status:	*Ongoing*
Type of incident		Injury or Ilness caused:	
Potential severity	Major [ ]	Serious [ ]	Minor [ ]
Recurrence Probability	High [ ]	Medium [X]	Low [ ]
Background Information			
Description of How Accident Occurred:			
Evidence/Media			
Insert here or refer to Appendices			
Incident Investigation			
Immediate causes **Contributory/Root Causes:**			
Supporting Documents			
The following supporting documents have been consulted in preparation of this accident investigation report (Also refer to Appendix C)			

Figure 1.5 Accident report form example. *Source:* Rosina Lillywhite.

Conclusion, Preventative and Corrective Actions

The following Immediate/Containment actions are recommended:

RIDDOR Report: complete necessary filing to local authority relating to the RIDDOR reportable event within 10 days of accident

The following Preventative actions are recommended for consideration:

Further Opportunities for improvement:

Completed by:

Name	Role/Position	Signed	Date

Appendix A – Evidence/Photos/Videos

Appendix B – Accident Report Form

Appendix C – Supporting Documentation

Figure 1.5 (Continued)

information on best practices for equipment care and assist with repairs or replacements when needed.

- Portable appliance testing (PAT): PAT is a process used to assess the safety of electrical appliances. The testing is typically performed by a competent person who inspects and tests the appliances for potential electrical faults or hazards. Various checks and tests are conducted on the appliance during a PAT test, including visual inspections, earth continuity testing, insulation resistance testing and functionality checks. The specific tests performed depend on the type of appliance and the level of risk associated with its use. PAT testing aims to ensure that electrical appliances are safe to use, especially in environments where they may pose a risk to the individuals using them or to the premises. This testing helps identify faults or defects that could lead to electrical shocks, fires or other hazards and should be carried out at least annually; some premises may be required to carry out testing every six months [13].

- Remember that the specific maintenance requirements may vary depending on the type of equipment in veterinary practice. Always consult the manufacturer's guidelines and seek professional assistance as necessary.

Identifying Faults in Equipment

It is important to remember that identifying faults in practice equipment is essential to prevent injury to staff, clients or visitors to the practice and to maintain practice equipment in good working order. Table 1.4 displays the possible

Table 1.4 Equipment faults and action required.

Equipment fault	Sign of fault	Action to take
Chemical and Biological Spills	Presence of spilled chemicals or biological agents, unusual odours, visible contamination.	• Ensure personal safety by wearing appropriate personal protective equipment (PPE) like gloves, goggles, and masks. • Isolate the area to prevent further contamination. • Follow established procedures for spill containment, clean-up, and disposal of hazardous materials. • Report the spill to the designated personnel responsible for handling such incidents, such as a supervisor or safety officer.
Glass Breakages	Shattered or broken glass, sharp edges, scattered glass fragments.	• Ensure personal safety by wearing gloves and taking precautions to avoid injury from glass shards. • Isolate the area to prevent access by others and minimise the risk of injury. • Safely clean up the broken glass using appropriate tools (e.g., broom, dustpan) and dispose of it properly. • If the breakage was due to a structural or safety issue, report it to maintenance personnel or the relevant department.
Infection and Infestation	Presence of pests, signs of infestation (e.g., droppings, nests), signs of infectious material or waste	• Avoid direct contact with infected or infested areas. • Notify the appropriate personnel responsible for pest control or facility maintenance. • Follow established procedures for cleaning, disinfection, and pest control. • Take necessary precautions to prevent the spread of infection or infestation, such as quarantining affected areas if required.
Electrical Faults and Equipment	Malfunctioning or non-operational equipment, tripped circuit breakers, power outages, burning smells, sparks, overheating.	• Ensure personal safety by disconnecting or switching off the equipment and isolating the power source if possible. • If there is an immediate danger, evacuate the area and contact emergency services if necessary. • Report the fault to the appropriate personnel responsible for maintenance or repair of electrical equipment. • Tag or label the faulty equipment to prevent further use until it has been repaired or replaced by qualified personnel.
Fire and Gaseous Leaks	Smoke, flames, burning smells, activated fire alarms, hissing sounds, and strong odours from gas leaks	• In the event of fire, follow established emergency evacuation procedures, activate fire alarms, and contact emergency services. • If there is a gas leak, evacuate the area immediately, avoid creating sparks, and notify emergency services and relevant authorities. • Report the incident to the appropriate personnel, such as the fire marshal or safety officer, and follow the organisation's reporting procedures for fire or gas-related incidents.

Source: Rosina Lillywhite.

faults to look out for in practice equipment and the relevant action to take if a fault is identified.

1.8 Emergency First Aid

Emergency first aid in the workplace refers to the provision of immediate and basic medical assistance to an injured or ill person until professional medical help arrives. Key points to consider in relation to emergency first aid in the workplace are as follows [14]: cardiopulmonary cerebral resuscitation (CPCR), choking, wounds, fractures and burns.

Appointing First Aiders

The number of first aiders required in a workplace depends on the size of the workplace, nature of the work and the level of risk involved. The HSE provides guidelines on the recommended ratios of first aiders to employees. First aiders should receive appropriate training to provide first aid in the workplace. The training should cover topics such as CPCR, bandaging, treating burns and fractures and handling medical emergencies [14].

First Aid Training

- Employers should ensure that there are an adequate number of trained first aiders available at all times, taking into account shift patterns, absences and other factors.
- First aid training should be provided by competent training providers who follow recognised standards and guidelines.
- First-aiders may need to undergo refresher training periodically, typically every three years, to keep their skills and knowledge up to date.

Responsibilities of First Aiders [15]

- First aiders should be familiar with the first aid facilities and equipment available in the workplace.
- They should assess the situation, provide appropriate first aid and seek professional medical help when necessary.
- First aiders should maintain confidentiality and treat individuals with respect and dignity.

First Aid Kits and Equipment

Ensure that the workplace is equipped with a well-stocked first aid kit that is easily accessible to all employees. Regularly check the contents and replenish supplies as needed. Additionally, workplaces may require specific first aid equipment based on their nature of work or industry such as eye wash stations or a defibrillator.

First Aid Kits

Availability and accessibility [16]:

- Employers are required to provide suitable and sufficient first aid equipment in the workplace.
- First aid kits should be easily accessible to all employees, and their locations should be clearly marked.
- The number and size of first aid kits needed will depend on the size and nature of the workplace and the level of risk identified in the risk assessment.

Contents of First Aid Kits [16]

- First aid kits should contain a range of items suitable for treating common workplace injuries and illnesses.
- The contents of the first aid kit should be based on the findings of the workplace risk assessment.
- Typical items that may be included in a first aid kit are adhesive dressings, sterile eye pads, bandages, disposable gloves, scissors, resuscitation face shields and guidance on first aid.

Regular Inspection and Restocking

- The person responsible for first aid arrangements in the workplace should regularly check and restock the first aid kits.
- The contents should be maintained in good condition, with items in date and sealed properly.
- Records should be kept of inspections, including dates, details of items checked and any replenishments made.

It is important to note that specific requirements for first aiders and first aid kits may vary based on the country, industry and regulatory authorities. It is advisable to consult the local health and safety regulations and guidelines relevant to practice to ensure compliance with the specific requirements.

Documentation and Reporting

Maintain accurate records of any incidents, injuries or illnesses that occur in the workplace. Follow the reporting procedures set by the practice which may include completing incident reports and notifying relevant personnel or authorities. Remember, while emergency first aid is important, it should never replace the need for professional medical care. Once professional help arrives, provide them with all relevant information and cooperate with their instructions [4].

1.9 Working Time Requirements and Pay

The Working Time Regulations (WTRs) in the United Kingdom provide legal provisions to protect workers' health, safety and well-being by establishing limits on working hours, rest breaks and annual leave entitlement. The key points to understand about the Working Time Regulations include [17]:

Maximum weekly working hours: The WTR limits most workers' average working time to 48 hours per week. This average is typically calculated over a reference period of 17 weeks. Workers can voluntarily choose to work longer hours by signing an opt-out agreement, but they cannot be forced or pressured into doing so. Some categories of workers, such as certain mobile workers and those in certain industries, may have different rules and exemptions regarding maximum working hours. Other requirements include the following [17]:

- Rest breaks and rest periods: Workers aged 18 and above are entitled to a minimum 20-minute uninterrupted rest break if their working day exceeds six hours.
- Workers under the age of 18 are entitled to a 30-minute uninterrupted rest break if their working day exceeds 4.5 hours.
- Workers are entitled to a daily rest period of 11 consecutive hours in each 24-hour period.
- Workers are entitled to a weekly rest period of at least 24 consecutive hours in each 7-day period or at least 48 consecutive hours in each 14-day period.

Annual Leave Entitlement [17]

- Full-time workers are entitled to a minimum of 5.6 weeks (or 28 days) of paid annual leave per year (including bank holidays).
- Part-time workers' leave entitlement is calculated pro-rata, depending on the number of days or hours they work in a week.
- Public holidays can be included as part of the annual leave entitlement if stated in the employment contract.

Night Work

The WTR includes specific provisions for night workers, defined as those who regularly work at least three hours during the night period, typically between 11 p.m. and 6 a.m. Night workers are entitled to receive regular health assessments and have the right to transfer to day work if deemed necessary for health reasons. There are additional restrictions on the average weekly working hours for night workers, and they should not exceed eight hours on average over a 17-week reference period [17].

Record Keeping and Enforcement

Employers are required to maintain records of workers' working hours, including any opt-out agreements, for at least two years. The HSE is responsible for enforcing the WTR in relation to working time and rest breaks, while the employment tribunals deal with disputes related to annual leave entitlement. It is important to note that there are certain exceptions and variations to the WTRs for specific sectors, such as veterinary, healthcare, emergency services and armed forces. It is advisable to consult the official United Kingdom government resources or seek legal advice to understand the specific application of the WTR to a particular industry or employment situation [17].

Refer to the United Kingdom government's official website or consult the advisory, conciliation and arbitration service (ACAS) guidelines for detailed and up-to-date information on the WTRs.

National Minimum Wage (NMW)

In the United Kingdom, the government sets the minimum pay requirements to ensure workers receive a fair minimum wage for their work [18]. The NMW is the minimum hourly rate that most workers in the United Kingdom are entitled to receive varies, depending on the worker's age and whether they are an apprentice. The rates are updated annually [19].

National Living Wage (NLW)

The NLW as of April 2024 has been made available to all those 21 years old and above, previously this has only been available to those 23 years old and above. The NMW and the NLW are reviewed by the government each year and updated in April, so it is important that the most up to date figures are referred to [19].

Additional Considerations

It is important to note that the minimum pay requirements may differ for certain groups or circumstances, such as workers in specific industries, those on apprenticeships or individuals with disabilities. Some workers, such as those who are self-employed, volunteers or in certain educational or training programs, may not be entitled to the NMW or NLW. However, specific rules and exceptions apply, so it is advisable to consult official guidance or seek legal advice for individual circumstances. Employers are legally obligated to pay their workers at least the minimum wage rates applicable to their age and employment status.

The rates are periodically reviewed and updated by the government. It is essential for employers to stay informed about the current rates to ensure compliance with the minimum pay requirements.

For the most up-to-date information on the NMW and NLW rates, it is recommended to refer to the official United Kingdom government website or consult the HM Revenue and Customs (HMRC) guidance on minimum wage compliance.

References

1 Hazard Definitions | IFRC [Internet]. [cited 2023 Jun 23]. Available from: https://www.ifrc.org/document/hazard-definitions.

2 The Management of Health and Safety at Work Regulations 1999 [Internet]. King's Printer of Acts of Parliament; [cited 2023 Jul 17]. Available from: www.legislation.gov.United Kingdom/United Kingdomsi/1999/3242/contents/made.

3 Cooper, B., Mullineaux, E., and Turner, L. (2021). *BSAVA Textbook of Veterinary Nursing*, 6e, 429–490. Gloucester: British Small Animal Veterinary Association.

4 COSHH CLP and REACH – COSHH [Internet]. [cited 2023 Jul 17]. Available from: www.hse.gov.United Kingdom/coshh/detail/coshh-clp-reach.htm.

5 Lifting Operations and Lifting Equipment Regulations (LOLER) [Internet]. [cited 2023 Jul 17]. Available from: www.hse.gov.United Kingdom/work-equipment-machinery/loler.htm.

6 Working Safely with Display Screen Equipment: Overview – HSE [Internet]. [cited 2023 Jul 22]. Available from: www.hse.gov.United Kingdom/msd/dse.

7 Legionnaires' Disease. The control of legionella bacteria in water systems [Internet]. [cited 2023 Jul 17]. Available from: www.hse.gov.United Kingdom/pubns/books/l8.htm.

8 Asbestos – HSE [Internet]. [cited 2023 Jul 22]. Available from: www.hse.gov.United Kingdom/asbestos.

9 Managing Risks and Risk Assessment at Work – Overview – HSE [Internet]. [cited 2023 Jul 17]. Available from: www.hse.gov.United Kingdom/simple-health-safety/risk/index.htm.

10 GOV.UNITED KINGDOM [Internet]. [cited 2023 Jul 17]. The Regulatory Reform (Fire Safety) Order 2005: summary of responses (accessible version). Available from: https://www.gov.United Kingdom/government/consultations/the-regulatory-reform-fire-safety-order-2005-call-for-evidence/outcome/the-regulatory-reform-fire-safety-order-2005-summary-of-responses-accessible-version.

11 Manso-Diaz, G., Lopez-Sanroman, J., and Weller, R. (2018). *A Practical Guide to Equine Radiography*, 1e, 1–17. Sheffield: 5M Publishing Ltd.

12 Reporting Accidents and Incidents at Work [Internet]. [cited 2023 Jul 17]. Available from: www.hse.gov.United Kingdom/pubns/indg453.htm.

13 Maintenance of Work Equipment – Work Equipment and Machinery [Internet]. [cited 2023 Jul 17]. Available from: www.hse.gov.United Kingdom/work-equipment-machinery/maintenance.htm.

14 PAT (Portable Appliance Testing) – HSE's answers to popular questions [Internet]. [cited 2023 Jul 17]. Available from: www.hse.gov.United Kingdom/electricity/faq-portable-appliance-testing.htm.

15 Legislation – First aid at work [Internet]. [cited 2023 Jul 18]. Available from: www.hse.gov.United Kingdom/firstaid/legislation.htm.

16 Workplace First Aid Training Courses [Internet]. [cited 2023 Jul 18]. Available from: www.sja.org.United Kingdom/courses/workplace-first-aid.

17 Workplace First Aid Kits – Small, Large & More [Internet]. [cited 2023 Jul 18]. Available from: www.sja.org.United Kingdom/first-aid-supplies/first-aid-kits/workplace-first-aid-kits.

18 GOV.UNITED KINGDOM [Internet]. [cited 2023 Jul 18]. National minimum wage and National living wage rates. Available from: https://www.gov.United Kingdom/national-minimum-wage-rates.

19 Acas [Internet]. Acas; [cited 2023 Jul 18]. Acas | Making working life better for everyone in Britain. Available from: www.acas.org.United Kingdom.

2

Professional Relationships and Communication

Marie Rippingale[1], Sophie Pearson[1], and Rosina Lillywhite[2]

[1] Bottle Green Training Ltd, Derby, United Kingdom
[2] VetPartners Nursing School, Petersfield, United Kingdom

Introduction

Good communication skills are vital for the smooth and efficient functioning of a veterinary practice. Communication is important not only to send and receive messages but also to build and maintain positive relationships with work colleagues and clients. Communication takes many forms but is basically a two-way process whereby a message is sent, received and responded to [1]. Effective communication is also a requirement of The Royal College of Veterinary Surgeons (RCVS) Code of Professional Conduct for Veterinary Nurses [2]. Therefore, effective communication skills are essential for registered veterinary nurses (RVNs) in order to progress their professional development.

2.1 The Dynamics of Communication

The Communication Process

The communication process refers to the exchange of information, ideas, thoughts and feelings between individuals or groups. It involves a sender, a message, a channel, a receiver and feedback.

The process works as follows [3]:

1) Sender: The sender is the person or entity who initiates the communication process. They have a message or information they want to convey to the receiver. The sender encodes the message into a format that can be understood by the receiver.
2) Message: The message is the information, idea or emotion that the sender wants to communicate. It can be in the form of spoken words, written text, gestures, facial expressions or any other means of expression.

3) Encoding: Encoding is the process of converting the message into a form that can be transmitted through a communication channel. It involves choosing words, symbols or non-verbal cues to convey the intended meaning.
4) Channel: The channel is the medium through which the message is transmitted from the sender to the receiver. This can be through face-to-face conversations, phone calls, emails, text messages, video conferences or any other means of communication.
5) Receiver: The receiver is the person or group to whom the message is directed. They decode the message by interpreting the words, tone, body language and other cues to understand the sender's intended meaning.
6) Decoding: Decoding is the process of interpreting and understanding the message by the receiver. It involves extracting meaning from the encoded message using the receiver's knowledge, context and cultural background.
7) Feedback: Feedback is the response or reaction given by the receiver to the sender. It indicates whether the message was understood, how it was interpreted and provides an opportunity for clarification or further communication.
8) Noise: Noise refers to any interference or disruption in the communication process that hinders the accurate transmission or reception of the message. This can be external factors such as background noise, technical issues or internal factors such as language barriers, distractions or biases.

The communication process is a dynamic and iterative cycle, where both the sender and receiver play active roles. It is essential for effective communication to ensure that the message is accurately encoded, transmitted through an appropriate channel, received and properly decoded by the intended receiver. Feedback helps in confirming understanding and addressing any misunderstandings or barriers that may arise. Figure 2.1 displays the steps involved in the communication process.

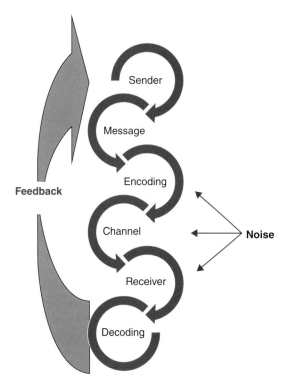

Figure 2.1   The communication process [3]. *Source:* Rosina Lillywhite.

Communication Categories

Verbal Communication

Communication can be categorised as either verbal or non-verbal. Spoken and oral communication is used for telephone and face-to-face communication. This form of communication can be used in digital marketing videos that can be posted on social media. With verbal communication, the choice of words used is important. Other important factors are the way and the speed at which the words are spoken [1]. Communication with clients takes practice, and experience can be gained from observing interactions between experienced colleagues and clients [1]. Written communication can be considered to be a type of verbal communication as it also uses words (or verbatim). Information relating to written communication can be found in Table 2.1.

Non-verbal Communication

It has been suggested that 93% of the meaning of a message is transmitted non-verbally; this can be broken down into the following [4]:

- 55% of meaning is transmitted by facial expression or body language
- 38% by vocal tone
- 7% of the meaning of a message is transmitted by the actual words spoken.

Non-verbal communication can include the following aspects [1]:

- Posture and body position – also known as body language
- Eye contact

Table 2.1   Examples of written communication used in veterinary practice [1].

Example of written communication	Points to consider
Clinical notes	These should be accurate, legible and completed in full with the author clearly identified. Preferably typed up rather than handwritten
Letters to clients	Any form of written communication from the practice should be on headed paper and preferably printed rather than handwritten. Letters should be clearly signed with the name of the author and their position in the practice. Correct grammar and punctuation should be used
Emails to clients, colleagues and allied professionals	Emails should be written with the same care and thought as a written letter. Correct grammar and punctuation should be used. Disputes should never be carried out over email, text, memos or social media
In-house forms, e.g. clinical parameter sheets, critical care sheets, care plans and anaesthetic monitoring records	These should be accurate, legible and completed in full with the author clearly identified
Official documents, e.g. laboratory submission forms, insurance claim forms, admit and discharge forms	These should be accurate, legible and completed in full with the author clearly identified
Flyers and information sheets for promotional purposes	These should be well considered and contain only accurate information. Input should be included from different members of the team. Correct grammar and punctuation should be used. Any information should be proofread before being published
Notes and memos	These should be professional and convey a clear message. Disputes should never be carried out over email, text, memos or social media

Source: Marie Rippingale.

- Facial expressions
- Paralanguage
- Proxemics and haptics
- Appearance

Posture and Body Language

Posture and body language can convey mood and the type of attitude that one person has towards another person and can therefore give the client a powerful message [5]. Communication is more effective when an open body posture is used, so folded arms and crossed legs should be avoided [1]. The communicator should face the person they are talking to and use appropriate eye contact. Standing behind barriers such as reception desks and computer stations should be avoided [1]. If the communicator needs to use the computer during the conversation, they should tell the client that this is what they are doing [1]. This will prevent the client from feeling like they are being ignored or unattended.

Eye Contact

Making eye contact is one of several skills known as an attending skill. Attending behaviours let other people know that you are focused on understanding them and ready to listen [4]. Making eye contact should not be confused with staring or a fixed eye gaze, as this can be unnerving. Eye contact should be maintained at a comfortable level for both the sender (communicator) and the receiver (client) [5].

Facial Expressions

Facial expressions provide a good source of non-verbal information and are especially useful when conveying emotion [5]. According to research, the face reveals six primary emotions [5]:

- Surprise
- Fear
- Anger
- Disgust
- Happiness
- Sadness

Facial expressions can be used as cues to help to evaluate emotions and to determine if the message was received correctly [5]. When communicating with clients, it is important that the communicator is aware of their facial expressions and an open and friendly approach is recommended [1]. Expressions must be appropriate to the situation for example conveying concern if the client is worried or upset [1]. It has been suggested that the power of facial expressions far outweighs the power of the actual words used [4]. Facial expressions are therefore an important part of communication and should be considered and used carefully.

Paralanguage

Paralanguage refers to aspects such as the tone, volume, pitch, timbre (quality of a voice distinct from its pitch and intensity) and intonation (the rise and fall of the voice in speaking) emphasis and fluency which accompanies speech [5]. Paralanguage can accompany words to make up the true meaning, and these features can help in the interpretation of the message by giving the receiver clues about the state of mind of the sender [5]. The tone of voice used can be influenced by the emotional state of the person. Therefore, in practice, it is important to be aware of your own individual emotional state and to manage this carefully when communicating with others. This is especially relevant in high-pressure and time-poor situations, as there may be a tendency to rush communication, which will then not be effective. Paralanguage also includes 'non-lexical' aspects that can be added to speech, including marks of encouragement such as 'ah', 'hmmm' and 'uh-huh' [1]. These marks can be used to encourage someone to keep speaking and also make up an important component of listening skills.

Proxemics and Haptics

These terms relate to the proximity to a person and touch [1]. The intimate space of a person is generally up to 45 cm and is reserved for intimate thoughts and feelings. The personal distance ranges from 45 to 120 cm and is used for less intense personal exchanges [5]. Both intimate space and personal distance for individuals are influenced by age, sex and culture [5]. In practice, it is important to read the response of the client to your proximity and adapt accordingly. Touch can be used to communicate affection, familiarity and sympathy [1]. Touch can, however, be a controversial subject and it is important to be aware that not all clients will respond well to being touched. There may be important cultural issues relating to touch that need to be understood [1].

Appearance

The clothes that someone wears, their hairstyle and the colours chosen can all be considered forms of non-verbal communication. In veterinary practice, the choice of uniform worn can affect physiological reactions, judgements and interpretations [5]. People form impressions of each other within 20 seconds to a few minutes [5], so it is important to convey a professional appearance at all times.

Table 2.2 displays some key points relating to non-verbal communication.

Listening Skills

Listening is an important communication skill. Poor listening skills have been cited in a large percentage of medical negligence cases and have been identified as one of the main reasons why individuals take legal action against

Table 2.2 Key points relating to non-verbal communication [6, 7].

Non-verbal communication type	Things to do	Things to avoid
Posture and body position (Body language)	Maintain an open and approachable posture: Stand or sit upright with an open stance, facing the client directly. This conveys attentiveness and willingness to listen	Avoid crossing your arms or legs: Crossing your arms or legs can create a barrier between you and the client, making you appear defensive or disinterested. Keep your arms relaxed at your sides or lightly resting on a desk or table
	Maintain appropriate eye contact: Make regular eye contact with the client to demonstrate active engagement and interest in the conversation. However, be mindful not to stare excessively, as it can make the client uncomfortable	Avoid fidgeting or nervous movements: Excessive fidgeting, such as tapping fingers or shifting weight, can convey nervousness or lack of confidence. Try to maintain a calm and composed demeanour
	Use open and welcoming gestures: Use open hand gestures, such as keeping your palms facing upward or loosely clasping your hands in front of you. This encourages a sense of openness and approachability	Do not invade personal space: Respect the client's personal space by maintaining an appropriate distance. Invading personal space can make them feel uncomfortable or threatened
	Lean slightly towards the client: Leaning slightly forward demonstrates interest and involvement in the conversation. It shows that you are focused on understanding their concerns and needs	Avoid turning away or distractions: Face the client directly and give them your undivided attention. Avoid turning away, checking your phone or engaging in other distracting activities, as it can undermine the client's perception of your attentiveness
	Mirror the client's body language: Subtly mirroring the client's body language can help establish rapport and create a sense of connection. However, be cautious not to mimic them too closely, as it may appear insincere	Do not display negative body language: Avoid negative body language such as rolling your eyes, sighing or showing impatience. These gestures can create a negative impression and damage the client's trust in your professionalism
Eye contact	Establish regular eye contact: Maintain regular eye contact with the client throughout the conversation. It shows that you are actively listening and engaged in the discussion	Avoid staring excessively: While maintaining eye contact is essential, avoid staring for prolonged periods, as it can make the client uncomfortable. Use natural breaks in the conversation to briefly glance away or focus on other aspects of the consultation
	Show interest and attentiveness: Demonstrate your interest in the client's concerns by maintaining focused eye contact. This conveys that their opinions and questions are valued	Do not constantly break eye contact: On the other hand, avoid constantly breaking eye contact, as it may convey disinterest or distractibility. Find a balance between maintaining eye contact and looking away occasionally
	Use eye contact to convey empathy: Eye contact can help convey empathy and understanding. It shows that you genuinely care about the client's feelings and their pet's well-being	Do not use eye contact to intimidate: Eye contact should be warm and inviting, not intimidating. Avoid using intense or aggressive eye contact that may make the client feel uncomfortable or defensive
	Match the client's eye contact: Mirror the client's eye contact to create a sense of connection and rapport. If the client maintains strong eye contact, reciprocate by doing the same. However, be mindful not to make the client uncomfortable by staring excessively	Avoid distractions during eye contact: When engaging in eye contact, minimise distractions and focus solely on the client. Avoid looking at other things or checking your phone, as it can give the impression of disengagement
Facial expressions	Maintain a friendly and welcoming expression: Keep your facial expression warm, friendly and approachable. Smile genuinely to create a positive and welcoming atmosphere	Avoid displaying negative or judgmental expressions: Be mindful of your facial expressions to ensure you do not unintentionally convey negative emotions or judgments. Avoid frowning, rolling your eyes or displaying impatience, as these can make clients feel uneasy or misunderstood

Table 2.2 (Continued)

Non-verbal communication type	Things to do	Things to avoid
	Show empathy and understanding: Use facial expressions to convey empathy and understanding towards the client's concerns. Displaying a compassionate expression can help reassure clients that their pets are in good hands	Do not overuse or fake expressions: Authenticity is crucial when using facial expressions. Avoid overusing or faking expressions, as they may appear insincere or manipulative. Let your expressions be a genuine reflection of your emotions and intentions
	Use facial expressions to reflect active listening: Show your engagement and attentiveness through facial expressions. Nodding your head occasionally and maintaining an interested and focused expression can communicate that you are actively listening and processing the information	Do not let facial expressions overshadow verbal communication: While facial expressions are essential, ensure they complement your verbal communication rather than overpower it. Maintaining a balance between facial expressions and spoken words ensures clear and effective communication
	Use appropriate facial expressions for different situations: Adjust your facial expressions based on the context. For example, you may display concern or sympathy when discussing a patient's health issue or show excitement and happiness when delivering good news or positive outcomes	Avoid inappropriate or excessive smiling: While a warm and friendly smile is encouraged, be mindful of the context. Excessive or constant smiling without considering the seriousness of the situation may be perceived as unprofessional or insensitive
Paralanguage	Use a warm and friendly tone: Maintain a pleasant and inviting tone of voice when speaking to clients. A warm and friendly tone helps create a positive and comforting conversation atmosphere	Avoid speaking too loudly or softly: Be mindful of your volume and avoid speaking too loudly or softly. Speaking too loudly may come across as aggressive, while speaking too softly may make it difficult for clients to hear and understand you
	Vary your pitch and intonation: Utilise appropriate variations in pitch and intonation to convey meaning and emphasise important points. Modulate your voice to express empathy, enthusiasm or concern as needed	Do not rush through your words: Avoid speaking too quickly or rushing through your words. Rapid speech can make it challenging for clients to follow along or comprehend the information being conveyed
	Speak clearly and articulately: Enunciate your words clearly and avoid mumbling or speaking too quickly. Clear and precise speech helps clients understand you better and fosters effective communication	Avoid a monotone voice: A monotone voice lacks enthusiasm and engagement, which can make the conversation dull and uninteresting. Vary your tone and inflexion to keep clients engaged and convey genuine interest
	Use a calm and reassuring voice: When discussing sensitive or difficult topics, employ a calm and reassuring voice to instil confidence and provide emotional support to clients. This can help alleviate their concerns and create a sense of trust	Do not sound condescending or patronising: Be conscious of your tone to ensure it does not come across as condescending or patronising. Treat clients respectfully and maintain a professional and courteous tone throughout the conversation
Proxemics	Respect personal space: Be mindful of personal space and maintain an appropriate distance when interacting with clients. Respect their comfort zone and avoid invading their personal space unless necessary	Avoid invading personal space: Invading a client's personal space without their consent can make them feel uncomfortable or threatened. Maintain a respectful distance and allow them to dictate their desired level of closeness
	Use proximity to convey attentiveness: During conversations, leaning slightly towards the client can indicate attentiveness and active engagement. It demonstrates that you are focused on understanding their concerns and needs	Do not stand too far away: Standing too far away from the client can create a sense of emotional distance or detachment. Find an appropriate balance between personal space and proximity to establish a comfortable and connected environment
	Adapt to cultural norms: Different cultures have varying expectations regarding personal space. Be aware of cultural differences and adapt your proximity accordingly to ensure you respect and accommodate diverse cultural norms	

Table 2.2 (Continued)

Non-verbal communication type	Things to do	Things to avoid
Haptics	Use a gentle touch with consent: In certain situations, gentle touch can comfort and reassure clients. However, always seek consent before initiating any form of touch, such as a handshake or pat on the shoulder	Avoid intrusive or inappropriate touch: Respect personal boundaries and refrain from intrusive or inappropriate touching. Be cautious and sensitive to cultural and individual preferences regarding touch
	Use touch to soothe animals: Touch can be beneficial in soothing and comforting animals. Employ gentle touch while handling and examining animals, ensuring it is appropriate and respectful to the animal's needs and behaviour	Do not assume comfort with touch: Not everyone may be comfortable with physical contact, so it is important to be mindful and respectful of individual preferences. Always seek permission and respect their boundaries
Appearance	Dress appropriately: Wear clean, professional attire that is suitable for a veterinary practice. Follow any dress code guidelines your workplace sets and ensure your clothing is well-fitted and neat	Avoid wearing inappropriate attire: Refrain from wearing clothing that is too casual, revealing or inappropriate for a professional setting. This includes items such as overly casual t-shirts, shorts or clothing with offensive or controversial graphics
	Maintain personal hygiene: Pay attention to personal grooming, including cleanliness, hairstyle and hygiene practices. Maintaining good personal hygiene helps convey professionalism and attention to detail	Do not neglect personal grooming: Ensure that your hair is well-groomed, your nails are clean and trimmed, and any facial hair is well-maintained. Neglecting personal grooming may give the impression of a lack of professionalism or attention to detail
	Wear a name badge: Consider wearing a name badge that clearly displays your name and position within the veterinary practice. This can help clients easily identify and address you during interactions	Minimise strong or overpowering scents: Be mindful of using strong perfumes, colognes or body sprays, as they may be overpowering or cause discomfort for clients with sensitivities or allergies. Opt for subtle scents or avoid them altogether
	Pay attention to accessories and jewellery: Choose accessories and jewellery that are tasteful and minimal. Avoid wearing excessive or distracting accessories that may draw attention away from the conversation	Avoid excessive or distracting makeup: Keep your makeup natural and professional. Excessive or distracting makeup can draw attention away from the conversation and may not be appropriate in a veterinary practice setting

Source: Rosina Lillywhite.

healthcare professionals [4]. Attentive listening is considered to be one of the most important elements of therapeutic communication and requires an understanding of verbal and non-verbal cues such as eye contact and paralanguage [5].

Attentive listening requires four main components [1]:

- Time to respond: Adequate pauses should be left after a question or statement to give the client time to think and respond in their own time.
- Facilitative responses such as mirroring and eye contact: Consideration should be given to height differences when mirroring clients. For example, if the client is sitting, then the communicator should sit down also. The communicator should not talk down to the client from a height, as this could be intimidating and negatively affect communication and understanding.
- Non-verbal skills: It is important to use body language and facial expressions appropriate for conversational

topics, such as expressing concern if a patient has deteriorated or euthanasia needs to be discussed.
- Picking up on verbal and non-verbal cues: It is important to pick up on the client's body language, facial expressions and tone of voice and adapt your communication style accordingly.

The following are suggestions for achieving effective listening in a veterinary practice setting [1]:

- Appropriate eye contact should be maintained
- Appropriate facial expressions should be used
- Body language should be considered
- Paralanguage includes cues such as 'ah', 'hmmm' and 'uh-huh' to encourage the client to continue speaking.
- Interruptions should be resisted, and silence should be allowed where appropriate
- Reflective statements should be used, such as saying, 'You were saying you think that Boris is not eating as much as normal; let's talk a bit more about that'.

- Summaries can be used to demonstrate effective listening. This helps to bring information together and allows the client the opportunity to add anything they may have missed out.

Questioning Skills

Effective questioning is an important skill to learn. RVNs are required to ask many questions during a working day, whether during a client consultation, for example, admissions or discharges or with colleagues when contributing to the formation of a patient care plan. Different types of questions may be asked, and these can be categorised as follows [5].

- **Closed questions:** These questions are used when only a 'yes' or 'no' answer is required. This type of question can elicit a concise answer but limits explanation.

Example question: 'Did the injection work?'
Answer: 'Yes'

- **Open questions:** These questions aim to get the client to tell a story. Open questions will allow the client to describe their experiences, feelings and understanding of an issue.

Example question: 'What seems to be the problem with Tilly?'
Answer: 'She seems very quiet and is not eating properly ....'

These questions give the listener the opportunity to follow up to get more details.

The advantages and disadvantages of open and closed questions are displayed in Table 2.3.

Sub-categories of open and closed questions are as follows [5]:

Table 2.3 The advantages and disadvantages of open and closed questions [8].

Type of questioning	Advantages	Disadvantages
Closed	Efficiency: Closed questions typically require a short and specific answer, which allows veterinarians to gather information quickly. This can be particularly useful when time is limited and there is a need to collect important details efficiently	Limited information: Closed questions tend to elicit brief, specific responses and may not allow clients to provide additional details or elaborate on their concerns. This can restrict the amount of information gathered, potentially overlooking important factors that could contribute to a more comprehensive understanding of the animal's condition
	Clarification: Closed questions can help veterinarians clarify specific information or details about the animal's condition or history. This can lead to a better understanding of the situation and enable the veterinarian to make more accurate diagnoses and treatment decisions	Lack of client engagement: Closed questions can create a one-sided conversation, with clients feeling like passive recipients of questions rather than active participants in the decision-making process. This may reduce client engagement and their overall satisfaction with the veterinary consultation
	Control over conversation flow: Closed questions allow veterinarians to guide the conversation and control the direction of the consultation. This can help ensure that essential information is obtained and prevent the conversation from straying off-topic	Potential for misinterpretation: Closed questions may not provide enough context or opportunity for clients to express themselves fully, potentially leading to misinterpretation of their responses. This can hinder accurate diagnosis or treatment planning if critical information is overlooked or misunderstood
	Limited response options: Closed questions typically provide a limited set of response options (such as 'yes' or 'no' or selecting from a predetermined list). This can simplify decision-making and allow for more structured data collection and analysis	Restrictive communication: Closed questions can limit the flow of conversation and inhibit open communication between the veterinarian and the client. This may hinder the development of a trusting relationship and prevent clients from fully expressing their concerns or asking questions that could provide valuable insights
Open	Comprehensive information: Open questions encourage clients to provide detailed and descriptive responses, allowing veterinarians to gather a more comprehensive understanding of the animal's condition, history and any related concerns. This can facilitate accurate diagnoses and tailored treatment plans	Time-consuming: Open questions often result in longer responses, requiring more time to elicit and listen to the client's answers. In a busy veterinary practice, this may limit the number of cases that can be seen or lead to delays in appointment schedules

(Continued)

Table 2.3 (Continued)

Type of questioning	Advantages	Disadvantages
	Client engagement and satisfaction: Open questions promote active client participation in the conversation, making them feel heard and involved in the decision-making process. This can lead to increased client engagement, satisfaction and a stronger veterinarian–client relationship	Tangential information: Open questions sometimes elicit off-topic responses or provide excessive and unrelated information. This can make it challenging for veterinarians to extract the relevant details and may require additional clarification or redirection
	Exploration of client perspectives: Open questions allow clients to express their thoughts, concerns and observations in their own words. This can provide valuable insights into the animal's behaviour, environment and other factors that may be relevant to their health. It also allows veterinarians to better understand the client's perspective and address any specific needs or preferences	Lack of structure: Open questions do not provide a predetermined set of response options, potentially making it more difficult to categorise or quantify the information gathered. This can impact data analysis and may require additional effort to organise and make sense of the collected data
	Flexibility and adaptability: Open questions provide flexibility in the conversation, allowing it to flow naturally and adapt to the client's responses. This can lead to unexpected but relevant information being shared, leading to a more nuanced understanding of the situation	Potential for information overload: Open questions can encourage clients to provide extensive information, which can overwhelm both the client and RVN. It may require active listening skills and the ability to filter and prioritise relevant information to avoid getting bogged down in excessive details

Source: Rosina Lillywhite.

- **Reflective questions:** This type of question is useful if it is necessary to soften the questioning process. It also demonstrates to the client that you are listening. Reflective questioning generally involves summarising what the person said. It is important to do this correctly, as if the message changes during the summary, the communication may become ineffective.
- **Probing questions:** These are used as a follow-up to the initial question to elicit the scope of information required. Probing questions should be used with sensitivity, and non-verbal cues should be assessed to check if the client is feeling uncomfortable. Probes can take a non-verbal form, such as a raised eyebrow.
- **Focussed questions:** This type of question is neither open nor closed but includes characteristics of both. A focused question limits an area within which a client can respond but simultaneously encourages more than a 'yes' or 'no' answer.
- **Leading questions:** These questions lead to a predicted answer. Leading questions can be subtle and encourage the acceptance of ideas but may limit the possible replies.

Communication Styles

Communication styles vary between individuals, and this can lead to conflict and misunderstandings [9]. It is important to understand the characteristics and tendencies of different communication styles as this can help to facilitate positive interactions between people with differing styles [9]. There are four primary communication styles [9]:

- Passive
- Aggressive
- Passive–aggressive
- Assertive

See Table 2.4 for further information.

It is important to identify your own communication style and understand the advantages and disadvantages of this. Once your communication style has been identified, you can develop ways to adapt it not only to meet the needs of other people but to different situations. For example, the communication style adopted to deal with an aggressive client or conflict will need to be an assertive communication style. A passive communication style may be more appropriate in a sensitive situation, such as euthanasia. An awareness of communication style and possible adaptations that can be made, may also be useful when communicating with different colleagues. These factors can all help to contribute to a more efficient and productive working environment, and this will benefit all patients, colleagues and clients equally.

Telephone Communication

Communicating on the telephone presents a unique set of challenges as aspects of non-verbal communication cannot

Table 2.4 The four primary communication styles [9].

Communication style	Details	Identifying features	Methods of dealing with this communication style
Passive	Typically quiet and does not seek attention. May be indifferent during debates. Rarely take a strong stance or assert themselves. Do not usually share their needs or express their feelings	• Difficulty saying no • Poor posture • Easy-going attitude • Lack of eye contact • Soft voice • Apologetic demeanour • Fidgeting	**Take a direct approach:** Initiate one on one conversations, as private interactions may be more comfortable for a passive communicator **Ask for their opinions:** Allow plenty of time for them to think about their responses **Use open questions:** This will encourage some elaboration. Give the person time to think and respond
Aggressive	Frequently express their thoughts and feelings. Tend to dominate conversations. Can react before thinking, which can negatively affect relationships and decrease productivity. Can be intimidating to clients and colleagues	• Interrupting other people while they are speaking • Invading personal space • Presenting an overbearing posture • Using aggressive gestures • Maintaining intense eye contact	**Be calm and assertive:** Try not to be intimidated. Focus the conversation on an actionable approach to the problem **Keep conversations professional:** Direct the conversation away from personal issues or emotions **Know when to stop:** Leave the conversation if the aggressive communicator becomes too demanding or there is a lack of positive progress
Passive–aggressive	Appear passive on the surface but often have more aggressive motivations driving their actions. Their words might sound agreeable, but their actions do not always align. Tend to quietly manipulate a situation to benefit them	• Muttering • Using sarcasm • Exhibiting denial • Hiding their emotions • Giving people the silent treatment	**Make clear requests:** Try not to leave room for misinterpretation or confusion **Confront negative behaviour:** Talk to them directly about their behaviour and involve management if there is no progress **Ask them for feedback:** Do this in a one-to-one situation to try to encourage an honest response
Assertive	This style is typically the most productive in the workplace. Assertive communications confidently share their thoughts and ideas while being respectful and polite. They readily take on challenges but also know when to say no. They understand their limits and protect their boundaries without being overly aggressive or defensive	• Expansive gestures • Collaborative tendencies • Healthy expression of ideas and feelings • Good posture • A clear voice • Friendly eye contact	**Showcase this behaviour:** Encourage these people to share their ideas and thoughts **Place in a leadership position:** To act as an example to others **Enlist their help:** Get them to assist in dealing with passive, passive–aggressive and aggressive communicators

Source: Marie Rippingale.

be relied upon [1]. The person receiving the information can only receive information from what is said and how it is said. Many situations require RVNs to communicate via the telephone, such as triaging emergencies, taking query calls, making appointments, delivering patient updates and carrying out follow-up phone calls [1].

The following points are important to facilitate effective telephone communication [1]:

• When answering the phone, the operator should offer their name, the practice name and role in the practice so that the client knows who they are speaking to.

- Phone calls should be answered with a welcoming and warm demeanour. This will help to put the client at ease from the start.
- The operator should speak slowly and clearly. Frequent pauses should be made to give the client a chance to process the information given.
- Try to avoid using complicated veterinary terminology, as the client will not understand, and this can negatively affect the information being discussed.
- The operator should have access to the client database and clinical notes. However, General Data Protection Regulations (GDPR) should be considered at all times.
- The client should be allowed to speak without interruption.
- Important points should be repeated during the call.
- Client understanding can be checked by asking questions and checking the answer for accuracy.
- Notes should be taken to ensure there is something to refer back to.
- If the operator is unsure about something, they should ask another member of staff for advice.
- Ensure that any messages are passed on to the appropriate team member.

For information regarding triage and emergency calls, please see Chapter 14.

2.2 Communicating with Clients

Communication skills are important as they affect the client experience. Empathy is an essential quality to consider, and this is often at the forefront of our minds as RVNs are often animal owners themselves [1]. The human–animal bond will present itself in different forms in equine practice; however, the majority of clients will have an emotional attachment to their animal.

Nurse Clinics and Consultations

Nurse clinics and consultations are now growing in popularity in equine practice, especially with the development of the ambulatory nursing role. Therefore, RVNs must have knowledge of how to communicate effectively with clients and how to run a consultation successfully. In more formal interactions with clients, referring to a standard 'framework' is useful. For many years, the Calgary-Cambridge model (adapted for veterinary use) (Figure 2.2) has been used to teach, evaluate and practice veterinary communication skills [1].

Preparation

To provide a safe and professional service, good preparation is essential. The following should be considered [1]:

- **Environment:** If conducting the consultation at the practice, ensure that the clinical area is clean, safe and private. If conducting the consultation in a yard, try to talk to the client in a private area, away from the patient, to reduce possible distractions.
- **Patient history:** It is a good idea to check the patient's details beforehand, including the patient's name, sex, clinical history and any notes on adverse reactions or relevant behavioural traits.
- **Equipment:** Ensure all required equipment, paperwork and consumables are ready and easy to access.
- **Self-awareness:** First impressions are important, and RVNs should present a professional image to the client. Maintaining a clean uniform can be challenging, but every effort should be made to appear neat and tidy. An awareness of your emotions is important; it is essential to remain impartial even if you find the case difficult or upsetting to deal with. Each new consultation should be treated individually, and each client should be welcomed with a smile and a warm greeting, even if the previous consultation was upsetting or challenging.

Opening the Consultation

The consultation should be opened in a clear and professional manner. This includes a warm greeting, a friendly facial expression and a clear greeting to the client and the animal [1]. If the client is new, then an introduction will be required. The consultation should start with an open question such as 'How are things with Chaplin today?' This allows the client to provide some general information about their animal [1]. It is essential to allow the client to speak and not interrupt them. Attentive listening skills are important here.

Gathering Information

Effective history-taking will facilitate the gathering of detailed, relevant and accurate information. In equine practice, the veterinary surgeon (vet) or RVN will likely have seen the patient recently; however, it is still important to ask the client how they think the animal is getting on. A combination of techniques, such as attentive listening and effective questioning, are essential here.

Physical Examination

If time permits, it is better to take the patient's history first and then examine the patient afterwards [1]. It is essential to signpost what you are doing to the client by saying something such as, 'I am just going to check Chaplin over now'. It is important to include the client in the examination; for example, teach them to correctly use a weigh tape to assess the weight of their horse, letting them feel a lump that has been identified or demonstrate to them how to safely assess

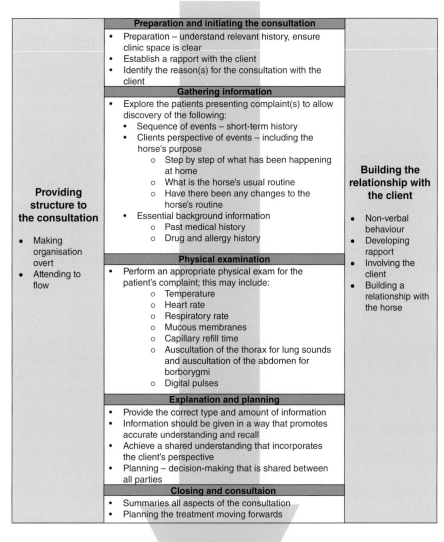

Providing structure to the consultation

- Making organisation overt
- Attending to flow

Preparation and initiating the consultation

- Preparation – understand relevant history, ensure clinic space is clear
- Establish a rapport with the client
- Identify the reason(s) for the consultation with the client

Gathering information

- Explore the patients presenting complaint(s) to allow discovery of the following:
  - Sequence of events – short-term history
  - Clients perspective of events – including the horse's purpose
    - o Step by step of what has been happening at home
    - o What is the horse's usual routine
    - o Have there been any changes to the horse's routine
  - Essential background information
    - o Past medical history
    - o Drug and allergy history

Physical examination

- Perform an appropriate physical exam for the patient's complaint; this may include:
  - o Temperature
  - o Heart rate
  - o Respiratory rate
  - o Mucous membranes
  - o Capillary refill time
  - o Auscultation of the thorax for lung sounds and auscultation of the abdomen for borborygmi
  - o Digital pulses

Explanation and planning

- Provide the correct type and amount of information
- Information should be given in a way that promotes accurate understanding and recall
- Achieve a shared understanding that incorporates the client's perspective
- Planning – decision-making that is shared between all parties

Closing and consultaion

- Summaries all aspects of the consultation
- Planning the treatment moving forwards

Building the relationship with the client

- Non-verbal behaviour
- Developing rapport
- Involving the client
- Building a relationship with the horse

OBSERVATION

Figure 2.2 The Calgary-Cambridge model (adapted for veterinary use) [1]. *Source:* Rosina Lillywhite.

the patient's normal clinical parameters such as temperature, pulse and respiration. These readings can then be used for reference in the future.

Giving Information, Explaining and Planning

The veterinary team should work towards achieving client concordance for treatment plans to be successful. To achieve this, it is important to understand the meaning of the following terms [1]:

- **Compliance:** This term suggests an approach whereby the client is given instructions that they are expected to comply with. However, it is now understood that for the treatment plan to be successful, the involvement and agreement of the client is vital.
- **Concordance:** This concept originated in human medicine. The term refers to an agreement being reached between the client and the vet or RVN. The agreement is expected to incorporate the wishes and beliefs of the

client in the decision-making process. This is what should be strived for in veterinary practice.

- **Adherence:** This term can be defined as the level to which a client follows recommendations of the vet or RVN or the agreed treatment plan. Lack of adherence should not be viewed as a failure on the client's behalf. It should provoke reflection as to how concordance was sought initially and lead to interventions being put in place to rectify any oversights. Adherence is an area where RVNs can help significantly by providing support, whether that be as a contact at the practice or by providing ambulatory support in the form of yard visits. This would be carried out under the direction of the case vet.

The success of the treatment plan will largely depend on how information is presented, how well it is understood and the extent to which the client has been involved in the decision-making process [1]. The veterinary team should strive to achieve concordance and adherence to the plan; otherwise, the plan will not be successful and patient welfare could be compromised. The following points are essential to consider when delivering information to clients [1]:

- Information should be clear, succinct and offered in an appropriate order.
- Give information in manageable amounts and ensure that each piece is understood.
- Information should be pitched at the correct level for the client to facilitate understanding.
- Appropriate aids should be used to facilitate client understanding, such as diagrams, models and practical demonstrations.
- Shared decision-making should should be incorporated if appropriate.
- Motivation and support should be given to the client to encourage concordance with the treatment plan.
- The cultural and religious beliefs and the socioeconomic and financial status of the client should be respected and considered throughout the consultation.

Closing the Consultation

The consultation should be closed professionally. A final discussion and treatment plan summary should be offered [1]. The client should be asked if they have any further concerns or final questions. The client should be clear on when the next appointment will be and who their contact point will be at the practice until then.

Safety Netting

Safety netting involves explaining to the client what to expect following the consultation and what to do if anything unexpected occurs [1]. For example, a weight loss diet for a patient with equine metabolic syndrome (EMS) may have been discussed in the yard. This would have included discussions and demonstrations relating to weight taping, weighing and soaking hay, applying a grazing muzzle, restricting grazing and (if appropriate) an exercise programme. Safety netting may include saying something like, 'Let's see how you and Chaplin get on with the new management programme. If you have any concerns at all, then contact me at the practice straight away'. The client should then be provided with the relevant contact details.

Follow Up

There should always be some form of follow-up after a consultation [1]. This could be a phone call, an email or another appointment either at the practice or out in the yard. If the client mentions at the follow-up that they are struggling with the treatment plan or contacts the practice to ask for help, this should be acted upon immediately. Sometimes, a chat on the phone will be enough to get the client back on track with the treatment programme. In some situations, a visit may be required, and new interventions discussed. It is important to involve the case vet if the treatment plan requires significant changes. The case vet should be kept fully updated regarding the progress and follow-up of each and every case.

Building Client Relationships

Trust is an important factor in building relationships with clients. If a bond of trust can be formed between the RVN and the client, the consultation will be more effective at achieving client concordance and adherence to treatment plans. This will then contribute to improved clinical outcomes and patient welfare, leading to job satisfaction for the RVN [1]. Trust can be built from something as simple as showing a genuine interest in the clients and their animals. This can take many forms, including greeting the patient on arrival, asking open questions such as 'How is Harry today?' and showing empathy for any concerns [1]. Body language should also be considered, such as maintaining appropriate eye contact, not standing in front of a barrier and maintaining an open body position.

Shared decision making (SDM) is an important part of communication in veterinary practice. SDM refers to a process where medical professionals seek the opinions, goals and wishes of their patients/clients and work with them to try and achieve these goals [1]. With SDM, all appropriate treatment options, benefits and contraindications should be discussed, and the decisions made together between the client and the veterinary professional [1]. Some clients may still prefer a more directive style where they are given instructions without being asked for any input [1]. It is important to gauge which approach the client would feel most comfortable with or ask them what they would prefer. SDM is thought to build relationships more effectively, so the client should be given the choice of having this approach where possible.

2.3 Factors Affecting Working Relationships with Clients

The Human–Animal Relationship

When considering how to communicate with clients, it is essential to acknowledge the importance of the human–animal relationship. When meeting a client for the first time, it is important to establish what type of relationship exists between them and their animal [4]. For example, an elite sport horse may have a different value and meaning to their owner than a companion pony who has been in the family for many years. Table 2.5 displays some examples of different client–animal relationships and how this may affect veterinary treatment and communication. These are intended as examples only. Each human–animal relationship is individual and unique; assumptions should not be made based on face value. The best way to approach the human–animal bond with each individual client is to ask an open question at the start of each consultation [4], such as 'Can you tell me all about Billy?'. This should be followed up by attentive listening.

Table 2.5 Examples of different client–animal relationships and how this may affect veterinary treatment and communication.

Animal type and use	Owner concerns	Financial considerations	Communication considerations
Elite competition horse	The horse needs to be sound and healthy to compete	Finances are unlimited as long as the horse can still compete. Euthanasia may be considered if the horse can no longer complete	Needs to be direct, honest and clear. Realistic expectations are given regarding the prognosis to compete
Racehorse	The horse needs to be sound and healthy to compete. Needs to earn money to pay for stabling and training	Money may be no object but only if likely to return to a competitive career. Maybe part of a syndicate so extra funding possible depending on career prospects. Euthanasia may be considered if the horse can no longer race competitively	Needs to be direct, honest and clear. Realistic expectations are given regarding the prognosis to race in the future. When dealing with a syndicate, communication may be more difficult as multiple owners need to be considered
Old companion pony	The owner is very attached to the pony as has owned it for many years. Happy to try any treatment	Finances may be limited, but the owner still wants to try all treatment options	Clear and honest communication. Must be realistic with treatment options. May need to broach euthanasia if treatment options are unlikely to be successful. This must be broached carefully and sensitively to respect the bond the owner has with the pony. If euthanasia is carried out, bereavement support should be offered
Retired competition horse and broodmare	Wants to continue the genetic line for this mare. Youngstock are valuable	Willing to invest in treatment as long as the mare can still breed. Euthanasia may be considered if the mare cannot be used for breeding	Needs to be direct, honest and clear. Realistic expectations are given regarding the prognosis to breed. Quality of life must be discussed if the mare is retired to pasture and still expected to be a broodmare. Embryo transfer could be discussed if the mare is physically unable to carry a foal to term
Two companion donkeys	Elderly owner. Not from a horsey background. Has the donkeys as companions	Finances may be limited, but the owner still wants to try all treatment options. The owner may not understand the condition and treatment options well as does not have much experience in keeping equids	Clear and honest communication. Time must be spent explaining the condition and treatment options and checking understanding. If euthanasia needs to be broached, this must be done with care and sensitivity, especially as this is an elderly person, and these animals may be their only company. If one donkey must be euthanised, the

(Continued)

Table 2.5 (Continued)

Animal type and use	Owner concerns	Financial considerations	Communication considerations
			idea of replacing them with a new companion must be broached to prevent complications with the surviving donkey. If euthanasia is carried out, bereavement support should be offered. Consider signposting to other support services
Middle-aged cob used for pleasure riding	The owner is attached to the horse and has little desire to compete	Finances may be limited, but the owner will want to try all treatment options. The horse needs to be sound enough to do low-level activity	Clear and honest communication. Must respect clients' bond with the horse. Must be realistic in terms of the patient returning to low-level activity

Source: Marie Rippingale.

Culture and Religion

When working in veterinary practice, clients with different cultural and religious beliefs will likely be encountered, and this must be considered when it comes to communication. Religion can be seen as an ethical code for many people [4]. Judaism and Christianity promote kindness to animals from the standpoint of the negative effect of cruelty to animals on the perpetrator and the animal owner [4]. Some Eastern religions, such as Jainism, Hinduism and Buddhism, will not allow euthanasia under any circumstances.

These religions apply an intrinsic value to the lives of animals, and as they believe in reincarnation, cruelty to animals, including ending their lives, is seen as potentially interfering with a fellow human in one of their other incarnations [4]. The refusal of a client to euthanise an animal on religious grounds is difficult to manage. In these situations, the needs of the animal and the needs of the client must both be discussed, respected and investigated so that an appropriate course of action can be taken for all involved. See Table 2.6 for further information.

Table 2.6 Different religious views on animal welfare and veterinary treatment [10].

Religion	Views on animal welfare and veterinary care	The use of blood products	Euthanasia of animals
Christianity	Christians generally believe that humans are responsible for being good stewards of God's creation, including animals. Many Christian denominations promote kindness and compassion towards animals, emphasising the importance of their welfare. However, opinions on veterinary care may differ, with some Christians advocating for responsible pet ownership and proper medical treatment, while others view veterinary interventions as optional	Most Christian denominations do not have explicit restrictions on the use of blood products. However, some Jehovah's Witnesses, a Christian sect, conscientiously object to blood transfusions based on their interpretation of biblical passages prohibiting blood consumption. Other Christians generally see the medical use of blood products as a matter of personal decision and rely on modern medical practices	Christian views on euthanasia in animals can vary. While many Christians believe in responsible stewardship of animals and promoting their welfare, there is no unified stance on euthanasia. Some Christians may support euthanasia for animals in cases of incurable suffering or to prevent further pain, while others may advocate for alternative approaches like palliative care
Islam	In Islam, animals are considered part of God's creation and should be treated with compassion and respect. Islamic teachings emphasise the concept of Halal, which includes guidelines for the humane slaughter of animals for food. Veterinary care is encouraged to maintain animals' health and well-being, including providing necessary medical treatment	Islamic teachings do not specifically address the use of blood products in animals. Muslims are generally encouraged to treat animals compassionately and avoid causing unnecessary harm or suffering. As long as the use of blood products is necessary for the health and well-being of the animal, it is likely to be considered permissible	Islamic teachings generally oppose euthanasia. Life is seen as a gift from Allah, and actively hastening death violates this belief. Palliative care and pain alleviation are encouraged to ensure comfort and dignity for the terminally ill

Table 2.6 (Continued)

Religion	Views on animal welfare and veterinary care	The use of blood products	Euthanasia of animals
Judaism	Judaism teaches that humans are responsible for treating animals with kindness and preventing unnecessary suffering. Jewish law, as outlined in the Torah, includes specific guidelines for animal welfare, such as the prohibition of causing animals unnecessary pain. Veterinary care is generally seen as an important aspect of fulfilling these responsibilities	In Judaism, the prohibition on consuming blood applies specifically to dietary practices for humans. There are no explicit restrictions on the use of blood products in animals. The well-being and health of animals are important in Jewish teachings and using blood products for veterinary purposes would generally be acceptable	In Judaism, there is a general obligation to prevent unnecessary animal suffering. Euthanasia for animals may be permissible when it is determined that the animal is experiencing severe or incurable pain or distress and is done humanely. However, some may feel that Jewish law values the preservation of life and considers euthanasia as interfering with the divine process of life and death
Hinduism	Hinduism promotes the idea of Ahimsa or non-violence, towards all living beings, including animals. Many Hindus follow a vegetarian or vegan diet as an expression of this principle. While veterinary care is not explicitly addressed in Hindu scriptures, the general sentiment of compassion towards animals would likely extend to the need for proper veterinary treatment	Hinduism promotes the principle of Ahimsa or non-violence, which extends to all living beings. Many Hindus interpret Ahimsa to mean refraining from causing harm or unnecessary suffering to animals. While there is no specific guidance on the use of blood products in animals, it is generally recommended to prioritise the well-being and welfare of animals. As such, using blood products for legitimate medical purposes in animals, if necessary for their health and survival, is likely to be seen as permissible	Hinduism places value on compassion and minimising suffering. While there is no direct mention of euthanasia in Hindu scriptures, the principles of Ahimsa and compassion would support the notion of relieving an animal's pain and suffering. In cases where an animal is experiencing incurable and extreme suffering, some Hindus may consider euthanasia a compassionate act to end the animal's distress
Buddhism	Buddhism emphasises compassion and respect for all living beings, including animals. Buddhists are encouraged to practice non-violence and to avoid causing harm to animals. While the specific approach to veterinary care may vary among Buddhist communities, the general principle of alleviating suffering and promoting well-being would likely support the provision of veterinary treatment	Buddhism promotes the principle of non-harming (Ahimsa) and compassion towards all sentient beings, including animals. While there are no specific guidelines regarding using blood products in animals, the general principle of minimising harm and promoting well-being would suggest that using blood products for medical purposes in animals may be considered acceptable if it is necessary to save or improve their lives	Buddhism strongly emphasises compassion and the avoidance of causing harm to all beings. While euthanasia is not directly addressed in Buddhist scriptures, the intention to alleviate suffering and prevent further pain is consistent with Buddhist teachings. In cases where an animal is experiencing severe and incurable suffering, some Buddhists may consider euthanasia a compassionate act to end their pain and distress
Jainism	Jainism strongly emphasises non-violence and respect for all forms of life, including animals. Jains follow a strict vegetarian or vegan lifestyle and often take great care to avoid causing harm to animals. In the context of veterinary care, Jains would likely support compassionate treatment and medical interventions to alleviate animal suffering	Jainism holds the principle of Ahimsa as a fundamental value, which prohibits causing harm or violence to any living being. Jains follow a strict vegetarian or vegan lifestyle, avoiding the consumption of animal products. While Jain scriptures do not explicitly address the use of blood products in animals, the principle of Ahimsa would generally guide Jains to minimise harm and cruelty towards animals. As a result, Jains would likely prefer alternatives to using blood products in animals whenever possible	Jainism advocates for avoiding harm and suffering to all living beings, including animals. Jains practice compassion and strive to minimise the pain and distress experienced by others. Regarding euthanasia in animals, Jainism does not have explicit guidelines in its scriptures. However, Jains prioritise non-violence and may consider euthanasia to prevent or alleviate severe and incurable suffering in animals, thereby reducing their pain and distress

It is important to note that the above summaries provide a general overview, and interpretations of religious teachings may vary among individuals and specific communities within each faith tradition. Additionally, religious views can evolve over time, so it is always advisable to consult religious leaders or scholars for more detailed and up-to-date information. Please consult the Further Reading section for more information.

Source: Rosina Lillywhite.

Socioeconomic Status

Clients may attempt to use animal ownership to elevate their social status. For example, someone with a high level of wealth may own an elite-competition horse even though they do not have a background in horse ownership. Other clients may want to own a certain breed of horse associated with competition success, such as an Arab, Thoroughbred or Warmblood. However, they may not have the necessary knowledge or experience to handle and care for these types of animals. Support and advice can be given where appropriate regarding handling, safety and husbandry. The clients can also be signposted to different charities and organisations to get support and advice if this is deemed appropriate. Clients must be allowed to decide how they would like to spend their own money. All healthcare options must be presented without preconceptions about the client's wealth [4].

Health Status

Animals can positively affect their owners' mental health just by providing companionship. Pet ownership has been associated with better health outcomes and increased social opportunities [4]. The association may extend beyond this with time, as the animal is associated with memories of loved ones, which can significantly affect decision making [4]. Animals may also have a negative effect on owners. With horses, this is mostly relevant to the potential to cause injury or accidents. There are also risks from zoonotic diseases such as dermatophytosis (ringworm) and salmonellosis. These effects should also be considered when communicating with clients.

Use of Appropriate Language

Verbal factors also present barriers to communication, including veterinary jargon. This may inhibit the client's understanding, putting them at risk of disengaging or becoming frustrated and dissatisfied. Communicating with clients may also be difficult if their first language is not English. In these cases, understanding should be confirmed, ideally with someone who can communicate with the client in their first language, for example, a family member or a friend.

Age-related Factors

Communicating with elderly clients requires the ability to adapt communication. The older population is more likely to have difficulties surrounding vision, hearing, mobilising or understanding the content of a conversation. With hearing difficulties, it is useful to speak clearly and loudly without shouting. For difficulties with sight, it is useful to provide printed information, such as consent forms or discharge notes, in a larger font. If clients have mobility difficulties, they may need to sit down, in which case, the communicator could also sit down to put them at ease. If a client has cognitive difficulties, it would be valuable for a friend, carer or family member to be present to facilitate communication. Special consideration must be given to communicating effectively with children. If children are present, it is useful to put them at ease by asking them about pets, hobbies or school. It is also important to be mindful of the terminology used when communicating in the presence of children (particularly terminology regarding euthanasia) to avoid causing distress.

Environment

It is important to consider the environment as a factor affecting communication with clients. Communication is more effective in a quiet environment with as few distractions as possible. This is not always easy to achieve in equine practice, as many consultations will be carried out in a yard setting. Where possible, the consultation could be carried out in a separate room, for example, the tack room or office. The client should be spoken to without the animal present to begin with, as the animal could serve as a distraction and make communication less effective. At the practice, the client could be spoken to in a designated room, to begin with and all relevant information gathered or relayed before taking the client to see their animal.

RCVS Practice Standards Scheme Requirements

The RCVS operate a practice standards scheme (PSS). This is a voluntary scheme where practices can achieve different levels of accreditation. As part of an effective means of communicating with clients, the PSS states that practices must provide information in alternative formats to accommodate disability, neurodiversity and learning differences [11]. Consideration should be given to font sizes and colours used. Web pages should be presented in an accessible format and written in plain English [11]. The PSS also requires practices to provide information regarding helping clients to cope with the loss of their horses and sources of support [11]. For more information regarding grief and support requirements for clients, see Chapter 17.

2.4 Relationships and Communication Within the Veterinary Team

Interprofessional Relationships

In veterinary practice, colleagues with a variety of different roles are required to work together as part of an interprofessional team. Good interprofessional practice is difficult to define; however, it could involve the following [12]:

- Effective communication. In an effective interprofessional team, different levels of communication are required. See Table 2.7 for further information.
- Knowledge of each other's roles and responsibilities.
- Respect between professions.
- Appropriate team structure.
- Set team processes between professions with complementary knowledge and skills.

The RCVS Code of Professional Conduct for Veterinary Nurses states, 'Veterinary nurses must work together with others in the veterinary team and business, to coordinate the care of animals and delivery of services' [14]. Therefore, some interprofessional practice is required in any veterinary practice setting. Vets are unique in their capacity to diagnose and treat disease. However, this does not mean they must make all decisions alone. It has been suggested that utilising different perspectives of professional groups can help to make decisions that any professional could not have made on their own [15]. Therefore, within a functioning interprofessional team, the vet can retain their role of diagnosing and prescribing, while also collaborating with colleagues to make decisions that benefit the patient, the client and the team overall.

Within a functioning interprofessional team, members are utilised according to their specific motivations and perspectives. Within the different roles in veterinary practice, the following preferences have been observed [15]:

- Vets tend to focus on diagnosing conditions and creating treatment strategies.
- RVNs tend to focus on patient welfare and well-being.
- Receptionists or client care advisors (CCAs) tend to focus on the client.
- Practice managers and administrators tend to focus on the practice and practice team.

This is not to say that individual professionals do not focus on other factors; however, making use of the naturally differing foci of the occupational groups within the veterinary practice, is a potential way to produce an expert team with distributed cognition rather than an unintegrated 'team of experts' [15]. Other members of the

Table 2.7 Levels of communication and their application to veterinary practice [13].

Level of communication	Details and application to veterinary practice
Interpersonal communication	Takes place between two or more individuals within the veterinary practice. It involves direct interaction, conversation and exchange of information. Interpersonal communication occurs between colleagues, such as vets, RVNs, receptionists and other staff members. It enables sharing of patient information, collaboration on cases, seeking advice and building relationships within the team
Vertical communication	Refers to the flow of information between different levels of personnel within the veterinary practice hierarchy. It involves communication between superiors and subordinates, such as vets, RVNs, practice managers and staff members. Vertical communication facilitates the dissemination of instructions, policies, feedback and performance evaluations
Horizontal communication	As mentioned earlier, horizontal communication involves communication among individuals at the same level within the veterinary practice. It occurs between colleagues with similar roles or responsibilities, such as vets communicating with other vets or RVNs collaborating with fellow RVNs. Horizontal communication facilitates teamwork, coordination, knowledge sharing and problem-solving
Diagonal communication	Refers to communication between individuals from different departments or levels within the veterinary practice. It involves cross-functional communication and collaboration to achieve common goals. For example, a vets may communicate with a receptionist to ensure proper scheduling and client communication, or RVNs may collaborate with laboratory personnel to discuss test results
External communication	Involves interaction between veterinary practice personnel and external parties, such as clients, referring vets, suppliers and regulatory bodies. This type of communication includes client consultations, discussions with referring vets, phone calls, emails and written correspondence with external stakeholders. External communication is crucial for client satisfaction, education and professional relationships

Effective communication at all these levels within a veterinary practice is essential for providing quality patient care, ensuring smooth operations and fostering a positive work environment. Clear and open communication promotes collaboration, enhances teamwork, reduces errors and ultimately benefits the well-being of the animals under the practice's care

Source: Rosina Lillywhite.

interprofessional team must also be considered, and these can include but are not limited to the following:

- Veterinary students
- Student veterinary nurses (SVNs)
- Patient care assistants (PCAs)
- Grooms

A good working environment is important for reducing errors and adverse events [12]. Medical errors can occur due to system errors such as work environment and organisation, human incompetence or acts of negligence [12]. It is, therefore, clear that there are patient and non-patient-related benefits to interprofessional practice. Achieving and maintaining good interprofessional practice is, however, challenging.

It is essential to understand the factors that may negatively affect interprofessional practice. Hierarchical structures produced by differences in traditional roles and responsibilities can negatively affect interprofessional practice [12]. Therefore, vets may find it difficult to delegate case responsibilities due to a lack of understanding of which tasks are appropriate to delegate to other team members. Conversely, individuals from traditionally lower-status occupations may feel oppressed if they are not allowed to fulfil the full range of their roles [12]. Ultimately, this could lead to performance issues and a reduction in the quality of patient care. The hierarchical structure can also prevent individuals in lower-status occupations from challenging the decisions made by their higher-status colleagues [12]. This concept can have effects on patient safety by errors not being challenged and therefore not being prevented.

Communication can be an overarching challenge that can affect interprofessional practice. Factors which could negatively affect communication between members of an interprofessional team are as follows [12]:

- Language – use of terminology and jargon
- Willingness to share specific professional knowledge
- Perceived unimportance of information to another professional
- Limited time
- Stress

If the challenges posed by hierarchy and communication are not addressed, stereotypical views regarding other professions can develop [12]. A potential means of addressing these issues is interprofessional education (IPE) and this is defined as 'when students from two or more professions learn about, from and with each other to enable effective collaboration and improve health outcomes' [12]. It is beyond the scope of this text to investigate the concept of IPE in detail; however, brief examples of application would be university students learning via a team project in a classroom or vets and other professionals completing teamwork simulations led by other professionals [12].

Ideally, all veterinary practices should look towards developing and maintaining functional, interprofessional teams. To start with, this may involve some inter-team education on the roles and responsibilities within the team. This could be enhanced by adopting a 'no blame culture' to encourage honesty and openness between colleagues. If a functional interprofessional team can be established and maintained, it would have significant positive benefits for the patients, clients, practice and team members overall.

Staff Wellbeing

Members of a veterinary team need to be able to identify when one of their colleagues is stressed and requires support. This may come in a simple form, such as offering a chat over tea or coffee, which would give the colleague a chance to talk about their problem. If the problem is more serious; however, a more structured approach is required, such as signposting the person to telephone helplines [4]. It is important to realise when the support required exceeds your level of expertise, and the person may require professional help [4]. Further information regarding mental health support agencies can be found in Chapter 3.

Staff Meetings

It is important to have regular formal communication between veterinary teams, and this can be achieved with team meetings. Meetings should be held at a fixed time and frequency [4]. They should be booked well in advance, so all staff know when to attend.

The following points are important to consider in relation to team meetings [4]:

- An agenda should be produced for each meeting. Time limits should be suggested for each item. This prevents one agenda item from being drawn out to the detriment of other items that must be discussed.
- Minutes should be taken and circulated as soon as possible following the meeting. Attendees should be asked to approve the minutes.
- Action points should be allocated to specific individuals, deadlines should be agreed upon and these should be followed up at subsequent meetings.

2.5 Operation of a Veterinary Reception Desk

In many veterinary practices, RVNs fulfil several roles, including that of a receptionist [16], and all RVNs must work collaboratively with colleagues in other roles in the practice. Good working relationships between those in nursing roles and those in reception roles facilitate the effective running of the practice and improve the client experience [12].

Greeting Clients

Those in a reception or client care role typically have a significant responsibility for creating a positive first impression of the practice [17]. Clients should always be greeted warmly, with a light and friendly tone of voice, by a member of staff who is dressed professionally. This greeting and a clean and tidy reception area, help to promote client confidence [18]. It is also beneficial to use the client's and patient's names when talking to the client so that they feel the service they are receiving is personalised to them [19]. When in a reception role, it is important to listen to the client's tone of voice/observe body language and respond appropriately, for example, displaying empathy or using a reassuring tone of voice if they sound concerned, so that they feel listened to and that the person they are talking to cares about their situation. Additionally, the reception team are usually the last people a client will interact with before leaving the practice. Maintaining a caring, professional image helps create a lasting positive impression for the client.

Making Appointments for Clients

When a client contacts the practice, careful use of open and closed questioning techniques alongside listening to the client carefully will help staff working at the reception desk to obtain key information. By using open questions and not interrupting the client, the nature of the client's needs can be determined. This can then be followed by closed questions, which will help obtain specific information. The reception team can then ensure that the client's needs are met appropriately [4].

When scheduling a first appointment, ensuring that the visit is as smooth as possible for the client is useful. If this is to take place at the practice, consider whether additional information regarding how to find the practice would be beneficial. It may also be helpful to give the client information regarding procedures once they arrive at the practice, such as where to park, reporting to reception and what to do while waiting for the RVN or vet. Clients should also be reminded to have their horse's passport to hand so that identity can be confirmed and medication declarations can be updated if necessary. Ensure that when the client has registered with the practice, contact information such as telephone numbers has been added to the record (with the client's permission) so that, if necessary, the vet can contact the client before the appointment. Providing patient information and clearly explaining the reason for

the appointment will help the vet prepare for the appointment appropriately and allow the day to run smoothly.

Regarding follow-up or regular appointments, receptionists or CCAs are often asked to call and book an appointment or send reminders. Call reminders are often considered a better alternative, but these can be very time-consuming, particularly if several attempts to reach the client are made. Pre-booking the next visit when the client is settling the bill for their current visit simplifies the process [20]. This should be followed by reminders to ensure the appointments translate into visits. Popular options for reminders include text and email.

Practices naturally have quieter and busier periods; it is helpful to offer appointments during the quieter periods first, so that those during busier periods are available to clients who are unable to come at another time. Many factors will need to be considered when prioritising appointments, including:

- Case urgency
- Staff availability
- Client preference
- The likelihood that the client may make an appointment elsewhere.

Regarding the latter factor, if the client books elsewhere, they may opt to remain with that practice, which would result in a significant loss of income over the lifetime of that particular patient [4]. Some practices may still use a hard-copy daybook for scheduling appointments, but many now use electronic systems. These allow multiple staff members to access the diary at any one time and for any amendments to be made easily. Some will also permit the automatic generation of reminders for clients.

All team members who are involved in booking appointments should ensure that the correct vet and appropriate length of time is allocated to the procedure. Ensuring sufficient time for each appointment will reduce the likelihood of appointments running late, which would likely result in client dissatisfaction [21]. Overbooking appointments can also cause stress in the clinical team and therefore, negatively affect their wellbeing [22].

A valuable skill to have as an RVN working on reception is the ability to recognise emergencies and when certain cases are more urgent than others. When an emergency arises, they should be seen as soon as possible, and this sometimes means that they need to be seen prior to existing appointments. If this is the case, clear and honest communication with clients who have existing appointments is crucial. When they are aware that the delay is due to an emergency, many will be happy to wait, but the opportunity to rebook may also be offered [4].

In some instances, communicating with other practice team members may be necessary when booking appointments. This may be due to further clarification regarding the urgency of a case, requesting a specific vet for a procedure which may require assistance with that particular procedure or if the client makes requests that are out of the norm for the practice. If requests are inappropriate, clear communication and education of the client is vital. For example, the client may request a vaccination appointment for the initial vaccination course on a date that does not fall within the necessary timeframe specified by the manufacturer.

Using Record-keeping Systems

A key aspect of communication in practice is good record-keeping [23]. The practice must keep certain records, including case records and consent forms [24]. Records can take many forms, including electronic and paper records. As practices are keeping and processing information about individuals, they must adhere to the Data Protection Act 2018, which is the UK's implementation of the GDPR. This requires them to ensure that the personal information that they hold is processed fairly and lawfully for specified purposes. The information should not be excessive, should be kept up to date, kept secure and should not be kept for longer than is necessary. It is recommended that medical records be kept for a minimum of six years so that they are available in the event of legal claims [4].

In addition to keeping records up to date, clarity and legibility are important, not only for giving a good impression but also for allowing ease of understanding by anyone required to access them. Abbreviations should only be used if they are commonly understood, handwritten notes should be easy to read and names should be spelt correctly [4]. All records should be stored securely. In the case of paper records, this may necessitate a lockable filing cabinet. A supply of temporary paper record sheets is useful to have available in the instance of a power failure. The record can then be scanned and stored electronically at a later date. Computer records should have an off-site backup system which will retain the records in the event of an interrupted power supply. Steps should be taken to prevent outside access to computer records, including using secure passwords [4].

Case records are the property of the veterinary practice; however, if the client has paid for reports specifically, such as radiographs, they are legally entitled to copies of them. The practice may, however, specify that the charge is for the diagnosis and subsequent advice and not for the images [4]. Client and practice confidentiality should be maintained at all times. In extreme circumstances, confidentiality may be breached and other organisations may be contacted if a vet or RVN believes that animal welfare

or public interest has been compromised. Permission may be sought to pass on information expressly (in writing or verbally) or implicitly. For example, if a client makes an insurance claim, the insurance company is entitled to receive information relevant to the claim [4].

In addition to the disposal of client records discussed previously, there are a variety of records within a veterinary practice that will require disposal. While there are no legal limits regarding document storage duration, regular disposal is recommended at different intervals for different records. Financial records should be kept for six years after the end of the financial year, and recruitment records should not be kept for longer than six months. Paper records may be disposed of via shredding, burning or professional confidential waste contractors. Sensitive data should be erased from computers prior to their disposal [4].

Taking Payments

RVNs working on reception may be required to take payments from clients. The most common forms of payment are cash, debit card, credit card and cheque [25]. Clients should be provided with an itemised invoice [4].

Debit and Credit Cards

It is important to be aware of how to use the card machine(s) in practice, including how to operate them successfully when taking payment in person and over the phone [26]. If transactions are declined, the client should be informed politely and discreetly. The payment method can be attempted again, or an alternative payment method can be requested [25].

Cash

There are risks associated with accepting cash, including acceptance of counterfeit money and the theft of money, particularly when large payments have been made. If a large sum of money has been paid, it is a good idea to have the amount checked by two members of staff before the client leaves. This will ensure that the amount of money accepted is accurate. The amount tendered should also be confirmed with the client before putting the cash in the till as the client may claim to have tendered a higher amount than has been given, and it is easy to make mistakes [4]. The drawers that cash is kept in should be lockable and closed immediately after putting the cash in them.

Insurance Claims

A large proportion of a practice's income can come from insurance payments. Clients will commonly ask a member of the reception team how to make a claim [26]. Some clients will pay as they go with treatment and then claim the fees back from their insurance company. Some practices will allow direct payments from insurance companies once the client has paid their 'excess' [4]. It is important that RVNs are aware of the individual practice policy regarding insurance claims.

Recording Payments

Historically, it was common practice to record payments in a daybook. Many practices now use computerised systems that automatically generate receipts. Any electronic payment slips should be kept securely in the till [4]. Many receptionists/CCAs are required to undertake a process known as 'reconciliation', typically at the end of each day. This is a process whereby receipts and cash accepted are matched with a sheet totalling the transactions from that day, allowing any discrepancies to be identified and errors rectified. The sheets must balance before closing the practice for the day [25]. The process of reconciliation helps prevent fraud and ensure that the client's payment records and accounts are accurate [4].

Communication in Relation to Second Opinions and Referrals

In some cases, clients may request a second opinion. The request may also be made by the vet. The purpose of doing so is to confirm the diagnosis [27]. Conversely, new clients to the practice should be asked whether the animal they are registering is currently being treated; this is not uncommon during treatment. These situations require the vet to adhere to guidelines set out in the 'RCVS Code of Professional Conduct for Veterinary Surgeons' which include not obstructing the client from seeking a second opinion and not obstructing them from changing or choosing a particular practice. If a change of practice has occurred or a second opinion is sought, the previous treating vet should be contacted promptly to obtain previous treatment and medication details. Not only is this in the patient's interest, it is also a professional courtesy to the previous veterinarian. The process of a second opinion or referral vet taking over the care of a patient without the knowledge of the original treating vet is called 'supersession' and is not acceptable practice [4].

In instances where the vet feels that a particular case is outside of their area of competence, they should refer it. The vet that accepts the referral will diagnose and treat the case before referring it back to the original practice [27]. The process first requires a referral letter to be written, which details the status of the case, the reason for referral and, if applicable, the results of any diagnostic tests conducted. The vet that has accepted the referral should send a referral report to the referring vet to aid them when they re-assume responsibility of the case. While in some cases, patients are referred to a vet with further qualifications or specialism in a particular field, referrals may also be made to other professionals such as behaviourists, physiotherapists and other allied professionals [4].

Taking a Patient History

Whether admitting a patient to the practice or registering a new patient, RVNs are frequently required to take a patient history. This will typically start with obtaining or confirming the client's details and, where appropriate, updating any contact information. It is also important to verify that the client is over the age of 18 to be able to give consent to veterinary procedures legally [3]. After obtaining relevant client information, the RVN should ascertain the patient's name, sex (including castration status of males) and if the patient is a mare, whether they are pregnant or lactating. Notes should also be made on the patient's breed, age and weight if known. The practice can ascertain the latter if they have access to a weighbridge and the client is unsure of the patient's current weight. The insurance status of the patient should also be discussed.

Legally, passports should be kept with equine patients during transportation. Therefore, clients should always bring the patient's passport with them when attending the practice with their horse, pony, donkey or mule. This, along with scanning the microchip, will allow the confirmation of the patient's identity and also allow the RVN to ascertain the vaccination status, travel history and any medical declarations for the patient, such as the horse being signed out of the human food chain. Alternative methods of identifying patients include acquired marking methods such as brands, microchips and tattoos. The latter is rare in the UK but may be found on the inside of the upper lip. Microchips are a useful form of permanent identification and are part of the United Kingdom equine passport system [28]. See Chapter 5 for more information regarding equine identification methods.

If admitting the patient for investigations, it is important to obtain either verbally or in writing the nature of the condition history related to the condition and any tests that have been performed previously. The RVN should also ascertain whether the client has moved practice or has been referred for a second opinion; history from the previous/referring practice must be obtained. Once a detailed history has been obtained and the client has provided all relevant information required, the information should be communicated to the relevant veterinary colleague who will manage the case.

Producing Written Clinical Records

RVNs are often responsible for producing a wide range of written clinical records, such as:

- Admission forms
- Consent forms
- Clinical parameter sheets
- Critical care sheets
- Pain scoring sheets
- Care plans
- Home care plans
- Details of examinations
- Records of medication administered

It is important that records are filled in at the time of the event or as soon as possible after the event. When producing these records, it is important that they are accessible to other colleagues who may need to use them. This includes legible handwriting, clear meaning, sufficient detail and the use of correct veterinary terminology. When abbreviations are used, these should be limited to commonly used and understood ones. It is always useful to add a signature or the initials of the person filling in the record. This will allow other members of the team to identify the correct person to direct queries to if required.

2.6 Customer Service

Veterinary medicine is not just a profession; it is also a business. vets and their colleagues are expected to have a given level of expertise and skill; as such, one of the main features that can make a practice stand out is customer service. Customer service encompasses everything that contributes to the experience of the client [29]. One of the most valued aspects of customer service in veterinary medicine is the treatment of the patient, not only the treatment related to the condition or complaint, but the approach taken with the patient and attitude towards them. This may include talking to and engaging with the patient.

Factors of Good Customer Service

Good customer service includes not only meeting customer expectations but also exceeding them. Small actions/gestures can exceed client expectations, from follow-up phone calls, to helping to carry items to the client's vehicle. There are many things that clients expect as a minimum from their veterinary practice, including prompt service, appropriate and comfortable facilities, transparency regarding costs, flexibility and the ability to adapt to meet the client's needs and a variety of products and services [30]. Calls should be answered/emails responded to promptly, all areas of the practice should be clean, tidy and in good repair and costs should be conveyed clearly and in full, with estimates provided where necessary. Regarding the staff in the practice, clients value competency, availability and kindness [30]. Staff should be dressed in smart clothing, have appropriate training, hold the relevant qualifications for their role, engage in continued professional development (CPD) and create a warm, welcoming atmosphere.

Factors that may influence the client's selection of a practice include location/proximity, opening hours/availability, prices and recommendations [30]. The variety of services available in accordance with expertise and equipment/facilities may also be an influential factor in selection. If the practice is a member of the RCVS PSS, the achievement of different levels of accreditation can be promoted to clients. The PSS aims to maintain high standards of veterinary care by setting standards [11]. Customer service should always be consistent, and feedback on the service provided should be encouraged. This should also include any complaints which should be acted upon to improve the service and promptly retain a loyal client base [4].

The Value of Clients to Veterinary Practices

Clients now typically have the choice of several practices to register at. With more choices available, practices must deliver an excellent service to gain and retain clients [31]; a satisfied client will return to the practice, which generates more income and keeps the practice in operation [31]. Furthermore, a satisfied client is more likely to recommend the practice to others, which helps the business to grow [31]. Profits can be utilised to invest in the practice, and therefore maintain or improve the service offered to clients.

When making the decision to choose or stay with a particular practice, money is rarely at the forefront of the client's mind. Clients are often willing to pay more for a better service. However, they ultimately tend to seek a balance between the cost and the service. Raising the profile of the practice via marketing should also be considered in order to gain new clients. This can take many forms, and the selection of the marketing strategy will often be guided by the allocated budget and the availability of time to dedicate to it. Marketing strategies may include:

- Television campaigns
- Radio campaigns
- Social media campaigns
- Flyers
- Branded merchandise
- Open days
- Attendance at events.
- Running client education evenings

Marketing can also be more effective when unique selling points are promoted [32]. This may include a particular piece of diagnostic equipment or an additional service that other practices in the area are not offering.

Handling Complaints

It is impossible to please all clients all of the time, so while it may be the ambition to prevent any complaints from occurring the in the first place, the occasional one is inevitable [33]. Furthermore, the work undertaken within a veterinary practice can be very technical and involve complex decisions being made and as such, human error may occur [34]. Objectivity is important when handling complaints to ensure that the procedure is not unduly influenced. An effective complaint-handling procedure is an important asset in veterinary practice; successfully managed complaints can restore a practice's reputation in the eyes of disgruntled or unhappy clients [33].

Complaints may be formal (such as a letter or email sent to the practice) or informal (such as a client complaining to a member of the reception team). The complaint should be acknowledged and recorded in line with the practice policy [4]. Clear records should also be kept of any responses given to the complainant, whether any action is taken (including when) and if the complainant has been referred to a different, more appropriate person within the practice. When complaints do arise, clients appreciate prompt handling and communication. Where investigations are necessary, this is not always possible. In this case, a realistic timescale should be discussed with the client to manage their expectations [33].

Complaints can be viewed as an opportunity not only to put things right but also to improve systems so that the issue does not occur again in the future. Excellent communication skills are vital to achieve a resolution. The complaint should be listened to carefully to ensure that no information is missed. If appropriate, an expression of regret that the client is not satisfied can be given and ideally, agreement on a way forward [4]. Staff handling complaints should always do so in a courteous manner and ensure that confidentiality is maintained at all times. Complaints cannot always be resolved in the client's favour. In these cases, offering a gesture of goodwill (such as a discount) may be beneficial to acknowledge their distress and show that they are valued as a client. When offering these gestures, care should be taken to ensure that they are not seen as an admission of guilt. Clients also appreciate a sincere apology from an empathetic practice team member [33].

In summary, the key points that can be followed to handle complaints in a veterinary practice effectively are as follows [33]:

1) Listen attentively: When a client approaches with a complaint, listen carefully to their concerns without interrupting. Let them express their feelings, frustrations and expectations fully. Show empathy and understanding throughout the conversation.

2) Stay calm and professional: It is important to remain calm and composed while addressing the complaint. Maintain a professional demeanour and avoid becoming defensive or argumentative. Remember that your primary goal is to resolve the issue and maintain a positive relationship with the client.

3) Apologise and take responsibility: If the complaint is valid, take responsibility for any mistakes or shortcomings. Offer a sincere apology for the inconvenience or dissatisfaction experienced by the client. This demonstrates your commitment to quality care and acknowledges their concerns.

4) Gather information: Ask relevant questions to gather all the necessary details about the complaint. Seek specific information about the incident, timing, personnel involved, and any supporting documentation or evidence. This will help in understanding the situation fully.

5) Investigate the complaint: Once you have gathered the necessary information, investigate the complaint thoroughly. Speak to staff members involved, review medical records or other relevant documents and examine the complaint's circumstances. This will help determine the facts and identify any areas needing improvement.

6) Respond promptly: Respond promptly to the complaint, preferably within a reasonable time frame. Inform the client that their complaint has been taken seriously and is being investigated. Offer an estimated time for when they can expect a detailed response.

7) Offer a resolution: Based on the findings of your investigation, propose a solution or resolution to address the client's concerns. If appropriate, provide options for compensation or remedies, such as a refund, additional treatment or future discounts. Ensure that the proposed resolution aligns with your practice's policies and ethical standards.

8) Communicate the outcome: Once a resolution has been determined, communicate it clearly and honestly to the client. Explain the steps taken to investigate the complaint, the outcome of the investigation and the actions being taken to prevent similar issues in the future. Be transparent and open in your communication.

9) Follow up: After resolving the complaint, follow up with the client to ensure their satisfaction and to address any remaining concerns. This demonstrates your commitment to their well-being and helps in maintaining a positive client–practice relationship.

10) Learn from the experience: Use the complaint as an opportunity to improve your veterinary practice. Reflect on the feedback received, identify any areas for improvement and implement necessary changes to prevent similar issues from recurring.

Handling complaints in a veterinary practice requires effective communication, active listening, empathy and a commitment to resolving the issue professionally and effectively.

References

1 Macdonald, J. (2020). Client communication and practice organisation. In: *BSAVA Textbook of Veterinary Nursing*, 6e (ed. B. Cooper, E. Mullineaux, and L. Turner), 232–251. British Small Animal Veterinary Association: Gloucester.

2 Pullen, S. (2012). The equine nurse's professional responsibilities. In: *Equine Veterinary Nursing* (ed. K. Coumbe), 186. London: Wiley-Blackwell.

3 Smith, J. (2023). The communication process [Online]. Available at: https://pressbooks.senecacollege.ca/buscomm/front-matter/introduction (accessed 7 July 2023).

4 Gray, C. and Clarke, C. (2012). Client communication and practice organisation. In: *BSAVA Textbook of Veterinary Nursing* (ed. B. Cooper, E. Mullineaux, L. Turner, and T. Greet), 207–227. British Small Animal Veterinary Association.

5 Kirwan, M. (2010). Basic communication skills. In: *Handbook of Veterinary Communication Skills* (ed. C. Gray and J. Moffett), 7–15. London: Wiley-Blackwell.

6 Fontanella, C. (2022). 13 body language tips that can make or break your customer service [Online]. Available at: https://blog.hubspot.com/service/body-language-in-customer-service (accessed 7 July 2023).

7 Skillsforcare. (2018). Communication skills in social care [Online]. Available at: www.skillsforcare.org.uk/resources/documents/Developing-your-workforce/Care-topics/Core-Skills/Communication-skills-in-social-care.pdf (accessed 7 July 2023).

8 Wolff, R. (2021). Advantages and disadvantages of open-ended and close-ended questions [Online]. Available at: https://monkeylearn.com/blog/advantages-of-open-ended-questions (accessed 7 July 2023).

9 Herrity, J. (2023). 4 Types of communication styles and how to improve yours [Online]. Available at: https://www.indeed.com/career-advice/career-development/communication-styles (accessed 19 June 2023).

10 Walker, A. (2019). Religion and the care, treatment and rights of animals [Online]. Available at: https://chaplaincy.tufts.edu/humanist/files/Religion-Animals.pdf (accessed 7 July 2023).

11 RCVS (2022). PSS equine modules and awards (V3.3) [Online]. Available at: www.rcvs.org.uk/document-library/equine-modules (accessed 25 June 2023).

12 Kinnison, T., May, S.A. & Guile, D. (2014). Inter-professional practice: from veterinarian to the veterinary team [Online]. Available at: https://jvme.utpjournals.press/doi/10.3138/jvme.0713-095R2 (accessed 25 June 2023).

13 Lumen Learning. (2023). Typical communication flows [Online]. Available at: https://courses.lumenlearning.com/suny-principlesmanagement/chapter/reading-barriers-to-effective-communication (accessed 7 July 2023).

14 RCVS. (2023). Code of professional conduct for veterinary nurses [Online]. Available at: www.rcvs.org.uk (accessed 25 June 2023).

15 Kinnison, T. and May, S.A. (2016). Evidence-based healthcare: the importance of effective interprofessional working for high quality veterinary services, a UK example [Online]. Available at: http://doi.org/10.18849/ve.v1i4.54 (accessed 25 June 2023).

16 Hamlin, J. (2013). Are VNs professionals or paraprofessionals. *The Veterinary Nurse* 4 (6): 315.

17 Sheridan, L. and Tottey, H. (2017). A compassionate journey part 3: the client experience. *The Veterinary Nurse* 8 (2): 66–73.

18 Fiskett, R.A.M. (2006). That first impression. *Journal of Exotic Pet Medicine* 15 (2): 84–90.

19 Lambert, A. (2015). The equine reception experience. *In Practice* 37 (2): 96–98.

20 Osborne, D. and Doherty, C. (2016). The benefits of pre-booking. *The Canadian Veterinary Journal* 57 (11): 1191.

21 White, B.J. (1994). Practice organisation. In: *Veterinary Nursing Book 1* (ed. D.R. Lane and B. Cooper), 195–206. Oxford: Elsevier.

22 Corah, L., Lambert, A., Cobb, K., and Mossop, L. (2019). Appointment scheduling and cost in first opinion small animal practice. *Heliyon* 5 (10): e02567.

23 Baldwin, S. (2021). Communication in veterinary practice. *Veterinary Nursing Journal* 36 (6): 195–197.

24 Orpet, H. and Welsh, P. (2011). *Handbook of Veterinary Nursing*, 2e. Chichester: Wiley-Blackwell.

25 Prendergast, H. (2014). *Front Office Management for the Veterinary Team-E-Book*, 2e. Elsevier Health Sciences.

26 Faulkner, B. (2015). The colourful receptionist©. *European Journal of Companion Animal Practice* 25 (1): 34–42.

27 Pullen, S. (2012). The equine nurse's professional responsibilities. In: *Equine Veterinary Nursing*, 2e (ed. K.M. Coumbe), 184–190. Chichester, UK: Wiley-Blackwell.

28 Linnenkohl, W. and Knottenbelt, D.C. (2012). Basic equine management. In: *Equine Veterinary Nursing*, 2e (ed. K.M. Coumbe), 184–190. Chichester, UK: Wiley-Blackwell.

29 Blach, E.L. (2009). Customer service in equine veterinary medicine. *Veterinary Clinics: Equine Practice* 25 (3): 421–432.

30 Moreau, P. (2012). Do you know your equine practice clients? *Veterinary Clinics: Equine Practice* 28 (1): 39–49.

31 Page, G. and Sadiwskyj, L. (2021). Valuing veterinary receptionists: setting the practice 'tone'. *In Practice* 43 (9): 536–539.

32 Lambert, A. (2016). Customer care and communication. In: *Aspinall's Complete Textbook of Veterinary Nursing*, 3e (ed. N. Ackerman), 11–20. Edinburgh, UK: Elsevier.

33 Coates, C.R. (2011). Practice—client relationships: handling complaints effectively. *The Veterinary Nurse* 2 (1): 42–45.

34 Kinnison, T., Guile, D., and May, S.A. (2015). Errors in veterinary practice: preliminary lessons for building better veterinary teams. *Veterinary Record* 177 (19): 492–494.

Further Reading

Mills, J.N., Volet, S., and Fozdar, F. (2011). Cultural Awareness in Veterinary Practice. *Journal of Veterinary Medicine Education* 38 (3): 288–297.

Johnson-Walker, Y. (2023). Understanding religious diversity. [Online]. Available at: https://www.journeyforteams.org/wp-content/uploads/2023/07/Topic-Overview_Topic-9_ReligiousDiversity.pdf (accessed 8 July 2024).

Szucs, E., Geers, R., Jezierski, T. et al. (2012). Animal welfare in different human cultures, traditions and religious faiths. *Asian-Australasian Journal of Animal Sciences* 25 (11): 1499–1506.

Wells, K. (2012). Accommodation cultural differences of opinion. *In Practice* 34: 310–311.

3

Professional Veterinary Nursing Responsibilities
Judith Parry

Bottle Green Training Ltd, Derby, United Kingdom

3.1 The Legal Framework for Veterinary Nursing Practice

Before looking at the laws relevant to veterinary nursing, it is important to understand where laws come from and the types of laws that exist.

Why Do We Have Laws?

Have you ever considered why laws are made and why we need them?

Hopefully, after a moment of reflection, you have considered that laws are required to enable society to run in some form of orderly manner and to provide protection. They provide rules and structure for dealing with situations and also provide a system of redress and punishment for any wrongdoing.

Where Do These Laws Come From?

Laws originate from legislation and can relate to a precedent system, that is, earlier laws or decisions that provide some examples or rules to guide decisions about a case. This guidance can be formalised through the legal system and from Acts of Parliament. An individual law or statute originates from a Bill. This Bill is passed through both the Houses of Parliament (the House of Lords and the House of Commons). Once the Bill has passed through both houses and been debated and voted upon, it ultimately passes to the Crown for Royal Assent. This is a very long and complicated process but ultimately if accepted by both houses, the Bill becomes a law [1].

Criminal Law

Any criminal offence is concerned with punishment by the state and is designed to protect society and individuals.

There are three types of criminal offence:

1) Indictable – these are serious offences and are tried in the Crown Court with a judge and a jury.
2) Summary – these are deemed to be more minor offences and are tried in a magistrate's court where the magistrate decides upon guilt. Animal welfare offences tend to fall into this category.
3) Triable either way – these offences fall somewhere between the two listed above and the defendant can opt for trial by a jury or a magistrate.

Civil Law

Civil law is more concerned with harm or loss suffered by an individual as the result of another person. In civil cases, an individual will take action against the person who has caused harm rather than the state.

'Tort', this is defined as a wrong against someone's personal safety, possessions or reputation. The most common civil actions seen within veterinary practice are as follows:

- Breach of Contract – not fulfilling the required action as agreed. For example, a surgical procedure has not been carried out.
- Negligence – causing injury by breach of duty of care. For example causing injury to a horse through lack of care during a procedure.
- Trespass – causing damage to someone else's property. For example, performing an unauthorised procedure.

The outcome of most civil cases results in financial compensation for damages or may lead to prohibitive measures such as an injunction (an official order given by a law court). The main differences between civil law and criminal law are displayed in Table 3.1.

Textbook of Equine Veterinary Nursing, First Edition. Edited by Rosina Lillywhite and Marie Rippingale.
© 2025 John Wiley & Sons Ltd. Published 2025 by John Wiley & Sons Ltd.
Companion website: www.wiley.com/go/equineveterinarynursing

Table 3.1 The main differences between civil law and criminal law.

Factors	Civil law	Criminal law
Redress (remedy or compensation for wrong doing or a grievance)	May be fines/damages or injunctions	Maybe a custodial sentence, fine or probation
Who is involved?	Person versus Person	Crown versus Accused
Laws which may be affected within the Veterinary field	Criminal Damages Act 1971 Contract Law	Animal Welfare Act 2006 Veterinary Surgeons Act 1966 Veterinary Medicines Regulations 2013
Decision	On the balance of probabilities	Beyond reasonable doubt

Source: Judith Parry.

Statutes

In the United Kingdom legal system, statutes are laws enacted by Parliament. They are also known as primary legislation or acts of Parliament. Statutes are considered the highest form of law and take precedence over other sources of law, such as common law and judicial precedent.

Which Statutes are Most Relevant to Me as a Veterinary Nurse?

Veterinary Surgeons Act 1966
Animal Welfare Act 2006
Data Protection Act 2018
Public Interest Disclosure Act 1998
Veterinary Medicines Regulations 2013
Ionising Radiation Regulations 2017

The Veterinary Surgeons Act (VSA) 1966

The Royal College of Veterinary Surgeons (RCVS) was established through the issuance of a Royal Charter in 1844. This Charter recognised the 'veterinary art' as a profession and gave the RCVS the power to administer examinations to the first recognised veterinary surgeons (vets). From this Charter, the VSA 1881 was developed to recognise qualified and unqualified practitioners. The VSA 1966 consolidated all earlier Charters and Acts into one single Act. This Act defines 'veterinary surgery' to mean the art and science of veterinary surgery and medicine.

This includes:

- Diagnosis of diseases in, and injuries to animals.
- Giving advice based on the diagnosis.
- Medical or surgical treatments of animals.
- Performance of surgical operations on animals [2].

Within the VSA 1966, there are several Schedules. Schedule 1 is concerned with provisions for the council, Schedule 2 is concerned with investigations and disciplinary committees, and Schedule 3 is concerned with what registered veterinary nurses (RVNs) and student veterinary nurses (SVNs) can and cannot do in practice.

The VSA 1966 (Schedule 3 Amendment) Order 2002

Schedule 3 of the VSA allows competent non-veterinarians to perform certain acts of veterinary surgery in order to maintain and promote animal welfare. These non-qualified persons may be the owner of the animal, household members or other people employed in the care of animals. It gives provision for the administration of first aid to preserve life or reduce pain and suffering.

In 1991, the VSA was first amended to recognise the role of the veterinary nurse in law. The VSA 1966 (Schedule 3 Amendment) Order 2002 made provision for vets to direct RVNs or SVNs who they employ to carry out limited acts of veterinary surgery. The RVN must be on the RCVS register for Veterinary Nurses, and the SVN must be officially enrolled as a Student Veterinary Nurse with the RCVS.

What Does This All Really Mean?

When looking at owners and animal caregivers, it allows them to administer medications and treatments in order to improve welfare. For example, it enables owners to give prescribed medications to their horses without the need for the vet to be present on site. Owners can perform first aid procedures whilst waiting for veterinary assistance if required.

The Schedule 3 amendment also allows for other equine professionals, such as farriers and physiotherapists, to perform certain procedures on horses in their care. However, if the patient is receiving non-routine care from these professionals, it is likely that a vet will need to delegate the task.

For RVNs and SVNs, Schedule 3 states that vets may direct RVNs or SVNs who they employ, to carry out limited veterinary surgery. Under this Schedule 3 exemption, the privilege of giving any medical treatment or carrying out minor surgery, not involving entry into a body cavity, is given to [2]:

- RVNs under the direction of their employer to animals under their employer's care. The directing vet must be satisfied that the veterinary nurse is qualified to carry out the medical treatment or minor surgery.
- SVNs under the direction of their employer to animals under their employer's care. In addition, medical treatment or minor surgery must be supervised by a vet or RVN and, in the case of minor surgery, the supervision must be direct, continuous and personal. The medical treatment or minor surgery must be carried out in the course of the SVN's training.

The RCVS has interpreted these terms as follows [2]:

- 'Direction' means that the vet instructs the RVN or SVN as to the tasks to be performed, but is not necessarily present.
- 'Supervision' means that the vet or RVN is present on the premises and able to respond to a request for assistance if needed.
- 'Direct, continuous and personal supervision' means that the vet or RVN is present and giving the SVN their undivided personal attention.

What RVNs and SVNs Cannot Do

- Perform medical treatment or minor surgery independently, without direction from a vet.
- Make a medical diagnosis.
- Administer medication to horses that are not under the care of their employing veterinary practice.
- Administer anaesthesia or sedation to effect.
- Perform surgical procedures that enter into a body cavity.
- Perform any procedure that is outside their competence regardless of whether it enters a body cavity or not [2].

Should RVNs and SVNs Perform Procedures that Fall Under the Remit of Schedule 3?

There is a general consensus that RVNs would like to improve recognition of their role and performing Schedule 3 procedures, which can help clarify the status and role of RVNs to the wider veterinary profession and the public. There is, however, no definitive list to describe what minor surgical and medical treatment is, and it is therefore vital that RVNs must always be aware of their level of competence in a task.

The pressures of veterinary practice do mean that when RVNs are allowed to perform Schedule 3 procedures, they can improve the smooth running of the practice. They often have the time to give their patients a more personal approach and perform tasks at a pace that maximises animal

welfare. This can improve job satisfaction as RVNs feel more fulfilled within their role. Performing these tasks does not, however, come without potential negative outcomes. RVNs are accountable and liable for their actions both within criminal and civil law. RVNs may not feel comfortable with the weight of responsibility associated with performing some of these tasks. This should be respected by the veterinary team. The safest RVN is one who is fully aware of their limitations, as well as their competencies, and is able to put patient welfare at the fore of their decision-making. The RCVS has produced a 'SUPERB' poster as guidance for vets on delegating Schedule 3 tasks to RVNs (Figure 3.1).

Lack of clarity surrounding Schedule 3 can often lead to vets being reluctant to delegate Schedule 3 procedures to RVNs. The British Equine Veterinary Association (BEVA) has produced a set of guidelines to help with the interpretation of Schedule 3, with a view to instilling confidence in vets to delegate more Schedule 3 procedures to RVNs in practice.

The BEVA Schedule 3 guidelines can be found here: https://www.beva.org.uk/Career-Support/Nurses/Schedule-Three

3.2 Professional Status and Accountability

The role of the veterinary nurse has advanced significantly over time and RVNs are now accountable and responsible for their actions. Veterinary nursing is now recognised as a profession in its own right. Therefore, it is assumed that RVNs must be professional and responsible people.

Professionalism

Before defining professionalism, it is important to understand what a professional is. The Oxford English Dictionary has multiple definitions of 'professional'; however, the keywords from these definitions are showing skill and being competent [3]. This therefore infers that all professionals should display particular characteristics and skills. It is often understood that a profession is a deliberate career choice, and this suggests a level of long-term commitment and training. This is certainly the case within the veterinary profession. vets and RVNs must achieve a licence to practice qualification that involves mastery of many body systems and behaviours. Not all professionals need to achieve qualifications to be a professional. There are many occupations where experience and commitment are enough.

A professional is recognised as having specialised knowledge that has been acquired through a commitment to develop and improve their skills. These skills are usually quantified through the achievement of qualifications within their field. This knowledge must be up-to-date to

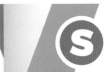

Is your delegation

S U P E R B ?

A six-point checklist for veterinary surgeons wishing to delegate work to registered/student veterinary nurses under Schedule 3*

(S)PECIFIC PROCEDURE?

Is the procedure medical treatment or minor surgery, not involving entry into a body cavity?

a. Remember, certain things are off-limits, including: independent medical treatment or minor surgery, major surgery, diagnosis, certification, castrations, spays, and dental extractions using instruments.

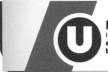

(U)NDER CARE?

Is the animal under your care?

a. Has the client given you responsibility for the animal's health?

b. Have you seen the animal immediately before delegation, or recently enough to have personal knowledge of its condition?

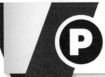

(P)ERSON?

Can you delegate to this person?

a. Under Schedule 3, you can only delegate medical treatment and minor surgery (not involving entry into a body cavity) to RVNs and SVNs, not to lay people.

(E)XPERIENCE?

Does the RVN/SVN feel capable, and have sufficient competence and experience?

a. Are they familiar with the species?

b. If they have not done this procedure before, have they had the right training and will they be supervised?

c. If there is a problem, do they know what to do?

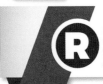

(R)ISKS?

Have you considered the risks specific to this case?

a. How difficult is the procedure?

b. How likely is it that something could go wrong?

c. Does the RVN/SVN understand the associated risks?

(B)E THERE!

Are you available to direct or supervise, as necessary?

a. RVNs must work under your direction, ie you have provided the necessary instructions about the task to be performed, but you do not have to be on the premises.

b. SVNs must work under your supervision
   i. For medical treatment, you need to be on the premises and available to assist.
   ii. For minor surgery (not involving entry into a body cavity), you must stay with the SVN and give them your undivided personal attention

www.rcvs.org.uk/schedule3

*Under Schedule 3 to the Veterinary Surgeons Act, only registered veterinary nurses and student veterinary nurses have the privilege to perform certain procedures in veterinary practice, as delegated to them by you, a veterinary surgeon colleague employed in the same practice. Make sure your delegation is SUPERB!

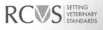 SETTING VETERINARY STANDARDS

superb poster a4.indd 1

31/10/2019 15:41:54

Figure 3.1 RCVS SUPERB poster (2023). *Source:* Reproduced with kind permission from the RCVS.

enable a professional to work to the best possible standard. A professional must be competent and reliable, and work with honesty and integrity.

What Makes a Professional RVN?

As far back as 1947, the role of the veterinary nurse was becoming more recognised and Phyllis Peake (vet and veterinary nurse) wrote that a good animal nurse needed 'a strong vocational call ... for self-sacrifice, tenderness and the ability to consider the patient as an individual' [4]. These sentiments still resonate with RVNs today. The recognition of veterinary nursing as a profession started with the first Animal Nursing Auxiliary training scheme being approved by the RCVS in 1961. The term 'veterinary nurse' was not used until 1984 as the title 'nurse' was protected within human medicine until then. Within 30 years of the first training scheme, the VSA was amended to recognise the role of the veterinary nurse in law. From this point, the profession has evolved very quickly with the introduction of further qualifications, such as the Diploma in Advanced Veterinary Nursing. In the year 2000, the very first equine veterinary nurses qualified, and this became a turning point for all veterinary nurses wanting to specialise in treating equine patients.

In 2002, the Veterinary Nurses Council was established, and in 2007, the non-statutory register was introduced. This was a voluntary register where qualified veterinary nurses could choose to sign up. Once on the register, veterinary nurses were able to perform procedures that fell under the remit of Schedule 3 and were accountable for their actions. Now, all newly qualified nurses apply to the RCVS Register to be able to practice as a veterinary nurse in the United Kingdom and make the following declaration:

> I PROMISE AND SOLEMNLY DECLARE that I will pursue the work of my profession with integrity and accept my responsibilities to the public, my clients, the profession and the Royal College of Veterinary Surgeons, and that, ABOVE ALL, my constant endeavour will be to ensure the health and welfare of animals committed to my care [5].

The RCVS continues to strive for more recognition of the role of the veterinary nurse and alongside the British Veterinary Nursing Association (BVNA), the Veterinary Nursing (VN) Futures project was launched in 2015. This project aimed to provide a view of the future of veterinary nursing and the progress of the profession.

Purpose and Principles of Professional Regulation

With the recognition of the RVN as a professional, there comes with it the need for regulation. This is to protect the people who use the professional services, to enhance the status of RVNs and to help to develop a sound knowledge base, as this is an integral part of professional status.

The regulation of veterinary nursing is statutory – this means it is required by law as set out in the VSA 1966. Voluntary regulation is where a code of practice is chosen but not required by law. The Royal Charter of 2015 confirmed the RCVS as the regulator of veterinary nurses.

What Does Statutory Regulation Mean?

- All veterinary nurses must now be on the RCVS Register for Veterinary Nurses.
- All nurses on the register can use the post-nominal RVN.
- RVNs are accountable for their conduct and are subject to the standards set by the RCVS Veterinary Nurses Council (VN Council).
- All RVNs will have to undertake compulsory continued professional development (CPD), which is now 15 hours every year.
- All RVNs will have to abide by the RCVS Professional Code of Conduct for Veterinary Nurses.
- All RVNs will be subject to the RCVS disciplinary procedures in cases of misconduct.

Because statutory regulation is required by law, the regulator has the force of the law to ensure its requirements are upheld. Non-statutory regulation does not require any Acts of Parliament/laws to ensure requirements are upheld. The RCVS VN Council replaced the Veterinary Nurses Committee in 2002.

It is responsible for:

- Setting education and training standards to enable nurses to enter the register.
- Reviewing post-qualification training to ensure professional development for veterinary nurses can be maintained.
- Setting the standards for behaviour, conduct and discipline for RVNs.

Whilst performing the above, the RCVS VN Council must keep animal welfare and good veterinary practice at the forefront of its values.

RCVS VN Council consists of:

- Six UK-based practising RVNs who are voted for by RVNs.
- Two UK-based practising vets who are appointed by the VN Council.
- Four lay members who are also appointed by the VN Council.

The RCVS VN Council is classed as self-regulating as it is run mostly by members of the profession but does endeavour to provide some balance with the appointment of lay members. It has been suggested that ideally, there should be a 50 : 50 split between members of the veterinary profession and lay people. An independently run regulatory body would comprise of members outside of the veterinary profession. This could be a government-run regulatory body. The structure of VN Council is currently under review. Readers are encouraged to check up to date sources for the most accurate information.

The General Dental Council and Nursing and Midwifery Council are independent regulatory bodies which comprise of multiple committees. These committees consist of members from both inside and outside of the profession. They have the same aims as the RCVS and core standards: they maintain the register of practitioners, set the standards for practitioners and education providers and investigate complaints. The advantage of self-regulation is that the regulators have a full understanding of the profession. Therefore, it is anticipated that decisions made would be in the best interests of the profession and its members. However, it could be said that independent regulation would lead to greater transparency and ensure that members are held fully accountable.

RCVS council is responsible for the governance of the RCVS college and its members as defined in Schedules 1 and 2 of the VSA 1966. It comprises of vets from veterinary universities, RVNs, lay members and the chief veterinary officer (CVO). The structure of RCVS Council is currently under review. Readers are encouraged to check up to date sources for the most accurate information.

In summary, the RCVS and VN Council are there to maintain the registers of vets and RVNs who are qualified to practice, and to guide and monitor the quality of education within the sector. They aim to ensure good ethical practice is adhered to, ensure continuous improvement in welfare of patients and protection for people who use veterinary services. The introduction of the RCVS practice standards scheme (PSS) aims to raise standards across the profession.

The RCVS has produced a Code of Professional Conduct for Veterinary Nurses. Within this code, there are five main principles of practice:

1) Professional Competence
2) Honesty and Integrity
3) Independence and Impartiality
4) Client Confidentiality and Trust
5) Professional Accountability [5]

These five principles are set to help RVNs protect and promote the health and welfare of patients within their care.

This code provides essential professional guidance for practising RVNs over six main themes:

1) Veterinary nurses and animals
2) Veterinary nurses and clients
3) Veterinary nurses and the profession
4) Veterinary nurses and the veterinary team
5) Veterinary nurses and the RCVS
6) Veterinary nurses and the public

There are also many additional supporting documents covering commonly encountered scenarios an RVN may experience and to provide a framework of best practices for an RVN to follow. Areas of practice covered include client confidentiality, referrals and second opinions and clinical governance.

The RCVS also has a veterinary nurse disciplinary procedures policy should any concerns be raised about an RVN. This involves a three-stage process which is comparable to the disciplinary process in place for vets:

1) Stage one is an assessment and investigation process. This is a fact-finding exercise to gain all of the facts relating to any concern that is raised. The decision from this process may be that there is no case to answer to, it may be that the RVN is given advice and the case is closed, or if there is a sufficient concern, then the case will progress to stage two.
2) In stage two, the case is reviewed by the Preliminary Investigation Committee (PIC). The facts are reviewed, and further investigations are carried out. A decision will be made as to whether the case should be referred to stage three and if the RVN's conduct may affect their fitness to practice.
3) Stage three involves an RVN disciplinary committee hearing. This is similar to a hearing in court, and a decision is made as to whether the RVN is guilty of serious misconduct and what formal action should be taken.

Potential courses of action:

- Not guilty – no action taken, or advice or guidance given
- Guilty of serious professional misconduct. This involves three possible sanctions:
  - Reprimand or warning
  - Suspension for up to two years
  - Removal from the register (may reapply after ten months to the committee to be reinstated).

Both stages one and two are confidential; however, stage three is usually public and may be listed on the RCVS website. The RCVS will only deal with serious concerns that affect a person's ability to practice as an RVN. For example, a serious breach of the code of professional conduct or serious criminal convictions [6].

RCVS VN Registration Rules 2017
The RCVS has a set of rules that have been approved by the VN Council and provide guidance for anyone wishing to register. These rules include:

- Completing and achieving a recognised educational programme and practical period of training.
- Make a disclosure that they are of 'good character' where they have declared any criminal convictions and if they have been removed from or refused to be registered by a professional organisation in the past.
- Pay a registration fee.

3.3 Ethical Principles

The Difference Between Ethics and Morals

What are ethics and where do they come from?

Why do we not all have the same ethical views when we are in the same profession?

Why do we even need to know about them to be RVNs?

These are some of the many questions that spring to mind when reflecting upon ethics and ethical theories. A simple way to describe the difference between morals and ethics is to say that morals allow us to quantify what is right and wrong, and ethics are the reasons as to why something is right or wrong. This creates new questions – where do they come from? How do we as individuals know what is right and wrong? There is no simple answer to these questions as our ethical views are continuously changing and evolving as we are exposed to different life experiences. As children, we learn basic ethical views from the adults and peers that we grow up with and look up to. There are the added influences of social media, the news and the people we work with as we move towards and through adulthood. We also have a strong instinct to protect ourselves and those closest to us. Alongside these influences, we need to follow relevant legislation and guidance to live and work effectively in society.

Ethical Theories

The most commonly recognised ethical schools of thought are:

- Utilitarianism
- Deontology
- Virtue ethics

Utilitarian Theory

This theory has been recognised in some form since the fifth century; however, it was more formally defined and recognised by two English philosophers, Jeremy Bentham in 1789 and further modified by John Stuart Mill in 1863. The theory itself is based upon the greatest benefit for the greatest number and is sometimes known as the 'happiness theory'. Bentham believed that the actions of a person were based upon the presence or absence of happiness.

If an action produced happiness, then it was right and if it created sadness, then it was wrong [7]. It can also be defined as the greatest happiness for the greatest number, as it is recognised that it is not possible to make everyone happy with every action. As it is based on the outcomes of a particular action or behaviour, it is also known as consequentialist theory. It is the outcome of the action and the amount of happiness it creates that make it right or wrong.

Sound good? Let us investigate it a little further ….

It is a useful theory to justify the morals of a person's actions. For example, it is justifiable under utilitarian theory to cause suffering to the few if the outcome will benefit the many. Therefore, from a utilitarian point of view, it is correct to test a drug on a small number of animals if the outcome is that the drug will save many more animals in the future. Under this theory, it is justifiable to cull a clinically well animal with an infectious disease to protect a herd, as is the case with equine infectious anaemia (EIA) [8].

However, can we always predict the consequences and outcomes of an action? How do we know we will get the result that will give the greatest happiness? What about the unhappiness of the few to please the majority – is this ok? Who gets to decide who the few are to be made unhappy? Why is their happiness any less important? What if perhaps the drug company in the example above has a big financial benefit for trialing this drug and is biased towards the outcomes?

So, perhaps it is not as perfect as we might think as the only ethical principle to apply to all situations.

Deontology

Deontology is very much in contrast to utilitarianism as it places the emphasis of an action on the duty of the individual to follow preset rules. The term itself is derived from the Greek 'deon' duty and 'logos' science [9]. This would therefore mean that the consequences of an action would not be considered. Immanuel Kant (1724–1804) was a German philosopher who believed that every person had certain duties, for example, do not lie and do not steal. He believed that everyone should follow the rules and do their duty [10]. Therefore, it can be summarised that an individual following deontological ethics would choose to follow the rules or laws. Within the field of veterinary medicine, there are many rules that should be followed, for example, the VSA 1966, The Animal Welfare Act 2006 and The RCVS Code of Professional Conduct for Veterinary Nurses. It could be assumed that this would be an ideal ethical principle to follow as these rules are set specifically for the profession and therefore are always going to be the correct course of action.

Sound good? Let's investigate it a little further ….

Deontology encourages us as veterinary professionals to follow the duties bestowed upon us within the profession. For example, to make animal welfare our first priority. Surely this is our main reason for being in this profession? So, if the example of the animal being used in a drug trial to save many more animals in the future were applied to deontology ethics, it is likely it would be a very different outcome. The welfare of the individual would be considered in this case and therefore, the trial would be deemed to be ethically wrong. It is a useful theory when considering the individual, as the consequences or outcomes are not relevant. However, when used alone, it does not always lead to the best outcome. Is it correct to trap rats and other rodents in a feed shed to protect the feed for horses? When applying the theory of deontology, the rights of the rats are equal to the rights of the horses and therefore, this would not be acceptable. But then the horse's welfare is potentially being compromised. Also, how do we know which rule we should apply? Sometimes, the rules can contradict themselves. For example, if you were presented with a pony with severe arthritic changes in its joints, which make it lame and unable to rise after lying down. It might be suggested that this patient should be euthanised for welfare reasons. One could argue that this is making animal welfare our first priority. However, what if the owner cannot agree to this outcome? What if they want to try absolutely every alternative they can? The RCVS Code of Professional Conduct states that 'veterinary nurses must be open and honest with clients and respect their needs and requirements' [11]. So, does this mean that the owner's wishes should be respected even though they are unlikely to lead to good welfare for the pony?

Perhaps we need to look towards virtue ethics instead?

Virtue Ethics

Virtue ethics is based upon the actions and decisions of the individual who is making them. If you are a good and nice person, you will make good decisions and therefore would be acting virtuously. Virtue ethics is an ancient theory that dates back to Aristotle and Plato in around 400 BCE [12]. So, what does it mean to be a good person? Surely a utilitarianist and a deontologist will believe that they are good people making good decisions? What does it mean to be a good person? Who can decide what is good? Does everyone within your veterinary practice have the same beliefs on what makes a person good?

Is a virtuous person someone who looks at all ethical theories and tries to understand the views of all parties involved prior to making a decision? When looking at the example of the arthritic pony, would a virtuous person try to understand why the owner does not feel ready to have their pet euthanised? Perhaps this pony is like a family member, and they want to feel they have tried everything possible to preserve the ponies' life. It could be suggested that a virtuous person might spend time with the owner ensuring they have a full understanding of their ponies' condition, and also ensuring adequate analgesia is given, so the owner's wishes can be respected whilst maintaining good animal welfare? This therefore suggests that rules are followed, and the consequences of any actions are considered equally.

None of the ethical theories would suggest that it is correct to hurt a horse intentionally; however, the theories would be applied from different perspectives:

- A utilitarianist would believe the action is wrong because the consequences would mean that the horse would be terrified and hurt.
- A deontologist would believe it is wrong because the rules are to make animal welfare a first priority, and it is against all animal welfare legislation.
- A virtue ethics theorist would believe it is wrong because they have respect for all living things and would therefore, not consider it to be right to inflict pain and suffering on any animal.

All three ethical theories have their own merits and value; however, it is difficult to decide which theory is best applied to scenarios encountered within veterinary practice. It is important to be mindful of each of them when considering an approach in a practical situation.

Medical Ethics in Human Medicine

Perhaps we need to look at other medical professionals? Within human medicine, there are medical ethics which might be of use to consider when making an ethical judgement.

These are:

- Non-maleficence
- Beneficence
- Autonomy
- Justice

Non-maleficence is best considered as 'first, do no harm'. This is an underpinning value of all RVNs; however, there is sometimes the need to inflict short-term harm for a positive long-term goal. For example, horses on box rest are not able to exhibit normal behaviours, but this is usually in the short term for rehabilitation of an injury and will ultimately lead to the patient having a better quality of life afterwards.

Beneficence is basically the promotion of good. Again, this is easily transferred to veterinary settings. Animals are given preventative medicines such as vaccinations to ensure protection from infectious and life-threatening diseases. This particular area is where RVNs can have a key role, as they can provide useful advice and guidance to owners on their pets' welfare and husbandry.

Autonomy is described as the ability to self-govern. This can be interpreted for animals in that they are able to act upon impulses and interests. For example, being able to decide when to graze and when to rest in the paddock.

Justice is interpreted as treating all animals equally and with respect. It is vital in veterinary medicine not to favour particular clients or animals based upon our own prejudices or preconceptions, but to give the same level of care to all. This can be particularly challenging with non-compliant patients [13].

Scenarios
Scenario 1
An owner has a 21-year-old Thoroughbred (Figure 3.2). This horse retired from racing as a four-year-old and has been retrained in most disciplines and achieved reasonable results, especially in dressage. Unfortunately, he has sustained multiple injuries during his working life and has always had weak and brittle hooves. As a result of this, he requires a special diet, remedial farriery and is now generally stiff and unable to compete. His demeanour is still bright, and despite losing some of his top line, he is comfortable with minimal veterinary treatment for stiffness. The owner however cannot afford to keep more than one horse and really enjoys competing.

The owner has approached your practice for advice.

Firstly, let's look at the possible options for this owner:

- Keep the horse and give up on any thoughts of competing for now.
- Sell the horse as a light hack/field companion.

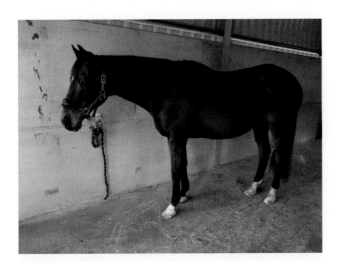

Figure 3.2 Scenario 1 – Retired Thoroughbred.
Source: Judith Parry.

- Rehome the horse to a retirement home/rescue centre.
- Have the horse euthanised to make space for another one.

Then, it is worth evaluating the effect of each action on the owner, the horse and the veterinary practice.

If the horse was kept, the owner would be able to make a judgement as to when the horse no longer had an acceptable standard of welfare. The owner knows the horses' normal behaviour and therefore, should be able to make a judgement regarding euthanasia. However, the owner will be unable to compete, and the horse has expensive and specialist needs. The owner would not feel guilty, as the horse has earned his retirement with them. The veterinary practice would be able to assist the owner in keeping the horse comfortable for as long as possible, and the horse should have a good quality of life for the foreseeable future. The owner may ultimately lose interest in the horse though and his welfare may suffer as a result.

If the horse was sold, there is the potential he could go on to have a comfortable life with a new sympathetic owner, who will enjoy a slower pace of life with the horse. The original owner will be able to buy a new competition horse. The veterinary practice may be able to help the new horse owner with managing an older horse and enable him to be comfortable. However, is it possible to predict what the new owner will be like? Will they just sell the horse once they realise the costs involved? This horse is a Thoroughbred and so might be too 'hot' for an inexperienced owner who just wants to hack.

If the horse was rehomed, this again would alleviate any financial pressures from the owner and leave them exempt from having to make the end-of-life decision. The horse may enjoy a quieter life at a retirement centre with other horses. But will the retirement home be able to maintain the expensive husbandry that this horse requires? What if the horses at this retirement yard are kept barefoot as they live collectively as a large herd? Might the horse end up with poor welfare as a result of lack of funds?

The final option is euthanasia, so the horse would no longer feel any discomfort or pain, the owner would be able to replace the horse with a new one, and the veterinary practice would receive the revenue from the euthanasia procedure. But does this sit well with all parties involved? Is this putting the horse's welfare as the first priority or the owner's?

Application of Ethical Theories
What Would a Utilitarianist Do?
They would look at which outcome would create the greatest happiness for all. So, this would likely be to advise that the owner keeps their horse until euthanasia is required, as then the horse's welfare is maximised and the practice is

not euthanising a healthy animal. The practice may want to assist the owner in judging the horse's welfare and quality of life over time.

What Would a Deontologist Do?

The deontologist may say that the owner has a duty of care to their horse and therefore opt for either the first or last option. They will not consider the owner's circumstances only their duty to animal welfare and their pet. If the owner is unable to maintain good welfare themselves then they would consider euthanasia, as this ensures the horse will not suffer. Therefore, the duty of maintaining welfare is upheld.

What Would a Virtuous Person Do?

This could be any of the options as a virtuous person may be able to assist with the rehoming/sale of the horse as they may know of a suitable owner for the horse. It is likely that a virtuous person will want to preserve the horse's life whilst trying to maintain the owner's happiness. They would try to keep all parties considered in the decision and try to find the most virtuous outcome for all.

The decision however, is ultimately with the owner.

Scenario 2

You have heard from an excited and long-standing client that they are getting their child's first pony and have contacted your practice to register. They have told you all about the stable yard where they will be and that they have been really lucky to find a perfect schoolmaster who can teach their child how to ride. They have stated that the pony will be mostly kept on field livery at the stables as they have very large fields, and therefore have plenty of grass. When you go to visit your horse after work, it comes to light that the client's new pony is actually one that you know from your stables. It is a well-behaved older Shetland pony (Figure 3.3) that has taught many children to ride over the years; however, you know that he has recently recovered from a severe bout of laminitis and has been box-rested during recovery.

What do you do?

Can you breach confidentiality for either client?

What about making animal welfare your first priority?

If you look at medical ethics in this case

- Non-maleficence – you cannot breach confidentiality, as it would bring the profession into disrepute should word get out that a member of the practice was passing on medical histories without consent.
- Beneficence – perhaps you could speak to the seller and ask them a little more about where the pony will be going and the new husbandry plans. You could perhaps ask

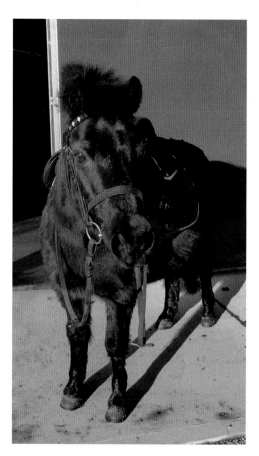

Figure 3.3 Scenario 2 – Shetland pony. *Source:* Judith Parry.

how they have advised the new owners regarding pasture management for a laminitic pony.

- Autonomy – in this case, it is ultimately up to the seller and the purchaser to find out about the pony and where it will be kept.
- Justice – all parties must be treated fairly and with respect and therefore you absolutely cannot breach confidentiality in this case to either the seller or the purchaser.

Scenario 3

In scenario number one, the owner decided to keep their horse. It is now at a point where the practice has been called out on several occasions to assist the fire brigade to lift the horse, as he keeps on getting stuck when lying down in his stable. The horse is still eating, but has significant muscle wastage of his hind limbs and is lame despite daily analgesia. The vet has suggested to the owner that they need to consider euthanasia for welfare reasons. The owner has refused.

What now?

As you know from reading this section so far, there is no correct answer here; however, it is worth considering what you would do after some reflection around the ethical theories and consideration of all affected parties.

Hopefully, these scenarios have helped to clarify why RVNs need to be aware of the different ethical theories and how they can be used to help to make a decision that can consider all affected parties and promote good overall patient care.

What about other ethical problems that may arise in veterinary practice, such as witnessing the poor practice of a colleague or substance abuse?

Can we use an ethical school of thought to justify any actions?

When faced with any of these suggested situations, the key is to speak up and take the issue to a responsible person in the practice. Whistleblowing is covered later in this chapter, but professionals must seek support and advice to ensure that our patients, our colleagues and the profession are protected from harm. All veterinary practices have procedures to follow when faced with such a problem and a deontological approach is often required. Guidance may be needed from an external source such as the RCVS confidential helpline or alternatively the Vetlife helpline, which is available 24 hours a day, every day of the week, to assist in making an ethical decision and provide the required support and guidance.

3.4 Consent

The Features of Consent

The word consent is taken from the Latin 'consentire', which means agree or allow.

It can further be defined as a deliberate or implied affirmation/compliance with a course of proposed action. For a person to be able to give consent, it must be given voluntarily and owners must never feel forced into a decision regarding the treatment of their animal [14].

Consent can be expressed in several ways:

- Express consent – this is when an owner directly gives consent for a specific procedure. This can be in writing or verbally.
- Verbal consent – this can be given directly in person, or over the telephone. Your practice might make a written record of the owner's wishes but the owner is not required to sign any paperwork.
- Written consent – this is the most common way of capturing consent in veterinary practice as the owner signs a consent form to give written consent for a procedure.

- Implied consent – this is when a person's actions indicate they are giving consent. For example, if an owner books an appointment for their horse at the practice. They arrive at the practice at the allocated time with their horse. This implies that they have arrived for their animal to have its treatment [15].

All of these types of consent are equally valid, but it must be considered that, just because someone has signed a consent form, it does not necessarily mean they have given consent. The main reason for gaining written consent is that it creates a permanent record of an owner's signature and therefore a record of their consent for a procedure. The consent form needs to contain enough detail to identify the owner, their animal and the veterinary practice. It needs to have a description of the proposed action and the risks associated. It should have space for an estimate of fees to be included and a reference to the use of any 'off licence' medications should they be necessary (Figure 3.4). It should be completed in its entirety with the owner.

What Makes a Good Consent Form?

This is a difficult question to answer, as the form needs to contain enough detail to outline the proposed procedure, list the risks and all of the details described above preferably on a single page of A4 paper. There also needs to be a breakdown of the costs that the owner is likely to incur for the procedure, including any expected aftercare costs. An owner is more likely to pay a bill if they are fully prepared and understand the need for those costs. Many owners have insurance for their horses, which they believe will cover all veterinary costs; however, there may be exclusions on their policy or limits that might be exceeded, plus the initial excess that the owner is liable for. Even if an owner declares their horse is insured, it is vital that they are still made aware of the cost of the proposed treatment in advance.

Informed Consent

The RCVS describes informed consent as 'an essential part of any contract that can only be given by a client who has had the opportunity to consider a range of reasonable treatment options with associated fee estimates and had the significance and main risks explained to them' [16].

How Much Information Is Enough?

This is an interesting question as the owner needs to be aware of all treatment options available and the risks; however, they may not be medically trained to understand the full details of a procedure. It is vital that they are made aware of the potential outcomes for any

SPECIMEN FORM OF CONSENT FOR ANAESTHESIA, CLINICAL AND SURGICAL PROCEDURES

Owner's Name _____

Address _____

_____

_____

Telephone: Home _____   Work _____

                    Mobile _____

NB: Please complete the section below if you have authority to act on behalf of the owner

Name _____

Address _____

_____

_____

Telephone: Home _____   Work _____

                    Mobile _____

Species and Breed _____

Name _____Colour _____

Age _____   Sex   M _____   F __

Neutered M   ___   Neutered F_____

Microchip/Tattoo/Brand _____

Details of the Operation/Procedure _____

_____

Figure 3.4   RCVS Specimen form of consent for anaesthesia and surgical procedures (2023). *Source:* Reproduced with kind permission from the RCVS.

- I hereby give permission for the administration of an anaesthetic to the above animal and to the surgical or other procedures detailed on this form together with any other procedures which may prove necessary.

- The nature of these procedures and of other such procedures as might prove necessary has been explained to me.

- I understand that there are some risks involved in all anaesthetic techniques and surgical procedures.

- I accept that the likely cost will be as detailed on the [attached] estimate and that in the event of further treatment being required or of complications occurring which will give rise to additional costs, I shall be contacted as soon as practicable so that my consent to such additional treatment and costs may be obtained.

- In the event that the veterinary surgeon is unable to contact me on the numbers provided, I understand the veterinary surgeon will act in the best interests of my animal.

- In order to protect the welfare of my animal, in the unlikely event of an emergency, or where additional pain relief or sedation may be required, I understand the veterinary surgeon may decide to use medicines that are not authorised for use in [state species].'

Notes and Instructions: _____

_____

_____

_____

The cost of the procedures described above (tick as appropriate)

☐   will be: £_____   OR

☐   will be within the range: £_____ to £_____

Inclusive of: VAT _____

☐ If you are NOT the owner, please tick the box to confirm you have the authority to act on behalf of the owner of the animal described above

☐ Please tick the box if you are UNDER the age of 18

*Signature _____

Date of Signature_____

*A copy of the form should be provided to the person signing and the original retained by the practice

Figure 3.4   (Continued)

Explanatory notes:

The purpose of the consent form is to record the client's agreement to treatment based on knowledge of what is involved and the likely consequences.

The client may be the owner of the animal, someone acting with the authority of the owner, or someone with statutory orother appropriate authority. Care should be taken when consent is given by a client who is not the owner of the animal. Practice staff should ensure they are satisfied that the person providing consent has both the authority and capacity to provide consent. For example, if the person providing consent is not the owner and has not confirmed his/her authority of the owner to act, only in exceptional circumstances, for example if the request is by the police, should the procedure be carried out.

Before being asked to sign a consent form, the person should be able to understand and retain the information provided and use it to come to a decision. The form should be seen as the culmination of discussions that have gone on before. If the practice uses standard information sheets, clients should be provided with an opportunity to read and ask questions before being asked to consent to the procedure/treatment.

A person may be mentally competent to sign but for reasons of physical disability is unable to provide a signature. An independent witness may be asked to confirm the client has given consent orally. If this is not practicable, then a professional colleague may be asked to confirm this.

A copy of the form should be provided to the person signing the form unless the circumstances render this impractical. Subsequent amendments to the form should be made in ink, initialled and dated. Where additional consent is required, a note of the conversation should be recorded on the clinical records.

Consent: *Veterinary surgeons must obtain the client's consent to treatment unless delay would adversely affect the animal's welfare (to give informed consent, clients must be aware of the risks)* Chapter 11 of the Supporting guidance to the RCVS Code of Professional Conduct on Communication and consent (paragraph 11.2 (i))

A person's understanding of the issues may be affected by a number of factors, such as impaired hearing or sight; mental incapacity; learning difficulties; difficulties with reading or language.

Age: Persons under the age of 18 are generally considered to lack the capacity to make binding contracts. They should not be made liable for any veterinary or associated fees. Persons under the age of 16 should not be asked to sign a consent form. Where they have provided a signature, parents or guardians should be asked to countersign. Where the person seeking veterinary services is 16 or 17, veterinary surgeons should, depending on the extent of the treatment, the likely costs involved and the welfare implications for the animal, consider whether consent should be sought from parents or guardians before the work is undertaken.

Has the client understood what has been said? Veterinary surgeons should consider their clients' language and communication needs. Clinical or technical terminology may need to be explained and clients may not wish to admit to a lack of understanding. Where there are language barriers, it may be helpful to arrange for a family member or friend to accompany the client. Additional time may be needed to ensure the client has understood everything and had an opportunity to ask questions. Veterinary surgeons should be alert to the possibility of misunderstandings concerning terminology used by the practice (eg 'euthanasia' and 'put to sleep').

Mental incapacity: The Mental Capacity Act 2005 (England and Wales) states: '*A person lacks capacity in relation to a matter if at the material time he is unable to make a decision for himself in relation to the matter because of an impairment of, or a disturbance in the functioning of, the mind or brain. It does not matter whether the impairment or disturbance is permanent or temporary. ...*'.
See Adults with Incapacity (Scotland) Act 2000
[There is no primary legislation dealing with mental incapacity in Northern Ireland as yet]

Where it appears a client lacks mental capacity to consent, veterinary surgeons should try to determine whether someone is legally entitled to act on that person's behalf, such as someone who may act under an enduring power of attorney. If not, veterinary surgeons should act in the best interests of the animal and seek to obtain consent from someone close to the client, such as a family member who is willing to provide consent on behalf of the person.

Fee estimates/Escalation of fees: *Veterinary surgeons should give realistic fee estimates based on treatment options and keep the client informed of progress, and of any escalation in costs once treatment has started (Chapter 11 of the Supporting guidance to the RCVS Code of Professional Conduct on Communication and Consent (paragraph 11.2 (g & i))*

Figure 3.4 (Continued)

proposed action, including the favourable and the unfavourable. It is also important for the owner to have knowledge of any aftercare requirements and costs involved. There are numerous complaints made by owners who have paid for surgical interventions and then find they cannot afford the multiple dressing changes and call-out fees required post-operatively. It might also be that they do not have the facilities to box rest or restrict exercise once the horse is discharged. These are all factors that the owner needs to consider before giving consent. This can prove to be more challenging in emergency situations where the owner is required to make a decision 'on the spot' regarding treatment options.

Can We Really List All of the Potential Side Effects?

It is important that owners are made aware of the most commonly encountered potential side effects of any procedure. Many owners do not consider that anything can go wrong and therefore it is vital to prepare the owner beforehand. The balance is to give them enough information to make an informed choice, whilst not scaring them out of a decision where patient welfare is then compromised. RVNs have a responsibility to ensure they are fully aware of what is involved in all proposed procedures and potential side effects, including the common side effects of any drugs used. RVNs can therefore ensure that the owner is given the best possible advice, before making a decision and giving informed consent.

Barriers to Informed Consent

There are multiple barriers to an owner being able to give informed consent.

These can include:

- Language barriers – this is not necessarily because the owner does not speak the same language, it might be that the person explaining the procedure has used veterinary terminology that the owner does not understand. The owner may feel that they cannot ask for clarification, as they do not want to appear unintelligent.
- Disabilities – the owner may have sensory disabilities; for example, they may be deaf or blind, or they could have additional learning needs that make it difficult for them to read or understand a consent form. The owner may lack the mental capacity to understand the procedure or aftercare requirements.
- Age – the owner may not be old enough to give consent. Anyone under the age of 18 years old is still classed as a child in the eyes of the law. It is therefore considered that they do not have the capacity to consent to veterinary procedures. Anyone under the age of 16 years old cannot

sign a consent form or give consent for veterinary treatment. The RCVS advises that the veterinary team should consider whether there is a need to gain consent from a parent or guardian for someone who is 17 or 18 years old [16].

- Time – this is particularly relevant should it be a major surgical procedure or an emergency situation. The owner needs to be given enough information to understand what they are consenting to whilst ensuring that any delays do not compromise a patient's welfare.
- Knowledge of the team – as discussed earlier, it is important that the person gaining consent has enough knowledge of the procedure to be able to give the owner sufficient and correct information. It might be that the operating vet is unavailable to discuss the procedure with the owner, and it will fall to the nursing team to explain the proposed treatment required.
- The owner might not be available to give consent – this could be because the owner has left the horse in the care of another party, or it might be that they have originally consented to a procedure but more interventions are required, and the owner is not contactable. It could also be that the horse has presented as a stray and therefore the owner has not been found. It is advisable to get the opinion of a second veterinary surgeon to confirm the course of treatment required or if there is no other veterinary surgeon available, then a police officer can be contacted to give consent in the absence of an owner. Seeking the opinion of another professional is the ideal course of action, as this protects all parties from accusations of unethical behaviour or conduct. In all cases, the patient's welfare must be made the main priority.

Do your admit procedures allow for enough time to be given to the owner to gain true, informed consent?

Scenarios

Scenario 4

You are attending a stable yard for a post-operative check and bandage change for a Welsh Section D pony who has had a suture repair to a wound on its left foreleg. The owner of the pony is 17 years old and has driven herself to the stable yard. Her parents do not live with her and there is no mobile phone service at the yard. On removal of the dressing, you notice that the wound has broken down towards the distal end and there is a purulent discharge present. The vet would like to administer an injectable antibiotic and analgesic whilst on site. Can this pony's owner give consent to this procedure?

Firstly, patient welfare should be considered. The best course of action from a welfare point of view is treat the pony immediately to prevent further harm. It might be that consent was gained at the initial treatment for aftercare requirements. The owner is over the age of 16 years, so could give consent but cannot enter into a contract for the fees. It is very likely that the vet will provide initial treatment, such as starting the course of treatment by injection and then should the pony require continued medication, the owner can be asked to collect it from the practice with a parent or suitable representative over the age of 18 who can give consent to the continued treatment. The pony is going to need repeat bandage changes, which again will provide suitable opportunities to ensure informed consent can be gained moving forward.

Scenario 5

You have been asked to admit a pony for routine dental work. On discussion with the elderly owner, it is becoming increasingly evident to you that they are confused and do not seem to understand the consent form. They have been a client at the practice for over 40 years and are well known to the team. What should you do?

Ideally in this situation, it would be best to speak to a senior member of the team who knows the owner, as they will be able to assist with assessing the owner's level of competence. It is likely that the practice will know of any relatives who can be contacted to help with explaining the procedure and gaining consent. Again, patient welfare may dictate that the pony needs the dental procedure for good welfare; however, the practice must prove that they have taken all reasonable steps to gain informed consent.

Scenario 6

An owner has booked their horse in for a booster vaccination to be administered at the practice to save a call-out fee. The horse arrives at the surgery with its passport. The person driving the lorry is a friend of the owner. The owner has a busy day at work and therefore cannot bring the horse themselves. Has the owner given implied consent for the vaccination to be administered by booking the appointment and arranging for the horse to arrive at the required time with its passport?

Yes. But have they given informed consent? This would really depend upon the details discussed during the booking of the appointment.

On a final thought regarding consent, how does your practice ensure they know who the owner of the patient presented is?

Does your practice register clients just as single owners or as married couples? Can a spouse give informed consent if their name is not registered on your system?

3.5 Legal and Ethical Duties to Self, Clients, Colleagues and Animals

Duty of Care

In simple terms, a duty of care is an obligation to ensure the safety or well-being of others. Within the veterinary field, we owe a duty of care to our colleagues within the industry, to our clients who use our services and to the animals we treat. We also owe a duty of care to ourselves. As RVNs, we deal with potentially life-threatening conditions and ethically challenging situations on a regular basis. It is vital that we feel we have provided a valuable and worthwhile service to our clients and our patients, whilst upholding the good name of the profession and our colleagues. The RCVS Code of Professional Conduct for Veterinary Nurses as discussed earlier, provides a valuable source of information and guidance for dealing with the most commonly encountered situations. It is a useful reference point as it outlines the duty of the RVN, taking all parties into consideration.

Another useful document for helping to guide a decision is the Animal Welfare Act 2006. This Act was designed to prevent animal suffering. It outlines the welfare needs for animals to prevent harm, which are:

- To be provided with a suitable environment and place to live
- To be fed a suitable diet
- To be able to express their normal behaviour
- To allow, any need to be housed with, or apart from, other animals
- To be protected from pain, injury, suffering and disease

Prior to this, legislation only provided a route of redress to punish should an animal suffer at the hands of an individual. The Animal Welfare Act 2006 has been further interpreted by the Department for the Environment, Food and Rural Affairs (DEFRA), who, have produced codes of practice from this Act and have created a Code of Practice for the Welfare of Horses, Ponies, Donkeys and Hybrids [17]. This code includes advice regarding housing, feeding, company and preventing pain, distress and suffering. Should anyone who is responsible for the care of an equid breach this code, they may face prosecution.

It can be challenging to interpret an animal's welfare needs, as such, should all owners who fail to vaccinate their horses face prosecution for not preventing disease? What about the patients who are on box rest? Are they able to express normal behaviour? It is therefore important to consider if the action is in the best interests of the patient when faced with these situations.

Negligence

Negligence is described as causing injury or distress due to a lack of proper care. Veterinary practices can be extremely busy and short staffed. Does this then lead to negligence with patient care? Do patients have sufficient catheter checks, hand walking for long enough, or even at all, or cold hosing even on the busiest of days? Could this be considered to be a lack of proper care?

As RVNs, we have a duty of care to ensure that patients do have proper care and nursing on such occasions. We must act as an advocate for the patient, and maintain and exemplify good nursing practices as part of our duty of care. In order that we can carry out this level of nursing, it is imperative that RVNs maintain their professional competence. This extends beyond achieving the veterinary nursing qualification and should be continuous throughout an RVN's career. To maintain this level of competence, it may be that formal CPD is undertaken, but it can also be that informal learning can take place within the working environment. The best way to become competent at any practical task is to learn how to do it and then keep practising it.

Dr Benner [18] discussed that continuous development was needed within general nursing to maintain career development with such a complex profession. She introduced the novice to expert model, which discussed how nurses develop their patient care skills and understanding over time. It comprises five key stages:

1) Novice – at this stage the individual has no previous knowledge or skills and needs to be taught simple and measurable skills. The novice is unable to prioritise which skills are most important and therefore requires support and guidance from an experienced person.
2) Advanced beginner – as the novice gains skills and experience, they progress onto this stage. They should be able to carry out tasks but will still need guidance and support.
3) Competent – at this stage, the nurse is able to reproduce taught skills without guidance and prioritise tasks.
4) Proficient – at the proficient stage, the nurse progresses to have a clear understanding of the skills and is able to plan and prioritise tasks based on that knowledge.
5) Expert – this is the final stage where the nurse has the confidence and intuition to fully understand a task and is able to grasp complicated patient care situations [18].

These stages of competence translate as well to veterinary nursing as they do to human nursing.

Whistleblowing

But what if it goes wrong?

What should we do when mistakes are made?

It is worth noting at this point, that mistakes will always be made within veterinary practice, and it is important to acknowledge and learn from these mistakes. As part of our duty of care and as professionals, we must be open, honest and conduct ourselves with integrity. It is vital that all members of the veterinary team continuously reflect upon successes and failures to maximise patient and client care. Regular clinical audits are invaluable tools for this and representatives from all areas of veterinary practice should contribute to them (See Chapter 6 for further information). However, there are occasions where individuals may knowingly attempt to conceal mistakes or unethical practices. We know we have a duty of care to our colleagues and to the profession, so what can we do in these situations? We do not want the whole profession to be brought into disrepute because of the actions of one single person.

To 'blow the whistle' is to disclose an action of wrongdoing that you have witnessed. The RCVS has provided guidance on how to whistleblow should this be required. The first recommendation is to try to resolve the matter internally. This is not to 'hush up' the concern, but it might be that it is something that can be resolved easily. All veterinary practices should have a clear policy on this, but in the first instance, it must be reported to a line manager or appropriate senior member of the management team. It is vital that internal processes are followed initially. Should an individual believe that the matter has not been effectively resolved internally, then they should report their concern to the RCVS Professional Conduct Department, who will be able to advise if the matter needs to be taken to another relevant body, or if they can investigate it themselves. It is vital to remember that client confidentiality must be observed at all times when reporting these cases. The Public Interest Disclosure Act 1998 is in place to protect an employee who 'blows the whistle' from unfavourable treatment by their employer [19].

Scenario 7

You are required to assist a vet to perform a bilateral neurectomy on the proximal suspensory ligaments of a horse. On admission, the owner asks you if the surgery will be obviously detectable because they are intending to progress the horse from affiliated advanced medium to advanced level dressage once it becomes sound. You are aware that it is against Federation Equestre Internationale (FEI) rules to compete a horse following this particular surgery. You report what the owner has said the operating vet, who dismisses your comments and elects to continue with the surgery. The surgery proves to be successful and following a period of recovery, the horse displays no signs of lameness.

What should you do?

Firstly, you need to find out what the whistleblowing procedure is for your practice and try to follow it. It is likely that you will need to take your concerns to your Head Nurse or Head Vet at the surgery. It might be that the vet who performed the surgery has since spoken to the owner to ensure that they are aware of the FEI rules, and the owner has now agreed not to compete the horse following the surgery. If this is the case, the vet has acted in the best interests of patient welfare to reduce any pain and suffering.

What if it is the Head Vet who performed the surgery?

At this point, you will need to take your concern to another senior member of the practice team. This might be the practice manager or area manager. If you believe that your concern has been ignored, then you can seek advice from organisations such as BEVA, BVNA and the RCVS professional conduct department before making a formal disclosure.

3.6 The Professional Role of an Equine Registered Veterinary Nurse in Practice

When reflecting upon this chapter, it is worth noting that the role of the RVN is ever-growing and evolving both in equine and small animal practice. To maintain professional standards and patient safety, it is paramount that continued growth and knowledge is maintained, not just as a requirement of registration, but as a requirement to be a well-rounded RVN. When planning further learning, RVNs should look to cover a good range of topics to maintain a balance and not just concentrate on specific areas of interest.

To increase the recognition of the RVN, it is important to acknowledge that it comes with a level of responsibility and accountability in law. RVNs must always maintain professionalism whilst keeping animal welfare at the fore of any decision-making and nursing considerations. Ethical dilemmas will often present themselves and must be faced with a measured and structured approach. As RVNs, it is important to consider how we can be the best possible nurses and gain the best job satisfaction at the same time. Professionals must accept that there will be days when it does not all go to plan and then work to minimise the impact of this on themselves as well as their colleagues, the clients and the patients in their care. Resilience comes from working well within a team and being able to look after your own mental and physical health. Practising mindfulness and trying to keep a positive mindset when tackling dilemmas and conflicts is vital. Looking to always follow 'above the line thinking', which involves being curious, positive and having a commitment to learning, can help to improve morale for yourself and the team around you.

The value of reflection and clinical audits should not be underestimated in the ability to drive continuous improvement and to act as an aid to stress management and support resilience. It is very easy to underestimate the impact of making continuous ethical judgements. As there is a requirement for confidentiality within veterinary medicine, it can be difficult to talk to people from outside of the profession about any concerns, therefore meaning that most discussions are with people who are in the same situation. It is vital to remember that owners may not always fully understand the pressures of veterinary practice, which can lead to exasperation and potentially compassion fatigue. Compassion fatigue is a term used to describe the physical, emotional and psychological impact of helping others. It is often mistaken for burnout, which is a cumulative sense of fatigue or dissatisfaction. Compassion fatigue and burnout can have serious negative effects on the people experiencing them, their colleagues and their patients. This can effect levels of patient care and safety [20]. It is essential that RVNs and all members of the veterinary team are able to find healthy coping strategies and are able to practice them regularly.

RVNs should always feel able to ask for help if help is required, it is ok not to be ok. Vetlife is an excellent source of help and support for any veterinary professional who is struggling with their mental health. It is useful to have the Vetlife contact details displayed around the practice and team members should be made aware of how to access these services [21]. The RCVS runs a Mind Matters initiative that offers training courses and resources to support mental health and reduce stress in the workplace [21]. There is a legal requirement to carry out a stress-at-work risk assessment in the workplace. The Health and Safety Executive (HSE) Management Standards are a useful resource for this [21]. RVNs, SVNs and vets should never feel alone, rather that they are a part of a large and growing team of veterinary professionals who ultimately all have the same goals.

References

1 Gray, C. and Wilson, K. (2006). Introduction to the legal system. In: *Ethics Law and the Veterinary Nurse* (ed. S. Pullen and C. Gray), 24–28. Oxford: Elsevier.

2 RCVS (2021). Delegation to veterinary nurses 2021 [Online]. Available at: rcvs.org.uk (accessed 30 November 2022).

3 Pearson, J. and Trumble, B. (1996). *The Oxford English Reference Dictionary*, 2e, 1154. Oxford: Oxford University Press.

4 Jones B.V. (2011). Veterinary nursing history – the early years [Online]. Available at: veterinary-nursing-the-early-years-2018.pdf (accessed 30 November 2022).

5 RCVS (2019). Code of professional conduct for veterinary nurses [Online]. Available at: www.rcvs.org.uk (accessed 30 November 2022).

6 RCVS (2022). A concern has been raised about me, information for veterinary nurses [Online]. Available at: Information for veterinary nurses – Professionals (rcvs.org.uk) (accessed 30 November 2022).

7 West, H.R. (2021) Utilitarianism philosophy [Online]. Available at: britannica.com (accessed 30 November 2022).

8 DEFRA (2019). Equine infectious anaemia control strategy for Great Britain [Online]. Available at: assets.publishing.service.gov.uk/government/uploads/system/uploads/attachment_data/file/842206/equine-infectious-anaemia-control-strategy.pdf (accessed 30 November 2022).

9 Duignan, B. (2020). Deontological ethics, encyclopaedia Britannica [Online]. Available at: britannica.com (accessed 30 November 2022).

10 Guyer, P. and Wood, A. (1992). *The Cambridge Edition of the Works of Immanuel Kant*, 691–670. Cambridge University Press.

11 RCVS (2022). Code of professional conduct for veterinary nurses [Online]. Available at: rcvs.org.uk (accessed 30 November 2022).

12 Summers, H. (2022). What were Aristotle's four cardinal virtues? [Online]. Available at: www.thecollector.com/aristotle-four-cardinal-virtues/ (accessed 30 November 2022).

13 Mullan, S. (2006). Introduction to ethical principles. In: *Ethics Law and the Veterinary Nurse* (ed. S. Pullen and C. Gray), 11–19. Oxford: Elsevier.

14 Collins (2022). Collins English Dictionary | Definitions, translations, example sentences and pronunciations. Available at: collinsdictionary.com (accessed 30 November 2022).

15 Information Commissions Office (2022). What is consent? [Online]. Available at: ico.org.uk (accessed 30 November 2022).

16 RCVS (2022). Communication and consent [Online]. Available at: rcvs.org.uk (accessed 30 November 2022).

17 DEFRA (2018). Horse welfare code of practice [Online]. Available at: https://assets.publishing.service.gov.uk/government/uploads/system/uploads/attachment_data/file/700200/horses-welfare-codes-of-practice-april2018.pdf (accessed 30 November 2022).

18 Benner, P. (1982). From novice to expert. *American Journal of Nursing* 82 (3): 402–407.

19 RCVS (2020). Raising concerns about a colleague [Online]. Available at: https://www.rcvs.org.uk/setting-standards/advice-and-guidance/code-of-professional-conduct-for-veterinary-surgeons/supporting-guidance/whistle-blowing/ (accessed 30 November 2022).

20 Lloyd, C. and Campion, D.P. (2017). Occupational stress and the importance of self-care and resilience. *Veterinary Ireland Journal* 4 (9): 1–7.

21 Lawson, A. (2020). Principles of health and safety. In: *BSAVA Textbook of Veterinary Nursing*, 6e (ed. B. Cooper, E. Mullineaux, and L. Turner), 49. British Small Animal Veterinary Association: Gloucester.

Useful Websites

Mind Matters
www.vetmindmatters.org
The British Equine Veterinary Association (BEVA)
www.beva.org.uk
The British Veterinary Nursing Association (BVNA)
https://bvna.org.uk
Vetlife
www.vetlife.org.uk

4

Equine Anatomy and Physiology

Lucy Middlecote[1] and Sophie Pearson[2]

[1] *Linnaeus Veterinary Limited, West Midlands, UK*
[2] *Bottle Green Training Ltd, Derby, UK*

4.1 Veterinary Terminology

Veterinary terminology is the body of specialised words relating to the science of veterinary medicine.

Anatomy – the study of the physical structure of the body.

Physiology – the way in which the body functions and works.

Directional Terms

Directional terms are used to provide additional information about the position of organs and tissues (Table 4.1 and Figure 4.1). They are commonly used during diagnostic imaging.

Anatomical Planes

Anatomical planes are used to describe the location of parts of the animal (Table 4.2 and Figure 4.2).

Root Words, Prefixes and Suffixes

By learning the meanings of root words, prefix and suffix words can be broken down into components to determine their meanings (Table 4.3).

Commonly used root words are shown in Table 4.4. For commonly used prefixes and suffixes please refer to Table 4.5.

4.2 Anatomical Boundaries and Body Cavities

The body can be divided into different compartments known as body cavities (Figure 4.3), which include:

- Thoracic cavity
- Abdominal cavity
- Pelvic cavity

Each cavity is lined with connective tissue called serosa. The serosa that lines the cavity itself is known as parietal serosa, and the serosa that lines the organs is known as visceral serosa [1–3].

Thoracic Cavity

- Houses the heart, the lungs and associated structures
- Defined by the thoracic inlet (cranially), diaphragm (caudally), vertebrae (dorsally), sternum (ventrally) and ribs (laterally).
- Lined by a serous membrane known as the parietal pleura. Where this covers the lungs, it is known as the pulmonary pleura.
- Between the lungs and the parietal pleura is the pleural space
  - The pleural space has a negative pressure, which allows the lungs to inflate.
  - There is a small amount of fluid here known as pleural fluid, which allows the lungs to move freely against the ribcage [1–3].

Mediastinum

- The space in the anterior chest between the lungs. It contains the thymus, heart, aorta, trachea, oesophagus, a variety of nerves and blood vessels [1–3].

Textbook of Equine Veterinary Nursing, First Edition. Edited by Rosina Lillywhite and Marie Rippingale.
© 2025 John Wiley & Sons Ltd. Published 2025 by John Wiley & Sons Ltd.
Companion website: www.wiley.com/go/equineveterinarynursing

Table 4.1 Directional terms.

Directional term	Description
Cranial (anterior)	Towards the head
Caudal (posterior)	Towards the tail
Rostral	Towards the nose
Dorsal	Towards or near the back
Ventral	Towards the belly
Lateral	Away from the midline
Medial	Towards the midline
Proximal	Towards the point of attachment
Distal	Away from the point of attachment
Dorsal (in relation to the limb)	The front surface of the lower limb
Palmar	The back or under surface of the lower forelimb area
Plantar	The back or under surface of the lower hindlimb area
Ipsilateral	On the same side
Contralateral	On the opposite side
Superficial	Nearer the surface
Deep	Further from the surface

Source: Lucy Middlecote.

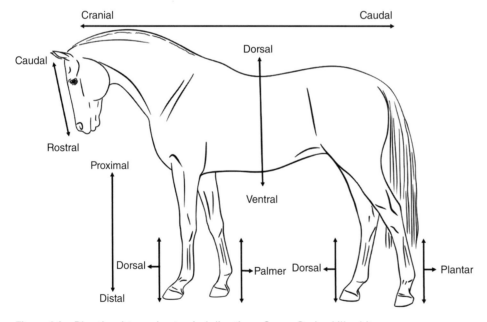

Figure 4.1 Directional terms/anatomical directions. *Source:* Rosina Lillywhite.

Table 4.2 Anatomical planes.

Anatomical plane	Description
Median plane	A line which divides the body along the mid-line into right and left halves
Sagittal plane	Any line parallel to the median plane
Dorsal plane/Frontal plane	A line parallel to the back of the animal
Transverse plane	A line perpendicular to the long axis of the animal

Source: Lucy Middlecote.

Figure 4.2 Anatomical planes. *Source:* Lucy Middlecote and Jennifer Farrar.

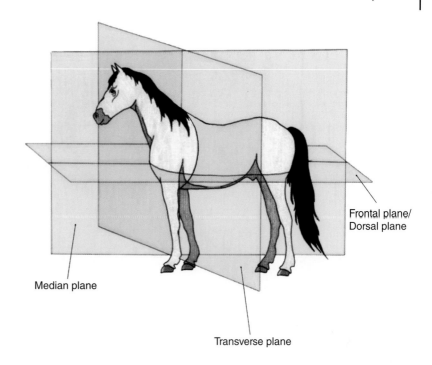

Frontal plane/ Dorsal plane

Median plane

Transverse plane

Table 4.3 Root words, prefixes and suffixes.

Component	Description	Example
Root	The essence of the word meaning; often relates to an organ, structure or disease	Cardium/Cardi(o) – relates to the heart
Prefix	Placed at the beginning of a word to alter or modify the meaning	Endocardium – within the heart
Suffix	Placed at the end of a word to alter or modify the meaning	Carditis – inflammation of the heart
Prefix + Root + Suffix – Endocarditis – inflammation within the heart		

Source: Lucy Middlecote.

Table 4.4 Root words.

Root word	Description	Example
Athro(o)	Joint; articulation	Arthritis – inflammation of a joint
Cardio(o)	Heart	Cardiology – the study of the heart and its function
Chondro	Cartilage	Chondrocyte – cartilage cell
Cyst(o)	Bladder	Cystotomy – incision into the bladder
Dermat(o)	Skin	Dermatitis – inflammation of the skin
Gloss(o)	Tongue	Hypoglossal – situated below the tongue
Haemat(o)/Haem(o)	Blood	Haemorrhage – bleeding from a ruptured vessel
Hepat(o)	Liver	Hepatocyte – liver cell
Hist(o)	Tissue	Histology – the study of tissues
Mamm(o)	Breast; mammary gland	Mammogram – radiograph of a mammary gland
Metra/Metro	Uterus	Endometrium – lining of the uterus

(Continued)

Table 4.4 (Continued)

Root word	Description	Example
Myo-	Muscle	Myositis – inflammation of a voluntary muscle
Neur(o)	Nerve	Neuralgia – pain in a nerve
Opthalm(o)	Eye	Ophthalmoscope – instrument used to examine the eye
Orchi	Testis (testicle)	Orchitis – inflammation of a testis
Oste(o)	Bone	Osteomyelitis – inflammation of a bone
Pneum(o)	Air or gas; lung	Pneumonia – inflammation of the lung tissue
-pnoea	Respiration; breathing	Dyspnoea – difficulty in breathing
Ren-	Kidney	Renal artery – the artery that supplies the kidney with blood
Rhin(o)	Nose	Rhinitis – inflammation of the mucous membrane of the nose
Vas(o)	Vessel; duct	Vasoconstriction – a decrease in the diameter of a blood vessel

Source: Lucy Middlecote.

Table 4.5 Commonly used prefixes and suffixes.

	Prefix/Suffix	Meaning	Example
1	Ab-	Away	Abduction – moving a limb away from the midline Abrasion – scraping something away, e.g. graze Abnormal – deviating from the norm
2	Ad-	Towards	Adduction – moving a limb towards the midline Administer – application of a drug/therapy Admittance – allow entry
3	Ex-	Out from	Exocytosis – transport of substances out of a cell Exophthalmos – anterior displacement of the eye Exocrine gland – secrete substances onto a surface
4	Ecto-	Outside	Ectoparasite – parasite that lives on the outside of the host Ectocytic – outside a cell Ectocornea – the outer layer of the cornea
5	Endo-	Within	Endoscopy – viewing internal parts of the body Endothelium – layer of tissue lining the inside of blood vessels and organs Endotracheal – within the trachea
6	Epi-	Upon	Epidermis – the superficial layer of skin Epiphysis – the end part of a long bone Epimysium – sheath of tissue surrounding a muscle
7	Hypo-	Under/Low	Hypoxia – low oxygen levels Hypothermia – low body temperature Hypotension – low blood pressure
8	Hyper-	Above/high	Hyperthermia – abnormally high body temperature Hypertension – abnormally high blood pressure Hypercapnia – abnormally high levels of carbon dioxide in the blood
9	Brady-	Slow	Bradycardia – slow heart rate Bradypnoea – slow respiratory rate Bradykinesia – slow movement
10	Tachy-	Fast	Tachycardia – fast heart rate Tachypnoea – fast respiratory rate Tachyphylaxis – rapid decrease in medication response
11	A/an	Lack of	Anaemia – insufficient red blood cells/haemoglobin in the blood to transport oxygen Anorexia – lack of appetite Apnoea – cessation of breathing

Table 4.5 (Continued)

	Prefix/Suffix	Meaning	Example
12	Inter-	Between	Intercellular – occurring between cells Interstitial – space between structures Intervertebral – between the vertebrae
13	Intra-	Within	Intracellular – occurring within a cell Intravascular – within a blood vessel Intraarticular – within a joint
14	Peri-	Around	Perivascular – around blood vessels Pericardium – serous membrane surrounding the heart Perimysium – sheath of connective tissue surrounding a bundle of muscle fibres
15	Post-	After	Postoperative – the period following surgery
16	Uni/mono-	One	Monorchid – having only one testicle Uniparous – producing only a single offspring Monogastric – having a stomach with a single compartment
17	Bi/di-	Two	Dichromatic – vision where only two of the three primary colours can be seen Biceps – a muscle comprising two heads
18	Tri-	Three	Triceps – a muscle comprising three heads
19	Quad/tetra-	Four	Tetralogy of Fallot – heart defect characterised by four specific defects occurring together Quadriceps – a muscle comprising four heads
20	Poly-	Many	Polyuria – excess urination Polyphagia – excess hunger Polypharmacy – use of multiple medicines at one time
21	Oligo-	Few	Oliguria – reduced urine output Oligodontia – less than the normal number of teeth
22	Macr-	Large	Macroscopic – visible to the eye
23	Micro-	Small	Microscopic – not visible to the eye Microscope – instrument used to visualise things that are too small to be seen by the eye
24	Hepato-	Liver	Hepatocyte – liver cell
25	Derm-	Skin	Dermatitis – irritation of the skin Dermatology – study of the skin
26	Pneumo-	Lung	Pneumothorax – air escaping the lungs into the thorax Pneumonia – infection of the lung(s) Pneumopathy – any disease of the lungs
27	Gastro-	Stomach	Gastroscopy – Viewing the inside of the stomach
28	Cyst-	Bladder	Cystoscopy – looking inside the bladder Cystitis – inflammation of the bladder Cystotomy – cutting into the bladder to remove intact urinary calculi
29	Nephro/reno-	Kidney	Nephrosplenic ligament – connects the kidney to the spleen Nephrotoxicity – dysfunction of the kidney caused by toxic chemicals Nephritis – inflammation of the kidney
30	Cardio-	Heart	Cardiology – study of the heart Cardiomyopathy – disease affecting the muscle of the heart Cardiogenic shock – condition caused by the inability of the heart to pump blood sufficiently
31	Entero-	Intestines	Enteropathy – disease of the intestines Enterology – study of the intestines
32	Optho-	Eye	Ophthalmology – study of the eyes Ophthalmoscope – instrument for visualising the eye
33	Thoraco-	Thorax/chest	Thoracocentesis – puncturing the thorax to remove air/fluid Thoracotomy – surgical procedure to gain access to the pleural space
34	Abdomino-	Abdomen	Abdominocentesis – puncturing the abdomen to obtain a fluid sample

(Continued)

Table 4.5 (Continued)

	Prefix/Suffix	Meaning	Example
35	Arthro-	Joint	Arthroscopy – procedure looking into a joint Arthrodesis – surgical immobilisation of a joint by fusing the bones
36	Teno-	Tendon	Tenocyte – mature tendon cell Tenoblast – immature tendon cell
37	Cyto-	Cell	Cytology – study of cells Cytotoxic – toxic to living cells Cytostatic – inhibits cell growth and multiplication
38	Haem-	Blood	Haematology – study of blood Haematoma – collection of blood outside of the vessels Haemopoiesis – production of blood cells
39	Erythro-	Red blood cell	Erythropenia – low red blood cell count Erythropoiesis – production of red blood cells Erythropoietin – hormone that stimulates red blood cell production
40	Leuco-	White	Leukocyte – white blood cell Leukopenia – low white blood cell count
41	Thrombo-	Blood clot	Thrombocyte – cell fragment responsible for clot formation (platelets) Thrombocytopenia – decreased number of platelets in the blood Thrombosis – formation of a clot in a vessel
42	Pyo-	Pus	Pyometra – pus in the uterus Pyothorax – pus in the thorax Pyonephritis – pus in the renal pelvis
43	Hydro-	Water	Hydrotherapy – use of water in treatment Hydrolysis – breaking a substance down using water Hydrocele – collection of fluid in the scrotum
44	Chrondro-	Cartilage	Chondrocyte – cell responsible for cartilage formation Chondropathy – disease of cartilage
45	Laryn-	Larynx	Laryngeal hemiplegia – paralysis of one or both arytenoid cartilages of the larynx Laryngeal nerve – nerve supplying the larynx
46	Myo-	Muscle	Myocardium – muscle of the heart Myopathy – disease affecting voluntary control of muscle Myology – study of muscles
47	Osteo-	Bone	Osteocyte – bone cell Osteology – study of bones Osteomyelitis – painful inflammation of bone
48	Dys-	Difficult	Dyspnoea – difficulty breathing Dysphagia – difficulty swallowing/eating Dysuria – difficulty urinating
49	Mal-	Bad/poor	Malabsorption – poor absorption of nutrients from food Malfunction – functioning badly Malpractice – poor practice
50	Iso-	Same	Isometric – equal dimensions Isotonic solution – has the same water/solute concentration as cells Isotonic contraction – tension remains the same in a muscle and the muscle shortens
51	Patho-	Disease	Pathology – the study of disease Pathogen – disease agent Pathogenesis – development of disease
52	Neo-	New	Neonate – new-born Neoplasia – new, abnormal growth Neonatology – medical specialism focussing on new-borns
53	-pathy	Disease	Myopathy – disease affecting the control of muscles Neuropathy – nerve damage that can cause pain, weakness or numbness Cardiomyopathy – disease of the heart muscle
54	-scopy	View	Arthroscopy – procedure looking in a joint Gastroscopy – procedure looking in the stomach Laparoscopy – procedure looking in the abdomen

Table 4.5 (Continued)

	Prefix/Suffix	Meaning	Example
55	-otomy	Cut into	Laparotomy – incision through the abdominal wall Hysterotomy – incision into the uterus Thoracotomy – incision into the pleural space
56	-ectomy	Cut out	Ovariectomy – surgical removal of an ovary/ovaries Neurectomy – surgical removal of all/ part of a nerve Hysterectomy – surgical removal of all/part of the uterus
57	-ostomy	Form an opening	Tracheostomy – incision into the trachea to create an opening Urethrostomy – creating a temporary opening for diversion of urine when the urethra is blocked Thoracostomy – incision in the chest wall with maintenance of the opening for drainage
58	-plasty	Repair/reform	Vulvoplasty – procedure altering the construction of the vulva, i.e. Caslick's procedure Hernioplasty – surgical reshaping of a hernia Tendoplasty – reparative surgery on a tendon
59	-centesis	Puncture	Abdominocentesis – puncturing the abdomen to obtain a fluid sample Thoracocentesis – puncturing the thorax to remove air/fluid
60	-algia	Pain	Neuralgia – pain along the course of a nerve Myalgia – pain in a muscle Arthralgia – joint pain
61	-itis	Inflammation	Nephritis – inflammation of the kidney Carditis – inflammation of the heart Arthritis – inflammation of the joints
62	-osis	Condition	Cyanosis – blue colouration caused by hypoxia Salmonellosis – infection of the salmonella bacteria Acidosis – build-up of acid
63	-ology	Study	Histology – study of tissues Cytology – study of cells Pathology – study of disease
64	-graphy	Record	Radiography – taking X-rays Ultrasonography – imaging the body with ultrasound waves Scintigraphy – imaging the body using a radioactive substance
65	-emia	Of the blood	Anaemia – insufficient RBCs/haemoglobin in the blood to transport oxygen Hypoxaemia – low oxygen levels in the blood Ischemia – restricted blood flow
66	-cyte	Cell	Osteocyte – mature bone cell Tenocyte – mature tendon cell Erythrocyte – red blood cell
67	-therapy	Course of treatment	Hydrotherapy – use of water as treatment Chemotherapy – use of cytotoxic drugs to treat cancer Cryotherapy – use of extreme cold treatment
68	-pnoea	Breathing	Apnoea – cessation of breathing Dyspnoea – difficulty breathing Tachypnoea – fast respiratory rate
69	-penia	Deficiency	Leukopenia – low white blood cell count Neutropenia – low neutrophil count in the blood Erythropenia – low red blood cell count
70	-oma	Swelling	Haematoma – a swelling of clotted blood Lipoma – benign tumour of fatty tissue Melanoma – a pigmented tumour
71	-lysis	Destruction	Haemolysis – destruction of red blood cells Bacteriolysis – rupture of bacterial cells Hydrolysis – breaking a substance down using water
72	-phagia	Eating	Dysphagia – difficulty eating/swallowing Polyphagia – excessive eating Aphagia – inability to swallow

Source: Sophie Pearson.

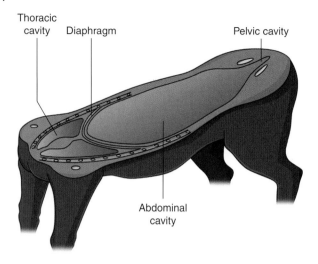

Figure 4.3 Body cavities. *Source:* Adapted from CABI.

Abdominal Cavity

- Houses the digestive system and some components of the urogenital system.
- Defined by the diaphragm (cranially), pelvic opening (caudally), vertebrae (dorsally) and abdominal muscles (laterally and ventrally). Lined by a serous membrane known as the peritoneum. This produces a small amount of peritoneal fluid, which enables the abdominal organs to move freely against each other [1–3].

Pelvic Cavity

- Anatomically but not physically separated from the abdomen.
- Houses the reproductive organs, the bladder and the rectum.
- Defined by the pelvic inlet (cranially), pelvic outlet (caudally), pelvic bones (dorsally) and muscles around the pelvic girdle (laterally) [1–3].

4.3 Cell Biology

Cell Structure

Cells are the individual units that make up tissues, organs and body systems. Cells are microscopic and carry out several basic functions, including taking in nutrients, excreting waste, respiring and reproducing. Depending on their location in the body and their function, some cells have specialised structures, but the basic structure of all cells is the same [1–3] (see Figure 4.4).

Cell membrane – composed of a phospholipid bilayer, the cell membrane is the semi-permeable outer covering that controls the entry and exit of materials/molecules in and out of the cell.

Nucleus – known as the cell's control centre, the nucleus contains deoxyribonucleic acid (DNA) in the form of chromosomes. The smaller nucleolus forms part of the nucleus

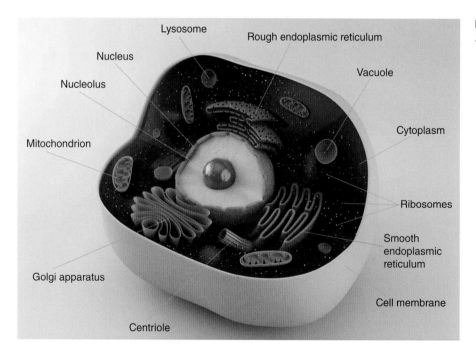

Figure 4.4 Cell structure. *Source:* Rosina Lillywhite.

and contains ribonucleic acid (RNA). The nucleolus is also responsible for the manufacturing of ribosomes.

Cytoplasm – the fluid component of the cell that contains the organelles.

Organelles – small structures located in the cytoplasm, to include:

- Centrosome – consists of two centrioles and is involved in cell replication.
- Mitochondria – produce energy via aerobic respiration, extract energy from food substances and store it as adenosine triphosphate (ATP), a form that the cell can use.
- Ribosomes – responsible for protein synthesis and often attached to the rough endoplasmic reticulum (RER).
- Rough endoplasmic reticulum (RER) – responsible for synthesising and transporting proteins along with the attached ribosomes.
- Smooth endoplasmic reticulum (SER) – responsible for the synthesis and transport of lipids.
- Golgi body/apparatus – flattened membrane sacs that are involved in the production of lysosomes, secretory granules and the plasma membrane. Responsible for the transport and modification of glycoproteins and other substances.
- Vacuole - The main function is to store substances, typically either waste or harmful substances, or useful substances the cell will need later on.
- Lysosomes – a collection of digestive enzymes in membrane sacs that form part of the defence mechanism of the cell [1, 3].

Cell Division

Cells reproduce by division, a process during which DNA is replicated. There are two types of division that can take place – mitosis and meiosis.

Mitosis

Somatic cells are the cells in the body other than germ cells (ova and sperm cells). Most of the cells in the body are somatic cells that divide by mitosis. During mitosis, somatic cells make identical copies of themselves; one parent cell divides into two identical daughter cells (Figure 4.5). The number of chromosomes in each resulting daughter cell is the same as the parent cell, known as the diploid number [3].

There are five stages involved in mitosis:

- Interphase – resting phase
- Prophase – chromosomes become apparent
- Metaphase – chromosomes line up along the middle of the cell
- Anaphase – chromatids separate
- Telophase – separation into the two new cells [1, 3].

Meiosis

Germ cells divide by meiosis in the gonads (ovaries and testes) to produce ova or sperm (Figure 4.6). During meiosis, one parent cell divides to create four daughter cells. The number of chromosomes in each resulting daughter cell is halved, known as the haploid number [1, 3].

The stages of meiosis are similar to mitotic division, but there are two cell divisions. The first division (meiosis I) is longer and more complicated, the process of the second cell division (meiosis II) is identical to mitosis:

Meiosis I – Interphase, Prophase I, Metaphase I, Anaphase I, Telophase I.
Meiosis II – Prophase II, Metaphase II, Anaphase II, Telophase II [1, 3].

Fluid

Fluid provides the medium in which the body's biochemical reactions take place. Water is essential for maintaining the body's internal environment and keeping it in a state of balance, known as homeostasis. The amount of water in the body will vary and is affected by age and how fat or thin the horse is, but it should make up approximately 60–70% of total body weight [1–3].

Each mammalian cell contains approximately 80% water. This is divided into intracellular fluid (ICF) and extracellular fluid (ECF). Intracellular fluid is found inside the cells and accounts for 40% of total body weight. ECF is the fluid which lies outside the cells and accounts for 20% of total body weight. Approximately 75% of ECF is interstitial fluid (fluid found around the cells), approximately 25% is plasma and a very small amount is transcellular fluid (includes lymphatic fluid, synovial fluid and cerebrospinal fluid (CSF) [1–3].

Body water is continually lost from the body and must be replaced to maintain total fluid balance. Water is taken in via drinking and eating, and is lost via urine, faeces, tears, secretions, sweat and respiration. Water that is lost via sweat and from the respiratory tract is termed insensible fluid loss. Fluid loss can lead to dehydration and hypovolaemic shock. Fluid losses will often be increased in sick horses via reflux, diarrhoea and blood loss [1–3].

Electrolytes

Fluid in the body is also made up of minerals that are dissolved in water, known as a solution. Solutions containing free ions are known as electrolytes. Free ions, which conduct electricity, can have a positive or a negative charge. Ions with a positive charge are referred to as cations, and ions with a negative charge are referred to as anions. The number of electrolytes present will increase or decrease

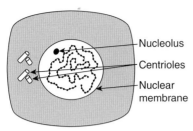

A Interphase
Cell has normal appearance of
non-dividing cell condition:
chromosomes too threadlike
for clear visibility.

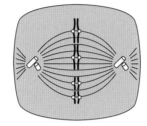

B Early prophase
Chromosomes become visible as
they contract, and nucleolus shrinks.
Centrioles at opposite sides of the
nucleus. Spindle fibres start to form.

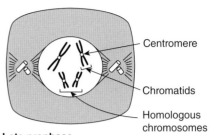

C Late prophase
Chromosomes become shorter and fatter – each seen
to consist of a pair of chromatids joined at the
centromere. Nucleolus disappears. Prophase ends
with breakdown of nuclear membrane.

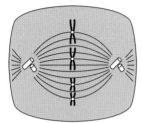

D Early metaphase
Chromosomes arrange themselves
on equator of spindle. Note that
homologous chromosomes do
not associate.

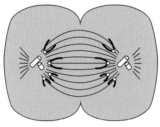

E Late metaphase
Chromatids draw apart at the
centromere region. Note that the
daughter centromeres are orientated
toward opposite poles of the spindle.

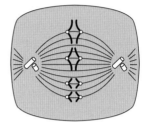

F Early anaphase
Spindle fibres contract and pull
the chromatids apart, moving
them to the opposite ends of
the cell.

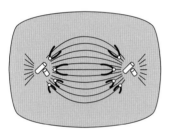

G Late anaphase
Chromosomes reach their destination.

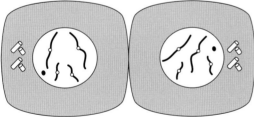

H Early telophase
The cell starts to constrict across the middle.

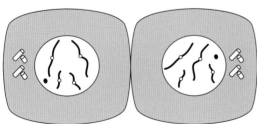

I Late telophase
Constriction continues. Nuclear membrane
and nucleolus reformed in each daughter
cell. Spindle apparatus degenerates.
Chromosomes eventually regain their
threadlike form and the cells return to
resting condition (interphase).
Note that the daughter cells have
precisely the same chromosome
constitution as the original parent cell.

Figure 4.5 Cell reproduction: mitosis. *Source:* Adapted from BSAVA and M.B.V Roberts.

the concentration of the solution, the more electrolytes, the greater the concentration.

The cations found in the intracellular fluid are potassium, magnesium and sodium. The anions are phosphate, bicarbonate and chloride. The cations found in the ECF are sodium, potassium, magnesium and calcium. The anions are chloride, bicarbonate and phosphate [1, 3].

Diffusion and Osmosis

To maintain homeostasis, body water and the associated chemical substances that it contains move around the body. The processes involved in this are diffusion, osmosis and active transport [1, 3].

Diffusion is a passive process that involves the movement of molecules/electrolytes from a solution where they are at

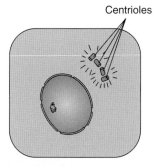

Centrioles

Interphase I

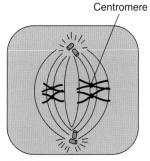

Spindle

Prophase I
This is divided into five stages: leptotene, zygotene, pachytene, diplotene and diakinesis. During this time the chromosomes contract and crossing over takes place.

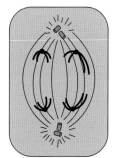

Centromere

Metaphase I
Homologous pairs of chromosomes lie side by side on the cell spindle so that there are two rows of chromosomes (unlike in mitosis when there is a single row).

Anaphase I
The spindle fibres contract and homologous chromosomes separate to opposite ends of the cell. The centromeres do not divide as in mitosis.

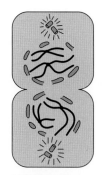

Telophase I
This is the stage of cytoplasmic division. In the female two separate cells are produced (the ovum and first polar body) but in the male cytoplasmic division is often incomplete and the cell has a dumb-bell shape with two sets of chromosomes.

Prophase II
The chromosomes remain contracted.

Metaphase II
This is like mitotic metaphase. The chromosomes line up one below the other on the equator of the spindle

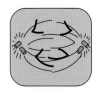

Anaphase II
Like mitotic anaphase. The spindle fibres contract, the centromere divides and the chromatids are pulled apart and move to opposite ends of the cell.

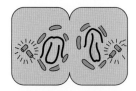
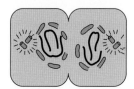

Telophase II
The cytoplasm divides. In the female this forms the ovum and second polar body and in the male the spermatids.

Figure 4.6 Meiosis. *Source:* Adapted from BSAVA.

a high concentration to a solution where they are at a low concentration and takes place where there is no barrier to the free movement of molecules (Figure 4.7). If the molecules are too big to pass through a cell membrane, then a different process takes place [1, 3].

Osmosis is a passive process that involves the movement of water from a solution of low concentration to one of a high concentration and takes place through a semi-permeable membrane (Figure 4.7). The pressure with which water molecules are drawn across a semi-permeable membrane is known as the osmotic pressure. Fluid that has the same osmotic pressure as plasma is known as isotonic.

Fluid with a higher osmotic pressure than plasma is known as hypertonic, and fluid with a lower osmotic pressure than plasma is known as hypotonic [1, 3].

If the plasma's osmotic pressure is high, water moves into the blood to equalise the concentration. If the plasma's osmotic pressure is low, water moves out of the blood and into the tissue spaces [1, 3].

Active transport is the movement of electrolytes against an osmotic gradient. Using energy, cells transport electrolytes across a cell membrane allowing them to move from a solution of low concentration to one of a high concentration [1, 3].

Diffusion

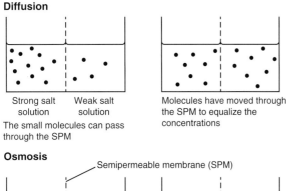

Strong salt solution   Weak salt solution

The small molecules can pass through the SPM

Molecules have moved through the SPM to equalize the concentrations

Osmosis

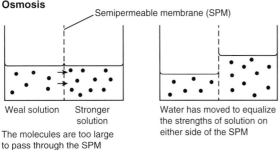

Semipermeable membrane (SPM)

Weal solution   Stronger solution

The molecules are too large to pass through the SPM

Water has moved to equalize the strengths of solution on either side of the SPM

Figure 4.7 Diffusion and osmosis. *Source:* Adapted from BSAVA.

Acid–base Balance

The concentration of hydrogen ions present within a solution is termed the pH.

- An acidic solution has a pH of less than 7.
- An alkaline solution has a pH of more than 7.
- A neutral solution has a pH of 7.

The normal pH of blood is 7.4. The body aims to maintain this level within a narrow range to ensure that it can function properly. To do this the body has mechanisms in place to include respiration, sodium and hydrogen ion exchange, and buffers. A buffer is a solution that resists changes in pH when acid or alkali is added to it [1, 3].

4.4 Basic Tissue Types

Similar cells found in one location are known as tissues. There are four main types found in the body:

- Epithelial tissue (epithelium)
- Connective tissue
- Muscle
- Nervous tissue

Epithelial Tissue

Epithelial tissue covers the internal and external surfaces of the body, providing absorption, secretion and protection for the underlying structures. The thicker the epithelium, the more protective it is and further protection may be provided by the presence of keratin. When epithelial tissue covers structures such as the lining of the heart, blood vessels and lymph vessels, it is known as endothelium. Epithelial tissue is classified according to the appearance of the cells (Table 4.6 and Figure 4.8) [1–3].

Table 4.6 Epithelial tissue.

Epithelial tissue	Description	Location
Simple squamous epithelium	Single layer of thin, flat cells Very delicate	Areas where diffusion occurs Examples: alveoli of lungs, lining blood vessels, glomerular capsule
Simple cuboidal epithelium	Square/cube shaped	Lining glands and ducts Lining parts of the kidney tubules
Simple columnar epithelium	Tall and rectangular/column shaped	Lining organs that have an absorptive function (for example, the intestine) or a secretory function (for example, digestive glands)
Stratified epithelium	Multiple layers Tough and protective Can be infiltrated with keratin for extra protection	Areas subjected to friction Examples: oesophagus, mouth, vagina Keratin Example: epidermis of the skin
Ciliated epithelium	Usually columnar in shape Cilia are present on the free surface of the cells	Lines tubes and cavities where material must be trapped and/or moved Examples: respiratory tract, oviducts
Transitional epithelium	Layers of cells that can stretch	In structures that need to stretch Examples: bladder, urethra, ureters
Glandular epithelium	Has secretory cells which secrete mucus/materials into the space they are lining	Examples: oral cavity, trachea

Source: Lucy Middlecote.

Connective Tissue

Connective tissue supports and holds the organs and tissues of the body in place (Table 4.7). It also provides a transport system, carrying nutrients to the body and waste products away. The basic structure consists of cells, fibres and a glycosaminoglycan matrix [1–3].

Muscle

Muscle tissue contains muscle cells that are arranged as fibres. Depending on the muscle type, it contracts and relaxes either voluntarily or involuntarily to bring about movement. There are three main types of muscle – smooth muscle, cardiac muscle and skeletal muscle (Table 4.8 and Figure 4.9) [1–3].

Nervous Tissue

Nervous tissue consists of many neurons which are responsible for the transmission of nervous impulses (signals).

Table 4.7 Connective tissue types.

Connective tissue type	Location
Blood	Circulating through the blood vessels
Haemopoietic tissue	Long bones
Areolar tissue (loose connective tissue)	All over the body Examples: beneath the skin, around blood vessels and nerves, between and connecting organs, and between muscle bundles
Adipose (fatty) tissue	In the dermis of the skin Around the kidneys
Dense connective tissue	**Parallel arrangement fibres** – tendons and ligaments **Irregularly interwoven fibres** – dermis of the skin, capsules of joints, testes, lymph nodes
Cartilage	**Hyaline cartilage** – between the epiphysis and diaphysis of growing long bones, at the articular surfaces of moving joints, walls of the respiratory tract, ventral ends of the ribs **Fibrocartilage** – in the intervertebral discs, the pubic symphysis, at the attachment points of ligaments and tendons **Elastic cartilage** – in the auricle of the ear, external auditory canal, Eustachian tube, epiglottis
Bone	The skeleton

Source: Lucy Middlecote.

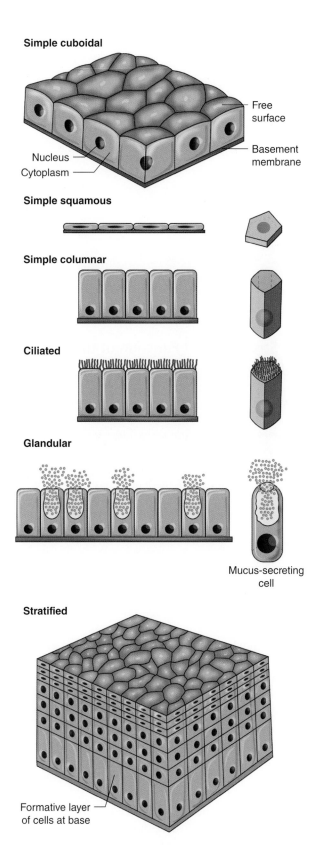

Figure 4.8 The different types of epithelial tissue found in the body. *Source:* Adapted from CABI.

Table 4.8 Different muscle types.

Muscle	Description	Control	Location
Smooth muscle (also called visceral muscle or involuntary muscle)	Unstriated (smooth) appearance Cells are long and spindle shaped, and surrounded by small amounts of connective tissue that binds the cells into sheets or layers The nucleus in each cell lies in its centre	Involuntary control	Walls of blood vessels, digestive tract, respiratory tract, bladder, uterus
Cardiac muscle	Striated (striped) appearance Cells are cylindrical in shape Branch to create a network of fibres which are linked by intercalated disks – these enable nerve impulses to be conveyed across the muscle producing a rapid response to any changes required by the body	Involuntary control	Heart Forms the myocardium
Skeletal muscle	Striated (striped) appearance Cells are long and cylindrical and lie parallel to each other Each fibre has several nuclei which lie on the outer surface	Voluntary control	Attached to the skeleton

Source: Lucy Middlecote.

Smooth muscle

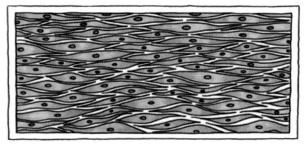

Cardiac muscle

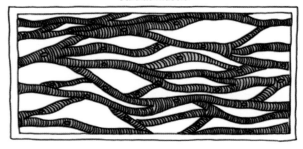

Skeletal muscle

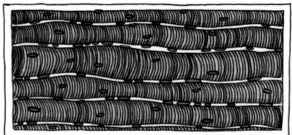

Figure 4.9 Muscle types. *Source:* Lucy Middlecote and Jennifer Farrar.

4.5 Structure and Function of the Integument

The term 'integument' refers to the outer covering of the body [1], specifically the skin (and associated glands), hair and hooves in equids. It forms a barrier against the external environment; the points at which it meets the natural openings of the body (e.g. mouth), it is continuous with the mucous membranes lining these openings [1].

Functions of the Skin

- Protection:
  - Protects underlying structures from physical injury [4].
  - Prevents entry of microorganisms [1].
  - Protection from ultraviolet (UV) radiation [4].
  - Protection against water loss [5].
- Thermoregulation
  - Sweat production cools the skin surface via evaporation [2].
  - Piloerection traps a layer of air, acting as insulation [3].
  - Vasoconstriction diverts blood away from the surface in cold temperature [3].
  - Vasodilation promotes heat loss [5].
  - Adipose tissue under the skin acts as insulation [5].
- Sensation
  - Skin is a sense organ for temperature, touch, pressure and pain [3].
  - Sensory nerve endings associated with hairs facilitate physical assessment of the environment and can trigger avoidance behaviours such as skin twitching to ward insects away [6].

- Production
  - Sebum is produced by sebaceous glands within the skin and is secreted onto the surface of the skin to form a water-resistant layer [5].
  - Vitamin D is synthesised from 7-dehydrocholesterol in the skin upon exposure to UV light. Vitamin D is required for the uptake of dietary calcium [1].
- Storage
  - Adipose tissue forms both an energy store and an insulating layer against cold weather [5].
- Communication
  - Pheromones are produced by specialised skin glands for intraspecific communication [1].

Skin Structure

The skin comprises two true layers: the epidermis and the dermis. The hypodermis lies beneath the skin [2]. The thickness of the skin varies in different regions of the body and is typically thicker in regions more prone to abrasion [5].

Epidermis

The epidermis is an avascular layer of stratified epithelium, composed of four layers [5]:

Stratum germinativum: Also known as the stratum basale [5]. This is the deepest layer of the epidermis and consists of a single layer of cells which divide rapidly via mitosis to replace cells lost from the more superficial layers.

Melanocytes, which are cells containing granules of melanin that give the skin its pigment are found in this layer [2].

Stratum granulosum: Cells begin to die as they move towards the surface. Development of keratin (keratinisation) occurs within the cells which gives them a granular appearance [3]. Keratin is a structural protein which provides protection [3]. The nuclei become shrunken in this layer [3].

Stratum lucidum: Cells have lost their nuclei when they reach this layer and develop a clear appearance [3].

Stratum corneum: The most superficial layer of the epidermis. It consists of many layers of dead, flattened, keratinised cells called corneocytes [3]. These cells continuously slough off and are replaced by the cells developing underneath [1].

Dermis

Otherwise known as the corium, this is the deeper layer of the skin [6], composed of dense connective tissue, with collagen and elastic fibres arranged in an irregular manner. Within the dermis are blood vessels, lymphatic vessels, nerves, sweat glands, sebaceous glands and hair follicles [3]. Arrector pili muscles associated with each hair are also present in this layer and permit the hair to stand to trap a layer of insulating air [1].

Hypodermis

The hypodermis is also known as the subcutis and is not a true layer of skin. It lies below the dermis (Figure 4.10) and contains connective and adipose tissue [3].

Figure 4.10 Structure of the skin.
Source: Sophie Pearson & Claire Hart.

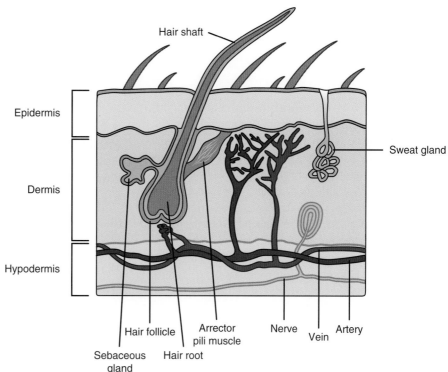

Glands

Sweat Glands

Also known as sudoriferous glands, these may be associated with hair follicles (apocrine) or independent of hair follicles (eccrine) [1].

Sebaceous Glands

Each hair follicle is associated with a sebaceous gland, which produces sebum. Sebum is an oily substance that is secreted onto the surface of the skin, forming a water-resistant layer. It also helps to retain moisture in the skin and acts as an antimicrobial [1].

Modified Sebaceous Glands
Ceruminous Glands

These line the external auditory canal of the ear and produce cerumen (ear wax) [3].

Meibomian Glands

These secrete the fatty component of the tear film onto the eyelids to moisten the eye [3].

Mammary Glands

These modified glands secrete milk for the nourishment of foals [5].

Hair

Structure

Hair is a keratinised structure that is important for insulation, protection and perception [2]. Each hair comprises an inner medulla, an outer cortex and an overlying cuticle [1]. They are produced by a follicle and the visible portion of the hair above the skin is referred to as the hair shaft, while the portion that lies within the follicle is referred to as the 'root' [3].

Growth

Follicles develop from epidermal cells and may be simple (a single follicle) or compound (grouped follicles). The follicles grow downwards into the dermis and form a hair cone, which overlies a hair papilla [1]. The papilla provides the growing hair with blood and nerve supply. Cells keratinise from the hair cone and form a hair. The hair grows up towards the surface of the epidermis and will grow continuously until it dies and becomes detached from the follicle. Hairs grow in different direction across the body and the direction of growth gives rise to hair tracts [3]. The growth of hair is cyclical, occurring in three phases:

- Anagen – rapid growth [2].
- Catagen – transitional phase [1].
- Telogen – resting phase, the follicle is inactive [2].

The shedding of hair is referred to as moulting and is influenced by changes in daylength and temperature with changing seasons. Hair growth varies between breeds; Arabs and Thoroughbreds for example do not develop coats as thick as native breeds [6].

Types
Guard Hairs

Also known as primary hairs [1], these form the outer coat. They are thicker, longer and stiffer than the hairs that form the undercoat [5]. Each hair grows from a single follicle and is associated with an arrector pili muscle, which contracts in cold weather [3].

Wool Hairs

Also known as secondary hairs [1], these form the undercoat. They are much softer, shorter and thinner than guard hairs. They are also more numerous as their number varies with changing seasons, becoming more numerous in winter. Many wool hairs may grow from one follicle and are associated with one guard hair. They act as a layer of insulation [3].

Vibrissae

Also known as tactile hairs, whiskers or sinus hairs. These hairs are thicker than guard hairs and may be found on the muzzle, eyelids and lips. Vibrissae grow from follicles deep in the hypodermis and protrude significantly beyond the coat. Nerve endings sensitive to mechanical stimuli surround the follicle and respond to the touch or movement of the hair, providing the equid with information about their surroundings [3].

Tylotrich Hairs

These are present across the body, scattered between guard and wool hairs. They are strong, thick, single hairs within a large follicle and act as fast-acting mechanoreceptors [1].

4.6 Structure and Function of the Musculoskeletal System

Physiology of Bone

Bone is a living tissue that continually changes throughout the horse's life [1]. Bone comprises an extracellular matrix that contains collagen fibres and the protein 'osteonectin', which are combined to form the organic material 'osteoid'. The osteoid forms the unmineralised aspect of the bone, but as the bone develops, calcium phosphate crystals are deposited within the bone. The crystals are insoluble and cause the bone tissue to become calcified; it is then referred to as 'mineralised bone' [3].

The osteoid is synthesised by osteoblasts, which are immature bone cells [1]. As bone becomes calcified, the osteocytes, which are mature bone cells, become trapped in spaces called 'lacunae' [3]. The osteocytes are responsible for maintaining bone structure. A third type of bone cell, called osteoclasts, are responsible for breaking down and remodelling bone [1].

Within the matrix of bone material are channels that carry blood vessels and nerves. These are called Haversian canals and each one is surrounded by lamellae, which are concentric cylinders of bone material [3]. Each canal and associated lamellae and lacunae are collectively called a 'Haversian System' or 'osteon' [1]. The outer surface of a bone is covered by a fibrous membrane called the periosteum [3].

The two types of bone are compact bone and cancellous bone. Compact bone is found in the cortices (outer surfaces) of all bones. The structure of the bone is very dense and regular [1], with Haversian systems tightly packed together

[3]. Cancellous bone is also known as 'spongy bone' and consists of interconnecting bars of bone called trabeculae with red bone marrow in the spaces [3]. The network of trabeculae means that cancellous bone is not as strong as compact bone [1].

Long Bone Structure

Long bones consist of a shaft and two ends (Figure 4.11), with separate regions that have differing characteristics [2]. The central shaft is known as the diaphysis [1], which has a dense cortex and an inner medulla [2]. Each end of the bone is known as the epiphysis and the region between the epiphyses and diaphysis is called the metaphysis. The metaphysis contains the epiphyseal growth plate, a region that is crucial in bone development [1].

Features of Bones

The shape of bones varies greatly and there are a variety of terms that can be used to describe features such as

Figure 4.11 Structure of a long bone.
Source: Sophie Pearson & Claire Hart.

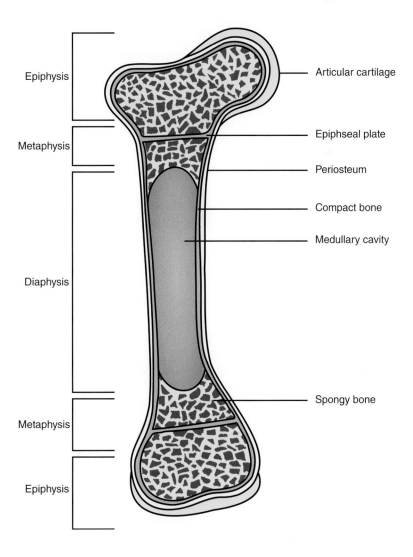

Epiphysis

Metaphysis

Diaphysis

Metaphysis

Epiphysis

Articular cartilage

Epiphseal plate

Periosteum

Compact bone

Medullary cavity

Spongy bone

prominences and depressions. Terms used to describe protuberances include tuberosity, trochanter and tubercle, which each typically act as a site for the attachment of muscles. Bones can also have grooves known as a trochleae (singular: trochlea), which tendons typically pass through or over, thus permitting the tendon to act as a pulley [3]. Condyles are rounded protuberances at the end of a bone [1], which are usually involved in the articulation with another bone. An epicondyle is a lateral projection on a bone, situated above the condyle [3]. Foramina (singular: foramen) are holes or openings in a bone and a sinus is a hollow cavity within a bone. A depression in a bone is referred to as a fossa, whereas a raised area is referred to as a crest. A process is a thin, elongated projection of bone [1].

Ossification

Ossification is the process by which bones are formed. There are two types of ossification: intramembranous ossification and endochondral ossification [3].

Intramembranous Ossification

Bone formed by intramembranous ossification does not have a cartilage precursor. Instead, bone cells are situated between two membranes [2] and the osteoblasts lay down bone material, replacing the fibrous connective tissue [1]. This is the process by which the flat bones of the skull are formed [3].

Endochondral Ossification

This type of ossification requires a cartilage model [5]. The model is present within the embryo and comprises hyaline cartilage, which is gradually replaced [2]; a process which continues after birth. Long bones develop by endochondral ossification [3]. The stages of endochondral ossification are outlined below:

1) A hyaline cartilage model develops within the embryo [3].
2) Primary ossification centres appear in the diaphysis, where osteoblasts lay down new bone material that replaces the cartilage and extends towards the end of the bone [3].
3) Secondary ossification centres appear in the epiphyses of the bone [3].
4) The primary and secondary ossification centres meet at the epiphyseal growth plate [1], which is a narrow band of persisting cartilage [3] that is radiolucent when radiographed.
5) On the epiphysis side of the growth plate, new cartilage is produced, which results in the lengthening of the bone at each end [1].
6) Eventually, the cartilage on the side of the plate nearest to the diaphysis is replaced with bone material laid down by osteoblasts [1].
7) The interior of the diaphysis is remodelled by osteoclasts; the medullary cavity is created during this process [1].
8) When the horse has reached its final size, the cartilage cells stop dividing and all remaining cartilage is ossified [1] and the epiphyseal plate is described as 'closed' [3].

Classification of Bone

Bones can be classified into the following shapes.

Long Bones

Long bones comprise an outer cortex of bone material [1] and a shaft that contains a central medullary cavity, containing bone marrow [3]. Examples include the femur, tibia and humerus.

Short Bones

These comprise an outer layer of compact bone and an inner layer of cancellous bone. They do not possess a medullary cavity. Examples of short bones include the carpal and tarsal bones [3], which develop from a single centre of ossification [1].

Flat Bones

Flat bones comprise an outer layer of compact bone and contain cancellous bone in the centre. They do not possess a medullary cavity [3] and stretch in two directions as they grow [1]. Examples of flat bones include the ribs and scapula.

Irregular Bones

Their structure is similar to that of short bones as they have an outer layer of compact bone, a core of cancellous bone and no medullary cavity. They do not fit easily into other categories however as their shape is less uniform and they are unpaired [3]. An example of irregular bones is the vertebrae.

Sesamoid Bones

The name 'sesamoid bone' is derived from the Arabic word for 'sesame seed', with which they share a shape. They are typically located near a tendon that runs over a bony prominence. The presence of the sesamoid bone changes the angle at which the tendon passes over the bone, reducing wear and tear [3]. They are also similar in structure to short bones as they have an outer layer of compact bone and a core of cancellous bone. Examples of sesamoid bones are the patella and the navicular bone.

Pneumatic Bones

Pneumatic bones contain sinuses, which are air-filled spaces that lighten the bone. Examples of pneumatic bones include the frontal and the maxillary bones [3].

Joints

A joint occurs where two or more bones join together or articulate. Different joints types facilitate different degress of movement. Joints are classified as follows [1, 2]:

- Synovial (Figure 4.12a). – These joints have a wide range of movement are are also known as diarthroses. Synovial joints are formed when a synovial membrane connects two bones and there is a space between the ends of the bones or joint cavity that is filled with synovial fluid. The ends of the bone are covered in articular (hyaline) cartilage and this allows low-friction articulation between opposing bones. Synovial fluid is a viscous substance that is made from the fluid component of plasma and hyaluronic acid. Synovial fluid acts as a lubricant between the cartilage of the two bones ends and nutrients diffuse from the synovial fluid into the articular cartilage. The synovial membrane lines the joint and produces the synovial fluid. A joint capsule made of dense connective tissue surrounds the whole joint. Some joints contain a pad of fibrocartilage called a meniscus such as the stifle joint, which contains two menisci that are firmly attached by ligaments to the tibial plateau.
- Cartilaginous (Figure 4.12b) – These joints have little or no movement. These joints can present as synchondoses, which are joints between the epiphyses and diaphysis in growing animals, or as symphyses, which are joints between the mandible bones of the lower jaw and the pubic bones of the pelvis
- Fibrous (Figure 4.12c) – These joints have little or no movement. Fibrous joints as present as sutures in the skull, or syndesmoses between two areas of bone.

The range of movement of a joint can be described using the following terms [1]:

- Flexion – bending the limb by decreasing the angle of the joint
- Extension – straightening the limb by increasing the angle of the joint
- Adduction – moving the limb distal to the joint towards the midline/body
- Abduction – moving the limb distal to the joint away from the midline/body

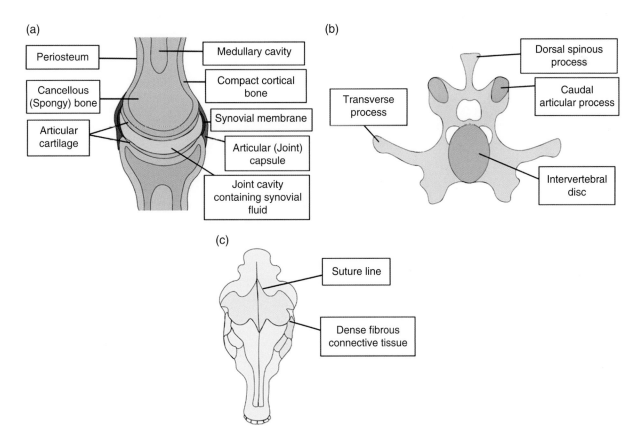

Figure 4.12 (a–c): Different joint types: (a) a synovial joint. (b) a cartilaginous joint. (c) a fibrous joint. *Source:* Rosina Lillywhite.

- Gliding – flat surfaces moving over each other e.g. in the carpus
- Rotation – movement shown by a pivot joint
- Circumduction – moving one end of a bone (usually the end distal to the joint) in a circular motion
- Protraction – lengthening the limb by moving the distal limb away from the body
- Retraction – shortening the limb by moving the distal limb towards the body

The Skeleton

Horses have approximately 205 bones. The skeleton has several functions in addition to acting as a framework for the horse. These include facilitation of movement, protection of soft organs and tissues, haemopoiesis and storage of minerals [1]. Figure 4.13 shows the skeleton of the horse.

The equine skeleton can be divided into two sections: the axial skeleton and the appendicular skeleton [7].

The Axial Skeleton

The axial skeleton comprises the skull, vertebrae, ribs and sternum [7].

The Skull

The main function of the skull is to protect the brain, inner ear, the eye and the nasal passages. The bones of the skull are joined by fibrous joints known as sutures [7], which give the skull a rigid structure. The region of the skull in which the brain is housed is called the cranium. There is one moveable joint in the skull (the temporomandibular joint) which facilitates chewing [3]. The bones of the skull are displayed in Figure 4.14.

The majority of the dorsal and lateral walls of the cranium are formed by the parietal bones. Situated below the parietal bones, on the caudolateral surface of the skull are the temporal bones. One each temporal bone is a rounded prominence at the ventral aspect. This is called the tympanic bulla and contains the structures of the middle ear. The floor of the cranial cavity is formed by the sphenoid bone, which has many foramina, permitting the passage of blood vessels and nerves [3].

The occipital bone is situated at the caudal aspect of the skull [3]. There is a hole in the occipital bone through which the spinal cord passes called the foramen magnum [2]. A pair of bony prominences called the occipital condyles are located on either side of the foramen magnum. The condyles articulate with the atlas, the first cervical

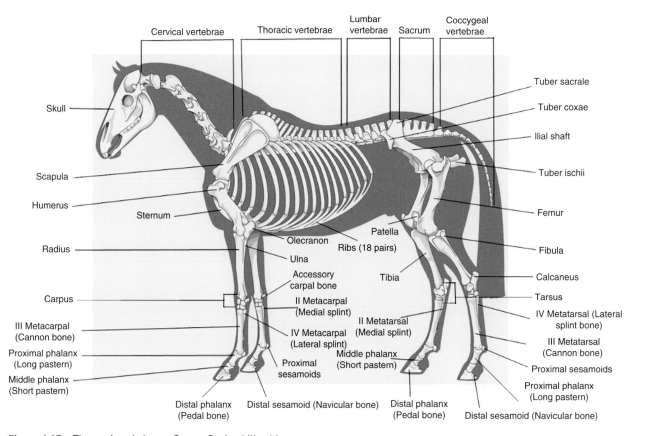

Figure 4.13 The equine skeleton. *Source:* Rosina Lillywhite.

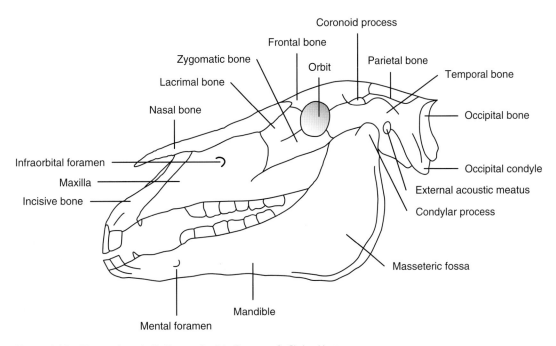

Figure 4.14 The equine skull. *Source:* Sophie Pearson & Claire Hart.

vertebra. Jugular processes are situated on either side of the occipital condyles and serve as attachment sites for muscles [3]. The equine skull has a prominent occipital ridge that the nuchal ligament attaches to [1].

The forehead is formed by the frontal bone, which also forms the front aspect of the cranium. The roof of the nasal cavity is formed by the nasal bone. The nasal septum, a cartilaginous plate, divides the nasal cavity into left and right halves. Each side is filled with nasal turbinates (also referred to as conchae), which are fine, delicate scrolls of bone, covered in ciliated mucous epithelium. At the caudal aspect of the nasal cavity, the ethmoid bone forms the boundary between the nasal cavity and the cranial cavity. The cribriform plate is located in the centre of the ethmoid bone, through which olfactory nerves pass, transmitting impulses from the mucosa in the nasal cavity to the olfactory bulbs within the brain [3].

The maxilla forms the upper jaw, and the lower jaw is formed by the mandible [7]. The mandible is divided into the horizontal and the vertical ramus. The vertical ramus has two processes: the condylar process and the coronoid process [2]. The condylar process contributes to the temporomandibular joint, where the mandible articulates with the rest of the skull. The coronoid process projects into the temporal fossa and is a site of muscle attachment for the temporalis muscle [3]. The lower cheek teeth are housed in the horizontal ramus of each mandible and each side is joined at the mandibular symphysis [2], which is a cartilaginous joint. On the lateral aspects of each mandible is a

depression called the masseteric fossa, where the masseter muscle is situated [3]. The upper incisors are housed in the incisive bone, the most rostral bone of the skull [3] which, in conjunction with the maxilla and palatine bone forms the hard palate and base of the nasal cavity [7].

Situated in the intermandibular space is the hyoid apparatus. This structure consists of a series of bones and cartilage, joined in a trapeze-shaped manner. The larynx and tongue are suspended from the skull by the hyoid apparatus, permitting movement of these structures when swallowing. The hyoid apparatus articulates with the skull via a cartilaginous joint in the temporal region [3].

The zygomatic bone projects laterally from the skull to form the 'cheekbone'. The prominent nature of this bone serves to protect the eye. The orbit, commonly referred to as the eye socket, is formed by aspects of several bones. At the base of the orbit is the lacrimal bone. Tears drain from the eye, through the lacrimal bone, into the nose [3].

The Teeth

Embedded within the maxilla, mandible and incisive bone are the teeth, adapted in equids for breaking down fibre. Horses have different types of teeth, suited to different jobs. The first type are the incisor teeth, situated at the rostral end of the oral cavity. The upper incisors are embedded in the incisive bone and the lower incisors are embedded in the mandible. They are referred to as central, lateral and corner incisors in accordance with their position (the central incisors are the most medial and the corners are the most lateral, with the lateral incisors positioned between the two). They are responsible for prehending food and cutting grass [3].

Caudal to the incisors are the canine teeth, also known as 'tushes'. Canine teeth erupt in the gap (diastema) between the incisors and cheek teeth; these often fail to erupt in mares, but males have four canines, which erupt at approximately five years of age. The lower canines are situated more rostrally than the upper canines, meaning that no contact occurs between these teeth (Figure 4.15) [2]. The premolars and molars are collectively referred to as the 'cheek teeth'. These are flattened to facilitate grinding food into smaller particles. In some horses, vestigial teeth known as 'wolf teeth' may develop in front of the pre-molars [3]. The wolf teeth are known as the first premolar. These are more commonly seen in the upper jaw than the lower jaw [2].

Similarly to other mammals, horses have two sets of teeth. The first set, which are smaller and seen in younger animals are referred to as deciduous teeth. The deciduous teeth are replaced by permanent teeth [1], a process which occurs from the age of two-and-a-half and is not complete until the horse is five [4]. Horses do not have deciduous molars or canine teeth. The timing of the eruption is as follows:

- Deciduous central incisors: by four weeks [4].
- Deciduous lateral incisors: between one and three months [4].
- Deciduous corner incisors: between eight and nine months [4].
- Permanent central incisors: at two-and-a-half years and in wear at three years [4].
- Permanent lateral incisors: at three-and-a-half years and in wear by four years [4].

- Permanent corner incisors: at four-and-a-half years and in wear by five years [4].
- Deciduous premolars: by three months [4].
- Permanent premolars: the first erupts at around two-and-a-half years, and the others at around three-and-a-half years [4].
- Permanent molars: the first erupts at approximately 9 months, followed by the second at 18 months. The final molar erupts at four-and-a-half years [4].
- Permanent canines: five years [4].

Dental formulae indicate the number of each tooth type present. The dental formulae for a full set of deciduous and permanent teeth are as follows:

Deciduous teeth in a male or female: (i3/3, pm3/3) = 24 teeth.
Permanent teeth in a male: (I3/3, C1/1, PM3–4/3, M3/3) × 2 = 40 (without wolf teeth) or 42 (with wolf teeth).
Permanent teeth in a female: (I3/3, C0/0, PM3–4/3, M3/3) × 2 = 36 (without wolf teeth) or 38 (with wolf teeth).

Each tooth is held in place in a socket, otherwise known as an alveolus. The outer part of the crown comprises enamel, while the outer aspect of the root comprises cementum. Dentine forms the inner aspect of each tooth, and a pulp cavity is present at the centre of each tooth (Figure 4.16). The pulp cavity contains, blood vessels, lymphatic vessels and nerves [1]. Equine teeth have adapted to a diet high in fibre and are referred to as hypsodont (long crowned). These teeth continue to erupt throughout the horse's life [2], which compensates for wear, which is approximately 2–3 mm per year [7]. A layer of enamel is not present over the occlusal surface (otherwise known as the 'table') of the teeth [3].

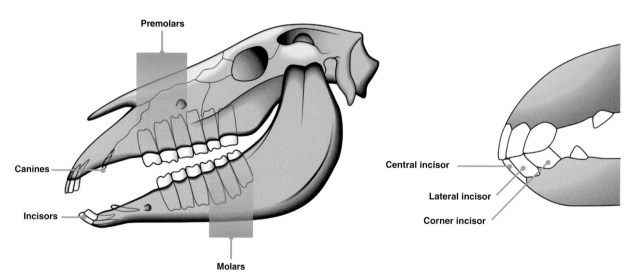

Mature horse - The adult horse has 12 incisors (for biting) and 12 premolars and 12 molars (for grinding).

Figure 4.15 Equine teeth. *Source:* Dechra Veterinary Products.

(a)

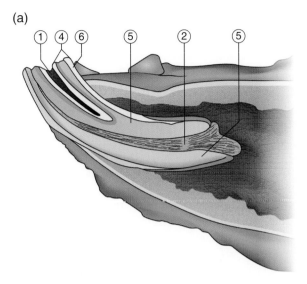

(b)   (c)   (d)   (e)

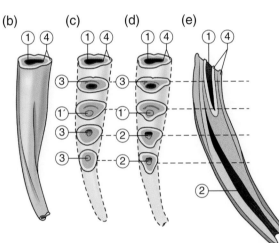

① Cup, black cavity in center of infundibulum
①′ Enamel spot, proximal end of infundibulum
② Dental cavity
③ Dental star, changing in shape from a linear to a rounded form
④ Outer and inner enamel rings
⑤ Cement
⑥ Lingual surface

Figure 4.16 The structure of a lower equine incisor. (a): In situ, sectioned longitudinally; the clinical crown is short in relation to the embedded part of the tooth. (b): Caudal view; the junction between the clinical crown and the rest of the tooth is not marked. (c): As a result of wear, the occlusal surface changes; the cup gets smaller and disappears, leaving for a time, the enamel spot: the dental start appears and changes from a line to a large round spot. (d): These are sawn sections of a young tooth for comparision. (e): Longitudinal section of an incisor, showing the relationship between the infundibulum and dental cavity; the latter is rostral. *Source:* Adapted from Elsevier.

The Vertebrae

The vertebrae collectively form the vertebral column, which forms a rod to support the body. It also houses and protects the spinal cord, provides sites of insertion for muscles and provides an attachment site for the ribs [3]. The vertebral column is divided into the following regions: cervical, thoracic, lumbar, sacral and coccygeal [1].

Basic Structure of Vertebrae

Vertebra all have the same basic structure with variations in accordance with differing functions [3]. A basic vertebra has a cylindrical body [2] at the ventral aspect. The cranial end of the body is convex, while the caudal end is concave. Above the vertebral body is the neural arch, forming the vertebral foramen. The vertebral foramina collectively form the spinal canal. Above the neural arch is the spinous process; the height of these processes differs in different regions of the vertebral column [3]. Transverse processes are situated on each side of each vertebra [6], the size of which also vary in different regions of the vertebral column. The transverse processes separate the muscles of the vertebral column into the epaxial muscles (situated above the processes) and the hypaxial muscles (situated below the processes) [3]. The vertebrae also have two pairs of articular processes [6], which are the cranial and caudal articular processes. The articular processes form synovial joints with adjacent vertebrae [3].

Adjacent to the body of each vertebra is an intervertebral disc [3], which permits slight compression [4], thereby acting as a shock absorber. The outside of each disc comprises a layer of fibrous connective tissue called the annulus fibrosus. Gelatinous material fills the centre of each disc and is called the nucleus pulposus [3].

Cervical Vertebrae

The horse, like all other mammals, has seven cervical vertebrae located in the neck (C1–C7). The first cervical vertebra is the atlas [4], which possesses large, wing-shaped processes [3]. The second cervical vertebra is the axis [7], which possesses a prominent cranial process called the dens [3], also known as the odontoid process [6]. The movement of the atlas and axis is not inhibited by spinous or transverse processes, which allows a large range of movement [3]. The joint between the skull and the axis permits the nodding movement of the head [4] and the articulation between the atlas and axis permits the rotation of the atlas around the odontoid process. Unlike the atlas and the axis, C3–C7 follow the basic vertebral structure [3].

Thoracic Vertebrae

The horse has 18 thoracic vertebrae (T1–T18) [7] which possess very prominent spinous processes [4]. The height of each process decreases slightly, moving towards the lumbar region and the withers are formed by T4–T9. The head of each rib articulates with the costal fovea of each corresponding thoracic vertebra, while the tubercle of the rib articulates with the transverse fovea [3].

Lumbar Vertebrae

The horse has six lumbar vertebrae (L1–L6) [4], with the exception of some Arab horses, which may have only five lumbar vertebrae. These vertebrae have smaller spinous processes than the thoracic vertebrae but possess large transverse processes. This restricts lateral movement but contributes to the protection of the kidneys [3].

Sacral Vertebrae

The horse has five sacral vertebrae (S1–S5) that are fused to form the sacrum [8], thus greatly restricting movement. An interosseous ligament joins the pelvis to the sacrum, forming the sacroiliac joint [3].

Coccygeal Vertebrae

The horse has between 15 and 20 coccygeal vertebrae (Cd1–Cd15–20) [5], but Arab horses typically have fewer coccygeal vertebrae. From Cd1 to the final coccygeal vertebra, each vertebra decreases in size and complexity [4]. The first few have very small spinous and transverse processes, which decrease in size further down the tail until they resemble a simple rod-shaped structure. The small processes permit a greater degree of movement in the tail [3].

Vertebral Formulae

The vertebral formula for the horse and the donkey differs as follows:

Horse: C7, T18, L6, S5, Cd15–20.
Donkey: C7, T18, L5, S5, Cd15–17.

The Ribs

The horse has 18 pairs of ribs [2], with the exception of Arab horses, which may have only 17 pairs. Each rib has a bony aspect that articulates with the thoracic vertebrae and the ventral part of each rib is made of cartilage, referred to as the costal cartilage. The region where the bony aspect of the rib meets the cartilaginous aspect is the costochondral junction [1]. The first eight pairs of ribs articulate directly with the sternum and are classified as 'true' ribs [7] or 'sternal' ribs. The remaining 10 pairs of ribs are referred to as 'false' or 'asternal' [3] and instead articulate with the rib in front, forming the costal arch. The space between each rib is called the 'intercostal space' [2].

The Sternum

The sternum supports the true ribs and forms the ventral boundary of the thoracic cavity [4]. The equine sternum is made up of eight bones called sternebrae. The manubrium is the most cranial sternebra and the xiphoid is the most caudal sternebra [1]. Situated between the sternebrae is a disc of cartilage called sternebral cartilage [3].

The Appendicular Skeleton

The appendicular skeleton comprises the bones of the limbs [7].

Bones of the Proximal Forelimb

The most dorsal bone of the forelimb is the scapula, commonly referred to as the shoulder blade [7]. This is a large, flat bone, divided in half on the lateral aspect by the scapular spine. This permits the insertion of the supraspinatus and infraspinatus muscles. At the proximal aspect of the scapula is a wing of cartilage, which also permits muscle attachment [3]. The horse does not possess a clavicle (collarbone); instead, the forelimb is connected to the trunk by a group of muscles referred to as the thoracic sling.

A shallow socket, called the glenoid cavity, is located at the distal end of the scapula. Here, the head of the humerus forms the shoulder joint with the scapula. On the craniolateral aspect of the humerus is a large prominence called the greater tubercle. A smaller prominence called the lesser tubercle is located medial to the each. The tubercles act as sites for muscle attachment. The shaft of the humerus is slightly twisted, and the condyle is situated on the distal aspect of the bone. On either side of the condyle are the medial and lateral epicondyles. The distal aspect of the humerus articulates with the radius and ulna to form the elbow joint [3].

The equine ulna and radius are fused to each other. The radius bears most of the weight and is situated medially. At the proximal end of the ulna, the olecranon process forms the point of elbow [3]. Articulating with the distal aspect of the radius are the carpal bones.

The carpal bones form the carpus, otherwise known as the knee. The horse has seven or eight carpal bones arranged in two rows [3]. The proximal row of carpal bones (from medial to lateral) consists of the radial carpal bone, the intermediate carpal bone, the ulnar carpal bone and the accessory carpal bone [7]. The accessory carpal bone is situated behind the ulnar carpal bone [2]. The distal row from medial to lateral are the first (not always present) [1], second, third and fourth carpal bones [7].

Bones of the Distal Forelimb

Distal to the carpus are the metacarpal bones. The horse has three metacarpal bones (the second, third and fourth metacarpal). The metacarpal bones are numbered as such due to the ancestors of the modern horse possessing five digits, which reduced with evolution. Only remnants of digits two, three and four remain. The majority of the horse's weight supported by the third metacarpal, otherwise known as the canon bone. The second (medial) and fourth (lateral) metacarpal bones are commonly called the splint bones and are fused to the third metacarpal bone [1].

The proximal aspect of the proximal phalanx articulates with the distal aspect of the third metacarpal bone [2]. This forms the metacarpophalangeal joint, commonly called the fetlock joint. Situated on the palmar aspect of this joint are two sesamoid bones called the proximal sesamoids [3]. The proximal phalanx is also referred to as the long pastern bone or P1 [7]. The distal aspect of the proximal phalanx articulates with the proximal aspect of the middle phalanx [2]. The middle phalanx is also called the short pastern bone or P2 [7]. The distal aspect of the middle phalanx articulates with the proximal aspect of the distal phalanx [2]. The distal phalanx is also called the pedal bone or P3 [7]. The joint between P1 and P2 is called the proximal interphalangeal joint but is commonly referred to as the pastern joint. The joint between P2 and P3 is called the distal interphalangeal joint but is commonly referred to as the coffin joint. The distal sesamoid is also part of this joint, situated at the palmar aspect of the joint. The distal sesamoid is commonly called the navicular bone [2].

Bones of the Proximal Hindlimb

The equine pelvis comprises three fused bones: the ilium, the ischium and the pubis [7]. At the top of the pelvis is the ilium, which is joined to the vertebral column at the sacroiliac joint. On the ilium is the tuber coxae, which forms the point of the hip [4]. The wings of the ilium (tuber sacrales) can be palpated at the croup [3]. The floor of the pelvis is formed by the pubis at the front and the ischium at the back [4]. The tuber ischii can be felt at the point of buttock [3]. On either side of the floor of the pelvis is a large hole called the obturator foramen [3], which reduces the weight of the pelvic girdle [3]. At the junction of the ilium, ischium and pubis is the acetabulum, the socket where the femur meets the pelvis [1].

The femur is a large bone that is a crucial point of attachment for key muscles of the hindlimb. The articular head is situated medially for articulation with the pelvis. The greater trochanter is positioned lateral to the head and the lesser trochanter is situated medially, both of which serve as points of muscle attachment. At the distal aspect of the femur are the medial and the lateral condyles that form part of the stifle joint, in articulation with the tibia. Situated between the condyles is a sesamoid bone called the patella, which sits in the trochlear groove [3].

The tibia and fibula are situated between the femur and the tarsus. The tibia is the larger of these two bones, whereas the fibula small, thin and is situated on the lateral aspect of the tibia. At the lower end of the tibia, the fibula tapers to a point and becomes fused to it [3].

The bones of the tarsus (commonly called the hock) are arranged in three rows. In the proximal row are the talus and the calcaneus [1]. The latter has an elongated proximal end (tuber calcis), which forms the point of hock [1]. A central tarsal bone is situated in the middle row, In the distal row are first, second, third and fourth tarsal bones. The first and second are fused but the third and fourth tarsal bones are separate [1].

Bones of the Distal Hindlimb

The bones of the distal hindlimb are similar to those of the forelimb. The key difference is the naming of the cannon and splint bones. The cannon bone of a forelimb is the third metacarpal whereas in the hindlimb, it is called the third metatarsal. Similarly, the splint bones which are called the second and fourth metacarpals in the forelimb are called the second and fourth metatarsals in the hindlimb. The arrangement and naming of the proximal, middle and distal phalanx, in addition to the proximal and distal sesamoids is the same as the forelimb.

Physiology of Skeletal Muscle, Tendons and Ligaments

Physiology of Muscle

Skeletal muscle consists of muscle cells called muscle fibres, which are surrounded by delicate connective tissue called endomysium. Individual fibres are grouped together in bundles known as fascicles, which are held together by connective tissue called perimysium. Many fascicles are held together to form the muscle and the entirety of the muscle surrounded by fibrous, elastic tissue called epimysium (Figure 4.17) [2]. In some instances, a bursa, which is a sac lined by synovial membrane and filled with synovial fluid, is present between a muscle/tendon/ligament and a bony prominence to reduce friction [3]. Such is the case with the navicular bursa which is located between the deep digital flexor tendon and the navicular bone in the distal limb.

Each muscle is made of bundles of microfilaments called myofibrils. These are the contractile elements of the muscles [4]. The thin filaments are called actin and the thick filaments are called myosin. The parallel arrangement of the actin and myosin allow the myofibrils to slide over each other. Areas of overlap give skeletal muscle a striped appearance under the microscope, which is why it is described as 'striated'. The bands are separated into sarcomeres; sarcomeres are the units of contraction. Skeletal muscle is under voluntary control and the process of muscle contraction requires energy in the form of ATP. The muscle also requires nervous stimulation; each nerve and the group of muscles fibres it stimulates

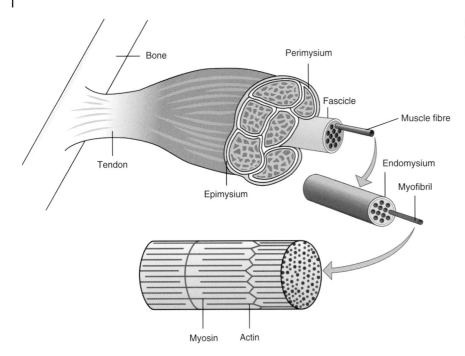

Figure 4.17 The microscopic structure of skeletal muscle. *Source:* Sophie Pearson & Claire Hart.

is referred to as a motor unit. The junction between the muscle and the nerve is called the neuromuscular junction [3].

Muscle Shapes

Muscles of the body differ in shape. A muscle with a thick central part (the belly) and tapered ends (the head) are considered a classically shaped muscle. The muscle is attached to the bone via tendons. The starting point of a muscle is the origin, and the insertion is situated at the opposite end. Some muscles have more than one head, with each head inserting at the same point. In some instances, muscles form rings that are responsible for controlling entry to/exit from a structure. These muscles are referred to as sphincters. In some instances, the muscle fibres form sheets of muscle, with the tendons also drawn out into sheets in an arrangement called an 'aponeurosis'. An example of this is the diaphragm. Muscles that lie completely in one region of the body are called intrinsic muscles. The origin and insertion of an intrinsic muscle are located in a single region and only act on a joint within the region. Conversely, extrinsic muscles have an insertion point in a different region to the origin. This alters the position of the whole region [3].

Physiology of Tendons and Ligaments

Tendons attach muscle to bone and serve to transfer the force of a muscle contraction to a bone, exerting pull on the bone. The point at which the tendon forms an attachment to the muscle is also known as the musculotendinous junction (MTJ). The point at which it attaches to the bone is known as the osteotendinous junction (OTJ).

Tenoblasts are immature tendon cells, which are fibroblasts of tendons that produce type 1 collagen. A number of fibrils form collagen fibres and a group of fibres forms a fascicle. Tenocytes are mature tendon cells that are responsible for maintaining the extracellular matrix and are arranged in rows between the collagen fibrils. A group of fascicles collectively form the tendon. Surrounding collagen bundles is the endotenon, which comprises loose connective tissue. Continuous with this sheath is the epitenon, which surrounds the entirety of the tendon. The paratenon consists of loose areolar tissue and is the outermost layer of the tendon. Fluid between the epitenon and paratenon serves to reduce friction. A bursa may completely surround a tendon to form a tendon sheath to reduce friction [3].

Ligaments connect bone to bone. Their structure is similar to that of tendons; however, they have less collagen, are more cellular and have a more limited supply of blood. The four types of ligaments are: supporting ligaments that support or suspend a structure, annular ligaments that wrap around joints, interosseus ligaments that link bones together and funicular ligaments that are cord-like ligaments, which help to hold bones together.

The horse possesses check ligaments, which are structures that serve to prevent over-extension of a joint. These include the radial check ligament, the carpal check ligament and the tarsal check ligament (Table 4.9).

Table 4.9 Muscles, tendons and ligaments of the forelimb of the horse.

Structure	Origin	Insertion	Action
Muscles			
Biceps brachii	Distal scapula	Radius	Flexion of the elbow
Brachiocephalicus	Cranial cervical vertebra	Proximal: shoulder Distal: humerus	Lateral movement of the head and neck; protraction of upper limb and extension of the shoulder
Deltoid	Scapula	Proximal humerus	Flexion and abduction of the shoulder
Extensor carpi radialis	Humerus	Metacarpal bones I, II and III	Extension of the carpus and flexion of the elbow
Flexor carpi radialis	Humerus	Metacarpal bone III	Flexion of the carpus and extension of the elbow
Latissimus dorsi	Caudal thoracic and cranial lumbar vertebrae	Caudal humerus	Retraction of the limb and flexion of the shoulder
Pectoral	Sternum and first four ribs	Scapular and humerus	Adducts, protracts and retracts the forelimb
Rhomboideus	Nuchal ligament	Scapular	Extends the shoulder; pulls scapular cranially and dorsally; raises the head
Supraspinatus	Cervical vertebrae deep to trapezius muscle	Scapular	Maintains shoulder extension
Triceps brachii	Scapular and proximal humerus	Ulna (olecranon process)	Extension of the elbow joint
Tendons			
Common digital extensor	Distal humerus and proximal radius	Phalangeal bones I, II and III	Extension of the carpus and joints between phalangeal bones I, II and III; flexion of the elbow
Deep digital flexor	Medial humerus and ulna (olecranon)	Palmar aspect of phalangeal bone III	Extension of the elbow; flexion of the carpus and phalangeal bones I, II and III
Lateral digital extensor	Lateral elbow	Phalangeal bone I	Extension of the carpus and phalangeal bones I, II and III
Superficial digital flexor	Medial humerus and caudal radius	Phalangeal bones I and II	Extension of the elbow; flexion of phalangeal bones I, II and III
Ligaments			
Carpal check	Distal carpus	Proximal deep digital flexor tendon	Extension of the elbow; flexion of the carpus and phalangeal bones I, II and III
Radial check	Distal radius	Proximal superficial flexor tendon	Extension of the elbow; flexion of phalangeal bones I, II and III
Suspensory	Proximal caudal metacarpus	Dorsal extensor tendon at the level of distal phalangeal bone II	Supports the fetlock joint

Source: Table reproduced with kind permission from BSAVA Textbook of Veterinary Nursing 5th Edition © BSAVA.

Major Muscles, Tendons and Ligaments of the Horse

Tables 4.9–4.11 show the origin and insertion points of the major muscles, tendons and ligaments. The action is the movement resulting from the contraction of that muscle.

Source: Table reproduced with kind permission from BSAVA Textbook of Veterinary Nursing 5th Edition © BSAVA

The Manica Flexoria

The manica flexoria is an extension or band like structure of the superficial flexor tendon that wraps around the deep digital flexor tendon just above the fetlock. The proximal manica flexoria is a collar of tendinous tissues which orginates from the medial and lateral borders of the superficial digital flexor tendon within the proximal aspect of the deep digital flexor tendon sheath. Within the proximal aspect of the digital flexor tendon sheath, the manica flexoria and the superficial digital flexor tendon create a ring through which the deep digital flexor tendon passes. The function of the manica flexoria is maintenance of the flexor tendons in alignment as they pass over the palmar/plantar aspect of the fetlock joint. The distal or digital manica flexoria is a similar tendinous band positioned on the dorsal surface of the deep digital flexor tendon in the mid-pastern region of the digital flexor tendon sheath.

The Stay and Suspensory Apparatus

The stay apparatus allows the horse to rest while remaining standing [2]. This is unique to equids, whereby muscles, tendons and ligaments of the forelimb and hindlimb work together to allow the horse to remain stood with minimal energy expenditure [1]. It consists of [2]:

- The medial patella ligament of the stifle
- The gastrocnemius and peroneus tertius
- The suspensory ligament, the sesamoid bones, distal sesamoidean ligaments and the other flexor tendons of the limb

Table 4.10 Muscles, tendons and ligaments of the hindlimb of the horse.

Structure	Origin	Insertion	Action
Muscles			
Gastrocnemius	Caudal distal femur	Calcanean tuber (point of the calcaneus)	Flexion of the stifle, extension of the hock
Peroneus tertius	Distal femur	Calcanean tuber, fourth tarsal bone, dorsal surface of third tarsal bone and metatarsal bone III	Ensures that the hock flexes when the stifle flexes
Semimembranosus	Tuber ischii of the pelvis and the sacrosciatic ligament	Distal femur	Extension of the hip; adduction of the hindlimb
Semitendinosus	Tuber ischii of the pelvis and the coccygeal vertebrae	Proximal tibia	Extension of the hip and hock joint
Superficial gluteal	Tuber coxae of the pelvis	Proximal femur	Flexion of the hip
Tendons			
Deep digital flexor	Proximal tibia	Plantar aspect of phalangeal bone III	Extension of the hock; flexion of the metatarsophalangeal joint and interphalangeal joints
Lateral digital flexor tendon	Lateral collateral ligament of the stifle and proximal tibia and fibula	Long extensor tendon and metatarsal bone III	Flexion of hock; extension of the metatarsophalangeal joint and interphalangeal joints
Long digital extensor tendon	Distal femur	Dorsal proximal surface of phalangeal bones I, II and III	Flexion of hock; extension of the metatarsophalangeal joint and interphalangeal joints
Superficial digital flexor	Distal femur	Calcanean tuber and plantar aspect of phalangeal bones I and II	Extension of the hock; flexion of the metatarsophalangeal joint and interphalangeal joints
Ligaments			
Tarsal check	Distal tarsus	Proximal deep digital flexor tendon	Extension of the hock; flexion of the metatarsophalangeal joint and interphalangeal joints

Source: Table reproduced with kind permission from BSAVA Textbook of Veterinary Nursing 5th Edition © BSAVA.

Table 4.11 Muscles and ligaments of the torso of the horse.

Structure	Origin	Insertion	Action
Muscles			
Abdominal oblique (external and internal)	Ribs	Pelvis	Abdominal wall support; aid to respiration
Intercostal	Rib to rib	Rib to rib	Lateral and medial movement of the chest wall
Longissimus dorsi	Pelvis (ilium) and sacral and thoracic vertebrae	Cervical (4-7), lumbar and thoracic vertebrae and ribs	Extension of the head and neck; lateroflexion of the spine
Rectus abdominis	Costal cartilage (4-9) and the sternum	Pubis of the pelvis	Abdominal wall support; aid to respiration
Sternocephalicus	Sternum	Mandible	Flexion of the head and neck
Transverse abdominis	Lumbar vertebrae and medial aspect of the last ribs	Linea alba	Abdominal wall support; aid to respiration
Ligaments			
Nuchal	Occipital protuberance of the skull	Cranial thoracic spinous process	Extension of the neck and head

Source: Table reproduced with kind permission from BSAVA Textbook of Veterinary Nursing 5th Edition © BSAVA.

Together, these structures prevent overextension of the fetlock and carpus or tarsus.

The Forelimb

In the forelimb, structures work to prevent flexion of the shoulder, elbow and carpal joints (Figure 4.18) [8]. The

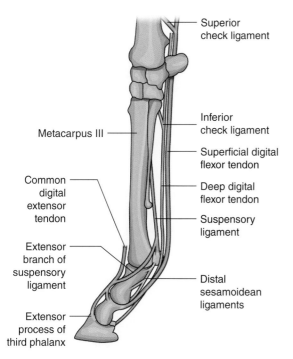

Figure 4.18 Suspensory apparatus in the forelimb. Adapted from Wiley.

Labels: Superior check ligament; Metacarpus III; Common digital extensor tendon; Extensor branch of suspensory ligament; Extensor process of third phalanx; Inferior check ligament; Superficial digital flexor tendon; Deep digital flexor tendon; Suspensory ligament; Distal sesamoidean ligaments

biceps tendon prevents flexion of the shoulder joint, while flexion of the carpus is prevented by the extensor carpi radialis [1]. The suspensory apparatus consists of the suspensory, intersesamoidean, collateral sesamoidean and distal sesamoidean ligaments. These ligaments support the fetlock and suspend the limb. They also prevent overextension and collapse of the fetlock [3]. The suspensory apparatus is reinforced by tension in the flexor tendons, including the accessory (or check) ligaments. The inferior or carpal check ligament runs from the palmar carpus to the deep digital flexor tendon and the superior or radial check ligament runs from the caudal radius to the superficial digital flexor tendon [2]. The structures that make up the suspensory apparatus are depicted in Figure 4.18.

The Hindlimb

In the hindlimb, the horse can utilise a stifle-locking mechanism. The horse has a total of three patellar ligaments: lateral, medial and middle. The medial patellar ligament is the longest and weakest of the three, originating on the parapatellar fibrocartilage and inserting onto the craniomedial aspect of the tibial tuberosity. When the horse needs to rest, they are able to contract the quadriceps muscle and the tensor fascia lata, which lifts the patella and twists it medially. This results in the medial patellar ligament becoming hooked over the medial condyle, which is then situated between the medial and middle patellar ligaments (Figure 4.19). This results in the stifle becoming locked [8]. In order to unlock the stifle, the horse must contract the quadriceps muscle, which causes the patella to move proximally before twisting laterally and returning to its

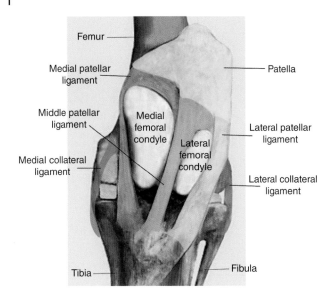

Figure 4.19 Patella in locked position. *Source:* Rosina Lillywhite

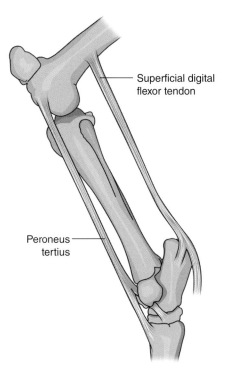

Figure 4.20 Reciprocal apparatus of the hindlimb.
Source: Adapted from Wiley.

original position. In some instances, the medial patellar ligament may fail to disengage during normal movement, a condition known as 'upward fixation of the patella' (UFP) [9], which prevents flexion of the limb.

Within the hindlimb, soft tissue structures form the reciprocal apparatus, which ensures that movement within the limb is coordinated. These structures include: the peroneus tertius muscle (which is a tendinous muscle) and the tendon of the superficial digital flexor muscle [10]. The arrangement ensures that the stifle and tarsus flex and extend at the same time and to the same degree (Figure 4.20) [8]. The fetlock is maintained in extension via the flexor tendons and suspensory apparatus.

The Hoof

The equine foot is colloquially referred to as the hoof. It can be divided into the internal structures and the external structures.

External Structures of the Hoof

The external structures of the hoof form a capsule, which is a covering of the horn. Horn is a tough epidermal tissue, made up of tubules bound together by intertubular horn. The hoof wall is divided into three areas: the toe, the quarters and the heel [6]. The wall grows from the coronary band at the proximal aspect of the hoof and extends downwards. The hoof grows at a rate of 2.5 cm (1 in.) every three months. Therefore, it can take 9–12 months to grow from the coronary band to the ground [4]. On the underside of the hoof is the sole, which is concave and serves to protect

the internal structures of the hoof. The periople forms an outer layer which maintains the moisture levels within the hoof [3].

At the back of the foot are the heel bulbs and where the hoof wall turns inwards at the heels are the bars, which prevent collapse of the heels [6]. The frog is a triangular wedge of tissue found on the underside of the hoof, which assists with circulation and absorbing concussion [3].

The white line marks the boundary between the insensitive external structures of the hoof and the sensitive internal structures (Figure 4.21) [6].

Internal Structures of the Hoof

The distal phalanx sits entirely within the hoof capsule. Projecting inwards from the hoof wall are the insensitive laminae which run vertically down the hoof wall. Projecting outwards from the distal phalanx are the sensitive laminae, which interlock with the insensitive laminae to suspend the distal phalanx within the capsule. Unlike the insensitive laminae, the sensitive laminae have an excellent blood and nerve supply [6]. Horses with certain endocrine disorders or inflammatory conditions are susceptible to a condition known as laminitis, whereby the sensitive laminae weaken and become damaged, resulting in instability of the distal phalanx.

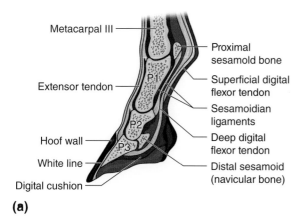

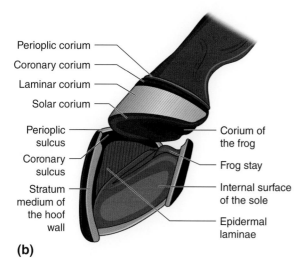

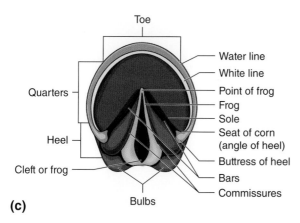

Figure 4.21 Parts of the equine foot. (a) Lateral view of the distal part of the forelimb. (b) Dissected view of the relationships of the hoof to the underlying regions of the corium and (c) weight-bearing surface. *Source:* Adapted from CABI.

Proximal to the frog is the digital cushion, a fibrous pad which assists with the absorption of concussion and aids circulation. On either side of the distal phalanx are the lateral cartilages, which work in conjunction with the digital cushion to aid shock absorption and circulation [3].

Running through the hoof capsule is the corium, which is continuous with the skin of the distal limb. It is named in accordance with the structures that it underruns and serves to nourish the structures of the hoof. This includes the perioplic corium, the coronary corium and the laminar corium [3].

4.7 Structure and Function of the Nervous System and the Special Senses

The function of the nervous system is to receive stimuli from the internal and external environment, analyse and integrate these stimuli, and bring about the necessary response [1, 2].

The nervous system is divided into two main parts: the central nervous system (CNS) comprising of the brain and spinal cord, and the peripheral nervous system (PNS) which comprises of all nerves arising from the CNS. The PNS includes the somatic nervous system (SONS) and autonomic nervous system (ANS). The ANS comprises the sympathetic nervous system (SNS) and parasympathetic nervous system (PSNS) (Figure 4.22) [1].

Neurons

Nerves are responsible for the transmission of nervous impulses throughout the nervous tissue (Figure 4.23). Each nerve consists of many neurons. A neuron is the main cell of the nervous system (Figure 4.24).

A neuron comprises:

- The cell body, which contains a nucleus.
- Thick dendrons or thin dendrites to carry nerve impulses towards the cell body.

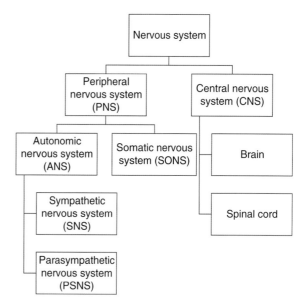

Figure 4.22 The nervous system. *Source:* Lucy Middlecote.

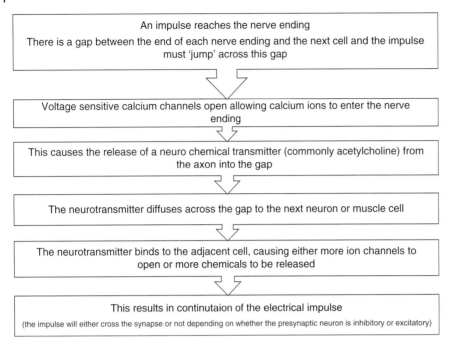

An impulse reaches the nerve ending
There is a gap between the end of each nerve ending and the next cell and the impulse must 'jump' across this gap

Voltage sensitive calcium channels open allowing calcium ions to enter the nerve ending

This causes the release of a neuro chemical transmitter (commonly acetylcholine) from the axon into the gap

The neurotransmitter diffuses across the gap to the next neuron or muscle cell

The neurotransmitter binds to the adjacent cell, causing either more ion channels to open or more chemicals to be released

This results in continutaion of the electrical impulse
(the impulse will either cross the synapse or not depending on whether the presynaptic neuron is inhibitory or excitatory)

Figure 4.23 Summary of nerve impulse conduction. *Source:* Lucy Middlecote.

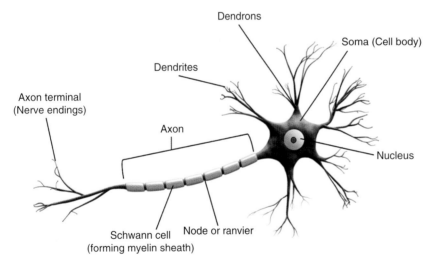

Dendrons

Soma (Cell body)

Dendrites

Axon terminal
(Nerve endings)

Axon

Nucleus

Schwann cell
(forming myelin sheath)

Node or ranvier

Figure 4.24 Myelinated neuron. *Source:* Rosina Lillywhite.

- A single axon to carry nerve impulses away from the cell body and towards other neurons. The axon will vary in length from a few millimetres to 1 m. In many neurons, a Schwann cell (insulating cell) produces a white lipoprotein myelin sheath around the axon. If the axon is surrounded by a Schwann cell then the neuron is termed as myelinated. Axons with a myelinated sheath have a rapid rate of impulse transmission in comparison to the less common non-myelinated neurons, which usually have a slower rate of impulse transmission. Small gaps between Schwann cells are known as nodes of Ranvier and allow nutrients to get to the axon.
- Nerve endings, which are located at the end of the axon and either connect a neuron with another neuron at a synapse or connect a neuron with a muscle at a neuromuscular junction. A synapse is a point of contact between neurons where information is passed from one neuron to the next [1, 3].

Central Nervous System (CNS)

The CNS comprises the brain and spinal cord. There are two types of tissue found in these areas: grey matter, which mainly consists of non-myelinated neurons, or a portion of the neuron not normally covered in myelin (e.g. the cell body), and white matter, which consists of myelinated neurons or the portions of the neuron that are normally covered in myelin (e.g. the axon) [1, 3].

The Brain

Housed in the cranium, the brain is divided into main areas: the forebrain, the midbrain (mesencephalon) and the hind brain.

The forebrain comprises the cerebrum which is the most obvious external feature of the brain and consists of a pair of lateral cerebral hemispheres, and the diencephalon which forms the most rostral part of the brain and includes three main areas: the thalamus, the hypothalamus and the epithalamus. On the ventral surface of the forebrain the pituitary gland, the olfactory bulbs and the optic chiasma can also be located. To enable the brain to increase its surface area without increasing its size, the surface of the cerebral hemispheres is highly folded. The tops of the folds are called gyri and the bottom of the folds are referred to as sulci [1–3].

The midbrain (mesencephalon) acts as a pathway for fibres running from the hindbrain to the forebrain, and has three main areas: the tectum, tegmentum (the main core of the mid brain) and the cerebral peduncle (crus cerebri) [1–3].

The hindbrain consists of the cerebellum, the medulla oblongata and the pons. The cerebellum is positioned caudal to the cerebral hemispheres and on the dorsal aspect of the pons and medulla oblongata. The outermost areas are comprised of grey matter and white matter is found in the central medulla. The cerebellum is responsible for CNS balance and co-ordination of movement. The pons and medulla oblongata are continuous of one another. The pons is the most rostral part of the hindbrain and has several functions, including the control of respiration. The medulla oblongata is caudal to the pons and is continuous with the spinal cord. Many of the cranial nerves (including V, VI, VII, VIII, IX, X, XI and XII) emerge from the CNS at this location [1–3].

Spinal Cord

The spinal cord extends from the medulla oblongata and leaves the cranium via the foramen magnum of the skull. It is predominantly housed in the vertebral canals of the spinal column and ends before the end of the spinal column in a series of fine nerves known as the cauda equina. The spinal cord has an outer cortical layer and a central butterfly shaped core. In contrast to the cerebellum, the outer layer consists of white matter and the central core consists of grey matter. In the centre of the spinal cord there is a central canal containing CSF, which connects the spinal cord with the ventricles (interconnecting tubes/cavities) of the brain (Figure 4.25) [1–3].

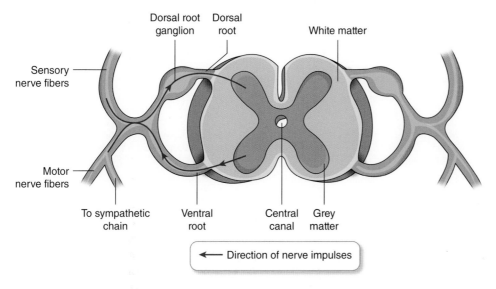

Figure 4.25 Cross-section through the spinal cord. *Source:* Adapted from the BSAVA.

Cerebrospinal Fluid (CSF) and the Meninges

The brain and spinal cord are protected by CSF and the meninges.

The CSF, which cushions and supplies nutrients to the nervous tissue of the brain and spinal cord, is produced by a series of blood capillaries known as choroid plexuses. The choroid plexuses lie in the ventricles (interconnecting tubes/cavities) in the brain. The four main ventricles are the two lateral ventricles in the forebrain, the third ventricle situated around the thalamus in the centre of the brain, and the fourth ventricle situated in the medulla oblongata [1–3].

The meninges consist of three membranes that protect the CNS and retain the CSF. Dura mater is the outermost membrane, which is attached to the periosteum of the inside of the cranium but separated from the periosteum of the vertebral bodies by epidural fat deposits, creating an epidural space (the epidural space is not found in the cranial cavity). The gap between the dura mater and the next arachnoid mater layer is the subdural space. The subdural space is filled with fat. Arachnoid mater is the middle membrane, which consists of large blood vessels supported by tough collagen fibres. The gap between the arachnoid mater and the next pia mater layer is the subarachnoid space. The subarachnoid space is filled with CSF. Pia mater is a thin fibrous membrane containing small blood vessels that supply nutrients to the nervous tissue [1–3].

Peripheral Nervous System (PNS)

The PNS comprises of all nerves arising from the CNS and includes the somatic nervous system and autonomic nervous system (ANS). The PNS is the system that enables the CNS system to communicate with the tissues and organs of the body. Peripheral nerves are either cranial nerves or spinal nerves. These nerves are either sensory (afferent) nerve fibres which collect information from the environment and transmit it to the central nervous system, or motor (efferent) nerve fibres which carry information from the CNS to tissues and organs, to control their activity. Some nerves have a mixed function in that they have both a sensory function and a motor function, and in this case, they are referred to as a mixed nerve [1–3].

Cranial Nerves

Many of the 12 cranial nerves originate in the hindbrain and exit the cranium through foramina. Some of the cranial nerves have a mixed function but most are responsible for either a sensory or a motor function (Table 4.12) [1].

Spinal Nerves

There are a pair of spinal nerves at each intervertebral junction, and each pair has a dorsal root and a ventral root. A spinal nerve is considered a mixed nerve because the dorsal route has a sensory function, and the motor root has a motor function. The dorsal root is where sensory (afferent) nerves enter the spinal cord transmitting information from the sensory bodies. The ventral root is where motor (efferent) nerves exit the spinal cord travelling to the somatic muscles and visceral organs. These motor nerve fibres supply the SNS [1].

Table 4.12 Cranial nerve numbers, names and functions.

Nerve number	Name	Function
I	Olfactory nerve	Sensory nerve that transmits the sense of smell
II	Optic nerve	Sensory nerve that transmits visual information to the brain
III	Oculomotor nerve	Motor nerve that supplies the muscles that collectively perform most eye movements
IV	Trochlear nerve	Motor nerve that supplies the dorsal oblique muscle of the eye
V	Trigeminal nerve	Mixed nerve that supplies many structures within the head. Sensory nerve of the head/face. Motor nerve that supplies various muscles of the head/face. Innervates the muscles of mastication
VI	Abducens nerve	Motor nerve that supplies the extrinsic muscles of the eye
VII	Facial nerve	Motor nerve that supplies a variety of muscles, including the ears, eyelids and lips
VIII	Vestibulocochlear nerve	Sensory nerve for balance (from the semi-circular canals) and hearing (from the cochlea)
IX	Glossopharyngeal nerve	Mixed nerve. Sensory nerve from the taste buds of the tongue and the pharynx. Motor nerve that supplies the pharynx, root of the tongue, palate and some salivary glands
X	Vagus nerve	Mixed nerve. Sensory nerve from the pharynx and larynx Motor nerve that supplies the larynx. Carries parasympathetic motor fibres to the heart and other visceral organs
XI	Accessory nerve	Motor nerve that supplies various muscles
XII	Hypoglossal nerve	Motor nerve that supplies the tongue

Source: Lucy Middlecote.

In the area of the forelimbs and the hindlimbs, there are a large number of nerves passing into and out of the spinal cord and as a result the spinal cord is thicker than normal in these areas. The spinal nerves here anastomose to form a plexus that supply the limbs; the brachial plexus is located deep beneath the scapula and supplies the forelimb, and the lumbosacral plexus supplies the hindlimb [1].

Clinically relevant peripheral nerves include the facial nerve, radial nerve, median nerve, ulnar nerve, sciatic nerve and femoral nerve [1, 3].

Spinal Reflexes

Due to the mixed function of spinal nerves, they can produce a reflex arc without going via the brain. A reflex arc is a fixed involuntary response to a certain stimulus and the response to stimuli is always the same, involving only nerve pathways in the spinal cord. This is a means of protection and produces a prompt response to potential damage. These reflexes can be used to assess damage at local level, although they do not indicate whether the spinal cord is intact above the reflex arc. Common reflex arcs include the panniculus reflex, patellar reflex, anal reflex, palpebral reflex and the thoracolaryngeal reflex [1–3].

Autonomic Nervous System (ANS)

The ANS is the unconscious/involuntary visceral nervous system that supplies motor innervation to many of the vital organs and systems. The ANS comprises the SNS and the PSNS (Figure 4.26).

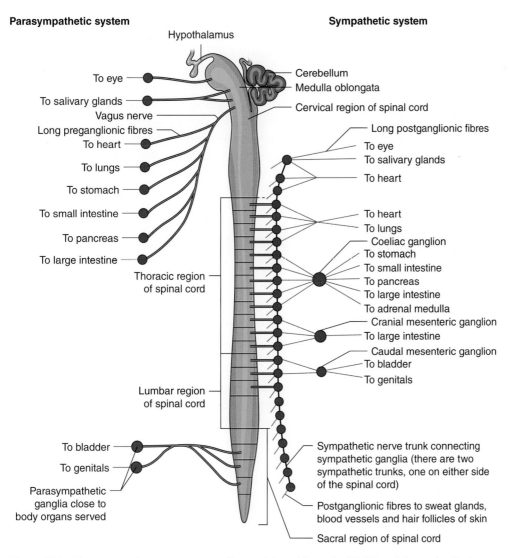

Figure 4.26 The autonomic nervous system. *Source:* Adapted from the BSAVA and Samantha Elmhurst.

Sympathetic Nervous System (SNS)

The SNS is often referred to as the system of 'fright, flight and fight'. The system is involved in maintaining homeostasis and enabling organisms to respond in the appropriate way to changes in their environment. Effects of the sympathetic nervous system include relaxation of bladder muscle and increase in bladder sphincter tone, vasodilation of blood vessels, dilation of the pupils, reduction in activity of the gastrointestinal tract, increase in heart rate, dilation of the bronchioles, increase in respiratory rate and piloerection [1–3].

Parasympathetic Nervous System (PSNS)

The PSNS gradually opposes the actions of the SNS. Effects of the parasympathetic nervous system include contraction of the bladder muscle and decrease in bladder sphincter tone, vasoconstriction of blood vessels, constriction of the pupils, increase in activity of the gastrointestinal tract, decrease in heart rate, constriction of the bronchioles and decrease in respiratory rate [1–3].

Preganglionic and Postganglionic Nerve Fibres

Ganglia are a group of nerve cells important in relaying signals. Preganglionic nerve fibres arise from the central nervous system and supply the ganglia, whereas postganglionic nerve fibres arise from the ganglia and supply the tissues. The preganglionic nerve fibres of the sympathetic nervous system are much shorter than the preganglionic nerve fibres of the parasympathetic nervous system. This is because the preganglionic nerve fibres of the sympathetic nervous system are located closer to the spinal cord than the preganglionic nerve fibres of the parasympathetic nervous system. The parasympathetic nervous system is more closely located to the effector organs [1, 3].

In the SNS, the preganglionic nerve fibres are short, and the postganglionic nerve fibres are long. Preganglionic nerves arise from vertebral spaces T1–L4, pass into the ventral roots of spinal nerves T1–L4, and exit where they then join the ganglia of the sympathetic trunk which runs parallel to the spinal cord along the length of the neck and back. In the PSNS, the preganglionic nerve fibres are long, and the postganglionic nerve fibres are short. The preganglionic neurons originate in the brainstem as discreet nuclei and are often dispersed within the cranial nerves. The PSNS also has a sacral outflow that innervates the pelvic organs and arises from vertebral spaces S1–S2 [1, 3].

Somatic Nervous System (SONS)

The SONS senses external stimuli and is responsible for conscious/voluntary body movement. All five of the senses are controlled by this system and there are two aspects: the afferent (sensory) aspect, which carries impulses from the sensory organs to the brain, and the efferent (motor) aspect, which carries impulses from the brain to the muscle to be moved [1, 3].

The Special Senses

The special senses are hearing, sight, smell, taste and touch.

Hearing

The main functions of the ear are hearing and balance.

External Ear

The ear position and movement in horses is an important indicator of expression. The external ear consists of the cone-shaped auricle (pinna) and the external auditory meatus (ear canal). The pinna comprises of cartilage covered with skin, is highly movable, and can be moved toward the source of a sound. The ear canal is surrounded by rings of cartilage [1–3].

Middle Ear

The middle ear is located within the temporal bone of the skull. Between the ear canal and the middle ear is the tympanic membrane (eardrum). The eardrum transmits sound vibrations to the middle ear containing three auditory ossicles known as the malleus (hammer; attached to the eardrum), incus (anvil) and stapes (stirrup). The ventral part of the temporal bone of the skull expands into the tympanic bulla, which is thought to improve hearing ability. The middle ear is connected to the nasopharynx by the auditory (Eustachian) tube which is responsible for ensuring equalisation of air pressure between the middle ear and the atmosphere. Between the nasopharynx and ventral skull, the auditory (Eustachian) tube is massively dilated to produce a diverticulum known as the guttural pouch. This has a volume of 300–500 ml. Each pouch is divided by the stylohyoid bone into a medial compartment and smaller lateral compartment by the bone. It is in close proximity to a number of the cranial nerves, the sympathetic nerve, the internal carotid artery in the medial compartment, and the maxillary artery in lateral compartment [1–3].

Inner Ear

The bony canals (labyrinth) containing perilymph are located within the inner ear and within these the more delicate membranous canals (labyrinth) which contain endolymph are located. The bony canals and the membranous canals form semi-circular ducts (canals) which allow the horse to maintain balance, and the cochlea, involved in hearing. In the semi-circular canals, the endolymph contains crystals which move in response to movement of the head resulting in stimulation of the hair that are also contained here. The hairs are connected to nerves which form the vestibulocochlear nerve (VIII), allowing transmission of movement to the brain. The three semi-circular canals are arranged at right angles which enables the brain to determine movement and position of the head more accurately. The snail shaped cochlea is filled with fluid which enables the reverberation of sound to stimulate nerve endings. The impulses are transmitted via the vestibulocochlear nerve (VIII) to the brain which then interprets them as sound. Between the semi-circular canals and the cochlea, are the utricle and saccule which help to control posture and balance [1–3].

Sight

The function of the eye is to provide sight. As the horse is a prey species, the eyes are on the side of the head to provide a greater field of vision. The anatomy of the eye is provided in Figure 4.27, and the structure and function of the components is outlined in Table 4.13.

Formation of an Image

The processes that lead to the formation of an image are summarised in Figure 4.28.

Smell (Olfaction)

Although not as highly developed as in other species, smell plays an important part in recognition. For smell to be detected molecules are trapped in the mucus lining of the caudal nasal passages and dissolved. This secretes a chemical reaction that stimulates the nerve endings. The olfactory lobe is located near to the nasal cavity and a number of olfactory nerves are responsible for transmitting smell to the brain. Nerves extend across small holes in the cribriform plate of the ethmoid bone and pass to the olfactory lobe [1, 3].

Flehmen

Flehmen is a visual behaviour displayed in response to odours/smells in which the upper lip is elevated and curled, exposing the incisor teeth (Figure 4.29). In addition, a horse usually extends the neck and raises the head. The inhalation that occurs during flehmen facilitates the movement of molecules into the specialised chemosensory vomeronasal organ to amplify odours. The vomeronasal organ is located near the palate and communicates with the ventral nasal meatus. Receptor cells in the vomeronasal organ transmit information to the accessory olfactory bulb of the brain via the vomeronasal nerve. Stallions tend exhibit this behaviour around mares, and mares will often demonstrate the response after giving birth or while in season.

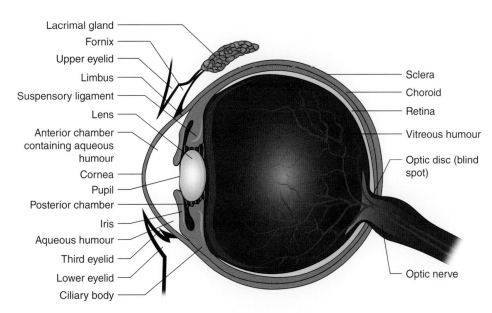

Figure 4.27 Longitudinal section through the eye. *Source:* Adapted from the BSAVA.

Table 4.13 Structure and function of the eye.

Anatomy	Structure and function
Sclera	Opaque outer protective 'white' coating The muscles controlling movement of the eye originate here and attach to the periosteum. These include the retractor bulbi muscle, dorsal rectus muscle, ventral rectus muscle, medial rectus muscle, lateral rectus muscle, dorsal oblique muscle and ventral oblique muscle The muscles are supplied by the oculomotor nerve (III), trochlear nerve (IV), trigeminal nerve (V), abducens nerve (VI) and facial nerve (VII)
Cornea	Transparent outer protective coating Numerous nerve endings make the cornea very sensitive to stimuli Light rays pass through the cornea, and it has a role in focusing light on to the retina

Uvea	Vascular layer beneath the outer connective tissue layer
	Consists of:
	
	• Choroid
	  – Underneath the sclera
	  – Contains blood vessels
	  – Tapetum lucidum on the dorsal part, which reflects light and aids night vision
	• Ciliary body
	  – Adjacent to the limbus
	  – Suspends the lens via zonular fibres (collectively known as the suspensory ligament)
	  – The shape of the lens is controlled by the ciliary muscle
	• Iris
	  – Anterior to the ciliary body
	  – Pigment cells which give colour to the eye
	  – Smooth muscle which contracts and dilates the pupil to control the amount of light entering the eye

Corpora nigra	Small group of roughened brown structures suspended from the pupil margin Pigmented extensions of the iris epithelium Involved in reducing glare from bright light to improve vision
Lens	Focuses light on the retina The shape of the lens is controlled by the ciliary muscle, however in the horse, the lens does not have a great ability to change shape and is not the only component responsible for focusing light on the retina
Vitreous body	Caudal to the lens and consists of the vitreous humour and connective fibres Maintains the shape of the eye
Anterior chamber	Space between the lens and the cornea Filled with aqueous humour
Posterior chamber	Space between the iris and the lens
Retina	Connected to the brain via the optic nerve Contains light-sensitive cells Comprises of different layers of cells: • Pigmented cells (outer layer) • Receptor cells (rods for black and white vision and cones for colour vision) • Bipolar ganglion cells • Multipolar ganglion cells Has a blind spot (the optic disc) situated at the area where the optic nerve exits the eye A series of blood vessels run across the surface, supply nutrients and oxygen to the cells of the retina The retina is not perfectly round which means that horses can detect a location on the retina where the light is in focus by raising or lowering the head
Eyelids	Each eyelid consists of a thin outer layer of skin over a muscular and fibrous layer The inner surface of the eyelids is lined by conjunctiva The upper and lower eyelids join at the medial and lateral canthi The tarsus which gives structure to the eyelid, is a fibrous area at the edge of the eyelid The third eyelid is a T-shaped piece of cartilage, the nictitating membrane, covered by conjunctiva. It provides protection for the eyeball and secretions from the Harderian gland
Lacrimal gland	Situated dorsolateral to the eye Responsible for tear production Lacrimal fluid is moved across the eye by blinking and drained by the punctum lacrimale which is connected to the nasolacrimal duct and drains into the nasal cavity

Source: Lucy Middlecote.

Figure 4.28 Formation of an image.
Source: Lucy Middlecote.

Light rays from an object pass through the cornea and the pupil to hit the lens

↓

Light rays pass through the lens to be focused on to the retina

↓

Light rays pass through the layers of the retina to the photoreceptor cells which generate nerve impulses

↓

Nerve impulses travel along the nerve fibres of the optic nerve to the brain

↓

On the ventral surface of the brain some nerve fibres cross via the optic chiasma to opposite side of the brain so that each cerebral hemisphere receives information from both eyes

↓

Information is carried to the visual cortex of the cerebral hemispheres, where it is interpreted as an image

↓

The image formed is smaller than the original and inverted but the brain modifies it

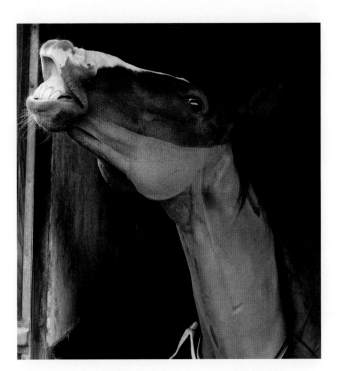

Figure 4.29 The flehmen response. *Source:* Dr Francis Boyer.

Other horses are more likely to demonstrate the flehmen response after sniffing faeces or urine, eating something unusual, or even if they are looking for the right place to roll in the field.

Taste

The taste buds detect flavour. Similar to smell, taste buds are stimulated when the chemical causes the 'taste' dissolves in the saliva. Depending on where the tastebud is located, sensory signals are then sent to the brainstem via the facial nerve (VII), glossopharyngeal nerve (IX) or vagus nerve (X) [1].

Touch

Tactile hairs on the muzzle (referred to as whiskers) play an important role in the sensory awareness of the horse [1]. Touch receptors are present in the skin and sense changes in temperature, pressure and pain. Horses have the ability to protect themselves against the threat of parasites such as flies, but also tolerate the weight of a rider and the pressure of being ridden [1].

4.8 Structure and Function of the Endocrine System

The endocrine system is a regulatory system, working in conjunction with the nervous system Endocrine glands are ductless and synthesise and secrete hormones. These are carried around the body in the circulation to target tissues; other tissues that the hormones encounter are unaffected. Endocrine glands secrete hormones in response to a stimulus; stimuli vary between glands and may include nerve impulses, other hormones and changes in levels of chemicals in the blood [3].

Feedback loops control hormone secretion. Where an increase in the levels of a hormone are detected, production of that hormone will decrease. This process is called negative feedback [3].

Endocrine Glands

There are seven endocrine glands that make up the endocrine system (Figure 4.30).

Pituitary Gland

This gland, also known as the hypophysis [2], is situated ventral to the hypothalamus, suspended from it by a stalk. It comprises two lobes that each act as separate glands [3].

The anterior pituitary gland is also known as the adenohypophysis [1]. The hormones produced by this lobe are outlined below:

- **Somatotrophin (growth hormone):** Acts on all tissues of the body to control the growth rate of young animals. Specifically, it controls the growth rate of bones, is involved in protein production and regulates energy use when food intake is low [3].
- **Thyroid stimulating hormone (TSH):** Acts on the thyroid gland [2]. It stimulates thyroxine (a thyroid hormone) release which controls metabolic rate [1].
- **Adrenocorticotrophic hormone (ACTH):** Acts on the cortex of the adrenal glands. It stimulates the release of hormones from these glands [2].

- **Prolactin:** Acts on the mammary glands during pregnancy. It stimulates the development of the mammary glands and the secretion of milk [1] (which also requires secretion of oxytocin) [3].
- **Follicle stimulating hormone (FSH):** In females, this hormone acts on the ovaries to stimulate development of follicles [5]. In males, this hormone acts on Sertoli cells to stimulate spermatogenesis.
- **Luteinising hormone (LH):** In females, this hormone acts on the ovaries to stimulate ovulation and development of the corpus luteum. Secretion of LH is stimulated by oestrogen in the blood [3].
- **Interstitial cell stimulating hormone (ICSH):** In males, this hormone acts on interstitial cells (cells of Leydig), stimulating them to secrete testosterone [3].

The posterior pituitary gland is also known as the neurohypophysis [1]. The hormones produced by this lobe are outlined below:

- **Antidiuretic hormone (ADH):** Acts on the collecting ducts of the kidneys. This hormone (also known as vasopressin, alters their permeability to water. This aids maintenance of homeostasis and is secreted in response to a change in levels of ECF [3].
- **Oxytocin:** During parturition, oxytocin stimulates uterine contraction [1]. When a neonate is suckling from the mare, oxytocin also stimulates myoepithelial cells of the udder, resulting in the release of milk [3].

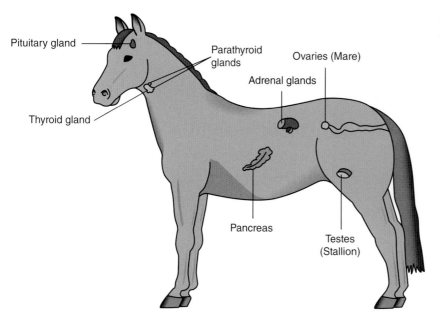

Figure 4.30 The endocrine glands. *Source:* Sophie Pearson & Claire Hart.

Thyroid Gland

This gland consists of two lobes situated on either side of the larynx [5]. Their secretions are under the control of TSH, secreted by the anterior pituitary [3]. The hormones produced by the thyroid gland are:

- **Calcitonin:** Produced by parafollicular cells. Calcitonin lowers the levels of calcium in the blood by reducing the rate or bone resorption and stimulating deposition of calcium in the bone. It also decreases calcium absorption in the gastrointestinal tract and increases calcium excretion via urine [3].
- **Thyroxin (T_4) and triiodothyronine (T_3):** Produced by follicular cells. These hormones act on most cells of the body and control metabolic rate [3]. These hormones are vital in ensuring normal growth [5].

Parathyroid Gland

Situated behind the thyroid gland are the parathyroid glands [2]. Each thyroid gland is associated with two parathyroid glands, resulting in four parathyroid glands in total [1]. These produce and secrete parathyroid hormone (PTH), otherwise known as parathormone, in response to a decrease in calcium levels in the blood [4]. Therefore, its action is antagonistic to that of calcitonin. It stimulates the increase in levels of calcium in the blood by increasing the absorption of calcium from the gastrointestinal tract, increasing resorption of calcium in the distal tubules of the kidneys and releasing calcium from bone. PTH is also involved in the management of phosphate levels by increasing the deposition of phosphate in bone [1].

Pancreas

This gland is positioned within the abdominal cavity, in the loop of the duodenum [5]. This gland has both exocrine and endocrine functions and is therefore termed a 'mixed gland'. The exocrine cells of the pancreas secrete digestive enzymes into the small intestine via the pancreatic duct. The endocrine secretions are produced by areas of exocrine tissue referred to as the islets of Langerhans [3]. These secretions comprise three hormones, each from different cell types:

- **Glucagon:** From the alpha cells. Low levels of glucose in the blood stimulate the secretion of glucagon [3]. This breaks down glycogen stores in the liver, which are converted to glucose and released into circulation, thus increasing blood glucose levels. This process is called glycogenolysis [5].
- **Insulin:** From the beta cells. High levels of glucose in the blood stimulate the secretion of insulin. This lowers blood glucose levels by increasing cellular uptake of glucose and stimulating glycogenesis [3]. Glycogenesis is the process of converting excess glucose into glycogen which is then stored in the liver [5].
- **Somatostatin:** From the delta cells [1]. Somatostatin is mildly inhibitory to both insulin and glucagon [3] to prevent large fluctuations in glucose levels in the blood [5]. Large fluctuations in blood glucose levels can damage tissues, decrease gut motility and decrease secretion of digestive juices.

Adrenal Glands

There are two adrenal glands, each one lying close to the cranial aspect of the kidneys. Each adrenal gland comprises two distinct regions: an outer cortex and inner medulla [4]. The cortex secretes steroid hormones and release of these is controlled by ACTH:

- **Glucocorticoids:** The main glucocorticoids are cortisol and corticosterone. Their levels increase in response to stress, and they increase the levels of glucose in the blood. This is achieved by gluconeogenesis, which is where amino acids are converted to glucose in the liver. Raised glucose levels are also achieved by preparing fatty acids for conversion to glucose by mobilising them from adipose tissue. If present in large quantities, these hormones may also depress inflammatory responses which can be used to reduce swelling and inflammation but also delays healing and repair [3].
- **Mineralocorticoids:** These hormones include aldosterone which acts on the distal convoluted tubules in the kidneys. This is produced by the renin–angiotensin–aldosterone pathway to control sodium and potassium levels in the blood [1]. It also regulates pH of ECF via the excretion of hydrogen ions [3].
- **Sex hormones:** Sex hormones include androgens and oestrogens. The significance of their production by the adrenal cortex remains unclear as these hormones are primarily produced by the gonads [1].

The adrenal medulla produces adrenaline (epinephrine) and noradrenaline (norepinephrine), each of which has similar actions. They are released in response to stress, hypoglycaemia, hypotension and hypothermia. The glands have a good vascular supply to prepare the body for emergency actions rapidly [2] including:

- Glycogenolysis increases the energy levels of the body by increasing blood glucose levels [3].
- Increasing heart rate [1].
- Increasing respiratory depth so that more oxygen can be transported to tissues [3].
- Vasodilation of vessels of skeletal muscles to improve the supply of oxygen and glucose [3].

- Decrease gastrointestinal tract and bladder activity [1].
- Pupil dilation [1].
- Sweat production [1].

Ovaries

Two ovaries are present in females that produce the following hormones at the onset of maturity:

- **Oestrogen:** This is produced by developing follicles [1] and has a negative feedback action on the anterior pituitary gland, inhibiting FSH secretion, thereby facilitating further follicular development [3]. Oestrogen causes behavioural changes and physical changes of the reproductive tract associated with the oestrus cycle [4].
- **Progesterone:** Following ovulation, a corpus luteum develops from the remaining follicular tissue. The corpus luteum secretes progesterone which prepares the reproductive tract for pregnancy and maintains pregnancy [3].

Testes

A pair of testes are present in males, situated in the scrotum which is external to the abdominal cavity. Following the onset of maturity, the following hormones are produced:

- **Testosterone:** This is produced by interstitial cells in response to stimulation by ICSH. Testosterone is responsible for development of spermatozoa, and development of male characteristics and behaviours [3].
- **Oestrogen:** Sertoli cells in the seminiferous tubules produce a small amount of oestrogen [1].

Other Endocrine Activity

- **Erythropoietin:** Produced by the kidneys to stimulate red blood cell production in bone marrow [1].
- **Melatonin:** Produced by the pineal gland within the brain. The rate of production is influenced by the length of daylight, more is produced during hours of darkness [1].
- **Gastrin:** Produced by the stomach to stimulate the release of gastric juices [3].
- **Secretin:** Produced by the small intestine (specifically S cells of the duodenum) [2] to stimulate the release of intestinal and pancreatic juices [3].
- **Chorionic gonadotrophin:** Produced by the ectodermal layer of the chorion around the conceptus to maintain the corpus luteum during gestation [3].
- **Relaxin:** Produced by the corpus luteum to relax pelvic ligaments pre-parturition [3].

- **Thymic hormone:** Produced by the thymus gland to stimulate lymphocyte development. This gland becomes relatively inactive following puberty [4].

4.9 Structure and Function of the Circulatory System

The circulatory system comprises the heart, blood vessels and blood. It is closely linked to the lymphatic system [4].

The Heart

The heart, located in the ventral mediastinum of the thoracic cavity is the conically shaped organ responsible for rhythmically pumping blood around the body [3]. It is situated slightly left of the midline [5] (between the second and sixth intercostal spaces) and is surrounded by the pericardium, a double layered serous membrane which contains pericardial fluid to allow the heart to contract freely [1]. The heart is separated into the left and right halves by the septum [2]. Each side has an atrium which receives blood from veins, and a ventricle which pumps blood out into the arteries, resulting in a total of four chambers (Figure 4.31). The left side of the heart pumps blood into the systemic circulation while the right-side pumps blood into the pulmonary circulation [3].

The walls of the heart comprise three layers. The inner layer is the endocardium which is continuous with the endothelial layer of the blood vessels. The middle layer is the myocardium which is made of cardiac muscle tissue. The outer layer is the epicardium which forms the inner serous layer of the pericardium [3].

The ventricles have a thicker muscular wall than the atria to facilitate pumping blood out of the heart. The left ventricle has the thickest myocardium as it must pump blood all around the body in the systemic circulation via the aorta [1].

Valves

To ensure the unidirectional flow of blood within the heart, valves are present to prevent backflow [1]. Between the atria and ventricles are the atrioventricular (AV) valves. The left AV valve is also known as the bicuspid or mitral valve and comprises two cusps. These are fibrous flaps attached to a ring of fibrous tissue that surrounds the entrance to the ventricle. The right AV valve is also known at the tricuspid valve and is composed of two cusps. Chordae tendineae (fibrous threads) attach the free edges of the atrioventricular valves to the papillary muscles of the ventricular walls. Blood is able to fill the ventricles from the

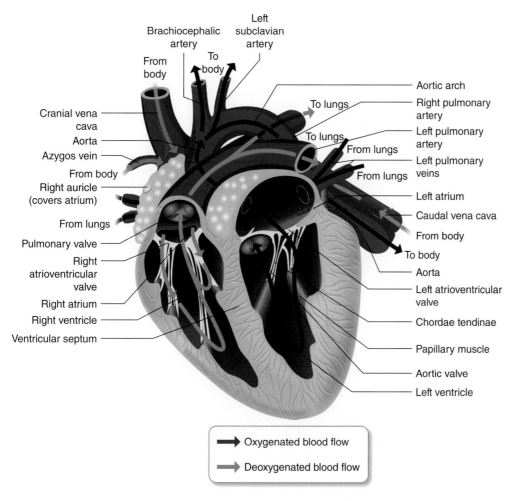

Figure 4.31 The structure of the heart. *Source:* Adapted from Elsevier.

atria when the valves are open. The valves then close when the ventricles are full, and eversion of the valves is prevented by the chordae tendineae [5].

Valves are also present at the base of the two major blood vessels that leave the heart; these are called semilunar valves due to the half-moon-shaped cusps. Each of the semilunar valves comprises three cusps. The pulmonary artery leaves the heart at the right ventricle and contains the pulmonary valve at the base. The aorta leaves the left ventricle and houses the aortic valve at its base [3].

The closing of the valves causes the heart sounds heart upon auscultation. The first heart sound ('lub') occurs when the AV valves close and the second heart sound ('dub') occurs when the semilunar valves close [1].

Circulation of Blood Through the Heart

Blood returns to the right side of the heart from the body via the cranial and caudal vena cava. This deoxygenated blood enters the right atrium which contracts when full, passing

the blood through the right AV valve into the right ventricle. The right ventricle contracts when full, pushing blood out of the heart through the pulmonary artery via the pulmonary valve. The blood is carried in the pulmonary circulation to the lungs where gaseous exchange occurs and the blood becomes oxygenated [3].

Oxygenated blood returns to the heart from the lungs via the pulmonary veins on the left-hand side. The pulmonary artery and the pulmonary vein are the only exception to the rule that oxygenated blood is carried in arteries and deoxygenated blood is carried in veins [4]. The blood enters the left atrium, which contracts at the same time as the right atrium. The blood is forced through the left AV valve into the left ventricle. The left ventricle contracts at the same time as the right ventricle and forces the blood through the aortic valve and out of the heart via the aorta [3].

The cardiac cycle is the contraction and relaxation of both atria followed by contraction and relaxation of both ventricles, a process which then repeats. The period of contraction within the cycle is called systole and the period of relaxation is called diastole [1].

Blood Pressure

Blood pressure within vessels changes constantly due to the constant contraction and relaxation of the heart. It is highest during systole (110–160 mmHg in healthy horses) and lowest during diastole (70–90 mmHg in healthy horses) [11]. Blood pressure is affected by the volume of blood in the body, heart rate, contractility of the ventricles and the tone of the blood vessels. Hypovolaemia (low blood volume) leads to a decrease in pressure while hypervolaemia (increased blood volume) increases blood pressure [3].

Baroreceptors located in the carotid sinus and aortic arch detect blood pressure, relaying this information to the brain [3]. Rapid detection of changes allows compensatory mechanisms such as change in heart rate to be implemented. Arterial blood pressure in the horse can be measured by placing a cuff around the tail (which measures the pressure in the middle coccygeal artery), via an inter-arterial catheter in a peripheral artery (such as the metatarsal, metacarpal, facial or transverse facial artery) or via a doppler [11].

Conduction System of the Heart

The myocardium is specialised muscular tissue that is able to contract automatically and rhythmically. The initiation and conduction of the heartbeat is controlled by the conduction system. This mechanism starts at the sinoatrial (SA) node which is often referred to as the pacemaker of the heart (Figure 4.32). This is a region of specialised cardiac muscle cells situated in the wall of the right atrium, close to the cranial vena cava. The impulse arises at this node which causes a wave of contraction across both atria (atrial systole) [3].

The AV node is another region of specialised cardiac muscle cells situated at the top of the interventricular

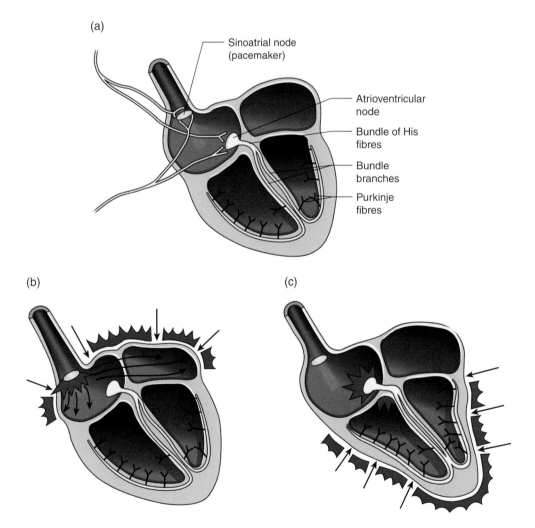

Figure 4.32 Conduction mechanism of the heart. (a) Heart at rest. (b) Sinoatrial node fires, action potentials spread through atria, which contract. (c) Atrioventricular node fires, sending impulse along conducting fibres; ventricles contract. *Source:* Adapted from the BSAVA.

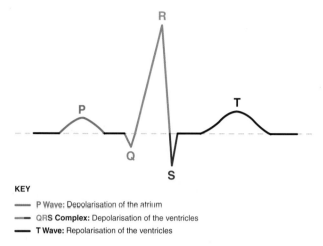

KEY

— P Wave: Depolarisation of the atrium
— QRS Complex: Depolarisation of the ventricles
— T Wave: Repolarisation of the ventricles

Figure 4.33 A PQRST wave. *Source:* Sophie Pearson & Claire Hart.

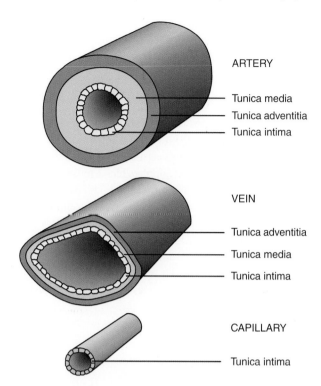

Figure 4.34 Blood vessel structure. *Source:* Sophie Pearson & Claire Hart.

septum. The impulse must pass to this node as the myocardium of the ventricular walls is not in electrical continuation with the atrial walls. The AV node conveys the impulse through specialised fibres within the intraventricular septum called the bundle of His. This bundle divides into the left and right bundles at the bottom of the septum which spread through the ventricles. The bundles are connected to Purkinje fibres (specialised neurons) which are spread throughout the ventricular myocardium. The wave of contraction (ventricular systole) commences at the apex of the heart, disseminating through the myocardium to push the blood up to the veins that leave the heart [3].

Cardiac electrical conductivity can be measured via electrocardiography (ECG) and is illustrated as a wave (PQRST wave) as depicted in Figure 4.33.

Fit horses can undergo a phenomenon at rest called second degree AV block. Their heart rate is normal but dropped beats occur (typically every fourth to sixth beat), which is completely normal in these horses. The phenomenon ceases when these horses start exercising [12].

Blood Vessels

The three major vessels that form the circulatory network are arteries, veins and capillaries [3] (Figure 4.34).

Arteries and Arterioles

Arteries transport oxygenated blood away from the heart, with the exception of the pulmonary artery which transports deoxygenated blood away from the heart. The walls are thick and comprise three layers. The innermost layer is the tunica intima (also called the tunica interna) which is an endothelial lining. The middle layer is the tunica media which is made of smooth muscle and elastic tissue [1]. The outermost layer is the tunica adventitia which

comprises collagen and elastic fibres. The walls are able to dilate and constrict, thereby withstanding the high pressure of the blood that leaves the heart due to the elastic properties [3].

The arteries divide into smaller vessels called arterioles. These connect the arteries to the capillaries.

Capillaries

Arterioles divide further into smaller blood vessels; at the point where the vessels are one cell thick, they become capillaries. The capillary wall comprises the tunica intima only to permit diffusion between the vessels and tissues. Capillaries form networks within the organs called capillary beds which permit the exchange of gasses, fluids and nutrients [3].

Venules and Veins

Blood that flows out of the capillary bed is collected in thin-walled vessels called venules. Venules transport the blood to the veins, whose general structure is similar to that of arteries, but the walls are thin and there is a lower proportion of elastic fibres and smooth muscle tissue. Veins transport deoxygenated blood to the heart, with the exception of the pulmonary vein which transports oxygenated blood to the heart from the lungs. Present within some veins are semilunar valves which ensure unidirectional flow of blood. The blood is also propelled along the vessels by contraction of surrounding skeletal muscle which compresses the veins [3].

Arterial Circulation

Oxygenated blood leaves the left ventricle of the heart via the aorta, which branches into several other arteries:

Coronary artery: Supplies cardiac tissue [1].

Brachiocephalic trunk: Supplies blood to the head via the carotid arteries. It is also connected to the right subclavian artery that supplies blood to the right forelimb. This continues within the limb as the right axillary artery and the right brachial artery. There is also a left subclavian artery that supplies the left forelimb and continues as the left axillary artery and the left brachial artery [4].

Spinal arteries: Supply muscles and structures of the vertebral column and thorax [3].

Renal arteries: Supply the kidneys and adrenal glands [3].

Ovarian/Testicular arteries: Supply the female/male gonads, respectively [3].

External iliac artery: Supplies the hindlimb and continues as the femoral artery [3].

Internal iliac artery: Supplies the pelvic viscera [3].

Cranial mesenteric artery: Supplies the small intestine [3].

Caudal mesenteric artery: Supplies the large intestine [3].

Coeliac artery: Divides into the left gastric, splenic and hepatic arteries to supply the stomach, spleen and liver, respectively [3].

Coccygeal artery: Supplies coccygeal muscles. Can be used to assess pulse in anaesthetised horses [13].

Lingual artery: Supplies the tongue [13].

Metatarsal/Metacarpal artery: Supplies the distal limbs. Can be used to assess pulse in anaesthetised horses [13].

Palmar digital artery: Supplies structures of the hoof. Palpable on the caudal aspect of the pastern, at the level of the proximal sesamoid bones [13].

Transverse facial artery: Supplies the lateral face. Palpable caudal to the eye [13].

Auricular artery: Situated on the dorsum of the ear, supplying the external ear. It is a potential site for placement of arterial catheters [14].

Hepatic Portal System

In addition to receiving blood from the hepatic artery, the liver receives blood directly from the digestive tract via the hepatic portal vein. This blood therefore passes through two capillary beds before draining into the hepatic vein which joins the caudal vena cava [3].

Venous Circulation

Deoxygenated blood drains into the right atrium via veins. Major veins include:

Coronary sinus: returns blood from the wall of the heart. Coronary veins join to form the sinus [1].

Cranial vena cava: returns blood from the head, neck and forelimbs [3].

Jugular veins: return blood from the head and drain into the cranial vena cava [3]. This vein is typically used when catheter placement is required.

Lingual vein: drains the tongue.

Subclavian veins: collect blood from the forelimbs and drain into the cranial vena cava. The brachial veins in the deeper tissues of the limbs and the cephalic veins within the superficial tissues drain into the subclavian veins [1].

Lateral thoracic vein: this is a tributary of the axillary vein and is a common site of catheterisation when the jugular vein cannot be used [11].

External iliac veins: return blood from the hindlimbs. The saphenous vein drains into the femoral vein, which leads to the external iliac vein [1].

Renal veins: return blood from the kidneys [3].

Azygous vein: returns blood from the thoracic body wall [3].

Coccygeal vein: returns blood from the coccygeal tissues.

Facial vein: returns blood from structures of the face and drains into the jugular vein.

Pulse

Pulse rate can be measured via palpation of an artery near the surface of the body. Arteries commonly used are the transverse facial and submandibular arteries. In a normal healthy horse, the pulse rate should be identical to the heart rate and the rhythm should be regular. The pulse should also feel strong and firm; weak pulses are indicative of reduced cardiac output and pulses with stronger than normal pressure are indicative of increased heart rate [13]. A pulse deficit (where the rate differs from the heart rate) is indicative of an arrhythmia [1]. Palmar digital arteries are often palpated to assess problems in the hoof [13].

Blood

Blood is the transport medium of the cardiovascular system that can be divided into the cellular components and the fluid component (plasma), which forms part of the ECF [3]. The functions of blood include:

- Transportation
- Thermoregulation
- Osmoregulation
- Maintenance of pH balance

- Immune defence
- Haemostasis via clot formation

Plasma

Plasma is the fluid fraction of blood seen when a sample is spun in a centrifuge and comprises approximately 90% water [3]. Within the water are dissolved substances being transported around the body including the following components:

- **Gases:** carbon dioxide and oxygen.
- **Electrolytes:** including sodium, potassium, magnesium, calcium and chloride ions.
- **Proteins:** including albumin, fibrinogen and globulin which aid maintenance of osmotic pressure due to their large size.
- **Nutrients:** glucose, amino acids and fatty acids.
- **Waste:** urea and creatinine.
- **Hormones**
- **Enzymes**
- **Antibodies**

Blood Cells

The blood cells can be divided into three categories: erythrocytes (red blood cells), leucocytes (white blood cells) and thrombocytes (platelets).

Erythrocytes

The most numerous blood cells are the erythrocytes, which carry oxygen and a small amount of carbon dioxide; the majority of carbon dioxide in the blood is dissolved in the plasma. Erythrocytes are biconcave discs without a nucleus, containing haemoglobin, a protein that contains iron. The lack of a nucleus enables maximal space for carrying haemoglobin, which binds to oxygen to become oxyhaemoglobin [5]. The cell membrane of an erythrocyte is relatively thin and flexible, allowing them to pass through narrow capillaries more easily and the shape of the cell increases the surface area for diffusion of oxygen [3].

Erythrocytes are formed in the bone marrow from stem cells. In young animals, this occurs in long bones, the pelvis, the sternum and the skull. In adult animals, it occurs in the epiphyses of the long bones, the sternum, the skull and the pelvis [1]. The stem cells first develop into erythroblasts. Erythroblasts then start to gain haemoglobin and the nucleus becomes smaller, at which point they are referred to as normoblasts. Normoblasts then develop into reticulocytes at which point the nucleus has disintegrated into fine threads called Howell–Jolly bodies. These then disappear entirely, and the cell then becomes a mature erythrocyte, which can be released into the circulating blood. The entire

process from stem cell through to becoming an erythrocyte takes 4–7 days [3]. Erythropoiesis is controlled by a hormone released from the kidney called erythropoietin. When oxygen levels in tissue are low, erythropoietin is released, which stimulates erythrocyte production in the bone marrow [5].

Once released, erythrocytes will remain in circulation for around 120 days before being broken down in either the spleen or lymph nodes [1]. In cases of erythrocyte shortage, such as a severe haemorrhage, reticulocytes will be released into the circulation to compensate for the deficit. When erythrocytes are broken down, iron is returned to the bone marrow. The haem content of haemoglobin is converted to bilirubin (a bile pigment) by the liver, which is then excreted in bile [3].

Leucocytes

Unlike erythrocytes, all leucocytes contain nuclei and there are far fewer in the circulation. Leucocytes can be divided into granulocytes and agranulocytes in accordance with the presence or lack of granules visible in the cytoplasm when observed with a microscope [5] (Figure 4.35).

Granulocytes

Neutrophils: the most numerous leucocytes, neutrophils have granules that stain purple when they take up neutral dyes. They also have a large, lobed nucleus [1]. Neutrophils engulf and break down invading bacteria and cell debris via

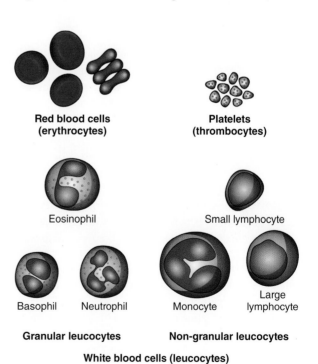

Figure 4.35 Blood cells. *Source:* Adapted from Elsevier.

phagocytosis. The presence of immature neutrophils (band cells) and an increase in circulating neutrophil numbers (neutrophilia) is indicative of infection, while a reduction (neutropenia) can occur with some viral infections [2].

Eosinophils: granules in the cytoplasm stain red when the cells take up acidic dyes [3]. The granules of equine eosinophils are large and may obscure the nuclei, which gives the cells a raspberry-like appearance [15]. Eosinophils are key cells in the defence against parasites and an increase in eosinophils (eosinophilia) is indicative of a parasitic infection. Eosinophils also regulate allergic and inflammatory responses, secreting enzymes that inactivate histamine [3].

Basophils: granules in the cytoplasm stain blue when the cells take up alkaline dyes. They contribute to allergic reactions by secreting histamine, increasing inflammation. They also secrete heparin, an anticoagulant, to prevent unnecessary blood clots forming [3].

Agranulocytes

Monocytes: these are the largest leucocytes and contribute to immunity via phagocytosis. They have a horseshoe/kidney bean-shaped nucleus. When monocytes migrate to tissues they mature, at which point they are called macrophages [3].

Lymphocytes: these are the second most common leucocyte after neutrophils. They have a round nucleus that almost fills the cell [5]. They are produced in lymphoid tissue and can be divided into two types. B-lymphocytes are involved in humoral immunity and produce antibodies, while T-lymphocytes destroy foreign cells [3].

Thrombocytes

Thrombocytes, commonly referred to as platelets are fragments of large cells called megakaryocytes. They are formed in bone marrow, do not possess a nucleus and are concerned with the formation of blood clots [5].

Coagulation

An important defence mechanism of the body is the formation of blood clots to prevent excessive blood loss from damaged vessels and to prevent the entry of pathogens into damaged vessels. The process of clot formation requires stages to occur in a specific order and is therefore termed the coagulation cascade. This process occurs as follows:

1) A seal is formed across the damaged blood vessel when platelets stick to the area and each other. This is termed primary aggregation.
2) Secondary aggregation occurs when the platelets release an enzyme called thromboplastin. In the presence of thromboplastin and calcium ions, prothrombin (a plasma protein) is converted to an active enzyme called thrombin.
3) Thrombin converts fibrinogen (a plasma protein) into fibrin, which is a network of insoluble fibres.
4) The fibrin network forms across the damaged area and traps blood cells, thus forming a clot. At this point, the vessel is sealed to prevent blood loss. It takes 3–5 minutes for the clot to form

Vitamin K is essential to the clotting process as it is required by the liver for the manufacture of prothrombin. Therefore, a lack of vitamin K can lead to an increase in clotting time. It can also be increased by liver disease, genetic disorders, some disease processes, a lack of thrombocytes (thrombocytopaenia) or a lack of calcium [3].

4.10 Structure and Function of the Lymphatic System

The lymphatic system works closely with the circulatory system [5], returning excess interstitial fluid to the circulation in the form of lymph [3]. Lymph is similar in composition to plasma but does not contain the larger plasma proteins [3] and contains more lymphocytes [3]. It comprises 2–3% of total body fluid and has a clear, yellow-tinged appearance [6].

The lymphatic system is also involved in immunity and transport of fatty acid molecules. The system comprises a network of lymphatic vessels and lymphoid tissue [5].

Lymphatic Capillaries, Vessels and Ducts

Vessels of the lymphatic system begin and blind-ended lymphatic capillaries, which are similar to the capillaries of the circulatory system. They have thin walls and merge to form the larger lymphatic vessels [1]. The lymphatic capillaries found within the villi of the small intestine are referred to as lacteals. These transport the fat that has been digested from the lumen of the gastrointestinal tract in the form of chyle [3].

The larger lymphatic vessels are similar in structure to veins and also possess numerous valves that are closely spaced to prevent backflow of lymph [1]. The movement of lymph through these vessels is predominantly passive; lymph is moved along the vessels by the contraction of surrounding muscles and pulsation of blood vessels adjacent to the lymphatic vessels [4]. The presence of valves prevents pooling of the lymph in the vessels [1].

The lymph vessels drain into lymphatic ducts, which return the lymph to circulation. The primary lymphatic ducts are:

The right lymphatic duct: This duct drains lymph from the right forelimb and the right side of the head, neck and thorax. Fluid is then returned to circulation via the right jugular vein or cranial vena cava, to the right side of the heart [3].

The cisterna chyli: This is the first part of the *thoracic duct*, situated in the abdomen, collecting lymph from pelvis, hind limbs and abdomen. The cisterna chyli passes through the aortic hiatus of the diaphragm, into the thorax. Here, it becomes known as the thoracic duct [3].

The thoracic duct: This duct is the main collecting duct for lymph. Lymph from the left forelimb and the left side of the head, neck and thorax drains into the thoracic duct. Fluid is then returned to circulation via the right jugular vein or cranial vena cava, to the right side of the heart [3].

Tracheal ducts: A pair of tracheal ducts drain lymph from the head and neck. These either drain lymph into the thoracic duct or directly into one of the large veins in close proximity to the heart [3].

Lymph Nodes

Spaced at intervals along the lymphatic vessels are masses of lymphoid tissue called lymph nodes [1]. Each node is bean-shaped and enclosed in a capsule of connective tissue (Figure 4.36). Within the capsule are trabeculae, a network of tissue, that support the node. The lymph flows through the spaces (sinuses) within the node. The network of tissue acts as a mesh to filter particles and bacteria, which are then destroyed via phagocytosis. All lymph passes through a minimum of a one lymph node before it is returned to

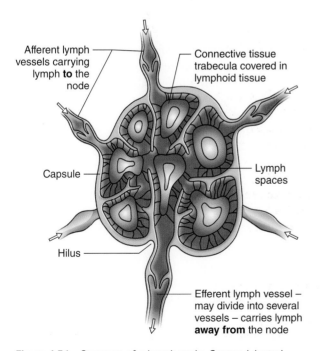

Figure 4.36 Structure of a lymph node. *Source:* Adapted from CABI.

the circulation. Multiple afferent lymph vessels carry lymph to a single lymph node. A single efferent vessel, situated at the hilus (indented region of the node) carries lymph away from the node [3].

The lymphoid tissue is divided into two regions: the outer region is the cortex and the inner region is the medulla [2]. The cortex contains follicles, otherwise known as germinal centres or lymph nodules, containing a high concentration of lymphocytes. When examined under a microscope, these areas appear darker than the rest of the node. The medulla drains lymph from the lymph node into the efferent vessel [1].

Lymphocytes are concerned with acquired immunity, one of the two types of immunity. The other type is natural immunity:

Natural immunity: Natural defence mechanisms of the body, including the mucous, sweat and skin [2].

Acquired immunity: The body is able to enhance natural defence mechanisms through recognition of antigens when repeat encounters occur. Acquired immunity can be subdivided into humoral immunity, where B-lymphocytes are conveyed and antibodies are produced, and cell-mediated immunity, where T-lymphocytes provide protection by destroying foreign cells [2].

When a horse has an infection, the lymph nodes may become enlarged. If the infection is generalised, lymph adenopathy may occur, which is where all of the lymph nodes become enlarged. Lymph nodes that are situated superficially may be palpated [3]. The nodes that may be palpated in the horse are:

Submandibular: These are the only nodes that are obviously palpable in a normal, healthy horse. The submandibular lymph nodes are situated in the intermandibular space, under the jaw. The nodes are arranged in a forward-pointing 'V' formation [2].

Prescapular: These are situated in front of the cranial border of the scapula and can be palpated when enlarged [1].

Subiliac: Also known as the pre-femoral or precrural lymph node, it is situated on the cranial border of the thigh, in the fold of the flank. It is positioned halfway between the tuber coxae and the patella.

Inguinal: When enlarged, the superficial inguinal lymph nodes can be palpated adjacent to the inguinal canal [2].

The parotid lymph nodes are not usually palpable but may be palpable when enlarged. They are situated adjacent to the parotid salivary gland [2].

Spleen

Situated within the left craniodorsal abdomen is the spleen, the largest lymphoid organ [1]. This is a highly vascularised organ [5] which is attached to the stomach, intestines, greater omentum and the left kidney (via the nephrosplenic ligament). It acts as both a lymph node and as a blood reservoir by storing blood, destroying aged blood cells, removing particles from circulation and producing lymphocytes [3]. The splenic artery supplies the spleen with blood, which is then carried away via the splenic veins. The spleen has a thick capsule, which contains a high proportion of smooth muscle, permitting splenic contraction and thus blood release at times of stress. The spleen becomes engorged when the muscle is relaxed, resulting in a size increase [2].

The tissue of the spleen can be divided into two regions: the red pulp and the white pulp. The white pulp consists of lymphoid tissue and contains a large number of lymphoid cells. The red pulp is the more vascular region and is the site of destruction of aged erythrocytes and red blood cell storage [1]. The erythrocytes are engulfed and destroyed by phagocytic cells, but any iron is preserved to be used again in the synthesis of haemoglobin [3].

Thymus

The thymus is situated in the thoracic cavity, cranial to the heart. It is an organ with greater significance in young animals, where it is at its largest. As animals age, the size of the thymus decreases. In early life, it is responsible for the production of T-lymphocytes, thus contributing to immunity [1].

4.11 Structure and Function of the Respiratory System

The Respiratory System

The respiratory system is responsible for conducting inspired air through the respiratory passages to facilitate gaseous exchange and conducting expired air to the environment [3]. The respiratory tract can be divided into the upper respiratory tract (comprising the nose, nasal cavities, pharynx, larynx and trachea) and the lower respiratory tract (comprising the lungs, bronchi, bronchioles and alveoli) [1].

The Upper Respiratory Tract

The Nostrils

The nostrils are also referred to as the external nares [5]. This is where inspired air enters the respiratory tract and passes through to the nasal cavity [3]. Equine nostrils are relatively large and able to dilate during exercise to facilitate increased airflow. The dorsal and lateral margins of each nostril are supported by alar cartilage. The alar fold divides the nostril into a dorsal and ventral section. The ventral aspect leads to the nasal cavity, while the dorsal aspect leads to a pouch called the false nostril [3]. It is a blind-ending pouch that is sometimes referred to as the nasal diverticulum [2].

The Nasal Cavity

The nasal cavity is a space that extends caudally from the nostrils. The cavity is divided down the middle into two halves by the nasal septum [5]. Each chamber is filled with fine scrolls of bone called the turbinate bones or conchae [3]. These project inwards from the dorsal and lateral aspects of the walls. At the rostral aspect of the cavity, dorsal and ventral conchae divide the chamber into three spaces called meati: dorsal meatus, middle meatus and ventral meatus. At the caudal aspect of the cavity, the bones form an intricate labyrinth called the ethmoidal labyrinth. The ethmoturbinates are covered in a mucous membrane called the olfactory mucosa. This helps to warm and moisten inhaled air in addition to cleaning it. The mucosa is also an important component in the sense of smell [2].

Paranasal Sinuses

Within the skull are air-filled cavities known as sinuses that are covered in respiratory epithelium, similar to the nasal cavity. The horse has seven paranasal sinuses that communicate with the nasal cavity via small openings [3]. The more caudal sinuses include the frontal, dorsal, conchal, ethmoidal, sphenopalatine and caudal maxillary sinus. Each of these sinuses drains via the caudal maxillary sinus, which opens via the nasomaxillary opening into the middle meatus. The two sinuses found more rostrally are the rostral maxillary sinus and the ventral conchal sinus. These sinuses drain via a different (but adjacent) nasomaxillary opening in the rostral maxillary sinus into the middle meatus. As the horse ages, the dimensions of the sinuses change as a consequence of eruption of the caudal four cheek teeth, which are embedded in the floor of the maxillary sinuses [2].

The Pharynx

Caudal to the nasal septum is the pharynx, which is divided into three regions. At the caudal aspect of the nasal cavity is the nasopharynx; this is situated above the soft palate. At the caudal aspect of the oral cavity is the oropharynx; this is situated below the soft palate. Finally, the laryngopharynx is the most caudal aspect of the pharynx and is a common passage for air and food [3].

The Larynx

The larynx forms the entrance to the trachea (Figure 4.37) and consists of cartilage, muscle and ligaments, covered in a mucous membrane [5]. It is suspended from the skull by the hyoid apparatus, which allows it to swing when the horse is swallowing and during respiration [2]. The hyoid apparatus is situated in the intermandibular space, comprising bones and cartilage in a trapeze-like arrangement. The four cartilages of the larynx give it a box-shaped structure. The epiglottis is the most rostral of the laryngeal cartilage and controls the movement of air into the larynx. When the horse swallows, the epiglottis covers the entrance to the larynx to prevent the entry of food [3]. The arytenoid cartilages are situated on either side of the midline and are attached to the vocal ligaments. These cartilages are able to move towards and away from the midline to control the flow of air into the larynx. The cricoid cartilage is the most caudal and is ring shaped. Finally, the largest of the laryngeal cartilages is the thyroid cartilage, which consists of two lateral plates. These meet ventrally to form the floor of the larynx [2].

Trachea

The trachea is a tube that passes through the thoracic inlet, conveying air from the larynx to the lungs. Incomplete rings of hyaline cartilage support the trachea, to prevent it collapsing [3]. The incomplete aspect of the cartilage rings facilitate expansion of the oesophagus when the horse swallows to ease the passage of a bolus. Each of the rings is connected by smooth muscle and fibrous tissue. The tracheal lumen is lined by ciliated mucous epithelium. The mucous is able to trap foreign particles that have entered the trachea. The cilia then transmit these particles towards the pharynx. They are then swallowed or exhaled [2].

Within the mediastinum of the thoracic cavity, the trachea terminates above the heart as a bifurcation [3].

The Lower Respiratory Tract

Bronchi

The trachea bifurcates into the bronchi; the left bronchus enters the left lung and the right bronchus enters the right lung. Within the lungs, the bronchi divide multiple times, the branches becoming smaller with each division. This is referred to as the bronchial tree (Figure 4.38). The bronchi are supported by rings of cartilage, which unlike the cartilage of the trachea, are complete rings. With each division of the bronchi, the support of the cartilage diminishes [3].

Bronchioles

Where cartilaginous support of the bronchi has diminished entirely, the passages are referred to as bronchioles. The walls of the smaller bronchi and the bronchioles contain smooth muscle that allows the passages to dilate to increase the volume of air that enters the lungs. This is under the control of the autonomic nervous system. Similarly to the bronchi, the bronchioles continue to branch into smaller passages. Terminal bronchi lead to alveolar ducts, which open into sacs called alveoli [3].

Alveoli

The arrangement of alveolar sacs is comparable to a bunch of grapes. The alveoli have very thin walls and a rich blood supply from capillary networks to facilitate gaseous exchange [1]. The epithelial lining (pulmonary membrane) does not possess cilia. Upon inspiration, oxygen from the inspired air diffuses across the pulmonary membrane into the capillaries. Carbon dioxide diffuses across the membrane from the capillaries into the alveoli, simultaneous

Figure 4.37 Airways of the head. *Source:* Rosina Lillywhite.

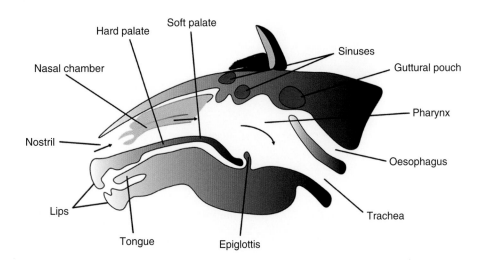

Soft palate
Hard palate
Sinuses
Nasal chamber
Guttural pouch
Pharynx
Nostril
Oesophagus
Lips
Trachea
Tongue
Epiglottis

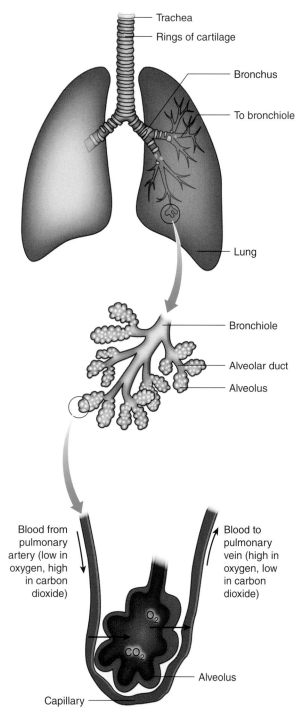

Trachea

Rings of cartilage

Bronchus

To bronchiole

Lung

Bronchiole

Alveolar duct

Alveolus

Blood from pulmonary artery (low in oxygen, high in carbon dioxide)

Blood to pulmonary vein (high in oxygen, low in carbon dioxide)

O_2

CO_2

Alveolus

Capillary

Figure 4.38 The structure of the lungs. *Source:* Adapted from Wiley.

with the diffusion of oxygen. This is then removed upon expiration. Millions of alveoli provide a large surface area for this exchange to occur, thus maximising the efficiency of exchange. The aspects of the tract leading up to the

pulmonary membranes, that are not involved in gaseous exchange, are referred to as dead space [3].

Lungs

Each lung is surrounded by a serous membrane called the pulmonary pleura, within the thoracic cavity, situated on either side of the mediastinum [1]. The lungs are divided into lobes by fissures. The left lung comprises three lobes: the cranial lobe (apical lobe), the middle lobe (cardiac lobe) and the caudal lobe (diaphragmatic lobe). The right lung possesses the same lobes and an additional lobe called the accessory lobe. This is smaller than the other lobes and is situated on the medial aspect of the caudal lobe. The shape of the lungs alters during a respiratory cycle [3]. The dimensions change in accordance with the changing dimensions of the thoracic cavity. The right lung is larger than the left [3].

Respiratory Mechanics

Respiration is dependent on changes in thoracic cavity volume, achieved by contraction of muscles. As the volume of the thoracic cavity increases, so does the volume of the lungs. This is brought about by negative pressure as each plural cavity forms a vacuum. Expansion of the lungs causes the air pressure within the alveoli to drop in comparison to atmospheric pressure, which results in air being drawn into the lungs [1].

Inspiration: Intercostal muscles are situated within the intercostal spaces. The external intercostal muscles assist with inspiration by lifting the ribs. The main muscle of inspiration is the diaphragm, which flattens when contracted, further increasing thoracic cavity volume and drawing air into the lungs [3].

Expiration: This process is predominantly passive; the diaphragm relaxes, returning to its domed shape. The external intercostal muscles relax to return the ribs to their normal position. These two passive movements reduce the volume of the thoracic cavity and therefore the volume of the lungs. This increases air pressure within the lungs, forcing air out of the respiratory tract. While the process is mainly passive, internal intercostal muscles can assist the process [3].

Control of Respiration

Respiratory movements are normally involuntary. Respiratory centres are situated in the pons and medulla of the brain, which send impulses to the phrenic nerves of the diaphragm, and to the intercostal muscles via the intercostal nerves [3]. Respiratory rate and depth are influenced by receptors:

Stretch receptors: These are situated within the bronchi and bronchioles, assessing the degree of stretch in the bronchial tree. They inhibit excessive inspiration and therefore over-inflation of the lungs. This is known as the Hering-Breuer reflex [1].

Chemoreceptors: Within the walls of the aortic and carotid arteries and in the walls of the medulla oblongata in the brain are chemoreceptors that detect changing proportions of oxygen and carbon dioxide. The changing proportions influence blood pH. When pH is too low, respiration is stimulated to remove the excess carbon dioxide [3].

Respiratory Terminology

Tidal volume: The volume of air that passes in and out of the lungs with each breath when the horse is at rest [1].

Inspiratory reserve volume: the additional volume of air that passes in and out of the lungs with each breath when the horse forces more air in during inspiration [3].

Expiratory reserve volume: the additional volume of air that is expired when forcibly exhaled [3].

Residual volume: the volume of air left in the lungs and airways following the most forced exhalation [1].

Functional residual capacity: the volume of air left in the lungs after a normal expiration [3].

Vital capacity: the functional capacity of the lungs (the volume of air that can be expired following the maximum inspiration) [3].

Respiratory rate: the number of breaths taken with one minute [3].

Minute volume: the volume of air inhaled and exhaled within one minute [16].

Dead space: the volume of the components of the respiratory tract that to not take part in gaseous exchange [2].

Equine Respiratory Specialisation

Horses are obligate nasal breathers [1], meaning that normal, healthy horses are unable to breathe through their mouth unlike many other species. They remain obligate nasal breathers when undertaking strenuous exercise and this is a consequence of the positioning of the soft palate and epiglottis. Normally, the equine epiglottis sits dorsally of the soft palate and the caudal free edge of the soft palate is in close contact with the larynx. Therefore, there is no communication between the nasopharynx and the oropharynx. However, this is disrupted in horses experiencing a condition known as 'dorsal displacement of the soft palate' (DDSP), which can occur during exercise. When a horse is experiencing DDSP, the caudal free edge of the soft palate becomes displaced and positioned dorsal of the epiglottis [17].

They are however able to expand the nostrils to inhale a greater volume of air with each breath [4]. It has been suggested that this could be an adaptation of the horse as a prey animal, allowing them to flee from predators without accidental aspiration of food if the horse were to detect a predator while grazing [18]. The previous theory was that obligate nasal breathing was an adaptation to allow horses to detect predators via olfaction while grazing. However, other grazing prey species that employ the Flehmen response such as cattle and deer are not obligate nasal breathers. Furthermore, the Flehmen response is counterproductive to the flight response as it requires breath holding [19].

The horse has developed a link between respiration and locomotion as a consequence of the thoracic muscles of respiration and locomotion creating anatomical and mechanical restraints [20]. At canter and gallop, the horse's respiratory rate becomes linked to their stride rate, and horses take one breath per stride. This is a process called locomotory–respiratory coupling. As the horse raises its head and lifts its limbs, the abdominal viscera move caudally in time with inspiration. The caudal movement of the abdominal viscera allows the lungs to expand to a greater volume than they otherwise would. Following this, the feet land and the horse lowers their head, causing the abdominal viscera to move cranially in synchronisation with expiration [4]. The cranial movement of the abdominal viscera aids expiration by increasing the pressure on the diaphragm.

4.12 Structure and Function of the Digestive System

The function of the digestive system is to receive and digest food to meet the nutritional requirements of the horse. The process of digestion involves the movement of ingesta along the gastrointestinal tract, the mechanical and enzymatic breakdown of food, the absorption of nutrients and the excretion of waste [1, 3].

The Physiology of Digestion

The act of eating involves three stages:

1) Prehension – taking food into the mouth
2) Mastication – chewing
3) Deglutition – swallowing

Once ingested, food needs to be broken down into smaller molecules so that it can be absorbed through the wall of the intestines and into the bloodstream. There are two types of muscular movement that break up and mix food – peristalsis, which pushes ingesta through the tract, and rhythmic segmentation, which breaks up and mixes the food boluses. The mechanical breakdown of food is initially carried out by chewing and followed by contractions of the stomach. Enzymatic breakdown involves enzymes and other agents breaking down ingested food material into easily absorbed substances. Absorption of nutrients into the bloodstream begins in the duodenum, with the highest levels of absorption taking place in the duodenum and jejunum [1–3].

Waste products are not required by the body and defecation is the process by which the body excretes solid waste products. Normal faeces should be the colour and smell characteristic of the species. Faeces should also be 'formed' and not watery, and contain water and fibre, dead and living bacteria, sloughed intestinal cells, mucus and stercobilin (a pigment derived from bile that gives faeces their colour) [1–3]. A summary of the process of digestion is provided in Figure 4.39.

The Digestive Tract

The digestive tract comprises of the mouth, the pharynx, the oesophagus, the stomach, the small intestine (duodenum, jejunum and ileum) and the large intestine (caecum, colon, rectum and anus) (Figures 4.40–4.42). The liver and the pancreas are also considered to be part of the digestive system and digestive process.

Mouth

The mouth includes the lips, the teeth, the tongue, the cheeks, the palate and the salivary glands.

Lips

The lips are particularly important in herbivore species, where they are used for prehension. They have an inner layer of mucosa and an outer covering of skin with underlying muscles and tendons. The skin is well supplied with sebaceous glands, which provide waterproofing and scent. The lips are innervated and controlled by the facial nerve [1].

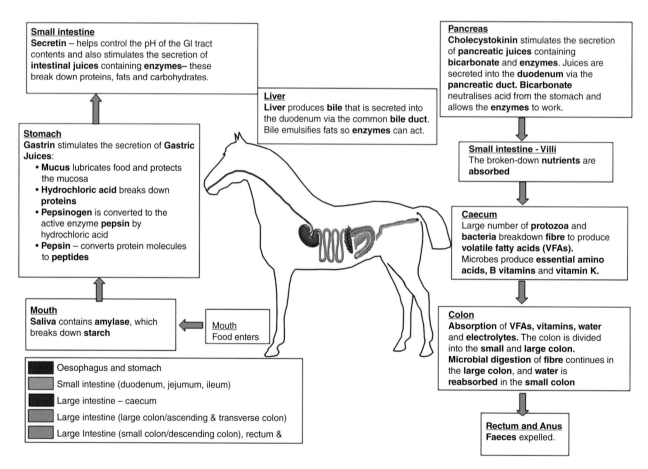

Figure 4.39 Summary of digestion. *Source:* Lucy Middlecote and Rosina Lillywhite.

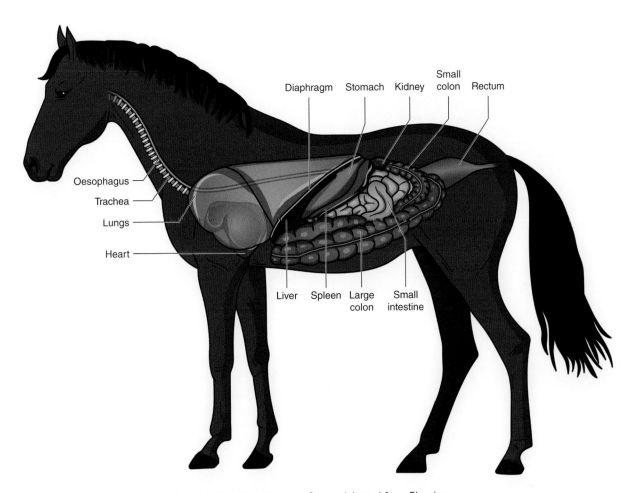

Figure 4.40 Left lateral view of the equine digestive tract. *Source:* Adapted from Elsevier.

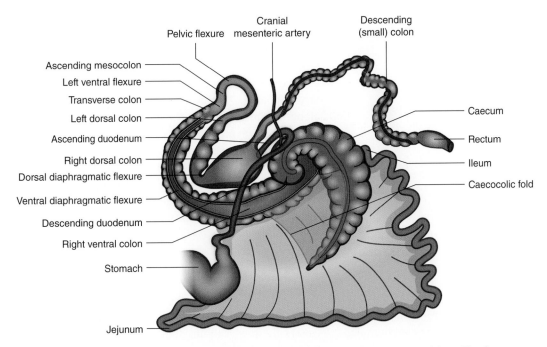

Figure 4.41 Diagrammatic representation of the equine digestive tract. *Source:* Adapted from Elsevier.

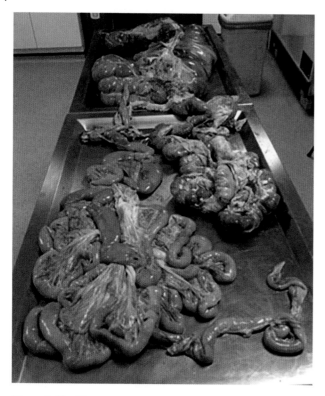

Figure 4.42 The equine digestive tract. *Source:* Lucy Middlecote.

Teeth

Teeth are covered in detail in Section 4.6 of this chapter. They are used for cutting and grinding food, the teeth are embedded in the maxilla and mandible. Horses have two sets of teeth in a lifetime – the deciduous dentition (temporary teeth), which are present at birth and the adult dentition (permanent teeth).

Tongue

The tongue is involved in prehension and helps with the formation of a food bolus. The tongue has numerous taste buds and consists of a number of parts:

- Apex – tip
- Body – main part
- Root – where the tongue attaches to the mouth
- Median groove – central depression in the dorsal surface
- Papillae – small projections on the surface
- Frenulum – tissue that connects the tongue to the floor of the mouth

The tongue is wider at the tip than at the base and is covered in keratinised mucosa to protect it from the process of mastication. It consists of skeletal muscle and is controlled by the hypoglossal nerve [1, 3].

Cheeks (Buccae)

The cheeks are lined with stratified squamous epithelium known as buccal mucosa. They are used to move a food bolus from one side of the mouth to the other during mastication, an action that is highly developed in horses. The cheeks are controlled by the buccinator muscle [1].

Palate

Forming the roof of the mouth, the hard palate is wide and ridged and consists of various bones covered in keratinised epithelium, which protects the underlying structures. Caudally, the hard palate merges into the soft palate. The soft palate is also lined with keratinised epithelium but comprises soft tissue rather than bone [1, 3].

Salivary Glands

Salivary glands secrete saliva and have ducts which open into the mouth. Saliva is 99% water and 1% mucus and is required to moisten the mouth and provide lubrication. Saliva continuously washes the mouth and reduces the level of bacteria. In horses, saliva also contains the enzyme amylase, which breaks down starch [1].

The main pairs of salivary glands are the parotid salivary glands (large and found at the base of the ear), the mandibular salivary glands (found at the angle of the jaw), the sublingual salivary glands (found underneath the tongue) and the buccal salivary glands (located in the cheeks). Small salivary glands are also present on the lips, tongue, cheeks, soft palate and pharynx [1, 2].

Pharynx

Before entering the oesophagus, food passes the pharynx. The pharynx is defined by the base of the skull, the mandible and the larynx. The pharynx comprises of the nasopharynx (connected to the caudal nasal cavities), the oropharynx (connected to the caudal oral cavity) and the laryngopharynx (connected to the oesophagus and lies alongside the larynx). Food material enters the oropharynx and then passes around each side of the larynx to enter the oesophagus. The passages around the sides of the oesophagus are known as the lateral food channels [2]. In the pharynx, there is a network of nerve impulses that stimulate the nasopharynx and larynx to close and the oropharynx to open, enabling the food bolus (moved by the tongue) to pass into the oesophagus. This is a swallowing reflex that ensures food enters the oesophagus and not the airway [1].

Oesophagus

The oesophagus is approximately 1.5 metres in length. It passes down the left side of the neck, enters the thorax, crosses the mediastinum above the heart and travels via the oesophageal hiatus of the diaphragm into the abdomen, where it joins the stomach at the cardiac sphincter. It has four layers (from outermost – connective tissue, muscle, submucosa and a layer of stratified squamous epithelium) and is formed of internal longitudinal folds. The cross-section of the oesophagus appears star shaped. The oesophagus is innervated by the vagus nerve, which controls peristalsis and pushes ingesta into the cardiac sphincter of the stomach. In horses, the cardiac sphincter is well developed and only opens with the pressure of a food bolus to allow passage of food into the stomach. It also prevents horses from being able to vomit [1, 2].

Stomach

The stomach acts as a collecting chamber for food and initiates the mechanical and enzymatic breakdown of food. Food moves through the stomach via the cardiac sphincter, fundus, body, antrum, pylorus and pyloric sphincter (Figure 4.43).

The stomach has a capacity of 9–15 l, small in relation to the size and body mass of the horse and is mainly situated on the left side of the abdomen. It has a curved appearance with a smaller cranial curve (the lesser curvature) and a larger caudal curve (the greater curvature) (Figure 4.44). Blood is supplied to the stomach via the coeliac artery,

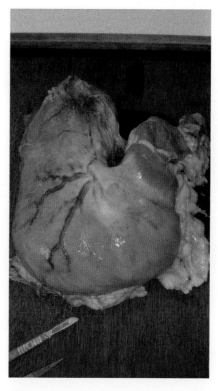

Figure 4.44 The equine stomach. *Source:* Lucy Middlecote.

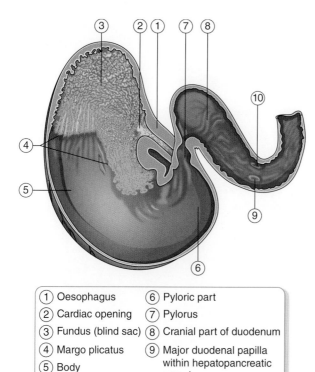

① Oesophagus	⑥ Pyloric part
② Cardiac opening	⑦ Pylorus
③ Fundus (blind sac)	⑧ Cranial part of duodenum
④ Margo plicatus	⑨ Major duodenal papilla
⑤ Body	within hepatopancreatic ampula
	⑩ Minor duodenal papilla

Figure 4.43 The interior of the equine stomach. *Source:* Adapted from Elsevier.

which arises directly from the aorta. Branches of the artery supply the curvatures of the stomach and then gradually spread out to the rest of the stomach. Venous drainage is via the portal vein [1, 2].

The stomach consists of six layers (from outermost – serosa, three layers of smooth muscle, submucosa and mucosa consisting of glandular columnar epithelium covered with mucus). The muscular layers of the stomach contract to help break down food and move it towards the pyloric sphincter. Internally, the lining of the stomach has a defined marked step known as the margo plicatus. This divides the cranial non-glandular section of the stomach form the caudal glandular section (Figure 4.45). The gastric mucosa contains deep folds (rugae), which flatten when the stomach fills. In response to food, the hormone gastrin stimulates the secretion of gastric juices, which contain mucus (from goblet cells), hydrochloric acid (from parietal cells), pepsinogen (from chief cells) and pepsin. In the body of the stomach, food is mixed with saliva and gastric secretions. Mucus lubricates the food and protects the mucosa, hydrochloric acid breaks down proteins and converts pepsinogen to the active enzyme pepsin and pepsin converts protein molecules to peptides. Foodstuff passing from the stomach, via the pyloric sphincter, to the small intestine is a soup-like acidic liquid known as chyme [1–3].

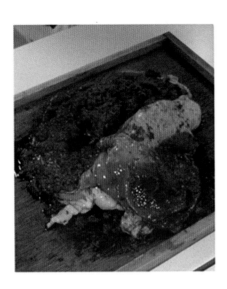
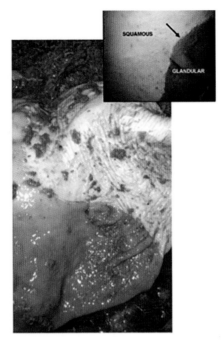

Figure 4.45 The interior of the equine stomach. *Source:* Lucy Middlecote.

Small Intestine

The function of the small intestine is the enzymatic breakdown of food and the absorption of nutrients following digestion.

The small intestine is attached to the dorsal abdominal wall via a thin, fibrous connection, known as the mesentery. It is approximately 25 metres in length and comprises the duodenum, the jejunum and the ileum. The duodenum begins ventral to the liver, where it forms a sigmoid flexure (bend) dorsally and then ventrally as it moves in a caudal direction. The jejunum is the longest part of the small intestine and, along with the duodenum, is where most of the absorption of nutrients takes place. The ileum is relatively short and has a much thicker wall than the rest of the small intestine. The ileum ends at the ileocaecal junction in the base of the caecum [1, 2].

The intestinal wall consists of four layers (from outermost – serosa, smooth muscle [longitudinal and circular], submucosa and mucosa) (Figure 4.46).

Blood is supplied to part of the duodenum via the coeliac artery. The remainder of the duodenum and the rest of the small intestine are supplied via the mesenteric artery. Venous drainage is via the cranial and caudal mesenteric veins. Lymphatic vessels drain into the cysterna chyli (which forms part of the thoracic duct) and returns lymphatic fluid to the venous bloodstream [1, 2].

The passage of chyme through the pyloric sphincter initiates the production of the hormone secretin, which helps to

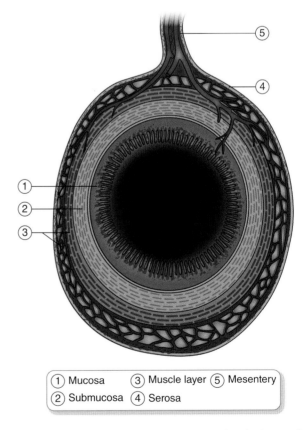

| ① Mucosa | ③ Muscle layer | ⑤ Mesentery |
| ② Submucosa | ④ Serosa | |

Figure 4.46 Cross-sectional diagram showing the layers of the small intestine. *Source:* Adapted from Elsevier.

control the pH of the gastrointestinal tract contents and stimulates the secretion of intestinal juices from Brunner's glands located in the submucosa. Enzymes in the intestinal juices help to breakdown proteins, fats and carbohydrates into smaller molecules. In addition, Brunner's glands also produce a mucus to protect the duodenum from the acidic content of chyme, provide an alkaline condition for the intestinal enzymes to be active, and lubricate the intestinal walls [1, 3].

Located in the inner mucosa layer are finger-like projections known as villi, which increase the surface area of the small intestine. Along the villi, there are even smaller projections known as microvilli, which are collectively called the brush border. Within the villi, there are capillaries, which absorb nutrients into the bloodstream and lacteals, which absorb chyle (a milky liquid containing digested fats) [1–3].

Special Considerations

Immunoglobulins are the main antibodies in colostrum. Neonatal foals have specialised cells in their small intestine that enable these large molecules to pass directly into the bloodstream for a few hours after birth. This results in the transfer of immunity from the dam to the foal. The absorption of colostral immunoglobulins is greatest during the first 6–8 hours after birth, but after 24 hours absorption of immunoglobulins across the intestinal wall is no longer possible due to changes that take place in the intestine. It is therefore imperative that neonates suck and take in colostrum as soon as possible following birth [1, 2].

Associated Organs
Liver

With reference to the digestive system, the liver is responsible for the metabolism of proteins, fats and carbohydrates absorbed from the small intestine and for the production of approximately 10 l per day of bile. Located between the hepatocytes are bile canaliculi that secrete bile. Bile emulsifies fats so that enzymes can work effectively. Horses have no gallbladder for the storage of bile, and it is transported directly to the duodenum via the biliary system and bile duct [1–3].

Predominantly located on the right side of the abdomen, the liver is a solid deep red organ located between the stomach and the diaphragm. It weighs approximately 5 kg and is divided into four main lobes – left lobe, right lobe, caudate lobe and quadrate lobe. The liver receives blood from both the hepatic artery, which supplies the liver cells, and the hepatic portal vein, which transports absorbed products of digestion from the gastrointestinal tract directly to the liver for metabolism [1–3].

Pancreas

The pancreas is a glandular structure with both endocrine and exocrine components; therefore, it is known as a mixed gland. The exocrine section of the pancreas secretes pancreatic juices, which contain enzymes and bicarbonate, into the duodenum via the pancreatic duct. Pancreatic juices occur in response to hormones cholecystokinin, secretin, gastrin and stimuli from the autonomic nervous system. The enzymes present in pancreatic juices are proteases (act on proteins and convert them to amino acids), lipases (activated by bile salts and convert fats to fatty acids and glycerol) and amylases (act on starches and convert them to maltose). Bicarbonate neutralises the acid from the stomach and ensures that ingesta moving into the small intestine is less acidic and allows other enzymes to work [1–3].

Large Intestine

The large intestine comprises the caecum, the colon, the rectum and the anus.

Caecum

The caecum is a blind-ending diverticulum shaped like a giant comma. It has a capacity of up to 35 l and is approximately 1 metre in length. There are four longitudinal muscles, known as taeniae, situated over the length of the caecum, which cause sacculation and pull the caecum into a series of non-permanent pouch-like formations known as haustrae. The caecum is a large chamber for microbial fermentation of fibre and is responsible for microbial digestion. Large numbers of protozoa and bacteria break down fibre to produce volatile fatty acids (VFAs), and microbes produce essential amino acids, B vitamins and vitamin K. On average, food is retained in the caecum for about five hours [1–3].

Colon

The colon is responsible for the absorption of VFAs, vitamins, water and electrolytes. It consists of an ascending portion, a transverse portion and a descending portion. The descending colon is held close to the dorsal wall by the mesocolon.

In horses, the colon is often divided into the large and small colons. Microbial digestion of fibre continues in the large colon and water is reabsorbed in the small colon. The large colon is equivalent to the ascending colon and the transverse colon. It has capacity of up to 80 l and is approximately 4 m in length. On average, food is retained in the large colon for about 50 hours. Apart from its origin and termination, the ascending colon is free to move within the abdomen. It is folded which giving rise to four distinct parallel areas and flexures, situated in the following order – right ventral colon, sternal flexure, left ventral colon, pelvic flexure, left dorsal colon, diaphragmatic flexure and right dorsal colon. The pelvic flexure is a common site for obstructions to occur because this is where the tract narrows, the number of taeniae reduces from four to three and the consistency of the ingesta becomes less fluid. The small colon is equivalent to the descending colon. It has a similar diameter to the small intestine and is about 3 m long. Blood is supplied to the ascending and transverse colon (large colon) by the cranial mesenteric artery and to the descending colon (small colon) by the caudal mesenteric artery [1–3].

Rectum and Anus

The remaining waste moves from the colon to the rectum. The rectum is a collection chamber that is held close to the dorsal wall by connective tissue and muscle. It is about 30 cm in length. The movement of faeces out of the rectum is controlled by the muscular anal sphincter, which is usually in a state of constriction to ensure that the opening to the large intestine is closed. When faeces move into the pelvic cavity, stretching of the rectal wall stimulates voluntary straining as result of abdominal contractions. This causes relaxation of the anal sphincter, and the waste is forced out. Increased pressure will also result in excretion [1–3].

4.13 Structure and Function of the Urinary System

The urinary system is responsible for osmoregulation and excretion.

Osmoregulation – regulation of the chemical makeup and volume of body fluids.

Excretion – removal of waste products and excess water [1, 3].

The urinary system comprises two kidneys, two ureters, the urinary bladder, the urethra and the penis or vestibule.

Kidney

The equine kidneys are brown-red in colour with a flat, smooth surface (Figure 4.47). The right kidney is situated in a slightly more cranial position than the left kidney, is heart shaped and sits in a depression of the liver. The right kidney is approximately 15 cm in length and 15 cm in width. It is attached to the pancreas and base of the caecum. The right kidney is inaccessible and impalpable on rectal examination. The left kidney is more bean shaped, lies ventral to the last rib and the first three lumbar processes and is very slightly mobile. The left kidney is approximately 18 cm long and 10–12 cm wide. Laterally, the left kidney borders the spleen with which it is connected via the nephrosplenic ligament. The left kidney can be palpated during a rectal examination. Each kidney receives oxygenated blood from a renal artery and is drained by a renal vein. The renal artery enters the kidney, and the renal vein exits the kidney at the area known as the hilus (Figure 4.48). The kidneys have a good blood supply with each kidney receiving more than 20% of cardiac output at any one time [1–3].

The kidney is surrounded by an outer capsule and consists of three main areas:

- The outer cortex
- The inner medulla
- The renal pelvis

Nephron

The nephron is the functional unit of the kidney responsible for the formation of urine. At birth, a healthy kidney has approximately one million nephrons, which gradually

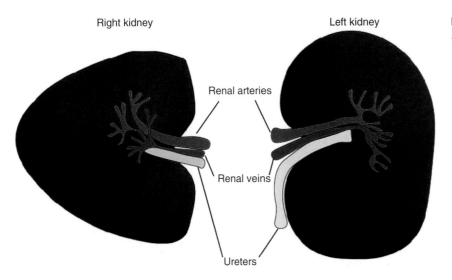

Right kidney

Left kidney

Renal arteries

Renal veins

Ureters

Figure 4.47 The equine kidneys. *Source:* Rosina Lillywhite.

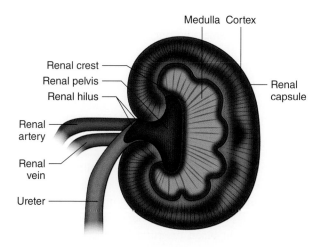

Figure 4.48 Section through an equine kidney. *Source:* Adapted from the BSAVA and Samantha Elmhurst.

degenerate throughout life. Each nephron comprises the glomerulus, the proximal convoluted tubule, the Loop of Henle, the distal convoluted tubule and the collecting duct [1–3].

Urine Formation

The process of urine formation plays a key role in home-ostasis. Urine is an indicator of the health status of the animal and normal urine should only contain water, salts and urea. The act of passing urine is termed micturition and normal urine output is 1–2 mls/kg/hour. In a healthy horse the volume and concentration of urine are affected by diet, exercise and environmental conditions [1–3].

Each part of the nephron is involved in the formation of urine. Urine is an ultra-filtrate of plasma, and the filtrate is modified and concentrated by the different parts of the nephron to produce urine. As the process is not selective for any substances, the kidney needs to reabsorb any substances that are important for the body. Reabsorption of water, electrolytes and other substances will take place in the tubules so that the body can retain sufficient water to maintain balance, but as well as reabsorption, the secretion of some substances is important to dispose of foreign substances. The changes made will depend on the status of the ECF (Figure 4.49) [1–3].

Glomerulus

Located in the cortex of the kidney, the glomerulus is a knot of capillaries surrounded by the cup-shaped glomerular capsule (Bowman's capsule). Blood is supplied by an afferent arteriole and drained by an efferent arteriole. The glomerulus is a short distance from the aorta, which enables blood pressure within the glomerulus to be maintained at

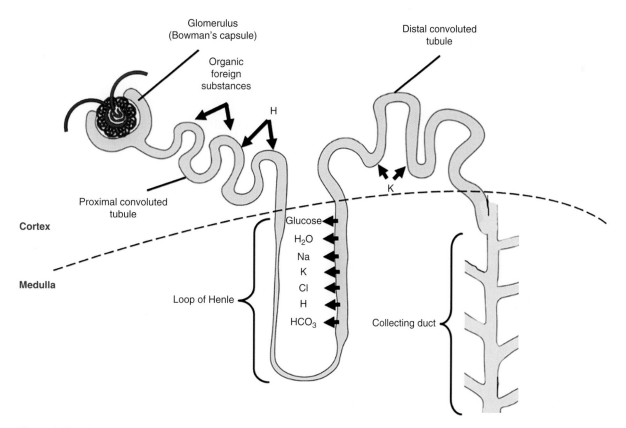

Figure 4.49 Kidney nephron function. *Source:* Rosina Lillywhite.

a high level. In addition, the hormone renin is secreted by the walls of the glomerulus and causes the efferent part of each glomerulus to constrict, which increases the pressure behind it, increasing blood pressure [1, 3].

The glomerular capsule is lined with a selectively permeable basement membrane perforated by tiny pores/holes. As blood flows through the glomerulus, the blood pressure forces water, electrolytes and other substances through the holes in the wall of the glomerulus and into the glomerular space. The holes are large enough to allow some small molecules (including urea, haemoglobin and simple sugars) but not large molecules (including proteins and larger blood cells) to leave the glomerulus. This process is known as ultrafiltration and means that plasma is filtered through the basement membrane of the glomerular capsule. The resulting filtrate is referred to as glomerular filtrate. From here, the filtrate passes into the proximal convoluted tubule [1, 3].

Proximal Convoluted Tubule

About 65% of all reabsorption of water, sodium (Na^+) and glucose takes place in the proximal convoluted tubule. The proximal convoluted tubule is a long-twisted tube lined by cuboidal epithelium with a brush border, which provides an increased surface area for the reabsorption of water and electrolytes. The reabsorption of sodium provides the osmotic potential for water reabsorption. To pump sodium out of the tubule and into the blood vessels, it is exchanged for potassium (K^+). In addition, the proximal convoluted tubule is responsible for the concentration of nitrogenous waste and the secretion of certain drugs and toxins [1, 3].

Loop of Henle

The loop of Henle is a U-shaped tube which dips down (descending limb) into the renal medulla and then back up (ascending limb) into the renal cortex. The fluid from the proximal convoluted tubule passes first into the descending limb of the loop of Henle. The descending limb consists of a thin layer of epithelium and is permeable to water but contains no pumps. The thin wall allows water to pass out of the lumen and into the interstitial tissue via osmosis. The fluid then passes into the ascending limb of the loop of Henle. The ascending limb consists of a thicker layer of epithelium and is impermeable to water, but the walls contain pumps that pump sodium, potassium and chloride (Cl^-) out into the interstitial tissue. Sodium ions pumped out from the ascending limb are then able to draw out water from the descending limb by osmosis [1, 3].

Distal Convoluted Tubule

The fluid from the loop of Henle passes into the distal convoluted tubule, a less twisted tube situated within the renal cortex. The distal convoluted tubule is lined with cuboidal epithelium but, unlike the proximal convoluted tubule, has no brush border. Fine adjustments are made here via the reabsorption of sodium and water; more sodium is reabsorbed, and more potassium and hydrogen are secreted. Hydrogen (H^+) secretion enables the body to maintain the acid–base balance. The secretion or reabsorption of hydrogen ions will depend on whether the blood pH is low or high [1, 3].

Sodium reabsorption and potassium secretion are regulated by the hormone aldosterone. In response to low blood pressure, the walls of the glomeruli release renin, a hormone that ultimately stimulates the release of aldosterone from the adrenal cortex. Aldosterone stimulates increased reabsorption of sodium, which results in increased water reabsorption and a rise in blood pressure. For every sodium ion that is reabsorbed back into the blood a potassium ion is secreted into the urine. Aldosterone is produced via the renin–angiotensin–aldosterone pathway (Figure 4.50) [1, 3].

Collecting Duct

The fluid from the proximal convoluted tubule passes into the collecting duct. Each collecting duct collects urine from several nephrons. Final adjustments to water content occurs in the collecting duct because, according to the status of the ECF, the walls can change their permeability to water. The process of increasing the reabsorption of water is controlled by antidiuretic hormone (ADH), which is released by the posterior pituitary gland in response to an increase in osmotic pressure or low blood pressure (Figure 4.51). Finally, the urine moves into the renal pelvis and then drains into the ureter [1, 3].

Ureter

Each kidney has a single ureter, which drains the renal pelvis and transports urine to the urinary bladder. Each ureter is 6–8 mm in diameter and 70 cm in length. The ureter is constructed of three layers (the innermost mucosal layer, the muscular layer and the outermost adventitia) lined with transitional epithelium and supported by a sheath of smooth muscle which helps to transport urine from the kidney to the bladder via peristalsis. In the horse, the ureter is wide as it leaves the kidney and narrows as it moves caudally. The ureters enter the urinary bladder at the trigone of the bladder [1–3].

Urinary Bladder

The bladder is a storage organ which is located in the pelvic cavity when it is empty and in the abdominal cavity when it is full. It is able to hold 3–4 l of urine before micturition is stimulated. Similar to the ureter, the wall of the bladder has three layers: it is lined with transitional epithelium, which allows expansion and contraction as urine collects and is

Figure 4.50 Summary of renin-angiotensin-aldosterone pathway. *Source:* Lucy Middlecote.

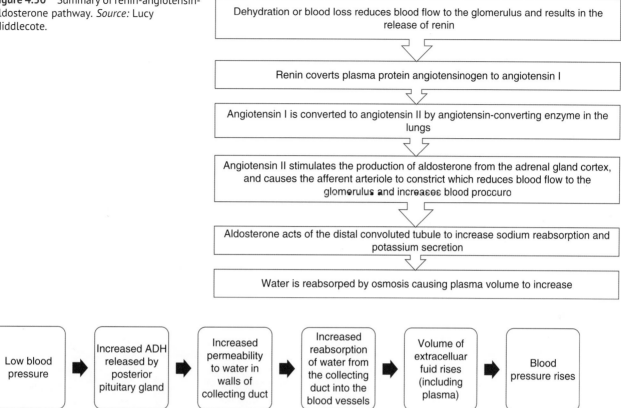

Figure 4.51 Control of water loss in the collecting duct. *Source:* Lucy Middlecote.

voided, and has layers of circular and longitudinal smooth muscle fibres. The bladder is cone shaped with a blunt end at the top, a body and a more pointed end (bladder neck) leading into the urethra. The trigone of the bladder is the area on the inside of the bladder neck where the ureters insert, and the urethra originates [1–3].

Bladder Sphincter

Located at the bladder neck, the bladder sphincter controls the flow of urine out of the bladder. The sphincter consists of two concentric rings of muscle: the inner sphincter is made of smooth muscle and is under involuntary control and the outer sphincter is made of skeletal/striated muscle and is under voluntary control. The bladder empties in response to a reflex stimulated by stretch receptors in the muscle wall; however, the brain can overcome the involuntary reflex until there is a more appropriate time to micturate [1, 3].

Urethra

The urethra is the tube, with the same structure as the ureter, which takes urine from the bladder to the outside environment. In male horses, the function of the urethra is to transport urine from the bladder, and sperm and spermatic fluid from the prostate gland to the penis for excretion. The urethra is long and measures approximately 75 cm. It runs caudally from the bladder, then ventrally over the rim of the caudal pelvis and cranially through the centre of the penis. In female horses, the urethra's only function is to transport urine from the bladder to the vestibule for excretion. The urethra is short at 2–3 cm long, and opens into the external urethral orifice in the vestibule caudal to the vagina [1–3].

4.14 Structure and Function of the Reproductive System

The reproductive system is housed within the abdominal and pelvic cavities. The system includes the external genitalia (penis and vulva) and the reproductive organs (testicles and ovaries), which work together for the purpose of reproduction. Fluids, hormones and pheromones are also important accessories to the reproductive system [1–3].

Reproduction and Hormones

Reproduction is defined as the transfer of genetic information via the process of mating. Specialised germ cells (spermatozoa and ova) fuse to form a single-celled zygote, which undergoes cell division to form an embryo. Once the major organs are formed, the embryo begins implantation and eventually becomes a foetus that develops during gestation. During parturition, the foetus is born and the newborn foal is known as a neonate [1–3].

Gonadotrophins, follicle-stimulating hormone (FSH) and luteinising hormone (LH) are released from the anterior pituitary gland and stimulate the reproductive organs. The hormones produced in response are testosterone, oestrogen and progesterone. Testosterone influences spermatogenesis and is responsible for the development of the male reproductive tract and male sexual characteristics. Oestrogen is responsible for many of the physical and behavioural changes associated with a mare being 'in season', and progesterone prepares the uterus to receive a fertilised ovum and maintains pregnancy. See Chapter 15 for more information on reproductive cycle of the mare [1–3].

Reproductive Anatomy of the Mare

The mare's reproductive organs include the ovaries, the uterine tubes, the uterus, the cervix, the vagina and vestibule, the vulva (Figure 4.52) and the mammary glands.

Ovaries

The function of the ovary is to produce ova (eggs) for fertilisation, and to act as an endocrine gland secreting oestrogen and progesterone. The ovaries are located in the dorsal abdomen, usually below the third/fourth lumbar vertebrae, and lie caudal to the kidneys. They are suspended from the abdominal wall via the mesovarium and attached to the dorsal body wall by the ovarian ligament. Blood is supplied via the ovarian artery [1–3].

In the mare, the ovaries are round or oval and vary in size. Although generally large, the ovaries are often smaller during the autumn and winter when they are hard with no follicles. During the spring and summer, in response to follicle-stimulating hormone (FSH), the ovary will often develop a follicle prior to ovulation, and then in response to a surge in luteinising hormone (LH) release an ovum from the follicle. Located close to each ovary is a funnel-shaped infundibulum (fringed with fimbriae), which catches the ovum and transports it through the uterine tube [1, 2].

Uterine Tubes

Also known as the fallopian tube or oviduct, the uterine tube is the site of fertilisation and where the early embryo resides before entering the uterus. The uterine tubes lie at the end of each uterine horn and are 20–30 cm in length. The uterotubular junction can determine whether an ovum is fertile, meaning that the mare has a unique ability to

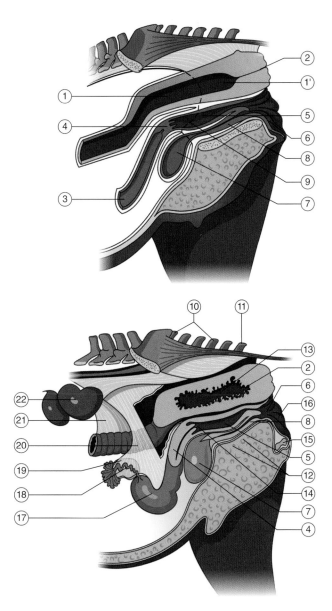

Figure 4.52 The reproductive tract of the mare. 1. Peritoneal part of the rectum, 1' Retroperitoneal parts of the rectum, 2. Anal canal, 3. Uterus, 4. Cervix, 5. Vagina, 6. Vestibule, 7. Bladder, 8. Urethra, 9. Caudal extent of peritoneum, 10. Sacrum, 11. Coccygeal vertebrae 2, 12. Floor of pelvis, 13. Rectum, 14. Vaginal part of cervix, 15. Clitoris, 16. Vulva, 17. Left uterine horn, 18. Uterine tube, 19. Ovary, 20. Broad ligament (largerly cut away), 21. Small colon, 22. Left kidney. *Source:* Adapted from Elsevier.

ensure that an unfertilised ovum does not enter the uterus by retaining it within the uterine tube [1, 2].

Uterus

The function of the uterus is to provide the correct environment for embryo survival and development, and to provide a means whereby developing embryos can receive nutrients via the placenta. The position of the uterus may change depending on how full the bladder or intestines might be. It is suspended within the pelvic cavity and abdomen by two large ligamentous sheets called the broad ligaments. These provide attachment to the body wall and an avenue for blood vessels, lymphatic vessels and nerves. The main blood supply is from the uterine artery. The uterus has a large cranial body and two short caudal uterine horns. The uterus consists of an outer layer of connective tissue (mesometrium), a central layer of muscle (myometrium) and a highly vascular inner layer (endometrium) lined by a secretory epithelium. Muscle layer changes are responsible for the differences in uterine tone at oestrus, dioestrus and early pregnancy [1–3].

Cervix

The cervix is the last line of defence between the uterus and the external environment. It is a thick-walled tubular sphincter that separates the uterus from the vagina and forms an important physical barrier for the uterus. Most of the time, the cervix remains closed but does open during oestrus and parturition. The cervix is short and projects caudally into the cranial vagina, which creates a space around the cervix known as the fornix [1–3].

Vagina and Vestibule

Mostly retroperitoneal, the vagina is a tubular structure that extends from the cervix to the external urethral orifice (where the urinary tract joins the reproductive tract). The vestibule leads from the external urethral orifice to the vulva. At the junction between the vagina and the vestibule, there is a fold of skin overlying the external urethral opening; this fold may continue on either side of the vagina to form the hymen (in maiden mares) [1–3].

Vulva

The vulva forms the external opening of the reproductive tract. It is directly ventral to the anus. There are two vulval lips, which should be full and firm and meet in the midline with the outer lips (labia) held closed to prevent entry of infection. Mares with abnormal anatomy can suck in air and foreign material to the vagina and uterus with the risk of causing infections detrimental to conception. At the lower end of the vulva, the clitoris is situated within a depression, known as the clitoral fossa. When a mare is in oestrus, the clitoris is repeatedly exposed in an act known as 'winking'. Certain bacteria can live on the clitoris and cause venereal infections. Infected mares show no clinical signs of disease, and it is only identified when a pre-breeding swab is taken and processed [1–3].

Mammary Glands

The mammary glands are modified skin glands found in pairs on either side of the midline. Each gland consists of glandular epithelium lined with secretory epithelium. Mares generally have one pair of mammary glands, each with one teat. Milk, produced in response to the hormone prolactin, drains into teat canals, which open on the surface at the teat orifices. Milk letdown or excretion in response to suckling is caused by muscular contractions induced by the hormone oxytocin [1–3].

Reproductive Anatomy of the Stallion

The stallion's reproductive organs include the testicles, the epididymis, the spermatic cord and deferent duct, the urethra, the penis and the accessory glands (Figure 4.53). See Chapter 15 for information on reproductive cycle of the stallion.

Testicles

The function of the testicle is to produce testosterone and oestrogen, as well as spermatozoa (sperm) and the fluid to transport it. Sperm is required to fertilise the ovum and produce offspring. Sperm comprises of the acrosome (a cap-like structure found on the head), the head (where the nucleus is located), the mid-piece (containing the mitochondria) and the tail (provides motion) [1–3].

The testicles (testes) are round to oval in shape, should be similar in size and are found outside the abdomen freely moving in the scrotum. They descend from the abdominal cavity through the inguinal canal and are wrapped in a double fold of peritoneum, forming the vaginal tunic/tunica vaginalis. Slightly lower than body temperature, the temperature in the scrotum is optimal for spermatogenesis. Located in the wall of the scrotum, the dartos muscle is responsible for contraction and relaxation of the scrotal skin; contracting the skin reduces the surface area and decreases the amount of heat that can be lost, and relaxing the skin increases the surface area, enables more heat to be lost and the temperature to be reduced [1–3].

Spermatogenesis occurs in the seminiferous tubules. These are small tubules that make up 70% of the testicles. The seminiferous tubules are lined with spermatogenic cells, which produce immature sperm (spermatids), and Sertoli cells that, under the influence of follicle-stimulating hormone (FSH) secrete oestrogen and nutrients to nourish and prolong the survival of the sperm. Lying between the seminiferous tubules are Leydig cells (interstitial cells) that secrete testosterone under the influence of luteinising hormone (LH). The seminiferous tubules drain into the epididymis [1–3].

Epididymis

Sperm are transported from the testicle to the epididymis in ducts. Even though it appears to be adhered to the testicle's outer surface, the epididymis is part of the testicle. The

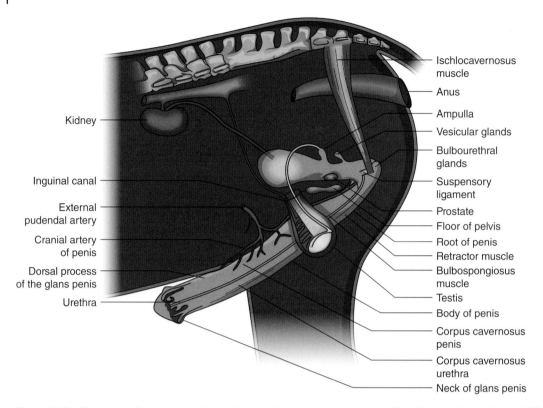

Figure 4.53 Diagrammatic representation of the reproductive system of the stallion. *Source:* Adapted from CABI.

cauda epididymis is attached to the caudal extremity of the testicle and, as this is where the temperature is at its lowest, sperm are stored here while they undergo a period of maturation. The epididymis is a lengthy convoluted duct which becomes narrower and tapers into the deferent duct within the spermatic cord [1–3].

Spermatic Cord and Deferent Duct

The spermatic cord travels from the epididymis and up into the abdomen. It contains the testicular artery and vein, nerves, lymphatic vessels, the cremaster muscle and the deferent duct. The cremaster muscle contracts or relaxes depending on ambient temperatures. This enables the testes to be either raised towards the body or lowered away from the body wall and ensures that sperm production is not impaired by inappropriate temperatures. Within the spermatic cord, sperm travels in the deferent duct (also known as the vas deferens or ductus deferens) and up into the urethra located at the bladder neck [1–3].

Urethra

The urethra is a tube that is common to both the urinary system and genital system. It transports sperm and spermatic fluid to the penis for excretion. The urethra is long and runs caudally from the bladder, then ventrally over the rim of the caudal pelvis, and cranially through the centre of the penis [1, 2].

Penis

The urethra runs through the centre of the penis to the tip. The terminal part of the penis is known as the glans penis. When retracted, the penis is housed and protected by the prepuce/sheath, which contains many glands that secrete smegma. The prepuce also has additional internal folds, which enable the penis to enlarge when it is engorged. The penis consists of erectile tissue, which has a profuse blood supply [1, 2].

Accessory Glands

The accessory glands are responsible for the production of spermatic fluid/seminal fluid, which transports and provides nutrition for sperm. The accessory glands include the seminal vesicles/vesicular glands, the prostate gland and the bulbourethral glands. The seminal vesicles are a pair of large (10–12 cm), smooth, elongated glands located on either side of the bladder and near to the prostate gland. The prostate gland is a single gland situated on both sides of the pelvic urethra. It provides a portion of fluid suspension for the sperm. The bulbourethral glands are a pair of glands located on the dorsal aspect of the urethra near the pelvic exit. They secrete clear fluid, which cleans and neutralises the pH of the urethra prior to ejaculation [1, 2].

References

1 Fraser, M. and Girling, S. (2011). Chapter 3 – Anatomy and physiology. In: *BSAVA Textbook of Veterinary Nursing*, 5e (ed. B. Cooper, E. Mullineaux, and L. Turner), 37–112. BSAVA: Gloucester.

2 Clegg, P.D., Townsend, N., and Conwell, R.C. (2012). Chapter 2 – Anatomy and Physiology. In: *Equine Veterinary Nursing Manual*, 2e (ed. K. Coumbe). Oxford: Blackwell Publishing.

3 Aspinall, V. and Capello, M. (2020). *Introduction to Animal and Veterinary Anatomy and Physiology*, 4e. Oxfordshire, UK: CABI.

4 Pilliner, S. and Davies, Z. (2004). *Equine Science*, 2e. Oxford, UK: Blackwell.

5 Dallas, S. and Ackerman, N. (2016). Canine and feline anatomy and physiology. In: *Aspinall's Complete Textbook of Veterinary Nursing*, 3e (ed. N. Ackerman), 65–113. Edinburgh, UK: Elsevier.

6 Hastie, P.S. (2012). *The BHS Veterinary Manual*, 2e. Shrewsbury, UK: Kenilworth Press.

7 Phillips, C. (2016). Equine anatomy and physiology. In: *Aspinall's Complete Textbook of Veterinary Nursing*, 3e (ed. N. Ackerman), 135–144. Edinburgh, UK: Elsevier.

8 Blignault, K. (2009). *Equine Biomechanics for Riders*. London, UK: J.A. Allen.

9 Andersen, C. and Tnibar, A. (2016). Medial patellar ligament splitting in horses with upward fixation of the patella: a long-term follow-up. *Equine Veterinary Journal* 48 (3): 312–314.

10 Van Weeren, P.R., Van den Bogert, A.J., Barneveld, A. et al. (1990). The role of the reciprocal apparatus in the hind limb of the horse investigated by a modified CODA-3 opto-electronic kinematic analysis system. *Equine Veterinary Journal* 22 (S9): 95–100.

11 Copas, V.E.N. and Boswell, J.C. (2012). Fluid therapy. In: *Equine Veterinary Nursing*, 2e (ed. K.M. Coumbe), 226–245. Chichester, UK: Wiley Blackwell.

12 Slater, J.D. and Knowles, E.J. (2012). Medical nursing. In: *Equine Veterinary Nursing*, 2e (ed. K.M. Coumbe), 246–285. Chichester, UK: Wiley Blackwell.

13 Snalune, K. and Paton, A. (2012). General nursing. In: *Equine Veterinary Nursing*, 2e (ed. K.M. Coumbe), 153–175. Chichester, UK: Wiley Blackwell.

14 McMillan, S. and Ackerman, N. (2016). Fluid therapy and nutritional support. In: *Aspinall's Complete Textbook of Veterinary Nursing*, 3e (ed. N. Ackerman), 477–504. Edinburgh, UK: Elsevier.

15 Kramer, J.W. (2000). Normal hematology of the horse. In: *Schalm's Veterinary Hematology*, 5e (ed. B.F. Feldman, J.G. Zinkl, and N.C. Jain), 1069–1074. Philadephlia, PA: Lippincott Williams & Wilkins.

16 Murrell, J. and Ford-Fennah, V. (2019). Anaesthesia and analgesia. In: *The BSAVA Textbook of Veterinary Nursing*, 5e (ed. B. Cooper, E. Mullineaux, L. Turner, and T. Greet), 663–737. Gloucester, UK: British Small Animal Veterinary Association.

17 Allen, K. (2015). Soft palate displacement in horses. *In Practice* 37 (8): 415–421.

18 Ahern, T.J. (1999). Pharyngeal dysfunction during exercise. *Journal of Equine Veterinary Science* 19 (4): 226–231.

19 Ahern, T. (2021). Horses are obligate nasal breathers: but does this obligation still apply when a horses 'Nasopharyngeal Air Supply' and with this its 'Defence through Flight', is compromised. *World Journal of Veterinary Science* 9: 27–30.

20 Cotrel, C., Leleu, C., and Courouce-Malblanc, A. (2006). Factors influencing variation in locomotor-respiratory coupling in Standardbred Trotters in the field. *Equine Veterinary Journal* 38 (S36): 562–566.

5

Applied Equine Welfare, Health and Husbandry

Nicola Smith[1], Louise Pailor[2], Lynn Irving[3], Kassie Hill[4], George Hunt[5], Cassie Woods[6], Bonny Millar[7], and Marie Rippingale[8]

[1] *Lantra Awards, Coventry, England, UK*
[2] *Wright and Morten Equine Clinic, Somerford Park Clinic, Somerford, England, UK*
[3] *Village Vet, Milton, England, UK*
[4] *Cliffe Equine Vets, Harbens Farm, East Sussex, England, UK*
[5] *E C Straiton & Partners LTD, The Veterinary Hospital, Penkridge, Stafford, UK*
[6] *Lower House Equine Clinic, Plas Cerrig Lane, Llanymynech, Oswestry, Shropshire, Llanymynech, UK*
[7] *Equicomms, CVS House, Norfolk, UK*
[8] *Bottle Green Training Ltd, Derby, UK*

Introduction

Over time, humans have manipulated equines, both in terms of their cosmetic appearance and performance ability, to accommodate our uses for them. As a result, many are now increasingly dependent on humans to ensure their welfare is maintained, as their natural ability to thrive has been compromised. Furthermore, some husbandry techniques may compromise welfare standards, exposure to unnatural conditions such as overcrowding or unsuitable housing may lead to injury or an increased risk of disease. Registered veterinary nurses (RVNs) should be able to recognise and reduce these risks through the delivery of good nursing care, ensuring good husbandry techniques are followed by those involved in care and the provision of advice where appropriate.

5.1 The Principles of Equine Welfare

Legislation and Codes of Practice

History of Legislation

The United Kingdom first implemented laws protecting animals in the nineteenth century, though it was not until the 1960s when public awareness increased, that an interest in animal welfare grew, in turn producing many changes resulting in improved conditions for animals of many species. In 1965 the Brambell committee produced a report of recommendations for the United Kingdom's government, which was developed by the Farm Animal Welfare Council.

A set of minimum standards for farm animals and intensive husbandry systems was introduced to define the physical and mental wellbeing of animals [1]. These were known as the 'FIVE FREEDOMS' [2].

Although originally developed for farm animals these 'five freedoms', now more correctly referred to as 'needs' were then recognised by the Animal Welfare Act 2006 after an overhaul of welfare legislation, replacing many outdated pieces of welfare legislation. This Act places a duty of care on owners to ensure their animal's welfare needs are met, gives more powers to those enforcing the legislation and allows tougher penalties [3].

Animal owners must always aim to provide the five 'needs' to their animals. The five welfare needs are as follows [3]:

- The need for a suitable diet: access to fresh water and diet to maintain health and vigour.
- The need for a suitable environment: providing an appropriate environment to include a shelter and a comfortable resting area.
- The need to be protected from pain, suffering, injury and disease: prevention of pain, injury or disease. If not possible, rapid diagnosis and treatment.
- The need to exhibit normal behaviour: by providing facilities with sufficient space and stimulation.
- The need to be housed with, or apart from, other animals: providing opportunities to interact with their own species where appropriate.

There must be some flexibility, especially in the provision of veterinary care where these needs cannot always be met.

Textbook of Equine Veterinary Nursing, First Edition. Edited by Rosina Lillywhite and Marie Rippingale.
© 2025 John Wiley & Sons Ltd. Published 2025 by John Wiley & Sons Ltd.
Companion website: www.wiley.com/go/equineveterinarynursing

There may be occasions where food may need to be withheld, or normal behaviour may not be possible and where turnout cannot be allowed, but RVNs should seek to minimise these restrictions and provide alternatives where possible, to minimise the impact on the physical and mental wellbeing of the equine patients in their care.

The Animal Welfare Act is the legislation that is used when it is believed there are shortfalls in welfare standards. Where there are clear breaches to the Act an improvement notice can be served if an animal's needs are not met based on the five needs. This 'notice' outlines the steps an owner must take to meet their animal's needs, within a given time period, this is to prevent any suffering to that animal. If the improvement notice is not adhered to, steps can be taken before any suffering occurs. This may involve removal of animals and subsequent bans to prevent ownership of animals for a length of time, may be served by the courts [3].

The Animal Welfare (Sentencing) Bill introduced in April 2021 has increased the maximum penalty for animal cruelty in England to five years in prison and unlimited fines [4].

The Five Domains Model of Animal Welfare was updated in 2020 and is becoming increasingly popular as a tool to assess the welfare of animals. This model includes a specific evaluation of the mental state of the animal and acknowledges the role that emotions may have to play in overall behaviour and welfare. For more information, please refer to the Futher Reading section at the end of this chapter.

Codes of Practice

The Department for Environment, Food and Rural Affairs (DEFRA) have produced Codes of Practice for dogs, cats and equines. These Codes interpret the five 'needs' into clear and constructive advice to ensure an animal's requirements are met. They summarise the legal responsibilities of the Act and provide guidance to owners on providing appropriate species-specific care [5, 6].

The DEFRA Code has then been further interpreted for the equine species by the National Equine Welfare Council who published their Equine Industry Welfare Guidelines Compendium 3rd edition in 2009. This aims to serve as a reference document for all activities relating to horses and is something that all those involved in the provision of care to horses should be aware of [7].

These texts are a good place to signpost owners so they can ensure they are meeting all the required welfare needs for their animals.

Veterinary Surgeons Act (VSA) 1966

The VSA 1966 was created to manage the veterinary profession in the United Kingdom by defining veterinary surgery and ensuring only those with the appropriate qualifications can practise, therefore protecting animal health and welfare. The Royal College of Veterinary Surgeons (RCVS) acts as the regulatory body for veterinary surgeons (vets) and RVNs in the United Kingdom in accordance with the Act. It controls the registration of vets and RVNs, regulates their professional code of conduct and education, and allows the suspension or cancellation of registration of any personnel in cases of misconduct.

The Act ensures that only vets can perform veterinary surgery and that they must hold appropriate qualifications and meet minimum standards in the United Kingdom. Vets from outside of the United Kingdom who wish to enter the United Kingdom register may need to undertake extra training and examinations if their country of training does not match the requirements of the RCVS [8].

In 1991 the Schedule 3 amendment to the VSA was added to make provision for RVNs. Under the current Schedule 3 amendment, RVNs are allowed to perform certain procedures but these must always be performed under the direction of a vet, and they must not undertake surgery entering into a body cavity. RVNs must be on the RCVS register, and must always work within their level of competence. In 2002 provision was added for student veterinary nurses (SVNs) to perform Schedule 3 tasks as part of their training but only while working under the employment of their registered training practice, under the direction of a vet and supervision by either a vet or an RVN [9–11].

The RCVS ensures that vets and RVNs keep up to date with their knowledge through continuing professional development (CPD). Current annual requirements are 35 hours for vets and 15 hours for RVNs [12].

The Act includes provision to allow members of the general public to administer first aid to save a life or relieve pain and suffering. Members of the public may administer medication to their own animals or those of their employer [8, 9].

For more information please refer to Chapter 3.

Farriery

The Farriers Registration Act 1975 (updated 2017) was developed to prevent and avoid suffering to horses arising from shoeing by unskilled people. The Farriers Registration Council now act as the regulatory body for farriers practising within the United Kingdom.

Farriery is defined as 'any act involving the preparation or treatment of the foot for the reception of a shoe, the fitting – by nailing or otherwise, or the finishing off of such work'. People allowed to shoe under the Act include registered farriers, apprentices under supervision, vets and veterinary students. As barefoot trimmers are not preparing the foot for a shoe, they are not liable under this act [13].

Farriers cannot diagnose, or penetrate the sensitive structures of the foot [11].

Equine Dentistry

There are some procedures that are covered by the VSA, that have been exempted for suitably qualified equine dental technicians (EDTs). Equine dentists must attend a DEFRA approved course and be held on a register in order to carry out these procedures. Dentists who have not attended these courses may only carry out routine treatments such as routine rasping, removal of loose caps and removal of calculus from above the gum margin.

Procedures permitted by registered EDTs (category 2 procedures) include tooth extraction including wolf tooth removal and the use of power tools. They are not allowed to perform surgical extractions involving incisions or repulsion and cannot administer sedatives or anaesthesia [14].

RVNs involvement in dentistry falls within the remit of the VSA. Specific guidance in the Code of Professional Conduct states they may, under the direction of a vet, carry out routine dental hygiene work. It specifically states that extraction of teeth using instruments is not considered within the meaning of minor surgery, therefore should not be carried out [11].

The Animal Welfare Act 2006 – The Impact on Veterinary Practice

The Animal Welfare Act states that mutilations involving alterations to soft tissue or bone structures must not be performed unless for medical reasons. There are however some permitted procedures in equine practice in the United Kingdom. These include:

- Castration, though anaesthetic must be used
- Microchipping/freeze branding
- Contraceptive or hormonal implants
- Embryo transfer and artificial insemination [11, 15]

Mutilations that are not allowed in the United Kingdom under the Act:

The Horse Nicking and Docking Act of 1949 banned docking unless due to injury or disease, and permission was needed to import docked horses [16]. This would now also come under the mutilations section of the Animal Welfare Act [3]. Docking was initially carried out on haulage horses as it was deemed to prevent injury and ensure cleanliness however it could be argued this could be produced by simply wrapping the tail. Later it was done purely for cosmetic appearance to give a 'bobbed' look which was fashionable for carriage horses, tails were also de-nerved to ensure a flat tail carriage. Nicking involves cutting the tail tendons to produce a fashionable high tail carriage. These procedures are deemed to interfere with welfare both due to the use of a tail to manage insects, but also as a way of demonstrating behaviour including oestrus [17].

On the subject of pin firing, there is no specific legislation covering this procedure, but the RCVS consider it to be unethical. It involves thermal burning of the skin overlying an injured tendon in the belief the scarring would improve healing. There is no evidence-based research to prove this is of any benefit [18]. This has been supported further by a 2016 study demonstrating controlled exercise was as effective as any other treatment for tendon injuries [19].

The Department for Environment, Food and Rural Affairs (DEFRA)

DEFRA is the government department responsible for environmental protection, food production and standards, agriculture, fisheries and rural communities in the United Kingdom including Northern Ireland [20]. The Animal and Plant Health Agency (APHA) is an executive agency of DEFRA and some of its activities which may impact on welfare include identifying and controlling notifiable endemic and exotic diseases in animals, researching diseases and vaccines, and regulating disposal of animal by-products to prevent dangerous substances entering the food chain. Notifiable diseases must be reported to APHA via the DEFRA rural helpline. They will investigate, take samples and have the power to put restrictions in place which may include culling [21]. See Chapter 6 for more information relating to notifiable diseases.

Other Animal Welfare Legislation

Welfare of Horses at Markets Order 1990

This Act applies to any location where equines are brought for sale. Some provisions include that unfit horses, or those likely to give birth must not be sold, there must be provision to avoid injury or suffering, foals under four months cannot be sold without a dam, excessive force must not be used and horses must be penned separately from other species and in a way to avoid injury including no overcrowding; stallions, rigs (a male horse with a retained testicle/s), and mares heavily in foal or with a foal at foot must be separate [22].

Licensing of Activities Involving Animals (England) Regulations 2018

This Act has five distinct licensable activities, mostly related to small animals, but there are elements covering equines where they are used to generate income.

Licensing by the local authority is required and minimum welfare standards must be maintained with all appropriate documentation maintained. This covers where horses are hired out for riding, where they are used in films or displays or used for entertainment purposes such as pony parties [23].

Control of Horses Act 2015

This Act was introduced in a bid to prevent abandonment and illegal grazing of horses which is becoming an increasing problem in some areas. This Act gives the landowner the right to detain a horse and to claim damages for any damages and expenses incurred. After 4 working days, ownership passes to the landowner who can then dispose of the horse as they see fit, as long as appropriate notices have been posted [24].

Animal Welfare Charities

Animal charities carry out vital work, increasing public awareness of welfare needs and providing care to animals in need. Individual charities each have a code of conduct which outlines their aims and objectives.

The Royal Society for the Prevention of Cruelty to Animals (RSPCA)

Founded in 1824, the RSPCA aims to protect animals through legislative change and improve welfare standards through the provision of evidence-based advice. Where required they will carry out animal welfare investigations and private prosecutions, though the charity does not have authority or legal powers in its own right [25].

British Horse Society

The British Horse Society is the largest equine charity in the United Kingdom. It was founded in 1947 and works to protect and promote the interests of all horses and those who care for them. Its core elements focus on education, welfare, access, and safety. Some of their initiatives include welfare services, campaigning for access to equestrian rights of way, road safety and qualifications for those caring for, and working with equines [26].

World Horse Welfare

Founded in 1927 under the title 'International League for Protection of Horses', by Ada Cole, World Horse Welfare are an international charity who aim to improve welfare standards for equines in the United Kingdom and worldwide. One of the primary campaigns of the charity was the provision of humane slaughter, and to stop the export of live equines for slaughter. They now rehabilitate and rehome horses across the United Kingdom [27].

The Blue Cross

Formed in 1897, The Blue Cross aims to help sick, injured, abandoned and homeless pets through the provision of veterinary care, rehoming and behavioural advice. They rehome animals including equids across the United Kingdom and offer support to pet owners including bereavement counselling [28].

The Donkey Sanctuary

Registered as a charity in 1973, the Donkey Sanctuary aims to help abused or homeless donkeys and provide education worldwide to improve welfare. They have a sister charity which provides riding therapy for children with special needs. With their own fully staffed veterinary hospital, they lead research into ways to improve the welfare and specialist health requirements for donkeys [29]. See Chapter 16 for more information regarding donkeys.

5.2 Essential Factors for Maintaining Equine Health

Housing

Generally, horses are stabled for human convenience however, stabling is sometimes essential for medical management of critically ill or injured horses. In a practice or equine hospital environment, the stables must be safe and secure, easy to clean, offer good ventilation but be free from drafts. They should be constructed of a strong, sturdy material with no sharp edges to prevent injury. Tie rings, racks and any other additions within the stable must be easy to disinfect, firmly attached and safe. Stables should be warm and dry. Floors should be non-slip and have an adequate drainage system, this is particularly important as drains can harbour bacteria. The size of the accommodation is also important as equine patients vary in size.

Stable Sizes

The BHS minimum stable size recommendations for horses are as follows [6]:

- Large horses (17 hh+): 3.65 m × 4.25 m (12 ft × 14 ft)
- Horses: 3.65 m × 3.65 m (12 ft × 12 ft)
- Large ponies (13.2 hh+): 3.05 m × 3.65 m (10 ft × 12 ft)
- Ponies: 3.05 m × 3.05 m (10 ft × 10 ft)
- Foaling box (horse): 4.25 m × 4.25 m (14 ft × 14 ft)

These sizes should enable a horse or pony to act as naturally as physically possible, to lie down and move around the stable if permitted to gain access to hay, feed and water. The foaling box should allow enough space for the mare and the foal at foot.

The Donkey Sanctuary minimum stable size recommendations for donkeys are as follows [6]:

- Mules: 3.65 m × 3.65 m (12 ft × 12 ft)
- Large donkeys: 3.05 m × 3.65 m (10 ft × 12 ft)
- Donkeys: 3.05 m × 3.05 m (10 ft × 10 ft)
- Average sized donkeys kept in pair: 9 m^2 (100 ft^2) of covered space.

Larger donkeys and mules will need more space, equivalent to that recommended for similar sized ponies and horses [6]. Please see Chapter 16 for more information about donkeys.

Figure 5.1 Stable doors may need to be adapted to cater for smaller patients. *Source:* Judith Parry.

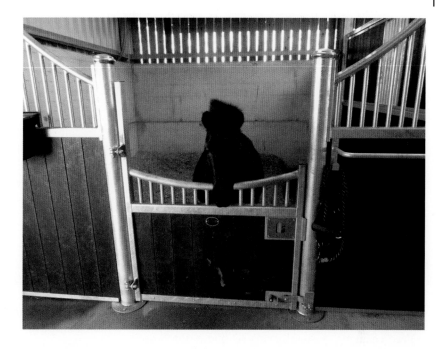

Horses are social animals and are generally happier and calmer if they can see other horses. Although it is not advisable to mix horses and ponies in the clinical environment, enabling them to look out over the stable doors will assist in their well-being while in the practice or hospital. Some stable doors may need adapting for Shetland ponies and donkeys so they can see over the top (Figure 5.1). Some stable doors can house a top grill if needed. Isolation facilities should be available for infectious patients (see Chapter 6).

Stable design is an important consideration. The four main types are:

- Stalls
- Loose boxes
- Barns
- Barn and loose box combination [30].

All stable design types have advantages and disadvantages. It is important to select the design that will work best for the type of yard being built. Building materials are also an important consideration. Wood is traditionally used as it is relatively cheap, however it can be damaged easily and can also be chewed. Brick is more expensive but is stronger and easier to disinfect. Detailed information on stable design is beyond the scope of this chapter. For further information please see the 'Further Reading' section at the end of this chapter.

Fixtures and Fittings

Some fittings are required for all stables however stables in an equine practice or hospital will require some more specific fittings and equipment, which are also discussed below. Care should be taken to ensure that all fittings are

secure and placed in an area that is convenient for staff but will not endanger the horse:

- **Hooks** – are required on the top and the bottom of the stable doors to hold them open and prevent them from slamming which will frighten the horses.
- **Bolts** – on both doors – one on the top door and two on the lower door. A kick bolt is advised on the lower door for extra security as some horses learn to open the top bolt.
- **Metal strips** – are required on the horizontal part of the lower door to prevent the horse from chewing the wood.
- **Tying rings** – should be placed at the front of the stable at the horse's eye-level.
- **Automatic water bowls** – are not usually used in an equine practice or hospital. While they do save on labour, the main disadvantage is that it is not possible to monitor how much the horse is drinking [30]. This is not ideal for RVNs when monitoring sick patients. Usually, a large water bucket is supplied as horses will drink approximately 20–40 l of water per day under normal circumstances [30]. Water should be changed frequently as it will absorb ammonia from the environment. The water bucket should be emptied and disinfected at least once daily for every patient.
- **Feed troughs and mangers** – may be made out of concrete, wood, or plastic. These fittings are useful for patients that cannot have a haynet such as foals and patients with eye ulcers. Feed troughs and mangers must be placed high enough for the horse to feed comfortably, but not so high that the horse cannot reach the food.

Containers must be cleaned out and disinfected regularly to reduce contamination [30].

- **Hay racks and haynets** – hay racks and haynets keep forage in one place, but do not mimic the natural feeding posture of the horse. Ideally, horses suffering with sinus or spinal conditions would be fed from the floor. Haynets must be tied high enough to avoid patients getting their feet caught if they were to paw at the haynet.
- **Feed buckets** – are suitable for use in an equine practice or hospital, as they are easy to clean, and prove to be less of a fomite than mangers. Feed buckets should be placed on the floor to allow for a more natural feeding position for the horse. Door buckets can be beneficial in some patients that need to feed from a raised surface, for example, following dorsal spinous process removal.
- **Fluid hangers** – are hooks attached to the celling for suspending fluid bags for intravenous (IV) administration and other medications. Ideally, an overhead pulley system is used to raise and lower the fluids when the bags need changing. A spiral giving set allows the horse to move freely around the stable [30].
- **Door grills** – These are used to prevent the horse from being able to get their head over the stable door. These are used for patients with indwelling IV catheters. As the jugular vein is most commonly used for IV catheters in horses, the grill is used to prevent the horse from rubbing the catheter on the door and/or pulling it out.

Bedding

Bedding is used to provide warmth and comfort to the horse. A bank of bedding can be built up around the edge of the stable to reduce draughts, provide comfort and to help prevent the horse getting cast (stuck against the wall). The ideal bedding material would have the following properties [30]:

- Warm
- Absorbent
- Soft
- Easily managed
- Nontoxic
- Dust/damp free
- Readily available
- Easily disposable [30]

Table 5.1 shows the types of bedding available for equine patients, and the advantages and disadvantages associated with each.

Table 5.1 Types of equine bedding and the advantages and disadvantages of each.

Type of bedding	Comments	Advantages	Disadvantages
Straw	Barley straw may be eaten so wheat straw is more commonly used as it is less palatable	Good insulating properties. Inexpensive to buy. Easy disposed of and recycled	Dusty and therefore can increase the risk of severe equine asthma (formerly known as recurrent airway obstruction or RAO). Can harbour spores. Barley and oat straw can be eaten and may cause impactions
Shavings	Used as an alternative to straw. Bought in bales	Absorbent and can be bought dust-extracted so better for horses with severe equine asthma. Provides warmth	More expensive than straw. More difficult to dispose of waste. Will compost down in time
Sawdust	Used as an alternative to straw. Bought in bales	Absorbent and provides warmth	More expensive than straw. More difficult to dispose of waste. Will compost down in time. More dusty than savings
Paper	Can buy in bales or shred newspapers yourself	Absorbent and dust free. Reasonably warm	More expensive than straw. More difficult to dispose of waste. Will compost down in time
Peat moss	Used as an alternative to straw. Bought in bales	Inedible. Dust free. Easily recycled. Reasonably warm	More expensive than straw. Can soften the feet. Environmental issues – becoming less readily available
Hemp	Used as an alternative to straw. Bought in bales	Dust and mould free. Warm	Expensive and can be eaten
Rubber matting	Surface is anti-slip and lower surface has drainage channels. Bought as mats	Cheap to maintain after initial purchase. Good drainage and supports horse's feet. Can provide warmth	Initial cost is expensive. Little warmth if used alone therefore will need to purchase additional bedding

Source: Marie Rippingale.

If rubber mats are not being used, a substantial bed must be provided to prevent decubitus ulcers (pressure sores) from developing. The calcaneus, elbows and tuber coxae are the areas that are most at risk for this, especially in a lean or emaciated patient.

Bedding Requirements for Special Cases

Patients often have specific bedding requirements according to their condition. It is important that RVNs understand the different requirements of these patients, to prepare appropriate accommodation quickly and effectively.

Severe equine asthma (see Chapter 13):

- The most important aspect of treating severe equine asthma is to remove the cause of the problem, i.e. dust, mould and or pollen usually found in hay and straw [30].
- Straw should be substituted for hardwood dust-extracted shavings, paper, peat or rubber matting.

Laminitis (see Chapter 13):

- Horses with laminitis need to be stabled and will require soft, supportive bedding such as shavings. As these horses also like to lie down frequently, rubber matting should be used with a deep bed on top [30]. The bedding should be continued all the way up to the door and food and water situated close together.

Colic (see Chapter 13):

- It is vital that these patients do not have access to edible bedding, as they may need to be starved.
- Shavings, peat or paper can be used.
- A deep bed should be supplied, with banks as the horse is likely to want to get down and roll [30].

Utilities

There should be utilities within close proximity of the stables to include hot and cold running water and an electricity supply. This would facilitate clinical treatments and assessments that need to be carried should the horse be unable to leave the stable. This is also beneficial when disinfecting the stable after each inpatient. The electricity supply must be inaccessible to horses, and any sinks must be earthed to reduce the risk of electric shocks or electrocution should a horse interfere with them. The need for hot running water is to facilitate good hygiene practices both for staff and the cleansing of patient receptacles and stable tools.

Fire Safety

Fires will also be of high risk in the stable environment. A fire evacuation plan must be implemented. The premises should be designed to incorporate the fire safety recommendations set out in the Communities and Local Government's 'Fire Safety Risk Assessment – Animal Premises and Stables'. Advice should be sought from the local Fire Prevention Officer in relation to statutory requirements. Highly flammable liquid material or combustible material should not be stored in or close to stables where horses are housed. Smoking in stable areas should be prohibited [6].

Ventilation

Ventilation is important to avoid draughts at ground level, which can cause a chill, but maintain a through flow of air to prevent a build-up of bacteria and reduce the transmission of airborne infection [30]. There are two types of ventilation:

- Passive ventilation:
  - Can be achieved by keeping the top door of the stable open to allow air to pass through and up into the apex of the roof.
  - Air vents allow the air to pass out and fresh air is then drawn in through the door, maintaining a cycle.
  - The heat from the horse rises upwards and further encourages this cycle.
  - This is called the stack effect.
  - Windows should be located on the same side as the door to prevent through draughts but provide light.
  - They should be hinged at the bottom and open outwards. There should be a wire mesh or iron bars covering the glass to prevent the horse from injuring themselves on the glass.
  - The glass itself should be wired safety glass [30].
- Active ventilation:
  - Mechanically pulls air into and/or out of the stable, using an extractor or air-conditioning system [30].
  - Due to the expense of installing active ventilation for stables, it is very rarely seen in equine accommodation.

Lighting

This may be natural or artificial. Natural lighting is achieved by installing windows, skylights and leaving the top half of the stable door open. To ensure that owners and staff can see adequately, some form of artificial lighting must be available [30]. The most common form of artificial lighting is a fluorescent strip light attached to the eaves of the roof. Hanging light bulbs are not ideal as the horse may be able to reach them. Light switches should be placed outside the stable and protected from moisture with a waterproof cover. All cables inside or outside the stable should have sufficient waterproof coverings [30].

Heating

Healthy horses can tolerate a wide range of temperatures if the air remains dry and draught free. However critically ill or injured horses and neonatal foals may require the use of supplementary heating, examples of which are listed below:

- Rugs and bandages – indoor and outdoor rugs are available for all shapes and sizes of horse, pony or foal. Bandages should be applied securely. The use of gamgee underneath will reduce the risk of the patient developing bandage sores.
- Duvets – commonly put under a stable rug to add extra warmth.
- Central heating – effective but very expensive so are rarely used. Heating units should be kept out of horse's reach.
- Electric fans – can be noisy and create dust. Ensure that the unit is kept out of the horse's reach.
- Infrared heat lamps – can be small, portable lamps or permanent lamps fixed to the wall. Either must be a safe distance away from the horse [30].

Cleaning Stables

It is very important that stables are mucked out regularly and correctly to preserve the health of the inpatients and to prevent the spread of disease. As a rule, stables are mucked out properly once daily in the morning and then 'skipped out' (all the faeces are removed but none of the urine) in the afternoon. Each yard should have designated equipment such as a wheelbarrow, fork, yard brush and skip and these can be colour coded for easy identification. This equipment should be disinfected daily.

The Mucking Out Process

1) The horse should be removed from the stable and either tied up outside or put in another stable. This is safer for the person mucking out and safer for the horse as it reduces the risk of injury.
2) Water buckets should be removed and disinfected before being refilled and put back once the stable has been mucked out.
3) Haynets and discarded/uneaten hay should be removed.
4) Starting at the front of the stable, any droppings should be removed and put in the wheelbarrow.
5) The remaining bedding should be forked up so that any further droppings can fall down. These should be removed.
6) Any urine-soaked bedding should then be removed. Clean bedding should be put to one side to be re-used.

7) The floor should be swept and left to dry before the clean bedding is spread back on to the floor. Fresh bedding should be applied on top if required.
8) Banks can be built if required and the front of the bed should be swept back in to a straight line. The bed should be thick enough so that if a fork is stabbed in to it, the floor cannot be felt.
9) The walls, fixtures and fittings should be scrubbed with an appropriate disinfectant and then dried with a clean towel.
10) The clean water bucket and fresh haynet can then be replaced.
11) The patient can then be returned to the stable [31].

Disinfecting Stables

After each horse is discharged, its stable should be emptied of all bedding, cleaned using a suitable detergent, and then disinfected with an appropriate solution. In the case of horses with an infection, the stable should then be swabbed for culture, and cleaning repeated as necessary [31]. All rugs, brushes, headcollars and leadropes, haynets and water buckets used on the horse should be thoroughly washed and disinfected. It is very important that protocols are in place for the mucking out, maintenance and disinfection of stables and equipment. See Chapter 6 for more information on cleaning and disinfecting stables.

Exercise

Horses need adequate exercise to keep them fit and healthy. Turnout allows the 'three Fs' of equine welfare to be fulfilled and these are as follows:

- Freedom: The freedom to move around and act as naturally as possible.
- Friends: The opportunity to socialise with members of their own species. Social interaction is important for the horse as they are herd animals.
- Forage: Turnout allows ab lib access to grazing which satisfies many physical and mental needs of the horse.

Each horse requires approximately 1.25–2.5 acres of grazing of a suitable quality if no supplementary feeding is provided [6]. A smaller area may be adequate where a horse is mostly stabled and grazing areas are only used for turnout [6]. If turnout is not available, ridden or groundwork exercise should be carried out. This could include hacking which is good for a horse returning to work, as hacking is normally carried out on the roads in walk and trot. The intensity can be increased overtime as required. Schooling the horse in an arena with a good quality surface is also a good choice of exercise as the walk, trot and canter gaits can be incorporated into the session. Pole work exercises, lunging, long reining, and the use of other training aids can also be incorporated and can also be carried out from the ground. The amount of exercise given can vary due to age, fitness levels, orthopaedic issues and time factors but is important for health and well-being. The workload should gradually be increased with at least one day off per week. Turnout and exercise are important for the psychological health of the horse and can help to prevent the development of stable vices such as windsucking, cribbiting and weaving.

Grooming

Grooming should be carried out at least once daily in an equine practice as it is an important form of enrichment for horses on box rest. Grooming the horse's coat, mane and tail will keep them free from dirt and grease and will also be an ideal opportunity to check the patient over for heat, swelling, skin disorders, general body condition and rubs. See Table 5.2 for the contents of a basic grooming kit.

Table 5.2 The contents of a basic equine grooming kit.

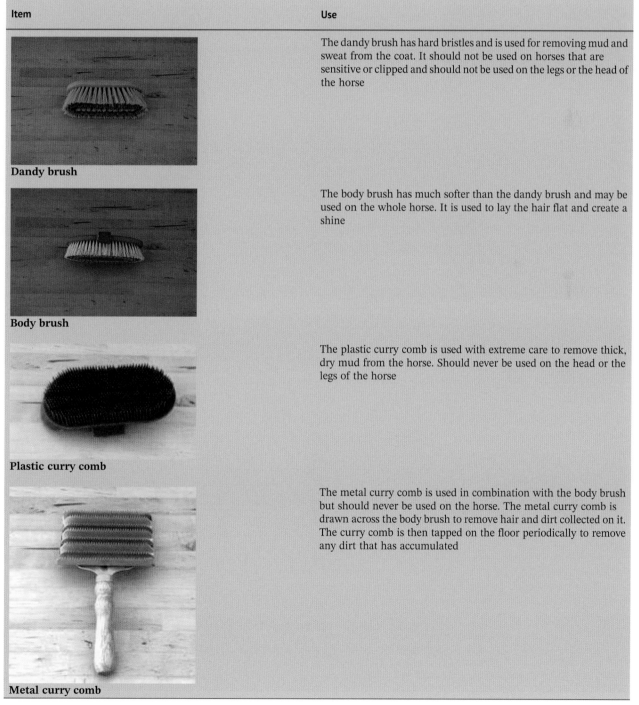

Item	Use
Dandy brush	The dandy brush has hard bristles and is used for removing mud and sweat from the coat. It should not be used on horses that are sensitive or clipped and should not be used on the legs or the head of the horse
Body brush	The body brush has much softer than the dandy brush and may be used on the whole horse. It is used to lay the hair flat and create a shine
Plastic curry comb	The plastic curry comb is used with extreme care to remove thick, dry mud from the horse. Should never be used on the head or the legs of the horse
Metal curry comb	The metal curry comb is used in combination with the body brush but should never be used on the horse. The metal curry comb is drawn across the body brush to remove hair and dirt collected on it. The curry comb is then tapped on the floor periodically to remove any dirt that has accumulated

(Continued)

Table 5.2 (Continued)

Item	Use
Rubber curry comb	The rubber curry comb is used in a circular motion to remove any loose hair and to give a massage
Shedding blade	The shedding blade is used to remove large amounts of hair when the horse moults. Should only be used on the body and never on the legs or face
Sponge	Three separate sponges should be available: one for the eyes, one for the nose and one for the anus. These areas should be cleaned using a sponge and clean water once daily
Mane comb	The mane comb may be made of metal or plastic. It is used to separate the mane and tail hairs. Mane and tail conditioner can be used to ease the separation of the hair and add shine
Sweat scraper	The sweat scraper is used to squeeze excess water out of the coat after bathing or hosing down. Should be used rubber side to the horse and only used on the body, not the head or legs

Table 5.2 (Continued)

Item	Use
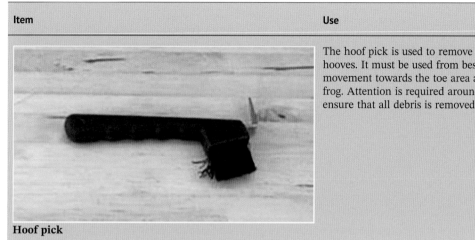 **Hoof pick**	The hoof pick is used to remove dirt and stones from the horse's hooves. It must be used from beside the bulb of the heel in a movement towards the toe area avoiding damage to the sensitive frog. Attention is required around the central and lateral clefts to ensure that all debris is removed

Source: Marie Rippingale. Images used with permission from Dr Francis Boyer.

The adage 'no *foot, no horse*' is a reminder that horses need regular hoof care. The feet must be picked out at least twice daily with a hoof pick. This should still be carried out if the horse is on box rest to prevent problems such as thrush developing. By carrying out good foot care, not only can the RVN discover foreign bodies, but the feet can be checked for any ailments or loose shoes. Regular farriery must also be carried out by a registered farrier, and horse's hooves need regular trimming regardless of whether they are shod or not. The usual interval for trimming and shoeing is 6–8 weeks. This routine should be continued even if the horse is in an equine practice on box rest.

Sheath Hygiene

Many geldings and stallions only exteriorise their penis to urinate or when excited. It is important to check the health status of the horse's sheath to detect any abnormal lesions, lumps or infection. Some horses are amenable to having their penis exteriorised and cleansed while others are not. This can be a health and safety issue for the handler and great care must be taken if trying to do so in the un-sedated or conscious horse. Acepromazine can be prescribed by a vet and administered to encourage horse to exteriorise the penis to facilitate cleaning. Sheath cleaning should only be performed if there is an indication to do so. Indications may include:

- Excessive smegma on the outside of the sheath or inside of hind legs
- Change in urine stream
- Reluctance to urinate
- Swollen sheath
- Swollen penis
- Any apparent discomfort while posturing

Gloves should be worn when carrying out this process. To clean the sheath and penis safely, a small stream of warm water can be run over the penis and the horse can be observed for a reaction. If the horse does not react, cleaning can continue with caution. Health and safety should be a priority, and sedation should be considered if persistent resistance is seen. Skin antiseptic solutions such as chlorhexidine or iodine should be avoided. Once clean, the penis should be dried carefully with paper towel.

Dental Care

Equine dentition consists of incisors, premolars and molars. The premolars and molars are also known as cheek teeth. Horse's teeth permanently erupt throughout its life and problems may arise if not checked regularly. Please see Chapter 4 for information regarding dental anatomy.

Clinical signs of dental disease include:

- Quidding (chewing food then spitting it out)
- Halitosis (bad breath)
- Long fibre strands in faeces
- Anorexia
- Weight loss
- Poor performance

Dental examinations should be routinely performed at least every six months by a vet or a qualified EDT. This would usually involve sedating the horse although this is not always necessary, but it is preferred by most vets as a more thorough examination can be conducted and is a more comfortable experience for the horse. A Hausmann's gag should be placed between the teeth to facilitate the opening of the mouth for the procedure, and to enable the EDT or vet to examine the entire mouth effectively and safely.

Motorised dental power tools are now used to correct the dental arcades. Old handheld rasps can still be used, but these can blunt quickly and require a considerable manual effort to use. A dental chart should be filled in for each horse to document their dental health and any treatment carried out (Figure 5.2). For more information see Chapter 12.

Vaccination

Equids are susceptible to certain pathogens which can be vaccinated against (Table 5.3). The most common are equine influenza and *Clostridium tetani* (tetanus). Vaccinated pregnant mares should have a tetanus toxoid booster 4–6 weeks prior to foaling. This ensures the foal receives maximum protection from the antibodies in the colostrum. Foals of unvaccinated mares or those who do not receive adequate colostrum for any reason should be given tetanus antitoxin at birth. All equids should receive a primary vaccination course then boosted according to the manufacturer's instructions.

Other diseases may also be vaccinated against although not so routinely, and vaccine regimes vary internationally. Vets should always refer to the vaccine data sheet for correct protocols and product information before administering a vaccine as these may not always be consistent with certain equine governing bodies and current epidemiology.

Adverse Reactions

Administering a vaccine, which is a foreign substance, into the body carries a risk of an allergic reaction. Owners should be made aware that an allergic reaction may occur, and they should be advised to report this to the vet if this is observed. Symptoms can range from mild lethargy to severe shock and may include:

- Swelling of the injections site
- Muscle soreness at the injection site
- Urticaria
- Diarrhoea
- Depression
- Ataxia
- Shivering
- Collapse

Non-steroidal anti-inflammatory drugs (NSAIDs) are the most common treatment given although, steroids and supportive therapy may be given for more severe reactions. The reaction should be noted on the patient's clinical records. The reaction should be reported to the Veterinary Medicines Directorate (VMD) via the suspected adverse reaction surveillance scheme (SARSS). See Chapter 9 for further information. A different type of vaccine should be given in future [38].

Parasitology

Endoparasites

There are numerous types of endoparasites (internal parasites) that use the horse as a host during their lifecycle (Table 5.4). Most horses acquire an endoparasite burden from the pasture they graze. Eggs passed in the faeces hatch into L3 stage larvae on the pasture which the horse will then ingest. These larvae then enter the intestinal mucosa where they eventually develop into fourth stage larvae, moult to adults which in turn then lay eggs which are passed out in the faeces thus completing the cycle. The degree of damage done to the horse depends on the type of worm, its lifecycle (whether it remains inside the gut or migrates around the body), the number of worms present, and the health and immune status of the horse (Figures 5.3 and 5.4).

Management of Endoparasites
Pasture Management

Pasture management strategies can be implemented to try to break the lifecycle of the worm burden. These include techniques such as the following:

- Poo picking – removing the faeces daily from the pasture will significantly reduce the amount of worm eggs being ingested, although this is not always possible due to time and weather constraints.
- Chain harrowing – this is not considered effective as a pasture management strategy as it actively spreads worm eggs and larvae around the pasture.
- Resting the pasture – from late summer until the following spring. This aids worm control because most of the larvae on the pasture will die-off over the winter. However, certain species such as large roundworm eggs, can survive in the soil for years.
- Cross grazing equids with other species – such as sheep. This is an excellent way to reduce the worm burden on the pasture. Sheep are not affected by equine endoparasites and are known as 'biological hoovers' for the land.
- Reducing the stocking density of equids on the land. Overstocking results in pasture with a high concentration of faeces and therefore great potential to infect the grazing animal if these faeces contain parasites or eggs.

Worming Strategies

There are three main strategies which are employed when considering the administration of anthelmintics to equine patients.

Interval Dosing   This is the administration of a specific drug at the yearly time interval recommended by the wormer manufacturer [40]. Interval dosing encourages increased use of anthelmintics at lower risk times, such

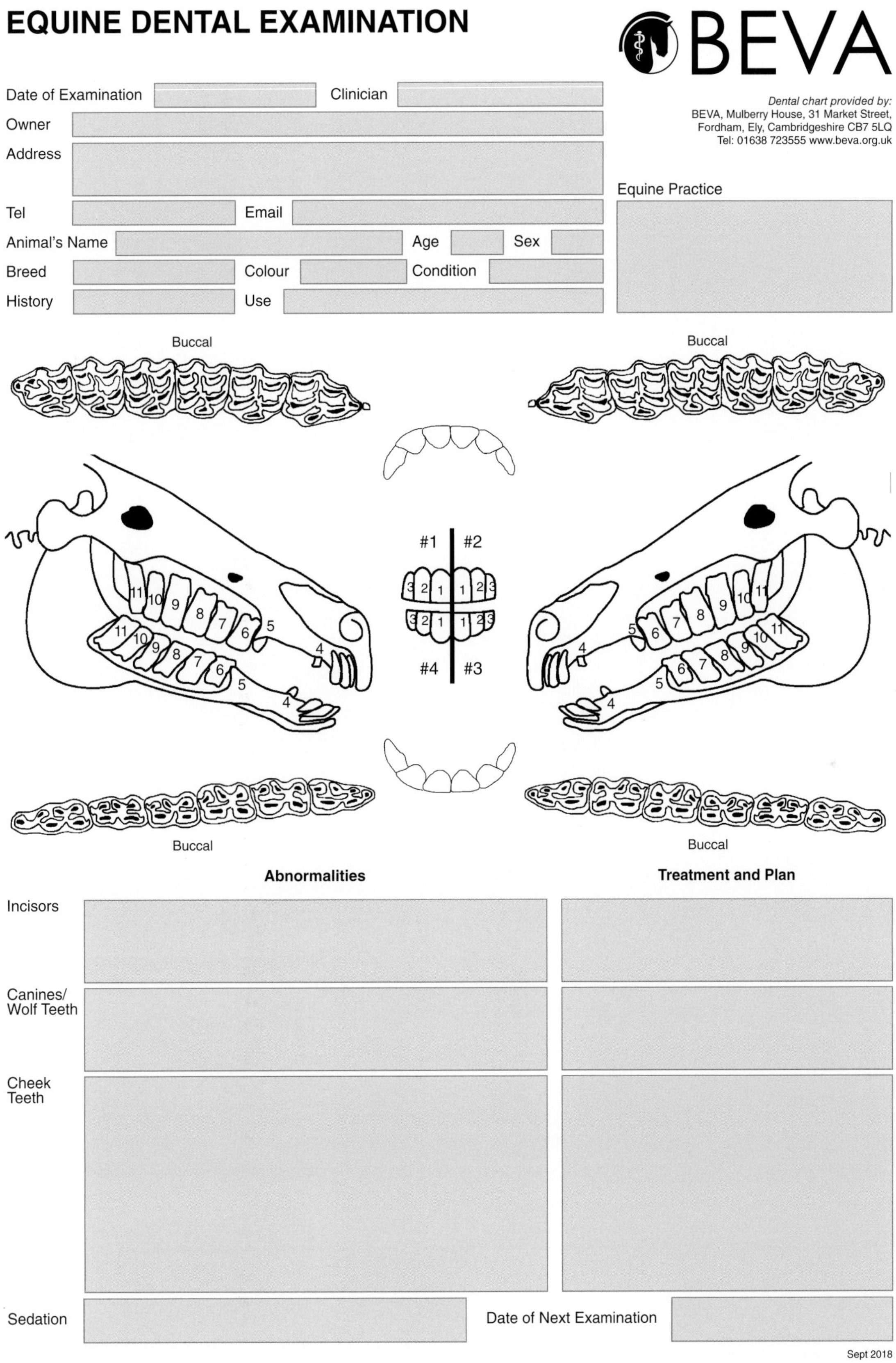

EQUINE DENTAL EXAMINATION

BEVA

Dental chart provided by:
BEVA, Mulberry House, 31 Market Street,
Fordham, Ely, Cambridgeshire CB7 5LQ
Tel: 01638 723555 www.beva.org.uk

Date of Examination _____ Clinician _____

Owner _____

Address _____

Tel _____ Email _____

Animal's Name _____ Age ___ Sex ___

Breed _____ Colour _____ Condition _____

History _____ Use _____

Equine Practice _____

Buccal

Buccal

#1 | #2

#4 | #3

Buccal

Buccal

	Abnormalities	**Treatment and Plan**
Incisors		
Canines/Wolf Teeth		
Cheek Teeth		
Sedation		Date of Next Examination

Sept 2018

Figure 5.2 Dental chart produced by The British Equine Veterinary Association (BEVA). *Source:* Used with kind permission from BEVA.

Table 5.3 Vaccination protocols available for equids.

Disease	Vaccine protocol	Special warnings for each target species
Equine influenza	• Primary course: From six months of age – 1 × 1 ml dose by intramuscular injection. Second dose four weeks later. Third dose (revaccination dose) five months after primary course. This revaccination results in immunity to equine influenza lasting at least 12 months • Yearly booster[a] [32]	• Foals should not be vaccinated before the age of six months, especially when born to mares that were revaccinated in the last two months of gestation, because of possible interference by maternally derived antibodies • Vaccinate healthy animals only [32]
Clostridium tetani	• Primary course: From six months of age – 1 × 1 ml dose by intramuscular injection. Second dose four weeks later • The first revaccination is given not later than 17 months after the primary course. • Thereafter, a maximum interval of two years is recommended [33].	• Foals should not be vaccinated before the age of six months, especially when born to mares that were revaccinated in the last two months of gestation, because of possible interference by maternally derived antibodies • Vaccinate healthy animals only [33]
Equine influenza and clostridium tetani (combination vaccine)	*Influenza:* • Primary vaccination course: From six months of age – 1 × 1 ml dose by intramuscular injection. Second dose four weeks later. Third dose (revaccination dose) five months after primary course. This revaccination results in immunity to equine influenza lasting at least 12 months • The second revaccination is given 12 months after the first revaccination • The alternate use, at 12 months interval of a suitable vaccine against equine influenza, containing the strains A/equine-2/South Africa/4/03 and A/equine-2/Newmarket-2/93, is recommended to maintain immunity levels for the influenza component* *Tetanus:* • The first revaccination is given no later than 17 months after the primary vaccination course • Thereafter, a maximum interval of two years is recommended *Other comments:* In case of increased infection risk or insufficient colostrum intake, an additional initial injection can be given at the age of four months, followed by the full vaccination programme (primary vaccination course at six months of age and four weeks later) [34].	• Foals should not be vaccinated before the age of six months, especially when born to mares that were revaccinated in the last two months of gestation, because of possible interference by maternally derived antibodies • Vaccinate healthy animals only [34]
Strangles	• Primary vaccination course: Administer one dose (2 ml) by intramuscular injection, followed by a second dose (2 ml) 4 weeks later. • Revaccination: In horses at high risk of S. equi infections it is recommended to repeat the primary vaccination regimen after two months [35]	• Vaccinate healthy animals only • Effect of vaccination on further stages of the infection, rupture of developed lymph node abscesses, prevalence of subsequent carrier status, bastard strangles (metastatic abscessation), purpura haemorrhagica and myositis and recovery, is not known • Efficacy has been demonstrated for the individual horse to reduce clinical signs of disease in the acute stage of the infection. Vaccinated horses can be infected and shed S. equi [35]

Equine herpes	• Primary course: A single dose should be administered from five months of age followed by a second injection after an interval of 4–6 weeks • In the event of increased infection risk, for example when a foal has consumed insufficient colostrum or there is a risk of early exposure to field infections with EHV-1 or EHV-4, earlier vaccination may be given • In these circumstances the foal should receive a single dose from three months of age followed by the above mentioned full primary vaccination course • Revaccination: Following completion of the primary course, a single dose should be administered every six months • Use in pregnant mares: To reduce abortion due to EHV-1 infection, pregnant mares should be vaccinated during the 5th, 7th and 9th month of pregnancy with a single 1.5 ml dose on each occasion [36]	• Vaccinate healthy animals only [36]
Equine viral arteritis (Notifiable disease)	• Primary course: administer dose (1 ml) by intramuscular injection followed by a second 1 ml dose 3–6 weeks • Horses can be vaccinated form the age of nine months onwards • Revaccination: Recommended every six months [37]	• Vaccinate healthy animals only • Vaccination does not prevent infection • Vaccination does not have an effect on the shedding of EAV by previously infected carrier stallions • The effect of the vaccine on the fertility of breeding stallions has not been investigated. Under some national legislation EVA is a notifiable disease (UK). Please refer to the national product literature for recommendations on vaccination to comply with this legislation • Equine viral arteritis (EVA) is a notifiable disease in the United Kingdom. Vaccinated horses will become seropositive and therefore it is recommended that they are blood tested prior to primary vaccination to demonstrate that they were previously seronegative. Details of blood testing and vaccination schedule should be recorded in the horse passport • Do not use in pregnant mares [37]

a In January 2024, vaccination rules for equine influenza changed for many equestrian disciplines in accordance with advice from the British Equestrian Federation (BEF). Vaccination rules differ between different sporting bodies, but a summary is as follows. The interval between the 1st and second vaccination has changed from 21 to 60 days. The interval between the second and third vaccination has changed from 150-215 days to 120-180 days. Booster vaccinations are to be given within 6 or 12 months depending on the requirements of the relevant governing body. Readers are encouraged to check the most up to date guidelines.
Source: Louise Pailor and Marie Rippingale.

Table 5.4 Endoparasites that affect equids.

Type of parasite	Species	Clinical particulars	Diagnosis method
Small red worms	Cyathostomes	The normal lifecycle takes place over a few weeks from ingestion of larvae to adult egg laying worms (Figure 5.3). However, these worms have the ability to hibernate within the gut wall in small cysts. The emergence of large numbers of larvae all at the same time (usually during the late winter) can cause huge damage to the gut lining. This can cause inflammation, diarrhoea, colic and death in up to 50% of affected horses [39]. This condition is known as cyathostominosis	Faecal worm egg count (adults only). Blood test (encysted larvae)
Large red worms	Strongyles – *Strongylus spp.*	Larval stage of Stongylus vulgaris can migrate through blood vessels to develop within the major artery supplying blood to the intestinal tract (Figure 5.4). This migration not only damages the blood vessel walls, but can also lead to blood clots and a weakening of the blood vessels. Some species damage the liver and other internal organs with disruption to the blood supply that can cause colic and, in rare cases, death [39]	Faecal worm egg count
Adult roundworms	*Parascaris equorum*	Adult large roundworms can reach up to 50 cm in length. Large roundworms typically only affect foals and young horses, as older horses develop an immunity to them [39]. Adult ascarids and migrating larvae can cause poor growth, digestive and respiratory problems and occasional fatalities. The eggs of large roundworms can survive in the soil and in stables for many years. Young horses become infected by ingesting these eggs from the pasture and their surroundings. Clinical signs can include: coughing, a pot-bellied appearance and weight loss	Faecal worm egg count
Pinworms	*Oxyuris equi*	Pinworms inhabit the colon and are not thought to be harmful. However, pinworms can cause pruritus incited by the egg-laying behaviour of the female worms and by the sticky egg masses in the perianal region when drying, which can result in scratching and damage to the tail	Pinworm eggs are not normally found in faecal samples, diagnosis is normally made by microscopic examination of sticky tape preparations taken from around the anus [39]
Tapeworms	*Anoplocephala perfoliata*	The tapeworm requires a host in the form of the forage mite. Eggs develop within the mite which is then ingested by the horse. The eggs are then released during digestion into the intestines where they attach to the lining of the intestines and continue to develop into adult tapeworms. These tend to congregate around the narrow junction of the small intestine and the caecum (the ileocaecal junction). The presence of large numbers of worms here can cause an impaction to occur and the horse to display colic symptoms. Severe tapeworm infestations can cause digestive disturbances, loss of condition, colic and death. An antibody-based blood test (ELISA) or a saliva-based test, can be used to determine the level of exposure in individual horses	Blood or saliva test

Table 5.4 (Continued)

Type of parasite	Species	Clinical particulars	Diagnosis method
Lungworm	*Dictyocaulus arnfieldi*	Donkeys are thought to be the natural host of this parasite, but horses can also be infected with lungworms. This infection is likely to occur when horses share the same grazing as donkeys. Donkeys can tolerate a large infestation of lungworms without any obvious signs, whereas infected horses show obvious respiratory signs, such as persistent coughing, weight loss and poor performance. Horses and donkeys can live together safely as long as an appropriate worming programme is in place	Faecal worm egg count
Bots	*Gastrophilus intestinalis*	Bot flies are a common irritant to grazing horses during the summer months. The female flies lay their small, sticky yellow eggs on the coat of the horse, typically on the forelegs, shoulder or abdomen. As the horse licks itself, or is groomed by another horse, the eggs hatch and the larvae are transferred into the mouth of the horse, where they burrow into the tissues of the tongue and mouth before being swallowed. Once in the stomach, the larvae attach themselves to the gut lining to continue their development through the winter. The 'bots' eventually detach to continue unharmed through the digestive system to be passed out in the faeces. After pupating in the ground, they emerge as a new generation of flies. Advising clients to remove the eggs from the horse daily with a bot knife can help to disrupt the life cycle [39]	Bot eggs are visible on the coat of the horse. Bot fly larvae are occasionally seen in the stomach of the horse during unrelated gastroscope examinations

Source: Louise Pailor and Marie Rippingale.

as winter periods, when horses spend increased amounts of time stabled. This is expensive and often unnecessary. Also, many horse owners use anthelmintics at inappropriate intervals. The main disadvantage of this strategy is that horses may be dosed unnecessarily which may encourage the development of resistance [40]. Resistance occurs when parasites become tolerant to a drug used to kill them. It is an inherited trait that develops in response to selection pressure favouring survival of worms with the genetic ability to survive chemotherapy [39]. For this reason, it is essential that horses are dosed accurately according to bodyweight. Using too low a dose of wormer may speed up the development of resistance. On the other hand, frequent, unnecessary worming may also increase the potential for the development of resistance.

Strategic Dosing   This is the use of drugs at specific times of year to disrupt the seasonal cycle of transmission [40]. This helps to disrupt the seasonal cycle and transmission of parasites by reducing parasite egg output by horses. This also prevents the build-up of larvae on the pasture. However, problems can arise as a result of abnormal weather patterns. For example, wet, warm summers can lead to early or late peak pasture larval burdens [40].

Targeted Strategic Dosing   Faecal worm egg counts (FWECs) are measured prior to dosing (see Chapter 8 for further information). This is a test which counts the number of worm eggs (Figure 5.5) in a sample of faeces and gives a good idea of the horse's roundworm burden, if any. Only horses with FWECs over 200 eggs per gram (EPG) are wormed. This is the strategy best suited to minimise the problem of resistance to wormers. FWECs should be performed every 8–10 weeks. Diagnostic limitations mean that negative FWECs do not guarantee a horse is parasite-free as, for example, a horse may be harbouring immature parasites which have not yet started to produce eggs. Also, small redworms developing in the gut wall cannot be detected by this method. For this reason, it is recommended that a blood test is performed to determine the presence of small

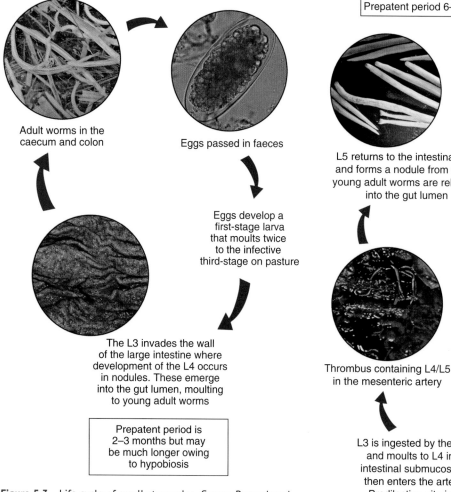

Figure 5.3 Life cycle of small strongyles. *Source:* Reproduced with permission from BSAVA Textbook of Veterinary Nursing 5th Edition © BSAVA (BSAVA Fig 7.44).

strongyles. If this is not possible, an anthelmintic capable of treating encysted cyathostomes should be administered to the horse in late autumn/early wintertime. Tapeworms are not detected by routine FWECs, so a enzyme-linked immunoassay (ELISA) (blood) test or tapeworm saliva test should be carried out in the spring and autumn [39].

If strongyle or ascarid related anthelmintic resistance is suspected, Faecal worm egg count reduction (FWECR) tests can be performed. FWECRT tests are performed by collecting a faecal sample prior to worming and performing an initial FWEC test. The anthelmintic in question is then administered and another faecal sample is collected 14 days following treatment. The following equation is then applied to calculate the percentage reduction in the faecal egg count for the horse individually [41].

$$\frac{\text{Eggs Per Gram (EPG)} - \text{EPG} (14 \text{ days post treatment}) \times 100}{\text{EPG (pre} - \text{treatment)}}$$

$$= \text{FECRT}$$

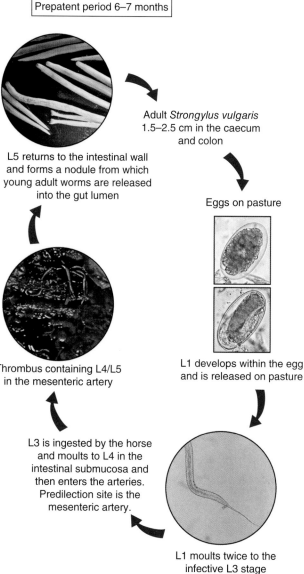

Figure 5.4 Life cycle of Strongylus vulgaris. *Source:* Reproduced with permission from BSAVA Textbook of Veterinary Nursing 5th Edition © BSAVA (BSAVA Fig 7.45).

This test can also be used to assess the presence of anthelmintic resistance in a group of horses. The results of the FECRT should inform the anthelmintic dosing strategy moving forwards.

Anthelmintics

There are different classes of anthelmintics which are available to treat and kill endoparasites. They are grouped into different classes for their effectiveness on targeted species. The four groups are:

- Pyrantels
- Macrocyclic lactones (Ivermectin/moxidectin)

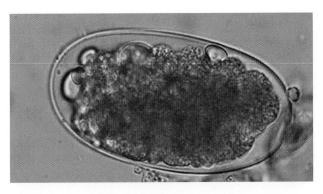

Figure 5.5 A typical cyathostomin/large strongyle egg. *Source:* Reproduced with permission BSAVA Textbook of Veterinary Nursing 5th Edition © BSAVA (BSAVA Fig 7.46).

- Benzimidazoles (fenbendazole)
- Praziquantel

The different active ingredients in the classes can be used alone or in combination to treat several different endoparasites (Table 5.5).

Prescription of Anthelmintics

All anthelmintics are licensed by the VMD and are given a pharmaceutical class. They are usually Prescription Only Medicines (POM) that can only be prescribed by a Vet, Pharmacist or Suitably Qualified Person (SQP) or Animal health Advisor (POM-VPS), who holds the qualification to prescribe equine anthelmintics. A clinical assessment of the animal is not required when prescribing this classification of veterinary medicine, and the animal does not have to be seen by the prescriber. However sufficient information about the animal and the way it is kept must be known to the prescriber in order to prescribe and supply appropriately [42]. See Chapter 9 for more information.

Owner Guidance

National Equine Health Survey (NEHS) 2015 results showed that many horse owners were not worming correctly. About one third of people who thought they had treated for encysted cyathostomins had used an unsuitable product, while around 7% used a product that resistance had been reported on, indicating some horse owners still did not know how to effectively control worms [39]. This is an area where RVNs and SQPs can play an important role in communicating best practice parasite control guidelines. Once a worming protocol has been selected, it is important to advise clients on how to estimate the dose of the wormer accurately. Under-dosing horses with wormers can contribute significantly to anthelmintic resistance. Conversely, over-dosing horses with wormers can cause some unpleasant side effects. The simplest way to

encourage clients to assess the bodyweight of their horse correctly is via the use of a weigh tape. These are cheap to purchase and easy to use. Ideally, an electronic weighbridge could be used to gain an accurate weight for each horse, but this is not always possible due to transport limitations. Some practices/feed companies will take the weighbridge out to yards and offer weighbridge clinics, which can also be very useful for clients. It is important that RVNs and SQPs make clients aware of all the options available, so that they can make an informed choice.

BEVA have produced a toolkit called protectMEtoo to assist vets, RVNs and practices to develop anthelmintic policies for the better, more responsible use of dewormers. More information can be found in the Further Reading section.

Ectoparasites

Ectoparasites are parasites found on the outside of the body within the skin and hair. They may be host specific and some can potentially affect other species. With any ectoparasitic infection it is important to observe good hygiene between patients so as not to initiate the spread of any parasites. Wearing gloves, washing and disinfecting grooming tools, feed and water buckets, and avoiding the sharing of stable tools will all help to limit the spread of disease. Horses that have an ectoparasitic infestation should be tended to last to avoid spreading the parasite to other patients in the practice.

Lice

Lice are a common ectoparasite that affect equids. A lice infestation is most common in groups of horses housed together in the winter months. There are two species of lice that affect equids:

- *Damalinia equi* – a biting louse (Figure 5.6a,c).
- *Haematopinus asini* – a sucking louse (Figure 5.6b–d).

Lice have six legs and are approximately 2 mm in length. The biting louse has distinguished mouth parts compared to the sucking louse. The eggs can be seen by the naked eye within the mane and hair and sometimes the lice themselves can be seen moving within the coat. Clinical signs may present as pruritis (itching), hair loss and in severe cases anaemia. Transmission is by direct contact or inanimate objects for example, feed or water buckets, grooming kits and rugs. Treatment is usually a diluted topical solution of Permethrin [43].

Mites

Chorioptes is a mite which causes chorioptic mange in horses (Figure 5.7). The mite has eight legs and resides on the skin surface. They are most commonly found on heavily feathered types such as cobs. A common presenting

Table 5.5 Equine anthelmintics and their different uses.

Active ingredient	Small red worm adults	Small redworm larval stage	Strongyles	Roundworms (Ascarids)	Pin worm	Tapeworm	Bots	Lungworm	Comments
Fenbendazole	✓	✓	✓	✓	✓	X	✓	✓	Five-day course can be used against inhibited mucosal stages of small redworms. Use in conjunction with FWEC and blood test for encysted small redworm larvae. There is widespread resistance to this wormer group against small redworms
Pyrantel	✓	X	✓	✓	✓	✓ (Double dose only)	X	X	Double dose in spring and autumn (March/April and September/October). Use in conjunction with FWEC, tapeworm ELISA and/or saliva tests
Ivermectin	✓	X	✓	✓	✓	X	✓	✓	Dose according to results of FWEC
Moxidectin	✓	✓	✓	✓	✓	X	✓	✓	Use in conjunction with FWEC or blood test for encysted small redworm larvae. If this is not possible, one single dose required in late autumn/early winter to treat encysted small redworms
Praziquantel	X	X	X	X	X	✓	X	X	Dose in spring and autumn. Dose based on the results of ELISA blood sample or saliva test
Ivermectin & praziquantel (combination wormer)	X	✓	✓	✓	✓	✓	✓	✓	Single dose in spring and autumn (March/April and September/October) for roundworms and tapeworms. Use in conjunction with FWEC and tapeworm ELISA/saliva test
Moxidectin & praziquantel (combination wormer)	✓	✓	✓	✓	✓	✓	✓	✓	Use in conjunction with FWEC, blood test for encysted small redworm larvae, and tapeworm ELISA tests. If this is not possible, one single dose required in late autumn/early winter to treat encysted small redworms. This is the newest equine wormer on the market. It must be used carefully and strategically to help to lower the risk of anthelmintic resistance developing

Source: Louise Pailor and Marie Rippingale.

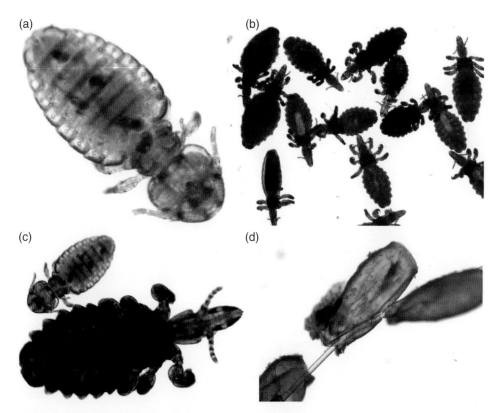

Figure 5.6 Ectoparasites: (a) Damalinia equi (biting louse), (b) Haematopinus asini (sucking louse), (c) Damalinia equi next to Haematopinus asini, and (d) nits of Haematopinus asini attached to a hair. *Source:* Costa et al. (2018) / John Wiley & Sons, Inc.

sign is that the horse will stamp their feet and rub their legs on objects in the stable due to local irritation. Chorioptes may be identified by a skin scrape. They are most prevalent in the winter months. Transmission is by direct and indirect contact. Treatments can be topical as for lice, or a more effective treatment is with an off-license course of the cattle wormer doramectin. Clipping of the feathers may aid in the prevention of infestation [43].

Sarcoptes scabiei are burrowing mites that affect domestic animals and humans. They are responsible for causing sarcoptic mange which is rare in the horse. Clinical signs include pruritis and severe self-trauma often accompanied by excoriation (self-trauma) and skin damage. Deep skin scrapings are required in order to identify this mite. They are smaller than other mites, measuring up to 0.4 mm in length. They are rounded in shape and are covered in distinctive ridges and scales on their dorsum [43].

Ticks

Ixodes ricinus is the species most common to affect horses, dogs and humans. They latch on to the horses' limbs from the grass, so can most commonly be found on the lower limbs. The mouthparts attach firmly, and their bodies enlarge as they feed. The female tick is approximately 1

cm in length, while the male may reach up to 3 cm when engorged with blood. Care must be taken on removal, as the mouthparts can be left behind in the skin and generate a foreign body reaction or infection [43].

Culicoides

Culicoides are small midges which cause intense irritation to most mammals and humans. Some horse and ponies develop a hypersensitivity to the saliva of the culicodes midge. Clinical signs include rubbing the mane and head of the tail until it is inflamed, bleeding, and hair loss occurs. This condition is more commonly referred to as 'sweet itch'. The midge is also a vector for spreading disease [43]. There are many topical remedies available however, prevention is better than cure. Management strategies include:

- Avoiding turnout near open water.
- Housing horses when midges are at their most active for example at dawn and dusk.
- Using fly rugs which cover the mane and tail.
- There is a ringworm vaccine which has been known to provide some relief when used off license for the prevention of sweet itch. Two doses are given two weeks apart in February before the midges start to populate.

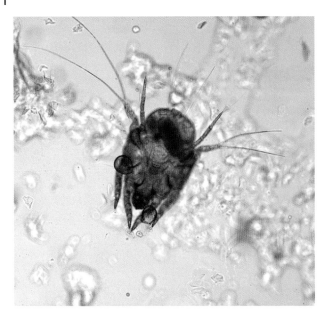

Figure 5.7 Example of a *Chorioptes* mite. *Source:* Costa et al. (2018) / John Wiley & Sons, Inc.

Stomoxys calcitrans

Stomoxys calcitrans is also known as the stable fly and looks similar to the house fly. It causes painful bites to the horse and is a source of great irritation. Management includes the use of topical fly repellent solutions, fly rugs and fly masks. Housing horses during the day in the summer may also help to prevent contact with these flies [43].

Normal and Abnormal Presentations in Equine Patients

Appearance

It is important to be aware of what is normal in terms of the appearance of the horse so that any abnormalities can be identified and addressed promptly.

- Eyes: The eyes should be open, clear and produce no discharge. The eyelids should close naturally.
- Ears: The pinna of the ear should be rigid and highly mobile. The horse will constantly move its ears to listen to the source of different sounds. Disorder affecting the ear are uncommon int the horse.
- Mouth: Incorporates the lips, teeth, tongue and oral cavity. The lips and incisors are responsible for taking food into the mouth. Lip injuries can occur from poor bitting and trauma.

The Nose

Tactile hairs on the muzzle (referred to as whiskers) play an important role in the sensory awareness of the horse. These hairs help the horse to navigate their surroundings. The Federation Equestre Internationale (FEI) outlawed the trimming of whiskers in competition horses in 2020. If this rule is breached it results in disqualification of the horse from the event. The nose should be able to move or twitch freely. A small amount of clear thin nasal discharge from either or both nostrils can be normal, however yellow or greenish purulent discharge from either one or both nostrils is abnormal, and may indicate a sinusitis, a tooth root infection or a number of respiratory diseases which present with an abnormal nasal discharge. Epistaxis (nosebleed) can also be an indication of abnormalities occurring from the nasal cavity, upper or lower respiratory tract.

Genitalia

The mare is more difficult to assess than the gelding as most of her genitalia is internal. The lips of the vulva should be firm, equal in shape and size, and meet in the middle to form an airtight seal. Abnormal defects can result in air being sucked in, and as it is positioned directly below the anus faeces may enter the vulval lips and result in recurring infections. The penis however can be easier to assess when exteriorised from its sheath to pass urine or during excitement in the stallion. The penis itself should be clean and free from any lumps or verrucose lesions. Some geldings and stallions may be reluctant to expose their penis for examination or cleansing, so may require sedation. Smegma beans may form in the male prepuce resulting in dysuria. These are a build-up of dead skin cells, moisture and oils which form into a ball like shape within the prepuce. They can be gently removed in the sedated horse with the aid of lubrication.

Mobility

The horse/pony should have room to manoeuvre whether that be in a stable environment or field. It should have enough room to lie down, rest and roll. These are the normal behaviours of the horse. The horse should be free from any lameness or stiffness and should any of these symptoms develop should be assessed by a vet.

Excretions

In the stabled horse it is easy to assess bodily excretions when mucking out. The normal horse will defaecate 8–12 times in any 24-hour period. The faeces should be soft and break apart on hitting the floor. The colour can vary from brown to green depending on the forage being ingested. A reduced amount of faeces or loose faeces may indicate a gastrointestinal upset and will generally progress to other clinical signs. Faecal output is more difficult to assess in the grass kept horse unless the faeces are removed from the field daily to reduce any endoparasite burden.

Urine should be yellow in appearance and may be clear or cloudy. The cloudy appearance to due to the high number of calcium carbonate crystals in equine urine. The depth of colour can depend on the hydration status of the horse. It can be difficult to assess the volume passed in a normal stable or grass environment.

Weight

Weight may be gained or lost either quickly or over a longer period. Weight gain is usually as a result of overfeeding and lack of exercise but can be linked to certain metabolic conditions such as equine metabolic syndrome (EMS). Weight loss however can be an indication for many clinical medical or dental issues and should be investigated. Body conditioning scoring is a system that can be used to assess body condition. See Section 5.3 for more information.

See Table 5.6 for further information about normal and abnormal presentations in equine patients. Further information on the conditions mentioned in Table 5.6 can be found in Chapter 13. Information regarding clinical examination can be found in Chapter 17.

The Principles of Introducing New Animal Stock

There are occasions when new horses will need to be introduced to an existing herd. This should be done carefully to reduce the chances of injury and the spread of infectious disease.

A new horse should be isolated on arrival to the yard and stabled separately from the rest of the horses. It should not be turned out with others [6]. Separate grooming and mucking out equipment should be used for the new horse. The isolation period will allow the horse to develop any clinical signs of disease that it may be incubating at the time of arrival, and this will allow time for veterinary advice to be sought before other horses on the yard become infected. The period of isolation and any testing for infectious diseases should be determined in consultation with a vet. It would also be a good idea to conduct a FWEC, to identify any existing endoparasite burden, which can then be treated before the new horse is turned out with other horses [6].

Horses need to be treated as individuals, even when they are kept in groups. When creating new groups, care should be taken to minimise fighting and stress, particularly when horses are to be mixed together for the first time. This risk can be reduced by grazing the new animal in an area immediately adjacent to the existing group for a short period prior to their introduction [6]. The turnout area can also be increased to allow for more room. Back shoes could be removed from all horses before a new horse is introduced. This will help to reduce the risk of injury. Plenty of food and water should be provided to ensure that horses

in the group do not feel the need to compete. This will minimise possible fighting and therefore the risk of injury. The group should be closely monitored after a new horse has been introduced [6]. Horses can also be grouped carefully depending on temperament or health status.

However the groups are put together, consideration should always be given to equine welfare. Horses are gregarious by nature and should be able to socialise with members of their own species. Isolating one horse from other horses can have a negative psychological impact [6]. Where this is not possible, to keep one horse with other horses, other animals such as donkeys, sheep and goats may be used to provide company. Horses may become distressed if separated from other horses, or from a horse with which they have formed a pair bond. Donkeys have specific socialisation needs. Please see Chapter 16 for more information.

5.3 Nutritional Requirements of Equine Patients

Introduction

It is important for RVNs to have a basic knowledge of nutrition, in order to provide a high standard of nursing care to equine patients. Providing a balanced diet aids in maintaining metabolic equilibrium which is achieved by the supply of key nutrients meeting daily requirements required to sustain the animal's life stage [44]. Equids are designed to be trickle feeders in the wild foraging for up to 16 hours a day, but due to domestication, their energy requirements have changed. Energy requirements are driven by several factors such as age, breed, temperament, workload and type, climate, overall health and for mares, pregnancy and lactation. The anatomy of the gastrointestinal tract and the process of digestion are covered in Chapter 4. This chapter section will focus on the nutritional requirements of horses. The nutritional requirements of donkeys are covered in Chapter 16.

Essential Nutrients

Nutrients are food components that help to support life [44]. An essential nutrient is one that is required and unable to be synthesised in the body and therefore must be provided as a dietary source. Nutrients are split into energy-producing nutrients and non-energy producing nutrients [44]:

- Energy producing nutrients: Carbohydrate, protein and fat
- Non-energy producing nutrients: Vitamins, minerals and water

Table 5.6 Normal and abnormal presentations in equine patients.

Observation	Normal amount	Abnormality	Associated conditions	Nursing care
Faeces	Average 8-12 piles per 24 h. Well formed	No faeces, very dry or diarrhoea	1) No faeces – colic, shock 2) Diarrhoea – salmonella, enteritis	1) Withhold food, give IV or oral fluids and electrolytes 2) Diarrhoea – clean area and apply barrier cream, tie tail up. Possible IV fluids
Urine	10 l per day. Horse will pass urine 4–6 times per day. Urine may be cloudy and light yellow in colour	1) +10 l dilute 2) −10 l concentrated 3) Red/brown colour (myogloburia)	1) Dilute – pituitary pars intermedia dysfunction (PPID) 2) Concentrated – kidney/bladder problems 3) Red/brown – Equine rhabomyolysis, post anaesthetic myopathy	1) Provide plenty of water, consider Pergolide 2) Provide plenty of water and IV fluids if necessary 3) IV fluids, anti-inflammatories, keep warm
Eyes	Normal horses have few secretions here	Yellow secretions	1) Conjunctivitis 2) Ophthalmic ulcer 3) Irritation from flies	1) Clean area BID, apply barrier cream under eye and give eye drops 2) As above 3) Clean area BID, apply barrier cream under eye and apply fly mask or fly repellent cream
Nose	Small amount, clear	1) Yellow secretion 2) Blood	1) Respiratory infection or strangles 2) Exercise induced pulmonary haemorrhage (EIPH) or 3) Guttural pouch mycosis (GPM)	1) Infection: clean nostrils BID, feed off floor, antibiotics 2) Strangles: isolate immediately, barrier nurse, clean nostrils, apply barrier cream, and bathe any other abscess sites BID 3) EIPH – clean nostrils, endoscope 4) GPM – endoscope, take to surgery
Reproductive	Mare – small amount when in season	Large amount, yellow or brown	Infection	Clean area BID, tie tail up, antibiotics. Check Equine herpes virus (EHV) status if in foal
Reflux	None	Any relux is abnormal	1) Colic 2) Equine dysautonomia	1) Stomach tube every 2 hours if necessary, IV fluids, surgery if required 2) Stomach tube every 2 hours if necessary, IV fluids, Total parenteral nutrition (TPN) may be required

Source: Marie Rippingale.

Macronutrients are needed in relatively large quantities and micronutrients are needed in smaller quantities.

Macronutrients

Carbohydrates

Carbohydrates are composed of the elements carbon, hydrogen and oxygen and serve to provides a major source of fibre and energy within the horse's diet. [44]. Carbohydrates can be classified as monosaccharides, disaccharides or polysaccharides:

- Monosaccharides: Are commonly referred to as simple sugars, are the simplest form of carbohydrate, and include glucose, fructose and galactose. They are found as components of large carbohydrate molecules in legumes and cereals grains. They are broken down in the stomach and small intestine. Fructans found in grasses are fermented in the hindgut. Excessive feeding of non-structural carbohydrates can lead to over production of lactic acid, a fall in pH. and destruction of microbes leading to the release of toxins implicated in laminitis, colic and endotoxaemia [44]. Glucose peaks at 1–3 hours after feeding which is associated with a rise in insulin. This may slow the release of free fatty acids (FFAs) into the circulation, so glycogen stores are used. If the equid is exercised at this stage, there may be a drop in blood glucose during the first stages of exercise, which may not be desirable because the brain can only use glucose as a fuel [45].
- Disaccharides are composed of two monosaccharide molecules linked together and include sucrose (glucose and fructose), commonly found in grass and legumes, maltose (glucose and glucose), which is produced as an intermediate in hydrolytic digestion of starch, and lactose (glucose and galactose), which is important for young foals [44].
- Polysaccharides are more commonly referred to as complex carbohydrates and consist of vast numbers of linked monosaccharide molecules [44]. Examples include starch, glycogen and fibre. Dietary fibre or roughage includes the polysaccharide cellulose (present in the cell walls of plant cells), pectin and lignin. Polysaccharides are fermented in the hindgut by microbes and volatile fatty acids (VFAs) are produced and absorbed into the bloodstream. The are then used as a source of energy immediately or stored as fat [44].

Protein

Protein is a molecule made up of chains of individual amino acids which are linked together by peptide bonds to make polypeptides, and when protein is consumed in the diet, these bonds are broken down so the amino acids can be absorbed for use in protein synthesis and metabolism. The protein or essential amino acids needed by the horse must be provided in the diet as they cannot be manufactured by the body. These include arginine, histidine, leucine, phenylalanine, methionine, isoleucine, lysine, threonine, tryptophan and valine. Important functions of protein in the body include structural enzymatic and hormonal roles, transport of nutrients across membranes and in the blood, and as a component of the immune system [46]. The mature horse requires only moderate amounts of protein approximately 8–10% of the daily ration. Higher amounts of protein, up to 16% of daily ration, are needed for the following horses: geriatric, pregnant, lactating, performance horses and youngstock. Protein is not an efficient energy source, and any excess will be converted into carbohydrates or broken down into urea. Protein is absorbed in the small intestine after being broken down into individual amino acids or small peptides [44].

Fats/Lipids

A typical forage-based equine ration should meet a horse's essential requirement for fatty acids, but additional fats may be required to aid in weight gain, managing inflammatory conditions like arthritis, or preventing and managing gastric ulcers. Performance horses require a large amount of digestible energy to support high-intensity performance, so feeding additional fat can increase the calorific density without increasing volume. Dietary sources of fat are available in commercial concentrate feeds, or feed grade oils such as vegetable, soya or corn. The amount to feed is based on the needs of the individual, or the required effects [45]. Any supplemental oil should be introduced slowly. 10% of the daily diet is suggested as an optimum level when incorporated in a complete and balance feed [44]. Adding oil to an existing feed has the potential to create multiple imbalances and therefore, levels of 5-8% in the total diet are more commonly recommended for high performance horses [44]. A good starting amount is around 0.1ml per kg bodyweight to gradually be increased to around 1ml/kg of bodyweight divided into daily doses.

Micronutrients

Vitamins

Additional vitamins and minerals should not be required if the diet being provided is well balanced. Although health status, individual needs, environmental conditions and workload may necessitate the need for supplementation, see Table 5.7 for guidance. The most common supplements are vitamins and minerals, salt, electrolytes and herbs. All of these are manufactured by feed companies and sold commercially in liquid, powder or pellet form.

All vitamins share certain characteristics, such as:

- They are essential for normal physiological function.
- An absence can cause a deficiency syndrome.
- They are synthesised in the body to level that supports normal function.

Vitamins are divided into fat soluble A, D, E and K and water-soluble groups B and C. Fat soluble vitamins require bile for their absorption and are stored in body fat which makes them more prone to surplus storage rather than deficiency. Water soluble vitamins are absorbed via active transport and are not stored therefore a deficiency in these vitamins is more likely [44]. Thiamine, riboflavin, folic acid are important B vitamins that are required in the horse's diet. Vitamin B12 is not believed to be required other than the amount provided by microbial synthesis and no deficiency has yet been observed in horses [45]. The vitamin C needs of healthy horses are met by tissue synthesis however, horses that have been subjected to trauma, disease or major surgery may require supplementation [45].

Minerals

Minerals are essential in the body for structural components, body fluids, and as catalysts and cofactors for enzymes and hormones. They are classified into macro minerals and micro minerals.

Macro minerals for horses include calcium, phosphorus, sodium, chloride, potassium, magnesium, and sulphur. These minerals are crucial for various bodily functions, including bone formation, nerve function, and muscle contraction. Although these minerals are generally available in a balanced diet, their absorption and utilisation are influenced by several factors, such as the mineral content in the diet, the individual horse's needs, physiological demands, and environmental conditions. Both deficiency and excess of any mineral can lead to health issues, making it essential to use supplements with caution. Over-supplementation can be as harmful as deficiencies, potentially leading to toxicity and other health problems. For more detailed information on the appropriate levels and sources for these minerals, refer to Table 5.8.

Microminerals, or trace elements essential for horses, include zinc, iron, copper, and selenium. These trace elements are vital for various metabolic processes, immune

Table 5.7 Essential vitamins for equine patients [44, 45].

Nutrient	Main function	Signs of deficiency	Signs of excess
Vitamin A	Growth, skin and epithelial maintenance, bone	Poor growth, reduced appetite, weak immune system, night blindness	Poor muscle tone, ataxia, loss of hair, lack of normal growth
Vitamin D	Bone growth, calcium phosphorus regulation, synthesised in skin by sunlight	Skeletal abnormalities, due to reduced calcium uptake, vitamin D may be destroyed by heavy metals and alkaline components of feed	Hypercalcaemia, bone resorption, anorexia, poor performance
Vitamin E	Normal growth, muscle metabolism, antioxidant, promote immune function	Effect on immune system, myodegeneration, poor performance	High vitamin E can interfere with absorption of vitamin A
Vitamin K	Blood clotting	Hindgut suppression, liver function compromise and, haemorrhage	Injectable can be toxic, depression, kidney failure, loss of appetite, laminitis
Thiamine (vitamin B1)	Growth, energy production, nerve function	Reduced growth, reduced appetite, muscle tremors	No records
Biotin (vitamin B7)	Maintenance of hoof, skin, hair and other tissues, metabolism	Poor quality hoof horn	No records
Ascorbic acid (vitamin C)	Formation of cartilage and bone. Biological antioxidant, normal growth, immune system and wound healing	Theoretically not needed in the diet but supplementation may help geriatric horses, those in intense work, under stress or those with lung disease	No records

Source: Lynn Irving.

Table 5.8 Essential minerals for equine patients [44, 45].

Nutrient	Main function	Signs of deficiency	Sign of excess
Sodium	Extracellular cation, nerve and muscle function, water balance	Salt craving, dehydration, decreased intake and production, disturbances in acid base and water balance	Rare unless a salt deprived horse is given free access and overindulges
Potassium	Intracellular cation, normal cellular function including heart and muscle	Reduced appetite, growth problems, weakness, muscles issues	Rare unless parentally excess due to error – cardiac issues
Chloride	Interrelated to sodium, osmotic pressure	Appetite loss, weight loss, poor performance	No records
Calcium	Bone formation, nerve and muscle function, blood clotting	Disturbance in bone quality and growth	Can affect absorption of other minerals such as zinc and magnesium
Phosphorus	Bone formation, energy metabolism, components of cell membrane, acid base buffer in blood and gastrointestinal tract	Skeletal abnormalities, abnormal appetite	Reduced calcium absorption
Magnesium	Bone, muscle contractions, metabolism	Ataxia, weakness, muscle tremors	No records

Source: Lynn Irving.

function, and overall health. A deficiency in these trace elements can have significant physiological effects, such as impaired growth, weakened immune response, and other metabolic disturbances. Therefore, monitoring and diagnosing any deficiencies accurately before initiating supplementation is important to avoid adverse effects associated with improper dosing. Proper diagnosis and targeted supplementation are key to maintaining optimal health in horses [44].

Water

Horses require a constant supply of clean, fresh water as it is a vital nutrient and makes up 60–70% of the body. As a general rule, horses require a minimum of 5 litres per 100kg bodyweight. Water requirements increase with environmental temperature, for example, a rise from 15°C to 20°C will increase water loss by 20% and will therefore increase an adult horse's water requirement by approximately 5 litres [44]. The effects will be greater in the foal, especially in the neonate as they have a greater surface to body mass ratio and an inability to efficiently concentrate urine.

The functions of water in the body are as follows [44]:

- Electrolyte balance
- Temperature regulation
- Removal of waste products
- Transport medium for nutrients
- Major component of blood and lymph
- Required for chemical reactions involving hydrolysis
- Regulates oncotic pressure

Water can be provided through an automatic water dispenser, water troughs and containers or via a natural free running source such as a stream. Monitoring the water intake of patients is an essential part of nursing care. Within a hospital or practice setting, automatic water drinkers are not suitable, as it is not possible to monitor water intake. Suitable containers should be used to allow for the amount of water consumed to be assessed. Such containers should be regularly checked refilled and cleaned. Extra water should always be provided during the warmer months. In the winter, ice should be thawed or removed from water buckets regularly.

The factors affecting water requirements include:

- Lactation
- Exercise
- Stress
- Illness
- Diarrhoea
- Reflux
- Environmental temperature
- Body temperature
- Type and amount of food ingested
- Water losses through excretion or evaporation

Water losses can be replaced through water derived from the metabolism of nutrients, by consumption of water or within the food ingested. High performance horses will lose large amounts of water and electrolytes in sweat. In these cases, access to water, salt blocks (or the use of added electrolytes) should be facilitated to assist in replenishing these losses [44].

The Effects of Balanced Nutrition on Bodily Functions

To maintain a consistent body weight and composition, a horse's maintenance nutritional requirement should be provided. An individual horse's nutritional requirements will depend on several factors including:

- Bodyweight
- Breed
- Age
- Growth
- Reproductive needs
- Exercise intensity
- Environmental factors
- Health status

Each horse has a differing metabolic efficiency, appetite, temperament, and health status, all of which influences their requirements alongside balancing intake with usage. Forage alone may be all an individual needs to achieve maintenance requirements, but if forage alone is not enough, concentrates and legumes can be added to satisfy their needs [45].

To ensure the appropriate and adequate supply of energy is provided to maintain health and vitality, the energy potential of feed needs to be determined and this is done using four pieces of information [44]:

- Gross energy (GE) refers to the total heat produced from the digestion of a food source.
- Digestible energy (DE) is the portion of the food's energy content that can be digested and absorbed by the horse.
- Metabolised energy (ME) is the energy remaining after subtracting the energy lost in urine and gases from the DE.
- Net energy (NE) is the GE minus the energy lost in faeces, urine, gases, and heat

Thermoregulatory mechanisms in horses are important to ensure they maintain a state or normothermia and do not develop either hypothermia or hyperthermia. Horses utilise convection, radiation, evaporation, and respiratory losses to remove heat from the body. To increase their internal temperature, they utilise their gastrointestinal tract. Food sources are digested in different parts of the gastrointestinal tract, but the main area of heat production occurs in the hindgut due to the fermentation that arises in the colon and caecum. Good quality forage will provide the maintenance energy requirement, but cereals maybe required to increase energy demands as they are more rapidly absorbed. Newborn foals have a poor ability to thermoregulate and maintain their body temperature through muscle activity, food intake and shivering. Therefore, a continual supply of milk during the early stages of life is imperative to maintain normothermia. As they develop into the weanling, yearling and youngster phase, their ability to thermoregulate is much improved but again, they need an adequate level of food intake to achieve this. Adult horses maintain their body temperature well if they are in good health and have a supply of forage and concentrates to supplement their energy requirements and allow thermoregulation to occur. In the geriatric or sick horse, thermoregulation can be assisted with the use of rugs, extra bedding, and heat lamps, which can all help to increase the body temperature of a hypothermic patient. Fans, cooling baths or clipping may be required to lower body temperature. Clipping may be required for patients with PPID or ECD, as they may struggle to thermoregulate due to the hirsutism (long, curly coat).

Monitoring of body weight and condition is important to ensure over feeding does not occur, as this will result in storage of excess as fat that can lead to obesity. This could lead to health issues such as insulin resistance, metabolic issues, laminitis, reproductive complications, liver conditions, lipomas, and gastrointestinal problems. Body condition scoring is a useful way of monitoring the condition of an animal and involves an assessment of fat stores on the horse's body. During a body condition score, different areas of the horse are felt to assess fat coverage and give the horse an overall body condition score. Fat feels soft and spongy, but dangerous amounts of fat in areas such as the crest of the neck feel hard and wobbly. In contrast, muscle feels firm but not hard. Regular body condition scoring allows the weight of the horse to be monitored over time and facilitates nutritional modification to ensure optimum health for each individual, which includes underweight horses as well as overweight ones. Figure 5.8 is a guide for body condition scoring in the horse. Body condition scoring in donkeys is different, please see Chapter 16 for more information.

Feeding according to the individual and its workload will ensure homeostasis is maintained. This is achieved by feeding according to energy requirement but also taking into consideration age, health, workload, the body condition required, and environmental conditions. If these factors are not considered, the result will be a under or overweight horse and both these conditions can lead to health implications. The implications associated with obesity have been mentioned previously and some of those conditions are also prevalent in underweight equids such as metabolic issues, gastrointestinal complaints, immunosuppression and gastric ulcers.

Metabolic processes within the body provides the energy required to sustain anabolic and catabolic reactions. Anabolic reactions use energy to build structural components

FAT SCORE CHART

Use the following guide to help you ascertain if your horse or pony is over weight. If you're not sure why not take a photo from the side and the rear then send them to our nutrition team who will be happy to help you? Make sure you score your horse or pony regularly to ensure you spot changes early.

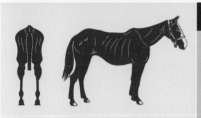

0 - EMACIATED

- No fatty tissue can be felt
- Skin tight over bones
- Shape of individual bones visible
- Marked ewe-neck
- Very prominent backbone and pelvis
- Very sunken rump
- Deep cavity under tall
- Large gap between thighs

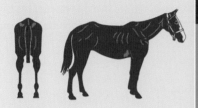

1 - THIN

- Barely any fatty tissue
- Skin more supple
- Shape of bones visible
- Narrow ewe-neck
- Ribs easily visable
- Prominent backbone, croup and tailhead
- Sunken rump; cavity under tail
- Gap between thighs

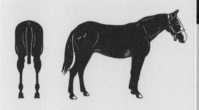

2 - LEAN

- A thin layer of fat under the skin
- Narrow neck; muscles sharply defined
- Backbone covered with a very thin layer of fat but still protruding
- Withers, shoulders and neck accentuated
- Ribs just visable
- Hip bones easily visable but rounded
- Rump usually sloping flat from backbone to point of hips, may be rounded if very fit
- May be small gap between thighs

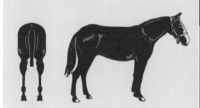

3 - MODERATE

- A thin layer of fat under the skin
- Top line developing and becoming more rounded
- Withers rounded over tips of bones
- Shoulders and neck blend smoothly into body
- Back is flat or forms only slight ridge
- Ribs not visible but easily felt
- Thin layer of fat building around tailhead
- Rump beginning to appear rounded
- Hip bones just visible

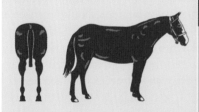

4 - FAT

- Muscles hard to determine beneath fat layer
- Spongy fat developing on crest
- Fat deposits along withers, behind shoulders and along neck
- Ribs covered by spongy fat
- Rump well rounded
- Spongy fat around tailhead
- Gutter along back
- From behind rump looks apple shaped

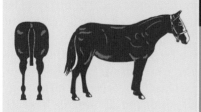

5 - OBESE

- Horse takes on a blocky, bloated look
- Muscles not visible as covered by layer of fat
- Pronounced crest with hard fat
- Pads of fat along withers and behind shoulders
- Extremely obvious gutter along back and rump
- Flank filled in flush
- Lumps of fat around tailhead
- Very bulging apple shaped rump
- Inner thighs pressing together

Figure 5.8 Dengie fat score chart. *Source:* Dengie Horse Feeds.

of the body such as muscle tissue. Whereas catabolic reactions break down large particles into smaller ones and produce energy. Most anabolic reactions occur shortly after feeding, while catabolic reactions tend to occur several hours if not a day after feeding, or after exercise when energy is required. If the metabolism is supported with a balanced diet, these reactions can occur with ease. If the body is lacking nourishment or exertion levels are high, the body cannot maintain the energy requirements, and this therefore puts stress upon the body system which can lead to health issues such as depression, dehydration, fatigue, poor performance [47].

Appetite is driven by several factors in horses which include routine, quality of feed, health, exercise, physical status, mental status, and hormonal status, all these factors can have a positive and negative effect on individuals. Horses thrive on routine and when this is disrupted, it can have a knock-on effect on wellbeing. This can include a reduction in appetite due to stress and anxiety. If left untreated, this could lead to health issues such as gastric ulcers. It is also important to provide good quality feed, and this has less to do with the cost of the feed, and more to do with how the feed is stored. The feed provided must be in date and stored in a dry cool container to ensure there is no damp, dust or mould within the feed. Such contaminants can make the feed unattractive and lead to inappetence and or health issues.

Hormonal factors can also affect appetite especially in breeding animals, stallions often become inappetent during the breeding season due to being so focused on procreating. This can also occur in mares when in season due to hormonal changes. Management in these situations is important to ensure good health is maintained. Studies have been carried out to assist feed companies to create the most attractive feed products for horses, but especially those in poor health as inappetence is commonly one of the first signs to occur. The studies have shown that blackcurrant, banana and mint are the most favoured flavours to be incorporated in commercial concentrates to increase their palatability.

Domestication has changed the nutritional requirements of horses in comparison to wild horses, mainly due to increased energy demands. Wild horses forage for high fibre diets, mainly eating grasses and other herbage which suit their gastrointestinal tracts. Domesticated equids have had to adapt to a change in their diet which includes the introduction of cereal grains alongside their daily forage. Sometimes, this causes complications within the gastrointestinal tract resulting in several types of colic such as colitis leading to diarrhoea, spasmodic colic, or laminitis. It is therefore imperative that any changes to the diet are carried out gradually and with caution. Wild horses are constantly on the move which helps promote gut motility. Domesticated horses are often stabled for long periods of time, and this can reduce gastrointestinal motility and make them more prone to developing impaction colic. This must be managed appropriately, and interventions should be tailored to the individual. This may include considerations such as the horse living out 24 hours a day.

Nutritional Requirements for Horses at Different Life Stages

The nutritional requirements for horses change throughout their lifespan depending on age and lifestyle. Essentially, the nutritional requirements should provide energy to support and maintain the body functions, to include any athletic exertion.

Pregnant and Lactating Mares

Pregnant mares should have their nutritional intake increased as follows to ensure both the mare and growing foetus are supported to an adequate standard:

- 9th month of pregnancy – 1.11 × maintenance.
- 10th month of pregnancy – 1.13 × maintenance.
- 11th month of pregnancy – 1.2 × maintenance.

For example, maintenance intake of a 500 kg mare at month 9 of gestation would be 2% of bodyweight in kilograms which is 10 kg × 1.11 = 11.1 kg. So, total nutritional intake would equate to 11.1 kg total in the form of forage or concentrates and would increase as the nutritional requirements increase through gestation [47].

The nutritional requirements of the mare increase during the lactation period and on average, will increase by 1.5–2 times maintenance but as always, every equid should be treated as an individual and adaptions should be made as required.

For example: 2% body weight is required for daily maintenance and an extra 2% is required to cover milk production, so a total of 4% body weight needs to be fed daily.

For a 500 kg mare, 2% bodyweight is 10 kg so that covers maintenance. Then the extra 2% to cover milk production is another 10 kg. So daily requirement is 20 kg in total of forage and concentrates to ensure nutritional requirements are met [44].

Consideration should be given in the lactating mare, to their increased water requirements. Lactating mares require a minimum of 12–14 lt of water per 100kg bodyweight to sustain good health and adequate milk production. Ideally, lactating mares should be given free access to a constant supply of clean water.

Foals

At birth, the foal is about 10% of its eventual mature body weight and will grow to approximately 30% of its mature weight by three months of age. Growth occurs quite rapidly at this time and relies mainly on the mare's milk as a source of energy and nutrients. Foals may consume 15–25% of their bodyweight per day during their first week of life [45]. The first milk the foal receives from the mare is colostrum which contains essential antibodies. Foals are born without circulating antibodies (agammaglobulinaemia), because the placenta prevents the transfer of antibodies (immunoglobulins) from mare to foetus. Therefore, it is essential that foals receive 2–3 l of good quality colostrum within the first 12 hours of life. In the last 3–4 weeks of pregnancy the mare concentrates antibodies in the colostrum ready for the arrival of the foal. Sometimes, mares can run milk early and unfortunately this can result in the loss of colostrum. Therefore, colostrum is often collected and stored from other mares, especially if the colostrum is of a good quality and quantity when the foal is born, or if the mare loses their foal soon after birth. An alternative option is to use commercially made colostrum, but the best quality is always to use natural colostrum from a mare. Newborn foals must have constant access to good quality milk to maintain their glucose and energy levels otherwise their body will breakdown and utilise other tissues. This is because newborn foals have a low volume of stored body fat. Foals will imitate the mare and start to eat the hay and feed that is made available for her, but this does not contribute much nutritionally until the foals are two to three months of age [48].

Weanlings

Weaning will normally occur when the foal is around six months of age. Sometimes, weaning may be required earlier, but should not occur in foals younger than three months old. As the foals grow, they become more nutritionally independent and ingest a larger quantity of forage and concentrates as they mature and develop.

The weaning process can occur in two different ways:

- A sudden weaning technique can be used which involves separating the mare and foal abruptly and ensuring that they cannot hear or see each other for 2-3 days. This can be quite a stressful process. If there are a number of foals on a stud together, the separated weanlings can be housed together to try to reduce stress.
- A gradual weaning technique can be used where a number of mares and foals are kept together on the same property e.g. a stud farm. The gradual weaning process involves one mare being removed from a herd of mares and foals every couple of days until only a nanny/baron mare remains. Their role is to guide and support the weanlings during this period. The stud team will constantly monitor the weanlings during this period to ensure no injuries or health concerns occur during the process (see Figure 5.9).

Once weaned, the foals are known as weanlings will receive creep feed which has been designed to ensure the appropriate amounts of protein, mineral, and trace elements are provided to support their growth and development. The term 'creep' refers to the enclosure where feed is placed so that only the foal and not the mare, has access to the feed [47]. After weaning, it is a lot easier for the stud

Figure 5.9 Mares and foals grazing. *Source:* Lynn Irving.

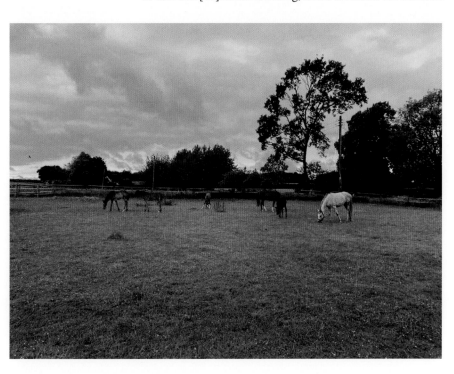

team or owner to control the weanling's nutrition as they can be fed individually, and their intake is more controlled. This is often required if a weanling has 'done well' off a mare and is overweight. The same applies if a weanling needs some extra help to gain a better body condition. Most creep feeds have feeding instructions on the packaging and weanlings should be fed according to their weight and individual requirements. Creep feeds are designed to be palatable and provide mineral and trace elements necessary for healthy growth and development. They come in small pellets and are easy to feed [48]. (see Figure 5.10). Each weanling should be assessed accordingly to ensure a good body score and a steady growth rate is achieved. This is paramount as the weanling continues through their growth period developing into yearlings (1 year old) and then into youngsters (2–5 years old).

Yearlings

Yearlings with free access to good-quality grass or hay may not require and additional feed. If extra nutrients as required, commercial feeds are available for yearlings and are commonly known as youngstock feeds. Again, these are complete feeds containing the correct amounts of protein, vitamins and trace elements required to ensure a healthy growth rate. Feed companies supply guidelines on the packaging to ensure that the yearlings receive the required amount according to body weight. However as

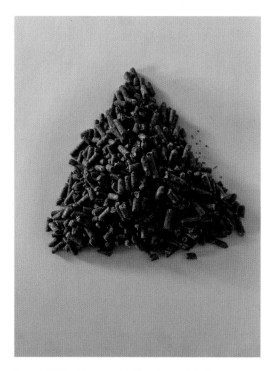

Figure 5.10 Creep feed. *Source:* Lynn Irving.

previously mentioned, each horse has its own metabolism and therefore should be treated as an individual to ensure no health concerns develop due to being over or under fed. It is very important especially in the larger breeds, for example, warmbloods that growth does not occur too quickly, as this can cause musculoskeletal and developmental complications such as:

- Cervical vertebrae stenotic myelopathy (CVSM) more commonly known as Wobblers syndrome.
- Flexure and angular limb deformities in foals
- Epiphysitis and physitis
- Osteochondrosis dessicans (OCD)

Athletic Horses

Increased athletic demands in performance and working horses may mean that the natural diet cannot satisfy the higher energy levels required by their workload. Higher energy demands can be met through feeding grain in the form of cereals. The non-structural carbohydrates from the grain (glucose, fructose and starch) are digested in the stomach and absorbed by the small intestine, making glucose available for anaerobic respiration [44]. When energy demand is very high, the quantity of cereals needed to meet requirements would overload the stomach and small intestine, allowing unabsorbed sugars to pass into the hindgut, where rapid fermentation would occur and lead to an overproduction of lactic acid, a fall in pH, destruction of microbes and the release of toxins. This sequence of events could lead to metabolic disturbances and the development of laminitis. Feeding fat is a safer way to meet energy requirements in these athletic horses. Fats are absorbed in the small intestine but are less likely to cause metabolic disturbances. Oil supplementation is a good way to introduce more fat into the diet. A source of high-quality protein (soyabean rather than oats) should also be provided for these horses. As mentioned previously, electrolyte supplementation should be considered for horses who have sweated excessively.

Geriatric Horses

Geriatric horses may be fed a normal maintenance ration if this allows them to maintain good body condition. However, conditions such as poor dentition may necessitate alterations to the diet, as poor mastication of forage will lead to lowered fibre digestibility and therefore, reduced intake. Where there is a loss of body condition but no other disease, a palatable, easily masticated diet that has a slightly higher protein content (12-16%) can be fed [44]. A 'hay replacer' diet may be offered which consists of short chop chaff, a compound feed such as grass nuts, and sugar beet all soaked down so that it is easy for the horse to chew. The hay replacer diet should be complied and fed according the horse's individual nutritional requirements. Oil can also be fed to increase the level of fat in the diet and encourage weight gain as mentioned earlier in this chapter section.

Nutritional Requirements

The basal metabolic rate (BMR) is the amount of energy expended by an animal while at rest, in a thermoneutral environment, with the digestive system inactive and in a post absorption state. The release of energy in this state is sufficient only for cellular processes such as respiration, circulation, and organ function. Factors that determine the BMR for an animal include:

- Species
- Bodyweight
- Age
- Hormonal status

Changes to these factors will, overtime alter the animal's BMR [44].

Nutritional requirements needed to maintain body weight in healthy, inactive adult horses have been calculated to be approximately 33–40 kcal/kg/day [6]. Gross energy (GE) is the total energy released by complete oxidation of food and is usually measured by burning food in an atmosphere of pure oxygen, in a calorimeter, an instrument that accurately measures heat released by combustion. No animal can utilise the gross energy content of its food, and the extent to which it can be digested and absorbed is known as the digestible energy (DE). Digestibility is measured as the difference between the amount eaten and the amount lost through faeces. Increased digestibility results in a reduced quantity of faeces being produced and reduced demands on the body system to eliminate waste. Only a portion of the DE is made available for tissues, the remainder is lost through faeces and methane production. The digestible energy amount required to meet maintenance energy needs in a normal active, non-working adult horse is the maintenance DE (DEM) and is calculated based on the bodyweight (BW) of the horse in kilograms as follows: DEM = (Mcal/day) = (BW) (0.03) + 1.4 [49].

The remaining portion is utilised by the tissues is metabolisable energy (ME). The digestible and metabolisable energy content of food varies according to the species and individual metabolic efficiency.

Maintenance energy requirements (MER) are the energy requirements of a moderately active adult equid in a thermoneutral environment. It includes the energy needed for obtaining, digesting, and absorbing nutrients in amounts to maintain bodyweight, as well as energy for spontaneous exercise. It does not include the energy required for additional work, gestation, lactation, growth, or repair, especially when illness or disease is present, so additional energy will be required in these situations [44]. Each individual horse requires a personalised feeding plan which should include regular monitoring of weight, body condition scoring and daily assessment to ensure that any extra energy requirements are met.

The amount of energy required for maintaining homeostasis while the animal rests in a stress free, nonfasted, thermoneutral environment is known as resting energy requirements (RER). There are two ways to work out the RER either by using kilograms or by using calories. An equid in lightwork requires 1.5–2% of its body weight in food per day and this increases depending on the workload, so 2–2.5% for moderate work and 2.5–3.5% heavy work.

Example 1 – Kilograms

500 kg horse in light work
500 kg ÷ 100 × 2 = **10 kg**
10 kg is then split 70% roughage – 7 kg
30% concentrates – 3 kg

Working out the RER utilising calories on the basis that in lightwork the equid requires 15,000 calories a day, moderate work 25,000 calories a day, heavy work 33,000 calories a day.

Example 2 – Calories

450 kg horse in moderate work requires **25,000 calories per day**
70% roughage – 17,500 calories
30% concentrates – 7500 calories

Utilising the feed information on the feed packaging, concentrates, forage, and supplements can be allocated according to the calorie allowance. These calculations are only broad guidelines, and every horse is an individual therefore, continuing assessment is required, and modification should be carried out if needed.

Energy density value of the feed is required, so the correct number of calories can be calculated. To calculate the energy density of a feed product, the total kilocalories from the fat, protein, and carbohydrates (carbon, hydrogen, and oxygen – CHO) information need to be added together. This will give the total energy density per 100 g.

For example:
Feed: Dengie Alfa-A Molasses Free

- Protein 14%
- Fats and oils – 8.5%
- CHO – 25.5%

Protein 14 + fats and oils 8.5 + CHO 25.5 = 48 kilocalories.

Therefore the total energy density = **48 kilocalories per 100 grams.**

For example:
Feed: Allen & Page Calm and Condition

- Protein 12%
- Fats and oils 6%
- CHO 58%

Protein 12 + fats and oils 6 + CHO 58 = 76 kilocalories.
Therefore the total energy density = **76 kilocalories per 100 grams.**

If the CHO are not available on the feed packaging, the protein, oil, ash, and fibre should be added together, and then this figure needs to be subtracted from 100. This will give the CHO percentage per 100 g to enable the energy density of the feed product to be calculated [44].

For Example:
Feed: Baileys Conditioning Cubes

- Protein = 12.5%
- Oil = 5.5%
- Ash = 6%
- Fibre = 9%

Protein 12.5% + oil 5.5% + ash 6% + fibre 9% = 33%
100–33% = 67% carbohydrates per 100 grams.

Roughage, Concentrates and Forage Replacers

Horses are hindgut fermenters who naturally live on a predominantly forage based diet, as the fibrous components act as a good source of energy. Forage also known as roughage, needs to be the main component of the diet, even for performance horses. Most sources of roughage come in the form of grass, hay, haylage, lucernes or beet pulp. On average, a horse should have access to 1.5–2% of their body weight in roughage and or grains and concentrates available every day. Most horses are fed at least 50% of their diet through a suitable source of roughage and the rest is made up with grains or concentrates depending on their energy requirements [45].

Grass is the most natural form of roughage for horses. It is also the best form because the horses must graze to gain each mouthful, so a constant trickle of food is entering the digestive tract (Figure 5.11). The nutritional value of grass changes through the seasons with it being most nutritious in the summer and the least nutritious in the winter.

Hay is harvested grass which is cut and left to dry outside for 2–3 days, and then baled and stored for later

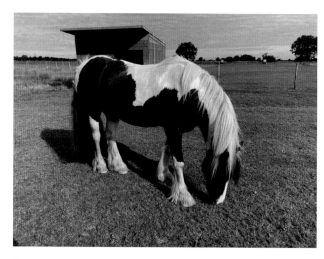

Figure 5.11 Horse grazing. *Source:* Lynn Irving.

use. Hay tends to contain more dust and fungal spores than haylage, and this can lead to respiratory irritation, and the development of a condition known as severe equine asthma. There are different types of hay depending on the seed used such as meadow, timothy, and oat. Different types of hay have different nutritional values, so they should be selected and fed depending on the individual requirements of each horse. Once harvested, if hay is stored in a dry barn with good airflow, it will retain its nutritional value for 2–3 years. Hay is typically 80–95% dry matter. Dry matter (DM) refers to the feed or roughage left after the moisture has been taken out whereas the term 'as fed' refers to a feed as it would be fed to a horse.

Haylage is grass that is harvested slightly earlier than hay, dried for 12–24 hours, and then baled so that it is 50–70% dry matter. Haylage production relies on an anaerobic environment, which is why it is wrapped in plastic and sealed to exclude as much air as possible. The fermentation progress inhibits the development of fungal spores., and this also helps to preserve the grass. Haylage has a high energy level and moisture content. It is also very palatable. As haylage contains fewer fungal spores than hay, it is less likely to cause respiratory irritation.

Silage is grass that is harvested, baled, and stored immediately. It is wrapped and sealed to exclude as much air as possible. This method of harvesting causes a rapid drop in pH, greater water activity and a decrease in available oxygen and soluble carbohydrates. As with haylage, the fermentation progress inhibits the development of fungal spores.

Table 5.9 Forage and forager replacers.

Type of forage	Comments
Chaff	Made from chopped straw or hay. Good source of fibre
Alfalfa (Figure 5.12)	Made from chopped alfalfa hay. Same plant family as peas and beans. Provides high levels of protein
Sugar Beet	Made from sugar beet plants. **MUST BE FED SOAKED.** High in fibre and low in sugar. Provides slow-release energy and is low in starch
Fibre Beet	**MUST BE FED SOAKED.** Combination of sugar beet, alfalfa, and oatfeed. Provides highly digestible fibre. Low in starch and sugar
Ready Grass (Figure 5.13)	Made from dried grass. Good source of forage if no grazing is available or the horse is on box rest
Lucerne Pellets	Good source of fibre and protein

Source: Lynn Irving.

The difference between haylage and silage is the moisture content but otherwise they are very similar with regards to harvest and storage. Most horses are fed hay or haylage, and sileage is more commonly fed to livestock such as cattle. Feeding silage carries a higher risk of botulism which is a paralysing disease caused by toxins from the anaerobic soil-borne bacteria *Clostridium botulinum*. Soil contamination within the bale can introduce botulinum bacteria which will produce botulinum toxin. When the contaminated silage is eaten, the toxin is absorbed and binds irreversibly to nerve/muscle junctions causing flaccid paralysis. Horses are extremely sensitive to the botulinum toxin and the prognosis for survival is guarded [50].

Legume hays such as alfalfa and lucerne are harvested like hay and stored in bales. Legume hay is different to grass hay as it uses bacteria in the nodules of its roots to acquire nitrogen from environment and use it to make protein. This makes legume hay higher in protein, energy, calcium, and vitamin A. It is fed to competition horses or horses requiring an increased energy supply. Care must be taken when feeding legume hay to young horses, as too much protein could lead to developmental diseases. This can affect bone development and overload the kidneys and liver due to excess levels of ammonia [44].

All roughage fed to horses should be of good quality and be free from dust, and fungal spores. The roughage must be visually inspected to check for mould and it should smell fresh. Mouldy haylage and sileage have a distinct pungent smell and should not be fed to horses, as it can cause colic and diarrhoea. A hay steamer can be used to remove a range of contaminants and airborne particles from hay while preserving the nutritional content. Although soaking the hay in water will reduce contaminants and air borne particles, it will also remove water soluble carbohydrates and sugars. Therefore, the nutritional requirements of the horse should be considered, as soaking the hay can drastically reduce the number of calories being fed. If dusty or spore contaminated roughage is fed to horses this can cause severe equine asthma, which may require veterinary treatment. Care should also be taken by personnel when handling roughage, wearing a mask is recommended to prevent the inhalation of dust or contaminants. If access to roughage is limited, good quality forage replacers are commercially available to ensure nutritional requirements are met (see Table 5.9 and Figures 5.12 and 5.13).

Roughage alone is not always enough to meet the nutritional requirements of domesticated horses. Other feed products can be utilised to bridge the energy gap. These can include compounds feeds which are complete feeds or concentrates which are complementary. Compounds feeds are available commercially through feed companies who produce a mixture of grains and cereals with added vitamins and minerals. Compound feeds tend to include a molasses binder which reduces dust and increases palatability. Molasses free options have been developed for use in horses who are prone to laminitis. Extruded or pelleted feeds also known as nuts, are often used. They are produced by grains and cereals that are cooked under high pressure, at a high temperature to produce a slurry that is made into nut pellets. The quality of compound feeds has increased over the years as feed companies use dedicated nutritionists to ensure that the feeds created can meet a large range of nutritional requirements.

Concentrates are used more for specific cases as the nutritional value for each of the separate concentrate needs to be

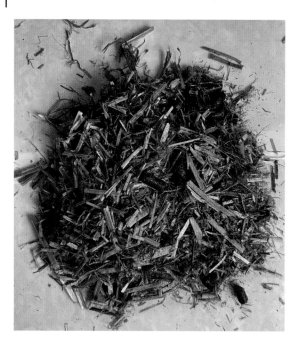

Figure 5.12 Dengie alfa-A molasses free *Source:* Marie Rippingale.

calculated. They can be fed whole or processed by cracking, rolling, or flaking and come in several forms such as the following [44]:

- Oats – these are a starch-based energy source and easy for horses to chew. Oats have the lowest digestible energy concentration of the commonly fed grains, due to the high crude fibre content (10%) in the outer hull. Oats are low in calcium but have a reasonably high level of phosphorous. They are a poor source of vitamins. Due to oats being deficient in some essential amino acids, the quality of protein they contain is poor.
- Maize – has the highest energy level of all commonly fed grains as it lacks an outer fibrous hull. Maize needs to be

crushed or cracked for optimum digestibility. Maize should make up no more than 25% of any grain mix fed, due to its fibre and high energy content. Feeding of maize should be reduced or avoided on rest days. Maize is a good source of vitamin A but is deficient in the amino acids lysine and tryptophan.

- Barley – this is less palatable than oats or maize and has a similar level of protein as oats and is in the middle in terms of energy value between oats and maize. Barley is low in fibre and should be mixed with sufficient roughage to avoid digestive upsets. To increase palatability and energy availability, barley should be rolled and heated before feeding.
- Bran – this is made up of the outer covering of the wheat grain and is a by-product of flour production. Bran is fed less commonly nowadays and in the past has been be used for its laxative properties and to make mashes. It has a poor amino acid balance, is low in calcium and high in phosphorous and this can lead to nutritional imbalances. Other, more nutritionally balanced alternatives are now available, however, if bran is fed, it should be limited to 10% of the feed.
- Sugar beet pulp – this is the by-product of the sugar refining industry. Most of the non-structural carbohydrate has been removed, leaving mostly structural carbohydrate or fibre. The energy value is between that of cereals and grass, but sugar beet pulp is better used as part of the forage component of the diet. **Dried sugar beet should always be soaked in water prior to feeding** as it swells in contact with water. If eaten dry, this swelling can cause a major obstruction.

Compound feed or concentrates are not a substitution for roughage they are to be used to provide extra energy or to complete a balanced diet [44]. A comparison of compound and concentrate feeds can be seen in Table 5.10.

As previously mentioned, dry matter basis (DM) refers to the feed or roughage after the moisture has been taken out

Table 5.10 Comparison of compound and concentrate feeds.

Compounds	Concentrates
Ready made	Separate feeds such as: oats, barley and bran
Come in a coarse mix or pellet/nut form	Need to calculate individual nutritional requirement for each horse before feeding and select different feeds to mix together
Includes vitamins and minerals	No vitamins and minerals included
Convenient and reasonably cheap	Can be time consuming and expensive to create a good quality feed
Palatable. Formulated by professionals	Can be bland. Formulated by the owner
Nutritionally balanced	May not be nutritionally balanced. Could cause laminitis or colic

Source: Lynn Irving.

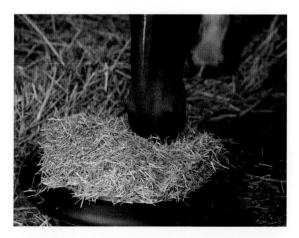

Figure 5.13 Dengie ready grass. *Source:* Dengie Horse Feeds.

whereas the term as fed refers to a feed as it would be fed to a horse. Only the DM contains nutrients therefore, if the feed contains more water, then a larger quantity will be required to meet the requirements. Requirements can be given in a variety of ways:

- Per kg DM feed intake
- Amounts per day on an as fed basis

To convert from as fed to a DM basis, the as fed value is divided by the DM percentage.

For example:
The pasture protein content on an as fed basis is 4% and the DM content is 40%.

The protein content on a DM basis would be 4 ÷ 40 × 100 = 10%.

To convert from DM to as fed basis, multiply the as fed value by the DM percentage:
Cereal protein content on a DM basis is 12% and the DM content is 90%.

The protein content on an as fed basis would be 12 × 90 ÷ 100 = 10.8% [45].

Supplements

There are a wide range of supplements available for horses. The most common supplements are oils, salt, vitamins, and minerals. If a compound feed or well-balanced concentrate diet and roughage is being provided, supplements should not be needed. However, if there is a health, environmental, or workload-based reason that the nutritional requirements of the horse are not being met, then supplementation may be required. Clients should be encouraged to consult an RVN or vet before feeding a supplement as they are costly and might not be necessary.

The Effects of Illness and Injury on Nutritional Requirements

Horses thrive on routine, both physically and mentally, and change, stress or illness may cause their nutritional requirements to change. If the horse is ill or injured, the metabolic rate may be affected because the body must work harder to repair damaged tissues and to create an immune response. Nutritional requirements will also be affected if the individual is hospitalised, as activity levels will be dramatically reduced. It is important to ensure adequate protein requirements in critically ill horses. Daily protein requirements in an adult horse equal 0.5–1.5 g protein/kg/day. However, in critically ill horses where protein catabolism can limit tissue healing, protein should be provided at 1–2 g/kg/day if hepatic function is adequate [49].

The feeding pattern of a horse may be disrupted due to anxiety and a change of environment if hospitalised. The diet may have to be altered due to the present condition, disease, or injury to assist in treating the ailment or to support and promote repair and recovery. The gastrointestinal tract may be affected if box rest or hospitalisation is required, and a laxative diet may be recommended to prevent a reduction in gut motility and reduce the risk of a pelvic flexure impaction occurring. If a disease or illness is diagnosed, nutritional requirements may have to change to aid in the recovery or as part of the treatment regime.

Liver Dysfunction

If a horse is diagnosed with liver dysfunction or damage, they will require a low protein, high carbohydrate diet to include a high percentage of forage such as hay and grass turnout alongside sugar beet, alfalfa, and ready grass. This diet being high in carbohydrates and starch will decrease the need for hepatic glucose synthesis, allowing the liver to recover and repair. Feeds need to be small in size and spread out throughout the day to minimise the burden on the hind gut. All these changes will have an effect on the horse, and this must be taken into consideration. For more examples of feeding for other specific conditions, see Table 5.11.

RVNs managing dietary changes in practice must take care to monitor patients closely for signs of secondary complications. RVNs also have a significant role to play in supporting clients who need to manage dietary changes in their horses. RVNs can help to guide and advise clients on dietary changes and even go out and provide follow up support on visits. This kind of follow up visit can help to increase client concordance with home care guidance and lead to a consistent provision of care. This will in turn increase the changes of a successful recovery for the patient.

Table 5.11 Examples of suggested diets for different clinical conditions.

Condition	Main considerations	Comments
Colic	Specific diets exist for different types of colic, and these should be followed where possible. In general, **guidance for equids prone to colic** are as follows: Reduce amount of starch fed in diet to <1 g/kg bodyweight (BW) per meal. Provide non-edible bedding. Feed little and often. Avoid rapid or major changes to diet. Ensure regular access to grazing. Ensure adlib access to roughage [51]	Medical treatment should be administered as required [51]
Equine gastric ulcer syndrome (EGUS)	Ensure adlib access to roughage. Starch intake should be restricted to <1 g/kg BW per meal and <2g/kg BW/day. Vegetable oil can be used to provide additional energy. Vitamin and mineral balance of diet should be checked and amended as required. Ensure regular access to grazing. Provide a probiotic supplement where appropriate. Ensure constant access to clean water, even when turned out [51]	Reduce stressful situations as much as possible, e.g. travelling, changing environments and long periods of confinement. Medical treatment should be administered as required [51]
Diarrhoea	Requirements vary however, additional protein is usually required. If diarrhoea is due primarily to small intestinal dysfunction, grain should be reduced, and grazing may be restricted. Highly digestible fibre should be provided for example, non-molassed sugar beet pulp, psyllium or soya hulls. Overtly mature, poorly digestible hays should be avoided. Once the diarrhoea has resolved, oil supplementation can be introduced gradually starting around 0.1 ml/kg BW and build up over approximately three weeks to around 1 ml/kg BW if weight gain is required. If small intestinal fat digestion is impaired for more than two weeks, parenteral administration of fat-soluble vitamins A, D, E and K is advised. Vitamin B supplementation may also be required. Probiotics may be useful [51]	Medical treatment should be administered as required. Electrolyte status should be monitored [51]
Laminitis	**General advice:** Prevention is better than cure. Equids prone to laminitis should be fed a diet based on forage with minimal/no cereals. If an energy source is required, oil should be used. Restrict access to grazing. Grazing muzzle may be useful. Forage analysis should be carried out. Ideally only forage with <10% Non-structural Carbohydrates (NSC) should be fed. Hay can be soaked in clean water to reduce the Water-Soluble Carbohydrate (WSC) content. However, results from this are variable so having forage analysed first is advisable. A broad-spectrum vitamin and mineral supplement can be provided. Make any dietary changes slowly and gradually. Do not starve obese patients and this can predispose them to hyperlipemia	Predisposing conditions should be tested for, e.g. PPID or EMS Maintain a regular exercise regime if appropriate, e.g. if no active laminitis is present. Avoid development of obesity by aiming for a body condition score of 5/9 Monitor weight changes regularly using an electronic weighbridge or weightage [51]

| EMS | **Turnout advice:** Turn out when levels of fructans/WSC levels are likely to be low, e.g. late at night or early in the morning. Avoid turnout during the middle part of the day. Co-graze with other species such as sheep to keep grass levels low. Restrict/avoid turnout when the grass undergoes rapid growth, e.g. early spring and autumn. Restrict/avoid turnout when the grass has been exposed to low temperatures, e.g. frost following by warm, sunny weather. Avoid pastures that have been 'stressed' through drought [51]

Initial diet: Restrict or eliminate grazing and do not feed grain. For weight loss feed grass hay with a low NSC content in amounts equivalent to 1.5% of current BW on an as fed basis daily. If weight loss is resistant, lower amount fed to a minimum of 1.2% BW [52]. Forage analysis should be carried out. Ideally only forage with <10% NSC should be fed [51]. Hay can be soaked in cold water for at least 60 minutes to reduce the WSC content [52]. A broad-spectrum vitamin and mineral supplement can be provided. Make any dietary changes slowly and gradually. Do not starve obese patients and this can predispose them to hyperlipemia [51]

Maintenance diet: Restrict grazing and do not feed grain. Maintain on initial hay amount unit body condition score 5/9 is achieved. Soak hay and provide a vitamin and mineral balancer. The decision to increase grazing should be made after clinical signs of laminitis have resolved and be based upon the results of follow up testing in consultation with the case vet. Grazing muzzles and strip grazing strategies should be employed to restrict the intake of grass [52] | Reassess BW every 30 days using an electronic weighbridge or weight tape. House in a dry-lot or small paddock with a companion. Keep stress to a minimum [52]. Exercise is recommended unless active laminitis is present. In previously laminitic horses that have fully recovered, the recommendations are low to moderate intensity exercise on a soft surface for >30 minutes, >3 times per week while monitoring for signs of lameness. For horses with no signs of lameness minimum recommendations are low to moderate intensity exercise >5 times per week [52] |

Source: Marie Rippingale.

5.4 Methods of Equine Identification

Introduction

There are many identifiers that can be used for equine patients, and these rely on not only using their individual features but also many acquired methods of identification.

Breeds

Although there are hundreds of different horse breed listed throughout the world. They can all be placed into the categories of cold, hot and warm-blooded. Cold-blooded horses refer to the gentler, large breeds such as the draft horses whereas, the hot-blooded horses are classified by being finely boned and higher spirited such as Arabians and Thoroughbreds. Warmbloods are therefore said to fall in between these two categories. It is beyond the scope of this chapter to discuss every equine breed. Tables 5.12–5.14 detail examples of some common horse, pony and donkey breeds. See Chapter 16 for further information regarding donkeys.

Coat Colours

Five basic coat colours exist for horses:

- Grey
- Black

Table 5.12 Examples of some common horse breeds.

Breed	Description	Relevant information
Thoroughbred	Refined head, deep chest, lean body, with well-angled shoulders and powerful hindquarters [53]. Height can range from 15hh to 17hh. Good, friendly temperament, but can be highly strung, nervous and sensitive [53]. Principle coat colours are: brown, bay, chestnut, black and grey [53]	Thoroughbreds are known and bred as racehorses. The breed was founded in England in the seventeenth and eighteenth centuries, when English mares were bred to the three imported founding stallions: the Byerley Turk, the Darley Arabian and the Godolphin Arabian [53]. To register to race through Weatherby's, foal must be bred by natural covering and not artificial insemination or embryo transfer
Warmblood	Well proportioned, deep chest, muscular neck, and powerful legs. Range in size from 15 to 17hh. Typically found in solid colours. Intelligent, easy-going, and even tempered	Warmbloods were bred to be a mix of the cold- and hot-blooded horses to provide a horse that can be suitable for all types of activities Commonly used for dressage or showjumping
Irish Draught	A pleasant head with good bone and a short cannon bones. Good ribcage with a strong, active, hindquarters. Ranging from 15.2 to 17hh Excellent temperament with a willing nature. All solid coat colours occur in this breed [53]	Developed to be a working horse on Irish farms with references to the breed dating back to the eighteenth century Now used for riding, hunting and driving
Irish Sports Horse	Well-proportioned muscular body with defined bone structure. Long neck and ears Ranging from 15 to 17hh Eager to please, friendly and intelligent	Irish sports horses are a cross between the Irish Draught horse and the Thoroughbred. They excel in may equestrian disciplines including eventing and hunting
Shire	Generally known by their large size, being muscular with feathering on their legs and a roman nose [53] Ranging from 16 to 20hh	Developed in the eighteenth century with a talent for weight pulling, the Shire was originally the work horse on farms carrying out tasks such as cart pulling, ploughing and even barge towing. They are now commonly used for cart-pulling and showing
Arab	Compact body. Small head with a dish shaped profile and a long, arched neck. High tail carriage [53] Ranging from 14.2 to 15 hh	Originally from the Arabian dessert, the Arab was used for transportation, hauling loads and war mounts. They were highly prized and can now commonly be found used for endurance due to their stamina. Arabs sometimes have 17 ribs and 5 lumbar vertebrae, in comparison to horses who have 18 ribs and 6 lumbar vertebrae
Suffolk Punch	A heavy draught horse Powerful arching neck and well-muscled shoulders. Legs are short with little to no feathering Tends to be shorter than other draught breeds ranging from 16.1 to 17.2hh. Suffolk Punch horses are always chestnut in colour. Seven colour shades are recognised by the Suffolk Horse Society ranging from a pale, mealy colour to a reddish chestnut, to a dark, almost brown chestnut [53]	Developed for farm work but since agriculture became more modernised the breed almost disappeared and is now a critical breed in the United Kingdom

Source: Kassie Hill and Marie Rippingale.

Table 5.13 Examples of some common pony breeds.

Breeds	Description	Relevant information
Shetland	The Shetland pony is a Scottish breed of pony originating in the Shetland Isles in the north of Scotland [53]. They range in height at the withers from approximately 70 cm (28 in) to a permitted maximum of 107 cm (42 in). They have a heavy coat and short legs. They are considered quite intelligent. In appearance, Shetlands have small heads, sometimes with dished faces, widely spaced eyes, and small and alert ears [53].	Shetland ponies are strong for their size, and are used for riding and driving. Due to their size, they are commonly ridden by children. They are sometimes used for racing in events known as 'The Shetland Pony Grand National'.
Connemara	Compact well balanced pony with a deep chest, strong back and short leg. They have a free movement and actively cover ground. They range in height from 12.2 to 14.2hh	Connemara ponies are a native breed that originates in the Connemara region of Ireland. They are prised for hardiness and agility making them popular ponies for young people for all activities
Welsh	Welsh ponies and cobs are divided into four sections – A, B, C and D. These sections are determined by the pony/cob's height They typically have a neat head with small pointy ears and prominent open nostrils. They have well-proportioned bodies with a quick, straight gait and powerful movement	The Welsh ponies and cobs have a wide range of uses and can be seen in many spheres of riding and driven work. Welsh ponies are also good at jumping
Exmoor	These ponies are stocky and strong with large girths and deep chests. They have wide chests with a broad back and loins. They also have prominent flesh around the eyes. They range in height from 11.2 to 13.2hh. The Exmoor ponies all fall with in a small coat colour range of bay, brown or dun with dark points. They are mealy coloured on the muzzle, around the eyes, on the inside of the flanks and thighs and under the belly [53]. No white markings are permissible [53]	There are still wild herds of Exmoor ponies running on the moors that are gathered in the summer where some are sold off to help control herd numbers

Source: Kassie Hill and Marie Rippingale.

Table 5.14 Donkey breeds and colours.

Equid	Description	Relevant information
Donkey	There are 17 different breeds of donkey known to exist in Europe [54]. Donkeys vary in size from 8.2 to 14.2hh and can have a lifespan of 30–50 years when not being used as working animals. The most common coat colour is grey, followed by brown, black, roan, skewbald and piebald. The rarest colour is pure white [54]. They have small limbs that are narrow set with a long back and a low set neck	Donkeys are not just little horse with big ears! They differ physically, mentally, and emotionally and as such should be cared for appropriately [54]. Donkeys are stoic in nature. They are typically used for carrying loads and pulling carts in hotter climates. They are now growing in popularity as pets in the United Kingdom. For more information see Chapter 16

Source: Kassie Hill and Marie Rippingale

- Brown
- Bay
- Chestnut

Identifying the true coat colour of an equid can sometimes be challenging, particularly in foals. The colour of the hairs on the muzzle can help to guide this decision [55].

Grey

A grey horse can be born any colour. The Lipizzaners are a prime example of this as the foals are born with a black coat colour which turns grey over time. The coat of a grey horse is made up of both white and dark coloured hairs with the skin having a dark pigmentation. Foals are rarely born grey but become grey once their foal coat is shed. As the animals age they tend to become whiter either becoming fully white or having a 'flea-bitten' coat, where the coat remains speckled with the horses' original colour. Horses can show a variety of grey coats over the period of lightening. A 'Steel' or 'Iron' grey coat is predominantly seen in younger horses as there is an even mix of light and dark hairs over the entire animal. As well as a 'Dapple' Grey where the grey coat has lighter rings of grey hairs scattered throughout [55].

Black

The coat, mane, tail, and skin are all black with no other colours permitted except white markings on the face and limbs [55].

Brown

The skin has a dark pigment with the coat a mix of both black or brown hairs. The mane, tail and limbs are either black or brown [55].

Bay

The coat of a is a dark red to a yellowish brown with the legs, mane and tail being black. Black hair on the limbs is referred to as black points [55].

Chestnut

The coat of a chestnut horse is made up of red hairs. The proportion of yellow hairs in the coat denotes the range in the chestnut colour from a dark reddish brown (liver chestnut) to a lighter reddish brown [55]. Chestnut horses often have a chestnut-coloured mane and tail. Some chestnut horses have what is known as a flaxen mane and tail. The flaxen mane and tail are often a golden blonde colour and are often seen in the Haflinger breed among others.

Palamino/Cremello

The coat of a palamino horse is a bright golden yellow colour with a mane and tail of white or flaxen. This coat can be considered a type of the basic chestnut colouration as they carry a genetic dilution of the chestnut gene. The coat of a cremello is a very pale golden colour due to them having a second dilution of the chestnut gene.

Dun

Dun coat colours are a dilution of the basic coat colour with the mane and tail remaining black [55]. The classic dun or bay dun is that where the underlying base coat is a bay colour and the body is a tan or golden colour. A red dun has a lighter tan coat with reddish instead of black points due to having a chestnut coat and thus no black to be affected. The blue dun or mouse dun is a smoky blue-grey to mousey brown colour with consistent black points and often have a dark head due to having a black coat as the base colour [56]. The dun will always have a dark dorsal strip along the horses' spine and there can often be stripping or 'Zebra Markings' on limbs. These coat colours do not get lighter with age. Dun is believed to be an ancient horse colour with many equids painted in caves appearing dun, and also being seen in the Przewalski horses.

Roan

The coat of a roan is made up of an approximately equal mix of white and coloured hairs. These horses tend to have solid colouring on the head and legs with the white hairs being dispersed on the body, giving the effect of the colour being lighter [55]. Unlike grey horses, this coat colour does get lighter with age. The different types of roan are dependent on the basic coat colours:

- Blue roan (black basic coat)
- Bay or red roan (bay or bay-brown basic coat)
- Chestnut or strawberry roan (chestnut basic coat) [56].

The roan coat colour does not lighten with age [55].

Skewbald

The coat of a skewbald consists of irregular well-defined patches of both white and any other colour except black [55]. Skewbald is mostly commonly thought to be brown and white, but it is not limited to this.

Other examples are:

- Chestnut and white (Figure 5.14)
- Palamino and white
- Blue roan and white

Piebald

The coat of a piebald horse consists of irregular well-defined patches of both white and black.

Albino

With the albino coat colour, there is no pigmentation of either the skin, hair or eyes which means the hair appears white and the eyes appear pink.

Appaloosa

The coat of an appaloosa is a combination of a base colour with an overlaid spotting pattern. There are a unique group of spotting patterns that people associate with the appaloosa horse.

These are:

- Spots: A horse that has white or dark spots all over a portion of its body.
- Blanket/snowcap: A solid white area normally over the hip area with a contrasting base colour.
- Blanket with spots: A white blanket which has dark spots within the white.
- Leopard: A white horse with dark spots that flow over the entire animal.
- Few spot Leopard: A mostly white horse with a bit of colour remaining around the flank, neck and head.
- Snowflake: A horse with white spots on a dark body.

Figure 5.14 A chestnut and white skewbald coat colour. *Source:* Dr Francis Boyer.

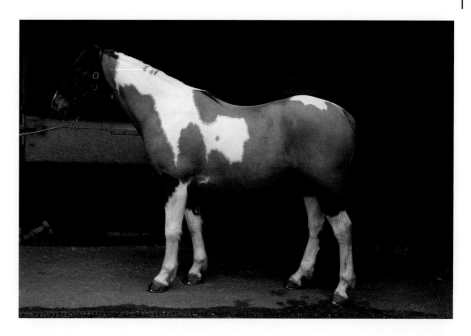

Base colours can be overlaid by a variety of spotting patterns and do not always fall neatly into a specific category. It is not always easy to predict a grown appaloosa's coat colour due to this, and the foals tend to be born with darker coats until they moult their foal coats.

Metallic

The coat of the Akhal-Teke breed is very distinctive and has a 'metallic' sheen which got them the nickname 'Golden Horses', although coat colours can vary widely dependent on the horses' base colour. The coat had a characteristic metallic sheen which with the dun variation can produce a golden effect, it is claimed that this is to provide camouflage within the dessert where they were originally found. A metallic silver colour also occurs [53].

Markings

Face Markings

Another useful identifier is the individual markings that each equid has on both their face and legs. These are described as, but not limited to:

- Blaze: A white marking covering almost the whole of the forehead between the eyes and extending beyond the width of the bridge of the nose onto the face, usually to the muzzle [56] (Figure 5.15).
- Stripe: A narrow white marking down the bridge of the nose [56].

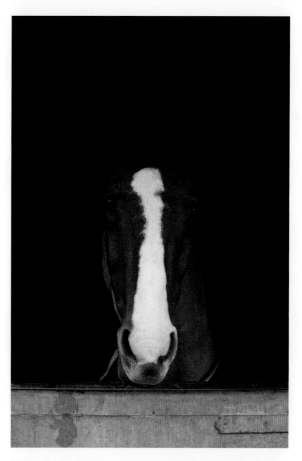

Figure 5.15 A blaze face marking. *Source:* Dr Francis Boyer.

- Star: Any white mark on the forehead.
- Snip: A white marking on the muzzle between the nostrils.
- White face: The most dramatic face marking covering most of the face and possibly covering the eyes. In incidences where the white extends over the eye, the horse can present with a wall eye. A wall eye is an eye that is blue in colour. The blue colour is created by a lack of pigment in the iris.

Leg Markings

Markings on the legs described according to the extent of white on the limb.

- Stocking: A white marking that extends to the bottom of the knee or hock.
- Sock: A white marking that extends higher that the fetlock but not as high as the fetlock/hock.
- Boot: The white marking extends up to the fetlock joint.
- Coronet: A white marking around the top of the hoof but does not extend onto the pastern.

Whorls

Whorls are also an important distinguishing feature in the horse and can sometimes be some of the only defining features on a block-coloured horse (Figure 5.16). They are commonly found on the head, neck, chest, abdomen, and stifles. Whorls are formed by the change in direction of flow of the hair and can be defined as simple, linear, and feathered [56]. These should always be recorded on the identification sketch in horse passports. As well as natural visual

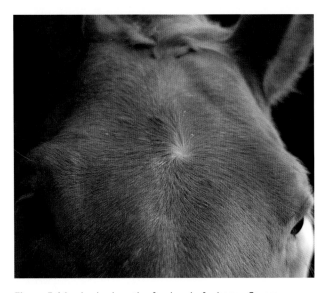

Figure 5.16 A whorl on the forehead of a horse. *Source:* Dr Francis Boyer.

difference in equids, there is also the need to record any acquired identification markers.

Microchipping

From October 2020, it was made compulsory for all horses to be microchipped, a microchip must be inserted, by a vet, into the ligamentum nuchae on the left-hand side of the animal, 2.5–3.75 cm from the dorsal midline [55]. The microchip is a small chip with a unique code. This code can be read by an electronic machine. The unique code is registered to both the equid and owners' details, and then recorded in the equids' passport. All foals must be microchipped by six months of age or 31st December of the year in which it was born, whichever is earlier.

Passports

All horses, ponies, donkeys and mules must have a passport with a valid microchip recorded. They also include a silhouette drawing of the equid which must have been completed by a vet. General information required is as follows:

- Any white marking on the horse must be outlined in red and cross hatched with diagonal lines.
- Flesh marks should be outlined and shaded completely in red. Any spots on the mark should be outlined in black and left unshaded.
- Any other marks shown in black for example, whorls.
- Whorls should be indicated by an X and feathered whorls have an X where the whorl starts and a line to indicate the direction and extent of the whorl.
- The Prophet's Thumb print is a natural dimple in the muscle usually found on the neck (Figure 5.17). This should be marked as a black triangle [56].
- Significant scars should be marked with the black arrow.
- An M in a circle should be placed at the location of the implantation of the microchip [56].
- If there are fewer than five distinguishing features listed on a passport application then it will not be accepted.

The horses' passport should be kept up to date with owners' details, a list of vaccinations and a declaration stating if the horse is, or is not, intended for human consumption. The passport should be kept with the horse at all times. This is a legal requirement, and also applies when the horse is being transported.

Height Measurements

The Joint Measurement Board is a non-profit organisation dedicated to measuring horses and ponies. These measurements are carried out by a list of vets who are official measurers of the board. A horse cannot be presented for a measurement until they are four years of age, and annual measurements are issued for horses and ponies at four, five,

Figure 5.17 A prophet's thumb mark. *Source:* Dr Francis Boyer.

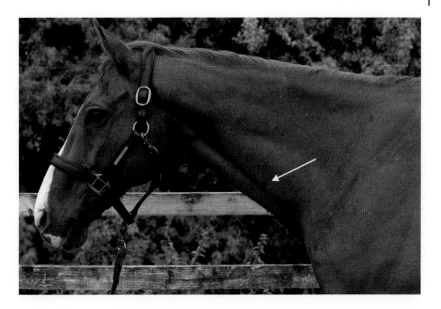

and six years of age. Any horse aged seven, or over having had at least one annual measurement, can be submitted for full measurement. The same official measurer is unable to complete consecutive measurements. A horse should be measured on a flat, level surface from the floor to the withers, without shoes on. Measurements should be carried out and recorded in centimetres. A pony is to measure fewer than 148 cm. It is useful for the horses and ponies to be trained to stand quietly and calmly throughout the measurement.

Tattooing

This is a rare form of identification method in the United Kingdom, but a tattoo can sometimes be found on the inside of the horses' upper lip.

Freeze Marking

A freeze mark occurs when a very cold blocks in the shape of letters and/or numbers are applied to the skin of the animal [55]. This in turn causes scarring to the area and the hair grows back white in colour. Freeze marks are commonly placed behind the withers on the back and can also be placed on both the shoulder or the neck. There is a national scheme to ensure that no two animals are marked with the same combination of numbers and letters [55]. Since microchipping has become compulsory, freeze marking is now less common.

Branding

Branding occurs using red hot irons that are applied directly to the skin to cause a scar in which the hair growth

is affected [55]. This is still used as an identification method for certain breeds such as Hanoverians, Trakehners, Warmbloods and Oldenburgs. Due to welfare concerns this is becoming less common.

Blood Typing

Genetic markers in the horses, as found on the red blood cells can be used for the identification or verification of parentage. The effectiveness of this relies on the number of genetic systems tested and is about 94–96% effective. The use of blood typing has been overtaken by deoxyribonucleic acid (DNA) testing as a more definitive method of parentage testing.

Deoxyribonucleic Acid (DNA) Testing

DNA testing is carried out commonly by breed associations, particularly where parentage or breed can be in question. A variety of samples can be collected from the animal to perform these tests, but most commonly hair plucks and blood samples are used. The accuracy of DNA sampling to determine parentage is good but this depends on having samples from both parents where the DNA is known.

Requirements of Passports and Record Keeping

Medicine Use and Passport Declaration Regarding the Fitness for Human Consumption

While all horses and other equids are legally required to have both a passport and a microchip, they are also legally defined as a food producing animal. This can be declared by the owner or agent of the animal in the passport by signing Part II of Section IX. In this section, the owner or agent signs a declaration as to whether the animal is in fact intended for human consumption or not. Where the animal is not intended for human consumption, there is no need for any record keeping of medications given to the animal other than any vaccines given. If the animal is intended for human consumption and are treated with medications and vaccinations, then there are complex record-requirements, some need to be recorded in the passport and others elsewhere. Some medications will need a withdrawal period prior to human consumption and more importantly some medications, for example phenylbutazone, will result in the horse being permanently being excluded from the human food chain. The requirements of record keeping in food producing animals are laid out by the VMD Veterinary Medicines Guidance Note 16 (see further reading). If the declaration has not been signed by an owner or agent, then the horse must be treated as if it is intended for the human food chain, unless the declaration is signed at the time. This legislation is intended to protect the human food chain and ensure that no potentially harmful medications enter into it.

Record Keeping in Relation to Animal Movements

Before exporting or moving a horse or other equine from the United Kingdom to the European Union (EU), the animal needs to be examined by an official vet and have an Export Health Certificate (EHC) completed. The EHC is an official document that confirms the horse meets the health requirements of the country of destination. Horses travelling to the EU must also be tested to prove they are free of equine infectious anaemia (EIA). If the horse is a registered horse, which means that it is registered with a national federation branch of an international body for sporting and competition purposes, this needs to be within 90 days of travel if the animals are staying in the EU, for fewer than 90 days, and within 30 days of travel for animals moving permanently. If the horse is not registered i.e. not a competition horse (usually registered with the FEI) then testing must be carried out within 30 days. All animals travelling must not only have an EHC but also a horse passport as means of identification and a microchip. The vet will also check Part II of Section XI in the passport to ensure that the horse has been signed out of the human food chain. All documentation will be inspected at an EU Border control post, and it is necessary to check with the border control post the noticed needed before transportation. When transporting equines from the United Kingdom to countries outside of the EU, a EHC will still need to be completed and there may be further health tests required depending on the destination.

5.5 Behaviour and Handling and Restraint Techniques

Introduction

As an RVN in practice, it is important to have a good knowledge of equine behaviour as this will facilitate an effective approach to handling and restraint techniques. A knowledgeable and sympathetic approach to handling equine patients will help to encourage the highest levels of safety and success for both the patients and personnel involved.

Equine Behaviour

Horses are prey animals and although now domesticated, their ethogram remains the same. They are most secure in stable herds, so safety is a priority for them. It is important to be aware of their normal behaviour patterns and factors that can influence them. Horses take a huge amount of security from being in their own environment and with a stable herd [57], so when bringing them into a hospital/practice environment, often on their own, it is important to know that they will not behave in the same way as they might at home. When placed in an unfamiliar environment, most horses will display a fight or flight response to anything aversive. The individual horses' temperament will determine which one of these responses they are likely to display when stressed. Horses often avoid conflict and prefer to escape however, if they have learnt from previous experience that this is not an option, they are more likely to display fear or defensive behaviour [58].

As an RVN, it is important to be familiar with basic equine body language. This ensures a better awareness of the horse's mental state and helps to inform an adjustment in handling techniques as required to ensure the health and safely of both the patient and staff. A quiet, confident approach is the best handling method for equine patients. For patients who are known to suffer with separation anxiety, a companion should be brought to the practice as this will make a huge difference to their stress levels. Considerations should also be given to positioning of stabling within the practice or hospital as this can also make a big difference to a horse's emotional state.

Aggressive Behaviour

It is rare for a normal, healthy horse to be truly aggressive and so it is important to recognise the signs of aggression and to be aware of the underlying causes [57]. In a practice setting, these underlying causes will commonly be pain, fear or learnt behaviour from a previous experience. There are other factors that can cause aggression in horses, but for the purpose of this section the ones most likely to be encountered in practice will be discussed.

Signs of aggression can include:

- Ears held flat back against the head
- Neck stretched out and threatening to bite
- Kicking with back legs
- Striking out with front legs.

When admitting horses, it is important to gain as much information from owners as possible to allow an understanding of the current temperament and to ensure safe handling. Known aggressive horses should be marked clearly on their stable to alert all staff and ensure that there are always two staff members present when entering the stable for safety. When entering stables, aggressive horses will often turn their back end towards the handler and threaten to kick when approached. The handler should stay by the open door to prevent them being trapped and potentially kicked. Often given a few minutes, these patients will begin to approach the handler and can be caught quietly using a headcollar. A bucket of feed can often be useful for encouraging the horse to approach. Aggressive horses may lunge and try to bite, so it is important that the handler does not turn their back on them. A hard hat and gloves should be worn by personnel and a headcollar should be left on the horse to facilitate catching. It is important that personnel speak quietly and move slowly around these horses to avoid escalating their behaviour. If an equine patient presents as aggressive, it is important to spend some time trying to identify the origin of the behaviour.

Aggression in horses is sometimes pain related. RVNs play a crucial part in the care and welfare of horses with the implementation of pain scoring and good observation skills. By recognising pain early as a cause of aggression, long term negative association with a veterinary setting can be minimised. Pain scoring of equine patients can be a useful tool for monitoring inpatients. Further information on pain scoring can be found in Chapter 14.

Handling the Equine Patient

RVNs are required to care for and handle a variety of horses on a daily basis.

Before approaching and handling horses, team members need to ensure that they are competent and safe to do so, and that appropriate personal protective equipment (PPE) is being worn, to include a hard hat, gloves and steel toe-capped boots.

Approaching a Horse

Horses use two forms of vision, monocular and binocular. This means horses can use their eyes independently

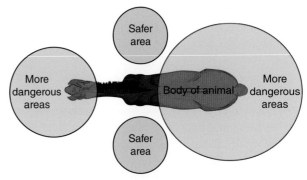

Safer approach area (left shoulder)
in the standing animal

Figure 5.18 Safe approach area. *Source:* Adapted from Wiley.

(monocular) and together (binocular) giving them a much larger field of vision. As a prey animal, this is crucial for their survival [59]. This does however mean that they have blind spots directly behind and in front of them and these are dangerous areas to approach a horse from (Figure 5.18). It is important not to startle them as this could lead to injury. It is safest to approach a horse from the left-hand side, near the shoulder. Body language should be always considered. Some horses may need to be approached more slowly than others. Voice aids can be used to alert the horse to the presence of the handler. For nervous horses, offering food may help in the initial approach of the patient. Once the handler is next to the horse, the leadrope should be placed over the neck with the right hand and the headcollar should be applied. Once the headcollar is in place, the leadrope should be held in the left hand just below the clip, and the end of the rope should be held in the right hand. The handler should face the horse and stand slightly to the side of their body to ensure that they cannot run into the handler if they move forward. This would be the basic restraint method for holding a horse while an examination is being performed.

When carrying out daily tasks around horses such as grooming and mucking out, it is advisable that horses are either held by a second person or tied up, if they are trained to do so. When tying a horse up, ensure that the area is safe and secure and that the horse can easily break away should it become distressed or panicked. Using thin bailing twine or an 'equi-ping' between the leadrope is recommended for this reason. When tying up a horse, always use a quick release knot.

Hoof Examination and Care

Prior to moving a horse from its stable, it is important to check the horses' feet and pick them out. This should also be carried out daily as part of the grooming routine. Not only is this crucial for ensuring that no compacted mud or stones affect a trot up, it is good for the overall good hygiene of the horse, and it also ensures good standards of cleanliness are kept around the in-patient yard and trot up area.

The hoof pick should be used from the side of the frog near the heel bulbs and the picking motion should move from the top of the heel area towards the toe. Care should be taken around the sensitive frog area. The handler should pick the foot out fully making sure that all stones, gravel, and mud is removed. The foot area should then be brushed thoroughly. The hoof wall should be examined for evidence of cracks. The frog and heel area should be checked for any signs of thrush. The shoe should also be checked to ensure that it is neither too loose nor too tight. This again is crucial prior to starting a lameness exam.

Leading the Horse

Prior to leading the horse, an assessment should be made as to what kind of restraining equipment may be most suitable. This could be simply the normal headcollar, a bridle or a chifney. A Chifney is an anti-rearing bit that is fitted with a head piece (Figure 5.19). When handling youngstock and stallions, a chifney is often recommended. A chifney should be used alongside a headcollar. Chifneys can be severe when used in the wrong hands, many pleasure horses may not have been trained in a chifney and therefore, care should be taken when first used. It is important not to pull on a chifney, instead its action should be used if the horse reacts, as an anti-rearing device.

Once the horse is caught and the headcollar/bridle is applied, the horse can be lead. The handler should stand on the left side, hold the leadrope close to the headcollar with the right hand, and place the left hand on the middle of the rope. The rope should not be knotted or wrapped around the hand, for safety reasons. The rope can be folded over to reduce any excess. The handler should remain at the shoulder of the horse and encourage it to walk forward by using their voice and a small amount of pressure with the right hand. Horses are often trained to response to the voice, pressure, and release, but not all horses will arrive in the practice 'trained'. Therefore, discussion with the owner and treating the horse as an individual is important.

Trotting up a Horse

Trotting up horses plays a large part of the role of the orthopaedic examination. Prior to the examination, the horse must be correctly restrained, and the handler should be wearing the correct PPE. Most clinics have a dedicated trot up area, this should be kept well swept and free of weeds. Droppings should be picked up. The area should be

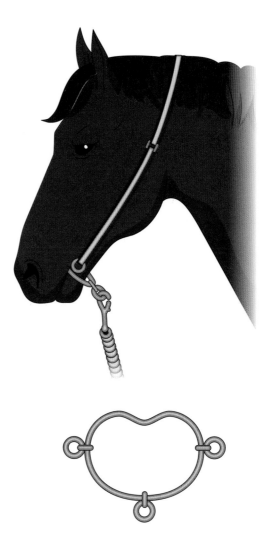

Figure 5.19 A chifney bit. *Source:* Adapted from Elsevier.

straight, and level and it should be situated a safe, enclosed space. Horses are initially seen walking away from the vet and then returning. The handler should walk on the left at the horse's shoulder and encourage a natural forward walk with a natural head movement and ensuring there is clear visibility of the limbs. A schooling whip may be carried in the left hand if required. When turning, the handler should remain on the outside of the horse. For a very lame horse in walk, the handler would be better positioned on the side of the sound leg, to avoid turning the horse onto the lame leg.

When trotting the horse, the same principles apply, with the handler needing to create a forward positive trot. The rein should be slightly loose, and the head should again, be allowed to move naturally, as head movement can be significant in the lameness evaluation. The horse should be halted at the end of the trot up, turned in walk and trotted back. Trotting up is often required following flexion tests. Here the handler needs to be aware of the horse's reaction to the flexing of the limb, as some horses can react unpredictably. The handler also needs to be ready to trot away on command immediately after the flexion test has been carried out. Therefore, both the handler and patient must be alert and ready to move.

Lunging

RVNs need to be confident in lunging a variety of horses, lunging is either carried out as part of the orthopaedic examination, or some in cases, with horses that have other conditions such as colic.

Equipment required includes:

- Patient
- Headcollar and leadrope
- Bridle or chifney
- Lunge rein
- Lunge whip
- PPE for handler

The handler should wear the correct PPE. Due to their length, lunge lines can pose a hazard, and many people prefer to lead the horse to the arena with a leadrope before transferring onto a lunge line. When lunging, it is advisable to use a bridle or lunge cavesson. For the purpose of a veterinary examination, it is preferred that training aids and boots are avoided as this may change the horse's natural way of going. However for young or excitable horses, this may be a requirement initially according to the owners' instructions.

Horses may be required to lunge on hard and soft surfaces. When on the desired surface, the handler should stand to the left of the horse, with the lunge line passed through the bit to the opposite side. The line can also be passed over the head of the horse if desired. The horse should be stand in the centre of the area. The lunge line should be gathered up to create a neat loop, but never wrapped around the hand or arm of the handler. The lunge line should be held in the most forward hand, with the excess in the opposite hand. The lunge whip should also be held in the opposite hand, creating a triangle between the handler, the lunge line, and the whip. Using the voice and body language, as well as encouragement from the whip, the horse should be sent forward onto a 20-metre circle. The horse can be kept on the circle by maintaining the triangle with the lunge line and the whip. The horse will need to be assessed on both reins.

When asking the horse to canter, the circle size may be increased in order to create room and a forward movement. When changing the rein (direction of travel), the lunge line will need to be attached to the bridle on the opposite side. Care should be taken when 'sending the horse out' on the lunge, as some horses may react by turning their hindquarters in towards the handler or pulling away. It is important to remember that during the lameness examination, the horse's temperament may change throughout. This could be after a prolonged period of box rest, or simply as it begins to feel better after following the administration of nerve or joint blocks.

Handling Specific Patients
Handling the Mare and Foal

Mares with foals at foot should be treated with caution, especially in the initial days post foaling and when dealing with a maiden mare. When dealing with a mare and foal, it is safer to catch the mare first and restrain her using a headcollar. Once the mare has been caught and is being held, a second person can then catch the foal. The mare must always be able to view the foal, and the person handling the mare should ensure she is positioned appropriately, so as not to cause distress. Foals should be touched and taught to feel comfortable and trust humans from as early as possible by the owners, but when admitting mares and foals to the practice this may not have always be possible. For more information regarding foals, see Chapter 15.

Handling Stallions

Stallions can be unpredictable and should always be treated with caution. A badly mannered stallion can be extremely dangerous to its handler. Many stallions, however, are well trained and well mannered. Stallions should be approached in a confident manner with appropriate restraint equipment ready if required. It is advisable to always work in twos when handling and working around stallions. Prior to admitting and moving stallions around the practice, a plan should be in place to avoid any unnecessary excitement, such as keeping stallions away from mares. All relevant members of staff should be aware when stallions are being moved. Where possible, stallions should be sedated in the stable prior to being moved to a treatment area.

Youngstock

Young horses can range from yearlings through to those who have not yet begun training, aged under five years old. With many sports horses now underdoing pre purchase screening radiographs, it is more common to see the admission of young horses for surgeries such as osteochondritis dissecans removal. These horses can require extra consideration as they may only have been briefly handled, but still require daily medication, examinations, and bandage changes. Therefore, from day one, the aim should be to build trust and confidence with the patient.

Restraint Methods Used in Equine Practice

Historically there are different ways to restrain a horse, but the most common ones used in a veterinary practice setting are described below. It is important to consider the health and safety of both the horse and the staff working at the practice when deciding on a method of restraint. Surveys have shown that equine veterinary staff have one of the highest risks of injury compared to other civilian occupations [59].

Before deciding on the most suitable method of restraint, it is important to assess the individual horse and the procedure being carried out. This should include an initial nursing assessment during the admission procedure, with the owner to determine any behavioural considerations while in the practice setting. Restraint with a chifney or bridle has already been mentioned and should be considered. Other methods of restraint will now be discussed.

Twitching
Nose Twitch

Nose twitching is a common method of restraint in equine practice. However, it is important that RVNs understand how the twitch works to ensure the welfare of the horse and to prevent harm and long-term behavioural issues from developing. A twitch is normally made from a pole with a loop of rope at one end (Figure 5.20). A thicker rope is more humane and causes less damage to soft tissues and nerves. Humane twitches are also available, these are made of metal and have a string that ties around the handles to keep it in place. The twitch works by exerting pressure on the nerve endings in the horse's nose. This causes a pain response in the central nervous system, which prompts the body to produce endorphins. These endorphins then produce an analgesic effect. Studies have shown that the initial application of the twitch does lower the heart rate of the horse for five minutes. After this time, it was shown that the heart increased which would indicate an increase in pain. **For this reason, twitches must not be left in place for any longer than five minutes as this could increase the risk of damage to the tissues** [60]. Many horses respond well to the twitch, and this makes it useful for short procedures. However, the twitch should only be used when absolutely necessary, other more positive methods of restraint should be attempted first. Repeated use of a twitch should be avoided where possible to avoid tissue damage and long-term behavioural problems, as patients may become head shy. Safety considerations when using a twitch include ensuring the person holding the horse

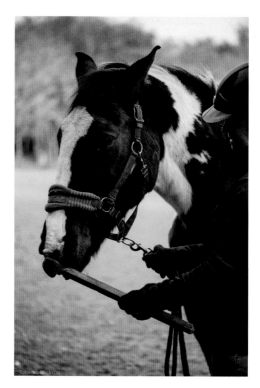

Figure 5.20 A nose twitch. *Source:* Rebecca Rockstro.

and twitch pole do so firmly. Both the handler and horse are at risk of injury if the pole becomes loose and the horse throws their head up.

Neck Twitch

Performing a neck twitch involves taking a large amount of skin from the base of the neck and pinching it tightly (Figure 5.21). This has a similar physiological effect as nose twitching and for some horses, a good response is seen. The main advantages of this method are the increased safety,

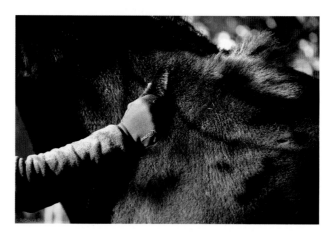

Figure 5.21 A neck twitch. *Source:* Rebecca Rockstro.

and it is often tolerated much better by the horse. The risks of tissue damage and long-term sensitisation are minimal. However, it should be considered that this will still be a negative experience for the horse and the use of this method should be minimised as much as possible.

Ear Twitch

Ear twitching involves taking a firm grip of the base of the ear and twisting it slightly. This method of restraint is contraindicated in adult horses, as it can result in injury to both the handler and the horse. It can also result in the horse becoming head shy. Ear twitching can be successfully used in foals however, all other methods of restraint should be attempted first, and the ear twitch should only be used as a last resort.

Stocks

Stocks are an essential piece of equipment when performing certain procedures to ensure the safety of patients and personnel. They are commonly used to restrain patients for procedures such as gastroscopy, upper airway scoping, radiography of the head and back, and dental procedures. Patients who are restrained in a set of stocks are commonly sedated as this lowers the risk of injury to both the horse and the staff present. Health and safety considerations are important when using stocks, as injury can still occur in sedated patients if they collapse, or on occasion, try and jump out of stocks, even while sedated. Taking this into consideration, horses should not be left tied up while in the stocks, a trained person should always be holding the horse, and sedation should be monitored closely to ensure it is adequate.

Chemical Restraint

Sedation is a common method of chemical restraint used to facilitate procedures in veterinary practice.

This is for two reasons:

- It provides some analgesia effect.
- It helps to ensure that the patient remains quiet enough to stand still while a procedure is performed.

The procedure could be anything from radiographs to standing surgery, where it is crucial that the horse does not move. There are implications with this as sedation carries risks, so it is important as an RVN that sedation is only administered under the direction of a vet. This method of restraint also requires a suitably trained person to monitor the horse in case of any complications such as the patient collapsing. For this reason, owners should not be left restraining sedated patients alone to avoid possible injury.

Many horses are needle shy or can become needle shy if care is not taken when injecting them. RVNs can play

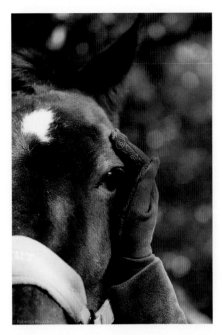

Figure 5.22 Horse's eye being covered. *Source:* Rebecca Rockstro.

an important role in keeping this risk to a minimum by taking time to ensure patients are as relaxed as possible. Covering the patient's eye on the side that is being injected often works well for nervous horses, as they are far more relaxed if they cannot see the administration (Figure 5.22). Often just giving patients a little longer to habituate to their environment will help them to relax and make the administration of injections less stressful and less painful.

Health and Safety Considerations

As RVNs, it is important to remember the risks involved when handling horses and performing procedures that often elicit pain. Safety of all staff should be a priority and it is important to ensure that everyone involved in handling patients has a good understanding of equine behaviour and body language, to help to avoid injury where possible.

For information relating to the handling and restraint of donkeys, see Chapter 16.

5.6 Transportation of Equine Patients

Introduction

It is important for RVNs to have a good knowledge of how to transport equine patients safely and correctly. This includes an awareness of relevant legislation, required safety checks for transportation vehicles, protective equipment for the patients and advice to give to clients regarding the transport of both healthy and injured patients.

Welfare of Animals (Transport) (England) Order 2006

Guidance from the United Kingdom government states that horses should not be transported if it might cause suffering or distress [61]. Movement of horses and ponies should always be in accordance with current rules and regulations (EU Council Regulation (EC) 1/2005, as implemented by The Welfare of Animals (Transport) (England) Order 2006). This applies to England, Scotland and Wales. The Welfare of Animals (Transport) (England) Order 2006 states it is illegal to travel any horse in a way that is likely to cause injury, harm, or unnecessary suffering. Before commencing the journey, any necessary arrangements must be in place to consider weather conditions, the length of the journey and meeting the animal's needs. All horses must be transported with their passports, this is required by law. The animal should be deemed fit to be transported. Any horses that fall ill during transportation should be separated from the other animals and receive treatment as soon as possible. Any horses older than eight months (except un-broken horses) must wear halters throughout transportation and those tethered must be able to be quickly released in the event of an emergency.

The space requirements for each animal are dependent on size and age:

- Adult horses: 1.75 m^2
- Young horses (6–24 months old) for journeys of up to 48 hours: 1.2 m^2
- Young horses (6–24 months old) for journeys over 48 hours: 2.4 m^2
- Ponies (under 144 cm): 1.0 m^2
- Foals (0–6 months): 1.4 m^2 [62].

Maximum journey times are designated as follows:

- Horses and ponies in a basic standard vehicle: 8 hours
- Horses and ponies in a higher standard vehicle: 24 hours (given liquid, and fed if necessary, every 8 hours).
- Unweaned foals in a basic standard vehicle: 8 hours
- Unweaned foals in a higher standard vehicle: Travel: 9 hours, Rest: 1 hour, Travel: 9 hours [62].

The vehicle used must be of an adequate standard that it will not cause stress or harm to any of the transported animals. The maximum ramp angle is 20°00 for horses which is a 36.4% slope equivalent to a rise of four over distance of 11 [62]. The temperature in the vehicle must not go below 0 °C during a journey of more than 8 hours. There should also be adequate personnel available to handle the animals during transportation. Anyone transporting horses for an 'economic activity' must have either long or short transporter authorisation from DEFRA dependant on the journey time.

If a client is transporting their own horse with a horsebox or trailer, according to United Kingdom Driver & Vehicle Standards Agency they must ensure that they:

- Have the right driving licence for the weight of the vehicle or trailer
- If required, have an operator licence
- Are qualified to transport horses if travelling for over 8 hours
- Perform regular safety checks
- Do not overload the horsebox or trailer
- Possess a valid ministry of transport (MOT) certificate for the vehicle or trailer
- Follow the necessary requirements for animal welfare

Drivers hired to transport horses to veterinary facilities on a commercial basis as part of their normal business, require a standard operator licence [63]. If they are moving horses across the European Union or other country borders, they must seek authorisation by the UK government Animal & Plant Health Agency (APHA). As the United Kingdom is a country that has easy accessibility to nations on the continent, it is not unusual for injured horses to be transported back to the United Kingdom for further treatment.

Many commercial transporters are experienced in shipping ill or injured horses to veterinary practices, and have lorries specially equipped for that purpose. They can accommodate any size equid and have adjustable partitions in padded stalls, non-slip flooring, electric low loading ramps, air conditioning, heating, closed-circuit television (CCTV), and air suspension to provide a stable ride. The drivers will know directions to several referral hospitals around the country and can liaise with the practice or the emergency services if a crisis arises during the journey.

Preparing the Patient for Travel

Horses are usually travelled in safety equipment which includes:

- Travel boots or bandages
- A tail guard or bandage
- Poll protector
- A rug (depending on the climate).

When using rugs for travel, care should be taken not to over rug and cause the horse to over-heat. A leather head-collar is often recommended as these are more likely to snap in the event of the horse getting caught on something and getting stuck. A leadrope with a safety clip is ideal so the horse can be released quickly in an emergency.

Preparing the Vehicle for Transport

A suggested vehicle safety check list is as follows [64]:

- Check that the vehicle is in good working order with no faults
- Check the flooring
- Check the fuel level, windscreen wash, water/coolant levels
- Check the tyres – pressure and appearance
- Check that all lights are working, including indicators
- Check the ramp
- For trailers, check the hitch is secure and the power is connected
- For trailers, check the quick release breast bar key
- Check the partitions and adjust depending on the horse
- Check the ventilation is adequate
- Stock enough water/hay/feed for the required journey plus extra
- Ensure that adequate insurance and breakdown policies are in place

The above is a basic list of checks that should be carried out prior to loading. Once it has been agreed that the vehicle is safe, appropriate bedding material should be placed on the floor (some horses prefer to travel and load on this) and a haynet should be provided if appropriate. A horse should never be loaded onto an unhitched trailer.

Things to consider when loading and unloading horses

- Anyone loading/unloading horses should be trained and confident to do so and wearing the correct PPE.
- Some horses may not be used to certain vehicles.
- Try to create more room by positioning the partitions to make the space more appealing to a horse than a dark, small area.
- Having an open front ramp may encourage a horse to load, but care should be taken that it does not barge through and escape.
- Position the trailer or lorry in a safe/secure area – alongside a wall or building.
- Horses may travel and load more easily with a companion. The companion horse should be loaded first and unloaded last.
- Select an appropriate surface to load on, avoid slippery or wet surfaces.
- When unloading, appropriate restraint should be used as some horses may try and rush down the ramp, which can be extremely dangerous for the handler.

Loading Ramps

Loading ramps are designed to make the entrance to the lorry or trailer more appealing by reducing the gradient of the ramp (Figure 5.23). Ramps of differing heights may be required for trailers and lorries. Either side of the ramp should have secure boarding in a funnelling style to encourage the horse to load. Loading ramps are particularly useful

Figure 5.23 Loading ramps.
Source: Rosina Lillywhite.

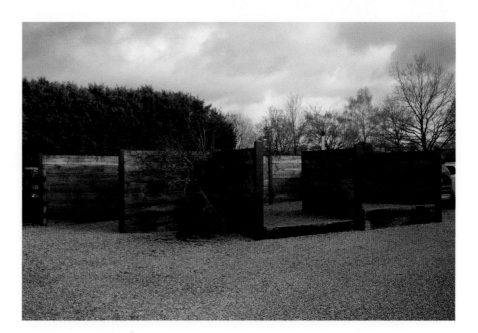

in veterinary settings when loading and unloading injured horses such as those with limb fractures.

Transporting Painful and Injured Patients

Horses that are being transported and admitted to the practice for more serious conditions may not conform to the stipulations mentioned above and should be transported at the discretion of the owner and the vet. The injured area of the horse's anatomy should be protected and immobilised adequately. A low ramp facilitates easier entry for the injured, sick, or weak horse. Loading must be carried out away from slippery surfaces and in an area that is clear of hazardous objects. In a trailer, the horse should be loaded on the side behind the driver. This helps to balance the trailer around turns and corners. In specially adapted trailers and boxes, a sling can be placed under the abdomen to help the horse to take some weight off an injured limb (Figure 5.24). Many horse boxes have standing stalls at 45 degree angles (slant load access), which help horses to balance when moving. Chest bars can be adjusted to allow the horse to lean on them for added stability and relief.

Most horses are willing to get off the lorry once at the destination. Using a well-lit loading ramp on arrival at the practice is preferable and will lessen the degree of a steep descent to the ground. It might be advisable to assess the

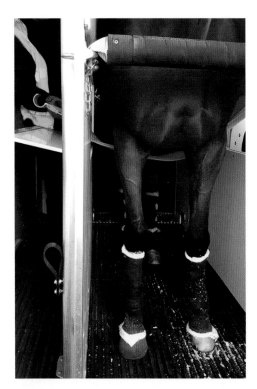

Figure 5.24 Injured horse having a sling fitted in an ambulance trailer prior to transportation. *Source:* Bonny Millar.

horse's condition prior to opening the doors and ramps. Care must be taken to prevent them rushing off and causing injury to themselves or the handler. A slow walk off, while guiding them on a short lead, is preferred to maintain control.

Limb Injuries and Fractures

A horse travelling with a leg injury, bandage or cast should, where possible, be loaded on a loading ramp to create a flat surface onto the lorry or trailer. This is not always possible at owner's premises, so parking in a way to reduce the gradient of the ramp even slightly, can be hugely beneficial, using what the owner has at home.

Horses who have a fracture should be correctly and appropriately bandaged/splinted prior to travel. The opposite leg should also be bandaged to support the limb. Horses with a fracture to their forelimb should travel facing backwards, and horses with a fracture to their hind limb should travel facing forwards [65]. This helps to keep the horse comfortable and balanced during breaking. Care must be taken when loading and unloading horses that have Robert Jones bandages and splints applied. The horse may not have adapted to moving in them, making them prone to stumbling. Help in the form of positioning heavily bandaged legs carefully for each step may be required by an assistant, while the handler keeps the walking pace steady. On arrival at the practice, the lorry or trailer should be backed up to the loading ramp.

Horses with Respiratory Disease

Horses with respiratory issues should avoid travelling unless necessary. For these horses it is important to allow them to have regular breaks to give them the opportunity to lower their head. Good ventilation should be maintained by opening windows, but care to be taken not to cause a draft that may cause the patient to become cold.

Horses with Colic

Travelling horses with colic can be extremely stressful for the owner and the driver, as horses may react violently due to pain and may lie down in the trailer or lorry. The treating vet will often administer some sedation before the horse travels to try to reduce the risks. Horses with colic when on route to a practice, should not be offered water or given a hay net. They may also have nasogastric tube secured in place by the vet for the journey. This is believed to help relieve any build-up of fluid and gas which can cause pressure in the stomach. Video surveillance installed in horse boxes and trailers is a safe way to monitor the horse while travelling. If a horse does lie down in the lorry, it is safer for the driver to continue their journey to the equine hospital. Under no circumstances should anyone go in with the horse on the side of the road when it is lying down.

Recumbent Horses

If a horse is severely injured and cannot stand, it may need be pulled onto the horsebox using large tarpaulins, mats, or even horse rugs. This will require a vet to be present to supervise, ensure safe practice and administer sedation. The horse may need continual monitoring and sedation while on the journey to prevent self-inflicted injuries as they naturally attempt to rise. Snug fitting bandages applied to the distal limbs can provide a good amount of protection against self-trauma. A head protector, or horse rugs can be placed under the head to protect the eyes and bony prominences. In these circumstances, veterinary expertise is essential and discussions with the owner might result in the journey being abandoned for safety reasons.

Mares and Foals

The transport of foals should be carefully considered to ensure the safety of both the mare and foal. While using a horse box is preferred, due to its integral stability, trailers may be the only available form of transport. Trailer partitions can be removed to enable the foal space to stay clear of an agitated or painful mare. This can come with a high risk of instability if the mare lurches from side to side, causing trailer sway due because of an unbalanced load.

Health and Safety Considerations

Considerations for RVNs

In practice, it is more appropriate that the client should load their own horse. The horse is familiar with the client and is more likely to load for them. There may be some occasions however, when RVNs are required to load a horse. This occurs if the owner is not able to do so for physical reasons, or if the horse is to be collected by a transporter. RVNs may also need to load horses onto horse ambulances at events. When tasked to load a horse, the correct PPE should be worn, this should include a hard hat, appropriate footwear, and gloves.

RVNs may need to assist with the loading horses who are reluctant to travel. This is where health and safety should be most rigorously considered. When assisting with loading, a lunge line can be used behind the horse to help to guide it onto the ramp and into the trailer or lorry. It is important to ensure no one stands directly behind the horse during this procedure. Using food at the front end is a good way to tempt the horse. Opening half of the partition or a front top door on a trailer can create a more open looking space and that may be more inviting. There are occasions when horses may need to be sedated to travel. When the horse is sedated, the feet can be carefully placed onto the ramp, but care must be taken when moving the limbs of a sedated horse. Pushing a sedated horse from behind, may look like a good solution, but this puts the handler in a dangerous area and so should be avoided. Once the horse has been successfully loaded, care should be taken when doing up the ramp as there is still a risk that the horse could be startled and so may kick out. Under no circumstances should a person travel inside a vehicle with a horse.

Considerations for Owners

Many veterinary practices provide detailed directions on how clients should travel to their location. The journey should be pre-planned, with the route and practice telephone numbers written down on paper in case a mobile network is unreliable or electronic navigational aids fail. Beginning with a full tank of fuel will alleviate some of the worry if a wrong route is taken. Horses must be supervised carefully while on the trip but under no circumstances should an owner travel in a trailer with a sick or injured the horse. The occasional stop to check the horse, is a safe way to monitor the condition of the horse.

References

1 Woods, A. (2012). From cruelty to welfare: the emergence of farm animal welfare in Britain, 1964–71. *Endeavour* 36 (1): 14–22.
2 Farm Animal Welfare Council (2009). *Farm Animal Welfare in Great Britain: Past, Present and Future.* Farm Animal Welfare Council.
3 UK Government. (2006). Animal welfare act 2006 [Online]. Available at: https://www.legislation.gov.uk/ukpga/2006/45/contents (accessed 27th August 2022).
4 UK Government. (2021). Animal welfare (sentencing) act 2021 [Online]. Available at: https://www.legislation.gov.uk/ukpga/2021/21/section/1/enacted (accessed 27th August 2022).
5 RSPCA. (2022). Animal Welfare Act [Online]. Available at: https://www.rspca.org.uk/whatwedo/endcruelty/changingthelaw/whatwechanged/animalwelfareact (accessed 27 August 2022).
6 DEFRA. (2017). Code of practice for the welfare of horses, ponies, donkeys and their hybrids [Online]. Available at: https://assets.publishing.service.gov.uk/government/uploads/system/uploads/attachment_data/file/700200/horses-welfare-codes-of-practice-april2018.pdf (accessed 15 October 2022).
7 National Equine Welfare Council (2009). *Equine Industry Welfare Guidelines for Horses, Ponies and Donkeys*, 3e. National Equine Welfare Council [Online]. Available

at: https://newc.co.uk/wp-content/uploads/2021/04/ NEWC-Compendium-front-cover.jpg (accessed 15 October 2022).

8 RCVS. (2022). How we work [Online]. Available at: https://www.rcvs.org.uk/how-we-work/ (accessed 27 August 2022).

9 UK Government. (2021). Veterinary surgeons act 1966 [Online]. Available at: https://www.legislation.gov.uk/ ukpga/1966/36 (accessed 27 August 2022).

10 RCVS. (2022). Code of professional conduct for veterinary nurses [Online]. Available at: https://www.rcvs.org.uk/ setting-standards/advice-and-guidance/code-of-professional-conduct-for-veterinary-nurses/ (accessed 27 August 2022).

11 RCVS. (2022). Code of professional conduct for veterinary surgeons [Online]. Available at: https://www.rcvs.org.uk/ setting-standards/advice-and-guidance/code-of-professional-conduct-for-veterinary-surgeons/ (accessed 27 August 2022).

12 RCVS. (2022). Continuing professional development (CPD) [Online]. Available at: https://www.rcvs.org.uk/lifelong-learning/continuing-professional-development-cpd/ (accessed 27 August 2022).

13 Farriers Registration Council. (2017). Farriery regulation [Online]. Available at: https://www.farrier-reg.gov.uk/ farriery-regulation (accessed 27 August 2022).

14 British Association of Equine Dental Technicians. (2019). Legislation [Online]. Available at: https://baedt.com/ performance/#legislationtop (accessed 27 August 2022).

15 UK Government. (2007). The mutilations (permitted procedures) (England) regulations 2007 [Online]. Available at: https://www.legislation.gov.uk/ukdsi/2007/ 9780110757797 (accessed 27 August 2022).

16 UK Government. (1991). Docking and nicking of horses act 1949 [Online]. Available at: https://www.legislation.gov. uk/ukpga/Geo6/12-13-14/70/2007-03-27 (accessed 27 August 2022).

17 Tozzini, S. (2003). Hair today, gone tomorrow: equine cosmetic crimes and other tails of woe. *Animal Law* 9: 159–181.

18 RCVS. (2011). Firing of horses. RCVS News Nov 2011 [Online]. Available at: https://www.rcvs.org.uk/news-and-views/publications/rcvs-news-november-2011/ (accessed 27 August 2022).

19 Witte, S., Dedman, C., Harriss, F. et al. (2016). Comparison of treatment outcomes for superficial digital flexor tendonitis in National Hunt racehorses. *The Veterinary Journal* 216: 157–163.

20 DEFRA. (2022). Who we are [Online]. Available at: https:// defrajobs.co.uk/who-we-are/ (accessed 27 August 2022).

21 UK Government. (2019). Notifiable diseases in animals [Online]. Available at: https://www.gov.uk/government/ collections/notifiable-diseases-in-animals (accessed 27 August 2022).

22 UK Government. (1990). The welfare of horses at markets (and other places of sale) order 1990 [Online]. Available at: https://www.legislation.gov.uk/uksi/1990/2627/contents/ made (accessed 27 August 2022).

23 UK Government. (2018). The animal welfare (licensing of activities involving animals) (England) regulations 2018 [Online]. Available at: https://www.legislation.gov. uk/ukdsi/2018/9780111165485 (accessed 27 August 2022).

24 UK Government. (2015). Control of horses act 2015 [Online]. Available at: https://www.legislation.gov.uk/ ukpga/2015/23/introduction/enacted (accessed 27 August 2022).

25 RSPCA. (2022). What we do to protect & improve animal welfare [Online]. Available at: https://www.rspca.org.uk/ whatwedo (accessed 27 August 2022).

26 British Horse Society. (2022). Our mission and values [Online]. Available at: https://www.bhs.org.uk/about-us/ our-mission-and-values/ (accessed 27 August 2022).

27 World Horse Welfare. (2022). Our history [Online]. Available at: https://www.worldhorsewelfare.org/ about-us/our-organisation/history (accessed 27 August 2022).

28 Blue Cross. (2022) Our history [Online]. Available at: https://www.bluecross.org.uk/our-history (accessed 27 August 2022).

29 The Donkey Sanctuary. (2022) Why donkeys matter [Online]. Available at: https://www.thedonkeysanctuary. org.uk/what-we-do/why-donkeys-matter?gclid= EAIaIQobChMIm7zfxsvQ-QIVlYBQBh0-bw2n EAAYASABEgIS-fD_BwE&gclsrc=aw.ds (accessed 27 August 2022).

30 Scorer, T. (2016). Stable design and management. In: *The Complete Textbook of Veterinary Nursing*, 3e (ed. V. Aspinall). London: Elsevier.

31 Monsey, L. and Devaney, J. (2012). Maintaining animal accommodation. In: *BSAVA Textbook of Veterinary Nursing*, 5e (ed. B. Cooper, E. Mullineaux, L. Turner, and T. Greet), 290. Gloucester: BSAVA.

32 NOAH. (2016). Equilis Prequenza, Suspension for injection for horses [Online]. Available at: URL:https://www. noahcompendium.co.uk/?id=-454672#A-454672_37 (accessed 05 December 2022).

33 NOAH. (2016). Equilis Te, Suspension for injection for horses [Online]. Available at: https://www. noahcompendium.co.uk/?id=-454714#undefined (accessed 05 December 2022).

34 NOAH. (2016). Equilis Prequenza Te, Suspension for injection for horses [Online]. Available at: https://www. noahcompendium.co.uk/?id=-454686#A-454686_41 (accessed 05 December 2022).

35 NOAH. (2015). Strangvac® Suspension for injection for horses and ponies [Online]. Available at: https://www. noahcompendium.co.uk/?id=-481567#A-481567_18, (accessed 05 December 2022).

36 NOAH. (2016). Equip EHV1,4 [Online]. Available at: https://www.noahcompendium.co.uk/?id=-457312#A-457312_35 (accessed 05 December 2022).

37 NOAH. (2016). Equip Artervac emulsion for injection for horses and ponies [Online]. Available at: https://www. noahcompendium.co.uk/?id=-457299#A-457299_35 (accessed 05 December 2022).

38 Harris, H. and Rock, A. (2016). Prevention of the spread of infectious diseases. In: *The Complete Textbook of Veterinary Nursing*, 3e (ed. V. Aspinall), 400. London: Elsevier.

39 Elsheikha, H. (2016). Equine internal and external parasites: identification, treatment and improving compliance. *The Veterinary Times Equine* 2 (2): 4–6.

40 Snalune, K. (2008). Equine internal parasites; their types and management. *VN Times* (7): 8–10.

41 NOAH (2022). Faecal egg count reduction testing (FECRT) and interpretation of results in equines [Online]. Available at: https://www.noah.co.uk/topics/equines/fecrt-testing/ (accessed 27 December 2022).

42 NOAH (2016). Controls on veterinary medicines [Online]. Available at: https://www.noah.co.uk/wp-content/ uploads/2022/06/NOAH-BD-Controls-on-Veterinary-Medicines-23-05-16.pdf (accessed 28th December 2022).

43 Naylor, R.J., Hillyer, L.L., and Hillyer, M.H. (2012). Laboratory diagnostics. In: *Equine Veterinary Nursing Manual*, 2e (ed. K. Coumbe), 219–220. Oxford: Blackwell Science.

44 Gajanayake, I., Lumbis, R., Greet, G. et al. (2011). Nutrition and feeding. In: *BSAVA Textbook of Veterinary Nursing*, 5e (ed. L. Turner, B. Cooper, and E. Mullineaux). Gloucester: BSAVA pp. 305–308, 310, 312, 320–322, 331.

45 Harris, P. (2001). Nutrition. In: *Equine Veterinary Nursing Manual* (ed. K. Coumbe). Oxford: Blackwell Science Ltd pp. 101,105–106, 110, 115.

46 Urschel, K. and Lawrence, L. (2013). Amino acids and protein. In: *Equine Applied and Clinical Nutrition* (ed. R. Geor, P. Harris, and M. Coenen), 113–114. London: Saunders Elsevier.

47 Urschel, K. and Lawrence, L. (2013). Feeding the growing horse. In: *Equine Applied and Clinical Nutrition* (ed. R. Geor, P. Harris, and M. Coenen), 243–254. London: Saunders Elsevier.

48 Stoneham, S.J. (2001). Foal nursing. In: *Equine Veterinary Nursing Manual* (ed. K. Coumbe), 284–287. Oxford: Blackwell Science Ltd.

49 Hart, K.A. and Epstein, K.L. (2013). Common problems and techniques in equine critical care. In: *Equine Medicine, Surgery and Reproduction*, 2e (ed. T.S. Mair, S. Love, J. chumacher, et al.), 572. London: Saunders Elsevier.

50 Slater, J.D. and Knowles, E.J. Medical nursing. In: *Equine Veterinary Nursing*, 2e (ed. K.M. Coumbe), 276. West Sussex: Wiley-Blackwell.

51 Harris, P.A. Clinical nutrition. In: *Equine Veterinary Nursing*, 2e (ed. K.M. Coumbe), 128–133. West Sussex: Wiley-Blackwell.

52 Frank, N., Bailey, S., Bertin, F. et al. (2020). Recommendations for the diagnosis and treatment of equine metabolic syndrome (EMS) [Online]. Available at: https://sites.tufts.edu/equineendogroup/files/2020/09/ 200592_EMS_Recommendations_Bro-FINAL.pdf (accessed 24 October 2022).

53 Hartley Edwards, H. (n.d.). *Ultimate Horse*, 40–41, 46–47, 106–108, 188–189, 214–215, 242–243. London: Dorling Kindersley.

54 The Donkey Sanctuary. (2023). About donkeys, breeds and cross breeds [Online]. Available at: https://www. thedonkeysanctuary.org.uk/what-we-do/knowledge-and-advice/about-donkeys (accessed 02 February 2023).

55 Linnenkohl, W. and Knottenbelt, D. (2012). Basic equine management. In: *Equine Veterinary Nursing*, 2e, 20, 21 (ed. K. Coumbe). Oxford: Wiley-Blackwell.

56 Weatherby's, (2008), Identification of Horses Booklet [Online]. Available at: https://www.weatherbys.co.uk/ Weatherbys/media/PDFs/Identification-of-Horses-Booklet.pdf (accessed 01 February 2023).

57 Simpson, H. (2004). *Teach Yourself Horse*, 4–5. Surrey: D J Murphy LTD.

58 Mills, D. and Nankervis, K. (1998). *Equine Behaviour Principles and Practice*, 5–6. London: Wiley-Blackwell.

59 Parkin, T.D.H., Brown, J., and Macdonald, E.B. (2018). Occupational risks of working with horses: a questionnaire survey of equine veterinary surgeons. *Equine Veterinary Education* 30 (4): 200–205.

60 Ahmed, B.F., AlicCarl, B., and Saabab, Y. (2017). Twitching in veterinary procedures. How does this technique subdue horses? *Journal of Veterinary Behaviour* 18: 23–28.

61 GOV.UK. (2023). Animal welfare. [Online]. Available at: https://www.gov.uk/guidance/animal-welfare#animal-welfare-during-transport (accessed 04 January 2023).

62 Welfare of Animals During Transport – Advice for Transporters of Horses, Ponies and Other Domestic Animals. (2007). [Online]. Available at: http://adlib. everysite.co.uk/resources/000/263/145/PB12544c.pdf, (accessed 02 October 2022).

63 GOV.UK. (2023), Transporting horses in horseboxes and trailers [Online]. Available at: https://www.gov.uk/ government/publications/guidance-for-horsebox-and-trailer-owners/transporting-horses-in-horseboxes-and-trailers (accessed 04 January 2023).

64 British Horse Society. (2022). Transporting your horse [Online]. Available at: https://www.bhs.org.uk/go-riding/riding-out-hacking/transporting-your-horse/ (accessed 22 July 2022).

65 Atkinson, T., Devaney, J., and Girling, S. (2012). Animal handling, restraint and transport. In: *BSAVA Textbook of Veterinary Nursing*, 5e (ed. E. Mullineaux, L. Turner, B. Cooper, and T. Greet), 236–244. Gloucester: British Small Animal Veterinary Association.

66 Costa, L.R.R. and Paradis. M.R. (Eds), (2018). Manual of Clinical Procedures in the Horse, John Wiley & Sons: Hoboken.

Further Reading

BEVA (2024). ProtectMEtoo toolkit. Available at: https://www.beva.org.uk/Resources/Medicines/Anthelmintic-Toolkit#:~:text=protectMEtoo,more%20responsible%20use%20of%20dewormers.&text=Develop%20practice%20guidance%20based%20on%20current%20best%20evidence (accessed 24 June 2024).

Mellor, D.J., Beausoleil, N.J., Littlewood, K.E. et al. (2020). The 2020 five domains model: including human-animal interactions in assessments of animal welfare. *Animals (Basel)* 10 (10): 1870.

Scorer, T. (2016). Stable design and management. In: *The Complete Textbook of Veterinary Nursing*, 3e (ed. V. Aspinall). London: Elsevier.

VMD. (2011). Veterinary medicines guidance note 16 [Online]. Available at: https://www.gov.je/SiteCollectionDocuments/Industry%20and%20finance/ID%20Veterinary%20medicines%20guidance%20note%20no.16%202020130605%20DEFRA.pdf (accessed 31 January 2023).

6

Infection Control

Jane Devaney

Philip Leverhulme Equine Hospital, University of Liverpool, Wirral, United Kingdom

6.1 Disease Transmission

To understand how infectious diseases are established and spread, the following definitions must be taken into account:

- **Infection** is the **colonisation** of an individual host by a foreign microorganism. Infectious agents that cause harm are called pathogens.
- **Disease** occurs when normal body processes are sufficiently impaired that a reduction in performance occurs. This leads to the development of clinical signs.
- A **contagious disease** is a communicable disease that can be spread rapidly from horse to horse through direct contact (touching another horse who has the infection), indirect contact, (touching a contaminated object), or droplet contact (inhaling droplets produced by an infected horse when they cough or sneeze).
- **Nosocomial** infections are also known as hospital-acquired infections. These are a subset of diseases that are acquired in a healthcare setting, such as a veterinary hospital.
- **Carriers** are infected animals which continue to shed infective agents despite showing minimal or no signs of the disease [1].
- A **zoonotic disease** is a disease that is transferable from animals to humans.
- The **incubation period** is the time lag between the exposure to a pathogenic organism and the onset of symptoms.
- A **notifiable disease** is a disease that must be reported to the Animal and Plant Health Agency (APHA). Failure to do so is an offence. Table 6.1 displays a selection of equine notifiable diseases.

Transmission

In order for pathogens to succeed and spread, they need to successfully infect a host. Pathogens spread between hosts via a number of different methods [1]:

- **Direct transmission:** This involves the spread of pathogens by direct contact. For example, equine influenza is spread via aerosol droplets, which are coughed out by infected horses and inhaled by non-infected horses.
- **Indirect transmission:** This occurs if an infection is acquired from a contaminated environment or via a vector.
- **Mechanical vectors:** Also known as fomites. These may be inanimate objects such as bedding, grooming equipment, feed buckets and haynets.
- **Biological vectors:** These are organisms that may convey infectious agents from one host to another, but do not cause disease themselves. For example, WNV is spread by mosquitoes, and so they are considered to be biological vectors.
- **Horizontal transmission:** Refers to the direct or indirect spread of infection between members of the same generation.
- **Vertical transmission:** Refers to the spread of infection from the dam to offspring. An example of this is the spread of EVA from a mare to her unborn foal.

Routes of Transmission

Different infective agents may be excreted by a variety of routes, including:

- **Saliva:** Rabies
- **Blood:** Equine infectious anaemia (EIA)

Textbook of Equine Veterinary Nursing, First Edition. Edited by Rosina Lillywhite and Marie Rippingale.
© 2025 John Wiley & Sons Ltd. Published 2025 by John Wiley & Sons Ltd.
Companion website: www.wiley.com/go/equineveterinarynursing

Table 6.1 Equine notifiable diseases.

Disease name	Causal agent	Clinical signs	Method of transmission	Prevention and control
Rabies (Zoonotic)	Virus	Affects all mammals. Behaviour changes: friendly animals may become cautious, shy animals may become bold. Hypersensitivity to noise or light. Increased aggression. Eyes taking on a staring expression. Drooping lower jaw and hypersalivation. Itching and increased thirst. In the final stages of rabies, clinical signs include weak muscles, dysphagia, drooping eyelids and saliva frothing at the mouth. General paralysis followed by convulsions and coma preceding death. Some animals will show no signs at all, so laboratory tests are required to confirm the diagnosis [2].	Infection is through bite/saliva from an infected animal [2].	Treatment not available for animals. Euthanasia is recommended [2].
Vesicular Stomatitis (Zoonotic)	Virus	Pyrexia, blisters on mouth and tongue. Lameness and hypersalivation [3].	Spread by flies and direct contact	Strict biosecurity and isolation of affected animals.
Equine Infectious Anaemia (EIA)	Virus	Some infected animals do not show signs. Clinical signs can include recurring pyrexia, lethargy, weakness and depression, loss of appetite and weight loss. Incubation period 1–3 weeks but can be up to 3 months [4].	Infection can be spread by large horse flies. It can also be spread by the venereal route and via vertical transmission. The virus can also be spread by iatrogenic transfer of blood, either in blood transfusions or on contaminated needles, surgical instruments and dental equipment [4].	There is currently no effective treatment for EIA and no vaccine available. All infected horses, including those that show mild or unapparent signs, become carriers and are considered potentially infectious for life. Infected animals must either be destroyed or remain permanently isolated from other equids to prevent transmission. A request to exempt an infected equine(s) from destruction will be considered taking into account the local situation and the need to preserve genetic diversity, or other characteristics, and the need to prevent exposure of other susceptible animals from potential infection both at the time and in future. Requests are considered on a case-by-case basis [4].

Table 6.1 (Continued)

Disease name	Causal agent	Clinical signs	Method of transmission	Prevention and control
Equine Viral Arteritis (EVA)	Virus	Clinical signs include abortion, conjunctivitis, watery eyes, swelling of testicles or udder, also around the eyes and lower legs, pyrexia, depression, anorexia, lethargy and stiff movement. Some infected horses will show no clinical signs. In rare cases, the disease can cause severe clinical signs and even death in young foals [5].	Spread via inhalation of respiratory particles. Can also be spread via the venereal route by either natural covering or artificial insemination (AI) and on fomites. Stallions can carry the disease for extended periods without showing clinical signs. Mares can spread the disease through vertical transmission to the foal or via the venereal route to a stallion [5].	Good biosecurity measures. Isolation of new horses, and testing all stallions, teasers and mares before breeding. Vaccination of breeding stallions should be considered. If EVA is confirmed in a stallion, it will remain under breeding restrictions until the risk is mitigated. This can be done through castration, export or repeated tests showing that it no longer has the virus. Until the risk has been mitigated, the stallion cannot be used for breeding except under licence from APHA. To mitigate the risk of disease spreading, the infected stallion may be named and its location publicised [5].
West Nile Virus (WNV)	Virus	Ataxia, pyrexia, listless/dullness, drooping lips, collapse, and inability to rise. Can lead to blindness, and seizure activity [6].	Spread by mosquitoes Incubation 3–15 days [6].	Vaccination can prevent encephalitis; supportive treatment can be given with varied success [6].
African Horse Sickness (AHS)	Virus	Respiratory form: Frothing and discharge from nostrils. Fever, slow, heavy breathing, coughing. Swollen face. Sudden death. Death rate 90% Incubation period 3–5 days Cardiac form: Swelling and redness around the eyes. Swelling of the head. Inability to swallow. Possible colic symptoms. Petechial haemorrhages on mucous membranes. Slow onset of death. Death rate 60% Mixed form: Mild respiratory signs. Swelling of head and eyes. Incubation period 2–14 days [7].	Spread by midges, no direct spread between horses.	If an outbreak were to occur the premises would be isolated and the affected animals destroyed, all other horses would be isolated. There is no vaccine for any serotype of AHS currently available in the United Kingdom or parts of Europe though research into safe and effective vaccines is on-going. Vaccines available in Africa are not suitable for use in the United Kingdom. A vaccine bank is being developed but will only be used in a strictly controlled manner, in an emergency situation [7].
Anthrax (Zoonotic)	Bacterial infection caused by *Bacillus anthracis*	Hot painful swellings of the throat and colic.	Inhaled, ingested, or contact with skin lesions. Spores can survive for decades or even centuries. Spores are found on infected animal carcasses, wool, hair and hides [8].	Strict isolation and biosecurity protocols.

(Continued)

Table 6.1 (Continued)

Disease name	Causal agent	Clinical signs	Method of transmission	Prevention and control
Glanders and Farcy (Zoonotic)	Bacterial infection caused by *Burkholderia mallei*	Coughing, nasal discharge, and fever. Ulcerated nodules on the skin or internal organs. Nodules on the nostrils, lungs and other internal organs are known as Glanders, those involving the limbs or body are known as Farcy. Chronic infection can last for years and result in death from chronic lung damage. Acute infections lead to death within days [9].	Infection is spread through contaminated food, water, or equipment. Animal to human infection is possible although rare and only possible when handling a case with obvious disease [9].	Isolation of infected animals and strict biosecurity measures including wearing masks, goggles, and gloves. Antibiotic treatment may be considered. Infected horses become carriers and must be isolated for life [9].
Contagious Equine Metritis (CEM)	Bacterial infection caused by *Taylorella equigenitalis*	CEM is a venereal disease. Stallions do not show clinical signs of the disease, but they can carry it. Mares will exhibit discharge from swollen genitals, especially 1–6 days after mating, lesions or damage to the skin, weakness/stiffness/lack of co-ordination and an inability to move [10].	Spread via the venereal route.	Pre-breeding swabs should be taken from the mare, the stallion should also be tested. Laboratories are legally required to report infection to APHA. Infected animals should be treated and retested as clear before breeding. Strict biosecurity controls should be adhered to. Treatment includes washing the affected area, and treatment with topical antibiotics.
Epizootic Lymphangitis	Fungal infection caused by *Histoplasma farciminosum*	Patches of damaged skin can appear anywhere on the body. Swollen and hard glands. Thick yellow scabs can form over patches of ulcers. Nasal discharge or ulcers in the nostrils. The likelihood of fatality increases with time, therefore earlier treatment is more effective. More commonly seen in equids younger than six years of age [11].	Infection is through wounds and equipment such as riding equipment that may contact open skin. It is also spread by flies. Can live in soil for up to 15 days [11].	Strict biosecurity on the premises, quarantine and euthanasia of infected animals.
Dourine	Parasitic infection of *Trypanosoma equiperdum*	Fever. Swelling of genital areas or udders and the surrounding skin. Fluid discharge from genitals (in mares). Lesions or damage to the skin. Stiffness and weakness. Lack of coordination. Inability to move. Dourine is often fatal, although some animals show no signs and recover from the disease [12].	Spread via the venereal route.	No treatment available, euthanasia recommended in affected animals.

Source: Jane Devaney and Marie Rippingale.

- **Urine:** Leptospirosis
- **Faeces:** *Salmonella*
- **Milk:** *Strongyloides westeri*
- **Across the placenta:** Equine viral arteritis (EVA)
- **By aerosol:** Equine influenza
- **By skin contact:** Dermatophytosis (ringworm)
- **During sexual contact:** Dourine
- **Via fomites:** *Streptococcus equi*

6.2 Microorganisms

It is beyond the scope of this chapter to discuss all microorganisms that cause disease. Therefore, only the main disease-producing microorganisms that affect equine patients will be discussed. Microorganisms vary in size and structure. The major similarities and differences are shown in Table 6.2.

Viruses

Shape and Structure

Viruses are much smaller than bacteria and consist of a single- or double-stranded nucleic acid (deoxyribonucleic acid (DNA) or ribonucleic acid (RNA) but never both) forming a central core, surrounded by a protein shell called a capsid. Together, these two parts form a nucleocapsid [13]. The different shapes of nucleocapsid are as follows:

- Helical
- Icosahedral
- Complex (poxvirus)
- Composite (some bacteriophages) [13]

Each helical or icosahedral shape of the nucleocapsid can be enveloped or non-enveloped (see Figure 6.1). This gives four basic shapes for viruses. There are no animal viruses

Table 6.2 Major similarities and differences between different types of microorganisms.

Characteristic	Bacteria	Viruses	Fungi	Protozoa	Algae
Size	0.5–5 µm	20–300 nm	3–8 µm (yeasts)	10–200 µm	Approximately 20 µm
Cell arrangement	Unicellular	Non-cellular	Unicellular or multicellular	Unicellular	Unicellular or multicellular
Cell wall	Present; mainly peptidoglycan	Absent	Present; mainly chitin	Absent	Present; mainly cellulose
Nucleus	No true membrane-bound nucleus	Absent	Membrane-bound nucleus	Membrane-bound nucleus	Membrane-bound nucleus
Nucleic acids	Deoxyribonucleic acid (DNA) and Ribonucleic acid (RNA)	DNA or RNA but never both	DNA and RNA	DNA and RNA	DNA and RNA
Reproduction	Asexual by binary fission	Replicate only within another living cell	Asexual and sexual by spores, budding in yeast	Asexual and sexual	Asexual and sexual

Source: Table reproduced with kind permission from BSAVA Textbook of Veterinary Nursing 5th Edition © BSAVA.

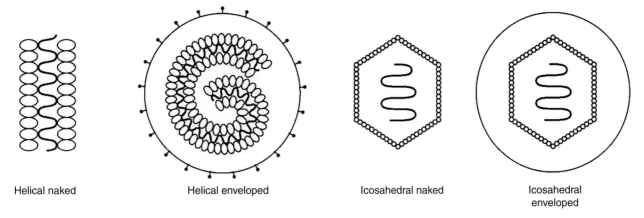

Helical naked   Helical enveloped   Icosahedral naked   Icosahedral enveloped

Figure 6.1 Helical and icosahedral viruses may be enveloped or non-enveloped (naked). *Source:* Figure reproduced with kind permission from BSAVA Textbook of Veterinary Nursing 5th Edition © BSAVA.

that are helical and non-enveloped, so viruses affecting equine patients can be grouped into the other three types [13].

Reproduction

Viruses are incapable of reproduction without a host cell and can only attach to cells that carry a compatible receptor. For example, influenza viruses can only attach to ciliated epithelial cells in the respiratory tract [13]. This specificity is known as tissue tropism. Viruses can only target a small number of host species, for example, the equine herpes virus cannot infect dogs.

Virus replication can take place via either the lytic or lysogenic cycles. These cycles differ in their mechanisms and outcomes.

Lytic Cycle:

- Attachment: The virus attaches to the host cell surface.
- Entry: The virus injects genetic material (DNA or RNA) into the host cell.
- Replication and Transcription: The viral genome takes over the host cell's machinery to produce viral components, including more viral genetic material and viral proteins.
- Assembly: New viral particles are assembled inside the host cell.
- Release: The host cell is often lysed (broken open), releasing newly formed viral particles, which can then infect neighbouring cells to repeat the cycle.
- In the lytic cycle, the virus immediately begins to replicate upon entering the host cell, leading to the rapid production of new viral particles and ultimately causing the destruction (lysis) of the host cell.

Lysogenic Cycle:

- Attachment and Entry: Similar to the lytic cycle, the virus attaches to the host cell and injects its genetic material.
- Integration: Instead of immediately hijacking the host cell's machinery, the viral DNA integrates into the host cell's genome, becoming a part of it. This integrated viral DNA is called a prophage.
- Replication: As the host cell replicates its own DNA, it also replicates the integrated viral DNA (prophage) along with it.
- Induction: Under certain conditions (such as environmental stress), the prophage may become active again.
- Entry into Lytic Cycle: The prophage excises itself from the host genome and enters the lytic cycle, leading to the production of new viral particles and lysis of the host cell, similar to the steps in the lytic cycle.
- The lysogenic cycle involves a period of dormancy where the virus's genetic material becomes part of the host cell's

genome without immediately causing harm. However, the virus can later re-enter the lytic cycle to produce more viral particles.

The key difference between the lytic and lysogenic cycles lies in their outcomes and the timing of viral replication. The lytic cycle involves immediate viral replication and destruction of the host cell, while the lysogenic cycle involves integration of the viral genome into the host cell's genome, followed by a period of dormancy before reactivation and subsequent lysis of the host cell.

Viral Diseases Affecting Equids
Equine Herpes Virus (EHV)
Strains 1–9 exist, with EHV-1, -3 and -4 known to cause the most serious health risks. EHV-1 causes four main health issues, including neurological disease, abortion in mares, neonatal death and respiratory disease. EHV-4 causes respiratory disease and occasional abortion in mares. Both EHV-1 and EHV-4 are spread directly via aerosol droplets in the air from coughing horses and indirectly via people, tack, feed and equipment. In the case of EHV-1, contact with aborted foetuses and placentae associated with abortions can spread the disease. The incubation period is from 24 hours to 14 days, typically around 4–6 days. Clinical signs of respiratory disease are fever, nasal discharge, dry cough, loss of appetite and lethargy. Neurological signs are incoordination of the limbs (mainly hind), ataxia, loss of bladder tone and recumbency. Isolation of all new arrivals on a yard for 21 days is essential. Treatment includes good nursing care, anti-inflammatories and, in some cases, intravenous (IV) fluids. Antibiotics will not treat the virus, but may be prescribed if a secondary infection occurs. A vaccine is available for EHV-1 and -4 (see Chapter 5), but it is seldom effective against neurological forms of the disease.

Equine Rhinitis Virus (ERV)
ERV should not be confused with rhinopneumonitis, which is caused by EHV. There are two forms of ERV: equine rhinitis A (ERA) and equine rhinitis B (ERB). Serologic studies show that ERV is distributed worldwide. Spread is by aerosol droplets as the horse sneezes, coughs, or snorts and by fomites such as grooming and feeding equipment. ERV causes mild to severe respiratory disease, which can affect the upper and lower airways. A vaccine is available in the United States. New horses should be quarantined. Treatment is the same as for EHV.

Information on equine influenza can be found in Chapter 13. See Table 6.1 for information regarding EIA, EVA, WNV and rabies. These are notifiable, viral diseases.

Bacteria

Shape and Structure

All bacteria are named according to the binomial system [13]. The first word starts with a capital letter and indicates the genus (plural: genera) to which they belong e.g. *Escherichia*. This is followed by the species name all written in lower case e.g. *coli*. Therefore, *Escherichia coli* is one of the species of the genus *Escherichia*, just as *Homo sapiens* (modern humans) is one of the species of the genus *Homo* [13]. The generic name is frequently shortened to initial letter, for example, *Escherichia coli* becomes *E. coli*; *Staphylococcus aureus* may be seen written as *Staph. aureus*. Both generic and specific names should be written in italics. The genus name can also be used with the abbreviation sp. (for one species) or spp. (denoting multiple species of the same genus) e.g. *Staphylococcus spp.* [13]. Many species of bacteria have characteristic arrangements that are useful in identification (Figure 6.2).

Bacteria can be classified according to their shape. The different shapes of bacteria include:

- **Bacilli** (or bacillus for a single cell) are cylindrical or rod-shaped cells. Some bacilli are curved, and these are known as vibrios [13].
- **Cocci** (or coccus for a single cell) are spherical cells, sometimes slightly flattened when they are adjacent to one another.
  - Pairs of cocci are called diplococci.
  - Rows or chains of such cells are called streptococci.
  - Grape-like clusters of cells are called staphylococci.
  - Packets of eight or more cells are called sarcinae.
  - Groups of four cells in a square arrangement are called tetrads.
- **Spirilla** (or spirillum for a single cell) are curved bacteria which can range from a gently curved shape to a corkscrew-like spiral. Many spirilla are rigid and capable of movement. A special group of spirilla known as spirochaetes are long, slender and flexible.

The structure of a generalised bacterial cell is depicted in Figure 6.3. Some of the structures depicted in Figure 6.3 are common to all bacterial cells; however, some are only present in certain species or under certain environmental conditions [13]. Bacteria are generally encased in a cell wall, which can vary in thickness and composition [14]. A capsule usually sits on the outside of the cell wall for protection purposes. Within the cell wall sits the cell membrane, which surrounds the cytoplasm. The bacterial chromosome contains the genetic material of the cell, and this is housed within the cytoplasm. Each cell may have one or more plasmids, which play an important role in antimicrobial resistance. Some bacteria possess other structures outside the cell as follows:

- **Flagella:** These help with the movement of the cell
- **Pili:** These are involved in cell reproduction
- **Fimbriae:** These are involved in the adherence of the bacteria to host cells [14]

The key differences in cell wall structure between gram-positive and gram negative bacteria result in their differential staining patterns:

Gram Positive Bacteria:

- These bacteria have a thick layer of peptidoglycan in their cell wall, which retains the crystal violet-iodine complex during the decolourisation step.
- They lack an outer membrane.
- After staining, gram positive bacteria appear purple or blue under the microscope.

Gram Negative Bacteria:

- These bacteria have a thinner layer of peptidoglycan in their cell wall, which does not retain the crystal violet-iodine complex well during decolourisation.
- They possess an outer membrane composed of lipopolysaccharides (LPS) that act as a permeability barrier.
- During the decolourisation step, the outer membrane is disrupted, allowing the crystal violet-iodine complex to be washed away more easily.
- After staining with the counterstain, gram-negative bacteria appear pink or red under the microscope [14].

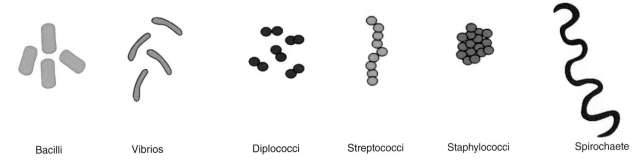

| Bacilli | Vibrios | Diplococci | Streptococci | Staphylococci | Spirochaete |

Figure 6.2 Different shapes of bacteria. *Source:* Rosina Lillywhite.

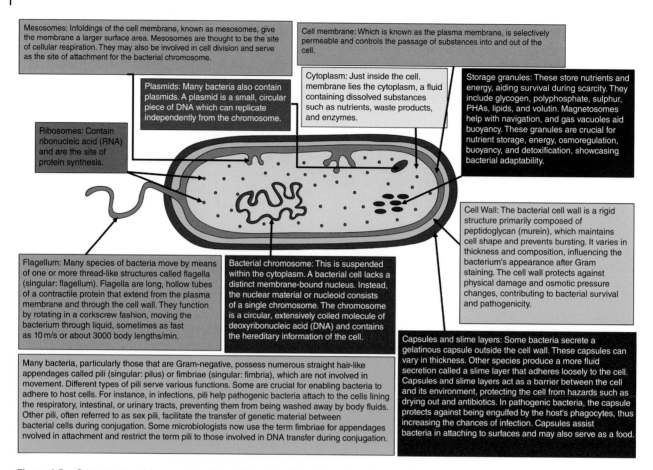

Figure 6.3 Components of a generalised bacterial cell and their functions. *Source:* Samantha Elmhurst and Rosina Lillywhite.

Growth

Bacteria can only grow and reproduce when environmental conditions are suitable [1]. Requirements for this are as follows:

- A suitable supply of adequate nutrients
- The correct temperature
- The correct pH (usually 7–7.4)
- Water
- The correct gaseous environment [13]

Aerobic bacteria can only be grown when oxygen is present. In contrast, anaerobic bacteria that do not need oxygen to survive [14].

Reproduction

In optimal conditions, bacteria can grow and reproduce rapidly [13]. Bacteria reproduce asexually by dividing into two identical daughter cells. This process is called binary fission (Figure 6.4). Gram-positive bacteria tend to favour reproduction via binary fission [14]. Replication of pathogenic bacteria usually takes place outside of the host's cells. This is in contrast to pathogenic viruses, where reproduction takes place inside the host's cells [1]. Bacterial reproduction can also be achieved by conjugation. This involves the transfer of DNA via a pilus from one bacterial cell to another [14]. Conjugation is important as during this process, the recipient cell acquires new genetic material, for example, resistance to an antibiotic. Gram-negative bacteria tend to favour reproduction by conjugation [14].

Endospores

Endospores are typically formed when a source of nutrients to the bacteria is exhausted, for example, when the environment dries out. More commonly seen in Gram-positive bacteria, the process is complex, but put simply, the bacteria produce a dormant, highly resistant cell that preserves the cell's genetic material. Endospores can remain viable for many years and can survive extremes of heat, pH, desiccation, ultraviolet radiation and exposure to toxic chemicals such as disinfectants [13]. As endospores are so difficult to kill, thought must be given in practice as to which sterilisation method is used, to ensure that the target organism and its spores are fully destroyed [13].

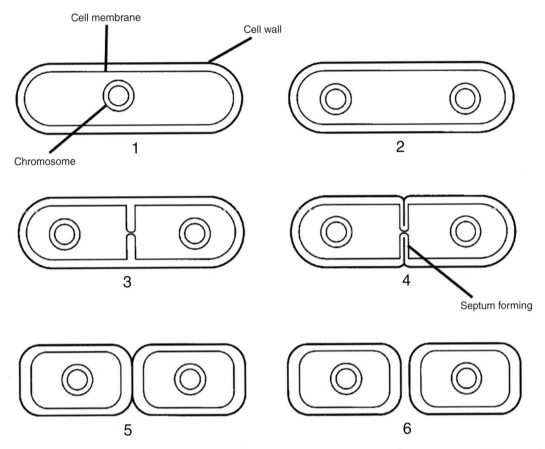

Cell membrane

Cell wall

Chromosome

1

2

3

4

Septum forming

5

6

Figure 6.4 Replication of bacteria by binary fission. (**1** and **2**) The cell grows, and the chromosome replicates to form two identical chromosomes. (**3**) As the cell enlarges, the chromosomes are separated, and the cell membrane grows inwards at the centre of the cell. (**4**) At the same time, new cell wall material grows inwards to form the septum. (**5** and **6**) The cell divides into two daughter cells. *Source:* Figure reproduced with kind permission from BSAVA Textbook of Veterinary Nursing 5th Edition © BSAVA.

Bacterial Diseases Affecting Equids

Campylobacteriosis (Zoonotic)

This is the most common bacterial cause of gastroenteritis in the human population worldwide. Campylobacter itself rarely causes enteritis in healthy horses; those compromised by other diseases may shed and display illness. It is spread by ingestion of contaminated food, water or by faecal ingestion. Clinical signs include colic, fever and diarrhoea, with possible blood visible. Treatment includes supportive therapy and antibiotics if required. Campylobacteriosis is rarely life-threatening in horses.

Escherichia coli (E. coli)

This is a common commensal organism in the gut of both healthy equids and equine patients with diarrhoea. It is not considered to be a primary source of morbidity in horses but should be considered a secondary source in sick patients. Treatment includes supportive therapy and antibiotics.

Rhodococcus equi (Zoonotic)

This is a source of morbidity and mortality in foals; initial infection is from inhalation of infected dust particles, progression can be slow until pneumonia exists; foals can then go on to swallow infected mucous, which sets up an infection in the gastrointestinal system; foals can also present with multiple sites of immune-mediated synovitis. Foals with abdominal involvement often present with fever, depression, anorexia, weight loss, colic and diarrhoea. Treatment of choice is with an antibiotic from the macrolide class, although secondary problems such as diarrhoea and hyperthermia can be seen following administration. *Rhodococcus equi* infection in humans is thought to be acquired by inhalation, inoculation into a wound or mucous membranes or ingestion.

Leptospirosis (Zoonotic)

This disease is caused by the gram negative spirochete bacteria *Leptospira* spp. *Leptospira* infection occurs through the membranes of a susceptible horse, and systemic bacteraemia ensues. The organism survives well in surface water, contamination is normally via contact with urine or urine-contaminated water/feed. The initial infection causes an immune response and transient fever, which may go unnoticed; however, the infection can then go on to infiltrate the kidneys, placenta and foetus in pregnant mares and more commonly recognised in, the eyes, where uveitis occurs, normally this can develop around 2–8 months post-infection and is thought to account for around 67% of uveitis seen in veterinary practice in the United Kingdom [15]. Uveitis is treated with antibiotics, anti-inflammatories and eye drops (see Chapter 13).

Methicillin-resistant Staphylococcus aureus (MRSA) (Zoonotic)

MRSA is a nosocomial infection that causes serious concern in the hospital setting for both humans and animals. *Staphylococcus aureus* is known to colonise the skin and has given a challenge to the management of post-operative wounds. Transmission from horses to humans is possible and vice versa; therefore, careful management of all wounds in the hospital or yard environment is essential. Transmission is through direct contact with an infected area, especially hand-to-nose contact, or through contact with a fomite. Non-healing wounds that exhibit excessive exudate should be swabbed and cultured immediately. Treatment can be challenging, but it starts with systemic antibiotics selected after carrying out culture and sensitivity testing.

See Chapter 13 for information on strangles, tetanus and salmonellosis.

Fungi

Fungi are parasitic, spore-producing organisms. Fungi grow aerobically and obtain their nourishment by absorbing food from the hosts on which they grow. They can be divided into two categories:

- **Moulds:** These are multicellular. An example is dermatophytes (ringworm).
- **Yeasts:** These are unicellular. An example is Candida spp. [13].

The primary source of most fungi infections is the soil. Fungal infections can be acquired by inhalation, ingestion, or through the skin, for example, through a cut or wound. Some fungal infections can cause disease in otherwise healthy animals, while others require a host that is incapacitated or immunocompromised by, such stresses as poor nutrition, viral infections, or cancer to establish infection. Prolonged use of antimicrobial drugs or immunosuppressive agents appears to increase the likelihood of some fungal infections. The infection itself may be localised or may affect the entire body.

Fungal Diseases Affecting Equids
Candidiasis

This is a localised fungal disease affecting the mucous membranes and the skin. It is distributed worldwide in a variety of animals and is most commonly caused by species of the yeast-like fungus, *Candida albicans*. Superficial infections limited to the mucous membranes of the intestinal tract have been described in foals. Widespread candidiasis has also been described in foals undergoing prolonged antibiotic or corticosteroid treatment. Infections are rare in horses. Signs are variable and nonspecific and may be associated more with the primary or predisposing conditions than with the candidiasis itself. Antifungal agents are required to treat this condition.

Pneumocystis

This is an opportunistic extracellular fungus. *Pneumocystis* pneumonia has been documented in several species, including humans, horses, foals, goats, pigs and dogs. Historically, disease has been thought to be a problem primarily in immunocompromised hosts. Recent evidence supports that *Pneumocystis* may be a component of the normal upper respiratory flora of immunocompetent animals [16]. Treatment includes antibiotics, anti-inflammatories and supportive care.

Information on guttural pouch mycosis and dermatophytosis can be found in Chapter 13.

Protozoa

Protozoa are a diverse group of single-celled eukaryotic microorganisms. They are classified under the kingdom Protista, although modern taxonomy considers this classification outdated. Protozoa exhibit a wide range of shapes, sizes, and lifestyles, and they play important roles in ecosystems as predators, parasites, and decomposers. Protozoa are unicellular organisms, meaning they are composed of a single cell. Despite being single-celled, protozoa can be quite complex in structure, often possessing specialised organelles for locomotion, feeding, and other functions.

Equine Protozoal Myeloencephalitis (EPM)

This disease affects the central nervous system. The name given to the protozoan organism shown to be the primary causative agent for EPM is *Sarcocystis neurona*. *S. neurona* is spread by grazing on land that has droppings from affected intermediate hosts; it cannot be transmitted from horse to horse [6]. EPM can affect any part of the nervous system from the cerebrum to the end of the spinal cord.

Clinical signs include incoordination, ataxia, muscle atrophy, lethargy, facial nerve paralysis, tongue paralysis difficulty swallowing; signs may not be symmetrical, in some cases, horses may stabilise and then relapse. Diagnosis is made through clinical exam, serum or cerebrospinal fluid examination for the presence of antibodies. Gold standard diagnosis relies on post-mortem examination of neural tissue. Treatment to control infection should include an FDA-approved anticoccidial drug (Ponazuril, Diclazuril, Sulfadiazine/Pyrimethamine) [6]. Non-steroidal anti-inflammatory drugs (NSAIDs), corticosteroids and dimethyl sulfoxide may be given. Vitamin E is sometimes used as an antioxidant treatment in infected horses, but the benefits of this practice, if any, have yet to be established. Treatment duration is mostly dependent on clinical improvement. Because of safety and efficacy concerns, compounded antiprotozoal drugs should not be used in horses with suspected EPM [17].

Cryptosporidiosis (Zoonotic)

Cryptosporidiosis parvum causes diarrhoea and weight loss in foals typically 1–4 weeks of age. Infection is via ingesting infected food or water, and to humans via surfaces or soil/water. Clinical signs are dehydration, diarrhoea and weight loss. Treatment is nursing support, and this is essential in immunocompromised foals.

Prions

Prions are misfolded proteins that can transmit their misfolded shape onto normal variants of the same protein. Prions cause several fatal neurodegenerative diseases in humans and many other animals. The word prion is from proteinaceous infectious particle. The role of a protein as an infectious agent is very different from all other known infectious agents, such as viruses, bacteria, fungi and parasites, all of which contain nucleic acids (DNA, RNA or both). The abnormal prion agent is not destroyed even if the material containing it is cooked or heat-treated.

Prion diseases include:

- Creutzfeldt–Jakob disease (CJD)
- Variant CJD (vCJD)
- Gerstmann–Straussler–Scheinker syndrome (GSS)
- Fatal Familial Insomnia (FFI)
- Kuru in humans
- Scrapie in sheep
- Bovine spongiform encephalopathy (BSE or 'mad-cow' disease)
- Chronic wasting disease (CWD) in cattle

Rabbits, dogs and horses are the only mammalian species reported to be resistant to infection from prion diseases isolated from other species. Infection occurs from eating products made from an infected animal. The disease has a long incubation process, typically 4–6 years and is progressive with worsening neurological signs, once signs develop, death normally occurs within 2–6 weeks.

Tick Bourne Disease

The Ixodes tick is common throughout the United Kingdom and can be a biological vector for the spread of disease.

Lyme Disease (Zoonotic)

This is caused by the spirochete *Borrelia burgdorferi*. Transmission occurs if horses are fed on by an infected tick. Clinical signs include intermittent leg shifting lameness, weight loss and low-grade fever. A rare form of neuroborrelias can cause ataxia, changed mentation or hyperaesthesia. Diagnosis under this circumstance is by sampling the cerebral spinal fluid. In the case of joint involvement, then serology for antibody titre may be helpful depending on the stage of infection. Prolonged antibiotics are required to treat this condition.

6.3 Antimicrobial Resistance

Antimicrobial resistance (AMR) threatens the effective prevention and treatment of an ever-increasing range of infections caused by bacteria, parasites, viruses and fungi. AMR occurs when bacteria, viruses, fungi and parasites change over time and no longer respond to medicines, making infections harder to treat and increasing the risk of disease spread, severe illness and death. As a result, medicines become ineffective and infections persist in the body, increasing the risk of spreading to others. Antimicrobials include medications such as antibiotics, antivirals, antifungals and antiparasitics. These medications are used to prevent and treat infections in humans, animals and plants [18]. Microorganisms that develop antimicrobial resistance are sometimes referred to as 'superbugs'. The process of becoming resistant to antimicrobials can occur in one of two ways:

- **Acquired resistance:** Describes the ability of the microorganism to adapt to antibiotics. These resistant bacteria can be exchanged between species by direct contact, the food chain and the environment.
- **Innate resistance** is the ability of a bacteria to have the characteristics through its structure to resist the activity of a particular antibiotic. Some examples of these characteristics are listed below:
  - Efflux pumps: Pathogens can possess efflux pumps, which are protein complexes that actively pump

antimicrobial agents out of the cell, thus reducing their intracellular concentration to sub-lethal levels. This mechanism is particularly common in bacteria and can confer resistance to multiple classes of antibiotics.

– Altered drug target: Pathogens may alter the target of antimicrobial drugs, such as enzymes or proteins essential for their growth or replication. By modifying these targets through mutations or other mechanisms, pathogens can render the antimicrobial ineffective while maintaining their essential biological functions.

– Enzymatic degradation: Some pathogens produce enzymes that can directly degrade or modify antimicrobial compounds. For example, β-lactamase enzymes produced by certain bacteria can hydrolyse β-lactam antibiotics like penicillin's and cephalosporins, rendering them inactive.

– Biofilm formation: Pathogens can form biofilms, which are structured communities of microorganisms embedded within a self-produced matrix of extracellular polymeric substances. Biofilms protect antimicrobials by physically shielding the pathogens within them and by creating a microenvironment that reduces the effectiveness of antimicrobial agents.

– Cell wall impermeability: Gram-negative bacteria possess an outer membrane that acts as a barrier to many antimicrobial compounds. Additionally, some bacteria can modify their cell wall components to reduce permeability to antimicrobials, thereby limiting their entry into the cell.

– Metabolic pathway bypass: Pathogens may bypass or alter metabolic pathways targeted by antimicrobial drugs, allowing them to continue essential metabolic processes even in the presence of the drug. This can involve upregulating alternative pathways or acquiring mutations that confer resistance to metabolic inhibitors.

– Quorum sensing: Certain pathogens use quorum sensing, a process by which they communicate and coordinate gene expression in response to population density. Quorum sensing can regulate the expression of genes involved in antimicrobial resistance mechanisms, allowing pathogens to mount a coordinated defence against antimicrobial agents.

– Antigenic variation: Some pathogens, particularly viruses and protozoa, can undergo antigenic variation by altering surface antigens targeted by the host immune system or antimicrobial drugs. This rapid genetic variation allows pathogens to evade recognition and neutralisation by the immune system or specific antimicrobial agents.

Antibiotic-resistant acquired infections exist in human and veterinary settings, the most notable in the veterinary situation is MRSA. The collaboration of many organisations recognises the need for change in the use of antibiotics in a responsible manner. One Health is a collaborative approach to health, which recognises that humans and animals live in a shared environment, and there is added value to be gained by working together on issues at the interface of different sectors. The World Health Organization (WHO) defines One Health as 'an approach to designing and implementing programmes, policies, legislation and research in which multiple sectors communicate and work together to achieve better public health outcomes'.

The British Equine Veterinary Association (BEVA) has produced a set of ProtectMe guidelines to help to prevent increasing antimicrobial resistance in equine practice (Figure 6.5). These guidelines can be downloaded and implemented in practice to ensure that best practice is adopted for the careful use of antimicrobials.

BEVA Protect Me guidance advises the following for establishing an antimicrobial policy in practice [19]:

1) Identify a list of common conditions.
2) For each condition, consider the likely pathogens.
3) Identify suitable **FIRST LINE** antimicrobials for treatment in these clinical scenarios. Based on an understanding of the likely pathogens, the spectrum of activity of the available drugs and the pharmacokinetics/pharmacodynamics of these agents as well as the 'cascade'.
4) Identify suitable **ALTERNATIVE** antimicrobials and protocols for their use. For example, there is a specific contraindication for the **FIRST LINE** antimicrobial in an individual, the disease has an unusual presentation and clinical experience suggests that **FIRST LINE** antimicrobials will be ineffective **OR** following initial treatment failure pending results of bacterial culture and sensitivity.
5) Identify drugs categorised as **PROTECTED** by the practice. As a minimum, these should include third- and fourth-generation cephalosporins and fluoroquinolones. Develop protocols to be followed prior to the use of these drugs.
6) Identify drugs categorised as **AVOIDED** by the practice. As a minimum, these should include novel drugs developed for the treatment of difficult infections in human patients, such as (i) Imipenem and (ii) Vancomycin.
7) Develop protocols for the use of prophylactic antimicrobials. (i) Clean surgery (e.g. periosteal strip). (ii) Contaminated surgery (e.g. colic surgery). (iii) High-risk surgery (e.g. synovial sepsis). (iv) Standing

ractice Policy: Develop protocols for antimicrobial usage
- Identify common clinical scenarios
- Formulate protocols for FIRST LINE and ALTERNATIVE antimicrobial therapy for these conditions
- Consider appropriate antimicrobial dosing using an evidence based approach
- Develop protocols for the use of PROTECTED ANTIMICROBIALS and AVOIDED ANTIMICROBIALS

 educe Prophylaxis: Develop rational protocols for prophylaxis
- Define surgical procedures as CLEAN, CONTAMINATED or HIGH RISK
- Rationalise disease control (e.g. the neonate, strangles)
- Discontinue use where the evidence indicates there is no clinical benefit (e.g. intraarticular medication)

 ther Options: Reduce or replace antimicrobials
- Wound debridement
- Topical preparations

 ypes of Drug and Bacteria: Select appropriate drugs
- Use cytology where possible
- Consider the dose and pharmacokinetics of the drugs selected
- Consider the suitability of the drug, compliance and risks of sub-therapeutic dosing that may accelerate the development of resistance

 mploy Narrow Spectrum Drugs:
- e.g. penicillin, rather than drug combinations.

 ulture and Susceptibility: Use bacterial culture promptly,
- Especially when clinical response is less than expected
- Or when long term therapy is suspected

 reat Effectively: Enough drug for long enough then stop
- Ensure dosing protocols provide therapeutic dosing
- Consider that marketing authorisations are sometimes at odds with research evidence

 onitor: Monitor the emergence of bacterial resistance
- Record use of PROTECTED antimicrobials
- Record when a cultured bacteria is not susceptible to the antimicrobials within your protocol
- Respond to emerging resistance and modify protocols
- Use this information as part of your clinical audit log

ducate: Inform your team and your clients
- Ensure that protocols and changes to protocols are communicated through the entire team
- Educate your clients to reduce pressure for antibiotics

Figure 6.5 BEVA ProtectMe. *Source:* Reproduced with kind permission from BEVA.

procedures (e.g. synovicentesis). (v) Disease prevention (strangles, high-risk foaling).

8) Develop protocols for **DOSE RATE, INTERVAL** and **ROUTE** for antimicrobials used by the practice. Note the inconsistencies between current marketing authorisations and the research literature. Monitor compliance and the emergence of resistance.

6.4 Infection Control Measures in Equine Practice

In a hospital setting, the following should be considered to help to reduce the transmission of disease between patients.

Hand Hygiene

There will be times when wearing gloves may be required for instance dealing with a sick foal or a post-operative infection. However, gloves can sometimes give the wearer a false sense of security. There is no replacement for hand washing or applying alcohol gel between patients. A handwashing procedure such as that recommended by the World Health Organisation (WHO) (see Figure 6.6) should be followed consistently by all staff. The WHO hand-rub procedure should be used by all staff when applying alcohol gel (Figure 6.7). Handwashing should always be carried out if hands are visibly soiled, but an alcohol rub can be used if hands are clean. In the hospital setting, facilities should be provided to do both. Alcohol gel stations should be situated three stables apart in stable blocks to facilitate compliance and regular use. A 'bare below the elbow' policy will ensure that sleeves and outer clothing do not pose a source of contamination.

Hands should be washed:

- Before and after touching a patient.
- Before and after touching a patient's environment or any potential fomites.
- Before gloving.
- Before performing any clean or aseptic task.
- Following any potential exposure to contaminated fluids or tissue, even if gloves have been worn.
- Between patients [1].

Equipment Cross Over

All patients should have their own headcollar, leadrope, rugs, bandages, tack and grooming kit associated with them; these should be labelled and should be washed as often as required. High-risk or isolated patients should also have their own thermometer, stethoscope and fob watch for checks.

Separate Stabling for Conditions

Low-risk patients can be grouped together in a stable block. Horses should not change stables during their stay. A record of the stable should be made on the patient records in the event of an infection being identified.

6.5 Antiseptics and Disinfectants

Sterilisation is the removal of microorganisms, including bacterial spores [20]. This process is paramount when it comes to performing surgical techniques in either a treatment room or an operating theatre. See Chapter 11 for more information.

Disinfection is the removal of microorganisms but not necessarily all pathogens and their spores [20]. Disinfection reduces the number of microbes but does not necessarily eradicate them all.

A **disinfectant** is a chemical agent that kills or prevents the reproduction of microorganisms on inanimate objects, for example, bleach [20].

An **antiseptic** is a disinfectant that is commonly used on living tissue, for example, a skin disinfectant such as chlorhexidine [20].

It is common for most practices to use different products for disinfection. It is important to understand the reason why different types are used, what pathogens they are effective against, the correct contact time to use and the correct concentration required. Product safety data sheets, Control of Substances Hazardous to Health (COSHH) documents and risk assessments should inform the creation and implementation of standard operating procedures (SOPs) so that every member of staff knows how to use each chemical safely within the hospital. Correct personal protective equipment (PPE) should always be worn by staff when using disinfectants. The main antiseptics and disinfectants used in veterinary practice are summarised in Table 6.3. This table should be used as a guide only, manufacturer's instructions should always be followed when using antiseptics and disinfectants.

6.6 Effective Clinical Cleaning

Disinfection is an important method to use to control the spread of disease in a clinical environment. Disinfection can be achieved via two methods:

- **Physical methods:** Include scrubbing and cleaning.
- **Chemical methods:** Correct use of chemical disinfectants.

How to Handwash?

WASH HANDS WHEN VISIBLY SOILED! OTHERWISE, USE HANDRUB

Duration of the entire procedure: 40–60 seconds

0

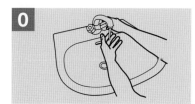

Wet hands with water;

1

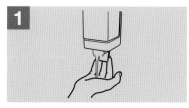

Apply enough soap to cover all hand surfaces;

2

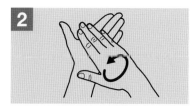

Rub hands palm to palm;

3

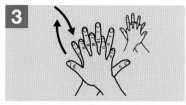

Right palm over left dorsum with interlaced fingers and vice versa;

4

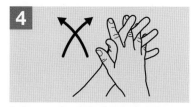

Palm to palm with fingers interlaced;

5

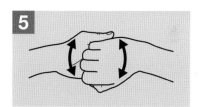

Backs of fingers to opposing palms with fingers interlocked;

6

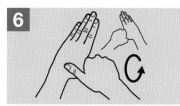

Rotational rubbing of left thumb clasped in right palm and vice versa;

7

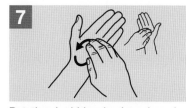

Rotational rubbing, backwards and forwards with clasped fingers of right hand in left palm and vice versa;

8

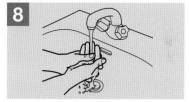

Rinse hands with water;

9

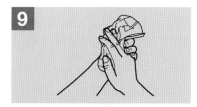

Dry hands thoroughly with a single use towel;

10

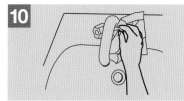

Use towel to turn off faucet;

11

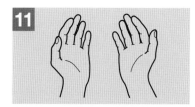

Your hands are now safe.

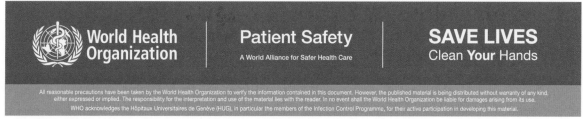

World Health Organization

Patient Safety
A World Alliance for Safer Health Care

SAVE LIVES
Clean **Your** Hands

Figure 6.6 World Health Organisation (WHO) poster providing guidance on how to wash hands effectively. *Source:* © World Health Organisation 2009.

How to Handrub?

RUB HANDS FOR HAND HYGIENE! WASH HANDS WHEN VISIBLY SOILED

Duration of the entire procedure: 20-30 seconds

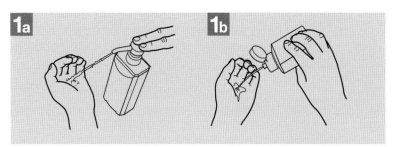 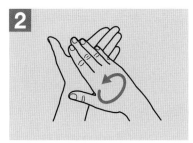

Apply a palmful of the product in a cupped hand, covering all surfaces;

Rub hands palm to palm;

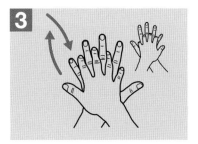 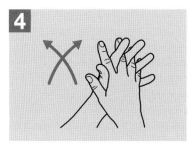 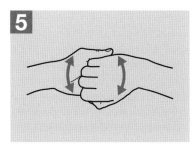

Right palm over left dorsum with interlaced fingers and vice versa;

Palm to palm with fingers interlaced;

Backs of fingers to opposing palms with fingers interlocked;

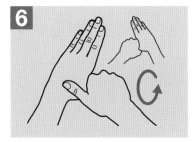 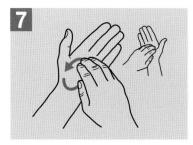 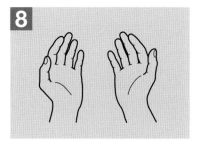

Rotational rubbing of left thumb clasped in right palm and vice versa;

Rotational rubbing, backwards and forwards with clasped fingers of right hand in left palm and vice versa;

Once dry, your hands are safe.

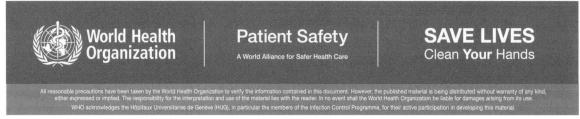

World Health Organization | **Patient Safety** A World Alliance for Safer Health Care | **SAVE LIVES** Clean **Your** Hands

All reasonable precautions have been taken by the World Health Organization to verify the information contained in this document. However, the published material is being distributed without warranty of any kind, either expressed or implied. The responsibility for the interpretation and use of the material lies with the reader. In no event shall the World Health Organization be liable for damages arising from its use.
WHO acknowledges the Hôpitaux Universitaires de Genève (HUG), in particular the members of the Infection Control Programme, for their active participation in developing this material.

May 2009

Figure 6.7 World Health Organisation (WHO) poster providing guidance on how to apply alcohol gel to hands effectively. *Source:* © World Health Organisation 2009.

Table 6.3 The main antiseptics and disinfectants used in veterinary practice.

Name	Effectiveness against pathogens	Precautions
Alcohol (Ethanol and isopropyl alcohol)	Effective against bacteria and fungi. No activity against bacterial spores [21]. Effective against enveloped viruses. Poor effect against non-enveloped viruses [22].	Must be used at high concentrations (60–91% solution) [22]. Should be applied evenly. Often used as the final step in a surgical skin scrub preparation. Can cause hypothermia in neonates if used in large quantities.
Cationic biguanides (Chlorhexidine)	Effective against most gram-positive bacteria, some gram negative, some fungicidal activity but limited activity against viruses [22]. No activity against bacterial spores [21].	Can be used as a skin antiseptic preparation. Contact dermatitis has been reported in up to 8% of human patients after repeated topical exposure. Displays a better activity in the presence of organic matter when compared to povidone iodine. Has a residual effect of up to six hours.
Idophors (Povidone Iodine)	Effective against bacteria, fungi, and viruses. Some action against bacterial spores [21].	Inactivated by organic matter. Potential to stain contact areas. Less irritant to mucous membranes than chlorhexidine, so more commonly used as skin prep for surgeries involving the oral cavity, respiratory tract, and the eye.
Phenols (Dettol)	Gram-positive and Gram-negative bacteria, enveloped viruses, and fungi [22]. Poor action against bacterial spores [21].	Highly toxic to cats and reptiles, may leave residue on porous materials. Can affect condition of rubber or synthetic items [22]. Remain viable in the presence of organic matter. Should be used immediately after dilution as this reduces stability.
Quaternary ammonium compounds (QACS) (Anigene, Safe4, Anistel, Distel)	Good effect against Gram-positive but less effective against Gram-negative bacteria. Fair antifungal action. Variable antiviral activity [21].	Inactivated by soap, hard water, and organic matter.
Aldehydes (formaldehyde, glutaraldehyde) Cidex	Effective against bacteria, fungi, and viruses. Good but slow activity against bacterial spores [22].	Irritant to eyes, skin, and airways. Used in the farming industry.
Chlorines (Bleach)	Effective against all pathogens including spores [22].	Reacts with other chemicals. Biocidal properties are inactivated by organic matter [22]. Irritant to mucous membranes, airways, and skin. Decomposes in light and heat. Is corrosive.
Peroxide compounds (Virkon S, hydrogen peroxide)	Effective against all pathogens [22]. Variable action against bacterial spores [21].	Irritant to skin and airways. Can cause corrosion to metal. Efficacy is reduced in the presence of organic material.

Source: Jane Devaney.

The efficacy of disinfectants can be negatively affected by the presence of organic material such as blood, faeces and soil. Physical cleaning methods are important to remove this organic matter and allow the disinfectant to have direct contact with the microorganisms present. Chemical disinfectants should always be used after physical cleaning methods have taken place to allow for maximum efficacy [20]. All areas of the practice or hospital will require regular disinfection. Each area of the practice should be assessed for risk according to the risk of cross-infection. SOPs should then be established for the cleaning and disinfection of each area [20]. Low-risk areas include offices and corridors. High-risk areas include examination rooms, stables and operating theatres.

Examination Rooms

Examination rooms can be the busiest places in the practice and are used for many procedures and treatments. They should have a tick list that covers all areas. Daily, the room should be emptied of all removable equipment and bins. All surfaces, walls and stocks should be disinfected, bins should be emptied and wiped over with disinfectant, and sinks should be cleaned. Clippers and shoe removal kits should be cleaned. The use of a disinfectant room fogger/bomb should be considered as part of a cleaning regime. SOPs should be followed.

Stables

As a minimum, all stables should be mucked out twice daily (see Chapter 5). In the hospital environment, each stable should be cleaned between patients. All bedding should be removed and the stable should be steam cleaned and then disinfected with a suitable solution [21]. Attention should be given to any fixtures and fittings, including hosepipes, as they can often drag onto the floor and become contaminated. Feed and water buckets should also be soaked in disinfectant for the described length of time as per manufacturer's instructions. In the case of a horse with a known infection, the stable should be swabbed for culture following the disinfection process [21]. If necessary, the disinfection process should be repeated before the stable is used again. Creating a tick list and following a SOP will help to ensure that a thorough and repeatable technique is adopted.

Feed areas should be emptied at designated intervals and disinfected with a suitable solution; bins should be emptied, disinfected, rinsed and allowed to dry before refilling; scoops and stirrers should also be disinfected. Warm and humid weather can increase the replication of mould and bacteria, so the room should be kept cool and dry with good ventilation. Feed bins should not be continually topped up. They should be emptied fully and then refilled with a new bag of feed. Pest control should be considered as rodents are a source of infection, including salmonellosis and leptospirosis, both of which are zoonotic. All tack, leadropes and headcollars should be disinfected, even if they have not been used. Any other areas, such as round pens, horse walkers or forges should be part of a regular rota for disinfection.

The Laboratory

Areas within the hospital that could be considered the highest risk of contamination are often the cleanest due to high levels of compliance. The lab will take samples from multiple patients, including blood, urine, bodily fluids, washes and faeces, which may be tested due to suspected infection. As a result, meticulous levels of hygiene are strict biosecurity when handling samples are imperative. Any suspected samples should be clearly labelled as such and therefore handled appropriately. As described in other areas, the lab should have a daily cleaning checklist. The cleaning regime should include wiping over the fridge and checking for old samples which should be discarded. All equipment, sink, work surfaces, bins, storage containers for consumables and shelving should be cleaned daily. Other items such as lighting and dispensers should be part of the cleaning regime. See Chapter 8 for more information.

The Operating Theatre

The operating theatre should be cleaned every morning before surgery starts regardless of use overnight. All surfaces and equipment, including anaesthetic equipment, theatre lighting, and waste bins and lifting equipment such as the hoist, should be wiped down with pH-neutral soap and then rinsed before being wiped with a suitable surface disinfectant at the correct dilution. Floors should be mopped with a designated mop and bucket, and the mop head changed after each use. Between each patient, all equipment should be wiped over, the Y piece from the anaesthetic circuit should be soaked in a suitable disinfectant, rinsed and hung to dry. Scrub bowls should be changed between patients, alongside clipper blades. Scrub sinks and taps should also be disinfected between patients. Recovery/induction boxes can be overlooked and require attention; they should be thoroughly disinfected after every patient and be included in the environmental surveillance, any damage to surfaces should be repaired immediately as bacteria can harbour in cracks. Stethoscopes and thermometers can be a source of infection and should be cleaned with an alcohol wipe between patients. Theatre cleaning checklists should be on display, they should be dated and initialled for daily, weekly and monthly tasks. SOPs should be followed. See Chapter 11 for more information.

Practice Vehicles

The Royal College of Veterinary Surgeons (RCVS) practice standards scheme (PPS) dictates the following in relation to infection control and biosecurity for practice vehicles:

- Vehicles must be clean, tidy and well-maintained.
- Vehicles must be equipped sufficiently to enable procedures to be performed out on yards.
- There must be clear segregation of clean and contaminated items.
- Protective clothing should be available.

- There should be the provision of safe storage and transport for waste materials, including sharps.
- Written cleaning protocols are required for all vehicles, and these must be regularly audited and recorded [23].

Registered veterinary nurses (RVNs) have an important role in assisting veterinary surgeons to ensure that practice vehicles are clean and well-stocked. This includes the facility to store contaminated sharps and waste safely, but also to include the facility to transport contaminated clothing, endoscopes or other diagnostic equipment. Dedicated clean clothing should be used for consulting and changed as required. Gloves and aprons must be readily available and used where appropriate. The vehicle should have a minimum stock checklist to ensure that everything is provided to facilitate correct biosecurity when visiting yards. In the event of an outbreak of infectious disease, regulations are governed by The Department for Environment, Food & Rural Affairs (DEFRA) but should include the donning of protective overalls (CE5/6) that are chemical and dustproof and must be discarded after use, gloves and close-fitting goggles and wellies that must be washed before and after each visit.

6.7 Isolation and Barrier Nursing

When managing patients with a contagious disease, it may be necessary to implement isolation or barrier nursing measures to prevent the spread of disease to other patients and members of staff. If there is any doubt as to whether a patient is infectious or not, the procedure should be to **isolate first and confirm the diagnosis later** [24].

Key definitions are as follows:

- **Isolation:** This is the physical separation of an animal reducing the risk of contamination from a proven or suspected infectious disease [20].
- **Quarantine:** This is the compulsory isolation of animals with, or suspected exposure to infectious disease. Strict protocols are in place for animals in quarantine [20].
- **Barrier nursing:** This creates a physical barrier between an infectious animal, other animals in the practice and veterinary staff members [20]. Barrier nursing often involves the donning of PPE such as overalls, aprons, gloves, hats, wellies or shoe covers.
- **Protective isolation or reverse barrier nursing:** This is the isolation of susceptible animals in an attempt to protect them from potential sources of infection [20]. Examples of relevant patients are neonates, geriatrics and immunosuppressed patients. Neonatal foals with failure of passive transfer are commonly put in protective isolation. See Chapter 15 for more information.

Isolation Accommodation

An isolation unit is an area specifically dedicated to housing patients who have or are suspected of having an infectious disease. The ideal attributes of such a unit are as follows:

- A separate building away from other stable blocks with an approach distance of at least 35 metres [24] (see Figure 6.8).
- The unit should have its own water supply and separate drainage.
- A completely separate set of equipment should be stored at the unit, including feed and water buckets, mucking out tools, grooming kits and veterinary equipment [24].
- Floors should be roughened concrete or sealed rubber mats. Walls should be impervious and central floor drains should be present [24].
- In the stable itself, there should be the facility to hang fluids and to observe the patient remotely through closed-circuit television (CCTV) (Figure 6.9).
- There should be the facility to provide heat in the isolation stable, for example, with heat lamps.

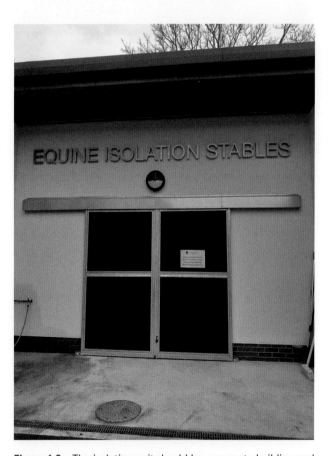

Figure 6.8 The isolation unit should be a separate building and clearly identified. *Source:* Jane Devaney.

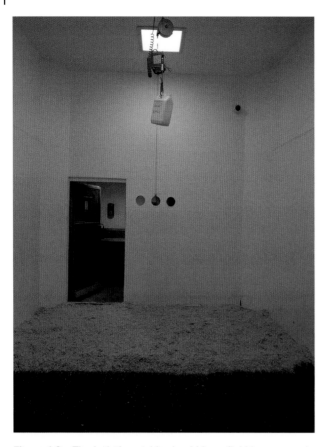

Figure 6.9 The isolation stable should have fluid hangers and CCTV. *Source:* Jane Devaney.

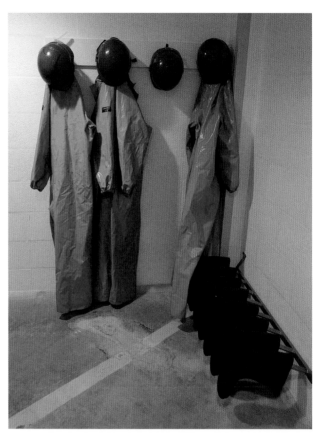

Figure 6.10 The isolation unit should have separate changing facilities. *Source:* Jane Devaney.

- There should be a separate area to store bags of contaminated bedding until tests confirm whether it is to be disposed of as non-hazardous waste, or as hazardous waste if it is confirmed to be infectious [21].
- Foot dips and disinfectant mats should be present.
- Ideally, there should be a separate set of stocks and exam rooms within the building to facilitate the examination and treatment of patients.
- Changing facilities should be present so that staff can change into separate isolation attire, including suits, wellies, gloves, masks and goggles if required (Figure 6.10).
- There should be a sink for washing hands, contaminated equipment and making up medication (Figure 6.11).
- Alcohol hand gel dispensers should be present at regular intervals.
- The isolation unit should be clearly identified with signs.

If it is not possible to set up a separate isolation unit in the hospital or practice, then the next best thing is a yard that can be identified as suitable and demarcated as such. The patient should be housed alone, or if this is not possible, the area must be identified as infectious, and an obvious barrier must be in place to prevent access. A disinfectant foot mat should be placed at the entrance to the stable and be impregnated with a suitable disinfectant effective against the pathogen being treated. Ideally, there should be a one-way system in place, where members of staff can change into isolation clothing, go into the stable, nurse the patient and then exit without retracing their steps. Staff members must ensure that they have disinfected themselves thoroughly before returning to the main yard.

Ideally, one member of the nursing team should be assigned to an isolation case for the duration of their stay. This designated member of staff should avoid contact with other patients until the isolated patient has been discharged. If this is not possible, the isolated horse should be treated last. The isolated horse should, however, still receive the same level of care as the other horses at the hospital. They should not be under-prioritised just because they are in isolation. Intensive nursing care is important for isolation patients, as horses are gregarious in nature and can become depressed when living alone. Interactions such as grooming and providing environmental enrichment are extremely important factors in the recovery of an isolation patient.

Depending on the type of infection and the facilities available, the owner may need to nurse the patient at home.

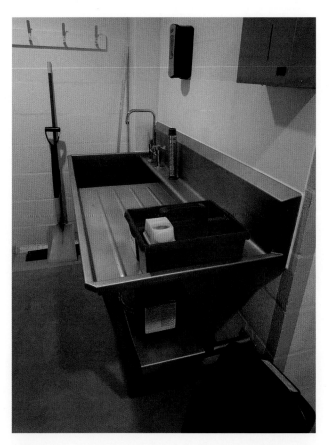

Figure 6.11 The isolation unit should have a separate sink area for the washing of hands and equipment. *Source:* Jane Devaney.

This should only be done when a suitable setup can be provided. This should be prepared before the patient is discharged. The RVN can play an important role here by going out to the yard and helping the owner to set up an isolation facility. The RVN can then remain as a point of contact for the owner to ask questions and get advice post-discharge. The risk to the owner should be considered, and thorough instructions given, alongside sufficient PPE. Owners with high morbidity (elderly or immunocompromised) should not be considered to nurse cases with MRSA at home.

An isolation stable that has housed a patient with a diagnosed infection will have to undergo a deep clean regime once the patient has been discharged. This includes removing and appropriately disposing of all bedding. The walls, floor, windows, door and any additional fixtures should be scrubbed with detergent, followed by a disinfectant. A high-temperature power washer is preferable for chemical disinfection [24]. Environmental swabbing should take place to confirm that the disinfection process has been successful. All equipment used for the patient should be cleaned and thoroughly disinfected. Following an SOP will ensure that a consistent and effective regime is maintained, and this will contribute to a successful infection control programme.

6.8 Clinical Audits

Clinical audits should be carried out regularly in equine practice. A clinical audit will help to identify where things are being done well and where improvements may be required [25]. Clinical audits can be used to assess many factors in the hospital and RVNs can play a very important role in developing concepts to improve client satisfaction, patient welfare, staff morale and profit. To begin, an area of interest needs to be identified, such as a recent disease outbreak or the incidence of surgical site infections. Data from the hospital or practice is then collected. This can take time to achieve but can be a rewarding and team-building experience. This data is then compared with current research and decisions are then made based on the outcomes [25]. The reader is directed to the further reading list for more information.

Clinical audits are a part of the bigger concept of clinical governance. The concept of clinical governance is about creating a 'whole system' cultural change that involves not only clinical audits, but also risk management, staffing and staff management, patient–client involvement, education training, Continued professional development (CPD) and clinical effectiveness [26]. Clinical governance is something that all RVNs should be involved with as it is vital to improve clinical standards and patient welfare. It is also a requirement in the guidance notes of The RCVS Code of Professional Conduct for Veterinary Nurses.

Acknowledgement

Thanks to The Philip Leverhulme Equine Hospital for their assistance in gaining images for this chapter.

References

1 Helps, J., Coyne, K., and Dawson, S. (2012). Infection and immunity. In: *BSAVA Textbook of Veterinary Nursing*, 5e (ed. B. Cooper, E. Mullineaux, and L. Turner), 127. Gloucester: British Small Animal Veterinary Association.

2 Gov.uk (2022). Rabies: how to spot and report the disease [Online]. Available at: https://www.gov.uk/guidance/rabies (accessed 01 January 2023).

3 Gov.uk (2018). Vesicular stomatitis: how to spot and report the disease [Online]. Available at: https://www.gov.uk/guidance/vesicular-stomatitis (accessed 01 January 2023).

4 Gov.uk (2018). Equine infectious anemia (swamp fever): how to spot and report the disease [Online]. Available at: https://www.gov.uk/guidance/equine-infectious-anaemia-swamp-fever (accessed 01 January 2023).

5 Gov.uk (2019). Equine viral arteritis: how to spot and report the disease [Online]. Available at: https://www.gov.uk/guidance/equine-viral-arteritis (accessed 01 January 2023).

6 Gov.uk (2018). West Nile Virus: how to spot and report the disease [Online]. Available at: https://www.gov.uk/guidance/west-nile-fever (accessed 01 January 2023).

7 DEFRA (2012). African Horse Sickness Control Strategy for Great Britain [Online]. Available at: https://assets.publishing.service.gov.uk/government/uploads/system/uploads/attachment_data/file/244348/pb13831-ahs-control-strategy-20130923.pdf (accessed 01 January 2023).

8 Legislation.Gov.UK (1991). The Anthrax Order 1991 [Online]. Available at: https://www.legislation.gov.uk/uksi/1991/2814/contents/made (accessed 01 January 2023).

9 Gov.uk (2021). Glanders and farcy: how to spot and report the disease [Online]. Available at: https://www.gov.uk/guidance/glanders-and-farcy (accessed 01 January 2023).

10 HBLB (2023). Contagious equine metritis – CEM [Online]. Available at: https://codes.hblb.org.uk/index.php/page/19 (accessed 01 January 2023).

11 Gov.uk (2018). Epizootic lymphagitis: how to spot and report the disease [Online]. Available at: https://www.gov.uk/guidance/epizootic-lymphangitis (accessed 01 January 2023).

12 Gov.uk (2018). Dourine: how to spot and report the disease [Online]. Available at: https://www.gov.uk/guidance/dourine (accessed 01 January 2023).

13 Fisher, M. (2020). Elementary microbiology. In: *BSAVA Textbook of Veterinary Nursing*, 6e (ed. B. Cooper, E. Mullineaux, and L. Turner), 136–143. Gloucester: British Small Animal Veterinary Association.

14 Naylor, R.J., Hillyer, L.L., and Hillyer, M.H. (2012). Laboratory diagnostics. In: *Equine Veterinary Nursing Manual*, 2e (ed. K. Coumbe), 216–217. Oxford: Blackwell Science.

15 Divers, T. J. (2022). Leptospirosis in Horses [Online]. Available at: https://www.msdvetmanual.com/generalized-conditions/leptospirosis/leptospirosis-in-horses (accessed 10 October 2022).

16 Ruotsalo, K. (2021). Pneumocytis pneumonia in a Thoroughbred colt [Online]. Available at: https://www.uoguelph.ca/ahl/pneumocystis-pneumonia-thoroughbred-colt (accessed 10 October 2022).

17 Young, A. (2019). Equine protozoal myeloencephalitis (EPM) [Online]. Available at: https://ceh.vetmed.ucdavis.edu/health-topics/equine-protozoal-myeloencephalitis-epm (accessed 10 October 2022).

18 Wright, E. (2020). Medicines, pharmacology, therapeutics and dispensing. In: *BSAVA Textbook of Veterinary Nursing*, 6e (ed. B. Cooper, E. Mullineaux, and L. Turner), 203. Gloucester: British Small Animal Veterinary Association.

19 BEVA (2012). Protect me toolkit [Online]. Available at: https://www.beva.org.uk/Protect-Me (accessed 02 January 2023).

20 Bowes, V. (2016). Managing the hospital ward and basic patient care. In: *BSAVA Textbook of Veterinary Nursing*, 5e (ed. B. Cooper, E. Mullineaux, and L. Turner), 352–353. Gloucester: British Small Animal Veterinary Association.

21 Monsey, L. and Devaney, J. (2012). Maintaining animal accommodation. In: *BSAVA Textbook of Veterinary Nursing*, 5e (ed. B. Cooper, E. Mullineaux, L. Turner, and T. Greet) p. 290, 297, 299, 303. Gloucester: BSAVA.

22 Wild, S. (2020). Infection control and disinfectant types [Online]. Available at: https://knowledge.rcvs.org.uk/quality-improvement/tools-and-resources/qi-cpd/#infection (accessed 29 January 2023).

23 RCVS (2022). PSS equine modules and awards (V3.3) [Online]. Available at: https://www.rcvs.org.uk/document-library/equine-modules/ (accessed 28 January 2023).

24 Linnenkohl, W. and Knottenbelt, D.C. (2012). *Equine Veterinary Nursing*, 2e (ed. K. Coumbe), 10. Oxford: Wiley-Blackwell.

25 McDonald, J. (2020). Client communication and practice organisation. In: *BSAVA Textbook of Veterinary Nursing*, 5e (ed. B. Cooper, E. Mullineaux, and L. Turner), 243. Gloucester: British Small Animal Veterinary Association.

26 RCVS (2018). Clinical audit: what is it and what can you do right now? [Online]. Available at: https://knowledge.rcvs.org.uk/document-library/clinical-audit-what-is-it-and-what-practices-and-individuals/ (accessed 28 January 2023).

Further Reading

RCVS (2023). Code of professional conduct for veterinary nurses [Online]. Available at: https://www.rcvs.org.uk/setting-standards/advice-and-guidance/code-of-professional-conduct-for-veterinary-nurses/ (accessed 28 January 2023).

RCVS (2022). PSS equine modules and awards (V3.3) – Section 6 Infection control and biosecurity [Online]. Available at: https://www.rcvs.org.uk/document-library/equine-modules/ (accessed 28 January 2023).

Mosedale, P. (2021). Infection control and biosecurity: auditing infection control measures [Online]. Available at: https://knowledge.rcvs.org.uk/quality-improvement/tools-and-resources/clinical-audit/ (accessed 28 January 2023).

7

Diagnostic Imaging

Rosina Lillywhite[1] and Cassie Woods[2]

[1] VetPartners Nursing School, Petersfield, UK
[2] Lower House Equine Clinic, Llanymynech, UK

Glossary

Anode The positive electrode to which negative ions transfer in the X-ray tube head (from the cathode) when high-voltage current acts [1].

Atom The smallest particle that forms an element [1].

Cathode The negative electrode of the X-ray tube head from which electrons are emitted [1].

Electron An elementary particle that carries a negative charge and circles around the nucleus of an atom; electricity results from a flow of electrons [1].

Kilovoltage (kV) Refers to how many thousands of volts are applied across the tube head.

Milliamperage (mA) Refers to the current flowing through the tube head.

Milliampere-second (mAs) The amount of current and the exposure time required to calculate the number of X-rays produced.

Neutron Particle in the atom with neutral charge [1].

Proton An elemental particle carrying one positive charge; it is the equivalent of the nucleus of a hydrogen atom and is commonly represented as H1 [1].

Radiation protection adviser (RPA) Qualified person such as a holder of a Diploma in Veterinary Radiology who advises a practice on radiation procedures and safety, in line with the code of practice [1].

Radiation protection supervisor (RPS) Employee of the practice who is responsible for radiation safety on a daily basis [1].

Radiation The electromagnetic spectrum of rays such as radio waves, light, X-rays and gamma rays; the radiation of a short wavelength and high energy can penetrate tissue and ionise molecules [1].

Radiograph The developed and fixed X-ray film or digital image, showing the negative image of the object that has been radiographed [1].

Radiographer A technician trained and qualified to take radiographs and often other diagnostic images such as magnetic resonance imaging (MRI) and computed tomography (CT) scans [1].

Radiography Diagnostic imaging of a part of the body using X-radiation [1].

Radioisotope A molecule that spontaneously emits radiation, losing energy and changing to a more stable form [1].

Radiologist Specialist trained in the interpretation of radiographs and other diagnostic imaging techniques [1].

Radiology The science of the use of radiation for diagnosing and treating disease [1].

Radiolucent A substance that is able to be penetrated by X-rays; the more radiolucent a material is, the darker it will appear on the finished radiograph. gases are the most radiolucent substances [1].

Radiopaque A substance that X-rays find more difficult to penetrate. The more radiopaque a material is, the lighter it will appear on the finished radiograph. Bone and metal are the most radiopaque substances [1].

Ultrasound Sound waves of extremely high frequency, over 20,000 Hz real time, that are produced by an ultrasound machine and used to create and record images of internal anatomical structures; used as a diagnostic tool to guide medical and surgical interventions [1].

7.1 Key Features of Legislation and Radiation Safety

In equine veterinary practice, radiation safety is of the utmost importance and is tightly governed by the Health and Safety Executive (HSE) under the legal guidelines set out in the Ionising Radiation Regulations 2017 (IRR17).

Ionising Radiation Regulations

IRR17 sets out the legal minimum regulatory requirements that a veterinary practice must adhere in order to use radiation. The definition of ionising radiation is particles such as X-rays or gamma rays with sufficient energy to cause ionisation in the medium through which it passes. IRR17 came into force on 1 January 2018 and replaced the previous version of the regulation, which was called the Ionising Radiation Regulations 1999 (IRR99). The new regulations require veterinary practices to register with the HSE if they use diagnostic radiography. This new registration process is a graded approach which requires employers to inform the HSE in one of three ways:

- Notification – this covers any work meeting the following criteria [2]:
  - Work with under 100 kg of radioactive waste.
  - Work carried out in an atmosphere containing radon 222 gas at an annual level exceeding 300 Bq (see radon map (Figure 7.5).
  - Any work that involves X-ray generators needs to be in at least the registration category.
- Registration – this covers work that meets the following criteria [2]:
  - Work with an X-ray generator.
  - Work with over 1000 kg of radioactive material containing artificial radionuclides or radioactive material containing naturally occurring radionuclides which are processed for their radioactive, fissile (able to undergo nuclear fission) or fertile (fertile is a term used to describe an isotope that is not itself fissile).
- Consent – this covers work that meets the following criteria [2]:

  a) The deliberate administration of radioactive substances to persons and, in so far as the radiation protection of persons is concerned, animals for the purpose of medical or veterinary diagnosis, treatment or research.

  b) The exploitation and closure of uranium mines.
  c) The deliberate addition of radioactive substances in the production or manufacture of consumer products or other products, including medicinal products.
  d) The operation of an accelerator (except when operated as part of a practice within sub-paragraph (e) or (f) below and except an electron microscope).
  e) Industrial radiography.
  f) Industrial irradiation.
  g) Any practice involving a high-activity sealed source (other than one within sub-paragraph (e) or (f) above).
  h) The operation, decommissioning or closure of any facility for the long-term storage or disposal of radioactive waste (including facilities managing radioactive waste for this purpose) but not any such facility situated on a site licensed under section 1 of the Nuclear Installations Act 1965.
  i) Practices discharging significant amounts of radioactive material with airborne or liquid effluent into the environment.

Radiation Safety Roles

Although all employees have a role in maintaining safety for themselves and others when working with radiation, two positions in practice have additional control over the work carried out and ensure the safety of all who work with radiation.

The Radiation Protection Advisor (RPA)

The RPA is someone from outside the practice appointed by the practice to ensure that the practice complies with IRR17. This person must have specialist qualifications and have relevant veterinary experience [2].

The Radiation Protection Supervisor (RPS)

The RPS is a person/s appointed to ensure compliance with the IRRs regarding work carried out in an area subject to the local rules. In particular, supervising the safe working arrangements set out in the local rules. Suitability for appointment depends on a knowledge and understanding of the regulations, the local rules and the ability to exercise a supervisory role. People taking on the RPS role should be adequately trained by attending a certificated training course and attending refresher training as required.

These team members will work together to produce risk assessments that identify the risks when performing specific procedures such as radiography, CT and scintigraphy. They will also work together to create a set of local rules that should be displayed in all areas of practice where radiation is used, and they should be specific to that area; according to the HSE, local rules should include the following [2]:

a) The dose investigation level specified in the regulations.
b) Identification or summary of any contingency arrangements indicating the reasonably foreseeable accidents that are possible in practice.
c) Name(s) of the appointed RPS(s).
d) The identification and description of the area covered, with details of its designation.
e) A summary of the working instructions appropriate to the radiological risk associated with the source and operations involved, including the written arrangements relating to non-classified persons entering or working in controlled areas.
f) Where an employer has detailed written working instructions contained within operations manuals or work protocols, it will usually be sufficient for the local rules to refer to the relevant sections of these documents. However, the employer must make sure the way these are summarised in the local rules is adequate.

Local Rules

Local rules in relation to radiation typically refer to regulations, guidelines, or protocols established by local authorities or organisations to manage and control radiation safety within a specific jurisdiction or facility. These rules aim to ensure the safe handling, use and disposal of radioactive materials and protect individuals and the environment from potential radiation hazards. Some common aspects covered by local rules related to radiation are as follows [2]:

- Radiation protection standards: Local rules specify acceptable levels of radiation exposure for workers and the general public. These standards are typically based on national or international guidelines, such as those set by the International Commission on Radiological Protection (ICRP) or relevant regulatory agencies.
- Licensing and permitting: Local rules often outline the requirements and procedures for obtaining licenses or permits to possess, use, or handle radioactive materials. These rules ensure that individuals or organisations comply with specific criteria, training and safety measures to minimise radiation risks.
- Radiation safety training: Local rules may require individuals working with or around radioactive materials to undergo specific radiation safety training programs.

These programs provide education on radiation risks, safe handling techniques, personal protective equipment (PPE) usage and emergency procedures.
- Radiation monitoring and measurement: Local rules may establish requirements for regular monitoring and measurement of radiation levels in areas where radioactive materials are used or stored. This includes the use of radiation detection equipment, such as Geiger-Muller counters or scintillation detectors, to assess radiation levels and ensure compliance with safety standards.
- Waste management: Local rules often address the proper management and disposal of radioactive waste materials generated from medical, industrial or research activities. These rules outline procedures for waste segregation, packaging, storage, transportation and final disposal in accordance with applicable regulations and guidelines.
- Emergency preparedness and response: Local rules may include protocols for responding to radiation emergencies, such as accidental spills, leaks, or overexposures. These rules establish procedures for evacuation, notification of authorities, containment of radioactive materials, decontamination and medical assistance.
- Inspections and enforcement: Local authorities may conduct regular inspections and audits to ensure compliance with radiation safety regulations. These inspections assess the implementation of local rules, verify the proper use of protective measures, review records and documentation, and address any identified non-compliance issues.

It is important to note that the specific local rules regarding radiation can vary depending on the country, state or local jurisdiction. Organisations and individuals working with radioactive materials should familiarise themselves with the relevant local rules and regulations applicable to their specific location and activities. Consulting with local regulatory bodies or radiation safety experts can provide the most accurate and up-to-date information on local rules and compliance requirements [2].

Authorised Personnel

When managing any room that uses ionising radiation, it is important to understand which personnel can be in the room or a designated controlled area. In veterinary practice radiation, a controlled area refers to a designated space within the facility where radiation-producing equipment is used, such as X-ray machines or radioactive materials. This area is subject to specific regulations and safety measures to ensure the protection of personnel, patients and the public from unnecessary radiation exposure. Because a horse requires restraint as they are not always immobilised by sedation, procedures such as radiography require someone to handle the horse during the procedure. In practice, this would ideally be a trained member of staff such as a groom or a patient care assistant (PCA). In an ambulatory setting, the owner may be required to hold the horse. Personnel allowed in a controlled room or a controlled area must meet the following criteria [3]:

- No persons below the age of 18 may enter the controlled area.
- No person receiving radiotherapy may enter the controlled area.
- No pregnant persons may enter the controlled area.
- No person should operate the X-ray equipment without the correct training and authorisation.

Room Design

Most practices will have a designated X-ray room, which serves as the controlled area; there are specific requirements that need to be met; these include [4]:

- Floor – Dimensions should be no smaller than 1.5 m × 2 m. The control area will typically contain a viewing station. If using portable machines, this will form part of the machine.
- Walls – Appropriate wall protection must extend from the floor to a height of no less than 2 m. All joints should overlap alongside any necessary lead lining. Various recommended shielding for protective X-ray room walls includes the following:
  - General purpose radiography and fluoroscopy – The primary wall thickness should be 320 mm solid cement before a secondary layer of 230 mm.
  - CT – The minimum wall thickness must be equivalent to 320 mm of concrete or a solid cement block.
- Doors – Must provide a solid barrier with lead lining necessary for radiation protection. X-ray room doors can also include lead-lined windows. All doors should consist of no less than 1.5 mm of protective lead.
- Windows – Shielded windows need to contain lead glass or lead acrylic in the form of double glazing. Window framing should be shielded with suitable lead equivalent thickness and protected by lead blinds or shutters. As for unshielded windows, positioning them at least 2 m above the ground is recommended.

As well as these features, a controlled area must be demarcated and signed using appropriate signage. A controlled area should have a two-stage fail-safe light in use. All doors in a controlled area should be covered. Lights must have a dual bulb system so that if one bulb were to blow, the other bulb would still work. Lights should be inspected daily. The lights should light up a yellow 'controlled area X-rays' sign when the machine is switched on, and the red 'No entry' sign must illuminate when an exposure is taken; for this to be possible, the lights need to be wired into the X-ray machine. If this is not possible, both lights should be illuminated at all times when the room is in use. If the portable generators are used in a yard, an area should be set up as a controlled area, and all personnel should be informed of this to prevent anyone from entering the area. To create a controlled area in a yard, the following should be carried out [5]:

- Cordon off an area of at least 2 m²; black and yellow plastic chains and bollards can be used to achieve this.
- Use stand-up plastic signs that say 'Controlled area X-rays, No entry.'
- Ensure that personnel are not present in the adjoining stables; preferably, use a brick stable away from anyone else in the yard.

PPE

The use of PPE when dealing with ionising radiation is essential because, in equine practice, personnel are often present in the room when performing radiographs; the correct use of PPE is of paramount importance [3].

Lead Aprons/Gowns

Any person who is in the controlled area during exposure should wear a lead gown/apron; the minimal thickness is 0.25 mm lead equivalent. Most modern gowns will offer higher protection than this; however, this will also increase the weight of the gown. Details and considerations for 0.25 and 0.5 mm gowns are as follows [6]:

0.25 mm Lead Equivalence
- Weighs 1–5 kg ('lightweight gown/apron')
- Attenuates 75% of the X-ray beam at 50 kVp
- Attenuates 51% of the X-ray beam at 100 kVp

0.5 mm Lead Equivalence
- Weighs 3–7 kg ('heavy gown/apron')
- Attenuates 99.9% of the X-ray beam at 50 kVp
- Attenuates 75% of the X-ray beam at 100 kVp

Lead gowns should cover the trunk and gonads and extend to mid-thigh. Lead gowns should never be folded as this can damage the lead inside; ideally, they should be hung up on hangers when not in use. Gowns should be periodically radiographed (once a year) to check for any damage to the lead; if any damage is found, they must be removed from use immediately. It is important to remember that an X-ray gown will only protect from scatter radiation, NOT the primary beam [7].

Thyroid Shields

Thyroid shields should be worn whenever a lead gown/apron is used and should be worn quite tightly. Despite a general awareness that the thyroid gland is sensitive to radiation, studies have found there are no clear protocols for thyroid shield use [3].

Lead Gloves

Gloves should be at least 0.50 mm lead equivalency and protect the user from some of the primary beam; however, this should not be tested; users should stay as far away from the primary beam as possible. Lead gloves should always be worn when holding the cassette or a limb. Staff often find them bulky and difficult to use; however, this should not be a reason for avoiding their use [2].

Dose Monitoring – Dosimeters

All those regularly involved in radiography should wear monitoring devices, and each staff member should wear at least one badge. Staff that are responsible for the daily running of radiography units may require two badges: one to monitor the whole body placed on the inside of the gown at waist height and one placed on the outside of the gown at collar height to measure thyroid exposure [5]. The practice may also place dosimeters in the radiography room or adjacent areas to monitor environmental risk to staff. All readings are documented and retained by the practice, and any high exposures should be investigated before staff are allowed back in close proximity to ionising radiation. The dosimeters must remain at the practice so that the radiation reading is accurate. Dosimeters are usually changed every three months depending on the staff member's workload; this may be increased to monthly if at high risk. Staff should never expose themselves or others to the direct X-ray beam or leave personal dosimeters in the controlled area if they are not present [3].

Types of Dosimeter

Film Badges These contain small pieces of photographic film and various aluminium filters within the badge. After being worn for a period of time, the film is developed and the exposure can be calculated by the degree of film blackening under different filters [8].

Thermoluminescent Dosimeters (TLDs)

TLDs contain radiation-sensitive crystals, which confine the electrons in 'traps' within the crystals. When the material is heated to hundreds of degrees Celsius, the electrons escape from the traps, releasing their energy as visible light. TLDs are small and chemically inert, and the readings can be stored for long periods [9].

Real-time Personnel Monitors

These are electronic devices that continually monitor personnel exposure and have an alarm to warn the wearer if they are being exposed to high levels of radiation. These are designed to help modify behaviours surrounding radiation safety and are starting to be used more commonly in equine practice.

All dosimeters apart from the real-time monitors will need to be sent away for development and reading; the results are typically shared with the RPA as well as the practice.

It is worth noting that not all PPE is equal in efficacy, and the rating should be checked before use [4].

7.2 Principals and Production of Radiation

Atomic Structure

To understand the principles of radiation, the structure of the atom needs to be understood (Figure 7.1) [10]. Atoms contain three sub-atomic particles, positively charged protons and smaller structures called neutrons, which have no charge and electrons; these are negatively charged and orbit in different planes, sometimes known as 'shells' [3]. The

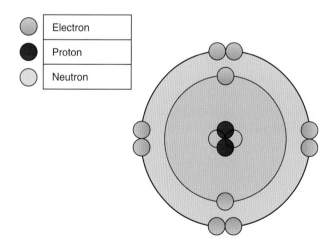

Figure 7.1 Structure of an atom. *Source:* Rosina Lillywhite.

protons and neutrons are found in the atom's nucleus, and the electrons are arranged in energy levels around the nucleus (planes/shells) [10].

Protons and electrons are typically equal in number, meaning that the atom is neutral. If an atom loses or gains an electron, it becomes a charged particle known as an ion. Whether this ion is positively or negatively charged depends on whether it gains or loses an electron [10].

- If an atom loses one or more electrons, it becomes a positively charged ion [10].
- If an atom gains one or more electrons, it becomes a negatively charged ion [10].

Atoms are displayed in the format shown in Figure 7.2. Neutrons and protons, known as the nucleons, are the atomic mass; in Figure 7.2, this is represented by the letter A. The atomic number is also referred to as the proton number and is represented by the letter Z. All the atoms of a particular element have the same atomic/proton number, i.e. all chlorine atoms will have the same atomic number. However, atoms from different elements will have different numbers. For example, oxygen has 8 compared with chlorine, which has 17. The letter X represents the chemical symbol for the element.

Using the information from the whole atomical structure in Figure 7.2, the number of neutrons an atom has can be worked out. Figure 7.3 shows the complete symbol for chlorine; the number at the bottom informs us that there are 17 protons, and we know that there will also be 17 electrons as this number is always the same. Therefore, a simple calculation can be performed to work out the number of neutrons present [10]:

$$35 \,(\text{Mass number (protons + neutrons)})$$
$$- 17 \,(\text{the number of electrons}) = 18 \,\text{neutrons}$$

The number of neutrons depends on the atoms of each element and is known as the atomic number. If an atom loses an electron, it becomes positively charged.

Types of Radiation

X-rays form part of the electromagnetic spectrum along with all types of electromagnetic (EM) radiation. These radiation types are found all around us in many forms;

A   A = Mass Number (Protons + Neutrons)

X   Z = Atomic Number (Protons)

Z   X = Chemical symbol of the atom

Figure 7.2 Atomical structure format [2]. *Source:* Rosina Lillywhite.

Figure 7.3 Complete symbol for chlorine [10]. *Source:* Rosina Lillywhite.

EM radiation is energy that spreads out as it travels from its source. Figure 7.4 shows the EM spectrum and the different types of EM radiation and wavelengths [10].

Although it is strange to see radio waves and visible light in the same spectrum as X-rays and gamma rays, they are not fundamentally different. Despite coming from various sources, they all find themselves on the EM spectrum because they are all EM radiation [11]. The different types of radiation are defined by the different amounts of energy found in the photons. Radio waves have low-energy photos denoted by a longer wavelength, whereas gamma rays have a shorter wavelength with high-energy photons. EM radiation can be expressed in three ways:

- Energy – Measured in electron volts
- Wavelength – Measured in meters (m)
- Frequency – Measured in cycles per second or Hertz

All three of these are precisely mathematically related [11].

Sources of Radiation

There are many sources of radiation, but these can be broken down into two different sections [10]:

- Natural sources
- Artificial sources

Natural Sources

Background radiation is naturally occurring and is all around us; many different sources contribute to it; these include [10]:

- Cosmic rays – the radiation that reaches the earth from space.
- Rocks and soils – some rocks and soils give off radiation and radioactive radon gas.
- Living things – plants will absorb radiation and then pass it up the food chain.
- Radon gas – Radon gas is a naturally occurring radioactive gas that is colourless, odourless and tasteless. It is formed from the decay of uranium, which is found in soil, rocks and water. Radon is considered a health hazard because it can accumulate in indoor environments and expose individuals to radiation.

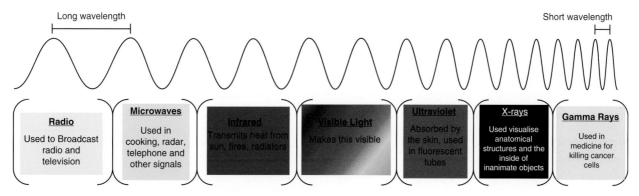

Figure 7.4 Electromagnetic spectrum. *Source:* Rosina Lillywhite.

Natural radiation levels cannot be controlled; however, they must be considered when working within veterinary medicine. The main problem that faces veterinary practice is radon gas; this naturally occurring gas emitted from the ground has been named the second largest cause of lung cancer in the United Kingdom after smoking by the HSE [12]. Practices must be aware of the radon level in their area; this information can be gathered by contacting the local authorities or searching Public Health England. Figure 7.5 shows a map of the United Kingdom and the radon risk ratings associated with each area (please note this Figure is a guide only and was compiled from information available at the time of publication; always check with authorities for up-to-date information).

Once armed with basic information on the local risk ratings practices, it is important to ensure that the recommended levels of $300\,Bq/m^3$ (becquerels per cubic metre) are not exceeded [12]. If radon levels are found to be high, and the practice does not have any preventative measures in place, a test kit should be ordered and used to monitor the levels over three months; this is due to the levels fluctuating over time. If the reading comes back as low, the practice is required by the HSE to monitor the levels again every 10 years [6]. If the reading comes back as high, the practice may be required to put in place the following measures:

- Installing a damp-proof membrane on the ground floor to provide a radon-proof barrier [6].
- Complete radon protection will require provision for a subfloor depressurisation (a radon slump) or ventilation (a ventilation subfloor void) [6].

Artificial Sources

Unlike natural sources, where interventions are limited, artificial sources are sources that humans have created and now contribute to background radiation. Artificial

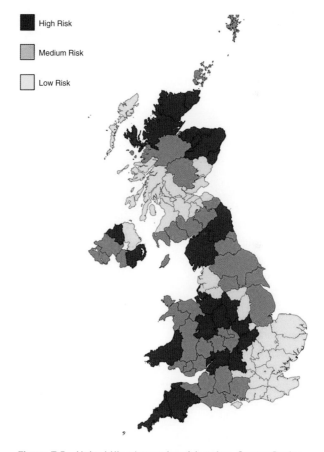

Figure 7.5 United Kingdom radon risk rating. *Source:* Rosina Lillywhite. This map is based on information gathered from relevant data available. For the most comprehensive upto date information visit: https://www.ukradon.org/information/ukmaps.

sources now contribute to around 15% of background radiation and include [2]:

- Medical X-rays and medical nuclear medicine
- Radioactive fallout from nuclear weapons testing
- Radioactive waste from nuclear power stations

Radioactive Emissions/Decay

There are three main types of ionising radiation; when a nuclide undergoes radioactive decay, it breaks down and falls into a lower energy state, and the energy expended is released as radiation [13]. There are three main types of ionising radiation that get emitted from an unstable radioactive atom; these are known as [10]:

- Alpha particles
- Beta Particles
- Gamma particles (or photons) [13]

Alpha Particles

- Are symbolised by α
- They are formed from two protons and two neutrons – the same nucleus as helium but without the electrons
- Are positively charged
- Are heavy
- Have a short range of travel

Beta Particles

- Are symbolised by β.
- Beta particles are high-energy electrons ($\beta-$) or positrons ($\beta+$).
- They have a charge of either −1 (for electrons) or +1 (for positrons) and a mass about 1/1836 times that of a proton or neutron.
- Beta particles have higher penetrating power compared to alpha particles but less than gamma radiation.
- They can be stopped by several millimetres of plastic or aluminium shielding.

Gamma Particles

- Are symbolised by γ.
- Have similar properties to X-rays except for the origin – X-rays originate from electron bombardment, whereas gamma particles are from radioactive atoms.
- Gamma radiation has a very short wavelength and high-frequency electromagnetic radiation.
- They have no charge and no mass.
- They can pass through several centimetres to several meters of material depending on their energy.

The process of a radioactive atom breaking down causes the atom to change into a completely different type of atom, this is known as radioactive decay. It is not possible to know how long it will take an individual atom to decay; however, it is possible to measure how long it will take for the nuclei of a piece of radioactive material to decay. This is known as the half-life of the radioactive isotope [4].

Different radioactive isotopes will have different half-lives, and there are two definitions used to describe how this is measured:

- The length of time it takes for the number of nuclei in a radioactive sample to halve.
- The length of time it takes for the count rate of a sample containing radioactive isotopes to halve from its initial start value [10].

The isotope used most commonly in equine veterinary medicine is called Technetium-99m (Tc-99m). It is primarily used for an imaging technique known as scintigraphy (see Section 7.3). Tc-99m is a rare radioactive metal found in the earth's crust, and because of this, it is predominately manufactured. Tc-99m is produced during nuclear reactor operations and is a by-product of nuclear weapons explosions, and it can also be found as a by-product of nuclear waste [14]. Tc-99m has a relatively short half-life, which is essential in veterinary medicine as it would not benefit the patient to have a long-acting isotope within the body for long periods of time. The half-life of Tc-99m is six hours; within three days, the radioactivity will have dropped to background levels as the Tc-99m changes to Tc-99, which emits soft beta rays [14]. Figure 7.6 shows how Tc-99m decays over time; it is essential to remember that external factors will affect decay, including the horse's metabolism, so practice safety measures should be in place to ensure that staff are not put at risk from handling patients following scintigraphy.

Properties and Effects of Radiation

As discussed, X-rays and gamma rays form part of the EM spectrum. All members of the EM spectrum have the following properties:

- They do not require a medium for transmission and can travel through a vacuum.
- They travel in straight lines.
- They travel at the same speed (3×10^8 m/s in a vacuum).
- They interact with matter either by absorption or scatter [3].

X-rays also have properties which mean in medicine, they can be utilised to image internal structures; these properties include [3]:

- **The direction of travel** – X-rays will always travel in straight lines, accurately representing the patient or objects they pass through. They can only change direction if they collide with an atom, and this may degrade the image [8].

Figure 7.6 Technetium 99m decay.
Source: Rosina Lillywhite.

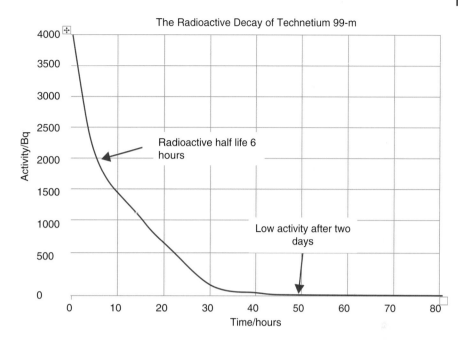

- **Ionisation** – X-rays can interact with tissues and cause ionisation, which occurs when atoms become positively or negatively charged by gaining or losing an electron. It is this effect that allows image production and absorption; however, it is also the reason that X-rays can damage cells and cause cancer [8].
- **Penetration** – Due to the high energy of X-rays, they can penetrate through substances. Photon absorption depends on the nature of the substance penetrated and the energy of the photons. This means some photons will pass through the patient completely, depending on the wavelength; the shorter this is, the higher the energy of the photons [3].
- **Divergence** – As the X-ray beam travels from the target, it will lose intensity and spread out, following the inverse square law (see below for more detail on inverse square law). This is used in radiation protection to reduce the risk and should be considered when setting up safe areas, and the focal film distance (FFD) to ensure consistent radiographs and safety has been considered [8].
- **Absorption** – As the X-rays pass through the patient, they may be stopped or slowed by the patient's tissue; if a dense tissue is being radiographed, for example, bone, the X-rays will be stopped; the term radiopaque is used to describe this. If an area of less density is being radiographed, for example, the sinus, the X-rays will not be stopped, and the term radiolucent is used. Figure 7.7 shows the different tissue types and the number of X-rays absorbed when X-rays pass through them. This image

also shows what colour will show up on the image to denote these different tissues [8].
- **Photographic effect** – X-rays interact with the silver halides within the X-ray film to form an image. They also cause certain phosphors to emit light or fluoresce, the principle used in intensifying screens. The more X-rays that strike the silver halide crystals within the radiographic film, the greater the reaction and the whiter the appearance on the processed radiograph. This interaction is also used in some types of personnel dosimeters [8].

The inverse square law is a fundamental principle in physics that describes how the intensity or strength of a physical quantity decreases with distance. It states that the intensity of a physical quantity is inversely proportional to the square of the distance from the source.

Here are the key points to understand about the inverse square law:

- Relationship: According to the inverse square law, if the distance from a source is doubled, the intensity of the physical quantity decreases to one-fourth ($1/2^2$) of its original value. Similarly, if the distance is tripled, the intensity decreases to one-ninth ($1/3^2$) of its original value and so on.
- Mathematical Formulation: Mathematically, the inverse square law can be expressed as:
- Intensity $\propto 1/\text{distance}^2$
- Where 'Intensity' represents the measured quantity, and 'distance' refers to the distance from the source.

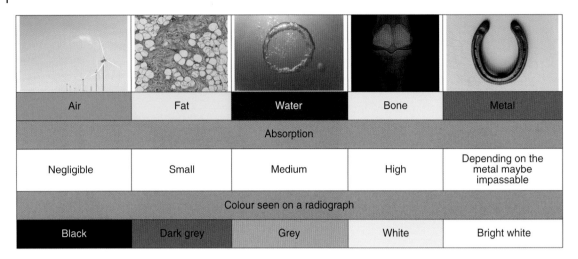

Air	Fat	Water	Bone	Metal
Negligible	Small	Medium	High	Depending on the metal maybe impassable

Absorption

Colour seen on a radiograph

Black	Dark grey	Grey	White	Bright white

Figure 7.7 Radiation absorption by different tissue types. *Source:* Rosina Lillywhite.

Examples: The inverse square law is applicable to various physical phenomena, including:

- Gravity: The gravitational force between two objects follows the inverse square law. As the distance between two masses increases, the gravitational force between them decreases proportionally.
- Light intensity: The intensity of light from a point source, such as a light bulb or a star, decreases with distance according to the inverse square law. This explains why objects appear dimmer as they move farther away from a light source.
- Electric and magnetic fields: The strength of electric and magnetic fields around a point charge or a current-carrying wire follows the inverse square law. As the distance from the source increases, the electric or magnetic field strength decreases.
- Application in radiological sciences: The inverse square law is particularly relevant in radiation safety and radiological sciences. It helps to determine the relationship between distance and radiation exposure. As an individual moves farther away from a radiation source, the exposure decreases in proportion to the square of the distance.

Understanding the inverse square law is important in various fields of science and engineering, including physics, astronomy, optics, radiation safety and wireless communication. It provides a fundamental understanding of how the intensity of a physical quantity changes with distance from a source

X-rays can produce biological changes in living tissue by altering the structure of atoms or molecules or causing chemical reactions. Although this can be used as a benefit, i.e. during cancer treatments, it can also cause harm to living tissue. Therefore, radiation safety should always be considered [3]. For more information on health and safety and PPE, see Section 7.1. Understanding the dangers surrounding the use of radiation can be difficult due to several factors:

- It is invisible.
- It is painless.
- It has cumulative effects.
- It has latent effects which may manifest at a later time.

The results of radiation on the human body can be split into two categories:

- **Somatic:** The somatic effects of radiation are seen on tissue immediately after exposure to a high dose (dose-dependent) of radiation. However, a low regular dose of radiation will have an accumulative effect, and any side effects may not be apparent for many years. The radiation harms rapidly dividing cells, meaning the most common body systems affected are the skin, gastrointestinal and reproductive systems.
- **Genetic:** The genetic effect is an effect that causes mutations in the chromosomes of germ cells in the ovaries and testes, affecting the offspring of the horse exposed.

Scatter Radiation

Scattered radiation or 'scatter' is a type of secondary radiation; as the primary beam leaves the tube head, the photons start to lose energy; as they interact with matter, they change direction instead of being absorbed. Each time scatter radiation hits an object, it changes direction. Not only does this have the potential to affect the image quality, but excess scatter also poses a risk to human health. Due to most equine practices using digital radiography, the detrimental effects to the image are not as readily seen as when using film; however, this should not mean that scatter radiation precautions to minimise it are not taken seriously. Scatter is produced for a number of different reasons. The following factors will alter the amount produced [2]:

- As the region under investigation gets denser – i.e. the patient's cervical spine there is more chance for the X-rays to interact with the electrons within the patient and result in scatter.
- If the collimator is not used effectively – the more open the collimator head is when the image is produced, the more chance there is to create scatter radiation. Making sure that images are collimated tightly not only benefits the image but also improves the safety of personnel. This is achieved through a collimator or light beam diaphragm, usually on the tube head mounting. This is constructed of a box containing a series of mirrors and a light source. The mirrors and light allow a beam of light to be projected onto the patient, representing the primary beam's area and position. The area of the primary beam can be adjusted using the collimator dials located on the top and/or the side of the collimator head. It is essential if this area gets knocked that, the collimation might be knocked out of alignment, causing the light to be misaligned from the primary beam.
- Higher voltages – The voltage should only be increased as the body part being imaged requires; the more energy used to produce an image, the more chance that the scatter will reach the plate; this could cause fogging on the plate (this is not seen as much in digital radiographs, but it can indicate an overexposed image).

Scatter radiation should be controlled to minimise the effect on the radiograph and ensure that staff are not exposed to any unnecessary harm. This can be done in several different ways [4]:

- If the structure that is being radiographed is dense, such as the shoulder, the limb can be manipulated, i.e. have a handler pull the limb forwards; this will bring the leg out, away from the body and reduce the amount of tissue that needs to be penetrated.
- Collimation of the primary beam will reduce the area exposed to radiation, improving safety and reducing tissue exposure and scatter. Collimation will enhance the quality and contrast of the image.
- Reducing the voltage as much as possible while achieving a diagnostic image.

As well as reducing the amount of scatter radiation produced, it is essential to reduce the amount reaching the film, as this will decrease image quality. Using a grid can be an effective tool to aid with this [6]. Depending on the type, a grid can remove 85–95% of all scattered radiation. A grid is constructed of alternating strips of a material able to absorb radiation, for example, lead. The gap between these strips (interspace) is made with a radiolucent material, usually aluminium or carbon plastic fibres. The interspace allows the primary beam to pass through to the film. However, the lead strips absorb the scatter radiation that does not hit the X-ray panel in a parallel orientation. Every grid has a grid ratio, which is determined by the lead strips' height and distance between them; this is used to calculate a grid factor. The grid factor influences the amount by which the mAs must be increased to compensate for the presence of the grid (typically, this is between 2 and 6). The introduction of digital radiography has meant that using a grid is not as necessary due to the computer's corrective software; it may still be advisable to use a grid when using higher exposures on areas such as necks and backs [7].

X-ray Tube Construction

Tube Structure

The tube head is responsible for producing X-rays and is comprised of an anode and cathode surrounded by a Pyrex tube. The purpose of the tube is to create a vacuum, preventing unwanted interactions during the production of X-rays. The anode and cathode have a high-tension electrical supply to create the necessary direct current to generate X-rays. Oil surrounds the Pyrex tube; this prevents the build-up of heat, and there is a lead surround to prevent X-rays from passing straight through the tube. Although a lead case surrounds the entire structure, a small window under the anode allows the primary beam to exit the tube. A small aluminium filter in the window removes any low-energy X-rays as this can be undesirable for image quality [8].

The Cathode

The negative side of the X-ray tube head is known as the cathode, and it comprises the following elements:

- A filament
- A focusing cap

The filament and its supporting wires are very fine wires that are heated to produce electrons in a similar way to which a toaster heats bread. To prevent the filament from melting, it is made from tungsten, which has a high melting point of around 6192°F (3422°C). The function of the focusing cap is to channel electrons in a narrow band towards the anode during exposure [15]. Both the electrons and focusing cup are negatively charged; this allows the electrons to be relayed to the centre, ensuring they remain in a narrow stream and are not spread, which means that no electrons fall beyond the boundaries of the anode [8].

The Anode

The anode is on the positive side of the X-ray tube and can be either stationary or rotating. As seen in Figure 7.8, the stationary anode is fixed, as the name may suggest. This type of anode is generally used in smaller portable units where a high tube current and power are not required [9].

Tubes that contain a rotating anode are used in larger, more high-powered machines that are required to produce a high-intensity beam quickly. Figure 7.9 shows the rotating anode in the tube head. Typically, most machines will have a rotating anode; stationary anodes are more common in small animal dental units.

The anode serves two principal functions [9]:

- It provides mechanical support for the target.
- It acts as a good thermal conductor for heat dissipation.

X-ray production results in 99% heat and 1% actual X-rays, so the heat must be removed to prevent the anode from melting. The target is the area where the electrons strike. In a rotating tube, this is a disc around the entire circle of the target disc. As the target rotates, the area that the electrons strike changes; this increases the area that the electrons can strike which in turn, increases the tube's lifespan [8]. If the anode is stationary, the whole surface is the target. The target is made of tungsten alloy embedded in a copper anode. In some tubes, the target is supported on molybdenum or graphite to make tube rotation easier. The area hit by the electrons is called the focal spot, which is the source of the radiation emitted from the X-ray tube. The effective focal spot emitted from the tube will alter depending on the angle of the target. This angle is usually between 7° and 20° to the vertical. The focal spot's effective size increases as the target angle increases (Figure 7.10) [8].

X-ray Production

The production of X-rays starts with the depression of the exposure button. This is typically a two-stage exposure button of which the first half depression rotates the anode and heats the cathode. A complete depression, after a short pause, causes actual radiographic exposure [8, 16]. Figure 7.11 shows the X-ray production process from the depression of the exposure button to the X-rays leaving the tube head. If the exposure button is released at any

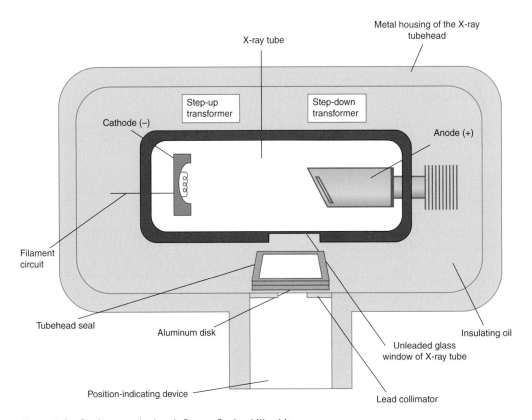

Figure 7.8 Stationary tube head. *Source:* Rosina Lillywhite.

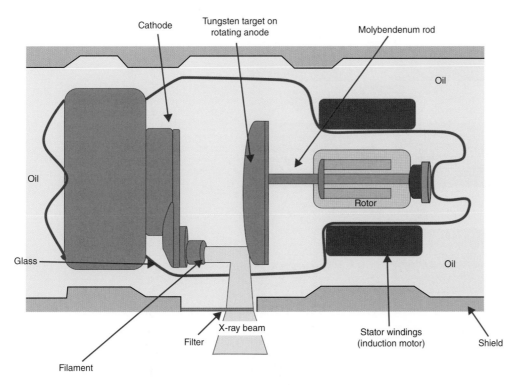

Figure 7.9 Rotating tube head. *Source:* Rosina Lillywhite.

Figure 7.10 The projected effective focal spot (seen on the target) is much smaller than the actual focal spot size (projected to the left). This provides a beam that has a small, effective focal spot size to produce images with high resolution while allowing for heat generated at the anode to be dissipated over the larger area [16]. *Source:* Rosina Lillywhite.

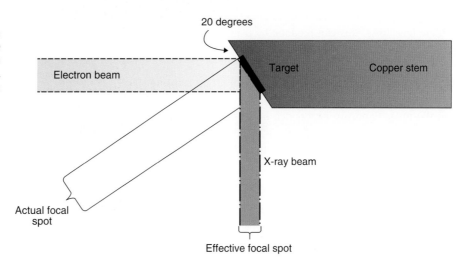

point before it is fully depressed, this will cease the exposure, and X-rays will not be produced.

- During the first stage of X-ray production, the filament at the cathode is heated and the selected milliamperage determines the heating amount. The higher the milliamperage, the higher the heat and the more electrons produced. Heating releases electrons from the surface of the filament wire. The electrons collect in the focusing cup. These electrons contain electrical potential and,

when a charge is applied, will flow from negative to positive (i.e. cathode to anode).

- During the second stage of X-ray production, a potential difference is applied between the cathode and anode, ensuring that the electrons flow to the anode. This is achieved by applying a kilovoltage selected when setting the exposure factors. The higher the chosen kilovoltage, the faster the electrons will move towards the target, resulting in higher-energy X-rays. The electrons are accelerated from the cathode to the anode and are

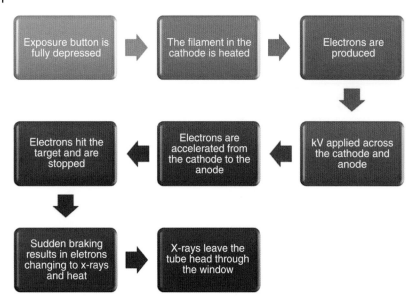

Figure 7.11 Flow diagram of the production of X-rays within the tube head [16]. *Source:* Rosina Lillywhite.

stopped as they strike the target. This sudden braking results in the electrons changing into X-rays, which are then released from the X-ray tube through the window [7].

Exposure Factors

When using a grid, it is essential to understand how to calculate new mAs; this can be done by using a simple grid calculation. But first, it may be necessary to work out the exposure factors [3].

Working out exposure factors can be important as some machines will work on the mA, whereas others will work on the mAs. Exposure factors can be worked out using a simple triangle calculation (Figure 7.12). Using this as a reference, try to solve the following maths questions (answers found at the end of the chapter):

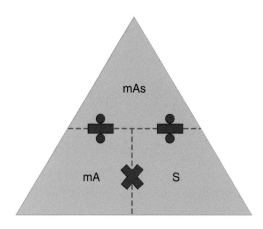

Figure 7.12 Calculation triangle for radiography. *Source:* Rosina Lillywhite.

Question 1:

- mAs = 10
- mA = 100

What are the seconds?
Answer:

Question 2:

- mA = 200
- S = 0.2

What is the mAs?
Answer:

Question 3:

- mAs = 20
- S = 0.1

What is the mA?
Answer:

Once the current and time of exposures have been worked out, it becomes easy to link the kV into the equation [6].

A simple rule links kV and mAs:

- Increasing the kV by 10 allows the mAs to be halved
- Decreasing the kV by 10 requires mAs to be doubled

Question 4:

- kV = 50
- mAs = 24
- The kV is changed to 60

What is the new mAs?

Question 5:

- kV = 40
- mAs = 12
- The kV is changed to 30

What is the new mAs?
Adding a grid:
The equation used for using a grid is:

$$new\ mAs = old\ mAs \times grid\ factor$$

Question 6:

- Old mAs = 12
- Grid factor = 3

What is the new mAs?

Types of Grid

There are several different types of grids:

Stationary grids – These can either be separate or built into the front of the cassette; they come in various sizes to fit the different plate sizes. As the name suggests, stationary grids do not move during exposure; they remain stationary. Types of stationary grids include [3]:

Parallel Type Grids

A grid where the absorbing strips are parallel to each other in their longitudinal axis. Also known as a non-focused linear grid, it has parallel strips when viewed in cross-section; this is why it is called a parallel grid [9].

Focused Type Grids

A grid in which the absorbing strips are slightly angled towards the focal spot. The grid can therefore be used only at a specified focal distance. Otherwise, the grid will absorb the primary radiation, and parts of the film are barely exposed. Focused grids may be linear or crossed [9].

Criss-cross Type Grids

A grid consisting of two superimposed parallel grids having the same focusing distance. Such grids efficiently remove scattered radiation but must be arranged at precisely right angles to the beam; this is, therefore, the limiting feature of these grids [9].

Tapered Type Grids

A grid in which the surface is tapered into the centre of the grid, functioning similarly to a focused grid. All of the strips are parallel to each other, and the tapered surface is towards the focal spot [17]. Figure 7.13 illustrates the different layouts of stationary grids.

Mobile grids, also known as 'Potter-Bucky', move during exposure and are integrated into an X-ray table, moving rapidly from side to side. The chance of grid lines can be eliminated when using a mobile grid. Due to this type of grid requiring a table and motor, this is not practical in equine practice [8].

Types of X-ray Generator

The fundamental principles of X-ray generators are the same; however, their powerfulness can differ. Generators

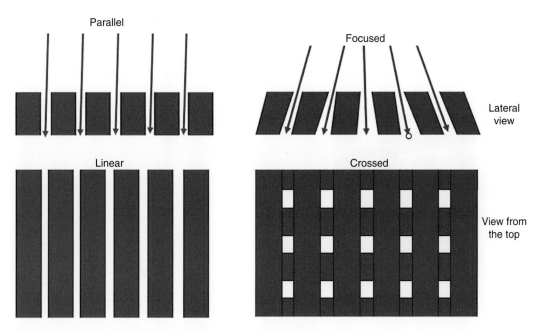

Figure 7.13 Types of stationary grid. *Source:* Rosina Lillywhite.

can be broken down into portable, mobile, fixed or static generators; which one is used will depend on the type of work that is done.

Portable

Portable generators are the most common in equine practice; they are convenient to fit into cars in their protective case and powerful enough to take good-quality radiographs. Modern portable generators are battery-powered, making it possible to radiograph a patient in a variety of situations. Older systems may still rely on a power cable, which limits their use to yards with a power supply. Due to their size and relatively low power, they are best suited to imaging lower limbs. However, some more modern units have increased in capacity, making it possible to image more proximal structures (it is important to remember that this can affect image quality as the exposure time is also higher, making it easier to get movement blur). Figure 7.14 shows a battery-powered portable generator currently on the market.

These generators should always be used with a stand. This statement from the HSE should be considered when using stands:

Here is a message from the community manager:

> It has been brought to the attention of HSE's Radiation Team that it has become common practice to carry out certain equine X-ray radiography examinations with the vet, or other person, holding the X-ray device. HSE are firmly of the opinion that it is reasonably practicable to use a stand or holder for the X-ray device for these types of exposures. Furthermore, an attempted justification that holding the X-ray device 'saves time and money or it's just easier' is simply not acceptable.

> *Holding an X-ray head/tube means that radiation exposures to the person holding it would not be As Low As Reasonably Practicable [ALARP] and there may also be a risk of serious, or fatal, electric shock. Additionally, there is the added risk of being very close to the horse if it were to kick out or move suddenly. In most cases HSE Radiation Specialist Inspectors will prohibit this practice if they become aware of it during an inspection, unless there was a very robust justification and it was fully considered in the radiation risk assessment with detailed safe systems of work in place [2].*

Therefore, hand-holding of the X-ray generator poses an unacceptable risk to the personnel involved from the standpoint of radiation safety. Because of this, many different types of generator stands are available on the market that can suit individual practice needs and prices. Figure 7.15 shows the Stat-X Espléndido sold by Podoblock; these stands are versatile and easy to use [18].

Mobile

These generators are rarely used in equine practice as they are bulky and have low ground clearance; historically, they were helpful in the operating theatre as they have a

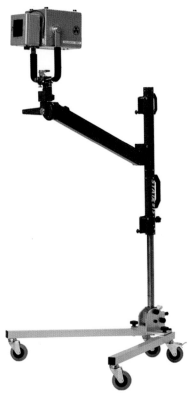

Figure 7.15 The Stat-X Espléndido X-ray generator stand.
Source: With permission from Podoblock; Rosina Lillywhite.

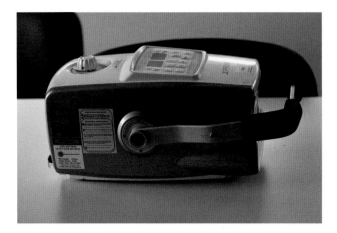

Figure 7.14 Battery-powered portable generator. *Source:* Rosina Lillywhite.

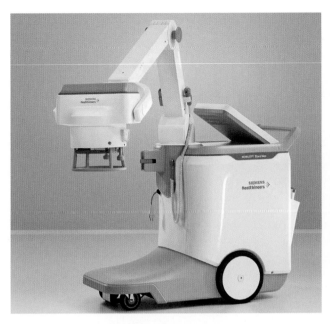

Figure 7.16 Mobile X-ray generator. *Source:* From Siemens Healthineers; Rosina Lillywhite.

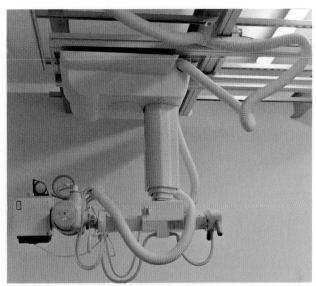

Figure 7.17 Gantry mounted generator. *Source:* Rosina Lillywhite.

higher-powered output and were better for the radiographic examination of the pelvis and intraoperative radiographs during fracture repair as the older portable machines had wires that could get in the way of the sterile field [7]. However, they have now largely been superseded by battery-operated portable units as the limitations of these machines outweigh the positives. Besides the poor manoeuvrability that this type of machine offers, it is also impossible to have the tube head reach the floor in most models, meaning it would be impossible to radiograph the horse's feet. These units are primarily used in human trauma units where moving the patient could cause further damage, and speed is essential. Figure 7.16 shows a modern DR mobile X-ray generator.

Fixed or Static

Fixed, sometimes known as static generators, are commonly used in equine referral practices and larger first-opinion practices. These high-output generators generally produce higher kVp (kilovoltage peak) and mAs compared with most portable machines. It is essential that the maximum kVp and mA are understood if using X-ray generators; this can be found in the technical specifications of the product. Figure 7.17 shows a gantry-mounted fixed generator [3].

Computed Radiography (CR) and Digital Radiography (DR)

Recent advancements in diagnostic imaging have replaced conventional film-screen systems with CR or DR systems (this textbook will not be covering film-screen systems or manual processing as these methods are becoming obsolete

in equine practice). CR and DR systems are now the mainstay systems used in equine practice [7]. CR and DR require the use of digital technologies which rely on computer networks and web facilities. DR uses flat panel detectors based on the direct or indirect conversion of X-rays to charge, which is then processed to produce a digital image [19]. CR uses cassette-based phosphor storage plates (PSP), which are scanned by the computerised system into a digital format for image processing, archiving and presentation. However, the procedure is digitised with DR from X-ray detection onward [19].

DR and CR systems produce digital images that can be manipulated and viewed on a computer. Care should be taken that the spatial and contrast resolution of the viewing screen does not compromise the image quality. CR and DR systems offer many options during and after image acquisition. Some image quality parameters are specific to the individual system [20]. This should be factored in if the system is changed so that the software works for the individual requirements of the practice. Personal preference plays a large role in what is considered to be the 'best image', and this will have an effect on the type of image system selected. Factors that should be taken into account are the type of imaging being performed and the types of cases being seen. The world of imaging technology is changing rapidly, and it is well worth checking standard procedures regularly; for example, DR plates are becoming more sensitive to X-rays; hence, exposures can be decreased, and areas where it was previously impossible to acquire diagnostic-quality radiographs with portable machines, might now be accessible. Table 7.1 highlights the advantages and disadvantages of CR and DR radiography; as

Table 7.1 Advantages and disadvantages of CR and DR radiography.

X-ray system	Advantages	Disadvantages
Digital (DR)	Speed and efficiency: DR systems provide immediate image acquisition and display, eliminating the need for manual processing steps. This significantly speeds up the workflow and allows for quicker patient throughput	Higher cost: DR systems generally have a higher upfront cost compared to CR systems. The cost of acquiring and maintaining the digital detectors can be a significant investment
	Image quality and consistency: DR detectors typically provide high-quality images with excellent spatial resolution and contrast. The images are digital from the start, reducing the chances of artefacts or degradation compared to CR systems	Limited flexibility: DR detectors are typically more rigid and less flexible than CR cassettes, making it challenging to use them in non-standard imaging positions or in portable imaging scenarios
	Lower radiation dose: DR systems generally require lower radiation doses to produce high-quality images compared to CR systems. This can be beneficial in terms of patient safety and dose reduction	Saturation and image clipping: DR detectors have a limited dynamic range compared to CR, which means that very high or very low exposure levels may result in saturated or clipped images, losing some details
	Integration and connectivity: DR systems are often more seamlessly integrated with picture archiving and communication systems (PACS) and radiology information systems (RIS), allowing for easy storage, retrieval and sharing of digital images	
Computed radiography (CR)	Cost-effective transition: CR systems can be a more affordable option compared to DR systems, especially when upgrading from traditional film-based radiography. CR technology allows the use of existing X-ray equipment with minor modifications, making it a cost-effective transition to digital imaging	Workflow speed: The process of digitising CR imaging plates takes longer compared to DR, as the plates need to be inserted into a separate reader and processed before the images are available for review. This can slow down the overall workflow in busy radiology departments
	Flexibility: CR imaging plates are reusable and can be used with multiple patients, making them more flexible than DR detectors. This can be advantageous in high-volume settings	Image quality variability: The image quality of CR radiography can be more susceptible to artefacts or degradation if the imaging plates are not handled properly or if there is dust or scratches on the plates
	Wide dynamic range: CR systems have a wide dynamic range, meaning they can capture a broad range of X-ray exposures. This allows for excellent image quality across different patient sizes and X-ray techniques	Higher radiation dose: CR systems may require a higher radiation dose compared to DR systems to achieve the same image quality
	Portability: CR cassettes are lightweight and portable, enabling easy transport between different X-ray rooms or facilities	

Source: Rosina Lillywhite [19].

highlighted in this table, the benefits far outweigh the drawbacks in favour of DR radiography, making it the most popular choice for equine practice [13].

CR Systems

Unlike traditional X-ray systems, which use film, CR systems use photostimulable phosphor imaging plates to capture images. Upon radiation exposure, the plate captures an image of the patient, which is CR's main similarity to traditional X-ray film capture. Instead of going through darkroom processing, the CR system uploads the image to a computer program for analysis [20]. This program allows the image to be adjusted and apply digital enhancements to make analysis easier.

Computed radiography systems comprise several hardware and software components that perform each part of the imaging process.

The main parts of a CR system include [21]:

- Radiographic generator: This device emits the necessary radiation to create an image on the plate.
- Imaging plates: CR systems use cassettes containing reusable phosphor plates rather than film. These can be erased and reused these plates thousands of times, significantly reducing the need for consumables.
- Image labeller: This labels the image with the correct patient details and views before processing; it is often connected to the workstation.
- Image reader or processor: The reader replaces the darkroom of conventional X-ray development. Rather than

applying chemical solutions to an exposure to reveal the image, CR readers scan the phosphor plate and digitise the image. They then transfer the image to the workstation.

- Workstation: Most CR radiography systems use a standard PC to view, evaluate and send digitised images.
- Software: Diagnostic imaging software provides a consolidated platform for storing, analysing and managing radiographs. This software streamlines file management and optimises analysis processes.

Proper system maintenance is critical for ensuring high-quality radiographs. For example, imaging plates must be erased after each use because residual energy can create ghost images in later exposures [15]. It is also essential to regularly erase unused cassettes, which can capture faint images even while not in use. CR cassettes need cleaning regularly (this should be done following the manufacturer's guidelines).

The CR Process

CR can be misleading because the imaging process includes minimal computations. It is more similar to traditional X-ray imaging than most computer processes [21].

The process works as follows:

1) Exposure

    First, using a generator, expose the imaging cassette and patient to radiation to capture a latent image. The energy from the radiation remains trapped in the cassette's phosphor layer [21].

    Exposure time and image quality can vary depending on the type of cassette used and other factors such as software, FFD, kV and mAs and the monitor used for viewing.

2) Labelling

    The cassette is then placed into a labeller that applies the patient details and view to the final computed image [21].

3) Digitisation

    The cassette is then placed into the CR reader, which scans the plate using a focused laser beam. The plate emits a bright blue light in response, allowing the reader to pick up the image on the plate [21].

    Using an analogue-to-digital converter (ADC), the scanner turns the light into a digital signal that transfers to the computer. Then, it wipes the image from the plate using a high-intensity light source [21].

4) Analysis

    Analysis can begin once the converter has transferred the image to the workstation. The computer software

allows image manipulation for more in-depth analysis. The cassette can be reused immediately after erasure if needed [21].

DR Systems

Flat panel detectors have become the modern favourite for X-ray imaging detecting systems. The reason can be attributed to its numerous benefits over other image-detecting systems, including image intensifiers and X-ray film plates [16].

The flat-panel detector is a modular composition of individual functioning units that combine to make detecting X-rays possible. These functional units are known as pixel arrays and are used to convert X-ray radiation to light energy, making up the image. These pixel arrays are the sensitive parts of the flat panel detector, which are usually square or rectangular shapes with varying dimensions depending on the size of the sample material under examination. However, depending on the desired spatial resolution, this array may include thousands of pixels, with each pixel having square shapes and micrometre-long sides. For every functional unit of the flat panel detector, very short radiation falls on the pixel array whenever an X-ray image is taken, while the pixels collect and store this radiation until it is read out. These pixels each include a photodiode that uses the impacting X-rays to generate an electrical charge. The pixels also have a switch with a thin-film transistor (TFT) or indium gallium zinc oxide (IGZO), often utilised as a display technology. However, IGZO is a more recent advancement than the TFT. The switch and the photodiode help generate the image by direct or indirect conversion of the X-rays [16].

Flat Panel Detector Working Principle

Generally, detectors are classified based on their method of conversion of X-rays to light energy during the creation of the image. According to this definition, two types of detectors, direct and indirect, are used in flat panel detectors [16].

Direct Detectors

The type of X-ray conversion used in direct detectors is the direct conversion method from which they derive their name. They establish their transformation using photoconductors like amorphous selenium (a-Se) or similar photoconductors to convert X-ray energies to an electric charge directly. Electron hole pairs are generated from the X-ray photons on the selenium layer using an internal photoelectric effect. Applying a bias voltage to the selenium layer depth allows the holes and electrons to be drawn to corresponding electrodes to generate a proportionate electric current to the radiation's intensity. In the TFT, array an electronic device is employed to read out the signals [16].

Indirect Detectors

Indirect detectors, on the other hand, employ a scintillating material layer such as gadolinium oxysulfide or caesium iodide to convert the X-ray energy to light with an amorphous silicon detector array embedded behind the scintillating layer. Like the image sensor chips found in a digital camera, photodiodes are included in every pixel that produces the electrical signals. These signals are comparable to the scintillator layer lights in front of the pixels used to generate a precise X-ray image [16].

Flat Panel Detector Process

To generate the images after an X-ray examination, the X-rays are converted into light energies that are also converted into electrical signals for each pixel's photodiodes. Furthermore, a thin-film transistor switch enables the readout of the electrical signals of each diode. Also, the photodiode and TFTs switch are connected using a signal wire with either an analogue or a digital conversion to generate an image after a low-noise amplification [22].

Image Quality

Image quality is a main parameter that influences the diagnostic success of an imaging procedure. The quality of the image is vital to ensure a correct diagnosis and avoid misinterpretation of an image. This is especially important concept to consider as registered veterinary nurses (RVNs) may be directed to acquire images for the veterinary surgeons (vets) to assess at a different time. Table 7.2 displays the different parameters that influence image quality [13].

Methods of Restraint for Radiographic Examination

The restraint of equine patients in preparation for radiographic examination is performed in two ways: manual and chemical. Special consideration needs to be given to manual restraint as this means radiation exposure for more personnel, and under IRR17, this should be limited where possible. Some patients cannot be chemically restrained due to the type of radiograph, for example, a barium swallow. However, most patients will be given a sedative to achieve chemical restraint; the correct restraint is essential to minimise the chances of injury to the horse or personnel during exposure and any damage to expensive equipment [9]. It is the responsibility of the case vet to assess the need for sedation and if required, to prescribe the correct type and dose of sedation to be administered.

When imaging patients with debilitating conditions, clinical considerations are essential to avoid causing a deterioration in the condition of the horse. Pain and suffering must be avoided as much as possible. With these patients,

depending on the area of interest, it may be helpful to use nerve or joint blocks to assist with good radiographic technique. This decision would be made by the case vet.

The implications of poor patient positioning can be detrimental to the diagnosis and therefore the prognosis of an injury. The best radiographic outcome can be achieved by ensuring the following [9]:

- There should be enough personnel available to carry out the procedure safely. Ideally, this should include a horse holder, a plate holder and a radiographer.
- The patient should be correctly restrained by a handler wearing appropriate PPE.
- The patient should be standing square, on a level surface.
- There should be enough room to manoeuvre around the patient with the radiographic equipment.

Figure 7.18 shows a horse positioned ready for a radiograph.

Radiographic Views

When radiographing a horse, the RVN must understand the requirements of the images to be captured. In order to achieve this, the RVN must have an understanding of anatomical projections and radiographic views. Figure 7.19 Displays nomenclature used to describe anatomical and radiological views. The direction of the X-ray beam is indicated by first describing the position of the tube in relation to the area of interest and then that of the X-ray cassette (Figure 7.19):

- In the head and trunk, 'left to right' and 'right to left' are the correct descriptions but may be referred to as 'lateral' on the radiograph (Figure 7.19).
- Dorsoventral and ventrodorsal are straightforward (Figure 7.19).
- Obliques should be described by starting with the closest standard projection and then adding the angle and direction in which the projection is altered (Figure 7.20). For example, a lateral view of the cervical vertebrae with the tube head tilted down by 30° would be described as a latero-dorsal lateroventral radiograph. In the limb, a view from the side is called a lateromedial or mediolateral. Above the carpus and tarsus, front-to-back views should be called craniocaudal or caudocranial. Below and including the carpus and tarsus, front-to-back views are called dorsopalmar or palmarodorsal in the forelimb, and dorsoplantar or plantarodorsal in the hindlimb.
- Obliques are constructed as described above but can be more complex.
- A view from between dorsal and lateral would be dorso – X° – lateral palmaromedial (Figure 7.20).

Table 7.2 Parameters that affect image quality in CR and DR radiography.

Parameter	Specific properties	Factors	Solutions
Image resolution	Image resolution quantifies how close structures can be to each other and still be visibly resolved and provides a measure of detail	Conventional radiography is usually expressed as line pairs/mm (10–15 lp/mm) – this book does not cover conventional radiography as it is not a process regularly used in equine practice	An essential factor in viewing a radiograph is the viewing screen; this needs a high-resolution screen; otherwise, the image taken as a high resolution will not be considered a high-resolution image, which means that the image will look poor in quality and this may affect the diagnosis
		In CR/DR radiography, the image is expressed in pixels, similar to photo cameras and smartphones	The resolution of an image is also impacted by how a file is sent; a jpeg (Joint Photographic Experts Group) which is a default setting for an image, compresses the file and reduces its quality; therefore, all diagnostic images sent to a vet should be sent as a DICOM (Digital Imaging and Communications in Medicine) image
		The manufacturer sets image resolution, which cannot be changed in DR systems; however, different plates with different resolution types are available in CR systems. While the standard plates are sufficient for most applications, high-resolution plates may be better for fine trabecular detail	Follow the manufacturer's guidelines, and if purchasing a new system, make sure these details are thought about
		In veterinary medicine, there are no minimum resolution guidelines, there are no minimum guidelines a system needs to have; however, they typically follow the ones set for human medicine	Contact the manufacturers to help make standard exposure charts that will be suitable for equine patients. Collaboration within the practice as the units are used will also enable this to happen
Image sharpness	Image sharpness describes how well the edges of a structure can be distinguished from other structures or the background. Image sharpness is affected by the equipment and the way radiographs are taken	Film-focus distance (FFD): try to ensure that the FFD is between 75 and 110 cm in modern units. This is marked with a laser that forms a cross on the patient at the correct distance; failing this, most units have an inbuilt tape measure	Using a generator stand should always be done for health and safety reasons; however, it also has an impact on movement blur as the holder often moves while holding
		Distance between the horse and the X-ray plate: try to keep the plate as close to the horse as possible, as this reduces the magnification of the image. If using a DR flat panel, be aware that the patient kicking the plate may cause costly damage	Using a plate stand rather than holding equipment by hand is also another way to reduce exposure to personnel
		Movement blur: movement blur can occur through all personnel involved in radiography	The use of a headstand may help steady the whole horse
			Adequate sedation, a combination of butorphanol and detomidine or romifidine, usually works well – over sedation is also undesirable, though, as this will increase movement blur

(Continued)

Table 7.2 (Continued)

Parameter	Specific properties	Factors	Solutions
			Exposure time should be as short as possible; however, this can be difficult in the smaller output machines radiographing denser tissues such as the neck and back. Where possible, try to keep exposure time below 0.2 s
			Post-processing: many systems have edge enhancement options. Beware that these can also lead to a false impression of sharpness
			Collimation: generally, the tighter an image is collimated, the sharper the image will be – however, it is essential to read the manufacturer's guidelines as this may not be the case with a DR system
Image contrast	Image contrast is the difference in radiodensity that makes an object distinguishable from another structure	The pixel depth (in bits per pixel) measures the image's contrast resolution (grey value). For example, a 1-bit image shows only black and white, an 8-bit image shows 256 greys and a 12-bit image 4096 greys It is expressed as contrast resolution and is a measure of the grey values. The more 'greys' an image displays, the more structures of different radiodensities it can distinguish	Image processing: DR and CR systems offer many post-processing and viewing options; good understanding and practical training are essential in getting the most out of a system
			Image display: ensure that the viewing screen has an adequate contrast range. When viewing an image, changing contrast and brightness will often facilitate a more accurate appraisal of the image
			Detector: different systems have different contrast, and this should be considered when buying a new system
			Object size and radiodensity: this is obviously out of the control of the operator
Signal-to-noise ratio	The signal-to-noise ratio is the ratio between the wanted information (for example, the image of a bone) and unwanted interference 'noise' (anything that hinders us from seeing the bone clearly)	Scatter: in the horse, the primary factor causing 'noise' in an image is scatter radiation, which is in turn influenced by the amount and radiodensity of the tissues. This is especially a problem in the proximal area of the horse	Collimation: the easiest way to decrease scatter is to collimate around the area of interest as tightly as possible
			Exposure values need to be set correctly using as low as reasonably possible (ALARP) protocols
			Detector and post-processing system: some systems are more sensitive to scatter than others
			Filter: this can be in the form of mechanical grids or digital filters. Grids can be used to reduce scatter to a certain degree. DR systems often reach the same scatter reduction as a grid through inbuilt filters. Grids need to be carefully chosen for the system used and require perfect alignment of the beam and an exact distance between the grid and the X-ray machine (required distance is usually shown on a label on the grid)

Exposures	Three parameters determine radiation exposure: kVp (peak kilovoltage), mA (milliamperes) and time (seconds)	kVp determines the energy of the X-ray beam and its penetration 'power'	Decreasing the kVp settings increases the image contrast and decreases the latitude. A kVp setting under 7) is desirable for good bone radiographs. The higher the kVp, the lower the contrast and the more scatter is generated
		mAs is the product of time and mA and determine the number of electrons and hence photons. It influences the 'blackness' of radiographs but not the contrast	Keeping the time under 0.2 s is a good way to avoid motion artefacts
		Exposure latitude is the extent to which a radiograph can be over- or underexposed and still achieve an acceptable result	CR and DR systems have a wide latitude, meaning that over- and underexposures can still result in a diagnostic image thanks to post-processing. The ALARA principle should always aim for the lowest exposure necessary for radiation safety
		Overexposure on CR and DR systems does not result in a black image like on conventional film–screen systems and to assess exposure. It is essential to understand the value range that an image should be within to be of the correct exposure; the manufacturer lists these values	Overexposure can result in an artificial blackness of the borders of bones ('blackout'). This may obscure lesions at bone margins, and care should be taken that the soft tissue envelope is visible on radiographs to ensure that the accurate margins of the bones are visible
		Underexposure often results in a very noisy image, which influences the vet's ability to see trabecular detail and may also obscure lesions	In these cases, an increase in mAs is indicated
		Portable X-ray machines are low-output generators. Their maximum output should be displayed on the machine (usually on a little sticker somewhere). machine generates lower outputs	Many of these machines will only generate the maximum output a few times in a short period before they either stop working for a while or image quality will deteriorate because the device will lower the output. If using a battery-operated generator, this will also require more battery power; therefore, the number of X-rays possible that day without changing may decrease
Image distortion and centring	Image distortion is influenced by the angle of the X-ray beam to the object and the angle of the X-ray beam to the plate. Ideally, the X-ray beam should be aligned at 90 degrees to the area of interest and the plate to avoid image distortion	In radiography, the general aim is to highlight small details that require the X-ray beam to be orientated tangential to the lesion, e.g. highlighting osteophytes at articular margins or subchondral bone changes. To avoid missing small lesions, four projections are used as standard in the horse's leg; in the case of the foot, even more. This inevitably means the X-ray beam hits the bone at a degree other than 90 degrees, resulting in distortion	Although this is impossible to change as the need for multiple angles outweighs the problems with distortion. However, it is important to remember that the angle of the plate and the generator should match to minimise this effect
		While the beam is often 90 degrees to the plate, this can be compromised, e.g. in a lateromedial stifle	In the case of the stifle, the position of the leg and the person holding the plate are essential for success
		Image distortion is also caused by suboptimal centring	It is essential to try and 'shoot' through joint spaces; if this is not possible, it may result in superimposition of the joint space

(Continued)

Table 7.2 (Continued)

Parameter	Specific properties	Factors	Solutions
		A horizontal beam is used for most cases in horses, which will work for horizontally orientated joints. Only the central beam is truly horizontal, while the other components of an X-ray beam diverge in a cone shape	The beam must be directly centred on the joint, or the divergence will result in the superimposition of the surrounding structures on the joint space
		Some joints are naturally sloped (e.g. the distal intertarsal and tarsometatarsal joints slope from lateroproximal to distomedial), and the beam has to be adjusted accordingly	Generally, this requires the beam angle to be 5 degrees dorsoventral for a lateral image
			It is vital to have the horse standing square and equally weight-bearing to standardise joint alignment as much as possible. Some horses' conformation requires the adjustment of the X-ray beam to their individual leg alignment
Post-processing artefacts	Post-processing artefacts are often system specific but include 'overzealous' edge enhancement or noise reduction, which may lead to misinterpretation of the trabecular pattern	Different practices have different requirements, e.g. a practice that primarily radiographs racehorses will want to put more emphasis on visualisation of changes in bone density and trabecular pattern, which requires 'harder' images with more bone detail and less soft tissue. Whereas a practice that deals with general riding horses may be more interested in visualising signs of osteoarthritis, such as joint effusion and periarticular osteophytes which require 'softer images' with good detail of joint margins	Discussing this with the vendor's applications technician can be beneficial
Other artefacts	Some of the most detrimental artefacts are found on the horse and are often relatively easy to address, for example, dirt on the skin or solar surface can mimic lesions		A good wire brush is beneficial in cleaning the hoof. A good body brush can be used to ensure the legs are clean, especially over the joints. In heavily feathered horses, feathers and the air between them, can obscure lesions and make it difficult to see the angles of the bones, so using water to flatten them or taping them up out of the way with a cohesive bandage is helpful to prevent this

Source: Rosina Lillywhite [13].

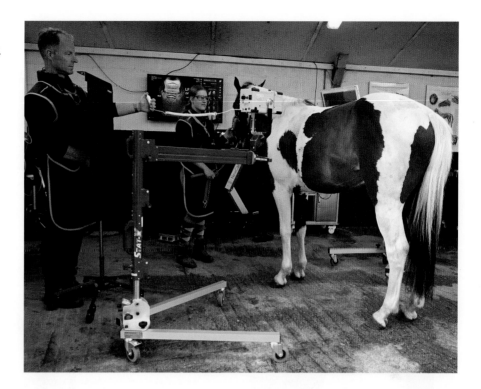

Figure 7.18 Horse correctly positioned for a radiograph. *Source:* With permission from Podoblock BV.

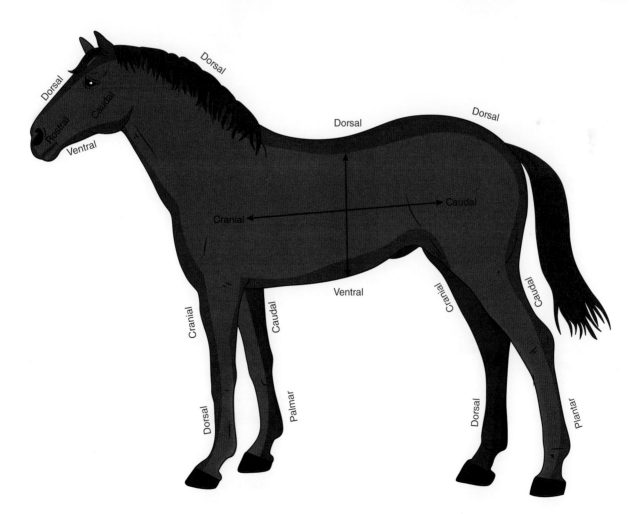

Figure 7.19 Nomenclature used to describe anatomical and radiological views. *Source:* Adapted from Wiley.

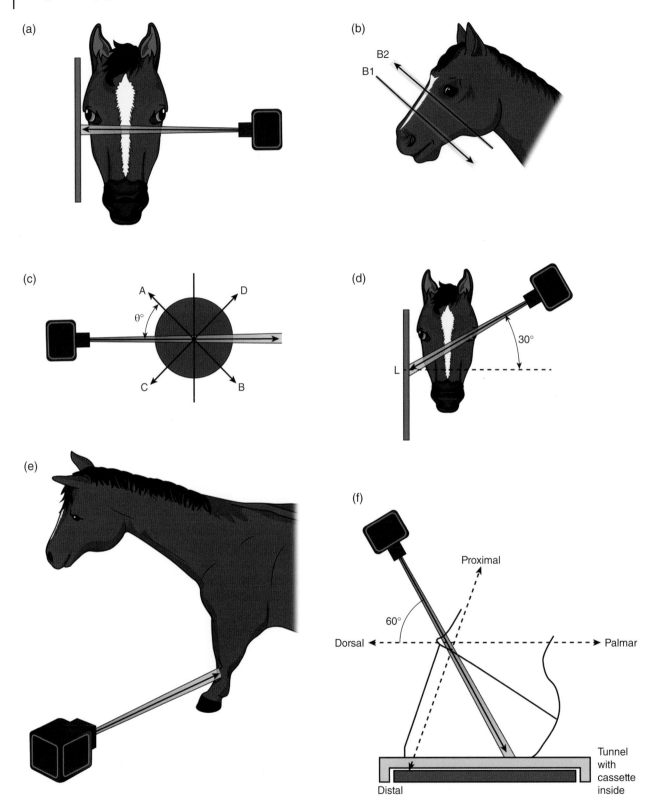

Figure 7.20 (a) Left to right lateral (lateral) view of the head. (b) Dorsoventral (b1) and ventrodorsal (b2) views of the head. (c) Description of oblique views A-θ-C to B–D. Both AB and CD are standard projections. (d) Latero-30°-dorsal lateroventral oblique view of the head. (e) Dorso-45°-lateral palmaromedial oblique view of the left forelimb. (f) Positioning landmarks for 'high coronary' (dorso-60°-proximal palmarodistal oblique) view of the foot. *Source:* Adapted from Wiley.

- An X-ray of the foot obtained by tilting the tube head down and placing it in front of the foot with the foot resting on a cassette is termed dorso – X° – proximal palmarodistal oblique radiograph (Figure 7.20).
- A radiograph of the point of the tarsus obtained by flexing the leg with the X-ray plate placed underneath the cannon bone and beam directed from behind the tibia down onto the plate would be called a caudoproximal plantarodistal view. These are often referred to as skyline views.

Table 7.3 lists the areas of the horse that can be X-rayed effectively, the possible views that can be taken, and possible reasons for the radiographs.

The Foot

One of the most common areas of the horse to be radiographed is the foot, which will form a large part of any radiographer's day. Preparing the equipment for all the required images is important with foot X-rays. Equipment required for standard foot X-rays includes:

- A generator – generally, this is easier with a portable unit rather than a mobile or gantry unit – however, as long as the tube head can reach the floor, it is possible to do the radiographs.
- Cassette or flat panel detector (DR plate).
- Farrier kit – the shoes will need removing, and the foot will need preparing.
- Scrubbing brush and water – foot X-rays require a clean foot to be of diagnostic quality (povidone iodine [PI] scrub can be added to the water to clean the foot; however, a neat solution should be avoided as this may show up on the radiograph).
- Play-Doh or something similar to pack the clefts of the frog – if using Play-Doh, avoid using anything coloured blue as this may contain cobalt blue and will show up on the radiograph.
- Flat blocks for the horse to stand on and raise the foot enough that the plate can capture the sole of the foot – ensure that the horse is raised using two of the same sized blocks – (Figure 7.21).
- Hickman blocks are used for upright pedal and navicular images, and tunnels are used for skyline navicular and allow for the patient to stand on a block that has the plate encased inside it (Figures 7.22 and 7.23a and b)
- Plate holder.
- Radiation safety equipment. See Section 7.1 for details.

Preparation

Generally, the shoes are removed for foot X-rays; however, in most cases, it is preferable to take the LM and DP radiograph with the shoes in place as this can help to see if the horse has an issue with foot balance. There are some reasons why the shoe may not be removed at all; these include:

- The horse has severe laminitis, and taking the shoes off would cause unnecessary pain and suffering to the patient.
- The horse has radiographs as part of vetting, and it is possible to get diagnostic images with them in situ.

The patient requires the hoof picking out, pairing and/or scrubbing to remove all loose horn and dirt to reduce the chances of artefacts appearing on the images. Once the feet are clean, they can be packed with Play-Doh; this ensures that there is no gas shadowing on the image, which can look like fracture lines (when the feet are packed, some practices may cover the floor with cling film or paper to prevent the packing from sticking to the floor).

Tips

- Ensure the horse is stood on a level surface with both feet on the same sized block; if the horse is not stood level and square, the joint spaces will overlap.
- For the LM, ensure that the beam is lined up with the heel bulbs, as this should aid a true lateral image.
- When taking a DP, ask the plate holder to rest the plate on the heel bulbs and then line with the plate ignoring the foot itself; this will ensure that the image is straight even if the foot is imbalanced.
- Inadequate foot preparation will produce artefacts in the pedal and navicular views, such as linear gas shadows mimicking fractures.
- The skyline navicular view is more difficult to obtain in small horses and ponies due to the difficulty in manoeuvring an X-ray machine partially under the abdomen; smaller tripod stands or stands with full manoeuvrability are ideal for these patients [6].
- For the skyline navicular, matching the angle of the beam to the angle of the dorsal wall will help with an accurate image; this can be done by looking from the side before the machine is taken under the horse.

Patient Preparation

From this point, on most patient preparation will be the same, especially for the limbs of the horse; this will include the following:

- The area needs to be groomed with a brush to remove any dirt or debris from the skin and to prevent artefacts from showing up on the radiograph.
- Sedation is recommended for radiographic procedures.

Table 7.3 Equine radiographic views [13, 17].

Area of horse	Indication	Common views	Collimation, centring and positioning aids
Foot	• Lameness localised to the foot by diagnostic analgesia • Positive response to hoof testers • Effusion of the distal interphalangeal joint • Increased digital pulses • Penetrating injuries to the sole • Clinical signs of laminitis • Assessment of foot conformation/in line with a farrier visit • Before a magnetic resonance (MR) scan • As part of a pre-purchase examination • Potential pedal bone fracture	Lateromedial (LM) Dorsopalmar (DP) Dorsoproximal-palmarodistal oblique (DPr-PaDiO) for the distal phalanx and sole Dorsoproximal-palmarodistal oblique (DPr-PaDiO) for the navicular bone Palmaroproximal-palmarodistal oblique (PaPr-PaDiO) or 'skyline' view of the navicular bone Additional views Dorso 45° lateral-palmaromedial oblique (D45L-PaMO) Dorso 45° medial-palmarolateral oblique (D45M-PaLO)	The beam is centred on the distal interphalangeal joint, 1 cm distal to the coronary band, midway between the heels and the dorsal hoof wall Positioning aids: Raised foot block (tip: to ensure a true foot balance ensure both feet are on blocks of equal height) The beam is centred on the dorsal hoof wall, midway between the sole and the coronary band. Positioning aids: Raised foot blocks (tip: same as for the LM however, make sure the plate can get close enough to the foot) When using the 'upright pedal' technique, the beam is horizontal; if using the 'high coronary' method, the beam is angled downward towards the weight-bearing foot at 65° from the horizontal. In both methods, the beam is centred on the midline just distal to the coronary band for the pedal bone Positioning aids: Either a Hickman block (Figure 7.22) for the 'upright technique' or a skyline tunnel (Figure 7.23a and b) (Tip: with modern radiography system, the foot may need to be packed with Play-Doh) The beam is centred on the midline approximately 2 cm proximal to the coronary band. For optimum image quality, the primary beam should be tightly collimated to the navicular bone; this means the margins should be just inside the medial and lateral aspect of the foot, and extending 3 cm proximally and distally Positioning aids: The Hickman block (Tip: the clefts of the frog need to be tightly packed) With the X-ray tube positioned directly behind the foot, the X-ray beam is centred between the heel bulbs at approximately 45° Positioning aids: The skyline tunnel allows a plate to be positioned inside so that the horse can stand on it without damaging the plate The horse needs to be stood with the limb to be imaged behind the contralateral limb (Figure 7.23a). Some modern blocks are angled slightly which reduces the need to position the limbs as described above, therefore the horse can stand more square (Figure 7.23b) For the lateral palmar process, the beam is centred on the lateral hoof wall, midway between dorsal and lateral (D45°L-PaMO). The cassette is placed perpendicular to the beam. To examine the medial palmar process, the beam is directed from dorsomedial (D45°M-PaLO) Position aids: Hickman block, some modern blocks have line to indicate where the plate should be positioned
Pastern	• Lameness localised to the pastern by diagnostic analgesia	Lateromedial (LM)	The beam is horizontal and centred on the lateral aspect of the pastern, midway between the coronet and the fetlock and aligned parallel to the heel bulbs Positioning aids: Small blocks for both limbs to ensure the distal joint is included in the image

Table 7.3 (Continued)

Area of horse	Indication	Common views	Collimation, centring and positioning aids
	• Positive flexion test • Soft tissue and bony swellings • Effusion of the pastern joint • Effusion of the digital flexor tendon sheath • Pastern lacerations • Pastern fracture	Dorsopalmar (DP) Dorso 45° lateral-palmaromedial oblique (D45L-PaMO) Dorso 45° medial-palmarolateral oblique (D45M-PaLO)	The beam is centred on the dorsal aspect of the pastern region, midway between the coronet and the fetlock joint and angled from proximal until perpendicular to the cassette. The exact angle will depend on the stance and conformation of the pastern Positioning aids: Small blocks for both limbs to ensure the distal joint is included in the image The horizontal beam is angled mid-way between dorsal and lateral (at 45°) for the dorsolateral oblique view and mid-way between dorsal and medial for the dorsomedial oblique view and centred on the mid-pastern Positioning aids: Small blocks for both limbs to ensure the distal joint is included in the image
Fetlock	• Lameness localised to the fetlock by diagnostic analgesia • Positive flexion test • Soft tissue swellings, including effusion of the fetlock joint and digital flexor tendon sheath • Signs of trauma, including wounds and swelling • As part of a pre-purchase or pre-sales • Examination • Fracture	Lateromedial (LM) Dorsopalmar (DP) Dorso 45° lateral-palmaromedial oblique (D45L-PaMO) Dorso 45° medial-palmarolateral oblique (D45M-PaLO) Addition views Flexed lateromedial (flexed LM)	The beam is centred on the lateral epicondyle of the distal metacarpus/metatarsus The beam is centred on the dorsal aspect of the joint space, angled proximally by approximately 10° and collimated to the fetlock joint The horizontal beam is angled mid-way between dorsal and lateral (45°) for the dorsolateral oblique view and mid-way between dorsal and medial for the dorsomedial oblique view and centred on the fetlock joint As for the weight-bearing LM view Positioning aids: A handler can be used to ensure the horses' fetlock is flexed or, a wedge block can be used to position the horses' fetlock into a flexed position
Third metacarpus/ metatarsus	• Lameness localised to this region by diagnostic analgesia • Signs of trauma, such as wounds and swellings • Bony swellings • Pain on palpation	Lateromedial (LM) Dorsopalmar (DP) Dorso 45° lateral-palmaromedial oblique (D45L-PaMO) Dorso 45° medial-palmarolateral oblique (D45M-PaLO)	The primary beam should be horizontal ard centred at the mid-point of the cannon bone or, alternatively, at the area of interest (wound, area of bony proliferation). Collimation of the primary beam should include the area of interest or the entire third metacarpal/metatarsal bone if fractures of the cannon are suspected The primary beam should be horizontal and centred at the midpoint of the cannon bone or, alternatively, at the area of interest (wound, area of bony proliferation). Collimation of the primary beam should include the area of interest or the entire third metacarpal/metatarsal bone if fractures of the cannon are suspected The primary beam should be horizontal and centred at the mid-point of the cannon bone or, alternatively, at the area of interest (wound, area of bony proliferation). Collimation of the primary beam should include the area of interest or the entire third metacarpal/metatarsal bone if fractures of the cannon are suspected Tips: For highlighting the splint bones the exposure will need to be reduced. A Dorso 45° lateral-palmaromedial oblique (D45L-PaMO) is used to highlight the lateral splint (metacarpus/metatarsus IV) A Dorso 45° medial-palmarolateral oblique (D45M-PaLO) is used to highlight the medial splint (metacarpus/metatarsus II)

(Continued)

Table 7.3 (Continued)

Area of horse	Indication	Common views	Collimation, centring and positioning aids
Carpus	• Lameness localised to the carpus by • Diagnostic analgesia • Soft tissue swellings, including effusion of the carpal joints or the carpal sheath • Signs of trauma, such as wounds or diffuse swelling	Lateromedial (LM)	The beam should be horizontal. Centre the beam on the middle carpal joint, which is level with the distal edge of the accessory carpal bone and collimate to include the distal radius and proximal metacarpus
		Dorsopalmar (DP)	Centre the beam on the intercarpal joint from dorsal to palmar. The cassette is held perpendicular to the horizontal primary beam, palmar to the carpus
		Dorso 45° lateral-palmaromedial oblique (D45L-PaMO)	Centre the beam on the intercarpal joint at an angle midway between dorsal and lateral (45° oblique). For the optimal view of the dorsomedial region of the joint most likely to show pathology, use an angle of 75° to dorsal. In both instances, the cassette should be positioned perpendicular to the direction of the primary beam
		Dorso 45° medial-palmarolateral oblique (D45M-PaLO)	
	• Assessment of ossification status of the carpal bones in premature or dysmature foals • Angular limb deformities of the carpal region • As part of a pre-purchase and pre-sales • Examination	Additional views Flexed lateromedial (flexed LM)	The limb being examined is raised with the carpus in approximately 2/3 of maximum flexion (the metacarpus perpendicular to the floor), and the beam is centred as for the weight-bearing LM view Positioning aids: Either a handler or a raised leg stand that is easily moved (will depend on horse temperament)
		Dorso 35°, 55°, 85° proximal–dorsodistal oblique (D85Pr-DDiO) or 'skyline' views	• Flexed D35° Pr-DDiO. This view skylines the dorsal aspect of the distal carpal row (mainly the third carpal bone). The limb is held in maximum flexion with the radius pushed forwards at approximately 60° to the ground • Flexed D55° Pr-DDiO. This view skylines the dorsal aspect of the proximal carpal row (radiocarpal and intermediate carpal bones). The limb is held in moderate flexion with the radius forward at approximately 45° to the ground (Figure 7.25) • Flexed D85° Pr-DDiO. This view skylines the dorsodistal radius. The limb is held with the radius vertical and the carpus in slight flexion adjacent to the contralateral carpus Positioning aids: Either a handler or a raised leg stand that is easily moved (will depend on horse temperament)
Elbow	• Clinical signs indicating a fracture in the region, e.g. a 'dropped' elbow appearance commonly associated with an olecranon fracture • Signs of trauma, such as wounds and swellings • Lameness localised to the elbow by diagnostic analgesia	Mediolateral (ML)	The primary beam should be horizontal, centred at the proximal aspect of the radius. Collimation of the primary beam should include the point of the elbow, the proximal third of the radius and a portion of the distal humerus Positioning aids: The limb will need to be pulled forward and upwards to ensure the olecranon is away from the body for visualisation
		Craniocaudal (CrCd)	The X-ray beam is directed horizontally from cranial to caudal, centred on the proximal radius. Collimation of the primary beam should include as much of the distal humerus as possible (usually, 3–4 cm of the humerus proximal to the point of the elbow can be radiographed) Positioning aids: The limb needs to be pulled forwards weight-bearing. If the horse resents this, the limb can held forward and low
		Additional views Cranio 45° medial–caudolateral oblique (Cr45M-CdLO)	The X-ray beam should be angled horizontally, centred at the proximal aspect of the radius. Collimation of the primary beam should include the point of the elbow and the distal humerus
Shoulder	• Lameness localised to the shoulder by	Mediolateral (ML)	The primary beam should be horizontal. The radiographer should palpate the distal aspect of the scapula of the contralateral limb (nearest the X-ray machine) and then centre the primary beam at a point 10 cm cranial and 10 cm proximal to this,

Table 7.3 (Continued)

Area of horse	Indication	Common views	Collimation, centring and positioning aids
	diagnostic analgesia • Soft tissue and bony swellings		to centre on the scapulohumeral joint on the opposing side. Collimation of the primary beam should include the proximal humerus and distal spine of the scapula
	• Signs of trauma • Lameness in Shetland ponies that cannot be attributed to other regions	Cranio 45° medial-caudolateral oblique (Cr45M-CdLO)	Positioning aids: The person holding the leg will need to ensure the limb is pulled forward and towards the floor, and the handler will need to ensure the head and neck are in a neutral position. This ensures the shoulder is away from the cervical spine and the other shoulder. The trachea should overlay the joint to allow for full visualisation The X-ray beam is directed horizontally from the craniomedial to the caudolateral and centred on the shoulder joint, which will be at approximately the same level as the distal spine of the scapula on the contralateral weight-bearing limb. Collimation of the primary beam should include the proximal humerus and distal aspect of the scapula spine Positioning aids: The person holding the leg will need to ensure the limb is pulled forward and towards the floor, and the handler will need to ensure the head and neck are in a neutral position. This ensures the shoulder is away from the cervical spine and the other shoulder. The trachea should overlay the joint to allow for full visualisation
		Additional views Cranioproximal–craniodistal oblique (CrPr–CrDiO) or 'skyline' view of the proximal aspect of the humerus	Position the X-ray machine above the shoulder. A 100 cm focus–film distance is usually impossible since the X-ray machine cannot be positioned high enough in relation to the humerus. Use a vertical X-ray beam. Centre the X-ray beam on the humeral tubercles. Collimate around the shoulder Positioning aids: The limb is held with the carpus flexed. The plate is held horizontally distal to the shoulder. The horse's head and neck are turned away from the limb to be examined
Tarsus	• Lameness localised to the tarsus by diagnostic analgesia • Soft tissue swellings, including effusion of synovial structures, e.g. the talocrural joint or the tarsal sheath	Lateromedial (LM)	The primary beam should be horizontal for a true lateromedial view. The beam is centred on either the tarsocrural or small hock joints. Alternatively, to avoid/reduce superimposition at the small hock joints, the X-ray beam may be angled slightly (5–10°) downwards (proximodistally). Collimation of the primary beam should include the point of the hock, the cranial aspect of the distal tibia and the proximal metatarsal bones
		Dorsoplantar (DP)	The primary beam is usually directed horizontally, but in some horses, directing the beam 5–10° proximo-distally will assist in imaging the medial aspects of the small hock joints more clearly. The beam should be centred on either the tarsocrural or small hock joints Collimation of the primary beam should include the point of the hock at the proximal limit, the proximal splint bones distally, and the medial and lateral malleoli of the tibia
		Dorso 45° lateral-plantaromedial oblique (D45L-PlMO)	The primary beam is directed horizontally and centred on either the tarsocrural or small hock joint. Collimation of the primary beam should include the point of the hock at the proximal limit, the proximal splint bones distally, the medial malleolus of the tibia and the plantar aspect of the calcaneus
	• Signs of trauma, such as wounds or diffuse swellings • Assessment of tarsal bone ossification in premature or dysmature foals	Dorso 45° medial-plantarolateral oblique (D45M-PlLO) or plantaro 45° lateral-dorsomedial oblique (Pl45L-DMO)	The primary beam is directed horizontally and centred on either the tarsocrural or small hock joints. Collimation of the primary beam should include the point of the hock at the proximal and plantar limits, the proximal splint bones distally, and the dorsal aspect of the distal tibia
	• Angular limb deformities of the tarsal region	Additional views Flexed lateromedial (flexed LM)	The X-ray beam should be horizontal, centred at the talus. Collimation of the primary beam should include the point of the hock, the distal tibia and the proximal metatarsal bones

(Continued)

Table 7.3 (Continued)

Area of horse	Indication	Common views	Collimation, centring and positioning aids
	• As part of a pre-purchase or pre-sales Examination		Positioning aids: The hind limb should be flexed. The plate is positioned on the medial aspect of the hock in a vertical plane
		Flexed dorsoplantar (flexed DPl) or 'skyline' view of the tuber calcanei/sustentaculum tali	The X-ray beam is directed as close to vertically (down) as possible while avoiding the musculature of the caudal aspect of the thigh. The X-ray beam can be collimated quite tightly to include only the most plantar aspect of the flexed hock, i.e. the calcaneus and sustentaculum tali Positioning aids: The hind limb should be flexed and held as caudally as possible. The plate is positioned horizontally, facing upwards, with its caudal aspect resting against the plantar aspect of the calcaneus/metatarsus
Stifle	• Lameness localised to the stifle by diagnostic analgesia • Soft tissue swelling, including joint effusion • Signs of trauma, such as wounds • Abnormal position of the patella • As part of a pre-purchase or pre-sales examination	Lateromedial (LM)	The primary beam should be horizontal, but the radiographer should take note of the mediolateral foot balance of the horse and adjust the beam to be parallel to this. The beam is centred at the level of the femorotibial joints Positioning aids: The plate will need to be placed into the groin area and be held as high as possible to ensure the patella is captured on the image
		Caudocranial (CdCr)	The X-ray beam is directed 10–15° proximodistally (downwards), centred on a line that divides the caudal aspect of the limb in half, and so that the exit point of the beam is at the proximal cranial tibia level (the radiographer can check this from the lateral aspect of the horse) Collimation of the primary beam should be wide proximo-distally to include the distal femur and proximal tibia, but the beam should be collimated tightly in a medial-lateral direction so that it includes the medial and lateral tibial condyles Position aids: The caudocranial view is more easily obtained if the horse is positioned with the leg being radiographed extended slightly caudal to the contralateral limb. The plate is held at the cranial aspect of the stifle, taking care when advancing it medially so as not to touch the horse's flank or sheath without warning
		Additional views	
		Caudo 60° lateral-craniomedial oblique (Cd60L-CrMO)	The X-ray beam should be angled 10° proximodistally (downwards) and centred at the level of the femorotibial joints, at the junction of the cranial 1/3 and caudal 2/3 of the limb Collimation of the primary beam should be wide proximo-distally to include the distal femur and proximal tibia, but the beam should be collimated tightly in a craniocaudal direction to include the medial and lateral tibial condyles Positioning aids: The plate will need to be placed into the groin area and extend as high as possible to ensure the patella is captured on the image
		Flexed lateromedial (flexed LM)	The primary beam should be horizontal and centred on the femorotibial joints. Collimation of the primary beam should include the distal femur and proximal tibia Positioning aids: The stifle is flexed by an assistant standing caudal to the horse and holding the distal limb in an elevated position. The degree of flexion can be varied according to the specific area of interest. The cassette is held as high up as possible in the groin region medial to the stifle

Table 7.3 (Continued)

Area of horse	Indication	Common views	Collimation, centring and positioning aids
		Cranioproximal-craniodistal oblique (CrPr-CrDiO) or 'skyline' view of the patella	The X-ray beam is directed distally (downwards), with a 10° lateral to medial angulation. The X-ray beam can be collimated quite tightly to include the most cranial aspect of the flexed stifle, i.e. the cranial patella Positioning aids: With the horse standing, the hindlimb should be flexed by an assistant and the distal part of the limb held so that the tibia is approximately horizontal (i.e. by lifting and then retracting the distal limb caudally and medially – to push the patella laterally). The plate is positioned horizontally, facing upwards with its caudal aspect touching the tibial crest
Pelvis	• Hind limb lameness that cannot be localised by diagnostic analgesia to other areas of the limb • External asymmetry or muscle atrophy of the pelvic region • Positive rectal examination: crepitus or asymmetry • Scintigraphic or ultrasonographic findings suggestive of pelvic disease	Ventrodorsal under general anaesthesia (GA VD)	Use a vertical X-ray beam. X-ray beam centring depends on the area of interest, as several overlapping views are required for a comprehensive radiographic examination of the pelvis. In a standard adult horse, seven separate views are described: • Anatomical landmarks: • Tubera ischii • Coxofemoral joints and obturadora • Foramina • Sacroiliac and lumbosacral joints • Tuber coxae • Coxofemoral joints: the limb to be radiographed is tilted nearer to the plate by slightly rolling the horse
		Cranioventral-caudodorsal oblique (CrVCdDO) in the standing horse	X-ray beam centring depends on the area of interest, as several overlapping views are required for a comprehensive radiographic examination of the pelvis. Collimate tightly around the area of interest to reduce scatter
		Right 30° dorsal-left ventral oblique (R30DLVO) Left 30° dorsal-right ventral oblique (L30D-RVO) for the coxofemoral joint	Centre the X-ray beam between the greater trochanter on the affected side and the base of the tail; an alternative method would be to centre on a spot that corresponds to two-thirds of the distance between the tuber sacrale and tuber ischii on the side of the X-ray machine Collimate around the area of interest
Cervical spine	• Ataxia and abnormal gait • Neck pain and stiffness • Cervical trauma • Abnormal head or neck carriage • Forelimb lameness unable to localised by diagnostic analgesia • Scintigraphic or ultrasonographic	**A standard radiographic examination of the cervical spine of an adult horse is composed of between four and 6, depending on plate size overlapping laterolateral (LL) views**	The most cranial view is centred on C1 ard should include the occipital bone. The subsequent views should include C1–C3, C3–C5 and C5–C7 respectively. In each case, the beam is centred on the body of the middle vertebra and collimated to the bones rather than the soft tissues of the neck. The cervical vertebrae are aligned in a slight S-shaped curve within the neck, and the caudal cervical vertebrae are located towards the ventral aspect of the neck. Palpation of the neck will aid in the precise localisation of the vertebrae Positioning aids: Ensure the head and neck are straight to the body and the head is on a head stand
		Additional views Ventrodorsal (VD) of the cranial neck	Orientate the X-ray beam obliquely upwards, perpendicular to the plate Centre the X-ray beam in the midline of the cranial neck at the level of the wings of the atlas. Collimate around the area of .nterest

(Continued)

Table 7.3 (Continued)

Area of horse	Indication	Common views	Collimation, centring and positioning aids
	• findings suggestive of cervical disease • Non-specific signs of neck problems, including poor performance and equitation problems • As part of a pre-purchase examination	Right ventral-left dorsal oblique (RV-LDO) and left ventral-right dorsal oblique (LV-RDO)	Positioning aids: Ensure the head and neck are straight to the body, and the head is on a head stand Centre the X-ray beam at the jugular groove. The level depends on the area of interest: • Cranial neck: C1–C2 • Mid neck: C3–C4 • Caudal neck: C5–C6 It is helpful to palpate the neck and use tape to mark the position of the plate/centring. Beware that some tape is radiodense and shows up on the radiograph. Align the field of view with the long axis of the cervical spine and collimate around the area of interest
Thoracic and lumbar spine	• Back pain and stiffness • Thoracolumbar trauma • Ataxia and abnormal gait • Positive response to regional analgesia • Hind limb lameness that cannot be localised to other anatomical regions by diagnostic analgesia • Scintigraphic findings suggestive of thoracolumbar disease • Non-specific clinical signs, including poor performance and equitation problems • As part of a pre-purchase examination	A series of several overlapping laterolateral (LL) views for the spinous processes and a separate series for the vertebral bodies Additional views Oblique projections are acquired to separate the left and right articular process ('facet') joints: Right 20° ventral-left dorsal oblique (R20VLDO) and Left 20° ventral-right dorsal oblique (L20V-RDO)	For the spinous processes, centre the X-ray beam approximately 10 cm ventral to the dorsal outline of the back using these markers as a reference: • Cranial thoracic spinous processes: first marker • Mid thoracic spinous processes: between first and second marker • Caudal thoracic spinous processes: between the second and third marker • Cranial lumbar spinous processes: between the third and fourth marker • Caudal lumbar spinous processes: fourth marker Align the field of view with the long axis of the thoracolumbar spine and collimate around the area of interest For the vertebral bodies centre, the X-ray beam is approximately 15–20 cm ventral to the dorsal outline of the back using these markers as a reference: • Cranial thoracic vertebral bodies: first marker • Mid thoracic vertebral bodies: between first and second marker • Caudal thoracic vertebral bodies: between the second and third marker • Lumbar vertebral bodies: between the third and fourth marker Align the field of view with the long axis of the thoracolumbar spine and collimate around the area of interest Positioning aids: Ensure the head and neck are straight to the body and the head is on a head stand Centre the X-ray beam approximately 20–25 cm ventral to the dorsal outline of the back using these markers as a reference: • Mid thoracic articular process joints: between first and second marker • Caudal thoracic articular process joints: between second and third marker Align the field of view with the long axis of the thoracolumbar spine and collimate around the area of interest Positioning aids: Ensure the head and neck are straight to the body and the head is on a head stand

Table 7.3 (Continued)

Area of horse	Indication	Common views	Collimation, centring and positioning aids
Thorax	• Clinical signs of lower respiratory or cardiac disease: cough, bilateral nasal discharge, tachypnoea and dyspnoea • Abnormal lung sounds • Exercise intolerance • Fever of unknown origin • Further evaluation of abnormal ultrasonographic findings	A standard radiographic examination of the thorax of an adult horse is composed of four overlapping laterolateral (LL) views. One or two views may be sufficient for ponies and small horses to cover the whole lung field. The radiographs should be obtained in full inspiration. Foals can be radiographed either in lateral recumbency or standing Additional views In foals ventrodorsal (VD)	Use a horizontal X-ray beam perpendicular to the long axis of the trunk. X-ray centring depends on the quadrant: • Craniodorsal: in the dorsal third of a line between the most caudal aspect of the scapula and the olecranon or in the dorsal third of the fourth intercostal space • Cranioventral: 10 cm caudal to the shoulder joint or in the middle third of the 2nd–3rd intercostal spaces • Caudodorsal: in the dorsal third of the 11th intercostal space • Caudoventral: in the middle third of the 6th–7th intercostal spaces Collimate to the edge of the plate Centre the X-ray beam in the midline just caudal to the xiphoid process Collimate to the edge of the plate
Abdomen	• Investigation of chronic and recurrent colic episodes • Suspected sand accumulation within the colon or the presence of enteroliths • Investigation of colic in foals, ponies and small horses • Investigation of meconium impactions in foals	Radiographic protocol of the abdomen of an adult horse is composed of several overlapping laterolateral (LL) radiographs. The number of views depends on the suspected disease, with the most commonly evaluated area being the cranioventral aspect of the abdomen	Use a horizontal X-ray beam perpendicular to the long axis of the trunk. X-ray centring depends on the area to be evaluated. Collimate to the edges of the plate
Head	• Nasal discharge • Soft tissue or osseous swellings • Clinical signs associated with dental disease (quidding, weight loss, discharging tracts, malodorous breath, etc.) • Lacerations or wounds	**Examination area** / **Radiographic projection** / **Structures evaluated** Premaxilla (incisor bone) and rostral mandible / Laterolateral (LL) / Incisive bone and rostral mandible	Collimation Use a horizontal X-ray beam perpendicular to the long axis of the head and plate X-ray beam centring depends on the area of interest: • Rostral head: corner of the mouth • Paranasal sinuses: dorsal to the rostral third of the facial crest • caudal head: the middle third of the caudal border of the mandibular ramus Align the field of view with the long axis of the nose for the rostral head and paranasal sinuses and collimate around the area of interest Positioning aids: Ensure the head is on a head stand

(Continued)

Table 7.3 (Continued)

Area of horse	Indication	Common views	Collimation, centring and positioning aids
	• Less specific clinical indications include poor performance, equitation issues, and headshaking	Dorsoventral (DV) — Incisive bone and rostral mandible	Orientate the X-ray beam perpendicular to the plate. Centre the X-ray beam in the midline of the head. Centring depends on the area of interest: • Rostral head: in the midline of the head at the level of the corner of the mouth • Paranasal sinuses: in the midline of the head at the level of the rostral third of the facial crest Collimate around the head
		Intraoral dorsoventral (DV) — Maxillary incisors and incisive bone	Orientate the X-ray beam obliquely downwards, directed 90 degrees to the plane that bisects the angle between the incisor reserve crown root and the plate. Centre the X-ray beam in the midline of the head on the central incisors. Collimate around the area of interest
		Intraoral ventrodorsal (VD) — Mandibular incisors and rostral mandible	Orientate the X-ray beam perpendicular to the plate. Centre the X-ray beam in the midline of the head at the level of the temporomandibular joint. Collimate around the head
		Nasal cavity and paranasal sinuses — Laterolateral (LL) — Nasal cavity and paranasal sinuses	As above with a reduced kV and mAs
		Dorsoventral (DV) — Nasal cavity, paranasal sinuses and zygomatic arch	As above, with a reduced kV and mAs
		Right 30° dorsal-left ventral oblique (R30D-LVO) and Left 30° dorsal-right ventral oblique (L30DRVO) — Maxillary cheek teeth, paranasal sinuses and orbit	Angle the X-ray beam so that the X-ray beam hits the dorsal plane (hard palate) at a 30-degree downward angle. Alternatively, the X-ray beam can be angled downwards 75 degrees when evaluation of the paranasal sinuses is required. Centre the X-ray beam dorsal to the rostral third of the facial crest. Align the field of view with the long axis of the nose by tilting the X-ray machine if necessary and collimating around the area of interest
		Mandible (body) — Laterolateral (LL) — Mandible (body)	
		Right 45° ventral-left dorsal oblique (R45V-LDO) and Left 45° ventral-right dorsal oblique (L45VRDO) — Mandible (body) and mandibular cheek teeth	Angle the X-ray beam so that the X-ray beam hits the dorsal plane (hard palate) at a 45-degree upward angle. Centre the X-ray beam in the middle of the body of the affected mandible. Align the field of view with the long axis of the mandible and collimate around the area of interest

Table 7.3 (Continued)

Area of horse	Indication	Common views		Collimation, centring and positioning aids
			Mandibular cheek teeth erupted crowns	Angle the X-ray beam so that the X-ray beam hits the dorsal plane (hard pa:ate) at a 10-degree downward angle. Centre the X-ray beam at the level of the rostral third of the facial crest. Collimate around the area of interest
		Open-mouth Right 10° dorsal-left ventral oblique (R10D-LVO) and Left 10° dorsal-right ventral oblique (L10D-RVO)		
	Caudal skull	Laterolateral (LL)	Cranial vault, temporomandibular joint, tympanohyoid articulation and vertical mandibular rami	As mentioned above, centring on the area of interest
		Ventrodorsal (VD)	Cranial vault, petrous temporal bone, stylohyoid bone, vertical mandibular rami, paracondylar processes, occipital condyles and zygomatic arch	As mentioned above, centring on the area of interest
		Rostro 35° latero 50° ventral-caudodorsal oblique (R35L50V-CdDO)	Temporomandibular joint	Angle the X-ray beam so that the X-ray beam hits the dorsal plane (hard palate) at a 50-degree upward angle Centre the X-ray beam at the level of the temporomandibular joint. Collimate around the area of interest
	Pharynx	Laterolateral (LL)	Pharynx, larynx, guttural pouches and soft palate	As mentioned above, centring on the area of interest

Source: Rosina Lillywhite.

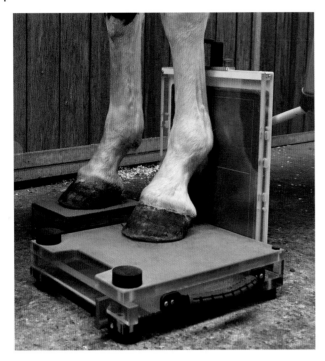

Figure 7.21 A horse stood level with both front feet in preparation for an X-ray. *Source:* With permission from Podoblock BV; Rosina Lillywhite.

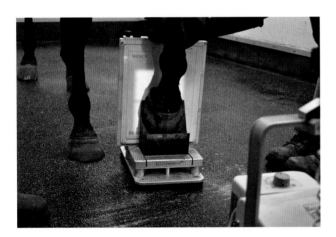

Figure 7.22 Use of a Hickman block for an upright pedal bone. *Source:* With permission from Liphook Equine Hospital; Rosina Lillywhite.

(a)

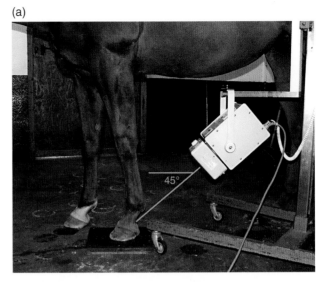

(b)

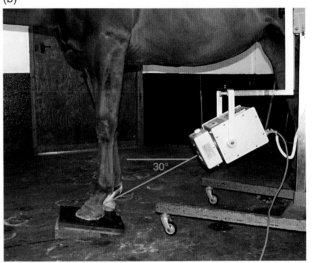

Figure 7.23 (a and b) Positioning to obtain the PaPr-PaDiO view of the navicular bone. (a) The foot is placed on a protective tunnel containing the cassette, caudal to the contralateral limb. The X-ray beam is angled 45 degrees down from the horizontal. (b) Alternatively, the horse is placed on a tunnel standing square. A wedge under the tunnel raises the toe of the foot, and the X-ray beam is angled down 30 degrees from the horizontal. *Source:* Figure used with kind permission from BSAVA Textbook of Veterinary Nursing 5th Edition © BSAVA.

- For the distal limbs, if the patient has heavily feathered legs, it may be necessary to wet the coat, plait the hair or tape with a self-cohesive bandage; this will enable the radiographer to have a good view of the limb without distorting it with the feathers.
- If the patient is in pain, try to minimise the amount the horse will need to move by ensuring that all equipment is pre-prepared and suitably placed.
- Have enough personnel available to help.

Pastern

Pastern radiographs are not commonly performed as most of the pastern is visible on the foot or fetlock images, and fewer problems are associated with the area. However, if images are required, the equipment needed for standard views (see Table 7.3) include:

- X-ray generator
- Foot blocks are still necessary to see the lower pastern joints

- Cassette or flat panel detector (DR plate)
- Plate holder
- Radiation safety equipment – see Section 7.1 for details
- Grooming brush

Tips

- On the DP image, if the horse is not weight-bearing correctly or the joint spaces will appear narrowed on one side of the leg.
- Both oblique views can also be obtained by reversing the beam direction, i.e. positioning from the palmar aspect of the limb instead of dorsal; this may be essential in a suspected fracture or severe lameness so that the patient does not have to be unnecessarily moved. However, it is essential to remember that the cassette will be positioned further from the joint, increasing geometric distortion. It is also essential that there is accurate labelling as the two views are alike [17].

Fetlock

Fetlocks are a common area to radiograph in the horse; however, gaining the perfect lateral can sometimes be challenging. Figure 7.24 shows the difference between a straight lateral and a misaligned lateral image of the fetlock. Figure 7.24a shows that the radiography has been taken either too caudally or cranially and has not aligned to allow for visualisation of the joint space. Figure 7.24b shows a correctly aligned image of the LM fetlock. Equipment required for fetlock images will include:

- X-ray generator
- Cassette or flat panel detector (DR plate)

- Plate holder
- Radiation safety equipment – see Section 7.1 for details
- Grooming brush
- Hickman block – if obtaining a flexed view

Tips

- When taking the lateral image, line up with the metacarpus/metatarsus for guidance on the angle of the beam from left to right – this is often more palmar/planter than if the heel bulbs are used as a guide.
- Although often referred to as a DP, this DP is actually a Dorsoproximal-palmarodistal oblique (DP10°-PaDO); by angling the beam, it ensures that this view does not have the sesamoid bone superimposed over the joint space, it is necessary to angle the beam distally by 15–20°.
- When doing a LM of the fetlock, it can be helpful to keep all equipment in place while the image is looked at this will allow for minor corrections to be made from the previous position. If the generator and detector are moved, it can be difficult to re-establish their original positions.
- Angulation of the beam by 60° from the dorsal instead of 45° in the oblique views gives a more complete projection of the dorsal articular margins of the proximal phalanx. The 45° oblique views are better for evaluating the insertion regions of the suspensory ligament branch on the abaxial surface of the proximal sesamoid bone.
- Both oblique views can also be obtained by reversing the beam direction, i.e. from palmar; this may be essential in a suspected fracture or severe lameness so that the patient is not moved unnecessarily. However, it is

Figure 7.24 The difference between an off-lateral fetlock image (a) compared to a true lateral image (b). *Source:* With permission from Liphook Equine Hospital and Rosina Lillywhite.

(a)

(b)

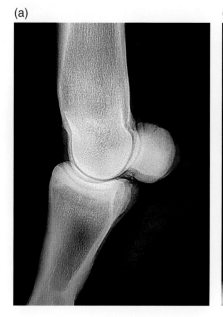
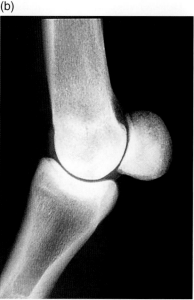

essential to remember that the cassette will be positioned further from the joint, increasing geometric distortion. It is also essential that there is accurate labelling as the two views are alike.

- Oblique views can be taken with a straight beam; however, for racehorse sales X-rays and if there is a suspected fracture to the condyle, it may be necessary to angle the beam distally. What is done routinely in practice will depend on case type and vet preference.

Metacarpus/Metatarsus

The main reason for radiography in this area is to examine the splint bone and/or the metacarpus or metatarsus post-traumatic injury. The equipment required for this radiograph includes:

- X-ray generator
- Cassette or flat panel detector (DR plate)
- Plate holder
- Radiation safety equipment – see Section 7.1 for details
- Grooming brush

Tips

- To ensure a true lateral, line the beam up with the metacarpus/metatarsus. If the heel line is used, most horses are toe in or out and this means that the limb higher up does not line up with the heel line.
- If the imaging is designed to look at the second and fourth metacarpal/tarsal bones (splint bones), the exposure will need to be reduced to prevent 'burning out' the splint bones.
- Remember that the splint bone closest to the detector is the splint bone that will be highlighted – for example, the DLPMO view will highlight the lateral splint bone or Metacarpal/metatarsal IV. The DMPLO will highlight the medial splint bone or Metacarpal/metatarsal II.
- When taking oblique images, it may be necessary to take multiple different angles to allow the area of interest to be highlighted.

Carpus

Carpal radiographs are standard if the practice sees a high number of performance horses, especially racehorses. In other areas of veterinary practice, they may be less commonly performed. The equipment required for carpal radiographs includes:

- X-ray generator
- Cassette or flat panel detector (DR plate)
- Plate holder
- Radiation safety equipment – see Section 7.1 for details
- Grooming brush
- If doing a flexed lateral view, another person holds the limb

Tips

- Due to the natural undulation of the articular surfaces, it is impossible to avoid superimposition to the opposing joint surfaces.
- A well-positioned DP will have a radiolucent space in the centre between the intermediate and radiocarpal bones.
- For a true lateral and to minimise the superimposition of the articular surface angle, the beam 5° distally for the lateral image.
- If doing a flexed image, ensure that the leg holder does not rotate the limb, as this will create obliquity in the image.

Figure 7.25 shows how to obtain a skyline carpus (Flexed D55° Pr-DDiO).

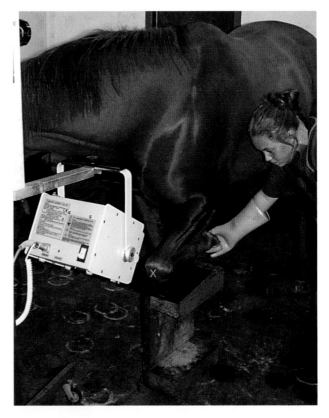

Figure 7.25 Positioning for a Pr-DDiO view of the carpus. Centre in the middle of the joint (X). The foot is placed vertically under the upper limb and restrained at the toe. The assistant stands to the side. *Source:* Figure used with kind permission from BSAVA Textbook of Veterinary Nursing 5th Edition © BSAVA.

Elbow

The elbow is an area that is not frequently imaged. Fractures are the most common indication for imaging this area; therefore, when imaging is required, the radiographs must be of diagnostic quality.

The necessary equipment includes:

- X-ray generator
- Cassette or flat panel detector (DR plate)
- Plate holder
- Radiation safety equipment – see Section 7.1 for details
- Grooming brush
- An assistant to hold the limb

Tips

- The lateral image is positioned mediolateral to allow the plate to go high enough up the limb. The limb will need pulling forwards – for best results, the assistant holding the limbs needs to pull the limb forwards, keeping the radius at 90° (perpendicular) to the floor.
- To obtain a lateral, first assess the position of the radius and line up with this; remember that often lateral is more caudal than it may seem.
- Try to make sure that everything is lined up as much as possible before the horse's limb is raised, as this can cause pain and increase movement.
- For the craniocaudal view, the limb can be placed on the floor slightly stretched forward, allowing the plate to be placed higher, getting more of the elbow in the image. The beam can then be angled to match this around 10–15°; be aware that this may cause distortion if the angles do not all match.
- For the craniocaudal view, the plate can be orientated into a diamond shape. This will ensure that most of the elbow is in the image; otherwise, getting the whole joint in the image will be challenging.

Shoulder

Shoulder radiographs are not that commonly taken in equine practice, as injuries to this area are relatively uncommon; however, when they are required, it is essential that they are of diagnostic quality. The following equipment is required:

- X-ray generator with a high-power output
- Cassette or flat panel detector (DR plate) – large-sized plate
- Plate holder
- Grid – should be used to reduce scatter radiation
- Backscatter lead – this helps to absorb any stray radiation
- Radiation safety equipment – see Section 7.1 for details
- Grooming brush
- An assistant to hold the limb

Tips

- The limb should be pulled forward and towards the floor to extend the shoulder away from the other shoulder and the cervical vertebrae.
- The distal aspect of the spine of the scapula on the contralateral limb can be palpated and also marked to aid in the identification of the correct centring point once the affected limb is protracted.
- The head and neck should be kept in a neutral position for the image to be diagnostic; the trachea must overlay the joint space to allow for correct visualisation of the joint.
- The lateral shoulder is often more caudal than it looks.
- The assistant that is pulling the limb forward needs to ensure that they are not pulling the limb either medially or laterally. It needs to remain straight to prevent superimposition of the joint space.

Tarsus

Disorders of the tarsus occur frequently in equine patients and are a common reason to radiograph this area. The equipment required includes:

- X-ray generator
- Cassette or flat panel detector (DR plate)
- Plate holder
- Radiation safety equipment – see Section 7.1 for details
- Grooming brush
- If doing a flexed lateral view, an assistant is required to hold the limb

Tips

- The small hock joints in normal horses slope slightly proximo-distally from lateral to medial. Therefore, to angle the X-ray beam directly through these narrow joint spaces, the X-ray beam can be directed 5–10° downwards.
- When lining up for the lateromedial, look at the metatarsus and line it up with this for the lateral. The heel bulbs are unlikely to be lateral with the hock joints.
- Taking a plantarolateral–dorsomedial oblique (PLDMO) projection will give approximately the same radiographic view as a dorsomedial–plantarolateral oblique (DMPLO) projection; however, there will be more magnification with the PLDMO because the cassette cannot be held as close to the limb due to the angulation of the distal tibia.

- When performing a flexed lateral, the limb should be held at 90° (perpendicular) to the floor. Care should be taken not to abduct the limb when flexing, as this will cause joint rotation.
- When performing a skyline, the assistant holding the limb needs to push the limb caudally to move the hock away from the thigh musculature.

Stifle

The stifle is routinely radiographed in equine practice, especially in sports horse medicine. The equipment required includes:

- Portable generators may be sufficient to radiograph the stifle; however, the caudocranial view may need a higher power
- Cassette or flat panel detector (DR plate)
- Plate holder
- Radiation safety equipment – see Section 7.1 for details
- Grooming brush
- If doing a flexed lateral view, an assistant is required to hold the limb

Tips

- Lining the beam up with the tibia will increase the chances of getting a lateral if the heel bulbs are used; this is unlikely to line up as lateral with the stifle.
- Desensitisation of the flank and medial aspect of the stifle should be carried out by gently stroking the area prior to putting the cassette in position. This can help to improve patient compliance as the horse becomes accustomed to physical contact in this region and is not startled by the sudden presence of the cassette.
- For the caudocranial view, the limb should be positioned behind the contralateral limb, opening up the joint space.
- To gain a straight caudocranial view, it is advisable to line up with the tarsus and then move the beam upwards.
- When doing a flexed lateral, the assistant holding the limb needs to make sure that they hold the limb with the tarsus at a neutral right angle and not rotate the limb, as this will affect the orientation of the image.
- For the skyline patella view of the stifle, the assistant holding the limb will need to push the limb cranially while medially pushing the distal aspect limb. Figure 7.26 shows a radiograph of the skyline patella; this patient had a chip fracture of the medial aspect.

Pelvis

The pelvis is not commonly radiographed in the equine patient because it can be challenging to perform due to the access of equipment and amount of tissue coverage.

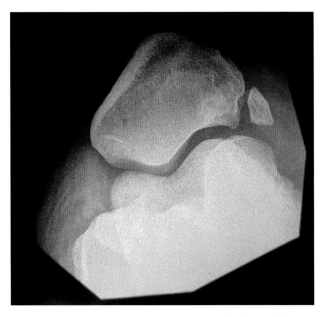

Figure 7.26 Radiograph of the skyline patella. *Source:* With permission from Liphook Equine Hospital and Rosina Lillywhite.

Horses do not commonly have issues in this area; however, radiographic examination may be essential for pelvic fractures and hip conditions seen in patients such as Shetlands.

The equipment required includes:

- X-ray generator with a high-power output
- Cassette or flat panel detector (DR plate) – large-sized plate
- Plate holder
- Grid – should be used to reduce scatter radiation
- Backscatter lead – this helps to absorb any stray radiation
- Radiation safety equipment – see Section 7.1 for details
- Grooming brush
- An assistant to hold the limb

Tips

- To reduce scattered radiation reaching the film, a grid should be used. Positioning the cassette accurately under the pelvis of a large horse can be challenging. Care must be taken to ensure the beam is centred on and perpendicular to the cassette.
- Faeces in the rectum may obscure regions of interest; rectal evacuation will assist in reducing this problem. The requirement for this will be decided by the case vet.
- It is now possible with a high-powered portable machine to obtain radiographs of the pelvis on a standing horse. To enable the hips to be radiographed, the legs will need to be abducted to allow for the positioning of the generator.

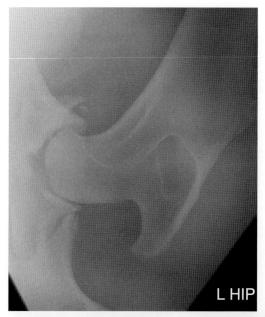

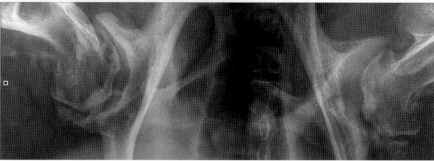

Figures 7.27 and 7.28   Show hip radiographs in the standing patient. Figure 7.27 shows an image of a hip in a standing horse. Figure 7.28 shows an image of both hips in a standing Shetland. *Source:* With permission from Liphook Equine Hospital and Rosina Lillywhite.

- Figure 7.27 shows a radiograph of an approximate 600 kg horse taken standing with the hip being radiographed and abducted. Figure 7.28 shows an image of a Shetland pony that was placed on foot blocks to give more height; no limb abduction was required as the generator could fit under the pony. Both of these radiographs show a clear image of the hip joints.

Head

The head is one of the most anatomically complicated areas of the horse and can be affected by many disorders. Radiography of the equine head has decreased in frequency due to the introduction of CT. However, in practices that do not have immediate access to CT, it is still an essential skill; the equipment required includes:

- X-ray generator
- Cassette or flat panel detector (DR plate) – large-sized plate

- Plate holder
- Radiation safety equipment – see Section 7.1 for details
- Grooming brush
- A rope headcollar
- Headstand
- Mouth gag – for some images

Tips
- When doing a laterolateral view of the head for sinus evaluation, it is easier to assess fluid lines with the head in an upright position as possible. If the oblique view is also taken, then this will mean that the angle of the beam does not need to be as steep.
- Using a rope headcollar is essential to prevent metal artefacts from being superimposed over the head. It should be noted that some rope headcollars have metal rings on them.

Cervical Spine

The radiographic imaging of the neck has become more valuable with the increases in image quality and capability. The equipment required includes:

- X-ray generator – a low output generator is sufficient for most neck radiographs; however, a higher power may be necessary for the caudal vertebrae
- Cassette or flat panel detector (DR plate) – large-sized plate
- Plate holder
- Radiation safety equipment – see Section 7.1 for details
- Grooming brush
- A rope headcollar for the imagers nearer the head
- Headstand
- Blinkers may help if the horse is head shy

Tips

- Lateral radiographs are usually obtained from one side only, but repeating the view from the other side can help localise an asymmetric lesion, as the lesion will be magnified when it is further from the cassette.
- Placing 2 or 3 radio-opaque markers at various positions along the neck dorsal to the vertebrae but still within the primary beam can help with positioning if repeat radiographs are required and with the identification of vertebrae.

It is important to remember that the head and neck need to be straight and not deviate from the midline.

Thoracic and Lumbar Spine

The thoracic and lumbar areas of the back are commonly radiographed, especially in the performance horse, and this means that high-quality imaging is essential. The equipment required includes:

- X-ray generator – a low output generator is sufficient for spinous processes; however, a higher power may be necessary for the vertebral bodies
- Cassette or flat panel detector (DR plate) – large-sized plate
- Plate holder
- Grid – should be used to reduce scatter radiation
- Backscatter lead – this helps to absorb any stray radiation
- Radiation safety equipment – see Section 7.1 for details
- Grooming brush
- A rope headcollar for the imagers nearer the head
- Headstand
- Blinkers may help if the horse is head shy

Preparation

Sedation of the patient is advised. The use of blinkers may be helpful. Divide the back according to the plate size so each view overlaps slightly. This is achieved by placing radiopaque markers (either using brought plastic or metal radiographic markers or by using barium paste) along the thoracolumbar spine, which will also enable the identification of specific vertebrae on the radiographs. Be aware that markers (especially if they are very radiodense or large) may affect image processing and cause artefacts. In standard adult horses, four markers are usually enough when using large plates:

- First marker: Withers (T6)
- Second marker: Mid thoracic spine (T11–T12)
- Third marker: Thoracolumbar junction (T18–L1)
- Fourth marker: Mid lumbar spine (L3).

Marker placement is helped by either palpating cranially from the lumbosacral junction, which can be felt as a dip or from the last (18th) rib [13].

Tips

- Several anatomic landmarks help identify individual vertebrae: the diaphragm attaches to the ventral surface of the 16th thoracic vertebra; the highest dorsal spinous process is that of T6; the anticlinal vertebra is normally T15.

Thorax

Radiographic examination of the thorax is often only performed in larger referral hospitals in adult patients. It can be useful for foals to assess for rib fractures post-foaling in smaller practices using a mobile generator; the equipment required includes:

- X-ray generator – high powered
- Cassette or flat panel detector (DR plate) – large-sized plate
- Plate holder
- Grid – should be used to reduce scatter radiation
- Backscatter lead – this helps to absorb any stray radiation
- Radiation safety equipment – see Section 7.1 for details
- Grooming brush

Preparation

Sedation of the patient is advised; some horses may benefit from the use of blinkers. It may also be helpful to divide the thorax according to the size of the plates so each view overlaps slightly. In the standard adult horse, the thorax is divided into four quadrants:

- Craniodorsal
- Cranioventral
- Caudodorsal
- Caudoventral

Tips

- If a grid is not used, scattered radiation can be reduced by leaving an air gap (15–30 cm) between the patient and the cassette. This technique causes the magnification of intrathoracic structures.
- The image should be taken when the horse is breathing in to increase the visualisation of the structures.

Abdomen

Abdomen radiographs are mainly taken in equine practice to assess the build-up of sand; in an adult horse, it is challenging to see anything other than sand. In the foal, abdominal radiographs can be more useful as structures are easily identifiable. Equipment required include:

- X-ray generator – high powered
- Cassette or flat panel detector (DR plate) – large-sized plate
- Plate holder
- Grid – should be used to reduce scatter radiation
- Backscatter lead – this helps to absorb any stray radiation
- Radiation safety equipment – see Section 7.1 for details
- Grooming brush

Tips

- The images should all overlap so that there is a complete idea of what is happening in the whole abdomen.
- Only the lower abdomen in an adult horse can be successfully radiographed.

Contrast Radiography

Contrast media that is required to perform contrast studies can be broken into two categories:

- Negative – These contrast media include gas and are not regularly used in equine patients.
- Positive – These contrast media include barium and iodine preparation and are more commonly used in equine patients.

Contrast media are used to highlight soft tissue that would not be visible on a plain radiograph. They can be used where contrast on radiographs is usually low, such as in the gastrointestinal tract, urogenital and vascular systems. Contrast media will either have a higher atomic number than the surrounding tissue, preventing the X-rays from passing through the structure that has the contrast media, which will appear white on the radiograph, or it will have a

lower atomic number and will let X-rays pass more freely, this will have a blackening effect on the radiograph. For a contrast media to be effective in equine patients, it must be:

- Easy to administer
- Non-toxic
- A stable compound that will not alter its state when administered
- Allow good contrast of the area of interest
- Be eliminated from the body quickly and easily without harming the patient's body
- Not cause harm to the patient or have carcinogenic properties
- Be cost-effective

Negative Contrast Media

- In equine practice, negative contrast agents are seldom used as they are not useful for the common contrast studies performed in equine practice. A negative agent will use a gas to fill an area of interest; due to this gas not absorbing much of the X-rays, the image will appear blackened. Three main gases can be utilised for these studies:
- Air
- Carbon dioxide
- Oxygen.

One of the only times that a negative agent may be seen is if air has infiltrated an area through a wound on the horse; this can then be seen as black areas on the radiograph.

Positive Contrast Agents

These contrast media are commonly used in equine patients for multiple studies, including myelography, barium swallows and joint and tendon sheath examinations. They have a higher atomic number than tissue and therefore look white in the image. Common positive agents include the following:

Barium Sulphate Suspension

These come in ready-made products such as Baritop® (Figure 7.29) or a powder form. The atomic number of barium sulphate is 56, and it is often used in barium swallows and helps test the function of the upper gastrointestinal tract (GIT) tract in horses. Due to the horse's size, it is impossible to radiograph further than the stomach effectively; however, the whole of a foal may be examined using this method. Barium powder can be mixed with a small amount of water to make a paste that can work as a marker on radiographs such as back images. Barium is a financially viable way of examining the function of the GIT tract or

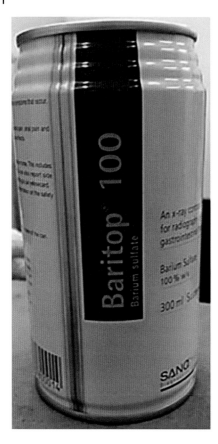

Figure 7.29 Baritop® can be used to perform a barium swallow examination on the horse. *Source:* Rosina Lillywhite.

placing markers on the horse for radiographic purposes; however, it should not be given if there is a suspected perforation as it can cause adhesions in the peritoneal cavity. Figure 7.30 shows a radiograph of the horse's pharynx after administering Baritop® orally, highlighting the horse's oesophagus.

Iodine-based Solutions

These contrast media have an atomic number of 35 and are water-soluble organic compounds; the most commonly used in equine practice is Omnipaque™. There are also non-soluble organic compounds seldom used in equine patients. The amount of iodine used in a product is expressed in milligrams per millilitre (mg/ml); for example, Omnipaque 300™ contains 300 mg/ml. Omnipaque™ is commonly used for myelography, where it is injected sterilely into the subarachnoid space to identify if a horse has spinal compression. It can also be injected into a joint space, tendon sheath or bursa to see if there is a penetration to that structure. Less commonly but also possible, it can be used to perform a venogram where a tourniquet is applied, and the vessels below are injected to see if there is sufficient

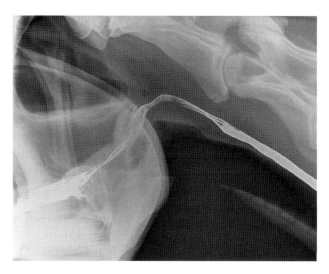

Figure 7.30 Radiograph of a horse following the administration of Baritop®. *Source:* With permission from Liphook Equine Hospital and Rosina Lillywhite.

blood flow to an area; this is most commonly used to assess blood flow to the foot in laminitic cases.

Archiving Image Data

Diagnostic imaging has undergone considerable changes over the last decade in human and veterinary medicine, largely caused by advancements in information technology (IT). Digital radiography has replaced film radiography in equine practice, and advances in computer and software systems mean that most equipment is now battery-powered and wireless. However, this has meant that with the increase in digital imaging, storage has also had to advance; this data uses vast amounts of storage space, and it all needs storing to meet GDPR guidelines (see Chapter 2 for more information). Before the widespread use of picture archiving and communication systems (PACS), data would need to be backed up onto disk, memory stick or internal servers; however, the PACS systems have made this all more efficient. Until recently, PACS was only affordable for large referral centres; however, there are more affordable cloud-based solutions for practices. These systems allow for central storage of large quantities of image data from any digital imaging and communications in medicine (DICOM) compatible imaging modality and easy retrieval to different computers (on-site or off-site). DICOM files store the image data and information about the patient, such as patient identification number, date of examination, breed, age and name. The stored data can be searched according to each of the included parameters. A PACS usually consists of a server for data storage and a workstation with dedicated software to retrieve and manipulate images.

Network infrastructure must be installed to send data from the various imaging modalities to the server and the workstation. The server should be housed remotely from the scanning facilities to ensure safe backup. The workstation should be placed for convenient access because it allows for displaying all images of a patient simultaneously. This facilitates reporting of studies and allows quick and easy access to images for viewing by both veterinary staff and clients. Most PACS also interlink to billing and clinical record systems, which can make workflow more efficient [23].

7.3 Scintigraphy

Scintigraphy, commonly known as bone scan, is a useful diagnostic imaging technique used in equine practice. Scintigraphy is used to identify skeletal problems anywhere in the body using a highly sensitive radioactive isotope. The images obtained represent physiology in contrast to morphology. They are picked up due to increased uptake of a suitable tracer where there is local metabolism of calcium and osteoblastic activity. The changes seen in the image represent increased bone turnover and/or increased blood flow; factors that affect this process include:

- Quantity of mineralised bone.
- Capillary permeability.
- Local acid-base balance.
- Fluid pressure within bones.
- Hormones.
- Dehydration.

Radiopharmaceutical Agent

The process of scintigraphy includes the use of a radiopharmaceutical, this is known as technetium -99m. This emits gamma rays that can be detected with a gamma camera and has a half-life of six hours. Technetium -99m needs to be combined with diphosphonate to enable it to bind to bone, such as methylene diphosphate (MDP) (99Tcm MDP) or hydroxymethylene diphosphate (HDP). Once the technetium -99m has been injected, the type of scan required will determine how long the horse needs to wait before scanning commences. 50–60% of the injected dose reaches the bones while the rest is excreted via the kidneys.

There are three possible scanning phases. The phase selected depends on the area of interest for each individual horse [24]:

- Phase I: An initial dynamic flow study (vascular phase) with rapid images 0–1 minute following injection – for these, the horse will need to be in position and injected so that scanning can start automatically after injection of the radioisotope.
- Phase II: The soft tissue image phase at 5–15 minutes when the tracer is still within the vascular compartment – these will still require injection of the radioisotope in the bone scan room so that scanning can start shortly after injection.
- Phase III: Static bone phase images at two to four hours – these can be injected with the radioisotope in the horse's stable.

Table 7.4 displays the phases and indications required for different scintigraphy scans.

Table 7.4 Phases and indications for different scintigraphy scans [17].

Phase	Use
Phase one – Vascular – Scan immediately	<ul><li>To evaluate blood flow to an area following degloving injuries</li><li>Aortoiliac thrombosis</li><li>Vascular infarcts</li><li>Detecting inflammatory processes</li></ul>
Phase two – Soft tissue – Start scanning 2–4 min after injection	<ul><li>Tendon/ligament injuries.</li><li>Synovitis, e.g. chronic proliferative synovitis</li><li>Digital sheath tenosynovitis</li><li>Carpal sheath tenosynovitis</li><li>Thoroughpin</li><li>Bog spavin</li><li>Bone spavin</li><li>Osteomyelitis, e.g. septic osteitis</li></ul>
Phase three – Bone – Start scanning 2–3 h after injection	<ul><li>Fractures</li><li>Degenerative joint disease (DJD)</li><li>Periosteal reactions, e.g. dorsal metacarpal disease</li><li>Enthesopathies</li><li>Myositis (altered muscle metabolism causes retention of the diphosphonate)</li></ul>

Source: Rosina Lillywhite.

The Detector

The detector is a camera with a head composed of sodium iodide crystals, which, once exposed to gamma rays, produce light flashes detected by a photomultiplier tube behind the crystals. This then emits an electrical pulse, which is monitored by electronic counting circuitry. The detector is an expensive piece of equipment to purchase, and it is also heat sensitive. This means that the room that it is placed in needs to be maintained at a constant temperature to avoid damaging the crystals in the head of the camera.

Table 7.5 displays the advantages and disadvantages of using gamma scintigraphy in the equine patient.

Patient Preparation

It is essential to remember that horses should not have had local anaesthetic injections before scintigraphy as this can affect the reading during the scan and create an inflammatory response. Nerve blocks should not affect a bone phase scan but will impact both vascular and soft tissue phase scans. However, intraarticular injections will impact a bone phase scan. It is recommended that the horse delay having a scan for 17 days following a local anaesthetic injection [17].

Diet

Before a scan, no dietary changes are required. However, post-scan, the horse will need to be treated as per practice policy regarding refeeding following the administration of large amounts of sedative medication. The horse should be well hydrated, though, as dehydration can impact the image quality, making the scanning process more challenging.

Site Preparation

Horses should have an intravenous (IV) catheter placed in one of the jugular veins to prevent extravascular injection of the isotope and aid with the administration of sedation during the scan. See Chapter 17 for information regarding IV catheter placement.

Other Preparations

- The horse should be rugged and have stable bandages applied to their legs for at least 12 hours.
- The horse can be exercised for 15 minutes before the scan to ensure adequate blood flow to the distal limbs; generally, this is done via lunging (both this and the bandaging help increase the uptake of the radioactive isotope within the skeleton enabling better image production).
- The above two points are critical in cold temperatures.
- Once the horse has been injected, the feet should be protected so they are not contaminated by radioactive urine splashes, which would introduce artefacts on the images. This can be achieved by covering the feet, for example, placing empty fluid bags over the feet and taping them in place.
- Diuretics may need to be administered if imaging of the pelvis or coxofemoral joints is required; otherwise, a full bladder may obscure the area of interest.

Equipment

- Gamma camera with motion detection
- Temperature controlled room
- Gantry-mounted system or floor mounted
- Computer for processing

Table 7.5 Advantages and disadvantages of using scintigraphy in the equine patient.

Advantages	Disadvantages
Can be helpful in detecting the early signs of disease such as fractures before they are detectable on a radiograph	Low specificity. It does not always provide a specific diagnosis
It is possible to bone scan the whole horse including the pelvis which is still difficult to image using other modalities	Results are only useful when considered in combination with a clinical examination and other imaging modalities
Can give an idea of the health status of the horse as a whole, rather than just one area	Equipment is expensive and requires a dedicated room that is temperature controlled. Fluctuations in temperature can damage the crystals in the camera head
Allows investigation and imaging in horses who have temperaments that are unsuitable for multiple nerve/joint blocks	Use of radioactive isotopes is tightly regulated by the HSE through the IRR17

Source: Rosina Lillywhite.

- Lead shielding for the contralateral leg – it is essential to shield the opposite leg when scanning the distal limbs to avoid superimposition
- Lead-lined storage box for storing waste such as IV catheters, once removed
- Syringe shields
- Handling forceps

Radioactive decontamination kit – all staff should know where this is and the protocol for use.

Dedicated Cleaning Materials

Electronic personal dosimeters are an excellent addition to scanning safety as they give a live reading and can alert the wearer if the dose rate of radiation exceeds set limits.

Drawing-up Technetium-99m Methylene Diphosphonate (99Tcm MDP)

In equine medicine, the drawing up process of 99Tcm MDP involves several steps to ensure the proper preparation and administration of the radiopharmaceutical. It is important to note that the specific protocols and procedures may vary between different veterinary practices or imaging facilities. The following is a general overview of the drawing-up process [24]:

1) Radiopharmaceutical preparation: The 99Tcm MDP is typically provided as a commercially prepared kit. The kit contains separate vials or components of the radiopharmaceutical, including the freeze-dried powder of 99Tcm MDP and a vial of sterile sodium pertechnetate (99mTcm) solution.
2) Reconstitution: The first step is to reconstitute the freeze-dried powder of 99Tcm MDP with the sterile sodium pertechnetate solution. The powder is typically dissolved in the solution by aseptically injecting the solution into the vial containing the powder. Care is taken to ensure aseptic technique and prevent contamination.
3) Mixing: Once the powder is reconstituted, the vial is gently agitated or rolled to ensure thorough mixing of the radiopharmaceutical solution. This step is important to achieve uniform distribution and proper labelling of the radioactive material.
4) Dose measurement: The final solution is then drawn up into a syringe, and the activity of the radiopharmaceutical is measured using a dose calibrator. The dose calibrator is a specialised instrument that measures the amount of radioactivity present in the syringe. This measurement ensures that the appropriate dose is being administered to the horse.

5) Shielding and handling: To minimise radiation exposure to personnel, appropriate shielding measures, such as lead-lined syringe shields or lead gloves, may be used during the drawing-up process. Careful handling of the syringe and adherence to radiation safety guidelines are essential.

It's important to note that the drawing up process of 99Tcm MDP should be performed by trained personnel who are familiar with radiation safety procedures and guidelines. The specific protocols may vary based on the manufacturer's instructions and the regulations of the country or region [14].

Patient Restraint

- Sedation is required following individual practice sedation protocols.
- An experienced handler is required.
- Depending on the horse's temperament, blinkers and cotton wool for the ears may be required.
- Some practices may use stocks; however, this is not essential and may hinder image acquisition.

Aftercare

Following the scintigraphy scan, the horse is considered to be a radiation hazard, and how they are treated and waste disposed of will depend on the practice of local rules and advice gained from the RPA in line with HSE guidelines and the IRR17. The most significant hazard associated with scintigraphy is urine; this makes the stable a designated temporary controlled area, protective clothing should be worn, and there should be minimal handling of the bedding for 48 hrs and, in some cases, longer following the administration of 99Tcm MDP [14]. Correct protocols must be followed when carrying out scintigraphy to prevent hazards to human health. Before a stable can be deemed safe to muck out, it should be assessed using a Geiger counter. These devices provide radiation readings in counts per minute (CPM) or counts per second (CPS). Some advanced models may also offer measurements in other units like microsieverts per hour (μSv/h) or millirems per hour (mR/h), which provide an estimation of the radiation dose rate [24].

7.4 Other Imaging Modalities

Computed Tomography (CT)

Computed tomography (CT) is a medical imaging technique that combines X-ray technology with computer processing to produce detailed cross-sectional images of the body. CT scans provide valuable information for diagnosing and monitoring various medical conditions. The principles of computed tomography involve several key aspects [3]:

X-ray Generation

CT scanners use X-ray tubes that emit a focused beam of X-rays. These X-rays pass through the body and are attenuated (absorbed or scattered) to varying degrees by different tissues based on their density and composition [7].

Detectors

A ring of detectors positioned opposite the X-ray tube captures the transmitted X-rays after they pass through the body. The detectors measure the intensity of the X-rays, which are used to create the image [3].

Data Acquisition

The X-ray tube and detectors are rotated around the patient's body during a CT scan. Multiple X-ray projections are acquired from different angles, typically in a 360-degree rotation or less. The data acquisition process is usually rapid, with modern scanners capable of capturing images in a matter of seconds [9].

Image Reconstruction

The collected data is processed by a computer to reconstruct cross-sectional images of the body. This reconstruction process involves complex mathematical algorithms, such as filtered back projection or iterative reconstruction, which use the acquired X-ray projections to generate a detailed image [25].

Hounsfield Units (HU)

The reconstructed CT images are represented in Hounsfield Units, named after Sir Godfrey Hounsfield, who pioneered CT imaging. HU values represent the tissue attenuation properties and are used to differentiate various structures within the body. Air is assigned a value of −1000 HU, water 0 HU and dense bone around +1000 HU [26].

Image Display and Analysis

The reconstructed CT images can be visualised on a computer monitor as cross-sectional slices of the body. These images provide detailed anatomical information and can be further manipulated, such as adjusting the window width and level to enhance specific tissue characteristics. Radiologists analyse the images to aid in the diagnosis and treatment planning [26].

Contrast Enhancement

Contrast agents, such as iodine-based or barium-based substances, can be administered to highlight certain structures or abnormalities during a CT scan. These contrast agents are typically injected intravenously, ingested or administered rectally, and they help differentiate various tissues based on their contrast uptake [26].

Multiplanar Reconstruction and 3D Visualisation

In addition to the standard cross-sectional images, CT data can be used to generate multiplanar reconstructions (MPR) and three-dimensional (3D) visualisations. MPR allows the images to be reformatted in different planes (e.g. sagittal, coronal) for better anatomical assessment. 3D visualisations provide a more comprehensive view of complex structures or aid in surgical planning [26].

There are primarily two types of CT scanners used in equine veterinary medicine: Helical (spiral) CT scanners and multidetector-row CT scanners.

Helical (Spiral) CT Scanners

Helical CT scanners were the first generation of CT scanners and are still commonly used in equine imaging. They consist of a rotating gantry that houses an X-ray tube and a detector array. The patient is placed on a moving table that advances through the gantry during the scanning process. This continuous movement allows for the acquisition of volumetric data in a helical pattern, resulting in faster scan times compared to conventional CT scanners [26].

Advantages of helical CT scanners include:

- Faster scanning times, reducing the risk of motion artefacts.
- Improved patient comfort as the table moves continuously, eliminating the need for multiple positioning adjustments.
- Ability to acquire volumetric data that can be reconstructed into high-quality images.
- A wide range of reconstruction algorithms to optimise image quality and diagnostic information are available.

Multidetector-row CT Scanners

Multidetector-row CT scanners, also known as multidetector computed tomography (MDCT) scanners, represent the latest advancement in CT technology. They feature an array of multiple detectors arranged in rows, allowing for the simultaneous acquisition of multiple slices (or detector rows) with each rotation of the gantry. Common configurations include 4-row, 16-row, 64-row and even higher numbers of detectors [26].

Advantages of multidetector-row CT scanners include [3]:

- Faster scanning times compared to helical CT scanners, as multiple slices are acquired simultaneously.

- Improved spatial resolution and image quality due to the high number of detectors.
- Ability to perform higher-resolution imaging and obtain thinner slices, allowing for more detailed evaluation of anatomical structures.
- Increased coverage area, enabling faster whole-body scanning or imaging of larger anatomical regions.

It is worth noting that the choice of CT scanner type depends on several factors, including the specific requirements of the clinical case, availability of equipment and financial considerations. Helical CT scanners are still widely used and provide excellent diagnostic capabilities. However, multidetector-row CT scanners offer improved speed, image quality and the ability to perform advanced imaging techniques such as dynamic or perfusion studies [26].

Both types of CT scanners can provide valuable diagnostic information in equine veterinary practice, allowing for accurate diagnosis, treatment planning and monitoring of equine patients [26].

Applications of CT for the Equine Patient

CT has a wide range of applications in the field of equine veterinary medicine. It provides detailed cross-sectional images of the equine body, allowing for precise anatomical evaluation and accurate diagnosis. Some key applications of equine CT are outlined below [26].

Musculoskeletal Imaging

Equine CT is particularly valuable for assessing musculoskeletal structures, including bones, joints and soft tissues. It aids in the identification and evaluation of fractures, bone abnormalities, joint diseases (such as osteoarthritis), tendon and ligament injuries, and the localisation of foreign bodies. CT can provide detailed three-dimensional reconstructions, allowing for a better understanding of complex skeletal and soft tissue pathologies [26].

Head and Neck Evaluation

CT plays a vital role in diagnosing and evaluating conditions affecting the equine head and neck region. It is useful in identifying dental disorders, sinus diseases, temporomandibular joint abnormalities, nasal and paranasal sinus tumours, guttural pouch infections and tumours affecting the skull or cervical vertebrae. CT imaging provides detailed information about the extent, location and characteristics of these conditions, aiding in treatment planning and surgical interventions [26].

Thoracic Imaging

CT scans of the equine thorax are valuable in evaluating respiratory diseases, pulmonary masses, pleural effusions and thoracic trauma. Equine CT provides high-resolution images of the lungs, allowing for the identification of subtle changes in lung parenchyma, bronchi and blood vessels. It also aids in the assessment of pulmonary nodules and masses, facilitating early detection and treatment. This is only possible though in small ponies and foals due to the size of the tube [26].

Abdominal Examinations

CT is increasingly used for evaluating abdominal conditions in horses. It allows for detailed visualisation of abdominal organs, such as the liver, spleen, kidneys, intestines and reproductive organs. Equine CT aids in the detection and characterisation of abdominal masses, abscesses, gastrointestinal obstructions and other intra-abdominal pathologies. Like thoracic imaging, this is only possible in small patients [26].

Treatment Planning and Surgical Procedures

Equine CT is an essential tool for treatment planning and guiding surgical interventions. It provides surgeons with detailed preoperative images, aiding in the precise localisation of lesions, assessment of tumour margins and planning of surgical approaches [26].

Lameness Evaluation

CT has revolutionised the evaluation of equine lameness by providing detailed imaging of bone and soft tissue structures. It helps identify subtle bone lesions, stress fractures, joint pathology and soft tissue injuries contributing to lameness. CT can provide a more accurate diagnosis and guide appropriate treatment options, including targeted therapies, surgical interventions and rehabilitation protocols [26].

In equine veterinary medicine, the two main approaches for performing CT scans on horses are standing CT and general anaesthesia (GA) CT. Each approach has its advantages and considerations, and the choice depends on the specific needs of the patient and the available resources [26].

Standing CT

Standing CT involves performing CT scans on a standing, sedated horse without the need for GA. This approach has gained popularity due to its advantages in terms of cost, reduced risks associated with GA and the ability to perform repeated scans or image-guided procedures [27].

Advantages of standing CT:

- Avoidance of GA: Some horses may have medical conditions or specific risks that make GA challenging. Standing CT allows for imaging without the need for GA, minimising the associated risks. See Chapter 10 for further information.

- Cost-effectiveness: Standing CT scans are typically less expensive compared to GA CT, as they do not require an anaesthetist or extensive monitoring equipment.
- Repeatability: If a follow-up scan or serial imaging is required, it can be easily performed on a standing horse without the need for repeated GA.

Considerations for standing CT [27]:

- Motion artefacts: Horses may move or shift during the scan, leading to motion artefacts and potentially affecting image quality. Sedation and proper positioning techniques are crucial to minimise motion artefacts.
- Limited access to certain anatomical regions: While standing CT can cover various anatomical regions, there may be limitations in accessing areas such as the head, neck or lower limbs due to the size and bulk of the equipment. In some cases, GA CT may be necessary for a comprehensive evaluation.
- Patient cooperation: Horses must be adequately sedated and trained to stand still during the scanning process, which may not be possible in all cases.

CT Under GA

GA CT involves performing CT scans on a horse under GA. This approach allows for precise patient positioning, reduces motion artefacts and provides access to anatomical regions that may be challenging to image with a standing horse [26].

Advantages of GA CT [26]:

- Precise patient positioning: Under GA, horses can be positioned more accurately, ensuring optimal alignment and reducing motion artefacts.
- Comprehensive evaluation: GA CT allows for imaging of all anatomical regions, including the head, neck and lower limbs, without limitations due to equipment size or patient movement.
- Higher image quality: The elimination of patient movement during GA leads to higher image quality and diagnostic accuracy.

Considerations for GA CT [26]:

- Anaesthetic risks: GA carries inherent risks, including the potential for complications and the need for specialised monitoring and support equipment.
- Cost and resources: GA CT involves additional costs associated with anaesthesia, monitoring equipment and personnel requirements, such as an anaesthetist.
- Recovery time: Horses undergoing GA CT require post-anaesthetic recovery, including monitoring until fully awake and stable. Recovery can take several hours.

The choice between standing CT and GA CT depends on various factors, such as the specific diagnostic question, anatomical region of interest, patient stability and available resources. Standing CT offers advantages in terms of cost, repeatability and avoidance of GA, whereas GA CT provides precise patient positioning, comprehensive imaging and higher image quality but involves anaesthesia-associated considerations. The decision should be made collaboratively between the veterinary team, considering the individual patient's needs and the available facilities and expertise [26].

Standing Distal Limb Imaging

Hallmarq Veterinary Imaging is a company that specialises in the development and production of standing equine computed tomography (CT) scanners. Their standing CT scanner, known as the Hallmarq Equine Standing Equine CT, is designed specifically for imaging the lower limbs of horses in a standing position [27].

The Hallmarq Equine Standing Equine CT scanner offers several benefits and features [27]:

- Convenience and safety: The scanner allows for CT imaging of the lower limbs while the horse remains standing, eliminating the need for GA. This minimises the risks associated with GA and can reduce stress for the horse.
- High-quality imaging: The scanner utilises advanced imaging technology to produce high-quality CT images of the equine lower limb. The detailed cross-sectional images aid in the diagnosis and evaluation of various musculoskeletal conditions, including lameness, fractures, osteoarthritis and soft tissue injuries.
- Ease of use: The scanner is designed to be user-friendly and efficient, with a streamlined workflow. It allows for quick and straightforward positioning of the limb and provides automated data acquisition for efficient image acquisition.
- Expert support and training: Hallmarq Veterinary Imaging provides comprehensive training and ongoing support for veterinary teams using their standing CT scanner. This ensures that users are properly trained in scanner operation, image acquisition and interpretation of CT images.

Patient Preparation

Patient preparation for a CT scan in equine patients involves several important steps to ensure a successful and safe imaging procedure. RVNs play a crucial role in preparing the patient and assisting in the overall process. The key aspects of patient preparation for a CT scan are outlined below [27]:

Pre-CT Assessment

Relevant patient history should be gathered, including previous medical conditions, medications, allergies and any specific concerns or symptoms.

A thorough physical examination should be performed to assess the patient's general health status and identify any potential issues that may affect the CT scan or anaesthesia, if applicable [27].

Fasting

Depending on the specific imaging requirements, fasting may be necessary prior to the CT scan. Follow the guidelines provided by the vet and practice policy on the fasting period and any specific dietary restrictions.

Sedation or Anaesthesia

The need for sedation or GA will be decided based on the patient's temperament, the specific imaging requirements, and the capabilities of the imaging facility. The sedative or anaesthetic drug protocol will be prescribed by the case vet. RVNs may administer sedation or anaesthesia as per the vet's instructions. It is not appropriate for RVNs to dose medication to effect. Therefore, any deviations from the agreed drug protocol must be discussed and agreed upon by the case vet before being administered [9].

Patient Positioning and Restraint

Assist in positioning the patient for the CT scan, ensuring proper alignment and immobilisation of the anatomical region of interest. Utilise appropriate restraint techniques, such as ropes, halters, or specialised equine positioning aids, to secure the patient in the desired position and prevent movement during the scan.

IV Access and Fluid Support

Establish IV access with a catheter if required, especially if contrast media administration or fluid support is required during the CT scan. Monitor and maintain the IV line during the procedure, ensuring the flow rate and integrity of the catheter [9].

Contrast Administration

If contrast media is indicated for the CT scan, the RVN will assist the vet with the administration of the contrast agent according to their instructions and guidance. The patient should be monitored for any adverse reactions or complications related to contrast administration. Any concerns should be promptly reported any concerns to the case vet [9].

Radiation Safety

Ensure appropriate radiation safety measures are in place, including wearing PPE such as lead aprons and gloves, and following radiation safety protocols established by the imaging facility.

Post-CT Care

Assist in the immediate post-CT care of the patient, such as monitoring vital signs, ensuring a smooth recovery from sedation or anaesthesia, and addressing any immediate post-procedural needs. Provide post-CT instructions to the owner or caretaker regarding medication administration, wound care (if applicable) and any activity restrictions or post-procedure monitoring requirements. Throughout the entire process, effective communication with the veterinary team, including the imaging facility personnel and the patient's owner or caretaker, is crucial to ensure a coordinated and safe patient experience [26].

It is important to note that specific patient preparation protocols may vary depending on the individual patient, the imaging facility's requirements and the specific imaging goals. Therefore, it is essential for RVNs to closely follow the instructions provided by the veterinary team and the imaging facility to ensure the best possible outcome for the patient's CT scan.

Overall, equine CT has significantly advanced diagnostic capabilities in equine veterinary medicine. Its applications span various anatomical regions and conditions, enabling more accurate diagnoses, improved treatment planning and better patient outcomes [26].

Magnetic Resonance Imaging (MRI)

MRI is a type of advanced imagining used in equine patients, predominately to assess problems associated with the foot and distal limb in standing horses and more proximal areas under GA. This non-invasive technology is able to produce three-dimensional detailed anatomical images providing a detailed and accurate diagnosis. MRI allows the evaluation of soft tissue (tendon and ligaments), joint capsules, joint fluid, bone and cartilage. It is therefore a valuable tool in lameness examinations [25].

Basic Principles of Image Production

MRI scanning is a valuable diagnostic tool used in veterinary medicine, including equine imaging. The basic principles of image production in MRI involve the interaction of magnetic fields and radiofrequency (RF) waves with the tissues of the equine patient. The fundamental principles involved in MRI image production are presented below [25].

Magnetic Field

MRI scanners generate a strong magnetic field by using superconducting magnets. This magnetic field aligns the protons within the body tissues of the equine patient [25].

RF Excitation

To produce an MRI image, RF waves are used to disrupt the alignment of the protons momentarily. The RF waves are emitted from a coil placed around the region of interest in the equine patient's body [25].

Resonance and Relaxation

When the RF waves interact with the protons, it causes them to resonate, or absorb and emit energy. This resonance is detected by the MRI scanner. After the RF excitation, the protons gradually return to their original alignment, which is called relaxation. The relaxation process involves two components: T1 relaxation (longitudinal) and T2 relaxation (transverse) [25].

Gradient Coils

Gradient coils are present within the MRI scanner. These coils produce a gradient magnetic field, which helps to encode spatial information. The gradient coils create a varying magnetic field strength along different directions, allowing differentiation of tissues based on their location within the equine patient's body [25].

Signal Detection

The MRI scanner detects the emitted RF signals from the resonating protons. These signals are converted into electrical signals by the receiver coil, which are then processed to generate an image [25].

Image Reconstruction

The acquired data from the MRI scanner is subjected to mathematical transformations to reconstruct a two-dimensional or three-dimensional image of the equine patient's anatomy. Various imaging sequences, such as T1-weighted, T2-weighted and proton density-weighted, can be used to provide different types of information about the tissues [25].

High-field equine MRI systems and low-field standing MRI systems are two different types of imaging technologies used in veterinary medicine for diagnosing and evaluating musculoskeletal conditions in horses. While they both serve the same purpose, there are significant differences between them in terms of image quality, capabilities and practicality [25].

Magnetic Field Strength

High-field Equine MRI High-field MRI systems typically have a magnetic field strength of 1.5 Tesla or higher, similar to the MRI systems used in human medicine. These systems generate a strong magnetic field, which allows for excellent image quality and spatial resolution [25].

Low-field Standing MRI Low-field standing MRI systems have a magnetic field strength of around 0.3 Tesla or lower. Although the magnetic field is weaker compared to high-field systems, it is still sufficient to obtain diagnostic images of the equine limb in a standing position [25].

Image Quality

- High-field MRI systems offer superior image quality due to their higher magnetic field strength. They provide detailed anatomical visualisation and better soft tissue contrast, enabling the detection of subtle abnormalities.
- Low-field standing MRI systems produce lower-resolution images compared to high-field systems. While they may not provide the same level of detail, they can still identify common musculoskeletal pathologies [25].

Imaging Capabilities

- High-field systems have the capability to perform a wide range of MRI sequences and protocols, allowing for comprehensive evaluation of various anatomical structures and pathologies. They can also be used for imaging other parts of the body besides the limbs.
- Low-field standing MRI systems are primarily designed for imaging the limbs of standing horses. They are specifically optimised for evaluating conditions such as lameness or injuries in the distal limb [25].

Practicality and Accessibility

- High-field MRI systems require the horse to be under GA as the horse is inserted into a tube similar to a CT. This can be costly, and there are limited facilities in the United Kingdom that offer this as a procedure.
- Low-field standing MRI systems offer the advantage of being performed on a standing horse, eliminating the need for GA. They can be installed in a practice or equine hospital, allowing for easier accessibility and more frequent use.

In summary, high-field equine MRI systems provide superior image quality and versatility but require general anaesthesia and specialised facilities. Low-field standing MRI systems, on the other hand, offer the advantage of imaging horses in a standing position without anaesthesia, making them more accessible and practical for routine evaluations of limb conditions. The choice between the two depends on factors such as specific clinical needs, available resources and the horse's condition [25].

MRI uses a magnetic field and does not damage tissue as it passes through. The body contains large amounts of water. Each water molecule is made up of 2 hydrogen atoms and 1 oxygen atom (H_2O). Inside each hydrogen atom, there is a central nucleus containing a proton.

Protons, which are positively charged, are abundant in the body and play a large part in obtaining images. All protons spin on their axis, creating a small magnetic charge. This takes place throughout the body and is known as precession.

MRI uses magnetic fields and radio waves, which it uses to detect water in tissues and uses this information to generate an image. Image detail is very high, because of the water content in the body [25].

When a large magnetic field is introduced via MRI close to the subject – e.g. equine or human, the protons will change their positions to align with the magnetic field.

During the process of image accusation, a radio frequency pulse sent from the MRI machine disrupts the alignment of protons. This radio frequency pulse is a weaker magnetic field, sent across the alignment. The protons become misaligned in either a 90-degree or 180-degree realignment [25].

As soon as the radio frequency stops (turned off by an MRI technician), the protons will realign to their original position, giving off electromagnetic energy as this occurs.

The MRI machine can detect this energy and obtain measurements. These energy bursts can help differentiate between the tissues, as different types of tissue give off different types of energy – enabling an image to be formed [25].

Standing MRI

Many practices now have the availability of standing MRIs. Standing MRI is used in lameness investigations and is readily available. It is often more appealing to an owner as it does not require the patient to undergo a general anaesthetic. However, the scope of areas that are imaged is limited to the distal limb. Therefore, it is more commonly used when lameness has been blocked to the foot or for emergencies such as solar penetration. Standing MRI can often be operated by two people. The horse is sedated during the examination [25].

MRI and GA

Under GA, MRI allows us to obtain images of areas other than just the foot, therefore allowing greater scope for diagnostic investigation. The following areas are suitable to be imaged by MRI under GA [25]:

- Distal limb
- Proximal suspensory
- Tarsus
- Stifles
- Head
- Neck
- Carpus

Equine MRI under GA enables a better-quality image, but carrying out GA for this may be challenging. This is due to the equipment required, patient access (positioning and due to health and safety) and patient monitoring. An equine theatre carrying out this procedure needs to be equipped with MRI-safe equipment. The procedure requires appropriate levels of personnel, and the initial set-up is costly, but overall obtaining the images may be more time efficient [25].

Equine practices carrying out MRIs will often use a separate operating theatre specifically designed for MRI use. This will include specialist monitoring and anaesthetic equipment as well as piped gas and specialist tables. There is also the risk of anaesthetic complications such as myopathy and as with any GA, the potential for mortality.

Patient Preparation

- Ensure the horse is clean and free from any mud and dirt
- Remove shoes
- Obtain radiographs of the feet to rule out any remnants of metal
- Place IV catheter for sedation
- Prepare equipment for a constant rate infusion (CRI) if practice protocol requires this
- Identify the area of interest for imaging
- Mark the lateral aspect of the limb either with a vitamin E capsule or oil in an extension set
- Ensure there is nothing on the horse that could be attracted to the magnet. This would include the use of a rope head collar if using a Highfield system.

Before any images are obtained, a thorough lameness work-up with a vet should take place [9]. Table 7.6 displays the advantages and disadvantages of MRI in the equine patient.

Health and Safety Considerations

Prior to entering the MRI room, staff members should have received appropriate training in the operations of and health and safety surrounding the MRI. Local rules for the MRI area/room should be in place and read and signed by all team members who are using the facility. Clear signage, restricted access and a lockable door are all required. Some practices have their MRI based in a self-contained unit adjacent to the main building, which enables control over access. Prior to entering the MRI examination area, team members should have removed all personal items (see list below). Any team member who is fitted with a pacemaker, vascular clip or any other type of implant should be assessed by an appropriate person as to their safety prior to working in the MRI unit [25].

Table 7.6 The advantages and disadvantages of MRI in the equine patient.

Advantages	Disadvantages
Accurate diagnosis: MRI provides high-resolution images that offer detailed information about the horse's anatomy, allowing veterinarians to make accurate diagnoses. It helps identify soft tissue injuries, bone abnormalities and joint problems that may not be easily detected through other imaging techniques	Costly: MRI is a relatively expensive imaging technique, and the equipment and maintenance costs are substantial. Additionally, specialised expertise is required to operate and interpret the MRI scans, which can further increase the overall cost
Non-invasive: MRI is a non-invasive imaging modality, meaning it does not require any surgical intervention. Horses can be examined without the need for anaesthesia or sedation in some cases, reducing the associated risks and complications	Limited availability: MRI machines are not as widely available as other imaging modalities like X-rays or ultrasounds. Access to equine MRI may be limited to certain specialised veterinary practices or hospitals, requiring the transportation of the horse to a different facility
Comprehensive imaging: Equine MRI provides multi-planar imaging capabilities, allowing veterinarians to view different anatomical structures from various angles. This comprehensive view aids in understanding the extent and location of injuries or abnormalities	Time-consuming: Equine MRI scans can take a considerable amount of time, typically ranging from 30 min to a few hours. The horse needs to remain still during the scanning process, which can be challenging, particularly for horses that are anxious or in pain
Early detection: MRI can detect conditions at an early stage, even before clinical signs are apparent. This early detection enables timely intervention and potentially more successful treatment outcomes	Anaesthesia or sedation: Although some horses can undergo MRI without anaesthesia or sedation, others may require it to ensure their safety and cooperation during the procedure. Anaesthesia carries inherent risks, and its administration should be carefully considered and managed
Safe for soft tissues: MRI does not use ionising radiation, making it a safe option for evaluating soft tissues like tendons, ligaments and muscles. It provides valuable information for assessing injuries and monitoring the healing process	Limited use for bony structures: While MRI is excellent for evaluating soft tissues, it has certain limitations when it comes to imaging bony structures. X-rays or CT scans are generally more effective for assessing bone abnormalities and fractures

Source: Cassie Woods and Rosina Lillywhite.

Those team members who are staying within the MRI field such as horse handlers or anaesthetists should wear MRI-specific headphones and earplugs. Horse handlers should not wear steel toe-capped boots in the MRI unit [25].

Patient Safety
- Standing horses should be adequately sedated. Sound-proofing ear covers and blinkers may help to keep the horse calm.
- Shoes should be removed, and feet X-rayed to ensure there are no nail remnants in the hoof.
- Thermodynamic burns are a risk to patients, caused by radiofrequency waves. Care should be taken to avoid any conducting materials placed within the magnetic field, which may cause a concentration of electrical current leading to heating and tissue damage.
- Post-procedure colic monitoring of the patient both when at the practice and once at home due to the levels of sedation used.
- Horses undergoing GA may be more at risk of myopathies due to the positioning of the limbs.

Equipment Choices for Use with a Magnetic Field
Equipment that is ferromagnetic should be avoided in the examination room. Items made of this type of material are likely to be attracted to the magnet, which may involve them moving towards the magnet at high speed and potentially oscillating within the magnetic bore. All metallic objects should be treated as hazardous [25].

Examples of items that should not be contained in the MRI suite are as follows:

- Gas cylinders
- Non-MRI safe anaesthetic equipment
- Trolleys
- Scalpels
- Instruments
- Clippers
- Hobbles
- Headcollars with metal fittings
- Mops and buckets

Personal Items
- Coins
- Jewellery

- Watches
- Hairpins
- Hearing aids
- Cameras
- Tape recorders
- Mobile phones
- Laptops

Endoscopy

An endoscope is a fibre optic instrument used for visualising the inside of viscera and other structures.

Endoscopy is a useful tool in equine practice and is used in a variety of situations to aid in diagnosis and surgical intervention. There are a variety of scopes available for different uses, and these are usually split into two categories: rigid or flexible, depending on their purpose. Table 7.7 displays the different types of endoscopes that are available in equine practice [28].

Endoscopes are expensive pieces of equipment and great care should be taken with handling, cleaning and maintenance.

Endoscopy of the Respiratory Tract

An airway examination may be required for a variety of reasons. The most common would be for horses that are displaying signs of respiratory disease such as equine asthma or pneumonia. Horses that are in training, such as racehorses, may be routinely examined as part of their

competition preparation [28]. Horses undergoing a poor performance examination may also receive an airway examination, particularly if an abnormal noise has been noted during exercise. Airway endoscopy enables the visualisation of anatomy and facilitates the retrieval of samples such as tracheal washes and guttural pouch washes. The airway endoscope is also a valuable tool for carrying out procedures such as laser airway surgery and visualising procedures such as catheterisation of the guttural pouch [28].

During examination of the airway, the nasal cavity, the ethmoid turbinates, the pharynx, the guttural pouches, the epiglottis, the arytenoid cartilages, the larynx, the trachea, carina and bronchi can all be visualised [29].

Preparation of the Patient for Airway Endoscopy

The patient should be adequately restrained. This could include a chifney or a bridle. A twitch should only be used if necessary. If twitching is used, it should be carried out with care. See Chapter 5 for further information. Often, for respiratory examinations, when looking at potential physiological abnormalities of the larynx and the pharynx, the horse will not be sedated. This will allow the function of the airway to be assessed. Horses undergoing this type of examination may be required to be worked immediately prior to the scope. PPE, including hard hats, should be worn, and care should be taken to avoid standing directly in front of the patient during the examination as un-sedated patients may resent this examination, and this could pose a

Table 7.7 Different types of endoscopes found in equine practice.

Type of endoscope	Flexible or rigid	Use
Bronchoscope	Flexible • 60 cm Upper airway • 100 cm Upper airway examination plus proximal tracheal examination • 150–200 cm for full respiratory examination	Airway examination, Cystoscopy, Hysteroscopy Sinoscopy, Proctoscopy Laser surgery Biopsies Sample collection
Gastroscope	Flexible • 3–3.5 m, depending on manufacturer	Gastroscopy – Biopsies Sample collection
Arthroscope	Rigid • 16–17 cm depending on manufacturer	Arthroscopy, Tenoscopy, Bursoscopy
Laparoscope	Rigid • 30–60 cm depending on the weight of the horse and vet preference	Laparoscopy
Dental scope	Rigid • 32–48 cm in length, depending on the manufacturer	Oral examination

Source: Cassie Woods.

health and safety risk to handlers. The passing of the scope into the lower airway can often cause the horse to cough. Therefore, once the functionality of the airway has been examined, sedation may then be administered according to the case vet's instructions [9].

It is important to have any equipment and consumables required to hand, to keep procedure time to a minimum. For those requiring a tracheal wash sample collection, it is helpful to have an endoscope flushing catheter pre-loaded into the scope prior to passing the scope [28].

Equipment Required for Respiratory Endoscopy Examination

- PPE, including a hard hat, steel toe-capped boots and disposable gloves
- Sedation
- Water-based lubricant
- Endoscope (for sizes, see Table 7.7)
- Light source
- Twitch (if necessary)

If guttural pouch examination is required:

- Guttural pouch guide wire/probe
- Endoscopic biopsy forceps (for examination of the guttural pouch)

Equipment Needed for Tracheal Wash Sampling

- As for respiratory endoscopy, with the addition of the following:
- Endoscope flushing catheter
- 2 × 30 ml pre-prepared syringes containing saline
- Sample collection tubes such as the anticoagulant ethylenediaminetetraacetic acid (EDTA), plain tubes and/or Cytospin, which is a fluid formulated with a mixture of alcohol and carbo-wax. This combination helps to maintain and enhance cellular embedded in fixated tissue, as well as guard it against airdrying artefacts. It is routinely used to fix aspirated cells and those obtained through bronchial washings.

Equipment Needed for a Bronchioalveolar Lavage (BAL)

- As for respiratory endoscopy, with the addition of the following:
- Endoscope flushing catheter
- 5 ml local anaesthetic
- 6 × 50 ml pre-prepared syringes containing saline
- BAL tube
- 5ml syringe for BAL tube cuff inflation
- Sample collection tubes: EDTA, plain tubes and cytospin

Technique for Passing the Endoscope for the Examination of the Respiratory Tract

1) The horse should be appropriately restrained.
2) Ensure all equipment is functioning and any additional equipment required is to hand.
3) Lubricate the end of the scope with water-based lubricant, avoiding the camera lens.
4) Place one hand on the horse's nose and hold the tip of the endoscope with the other hand.
5) Insert the endoscope into the nasal cavity, ensuring that the scope is placed ventrally into the ventral meatus.
6) Advance the scope slowly towards the pharynx, again ensuring a ventral line is taken.
7) The upper airway can then be assessed.
8) The function of the larynx may be assessed by occluding both nostrils, which can be done by pinching the nostrils, causing the horse to breathe in deeply.
9) The scope may then be passed into the trachea to examine the lower airways. At the end of the trachea, visualisation of the two major bronchi will be possible.
10) If a tracheal wash sample is to be obtained, this will be carried out in the upper trachea.

Obtaining BAL Samples

Performing a bronchoalveolar lavage (BAL) in an equine patient involves several steps. The personnel involved in the collection should be qualified and knowledgeable in the procedure; the procedure can be broken down into the following steps [28]:

Pre-procedure Assessment

- A thorough physical examination of the horse will be performed, including respiratory auscultation, to assess lung sounds and identify potential abnormalities.
- The horse's medical history will be evaluated, including any previous respiratory issues or treatments.

Preparation

- Gather necessary equipment: BAL tube/catheter or bronchoscope, sterile saline solution (the saline should be warmed to minimise the reaction from the horse), sterile containers for sample collection, syringes, gloves and PPE.
- Ensure the patient is properly restrained in a safe and quiet area.
- Administer sedation according to the vet's instructions.
- Local anaesthetic is administered via a catheter through a bronchoscope, following appropriate dosage guidelines and according to the vet's instructions.

Sample Collection

- A sterilised BAL tube/catheter is used to maintain an aseptic technique.
- The BAL catheter is inserted through one nostril, which can be used as a bronchoscope for visualisation and navigation.
- The catheter/bronchoscope is advanced through the nasal passages, past the larynx and into the trachea.
- The cuff on the BAL tube is inflated with saline.
- With the catheter/bronchoscope properly positioned within the trachea, the sterile saline solution is introduced slowly to avoid inducing coughing or respiratory distress.
- An appropriate volume of saline solution is gradually introduced (typically 60–240 mL) into the lungs.
- The saline solution is withdrawn by gentle suction or gravity flow using syringes or collection containers.
- The BAL fluid is collected into sterile containers, ensuring proper labelling for identification.
- Horses may find this procedure stressful, and violent coughing episodes may occur; it is therefore not always possible to carry out on every case, such as those with severe respiratory disease.

Post-procedure Care

- The horse's respiratory rate and overall condition should be monitored closely. Any immediate adverse reactions or complications should be recorded.
- Appropriate post-procedure treatments, such as bronchodilators or anti-inflammatory drugs should be administered, if directed by the case vet.
- A quiet and comfortable recovery area should be provided and the horse observed for any signs of respiratory distress or complications.
- The collected BAL fluid samples should be submitted to a diagnostic laboratory for analysis.

Examination of the Guttural Pouch

The guttural pouch is a unique structure found in horses and only a few other species. They are air-filled sacs that expand from the eustachian tube. The horse has one on each side of the head. An entrance to the pouch can be visualised using the scope and resembles a small slit (salpingopharyngeal fold) in the membrane. The lining of the pouches is a very thin membrane, and inside are some major/critical structures, which include cranial nerves and major arteries. Because of the presence of these crucial structures, care should be taken when advancing the scope into this area [29].

The guttural pouches may need to be examined when conditions such as *Streptococcus equi* (strangles) guttural pouch mycosis, guttural pouch empyema and guttural pouch tympany are suspected.

The endoscope should be pre-loaded with a guttural pouch guide wire prior to the start of the examination. This is advanced and used to initiate the opening of the pouch via the salpingopharyngeal fold prior to the insertion of the scope [28].

Endoscopy of the Gastrointestinal System

Gastroscopy is carried out routinely in equine practice. The most common reason for performing gastroscopy is to aid in the diagnosis of equine gastric ulcer syndrome (EGUS) [28]. Gastroscopy is also used for the diagnosis of other conditions, such as oesophageal obstructions, gastric impactions, gastric neoplasia and duodenal ulceration. Gastroscopy facilitates the visualisation of the oesophagus, the cardia, margo plicatus, the greater and lesser curvatures and the pylorus. Passing through the exit of the stomach (the pylorus) also allows visualisation of the most proximal part of the duodenum. While in the stomach and the duodenum the vet may also obtain samples or pinch biopsies [28].

Preparing the Patient for Gastroscopy

Starvation of the horse is essential in order to perform gastroscopy. Food is usually withheld for 12–16 hours, and water is withheld for 4 hours. However, many practices have their own protocols for this and therefore, it is important to confirm practice procedures when liaising with owners and formulating a plan for inpatients [9].

Horses may be starved at the owner's premises, or some often prefer to have them admitted to the practice for starvation the evening before. Horses should be bedded overnight on bedding they are unlikely to eat, therefore straw must be avoided. Remnants of hay and feed in the bedding should be removed from the bedding. A muzzle can be used if required [9].

The patient should be adequately restrained, which usually involves sedation. Three people are required to carry out this procedure: one to restrain the patient, one to pass the scope and one to drive the scope.

Once the patient is sedated, a Hausman's gag should be fitted. This is used to prevent the horse from chewing on the endoscope as it is advanced. A nasogastric tube is sometimes passed first; the gastroscope can then be passed through the lumen [28].

Equipment Needed for Equine Gastroscopy

- Gastroscope 3.0–3.6 m in length
- Camera processor/tower

- Light source
- Suction
- Air
- Water-based lubricant
- Hausman's gag
- Sedation
- Twitch (if necessary)

The Gastroscopy Examination

1) The horse should be appropriately restrained.
2) Ensure all equipment is functioning and any additional equipment required is to hand.
3) Place the Hausman's gag into the mouth or pass the length of the stomach tube if using this technique.
4) Lubricate the end of the scope with lubricant, avoiding the camera lens.
5) Place one hand on the horse's nose and hold the tip of the gastroscope with the other hand.
6) Insert the gastroscope into the nasal cavity ensuring that the scope is placed ventrally into the ventral meatus.
7) The scope should be advanced towards the larynx. Air and water can be used to initiate swallowing, and the tube should be advanced into the oesophagus in the same way as a nasogastric tube.
8) Visualisation of the oesophagus should confirm the gastroscope is in the correct place.
9) Air can then be used to dilate the oesophagus, providing an easier passage and visibility.
10) If resistance is encountered, the passing should be stopped and a vet should be alerted.
11) Once through the cardia, the air is then used to inflate the stomach.
12) The scope is then further advanced, keeping to the left, passing into the squamous region, following the curvature of the stomach advancing towards the margo plicatus and the pylorus.
13) Upon completion of the gastroscopic examination, suction should be used to deflate the stomach. The stomach walls can be visualised as they collapse. Air should be removed to avoid post-gastroscopy complications, such as colic.

Overground Endoscope

An overground endoscope is a type of video endoscope, and in equine patients, this allows for the visualisation and examination of the upper airway during exercise or other dynamic activities. It is a valuable tool for diagnosing respiratory conditions and assessing the performance of horses [28].

Setup

To use an overground scope, the following steps are typically involved:

- Sedation: Is seldom used as the horse is required to exercise after the scope is placed, and this would be counterproductive.
- Equipment preparation: The endoscope is connected to a video monitor or a portable recording device. The scope is usually flexible, allowing it to be easily and placed into the upper airway. The equipment should be checked prior to being used to ensure it is working properly.
- Insertion: The endoscope is carefully inserted through the nostril and into horse's ventral meatus. It is then advanced into the nasal passages, pharynx and larynx. This is then secured in place using specially designed head straps that form part of the scope system (Figure 7.31).
- Examination: Once the endoscope is in place, the structures in the upper airway can be visualised in real time. The video feed from the endoscope is displayed on the monitor or recorded for analysis following the examination.

Indications for Use

Overground endoscopy is commonly used in equine medicine for various purposes, including [28]:

- Evaluation of respiratory disorders: Overground endoscopy facilitates the examination of the upper airway to identify and diagnose conditions such as laryngeal hemiplegia (commonly known as 'roaring'), dorsal

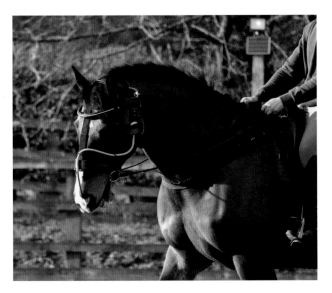

Figure 7.31 An overground scope in use. *Source:* Rosina Lillywhite.

displacement of the soft palate, pharyngeal collapse and other abnormalities.

- Assessment of performance issues: Horses that experience exercise intolerance or poor performance may undergo an overground scope to investigate potential respiratory problems that could be affecting their athletic ability.
- Pre-purchase examinations: In some cases, overground endoscopy forms part of a pre-purchase examination to assess the respiratory health of a horse before buying or selling it.
- Follow-up evaluations: Horses that have undergone surgical procedures or medical treatments for respiratory conditions may have periodic follow-up examinations. An overground scope is used to monitor their progress and assess the effectiveness of treatment.

It is important to note that the use of an overground scope should always be performed by a vet with experience in equine respiratory diagnostics. Manufacturer's guidelines and appropriate training should be followed to ensure correct and safe use of equipment [28].

Cleaning and Disinfecting of Endoscopes

Endoscopes should be cleaned after each use, and this should be carried out as soon as possible to avoid contaminates sitting in the biopsy channel and around the outside of the scope.

The endoscope will usually come with its own cleaning equipment, which should include a leak test pump, and a biopsy cleaning attachment. This will enable the scope to be fully submerged. Without this, the scope should not be submerged in water.

The leak test pump should be attached to the scope and inflated to check that the scope is safe to submerge. Usually, around 160 mmHg of pressure should be sufficient. A small amount of pressure may be lost initially (around 2 mmHg), which is normal. If there is any doubt that the pressure is not holding, the endoscope should be submerged [9].

Examination gloves should be worn when dealing with any cleaning chemicals. The scope buttons should be removed and cleaned. The biopsy flushing catheter should then be attached. The scope should first be submerged and flushed with an enzymatic cleaning solution. This enables any build-up such as mucous and blood to be broken down. The scope should be left in the solution for the time period according to the manufacturer's instructions. A channel cleaning brush can be used to remove any residue. The scope should then be removed and placed into a second disinfectant solution, diluted according to instruction. The flushing of the channel should be repeated, and the scope should be left submerged in the diluted disinfectant according to the manufacturer's instructions [9].

Finally, the scope should be flushed through with water to remove any chemical residue from the channel. The leak test pump should be disconnected and the biopsy flushing device removed. The outside of the scope should be wiped, and the lens should be gently cleaned with an alcohol wipe. The scope should then be hung to dry out. The scope buttons should be replaced when the scope is dry.

Cleaning the Endoscope in an Ambulatory Setting

Where it may not be possible to fully submerge the scope while in a yard, care should be taken to clean the scope between horses. There always remains the possibility that one or more horses in the yard are silent carriers for *Streptococcus equi*, and endoscopes may act as fomites in the transmission of this disease between animals [3]. Once the examination has ended, the scope can be rinsed through with both the enzymatic cleaner and the disinfectant using a 50 ml syringe to flush the biopsy channel. Water attached to the endoscope can then be pumped through. The outside of the scope should be wiped clean with a disinfectant wipe.

When using a twitch, it is important to also clean and disinfect this between patients; the safest way to avoid cross-contamination would be to change the twitch rope between cases [3].

Arthroscopy

An arthroscope is a small rigid endoscope that is connected to a video camera, used in equine surgery for the visualisation of joints, bursae and tendon sheaths. Arthroscopy can either be used as a diagnostic tool or to aid in surgical intervention. When carrying out arthroscopy, the image is produced via a video camera and projected onto a monitor [28].

Laparoscopy

Similar to an arthroscope, a laparoscope is a rigid endoscope attached to a fibre-optic camera, but much longer in length than the arthroscope. The laparoscopes are often custom made for the equine vet, as opposed to the arthroscope which is similar to that used in human surgery. Common procedures using laparoscopy in equine practice include ovariectomy, retained testicle removal, closure of the nephrosplenic space and nephrectomy [28].

Both the arthroscope and laparoscope enable surgeries to be performed using a 'keyhole' technique. This technique helps to reduce trauma, scaring and post-operative recovery time.

Care and maintenance of the arthroscope and laparoscope often become the responsibility of the RVN. Following surgery, the instruments should be cleaned as per normal surgical instruments, taking great care to avoid any damage to the camera lens. However, many arthroscopes and laparoscopes are not suitable for auto-clave sterilisation and are either sterilised using cold sterilisation or gas sterilisation with ethylene oxide [28].

Ultrasonography

Ultrasonography is a commonly used diagnostic imagining technique in equine practice. It is generally non-invasive and can usually be carried out on the same day. Ultrasonographic examination enables images to be obtained of internal organs and musculoskeletal structures. In equine practice, ultrasound plays a key role in diagnostics during lameness and poor performance examinations [30].

Ultrasound uses high-frequency sound waves to create real-time images of the body's internal structures. Ultrasound works in the following way [30]:

1) Transducer: The ultrasound machine consists of a hand-held device called a transducer. The transducer emits and receives sound waves.
2) Sound wave generation: The transducer contains piezoelectric crystals that generate sound waves when an electrical current passes through them. These crystals vibrate rapidly, producing sound waves at frequencies above the range of human hearing (typically between 2 and 18 MHz).
3) Sound wave transmission: The transducer is placed against the skin and covered with a gel to facilitate sound wave transmission. The gel helps eliminate air pockets that can interfere with the passage of sound waves.
4) Sound wave propagation: The transducer emits a brief pulse of sound waves into the body. These sound waves travel through the body, penetrating various tissues.
5) Reflection and echoes: When the sound waves encounter different tissues with varying densities, some of the waves are reflected back to the transducer. These reflected sound waves are called echoes.
6) Echo reception: The transducer detects the echoes as they return and converts them into electrical signals.
7) Signal processing: The electrical signals from the transducer are processed by the ultrasound machine. The machine analyses the timing and strength of the echoes

received to create a visual representation of the internal structures.
8) Image formation: The ultrasound machine uses the timing and strength of the echoes to determine the location and composition of the tissues. It constructs a two-dimensional or three-dimensional image based on this information.
9) Display: The ultrasound machine displays the generated image on a monitor in real-time, allowing the healthcare provider to observe the internal structures of the body.

Ultrasound is particularly useful for visualising soft tissues, such as organs, blood vessels and muscles. It can also provide information about motion and blood flow within the body. Additionally, Doppler ultrasound, a specialised technique, allows the assessment of blood flow patterns and velocities. Ultrasound imaging is safe, non-invasive, and does not involve the use of ionising radiation, making it widely used in equine practice. Table 7.8 displays the different modes found on an ultrasound machine and their indications for use in equine imaging [30].

Ultrasound Probes

Ultrasound transducers used in equine ultrasonography are essential components of the imaging system. They are handheld devices that emit and receive ultrasound waves to create images of the internal structures of a horse's body [30].

There are different types of ultrasound transducers used in equine ultrasonography, each with its own characteristics and applications. The commonly used transducers include [30]:

- Linear array transducers: Linear array transducers consist of multiple small crystal elements arranged in a line. They are versatile and commonly used for musculoskeletal imaging in horses. These transducers provide high-resolution images and are suitable for examining tendons, ligaments, joints and superficial structures, and they work on a frequency range of 3.0–17.0 MHz.

Table 7.8 Different ultrasonographic modes and indications for use.

Name	Definition	Description	Use
B-Mode	Brightness mode	The returning echo waves are represented by dots on a screen. The brightness of each dot is determined by the strength of the echo	Most equine ultrasonography is performed in this mode
M-Mode	Motion mode	Shows the movement of structures along a region of ultrasound image in relation to time	Cardiac ultrasonography
Doppler Mode	Doppler	For the assessment and visualisation of blood flow. Allows direction and velocity of blood flow to be visualised	Mainly cardiac but some use in reproductive and musculoskeletal

Source: Cassie Woods.

- Convex array transducers: Convex array transducers have a curved shape and are used for imaging large areas, such as the abdomen and thorax. They are ideal for evaluating organs like the liver, kidneys and heart in horses. The curved design allows for better visualisation of deep structures and improves the field of view, and they work on a frequency range between 1.0 and 7.0 MHz.
- Phased array transducers: Phased array transducers use multiple small elements that can be electronically controlled to steer and focus the ultrasound beam. They are commonly employed for cardiac imaging in horses to assess the heart's structure and function. Phased array transducers are also used for evaluating deep musculoskeletal structures, such as the back and pelvis, and they work on a frequency of 1.0–6.0 MHz.
- Endorectal transducers: Endorectal transducers are specialised probes designed for rectal examinations in horses. They are inserted into the rectum to obtain images of the reproductive organs, including the uterus, ovaries and prostate gland in males. These transducers are particularly useful for reproductive evaluations and monitoring during breeding and typically operate within a frequency range of 5–10 MHz.
- Microconvex transducers: Microconvex transducers have a small, rounded shape and are used for imaging small areas with limited access. They are commonly employed for equine ophthalmic examinations, allowing visualisation of the eye structures and detection of ocular conditions and typically operate within a frequency range from 5 to 12 MHz.

The choice of transducer depends on the specific imaging requirements and the area of interest. The appropriate transducer is selected based on the desired depth of penetration, field of view and resolution needed for accurate diagnosis in different clinical scenarios [30].

There are a variety of artefacts that can present during an ultrasound scan. Artefacts are objects seen on ultrasound that do not represent body tissue. They may obscure findings and serve to impede the correct diagnosis. The presence of artefacts may be due to the following being present at the examination site [30]:

- Dirt
- Grease
- Hair
- Scabs
- Air bubbles between the skin and transducer

RVNs can play a significant part in reducing the incidence of artefacts by performing careful and efficient skin preparation.

Preparing the Patient for Ultrasound Imaging

The patient should be restrained appropriately, including sedation; this is important for safety and also for quality image acquisition. The case vet will decide the type and dose of sedation to be administered. Once the patient has been sedated, the area of interest should first be brushed to remove any dirt and then clipped using No. 40 clipper blades. The contralateral limb may also need to be scanned to act as a comparison to the affected limb. It is important to check if this is the case, so that both limbs can be clipped at the same time if required [30].

Once clipped, the area should be cleaned with warm water and gauze to remove any grease, dirt and clipped hair. Then isopropyl alcohol is then applied, followed by ultrasound gel which can be massaged into the area. Care should be taken to avoid excessive amounts of gel as this can cause a lateral image artefact that may impair the structures being examined. Image quality can be improved greatly by allowing ultrasound gel to soak into the skin for at least five minutes prior to scanning [30].

There are some situations where patients may not require clipping; this could be due to the patient having fine or already clipped hair, horses that are bound for a competition where discreetness may be desired, or in some emergency situations. In these situations, the vet should make the owner aware that there may be a possible reduction in the quality of the image, which may reduce their ability to adequately visualise and diagnose subtle lesions. It may be possible to improve image quality without fully clipping, if the clippers are used in the direction of the hair coat to remove the ends of the hair; by doing this, the amount of air in the coat is reduced. When not clipping, it is essential to wet and clean the area and use copious amounts of isopropyl alcohol. However, some probes may be damaged by alcohol, so this must be clarified first [9].

There are certain breeds that may provide additional challenges when preparing the patient for ultrasonography; these include cobs and heavy horses. Preparing these patients in advance can be useful. Preparation includes clipping and cleaning the area thoroughly and applying copious amounts of ultrasound gel, then wrapping the leg in plastic wrap and applying an external bandage to hold the gel and plastic wrap in place. It has been found that this results in better penetration of the gel into the skin and improves image quality significantly. Following the ultrasound examination, the gel should be removed with warm water and legs where possible should be towel dried [31].

Use of a Stand-Off

In equine ultrasonography, a stand-off is used between the ultrasound transducer and the horse's skin during imaging. It helps create a consistent and reliable ultrasound image by reducing artefacts and improving image quality. The advantages of a stand-off include [31]:

- Image enhancement: A stand-off helps eliminate air gaps between the transducer and the horse's skin, ensuring better transmission of ultrasound waves. This improves image quality, reduces artefacts and enhances visualisation of internal structures.
- Distance control: The stand-off maintains a fixed distance between the transducer and the skin, which is particularly important when performing depth measurements or evaluating structures that require precise positioning.
- Thermal protection: In some cases, a stand-off can provide a barrier between the transducer and the horse's skin, reducing the risk of potential thermal injury from prolonged contact with the transducer.
- Improved ergonomics: Using a stand-off can enhance the ergonomics for the operator by providing a more stable surface and reducing strain on the hands and wrists during scanning.

Care of a Stand-off

Stand-offs are important pieces of equipment and should be cleaned and maintained correctly as follows [30, 31]:

- Cleanliness: Ensure that the stand-off is clean and free from debris or contaminants before each use. Wipe it down with a gentle disinfectant or warm, soapy water, following the manufacturer's instructions.
- Storage: Store the stand-off in a clean and dry environment to prevent contamination or damage. Some stand-offs may have specific storage requirements, so it's important to follow the manufacturer's recommendations.
- Inspection: Regularly inspect the stand-off for any signs of wear, cracks, or damage. If it becomes damaged, it may compromise the integrity of the coupling and reduce the effectiveness of the stand-off.
- Replacement: Over time, stand-offs may wear out or lose their effectiveness. Replace them as needed to ensure optimal image quality and performance during ultrasonography examinations.
- Compatibility: Choose a stand-off that is compatible with the ultrasound machine and transducer being used. Different transducers may have specific recommendations regarding the type and thickness of the stand-off to use.

It is important to note that the specific instructions for using and caring for a stand-off may vary depending on the manufacturer and the type of stand-off being used. Therefore, always refer to the manufacturer's guidelines and recommendations for the particular stand-off used in practice to ensure proper usage and maintenance [30].

Care and Maintenance of Ultrasound Equipment

Cleaning of the ultrasound machine must be carried out after each use. Not only does this help to maintain the equipment and promote a professional image, but it is also essential as part of the biosecurity program of the practice and to assist in infection control. This is particularly important as the ultrasound machine is often a useful tool for the diagnostic processes in neonatal foals where good hygiene is paramount [3].

Following use of the ultrasound machine, any excess dirt and debris should be removed gently using mild soap and warm water taking care not to get any electrical components wet. The machine can then be wiped over with a disinfectant wipe. The screen should be cleaned with a screen-specific wipe only and done gently. A hoover can be used to clean around the keyboard keys as these can become contaminated with dust and dirt. When not in use, the scanner should be kept in its box or stored safely on a designated hospital trolley. The temperature in the room should also be considered as a cold, damp or humid environment can have a detrimental effect on electronic equipment [3].

The use of ultrasound gel is necessary for obtaining images and should be used as part of the preparation and the examination. Ultrasound gel is used to replace air between the transducer and the patient's skin and is known as a coupling medium. Ultrasound waves have difficulty travelling through air, whereas the gel has the same acoustic properties as the soft tissue allowing passage and conduction of the ultrasound wave. Ultrasound gel also provides lubrication to the skin, allowing ease of movement of the transducer on the skin. A good tip to aid in the acquisition of good quality ultrasonography is to massage ultrasound gel as early as possible prior to the examination. A glove filled with water can also act as a coupling medium during some examinations, such as ophthalmic ultrasonography [31].

Ultrasound probes are a potential source of cross-contamination; however, they require careful care and cleaning. Firstly, ultrasound gel should be removed from the probe. This can be achieved by using a damp cloth. The presence of the gel can affect the function of any disinfectant. Disinfection of the probe is possible and can be carried out with a suitable disinfectant wipe. For more thorough disinfection, the probe may be cold sterilised; however, it is recommended to follow the instructions for the user's individual ultrasound machine as probes and systems may vary. Prior to storage, the probe should be dry. Each probe should be stored in its own padded storage bag [3].

Image Acquisition and Storage

When obtaining ultrasound images, key images are often captured that are then saved to the machine, a USB stick, transferred to a PACS server or transferred directly to the patient file depending on the software.

This is an important part of the imaging process as it enables the healing process to be monitored. It also enables colleagues or other veterinary practices to follow up on cases should the initial treating vet be unable to do so. Images are also useful for adding to referral reports. Ultrasound images are often saved as a JPEG or a DICOM file. Saving video files is also possible. Prior to the beginning of the ultrasound examination, patient information should be entered into the machine to ensure the images are saved accurately [30, 31].

During the ultrasound examination the anatomy is viewed in real time. When an area of interest has been identified, the screen can be 'frozen' and the image saved. Split screen mode is available on most machines and enables a 'frozen' image to be compared to a live image. This may be useful when comparing limbs [30].

Answers to Exposure Factor Questions (Section 7.2):

Question 1

- mAs = 10
- mA = 100

What are the seconds?
Answer: 10 mAs ÷ 100 mA = 0.1 S

Question 2

- mA = 200
- S = 0.2

What is the mAs?
Answer: 200 mA × 0.2 S = 40 mAs

Question 3

- mAs = 20
- S = 0.1

What is the mA?
Answer: 20 mAs ÷ 0.1 S = 200 mA

Question 4

- kV = 50
- mAs = 24
- The kV is changed to 60

What is the new mAs?
Answer: 24 ÷ 2 = 12 mAs

Question 5

- kV = 40
- mAs = 12
- The kV is changed to 30

What is the new mAs?
Answer: 12 mAs × 2 = 24 mAs

Question 6

- Old mAs = 12
- Grid factor = 3

What is the new mAs

Answer: 12 mAs × 3 = 36 mAs

References

1 Lane, D.R., Guthrie, S., and Griffith, S. (2016). *Dictionary of Veterinary Nursing*, 4e. Edinburgh: Elsevier.

2 Health and Safety Executive (2018). *Work with Ionising Radiation Approve Code of Practice and Guidance*, 2e, 7–173. Norwich: The Stationery Office.

3 Cooper, B., Mullineaux, E., and Turner, L. (2021). *BSAVA Textbook of Veterinary Nursing*, 6e, 429–490. Gloucester: British Small Animal Veterinary Association.

4 Health and Safety: Ionising Radiation [Internet]. [cited 2023 Jun 11]. Available from: https://www.hse.gov.uk/radiation/ionising/index.htm.

5 Butler, J.A., Colles, C.M., Dyson, S.J. et al. (2017). *Clinical Radiology of the Horse*, 4e. Oxford: Blackwell Science Ltd.

6 Weaver, M. and Barakzai, S. (2010). *Handbook of Equine Radiography*, 1e. Missouri: Elsevier Ltd.

7 Manso-Diaz, G., Lopez-Sanroman, J., and Weller, R. (2018). *A Practical Guide to Equine Radiography*, 1e, 1–17. Sheffield: 5M Publishing Ltd.

8 Ackerman, N. and Aspinall, V. (2016). *Aspinall's Complete Textbook of Veterinary Nursing*, 3e, 427–475. Edinburgh: Elsevier Ltd.

9 DeNotta, S., Mallicote, M., Miller, S., and Reeder, D. (2023). *AAEVT's Equine Manual for Veterinary Technicians*, 2e, 305–323. Hoboken: John Wiley and Sons Inc.

10 BBC Bitesize [Internet]. [cited 2023 Feb 8]. Atomic structure – Types of radiation – WJEC – GCSE Physics (Single Science) Revision – WJEC. Available from: https://www.bbc.co.uk/bitesize/guides/zcynv9q/revision/1.

11 Electromagnetic Spectrum – Introduction [Internet]. [cited 2023 Mar 1]. Available from: https://imagine.gsfc.nasa.gov/science/toolbox/emspectrum1.html.

12 Crook, L. (2019). Veterinary Practice. [cited 2023 Mar 2]. The importance of monitoring radon levels. Available

from: https://www.veterinary-practice.com/article/the-importance-of-monitoring-radon-levels.

13 Abdulla, S. and Clarke, C. (2020). *FRCR Physics Notes Medical Imaging Physics for First FRCR Examination*, 3e, 3–297. Nottingham: Radiology Cafe Publishing.

14 US EPA O. Radionuclide Basics: Technetium-99 [Internet]. 2015 [cited 2023 Mar 2]. Available from: https://www.epa.gov/radiation/radionuclide-basics-technetium-99.

15 Radiology [Internet]. [cited 2023 Mar 9]. Available from: https://www.vetmansoura.com/archive/Radiology/Productionofxray/Production2.html.

16 Themes UFO. 1. Plain Radiographic Imaging [Internet]. Radiology Key. 2016 [cited 2023 Mar 18]. Available from: https://radiologykey.com/1-plain-radiographic-imaging-2/.

17 What are X-Ray Grids? – JPI Healthcare [Internet]. 2022 [cited 2023 Mar 3]. Available from: https://www.jpihealthcare.com/what-are-x-ray-grids/.

18 Stat-X Espléndido [Internet]. Podoblock B.V. [cited 2023 Sep 7]. Available from: https://www.podoblock.com/product/stat-x-esplendido/.

19 News-Medical.net [Internet]. 2018 [cited 2023 Jun 11]. Digital Radiography versus Computed Radiography. Available from: https://www.news-medical.net/health/Digital-Radiography-versus-Computed-Radiography.aspx.

20 Nett, B. (2021). Digital Radiography (Direct Vs Indirect Flat Panels) • How Radiology Works [Internet]. [cited 2023 Jun 11]. Available from: https://howradiologyworks.com/direct-vs-indirect-digital-radiography/.

21 fujindtblog. FujiNDTBlog. 2023 [cited 2023 Jun 11]. What is CR Imaging & How Does it Work? | Complete Guide. Available from: https://ndtblog-us.fujifilm.com/blog/what-is-computed-radiography/.

22 Flat Panel Detector Working Principle [Internet]. Uni X-ray. 2021 [cited 2023 Jun 11]. Available from: https://unixray.com/flat-panel-detector-working-principle/.

23 Corley, K. and Stephen, J. (2008). *The Equine Hospital Manual*, 1e. Oxford: Blackwell Publishing Ltd.

24 Bone: Scintigraphy Technique in Horses | Vetlexicon Equis from Vetlexicon | Definitive Veterinary Intelligence [Internet]. [cited 2023 Jun 11]. Available from: https://www.vetlexicon.com/treat/equis/technique/bone-scintigraphy.

25 Murray, R.C. (2011). *Equine MRI*, 1e. Iowa: Blackwell Publishing Ltd.

26 Schwarz, T. and Saunders, J. (2011). *Veterinary Computed Tomography*, 1e. John Wiley and Sons ITD.

27 Standing CT Scanner for Horses [Internet]. Hallmarq Veterinary Imaging. [cited 2023 Sep 13]. Available from: https://hallmarq.net/products-solutions/standing-equine-leg-ct/.

28 Abutarbush, S.M. and Carmalt, J.L. (2008). *Equine Endoscopy and Arthroscopy*, 1e. Jackson: Teton NewMedia.

29 Davis, E.W. and Legendre, A.M. (1994). Successful treatment of guttural pouch mycosis with itraconazole and topical enilconazole in a horse. *Journal of Veterinary Internal Medicine [Internet]* **8** (4): 304–305. Available from: https://doi.org/10.1111/j.1939-1676.1994.tb03239.x.

30 Kidd, J.A., Lu, K.G., and Frazer, M.L. (2022). *Atlas of Equine Ultrasonography*, 2e. Oxford: John Wiley and Sons Inc.

31 Coumbe, K. (2012). *Equine Veterinary Nursing*, 2e, 385–431. Oxford: Blackwell Science Ltd.

Further Reading

Guidance for working with ionising radiation set out by the HSE can be found at: chrome-extension://efaidnbmnnnibpcajpcglclefindmkaj/https://www.hse.gov.uk/pubns/priced/l121.pdf.

8

Laboratory

Victoria Milne[1], Marie Rippingale[2], and Rosina Lillywhite[3]

[1] Lantra Awards, Stoneleigh Park, Coventry, UK
[2] Bottle Green Training Ltd, Derby, UK
[3] VetPartners Nursing School, Greenforde Business Park, Petersfield, UK

Introduction

Laboratory diagnostic tests are important tools used in equine practice to assist veterinary surgeons (vets) to make a definitive diagnosis. The majority of equine practices will have access to in-house laboratory facilities, as well as having access to external laboratories for the more specialised procedures with specialist clinical pathologists. It is important that registered veterinary nurses (RVNs) understand the skills required to work effectively and safely in the laboratory. These skills include preparation for sample collection, taking samples using a variety of methods, performing and recording the results of diagnostic tests, communicating results to both colleagues and clients and packaging and sending samples to external laboratories [1–3].

8.1 Safe Use of Laboratory Equipment

Operation and Maintenance

There are different pieces of legislation that are relevant to veterinary practice, and these serve to protect people, animals and the environment (Table 8.1). These pieces of legislation help to increase workplace safety by helping to minimise any potential risks [4].

A well-functioning laboratory, with equipment and systems that work effectively, contributes to the safety and efficiency of the work carried out. Maintenance is important in ensuring that the equipment used is in full working order and is reliable. Maintenance can be categorised as follows [1, 2]:

- Planned maintenance: This is used as a preventative effort to ensure that equipment is kept in the best possible working order.

- Unplanned maintenance: This is when equipment breaks down and requires repair.

Maintenance manuals should be available for all pieces of laboratory equipment. Regular maintenance, calibration and validation are needed to ensure all diagnostic results are accurate and reliable. Some maintenance will be carried out daily by personnel, but some may require specialist technicians such as employees from the manufacturing company. The frequency of such maintenance will be guided by the individual maintenance manual. Logbooks should be used to keep records of all maintenance that has been carried out and should include the following:

- The date and time that maintenance was carried out.
- The name/s of personnel that carried out the maintenance.
- A section for comments on any observations that have been noted [1, 2].

Calibration and Quality Control

Calibration and quality control are necessary to produce test results that are accurate and reliable. They are defined as follows:

- **Calibration:** Is the act of testing and adjusting the precision and accuracy of an instrument.
- **Quality control:** Is where procedures are used to continuously assess laboratory work and the results obtained, it looks at the precision and accuracy of all the processes associated within a laboratory.

Calibration and quality control allow for early detection of any system failures and possible inconsistencies due to

Table 8.1 Legislation relevant to working in a laboratory [4–9].

Legislation	Summary of the Act
Health and Safety at Work Act 1974	• This Act places duties on both employers and employees • Employers must protect the health and safety of their employees • Employees must take care of their own health and safety and also cooperate with their employer • This Act is designed to ensure that the working environment is safe and that hazards are dealt with to reduce any risk of injury [5]
Control of Substances Hazardous to Health 2002 (COSHH)	• This piece of legislation deals specifically with the risks posed by hazardous substances • Employers must assess risks created by hazardous substances and the appropriate control measures put in place. This could include risk assessments, standard operating procedures and staff training [6]
Reporting of Injuries, Diseases and Dangerous Occurrences Regulations 2013 (RIDDOR)	• This regulation requires employers to report deaths, accidents and serious injury and work-related diseases to the Health and Safety Executive (HSE) • RIDDOR is relevant to laboratories due to working with biological agents such as bacteria, viruses, fungi and other micro-organisms [4]
Environmental Protection Act 1990	• This Act is concerned with pollution on land and in air and water • It also covers waste disposal, including statutory nuisances (noise and odours) [7]
Hazardous Waste (England and Wales) Regulations 2005 (amended 2016)	• This regulation ensures that employers take responsibility for their hazardous waste that they produce and that the waste will cause no harm or damage • The regulation requires businesses that produce more than 500 kg of hazardous waste a year to register with the Environmental Agency. Hazardous waste includes all forms of clinical waste [8]
First Aid at Work Act 1981	• The First Aid at Work Act requires employers to provide adequate and appropriate equipment, personnel and facilities to ensure that employees can receive instant attention when required if taken ill or injured at work • This applies to all businesses, no matter how many employees they have [9]

Source: Vicky Milne.

environmental conditions. Calibration and quality control procedures should be carried out as follows:

- At the start of each shift.
- When an analyser has been serviced.
- As written in the maintenance manual for each piece of equipment.
- When results seem inconsistent with the clinical signs of a patient.
- When reagents are changed.

Quality control for analysers is usually run on a sample where the values are already known. The results are then checked to make sure they are as expected, and if not, the results produced should be reported to the manufacturer. If there is a concern with the validity of results, quality control would need to be carried out and the manufacturer alerted to the problem [1, 2].

Care and Hygiene Management

The cleanliness of a laboratory can have a huge impact on the results of diagnostic tests. It is crucial for all laboratories, of any size, to develop daily and weekly cleaning schedules. Having a schedule for staff to refer to when working in the laboratory will ensure that the laboratory is cleaned appropriately on a daily basis. This could include simple tasks such as disinfecting all workstations in the laboratory, sweeping and mopping floors, dusting and disinfecting surfaces and equipment. Setting some basic rules will also aid in maintaining the cleanliness and efficiency of the laboratory. Examples are as follows [10]:

- All equipment should be cleaned after use.
- All equipment should be put back in the correct place after use.
- Equipment function should be checked after use.
- Broken equipment should be repaired or replaced immediately.

Personal Protective Equipment (PPE)

Every laboratory should have PPE available for all staff in order to comply with relevant legislation. PPE, including masks, gloves, aprons and eye shields, must be worn by all staff when required. Eyewash stations should also be available in case chemicals accidentally come into contact with the eyes of personnel working in the laboratory. If there are employees who are at a greater risk in the laboratory, such as pregnant people or people who are immunosuppressed, additional risk assessments should be completed, which detail what additional measures should be put into place to ensure safety in the laboratory. See Chapter 1 for more information regarding risk assessments.

To work safely in the laboratory, staff must have access to the following [1]:

- The laboratory health and safety policy.
- Risk assessments.
- Standard operating procedures (SOPs).

The Use of Microscopes

Within a laboratory, a microscope is an essential piece of equipment. A microscope is a piece of equipment that is used to magnify small objects such as diagnostic samples, to allow them to be evaluated. A binocular microscope, which has a built-in light source, is the most suitable for a veterinary laboratory (Figure 8.1). Binocular microscopes have two eyepieces as opposed to one, the two eyepieces help to ease viewing and reduce eye strain. The components of a microscope and their functions are explained in Table 8.2.

Microscope Slides

Microscopes are often used with microscope slides. These are usually thin, flat pieces of glass typically measuring 75 × 26 mm and 1 mm thick [1]. Slides are used to hold samples in place for examination under a microscope and help to prevent the microscope and lenses from becoming contaminated. Plain slides can be used either way up, but some have a frosted area for labelling. When using these slides, the frosted side should be uppermost [1].

Cover Slips

Coverslips are flat pieces of glass measuring around 20 mm wide and fewer than 1 mm thick. Cover slips are placed over a specimen on a microscope slide to hold the specimen in place and to protect it from contamination. Cover slips also serve to protect the objective lenses from contamination and damage [1].

Microscope Care

Microscopes are expensive instruments that must be carefully stored and maintained. The following points should be considered [1, 2, 11]:

- The microscope must be turned off and covered when not in use.

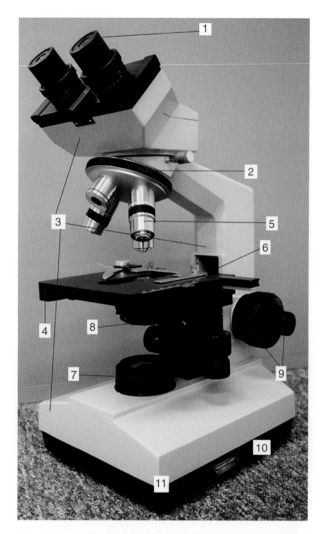

Figure 8.1 A binocular microscope. *Source:* Rosina Lillywhite.

- The microscope must be stored on a flat surface, away from water, excessive heat and vibrations.
- When moving the microscope, it should be lifted by the limb with one hand under the base.
- The stage should be cleaned after each use with disinfectant wipes.
- The eyepieces and the objective lenses should only be cleaned with lens tissue. Lens tissue is soft, lint-free tissue paper that will not scratch or damage the lens.
- Safety checks should be carried out regularly, including electrical testing.
- Immersion oil should be used sparingly with the X100 lens.
- When oil has been used, the oil immersion lens should be cleaned immediately after use with lens tissue. This will prevent the oil from solidifying and damaging the lens.
- The light should be switched off when not in use to prolong the life of the bulb and stop it from overheating. If

Table 8.2 Microscope components and functions [1–3, 11].

Microscope component	Function
1 Eyepiece	Monocular microscopes have one eyepiece; binocular microscopes have two. Eyepieces typically have a magnifying power of X10. They contain an ocular lens which magnifies the primary image for the operator to view
2 Objective turret	The objective turret holds the objective lenses and rotates in a clockwise direction allowing the operator to move from a lower-power objective lens, to a higher-power objective lens
3 Limb, body and base	The limb of the microscope connects the body and the base. A microscope should be carried by holding the limb with a second hand on the base of the microscope. The base includes the light source and the on/off switch
4 Stage (including mechanical stage)	The stage is a flat platform with a hole in the middle, which allows light from the condenser to illuminate the specimen. The microscope slide is placed on the stage and is held in place by clips. Once a specimen is placed onto the stage, using the focusing mechanisms the stage can be moved up and down to assist with focusing. The mechanical stage, attached on top of the stage, can then be used to move the microscope slide horizontally, or vertically
5 Objective lenses	The objective lenses are situated within the objective turret of the microscope. There are usually 4 objective lenses, starting at X4, which is the lowest power; X10, X40, which is the highest power for dry magnification; and X100, which would be used for oil immersion
6 Vernier scale	The Vernier scale is found on the mechanical stage. It consists of a horizontal and a vertical scale, which allows for the precise location of the specimen to be recorded and also relocated when required
7 Substage condenser	The substage condenser is situated below the stage and is made up of two lenses which condense the light from the light source and onto the specimen. The position of the condenser and the quantity of light passing through the specimen can be altered using the iris diaphragm
8 Iris diaphragm	The iris diaphragm regulates the amount of light that can pass through the substage condenser. Closing the diaphragm has advantages when examining parasites as it increases the contrast, which helps with visibility. Opening the diaphragm will help with visibility when examining cytological samples
9 Focusing mechanism (Fine and coarse)	Found on the side of a microscope, this mechanisms allows raising and lowering of the stage to help with the focus of the image. The larger wheel is the coarse focus; the smaller is the fine focus. To start with, the stage should be racked as high as possible (while watching the stage at all times) and then be lowered; this will prevent the objective lens from accidentally hitting the slide and potentially causing damage
10 Rheostat	The rheostat allows the level of light produced by the light source to be altered
11 On/off switch	The on/off switch is usually situated on the base of the microscope. Before turning the microscope on, the rheostat should be checked to make sure it is at its lowest setting; otherwise damage to the bulb could occur

Source: Vicky Milne.

the light does need to be left on, the light intensity switch (rheostat) should be turned down to the lowest setting.

- After use, the stage should be lowered, and the lowest power objective lens should be moved into position.

Magnification and Focusing

Most binocular microscopes have four objective lenses; each one has a different function [1, 2, 11]:

- X4 objective lens: This is a very low-power lens mainly used to obtain an initial focus on a sample. It can also be used for the examination of coat brushings and to scan a slide for an area of interest. When using this objective lens, the condenser and light should both be on a low setting.

- X10 objective lens: This is another low-power objective lens. This lens can be used for the identification of parasites and the assessment of urine sediment. It can also be used for locating areas of interest before increasing the magnification. When using this objective lens, the condenser and light should be on a low setting.

- X40 objective lens: This is a high-power objective lens. These lenses are mainly used to examine areas of interest in more detail, for example, when examining a pathological sample. When using this objective lens, the condenser and light should be on a medium setting.

- X100 objective lens: This is a high-power lens used with oil. This lens uses light that gets refracted through the thin layer of oil to the lens. It is used for cytology and to examine blood smears and fine needle aspirates. When using this objective lens, the condenser and light should be on a high setting.

Examining a Specimen on a Microscope Slide [1]

1) Use PPE if required.
2) Remove the microscope dust cover and ensure the microscope is plugged into an electrical socket.
3) Adjust the light beam diaphragm control so that it is in the middle position (to do this, look from the side, not down the eyepiece) and ensure the rheostat is turned down to its lowest setting.
4) Turn the microscope on. The power switch is usually on the base of the microscope.
5) Move the stage down to its lowest setting and secure the slide on the mechanical stage using the spring arm clips.
6) Rotate the objective turret (clockwise) and click the X4 or X10 objective lens into place (depending on the microscope).
7) Looking at the stage directly, move it back up until it almost touches the objective lens. Ensure that the lens does not touch the slide.
8) Look down the eyepieces and adjust the distance between them; only one field should be viewed (a single image) when the eyepieces are in the correct place.
9) Adjust the rheostat to a medium setting and adjust the substage condenser to a couple of millimetres below the stage.
10) While looking down the eyepieces, slowly move the stage downwards using the course focus until the image comes into view.
11) Once the specimen is visualised, the fine focus should be used to sharpen the image.
12) Rotate through the objectives lenses if a larger magnification is needed. If it was in focus at a low power, it should remain in focus at the higher power. Every time a larger objective lens is used, it should be observed during movement to ensure it does not touch the slide on the mechanical stage.

13) The Vernier scale should be read and recorded as this can be used to identify the position of interest and enable colleagues to examine the same area on the slide.

Oil Immersion Technique

The oil immersion technique is used when a detailed examination is required, for example, when looking at a blood smear. It works by refracting light through a thin layer of oil to the lens. Oil immersion must only be used with the oil immersion objective lens (X100). The oil immersion technique should be used during the final stage of an examination to prevent contamination of the other objective lenses.

When using oil immersion, the rheostat should be set to the highest value, as this will facilitate better visibility. The objective lenses should be rotated slightly so none are fixed into position; this leaves a space to drop a small amount of oil immersion directly onto the slide over the spot of light. If a coverslip is present, this will need to be removed. The oil immersion objective lens should be moved into place, ensuring it does not come into contact with the slide. Watching the stage position from the side, the stage should be raised slowly until the oil drop touches the lens. If the specimen was in focus with a smaller magnification, any adjustments should be made using the fine focus [1, 11].

The Battlement Technique

The battlement technique is used for a quantitative microscopic examination of blood when determining the number of cells seen. This differs from a qualitative examination used when assessing cellular morphology. When examining blood smears, a logical examination must occur to reduce the possibility of counting the same blood cell twice, which would give an inaccurate result. The battlement technique should begin on the left-hand side of a microscope slide and involves moving two fields to the right, two fields up, two fields to the right and then two fields down (see Figure 8.2). This pattern should be repeated across the slide until 100 cells have been counted. All cells in each field should be counted. For the most accurate count, the edge and the middle of the body of the smear should be examined. This is to compensate for the maldistribution of cells between the centre and the edge of the

Figure 8.2 The battlement technique.
Source: Vicky Milne.

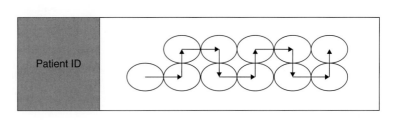

blood smear. The battlement technique is most commonly used when carrying out a differential white blood cell count where the percentages of the different cell types are determined [1–3].

Vernier Scale Readings

Vernier scale readings can be used to record the exact location of a specimen or a particular part of an image. Examples include an ectoparasite from a skin scrape or a white blood cell on a blood smear. There are two scales: the vertical Vernier scale (*Y*-axis, which runs from top to bottom) and the horizontal Vernier scale (*X*-axis, running from left to right). The main scale is marked on the stage, which gives half of the reading; the other half comes from the smaller Vernier scale. Both the vertical and horizontal Vernier scales must be read, and the readings must be recorded accurately.

The Method to Read the Vernier Scale is as Follows [1]:

1) The stage can be lowered if required to facilitate an accurate reading. The stage should not be touched again.
2) For each direction (vertical or horizontal), there is a main scale (marked on the stage) and a smaller, Vernier scale located next to the main stage.
3) For the main scale reading (which gives the first part of the scale), observe where the 0 on the Vernier scale aligns with the main scale. In Figure 8.3, it is 18. If this falls between two divisions, the lower number should be used.
4) For the Vernier scale reading, locate the number on the Vernier scale that is in closest coincidence with the main scale. In Figure 8.3, it is 4.
5) This will give the first complete reading of 18.4.
6) This procedure should then be repeated for the other axis.
7) Once both readings have been identified, they can be used to relocate an area of interest on a microscope slide.
8) All results should be recorded.

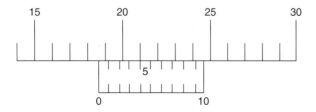

Figure 8.3 Vernier scale diagram. *Source:* Vicky Milne.

Analysers

An analyser is a laboratory machine that is used to quickly measure different chemicals and other characteristics in several biological samples, with minimal assistance. Most equine veterinary practices will have electronic analysers in the laboratory. In-house analysers allow for quick results and avoid the need to send samples externally. Analysers come in different forms, from large worktop machines to small handheld devices. To ensure the correct functioning of analysers and therefore accurate results, these machines must be cared for and maintained correctly.

The care and maintenance of analysers includes:

- Situating the machine in a safe and secure position, away from vibrations (such as the centrifuge). This will help to reduce the risk of damage to the analyser.
- Keeping the machine at an appropriate temperature, ideally between 20 and 22 °C.
- The machine should be switched off and covered when not in use.
- The machine should be used in accordance with the manufacturer's guidelines.
- Servicing should be carried out according to the manufacturer's guidelines.
- Quality control should be regularly undertaken to ensure accurate and valid results.

Haematology Analysers

Haematology analysers are used to count and characterise blood cells for the detection of diseases and monitoring purposes. They can carry out tests such as cell counts and coagulation tests, but in equine practice, they are most often used for their differential counts of both white and red blood cells. Most of these analysers work on either a coulter electrical impedance method or flow cytometry; both methods rely on the cells being passed rapidly through a laser beam (or a small aperture) to allow each cell to be counted and differentiated.

Haematology analysers provide more accurate cell counts than manual counts; for example, some of the analysers perform the differential white blood cell count on 10,000 rather than 100 cells. They are also much quicker; some analysers can perform 120 tests per hour. But for this to be accurate and timely, they need to be used correctly and serviced regularly. Haematology machines can help in the diagnosis of conditions such as anaemia, dehydration and different types of infections [1–3, 12, 13].

Biochemistry Analysers

Biochemistry analysers are used to measure the levels of various biochemical substances found within the blood,

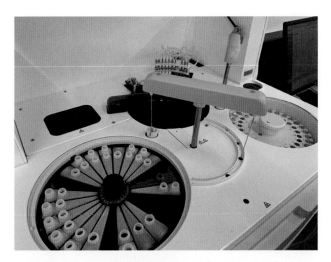

Figure 8.4 A biochemistry analyser. *Source:* Vicky Milne; With permission from B&W Equine Hospital.

for example, glucose and total protein (TP) (Figure 8.4). Results from biochemistry machines are compared to a reference range for each parameter; the results give information on the patient's clinical condition, and this facilitates a more accurate diagnosis and treatment plan. Biochemistry can help to diagnose conditions such as hepatopathy, bacterial infections and metabolic abnormalities. Often, biochemistry is initially used alongside haematology to get a full picture in relation to the health status of a patient.

There are two types of biochemistry machines [1–3, 14]:

- **Dry chemistry analysers:** These are the most commonly used analysers. The sample is dropped onto a series of chemical-impregnated slides, initiating a colour change. This colour change is then read and interpreted by the machine. The colour change reflects the amount of substance being tested.
- **Wet chemistry analysers:** These use wells of fluid rather than slides. Chemical reactions between the fluid and the blood create a colour change, which determines the biochemical levels in the individual sample.

Electrolyte and Blood Gas Analysers

These analysers read electrolyte levels in plasma and can give rapid results for tests such as sodium, chloride and calcium. They can be used for blood gas analysis in critical care patients and to monitor patients undergoing general anaesthesia. Handheld analysers can be used to measure glucose and lactate in blood samples.

Use of the Centrifuge

Centrifuges use centrifugal force to separate various substances. Centrifugal force is the apparent outward force applied to a mass when it is rotated. When centrifugal force is applied to a blood sample, the denser the particles, such as solids, will settle at the bottom of the sample, whereas the less dense, often liquid portion, will remain at the top on the surface.

There are three main types of centrifuge:

- Angle-head: This machine is the most commonly used, and the tubes are held in a fixed position, which is normally 40° from the vertical.
- Swing-out head: This starts the samples in a vertical position, and as the rotor turns, the samples swing out.
- Microhematocrit: This has a special type of rotor, which consists of small individual slots for holding blood microhematocrit or capillary tubes.

All types of centrifuge should be kept on a flat surface. When using a microhematocrit centrifuge, the safety plate in the lid should be screwed into place before starting the machine. Each centrifuge must be balanced when running, meaning two samples should always be spun together and placed at 180° to each other.

Depending on the type of sample to be centrifuged, the following speeds and times can be used [1]:

- Blood: 10,000 revolutions per minute (rpm) for five minutes.
- Urine: 1500–2000 rpm for five minutes.
- Faeces: 1000–1500 rpm for three minutes [1–3].

Use of a Refractometer

A refractometer is a scientific instrument which is used to determine the refractive index of a liquid (Figure 8.5). To determine the refractive index, a liquid sample is placed

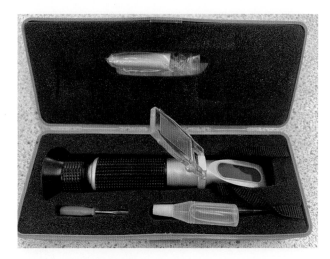

Figure 8.5 A refractometer. *Source:* Vicky Milne; With permission from B&W Equine Hospital.

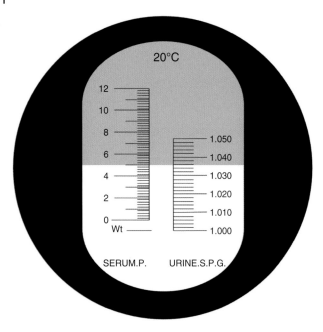

Figure 8.6 The scale used to read specific gravity is the one on the right-hand side of a refractometer. To read TP, the left-hand scale is used. *Source:* Vicky Milne.

onto a prism and light is allowed to pass through to create a line that is visible on an index or a scale (Figure 8.6). Each liquid will have its own refractive index. The scales seen on a refractometer will vary depending on the intended use. In veterinary medicine, refractometers are used to analyse urine specific gravity (USG) of urine samples and the TP concentration in blood samples [1, 2]. For further information, see the section on Haematology.

In order to gain accurate readings from the refractometer, it is essential that it is calibrated with distilled water before every use. A couple of drops of water should be placed onto the face of the prism. The refractometer should then be held up to the light. Once the scale has been focussed, the water should have a reading of 1.000. The scale adjustment screw can be used to align the reading to 1.000. Once calibration has successfully taken place, the refractometer is ready for use [2].

8.2 Sample Collection and Testing

PPE For Sample Collection

When setting up for sample collection, the need for PPE should always be considered. The handling of pathological specimens and some preservatives, such as formal saline, is classed as hazardous and precautions should be taken to ensure good health and safety standards. Some cases that require sampling could be classed as infectious or being treated as such until the sample results are known. Some infectious diseases may also be zoonotic, such as salmonella or dermatophytosis, so strict biosecurity measures will be

required to prevent the spread of infection to staff and other patients. PPE should include an apron or laboratory coat and gloves. Depending on the collection method used and the patient's disease state, PPE could also include a mask, hair cover, disposable boiler suit, foot covers and goggles [1–3].

Blood

Patient Preparation and Sample Collection

Horses may have blood samples taken for many reasons, including illness, monitoring responses to treatment and a yearly check-up. Patient preparation is hugely important, as well as making sure the sample is collected, handled and stored correctly. Mishandling of blood samples or using the incorrect blood tube or needle size, can negatively affect the diagnostic quality of the sample.

The equipment required for blood sample collection is as follows [1, 2]:

- Gloves.
- Clippers or scissors to remove hair (if appropriate).
- Clipper blades.
- Appropriate size syringe, depending on the sample needed.
- An appropriately sized needle (see Chapter 17 for further information).
- Skin antiseptic preparation.
- Swabs.
- Blood tubes (Figure 8.7).
- Vacutainer – these will be used with a specific needle, and a syringe would not be necessary. See Chapter 17 for further information.

Physical restraint is normally adequate when blood sampling a horse. Either a headcollar and leadrope or a bridle should be used. Stocks can also be used for such tests. The horse should be positioned so that the handler and sampler are on the same side of the horse and are not trapped, with easy access to the stable door. The jugular vein is most commonly used for blood sampling in equine patients [3]. See Chapter 17 for further details.

If a needle and syringe have been used to collect blood, the sample should be dispensed into an appropriate container quickly; this is especially important if clotting is undesirable for the sample. Anticoagulants are used to prevent clotting and are required for many diagnostic tests. The diagnostic test required will determine which anticoagulant is needed. If the incorrect one is chosen, the results from the tests may be invalidated. Table 8.3 displays the different colours of blood collection containers, including the anticoagulant used.

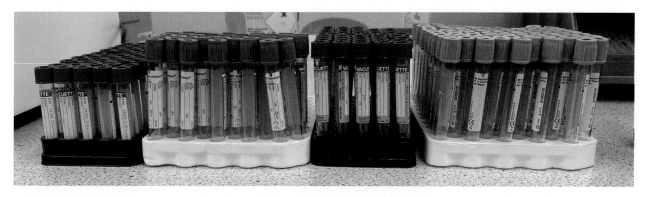

Figure 8.7 Different blood tubes used in equine practice. *Source:* Vicky Milne; With permission from B&W Equine Hospital.

Table 8.3 Different colours of blood collection containers and the corresponding anticoagulant used [1–3].

Anticoagulant	Blood tube cap colour	Vacutainer cap colour	Use
Lithium heparin	Orange	Green	Biochemistry
Ethylenediamine tetra-acetic acid (EDTA)	Pink	Purple	Haematology
Fluoride oxalate	Yellow	Grey	Glucose
Sodium/lithium citrate	Blue	Blue	Coagulation studies
No anticoagulant	White or brown	Red	Serum collection

Source: Vicky Milne.

All samples collected will degrade over time. The time taken to degrade will depend on the sample taken. Preservatives can be used to increase the 'life span', which is especially important if a sample is being sent to an external laboratory. It is also important to use the correct amount of sample to the preservative ratio for the preservative to work correctly. If there is a 'fill line' marked on a sample container, the sample should be filled to this line and not beyond it.

Blood should ideally be tested within four hours of being collected as it starts to degrade very quickly. If a lithium heparin sample is refrigerated, the plasma can be used for up to 48 hours. If an ethylenediamine tetra-acetic acid (EDTA) sample for haematology, is refrigerated, it can be used for up to 12 hours after being collected. Serum which has been obtained from a clotted sample can be frozen and thawed when required to stop the cells from degrading; otherwise, if kept refrigerated, it can be used for 48 hours.

Haematology

Blood forms about 10% of the body weight of the horse and consists of cells in plasma [3]. Plasma is the liquid part of blood, and this differs from serum, which is the substance that is left over once a clot has formed (see Chapter 4 for more information). Haematology is the study of blood and blood disorders. See Table 8.4 for examples of normal haematology and biochemistry reference ranges. The following tests are carried out as part of haematological analysis in the horse.

Blood Cell Counts

Blood cell counts are a quantitative examination of blood as they determine the number of blood cells seen. Within most practices, quantitative blood analysis is often carried out using a haematology machine. Such machines produce results within a quicker timeframe than manual blood cell counts and are often more accurate if used correctly. White blood cell counts are carried out on blood smears using the X10, X40 and then X100 oil immersion objective lenses. These are often performed to determine the quantities of each type of white blood cell, known as a differential white blood cell count (see section on blood smears). Red blood cell counts are commonly known as a packed cell volume (PCV) and are discussed below.

Table 8.4 Normal ranges for haematology and biochemistry laboratory results in equine practice.

Haematology or biochemistry	Lab test	Normal result		Vacutainer type and colour
Haematology	Total erythrocytes × 10^{12}/L		6.2–10.2	Ethylenediamine Tetra-acetic Acid (EDTA) (Purple) / Lithium heparin (Green)
	Mean cell volume (fl)		37–55	
	Mean cell haemoglobin (pg)		13–19	
	Mean cell haemoglobin concentration (%)		31–36	
	Haemoglobin (g/dl)		11–19	
	Packed cell volume (%)		32–53	
	Total leukocytes × 10^9/L		5.5–10	EDTA (Purple)
	Neutrophils × 10^9/L		2.7–7	
	Lymphocytes × 10^9/L		1.5–4	
	Monocytes × 10^9/L		0–0.5	
	Eosinophils × 10^9/L		0–0.6	
	Basophils × 10^9/L		0–0.29	
	Platelets × 10^9/L		100–350	EDTA (Purple) / Sodium/lithium citrate (Blue)
Biochemistry	Total protein (TP) (g/l)	Blood	53–75	Lithium heparin (Green) / Plain (Red)
		Synovial fluid	<20	
		Peritoneal fluid	<25	
		Pleural fluid	<25	
		Cerebral Spinal Fluid (CSF)	1–12	
	Albumin (g/l)		23–39	
	Globulins (g/l)		18–19	
	Glucose (mmol/l)	Adult horse:	4.3–6	Fluoride oxalate (Grey)
		24 hours old	6.7–12.9	
		One week old	6.7–10.6	
		One month old	7.2–12	
		Four months old	6.3–10.9	
		Yearling	5.8–9.2	
	Lactate (mmol/l)	Normal	<2	Plain (Red) / Lithium heparin (Green)
		Mild elevations	2–5	
		Marked elevations	5–8	
		Severe elevations	>8	

Table 8.4 (Continued)

Haematology or biochemistry	Lab test	Normal result		Vacutainer type and colour
	Serum Amyloid A (SAA) (mg/l)	0–20		
	Blood Urea Nitrogen (BUN) (mmol/l)	3–8		
	Creatine Phosphokinase (CK) international units (IU) per litre (L) (iu/l)	Adult Non-Thoroughbred Horses	110–250	
		Three-Year-Old Thoroughbred Horses in Training	156–875	
	Aspartate Aminotransferase (AST) (iu/l)	Adult Non-Thoroughbred Horses. Not liver specific	102–350	
		Three-Year-Old Thoroughbred Horses in Training. Not liver specific	289–630	
	Alkaline Phosphatase (ALP) (iu/l)	Not liver specific	86–285	
	Gamma-glutamyl Transferase (GGT) (iu/l)	Technically not liver specific but is a useful test in horses	1–40	
	Glutamate Dehydrogenase (GLDH) (ul/l)	Liver specific	0–11.8	
	Lactate Dehydrogenase (LDH) (iu/l)	Not liver specific	162–412	
	Sorbitol Dehydrogenase (SDH) (iu/l)	Liver-specific	0–8	
	Bilirubin (total) (μmol/L)	9–39 (up to 120 if starved >24 h)		
	Creatinine (μmol/L)	85–170		
	Calcium (mmol/l)	2.9–3.3		
	Phosphate (mmol/l)	0.9–1.9		
	Sodium (mmol/L)	134–142		
	Chloride (mmol/L)	91–104		
	Potassium (mmol/L)	3–5		Plain (Red)
	Adrenocorticotrophic Hormone (ACTH) (pg/ml)	November–July:	Negative: <30 pg/ml	
			Equivocal: 30–50 pg/ml	
			Positive: >50 pg/ml	
		July–November:	Negative: <50 pg/ml	
			Equivocal: 50–100 pg/ml	
			Positive: >100 pg/ml	EDTA (Purple)
	Insulin (iu/ml)	Resting insulin	<20	
			20–50 suggests the presence of insulin dysregulation	
			>50 confirms the presence of insulin dysregulation	Plain (Red)
	Immunoglobulin G (IgG) (g/l)	Normal	>8	
		Partial failure of colostral immunity	4–8	
		Failure of colostral immunity	<4	EDTA (Purple)

Also noted in the Vacutainer column: **Lithium heparin (Green)**

Source: Rosina Lillywhite and Marie Rippingale.

Table 8.5 Method for preparing a PCV sample.

Preparing a PCV sample
1   Put on appropriate PPE including gloves
2   Choose a sample of blood that has been collected into an EDTA tube
3   Gently mix the blood sample
4   Select a blue tipped microhaematocrit (capillary) tube and place it into the sample at an angle. Fill the capillary tube three-quarters full by capillary action (Figure 8.8)
5   As soon as the microhaematocrit tube is ¾ full, place a finger over the top of the tube and/or hold horizontally to prevent blood leaking out
6   Remove the tube from the sample and wipe the outside in a downwards stroke using a tissue
7   Plug one end of the microhaematocrit tube with a soft clay sealant such as Cristaseal (Figure 8.9). Repeat steps 4–7 to produce two PCV samples to balance the centrifuge
Using the centrifuge
8   Place the microhaematocrit tube into a microhaematocrit centrifuge, making sure the clay seal is closest to the rim of the centrifuge (sealed end outwards)
9   The centrifuge must be balanced with two filled capillary tube, hence why two PCV samples are normally made for one patient. The extra sample can also act as a comparison for accuracy testing. The two samples must be directly opposite each other (Figure 8.10)
10   Once the samples are in place, the inner safety lid must be screwed down over the samples before the centrifuge is started and then the main lid should be shut and locked
11   The centrifuge should be set at 10,000 revolutions per minute (rpm) for five minutes. (This does slightly depend on the make of the centrifuge)
12   The samples can now be read. All equipment and materials should be disposed of correctly

Source: Vicky Milne.

Packed Cell Volume (PCV)

PCV is a rapid test that can be performed in-house to determine a patient's hydration status, and the level of blood loss in patients who are or have been haemorrhaging. PCV is a measurement of the proportion of blood that is made up of cells. This value is expressed as a percentage. The PCV reference ranges in horses differ with age, fitness and breed. The normal reference ranges are as follows [3]:

- Neonates: 40–52%
- Six months of age: 29–41%
- Adults: 32–53%

To measure the PCV of a patient, blood is drawn into a microhematocrit or capillary tube from a blood sample. Microhematocrit tubes are thin tubes which are most commonly made from soda lime glass. There are two types of microhematocrit tubes [1]:

- Red-tipped tubes: Contain sodium heparin to prevent the sample from clotting. These tubes are used with plain blood samples.
- Blue-tipped tubes: Do not contain sodium heparin and so are used with blood samples that have been mixed with an anticoagulant.

The correct microhaematocrit tube should be selected for the sample being tested.

The method for preparing a PCV sample is displayed in Table 8.5.

When the microhaematocrit tube is removed from the centrifuge after spinning, the sample will have spun into layers. The red blood cells will be concentrated in a layer at the bottom of the tube next to the clay plug. Above this is the buffy coat containing white blood cells and platelets. Above this is the plasma (see Figure 8.11). A Hawksley haematocrit reader is most commonly used to read the %PCV of a sample (see Figure 8.12).

The Hawksley haematocrit reader is used as follows:

1) Place the capillary tube into the slot in the reader with the clay seal facing downwards (the capillary tube holder) (see Figure 8.13).
2) Align the top of the clay seal with the zero line on the reader, then move the capillary tube holder along until the very top of the plasma is aligned with the 100% line which is on the reader.
3) There is an adjustable reading line on the left side of the reader. This reading line should be moved until it is directly over the intersection between the red blood cells and the buffy coat layer.

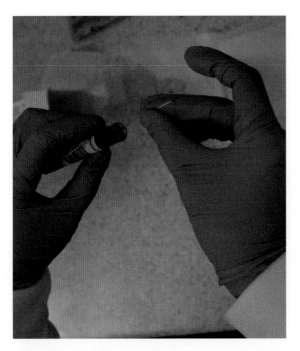

Figure 8.8 To fill the microhematocrit tube, it should be placed into the sample at an angle. *Source:* Rosina Lillywhite with permission from Liphook Equine Hospital.

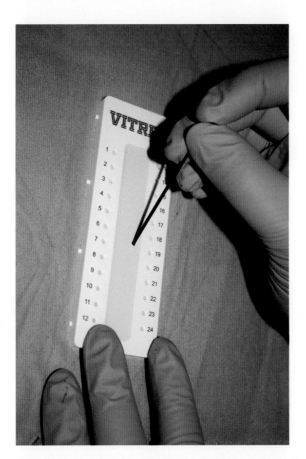

Figure 8.9 The microhematocrit tube should be plugged at one end with a soft clay sealant such as Cristaseal. *Source:* Rosina Lillywhite with permission from Liphook Equine Hospital.

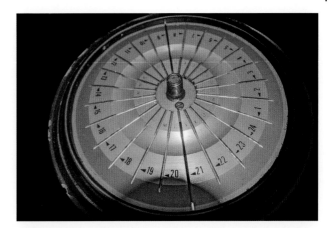

Figure 8.10 The centrifuge must be balanced with two filled microhematocrit capillary tubes. The two samples must be directly opposite each other. *Source:* Rosina Lillywhite with permission from Liphook Equine Hospital.

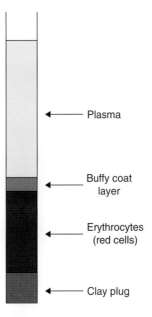

Figure 8.11 Different layers in a centrifuged microhaematocrit tube. *Source:* Rosina Lillywhite.

4) Once the adjustable reading line is in place, read the percentage it is lined up with on the right-hand side of the reader; this gives the PCV reading (see Figure 8.14).

If a Hawksley reader is unavailable, the following simple calculation can be used to manually identify the % PCV:

The length of the column of red blood cells divided by the length of the red blood cells, buffy coat and plasma combined X100. So, as an example, if the height of the red blood cells is 2.4 cm, this is divided by the height of all three layers, which is 4.8 cm [1–3]:

$$2.4\,cm \div 4.8\,cm \times 100 = 50\%\ PCV$$

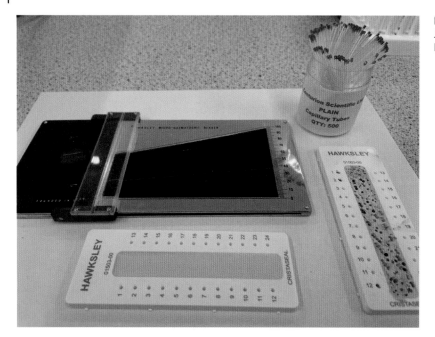

Figure 8.12 Hawksley haematocrit reader. *Source:* Vicky Milne with permission from B&W Equine Hospital.

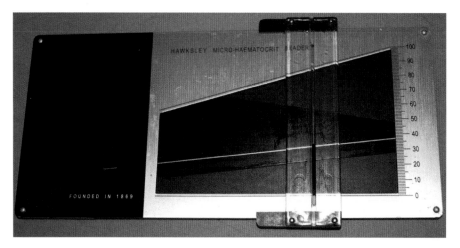

Figure 8.13 The microhaematocrit tube should be placed into the slot in the reader with the clay seal facing downwards (the microhaematocrit tube holder). *Source:* Rosina Lillywhite with permission from Liphook Equine Hospital.

Blood Smear

A blood smear is a method that is regularly used in veterinary practice, for in-house diagnostics and for sending samples to an external laboratory for examination. Blood smears comprise a layer of blood on a glass slide. They are useful to preserve blood, to examine the cellular content as well as investigate any abnormalities that an automatic analyser may not identify. Table 8.6 displays the types and functions of equine blood cells. Blood smears are very delicate, so they should always be handled with care, and if being sent to an external laboratory, time must be spent packing them correctly and safely.

Once the blood smear has been air dried rapidly, they are often stained with Diff-Quik® or Leishman's stain as this helps to facilitate the identification between different cells during microscopy and will also help to identify any abnormalities. The methods for performing and staining blood smears are displayed in Table 8.7.

Common Faults

Faults with blood smears should be identified quickly, as they can affect the results of the test. Common faults seen with blood smears are as follows [1–3]:

- Thickness of the blood smear – if the blood smear is too thick, it makes it difficult to see individual cells, whereas if it is too thin, there would be insufficient cells to see.
- If the blood smear is too short, it could be due to lack of blood, or the spreader slide being stopped too early.

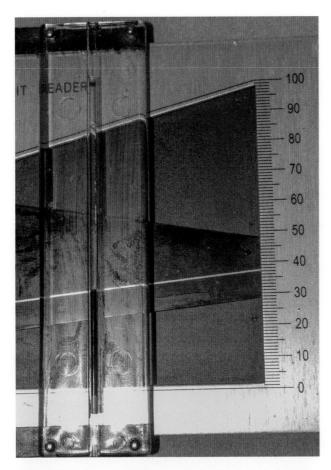

Figure 8.14 Once the adjustable reading line is in place, the percentage can be read on the right-hand side of the reader; this gives the PCV reading. *Source:* Rosina Lillywhite with permission from Liphook Equine Hospital.

- Hesitation bands where the spreader slide was not pushed in one smooth movement.
- Narrow, thick smear, often where the blood was not allowed to spread along the length of the spreader slide.
- Streaks and spots where blood is absent, due to grease on the slide.
- Crenation due to slow air drying of the smear.

Additional Haematological Analysis

The following parameters are commonly provided by auto-mated haematology analysers [1]:

- Mean Corpuscular Volume (MCV): Indicates the average size of red blood cells.
- Mean Corpuscular Haemoglobin Concentration (MCHC): Indicates the average haemoglobin concentration per red blood cell.
- Haemoglobin (Hb): These estimations indicate the level of haemoglobin found in red blood cells.

Red Blood Cell Morphology

The term crenation refers to the spikey of irregular margins of red cells seen on a blood smear. This usually results from cell shrinkage during the slow drying of the blood film. Howell-Jolly bodies are the basophilic remnants of the nucleus, and these may be visible in immature red blood cells [3]. Equine haematology differs from that of other species. Rouleaux formation is the stacking of red blood cells in columns and is readily seen in blood smears. This is a normal feature of equine blood [3].

Biochemistry

Blood biochemistry tests measure the concentrations of certain chemicals in the blood. Biochemical parameters are useful in the diagnosis of many conditions. Biochemical parameters can be assessed using a variety of methods, including [1]:

- In-house biochemistry analyser.
- External laboratory.
- Commercial test strips.
- Hand-held analyser.

Reference ranges vary between practices and laboratories. See Table 8.4 for examples of normal biochemical reference ranges.

Plasma Proteins
Total Protein (TP)

Total plasma protein measurements include fibrinogen; however, total serum protein levels do not as fibrinogen is used in the clotting process [1]. Elevated TP levels may occur as a result of dehydration, immune-mediated disease, lactation, neoplasia or infection [1]. Decreased TP levels may occur as a result of haemorrhage, protein-losing enteropathy, acute peritonitis and non-steroidal anti-inflammatory drug (NSAID) toxicity [15].

Refractometers can also be used to read TP levels in blood, peritoneal, pleural and synovial fluid.

Normal TP concentrations in different body fluids are as follows [15]:

- Blood 53–75 g per litre (g/L).
- Synovial fluid <20 g/L.
- Peritoneal fluid <25 g/L.
- Pleural fluid <25 g/L.
- Cerebral Spinal Fluid (CSF) 1–12 g/L.

The TP is read on the left-hand scale on the refractometer usually labelled 'Serum P'. The measurement will be in g/100 ml, so it will need to be multiplied by 10 to give the reading in g/l [1].

Table 8.6 Equine blood cell types and functions [1–3].

Cell type	Image	Description	Function
Erythrocyte		Red/pink, biconcave discs which contain no nucleus	Erythrocytes transport oxygen and a small amount of carbon dioxide around the body. They are biconcave discs without a nucleus, containing haemoglobin, a protein that contains iron. The lack of a nucleus enables maximal space for carrying haemoglobin, which binds to oxygen to become oxyhaemoglobin
Mature neutrophil		Granulocyte with a multi-lobed nucleus	Neutrophils are the most common white blood cells seen in equine blood. They are classed as granulocytes as they contain granules in their cytoplasm, which stain purple when they absorb a neutral dye. Neutrophils move quickly to sites of infection or inflammation around the body
Immature neutrophil		Granulocyte with a banded, or horseshoe shaped nucleus	**Neutropaenia** is a low number of neutrophils. This will be seen when there has been a sudden or overwhelming infectious or inflammatory process so the neutrophils get used up and there is a slight delay in the body producing more. **Neutrophilia** is an increase in neutrophils, and this is often seen due to infections, injury, stress or drug administration, including corticosteroid use
Eosinophil		Granulocyte which when stained with Diff-Quik, show multiple granules within the cell that are pink in colour. This gives them an appearance similar to a raspberry	Eosinophils are most often associated with parasitic disease and also allergic conditions. **Eosinophilia** is an increase in eosinophils and is often seen due to parasite infection and hypersensitivity (allergic reactions). **Eosinopaenia** is a reduced number of eosinophils, and this is not considered to be a significant finding in horses as eosinophils are often absent in clinically healthy horses
Basophil		Granulocyte that has multiple granules within the cell. Basophils differ from eosinophils as the granules often stain purple/blue	Basophils are rarely seen in equine blood samples. **Basophilia** is an increase in basophils, and this often indicates a long-standing allergic disease or also ongoing recovery from colic. **Basopenia** is a reduced number of basophils, and this is not considered to be a significant finding in horses as basophils are often absent in clinically healthy horses
Lymphocyte		Agranulocyte (no granules in the cytoplasm) where the nucleus takes up the majority of the cell	Lymphocytes try to remove foreign 'invaders' that cause disease. They manage the immune system (B cells and T cells). **Lymphocytosis** is an increase in lymphocytes, and this could be the result of excitement, exercise and an acute viral infection. **Lymphopenia** is a reduced number of lymphocytes, and this can be the result of stress, viral infections and severe bacterial infections. It is also associated with endotoxaemia
Monocyte		Large agranulocyte which has a bean-shaped nucleus	Monocytes are important in the breakdown of damaged tissues. **Monocytosis** is an increase in monocytes and may be seen with bacterial infections, chronic inflammation and stress. **Monocytopenia** is a low number of monocytes, and this is not considered to be a significant finding in horses as monocytes are often absent in clinically healthy horses

Table 8.6 (Continued)

Cell type	Image	Description	Function
Thrombocyte		Thrombocytes, commonly referred to as platelets are small fragments of large cells called megakaryocytes. They are formed in bone marrow, do not possess a nucleus and are concerned with the formation of blood clots	Thrombocytes are important for blood clotting. **Thrombocytopaenia** is a reduced number of platelets, and this is often seen due to an immune-mediated disease that causes platelet destruction. **Thrombocytosis** is an increase in thrombocytes, and this is rarely seen in equine blood

Source: Vicky Milne and Rosina Lillywhite.

Table 8.7 Methods for performing and staining blood smears.

Preparation of a blood smear

1) Put on a pair of gloves

2) Take a clean and grease-free microscope slide. Slides should be cleaned prior to being used, using ethanol or something similar, and then dried with a lint-free tissue

3) Select a spreader slide and clean and dry as above

4) Place the microscope slide onto a white background if possible, as this will aid in the visualisation of the smear

5) Using a microhaematocrit tube, draw a small sample of blood that has been well-mixed from an EDTA tube

6) Place a finger on the end of the capillary tube to prevent the blood from leaking

7) Place a small drop of blood at one end of the microscope slide, approximately 1 cm away from the edge (Figure 8.15a). If right-handed, it is often easier to place the drop of blood on the right-hand side of the microscope slide. If you are left-handed, place the drop of blood on the left-hand side

Spreading and drying a blood smear

8) Hold the spreader slide in your dominant hand between the thumb and index finger on the long sides, with the spreading edge closest to the microscope slide. Place it just in front of the drop of blood

9) Holding the blood sample slide on a firm surface to keep it still, draw the spreader back into the drop of blood, at a 45° angle (Figure 8.15b). Allow the blood to run along the length of the spreader slide; sometimes, gentle sideways movement will help with this. The wider the angle between the spreader slide and the blood sample slide, the thicker the blood smear; the thinner the angle between the spreader slide and the blood smear slide, the thinner the blood smear

10) With a single, smooth motion, push the spreader slide to the opposite end of the blood sample slide. This needs to be a rapid movement, and the spreader slide must stay in contact with the blood smear slide in order to produce a thin and even blood smear. Ideally, the resultant blood smear will cover two-thirds of the blood smear slide (Figure 8.15c)

11) Rapidly air dries the smear; heating the sample would distort the red blood cells

12) Label the blood smear slide accordingly and check the quality of the smear. The smear should have 'a head', where the drop of blood was placed, a 'body' between the head and tail, and 'a tail' which is the last section of the blood smear and is the feathered edge (Figure 8.16)

Staining a blood smear

Blood smears are routinely stained prior to microscopy in order to facilitate the examination of the blood cells (Figure 8.17). They help to identify blood cells and any abnormalities. The two most common types of stain used in veterinary practice are the Romanowsky stain, for example Leishman's, Giemsa and Diff-Quik and the Supravital stain, such as methylene blue. The difference between the two types would be that Romanowsky stains are used for differential white blood cell counts, Supravital stains are used for reticulocyte counts

Leishman's stain

1) Wear gloves
2) Place the blood smear onto a staining rack with the smear uppermost
3) Cover the blood smear with Leishman's stain and leave for two minutes
4) Add twice the stains volume of buffered distilled water (pH 6.8) and mix carefully with the Leishman's stain, leave for 15 minutes
5) Wash the slide well with buffered distilled water, both front and back, and prop upright to allow to dry

Diff-Quik stain

1) Wear gloves
2) Dip the blood smear into a fixative solution (methanol) 5 times (1 second each time) and then allow the excess fluid to drip off
3) Dip the blood smear into a stain (eosin) 5 times (1 second each time) and then allow the excess fluid to drip off
4) Dip the blood smear into a second stain (methylene blue) 5 times (1 second each time) and then allow the excess fluid to drip off
5) Rinse the slide with distilled water and allow to dry

Source: Vicky Milne.

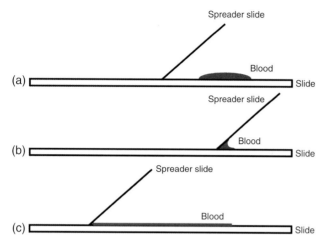

Figures 8.15 (a) A small drop of blood should be placed on the slide at one end of the microscope slide, approximately 1 cm away from the edge. (b) The blood sample slide should be held on a firm surface to keep it still; the spreader slide should be drawn backwards into the drop of blood, at a 45° angle. (c) With a single, smooth motion, the spreader slide should be pushed to the opposite end of the blood sample slide. *Source:* Vicky Milne.

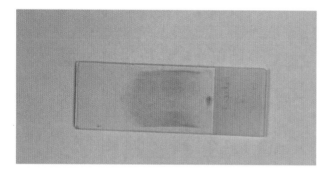

Figure 8.16 Blood smear showing the 'head', where the drop of blood was placed, the 'body' between the head and tail, and the 'tail', which is the last section of the blood smear and has a feathered edge. *Source:* Judith Parry & Marie Rippingale.

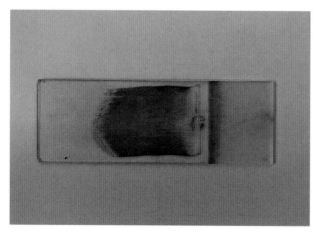

Figure 8.17 A correctly stained blood smear. *Source:* Judith Parry & Marie Rippingale.

Albumin

Albumin is one of the most important proteins in plasma or serum, making up 35–50% of the total plasma protein in most animals [1]. Hepatocytes synthesise albumin; therefore, levels can be affected by liver disease. Intestinal and kidney disease can also cause loss of albumin from the blood.

Globulins

Globulin concentration is usually calculated by subtracting albumin from TP. Specific measurements can be useful in determining the immune status of patients. Immunoglobulin (IgG) testing is particularly useful in assessing the immune status of neonatal foals with failure of passive transfer (see Section 8.4).

Ammonia

Ammonia is produced as a result of the metabolism of protein and should normally be excreted [1]. High concentrations of ammonia can cause neurological problems.

Blood Urea Nitrogen (BUN)

BUN is a waste product formed by the liver and excreted by the kidneys as a result of amino acid metabolism [16]. Elevated BUN can occur with infection, metabolic disease or corticosteroid therapy [16]. Decreases in BUN can occur as a result of a low-protein diet and liver failure. The normal BUN level for a horse is 3–8 millimoles per litre (mmol/l) [16].

Glucose

Glucose is the main source of energy for cells in the body, and its concentration is controlled by the hormones insulin and glucagon [16]. Glucose levels can be assessed using dipsticks or biochemistry analysers. Transient increases in blood glucose concentrations are common and may be due to insulin resistance, corticosteroid administration or alpha2 agonist administration [3]. Prolonged hyperglycaemia is rare in horses but can be seen with hyperadrenocorticism (equine Cushing's disease). Hypoglycaemia is uncommonly in adult horses but may be associated with anorexia or liver failure. It is important to monitor glucose levels in sick neonatal foals as these patients are particularly prone to hypoglycaemia.

Normal glucose reference ranges are as follows [15]:
Adult horse:

- 4.3-6 mmol/l.

Foals:

- 24 hours old: 6.7–12.9 mmol/l.
- One week old: 6.7–10.6 mmol/l.
- One month old: 7.2–12 mmol/l.

- Four months old: 6.3–10.9 mmol/l.
- Yearling: 5.8–9.2 mmol/l.

Lactate

Lactate is produced in anaerobic respiration, and its formation results in acidosis [1]. When the body fails to correct acidosis, blood lactate levels rise and this can be a result of a number of conditions, including [1]:

- Dehydration.
- Hypoperfusion.
- Hypoxia.
- Anaemia.
- Sepsis.

Blood lactate levels have been used as a significant prognostic indicator for survival in colic patients. Lactate ranges are as follows:

- Healthy adult horses: below 2 mmol/L.
- Mild elevations: 2–5 mmol/L.
- Marked elevations: 5–8 mmol/L.
- Severe elevations: Over 8 mmol/L.

Muscle Enzymes

When muscle cells are damaged, enzymes leak into the blood and this allows levels to be measured. Two clinically relevant muscle enzymes in horses are as follows [3]:

- Creatine Kinase (CK): High concentrations are found in skeletal muscle, cardiac muscle and the liver.
- Aspartate Aminotransferase (AST): This is found in skeletal muscle, cardiac muscle and the liver.

High concentrations of CPK and AST are seen with damage to skeletal tissues in conditions such as exertional rhabdomyolysis, atypical myopathy and post anaesthetic myopathy (see Chapter 13 for further details). The plasma concentration of CK peaks within six hours and rapidly decreases, whereas AST concentrations peak at 24 hours and remain high for 7–10 days. The values reached tend to be in thousands rather than hundreds [3].

Liver Enzymes and Liver Function Tests

Liver enzymes can be measured as part of biochemical analysis. Common hepatic biochemistry tests measure the following [3, 16]:

- Alkaline Phosphatase (ALP): Alterations in ALP may reflect chronic damage to the hepatobiliary tract. This test is not liver specific. The normal range is 86–285 IU/L.
- Aspartate Aminotransferase (AST) (see above also): AST is released from hepatocytes in acute liver disease. Elevation in blood AST levels can reflect muscle damage or

liver damage; therefore, this test is not liver specific. The normal range is 120–340 IU/L.
- Gamma-glutamyl Transferase (GGT): Alterations in GGT reflect damage to the hepatobiliary tract and can indicate acute and chronic liver disease. Technically, GGT is not liver specific as alterations can be seen in renal or pancreatic disease. However, as these are rare in horses, GGT is a useful indicator for both acute and chronic liver disease. The normal range is 1–40 IU/L.
- Glutamate Dehydrogenase (GLDH): Alterations indicate acute liver damage. This test is liver specific. It is worth noting that GLDH is unstable in transit and therefore requires assay shortly after collection. The normal range is 0–11.8 UL/L.
- Lactate Dehydrogenase (LDH): Elevations do not indicate specific liver disease, although elevations are more likely with hepatocellular conditions. 162–412 IU/L. LDH is useful when measured with other liver enzymes.
- Sorbitol Dehydrogenase (SDH). Indicates acute and current liver damage. It is worth noting that SDH is unstable in transit and therefore requires assay shortly after collection. SDH is liver specific. The normal range is 0–8 IU/L.

Serum Bilirubin

Serum bilirubin concentrations are of limited use in the horse compared with other species. Bilirubin is a breakdown product of haemoglobin, which is usually removed from the liver [3]. Concentrations are often not seen with liver disease but may be seen with biliary disease. The most common physiological reason for an increase in bilirubin concentrations is anorexia or inappetence [3]. If liver failure is suspected, a test of liver function, such as total serum bile acid estimation, should be carried out [3]. This is a useful test for monitoring the progression of liver disease in the horse. Blood ammonia concentrations may also be elevated with liver disease, especially in patients with encephalopathy [3]. Triglyceride levels may also be affected by liver disease, and these are particularly significant in hyperlipaemia (see Chapter 16 for further information).

Creatinine

Creatinine is formed from creatine, which is found in skeletal muscle. Creatinine diffuses out of the muscle cell and into most body fluids, including blood. In a healthy patient, creatinine is filtered through the glomeruli in the kidney and is eliminated in the urine. It is not an accurate indicator of early kidney disease as approximately 75% of the kidney tissue must be non-functional before elevated blood creatinine levels occur [16]. Increased creatinine can be an indication of hypovolemia, dehydration and acute/chronic renal failure [15]. The normal reference range for creatinine is 85–170 μmol/L.

Acid Base Balance

Hydrogen ions are produced by normal tissue metabolism, and concentrations are closely controlled by homeostatic mechanisms. Hydrogen ion concentrations can be measured on a pH scale of 1–14. In the normal horse, blood pH is slightly alkaline pH 7.35–7.45 [3]. Processes leading to a rise or fall in blood pH as known as alkalosis and acidosis. Blood pH is often measured in critical care patients and during general anaesthesia using handheld analysers.

Electrolytes

Electrolytes are the negative ions and positive ions found in body fluids. They are involved in managing water balance in the body. If small changes occur in the level of electrolytes in the body, serious consequences can follow [16]. Measurements of electrolyte concentrations are used in the diagnosis of many conditions, including renal, endocrine and metabolic disorders.

Calcium The majority of calcium is found in bone and is also involved in neuromuscular function. Calcium concentrations are usually related to phosphorus concentrations. The normal level for an adult horse is 2.9–3.3 mmol/l [15]. Increases in calcium occur with chronic renal disease and neoplasia. Decreases in calcium are seen with lactation or transport tetany and acute renal disease [15, 16].

Phosphate Phosphate levels are closely linked with calcium levels. The normal level for an adult horse is 0.9–1.9 mmol/l [15]. Reduced levels are seen with chronic renal failure and starvation. Increased levels are seen with acute renal failure [15].

Sodium Sodium is required for many vital functions in the body, including the regulation of blood pressure and volume and the transmission of nerve impulses [16]. An increased level of sodium in the blood is referred to as hypernatremia. This may occur along with dehydration. A reduced level of sodium in the blood is referred to as hyponatraemia and this may occur due to diarrhoea, excessive sweating, gastric reflux and renal disease [15]. The normal reference range for sodium is 134–142 mmol/L [15].

Chloride Chloride plays an important role in the normal balance of fluids in the body. A significant increase in chloride in the blood is referred to as hyperchloremia, and this may be associated with diarrhoea and kidney disease [16]. A decrease in chloride in the blood is known as hypochloraemia, and this is associated with excessive sweating, reflux and blood loss [15]. The normal reference range for chloride is 91–104 mmol/L.

Potassium Potassium has a key role in maintaining the electrical potential of the cell membrane [16]. An increase in potassium in the blood may be associated with acidaemia, uroperitoneum and oliguria. A decrease in the level of potassium in the blood may be associated with major surgery, anorexia and alkalaemia [15]. The normal reference range for potassium is 3–5 mmol/L.

Hormones

Adrenocorticotrophic Hormone (ACTH)

Adrenocorticotrophic Hormone (ACTH) testing is commonly carried out in the diagnosis of pituitary pars intermedia dysfunction (PPID) also known as equine Cushing's disease (ECD) (see Chapter 13). The recommended first-line test sampling protocol is as follows [17]:

- Collect a single EDTA blood sample at any time of day.
- Chill within three hours.
- Separate the plasma by centrifugation or gravity.
- Test in-house or ship to the laboratory overnight with cool packs (maximum delay 48 hours).
- If there is likely to be a delay between sample collection and analysis, centrifuged plasma can be frozen and sent or processed on a different day. Gravity-separated plasma should not be frozen as this will lead to a spurious increase in ACTH concentration and an inaccurate result.

This test has a high sensitivity and specificity when used in horses with advanced clinical disease. However, when used as a screening test, the positive predictive power of the test falls significantly and false positives can occur. Season (more specifically, day length) has a major impact on ACTH concentration in normal horses. Healthy horses have a significant increase in ACTH concentration in the Autumn months and so varying cut-off values have been proposed depending on the time of year the test is carried out. These values are as follows [17]:

November–July:

- Negative: <30 pg/ml
- Equivocal: 30–50 pg/ml
- Positive: >50 pg/ml

July–November:

- Negative: <50 pg/ml
- Equivocal: 50–100 pg/m
- Positive: >100 pg/ml

Further testing in the form of a thyrotropin releasing hormone stimulation test (TRHST) may be required if the results of the ACTH test are equivocal or in a case where PPID is still suspected despite a negative ACTH test result.

Insulin

Insulin testing is commonly carried out for the diagnosis of equine metabolic syndrome (EMS) (see Chapter 13). A single blood sample can be taken to assess insulin and glucose levels in the blood. Serum and fluoride oxalate samples are required for this. This test has low sensitivity, which means that a negative result does not rule out the presence of insulin dysregulation. Results can be interpreted as follows [18]:

- Resting insulin concentration of <20 IU/ml: This is considered to be within an acceptable range, although an oral Karo syrup test should be carried out to rule out insulin dysregulation.
- Resting insulin concentration of 20–50 IU/ml: Readings within this range suggest the presence of insulin dysregulation although, an oral Karo syrup test can still be useful to evaluate this further.
- Resting insulin concentration of >50 IU/ml: A resting insulin concentration in this range confirms the presence of insulin dysregulation.

Oral sugar testing can be used to further evaluate the insulin dysregulation status of a patient. Oral sugar testing works by either feeding the horse a normal feed and then taking a blood sample for insulin levels two hours afterwards or, administering at high sugar substance to the horse, e.g. Karo Light Cron Syrup and taking a blood sample for insulin and glucose levels after 60–90 minutes. For more information on PPID and EMS please refer to the Further Reading section.

Urine

Patient Preparation and Sample Collection

Analysis of urine samples can give a quick insight into the health status of a patient; for example, it can be used to detect nephritis, cystitis and bladder pathology. Urine collection can be carried out by catching a free-flow sample or via catheterisation.

Equipment required for free-flow urine collection:

- Gloves.
- Sterile collection container with or without preservative as required.

For a free-flow sample, a horse may not require restraint. Horses are more likely to urinate in a stable with fresh bedding, when unrestrained. However, the person collecting the sample should wear PPE in the form of a hard hat and steel-toe-capped boots. They should also be careful not to startle the horse by moving slowly and carefully. When collecting the sample, personnel should always stand to the side of the horse and never directly behind them. If a headcollar and leadrope are used, the horse would be positioned in a way that the person catching the urine would be able to do so by standing to one side of the horse with clear access to the door. When collecting a urine sample via the free flow method, a mid-stream sample should be collected.

Urine samples can be collected by passing a catheter through the urethra into the bladder. Equipment required for this method of urine collection includes:

- A suitable-sized sterile urinary catheter (this will vary between mares and geldings/stallions).
- 60 ml catheter-tip syringe.
- Sterile gloves.
- Sterile lubricant.
- Sterile container for sample collection.
- Cotton wool and a suitable skin antiseptic solution

Complications can occur following urinary catheterisation these can include bacterial cystitis and trauma. Urine collection via this method is the most accepted method for microbial testing as cystocentesis is impossible in the adult horse [1–3].

When placing a urinary catheter to obtain a sample, physical restraint (with either a headcollar and leadrope or a bridle) will be required. A set of stocks can also be used. The case vet will decide if the patient requires sedation. See Chapter 17 for more information regarding the placement of urinary catheters.

If a urine sample is going to be tested within a couple of hours of collection, a sterile universal container can be used and a preservative is not required. These containers can be used for urine samples for up to 24 hours post-sample collection if the urine is kept refrigerated. After 24 hours, bacterial counts will change, white blood cells will become unrecognisable and the pH may increase, meaning it would no longer be of diagnostic quality. Boric acid can be used as a preservative. It will prevent the multiplication of microorganisms for up to 72 hours, meaning the sample will remain of diagnostic quality for longer following sample collection. Thymol and formalin can also be used as preservatives for urine samples [1, 2].

Urinalysis

Measurement of Specific Gravity

Specific gravity is the density of a known fluid volume, for example, urine, compared with distilled water at an equal volume. Distilled water is used as it has a specific gravity of 1.000.

Normal USG readings are as follows [3, 19]:

- Adult horse: 1.020–1.050.
- Foal: 1.001–1.025.

The method for measuring specific gravity using a refractometer is displayed in Table 8.8.

Chemical Test Strips

Chemical test strips are mostly used in urinalysis. To ensure the results from chemical test strips are accurate, the following points should be considered:

- Ensure the tests strips are in date.
- Keep the tests in an airtight container.
- Check the strips are not damp or discoloured before use.
- The tests should be stored at a temperature that does not exceed 30 °C.
- Close the lid of the container immediately after removing a strip.
- Use urine that is fresh, not been centrifuged and has been thoroughly mixed.

In equine patients, chemical test strips or dipsticks are commonly used to measure urine pH. Equine urine is alkaline, with a pH range of 7.0–9.0. Often, the pH of a urine sample will reflect the diet the horse is on; for example, horses that graze pasture will often have more alkaline urine, whereas horses that are on a cereal-based performance-type diet will normally have more acidic urine.

The method for analysing urine using a urine dipstick is as follows:

1) On a piece of paper, write down all the chemicals that are listed on the outside of the container in order.
2) Put on a pair of gloves.
3) Gently mix the urine sample and draw up some urine using either a pipette or a small syringe.
4) Remove a test strip from the container (Figure 8.18).
5) Cover all test strip pads with urine (Figure 8.19) and note the time.
6) The test strip pads will change colour (Figure 8.20).
7) Wait for the appropriate time to start reading and recording the results (Figure 8.21). Each chemical test pad must be read at a specific time. Times will vary depending on the manufacturer.
8) Dispose of any used chemical test strips.

It is important to read the results at the correct time to ensure they are valid.

Urine dipsticks can also be used to test for proteinuria, which could cause inflammation to the kidneys and glucosuria, which can be seen in patients with PPID/ECD. Haematuria may be seen where there has been a traumatic injury [1–3].

Table 8.8 Method for the measurement of specific gravity using a refractometer.

Calibration of the refractometer
This should happen every time the refractometer is used
1) Make sure the prism surface of the refractometer is clean and then add a few drops of distilled water and close the cover
2) Holding the refractometer up to a light source, look down the eyepiece
3) Using the scale adjusting screw which is often found by the prism, calibrate the refractometer to 1.000 on the USG scale
4) Lift the cover and carefully dry the surface of the prism – the refractometer is then ready to use
Measuring the specific gravity
1) Put on a pair of gloves
2) Gently mix the urine sample
3) Apply a few drops of urine to the prism surface and close the cover
4) Holding the refractometer up to a light source, look down the eyepiece
5) Read the specific gravity off the appropriate scale and record the result
6) Clean the prism using water and dry
7) Dispose of all waste appropriately into hazardous waste

Source: Vicky Milne.

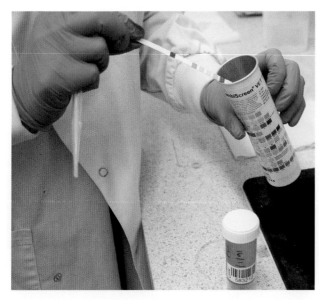

Figure 8.18 Remove a test strip from the container. *Source:* Rosina Lillywhite with permission from Liphook Equine Hospital.

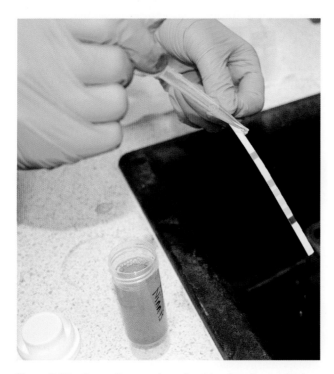

Figure 8.19 Cover all test strip pads with urine. *Source:* Rosina Lillywhite with permission from Liphook Equine Hospital.

Microscopic Examination of Urine

Microscopic examination of urine is inexpensive and can be carried out quickly in house.

The method for preparing a urine sample for microscopic analysis is as follows:

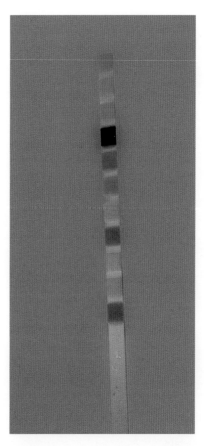

Figure 8.20 The test strip pads will change colour. *Source:* Rosina Lillywhite with permission from Liphook Equine Hospital.

1) The urine sample will need to be centrifuged at 1500–2000 rpm for five minutes. This allows the sediment to be separated from the supernatant (the liquid that remains above the sediment following centrifugation).
2) The supernatant should be removed as carefully as possible to avoid disturbing the sediment.
3) Once there is only a small amount of supernatant left and the sediment, re-suspend the sediment by mixing it with the supernatant that was left.
4) At this point, the sediment can be stained if required to assist with the examination of the urine.
5) Often 'Sedi-stain' is most commonly used but Leishman's and Gram stains can also be used.
6) The urine is then ready for microscopic examination.
7) Preparation of the sample for microscopy includes pipetting a small amount of sediment onto a clean microscope slide and carefully placing a coverslip on top, avoiding any air bubbles (this can be done by lowering the coverslip at an angle).

Microscopic examination of equine urine is often used to detect casts (cellular and protein casts), which will be seen

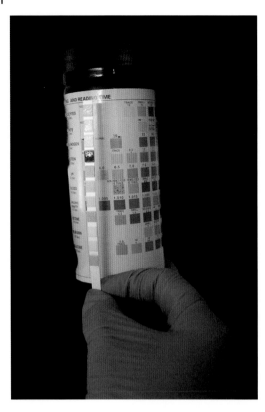

Figure 8.21 Wait for the appropriate time to start reading the results and record them. *Source:* Rosina Lillywhite with permission from Liphook Equine Hospital.

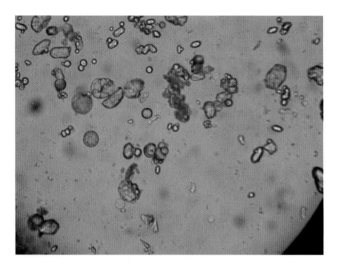

Figure 8.22 Calcium carbonate crystals are commonly seen in equine urine. *Source:* With permission from BSAVA Textbook of Veterinary Nursing 5th Edition. © BSAVA. Courtesy of Newmarket Equine Hospital.

with renal tubular damage. Leucocytes will be present during inflammation. If bacterial cells are seen accompanied by leucocytes, this may indicate an infection. Erythrocytes will indicate haemorrhage, trauma, inflammation or neoplasia. Equine urine will contain calcium carbonate crystals (Figure 8.22), and this is a normal finding, due to the urine being saturated with a solution of calcium carbonate. Struvite and calcium oxalate crystals can also be found in equine urine [1–3, 19].

Faeces

Laboratory testing of faeces is a common process in determining if a horse has an intestinal parasite burden. Faecal testing can also be used in the investigation of weight loss or persistent diarrhoea.

The equipment required for the collection of faeces is as follows:

- Gloves.
- Sterile universal container.
- Spatula – this can be used to aid the collection of the faeces.

The collection is simple in horses; the sample can be obtained from freshly voided faeces. A vet may carry out a rectal examination and obtain a faecal sample. If the sample is being collected in this manner, the horse will need to be physically restrained using a headcollar and a leadrope, or a bridle. Stocks could also be used for this procedure. Sedation is rarely required. If refrigerated, faecal samples can be kept for up to seven days. No preservative is required [1–3].

Microscopic Analysis of Faeces

Faecal analysis is carried out regularly in practice as it is used to detect endoparasites and monitor the success of anthelmintic programmes. Microscopic examination of faeces can be carried out in two ways: the faeces can be prepared using the 'flotation' method or the McMasters method.

The Flotation Method

For this method, 4 g of faeces is mixed with a chemical solution, primarily a sugar or salt solution such as zinc sulphate. The solution provides a specific gravity that will allow parasite eggs to float to the top of the sample and faecal debris to sink to the bottom. Once the faecal sample has been mixed with the solution, it is sieved through a fine gauze. The sample is then collected into a test tube covered with a cover slip. After 20 minutes, the coverslip is lifted off the test tube and a sample is placed straight onto a microscope slide ready for analysis.

The McMasters Method

This method uses a McMasters chamber (Figure 8.23) and involves mixing 4 g of faeces with 56 ml of flotation fluid, which is then placed through a sieve. The fluid that has been strained is stirred and using a pipette, a sample of the fluid is taken to fill the first compartment of the McMaster counting chamber. The fluid is stirred again, and another sample is taken to fill the second chamber. The counting chamber should be left to stand for five minutes to allow the eggs to float to the top before analysis begins.

The slides are examined using a lower-powered objective lens for both methods. When examining the sample, all eggs seen should be recorded and identified. If using the McMasters chamber, count all eggs within the engraved area.

To calculate the number of eggs per gram, add the number of eggs counted (in both chambers of the McMasters slide) and multiply by 50. For example, 10 eggs in chamber one plus 12 eggs in chamber two = 22 eggs × 50 = 1100 eggs per gram.

Large and small strongyle (cyathostomes) eggs, including Ascarid and Strongyloides spp., are easily identified during microscopic faecal analysis. Tapeworm segments may sometimes be seen microscopically but more are often seen during gross examination [1–3]. For more information

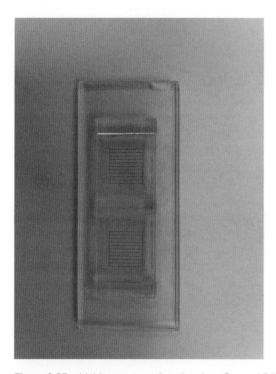

Figure 8.23 McMasters counting chamber. *Source:* Vicky Milne with permission from B&W Equine Hospital.

regarding worm egg identification and anthelmintic programmes, see Chapter 5.

Cytology

Cytology is a straightforward diagnostic technique used to examine cells from fluid or tissues to determine a diagnosis. For all samples, collection should be performed using a sterile technique as much as possible.

Samples that may require cytological examination could include:

- Tracheal washes.
- Synovial fluid.
- Peritoneal fluid.
- Pleural fluid.
- Cerebral spinal fluid (CSF).
- Fine needle aspirates (FNAs).
- Clitoral, vaginal or endometrial swabs.

The equipment required for the collection of cytology samples will vary according to the type of sample being collected. Various receptacles and preservatives are used, including EDTA, plain tubes, universal containers and cytospin fixation fluids. Fluid samples will often be placed into an EDTA tube as this will allow for nucleated cell counts. Plain tubes are often used for samples that require culture. Cytospin fixation fluid will preserve cells and is most commonly used for tracheal wash samples [1–3].

For tracheal washes, the patient will require suitable restraint with a headcollar and leadrope. The patient may be put in a set of stocks for extra restraint. Sedation is rarely used as this can interfere with the examination of physiological abnormalities of the larynx and the pharynx. See Chapter 7 for information regarding tracheal wash and bronchioalveolar lavage (BAL) sampling.

For synoviocentesis (joint fluid), abdominocentesis (peritoneal fluid) and thoracocentesis (pleural fluid), sampling is carried out under standing sedation. Clipping is required unless otherwise stipulated by the case vet. Areas to clip are as follows:

- Synoviocentesis: The clipped area should be around the joint of interest.
- Abdominocentesis: The clipped area should be at the lowest part of the abdomen on the ventral midline.
- Thoracocentesis: The clipped area is routinely situated between the sixth and seventh intercostal space [1–3, 20].

Once the site has been clipped, an aseptic skin preparation should be carried out as described in Chapter 12.

Sampling will then be carried out by a vet using an aseptic technique.

Synoviocentesis

Following adequate preparation and with the horse correctly restrained, a small bleb of local anaesthetic may placed subcutaneously over the sample site, to reduce the chances of the horse moving during the procedure [3]. The most suitable needle size will vary in relation to the joint being sampled. Once the vet has inserted the needle, synovial fluid should flow freely from the hub and can be easily collected. Occasionally, aspiration with a syringe may be required [3].

Abdominocentesis

Peritoneal fluid is most easily collected from a site 10–15 cm behind the xiphisternum in the ventral midline. Following adequate preparation and with the horse correctly restrained, the vet will place a needle through the skin and into the linea alba. The needle is slowly advanced until peritoneal fluid drips out. In most cases, an 18 g 1.5-in. needle is used. A teat canula may also be used following local anaesthetic infiltration and after making a stab incision with a number 11 blade [3]. In the neonate, sampling may take place with the patient in recumbency, but extra care must be taken to avoid inadvertent puncture of the intestines [3].

Thoracocentesis

Pleural fluid is collected through an intercostal space. Thoracic ultrasonography is invaluable in identifying the correct site for pleural fluid collection [3]. Following adequate preparation and with the horse correctly restrained, local anaesthetic is infiltrated into the intercostal tissues. The vet then inserts a needle immediately cranial to the rib and into the pleural space. The pleural cavity usually has a negative pressure, so entry will be accompanied by an influx of air [3]. Once this is identified, the needle should be closed off to prevent a pneumothorax from occurring [3]. A 19 g 2-in. needle is usually suitable for this procedure. If therapeutic pleural drainage is required, a large intravenous (IV) catheter, urinary catheter or human chest drain can be used [3].

CSF Collection

CSF can be collected in two ways: one from the atlantooccipital space carried out under general anaesthesia in adult horses, or via the lumbosacral space in which the patient would be restrained, standing and sedated. The patient would be chemically and physically restrained for a sample from the lumbosacral space. The skin over the tuber coxae would be clipped, and a surgical scrub would be performed (see Chapter 12); a bleb of local anaesthetic would be placed in the midline, and then a second surgical scrub would be completed. The patient should be stood square, with its weight distributed evenly on its hind limbs. A vet would then insert an 18 gauge 6-in. spinal needle with a stylet through the skin at the midline in the line bisecting the tuber coxae and down through the depression, which can be palpated caudal to the sixth lumbar spinous process. The patient is likely to flinch during this procedure, especially when the subarachnoid space is penetrated, which is often a sign to start aspirating the fluid into a syringe. Once a sufficient quantity of the sample has been obtained, the vet will withdraw the needle and decant the sample into a container with a suitable preservative (often EDTA or cytospin, although plain containers can also be used) [21].

FNAs

Samples for cytology may be collected from organs, lymph nodes and masses via a technique known as FNA and can provide information in some cases, although the level of diagnostic information can be limited. This technique sometimes used in equine practice but is more commonly performed in small animal practice. FNAs may confirm the presence of suppurative inflammation and causative organisms or may help identify seromas or haematomas. They may also provide information relating to melanomas and sarcoids. The procedure will be carried out by a vet but they may require assistance from an RVN [16]. The procedure is carried out as follows [22]:

- A 23 g needle and a 2–5 ml syringe is commonly used.
- The mass is stabilised using a hand, and the sterile needle is inserted.
- Negative pressure is created by attaching the syringe and pulling back on the plunger of the syringe.
- The needle is then removed from the mass and the syringe if used, is also removed.
- A syringe is then filled with air and attached to the needle. The plunger on the syringe is then depressed, and the sample is forced out onto a microscope slide.
- The slide is then air-dried.
- The sample may then be stained and examined in-house or sent to an external laboratory.

Reproductive Swabbing in Mares

Reproductive swabbing in mares is used to collect samples from the reproductive tract for various purposes, including breeding management, disease diagnosis and monitoring reproductive health. This procedure typically involves taking swabs from specific areas of the mare's reproductive tract, to collect samples of mucus, cells or other materials for analysis.

Clitoral Swabbing

Swabbing of the reproductive tract may take place as part of a breeding soundness examination (BSE). Although a BSE is not required for every mare who is intended for breeding, clitoral swabbing is recommended for any mare presented for breeding in the United Kingdom [23]. Examination of the internal reproductive tract and clitoral swabbing may only be carried out by a vet [23]. It is important to test all breeding mares for contagious equine metritis (CEM) and other venereal pathogens. The causal agents are found in the clitoral sinuses and fossa. The United Kingdom has a code of practice for CEM and other bacterial venereal diseases, which vets should follow [23]. CEM is a notifiable disease. Therefore, it is a statutory requirement to report any cases to the appropriate authorities. See Chapter 6 for more information on notifiable diseases. Swabs may also be taken from the vagina and the uterus in mares.

Method for Reproductive Swabbing in Mares [24]

Reproductive swabbing is typically performed by a vet, and involves the following steps:

1) Preparation: Before starting the procedure, the mare is restrained safely in a set of stocks. It's important to ensure the mare is calm to minimise stress.
2) Place a tail bandage.
3) Cleaning: The perineal area, including the vulva, is thoroughly cleaned to reduce the risk of contamination during the procedure.
4) Gloving: The vet will wear sterile gloves to prevent the introduction of any contaminants into the reproductive tract.
5) Examination: A vaginal speculum may be used to visualise the cervix if required. This helps the vet to locate the cervix and safely insert the swabs.

   Swab collection: Swabs designed for reproductive sampling are inserted either into the clitoral sinuses and fossa, into the vagina, or carefully advanced through the cervix into the uterus.

Swab Types

Different types of swabs may be used depending on the purpose of the sampling:

- Clitoral swabs: Sterile, narrow-tipped swabs should be used for sampling the clitoral sinus. Sterile, normal-tipped swabs can be used for sampling the clitoral fossa.
- Vaginal Swabs: These are usually sterile, normal-tipped swabs that are inserted into the vaginal vault to collect samples of vaginal mucus or secretions.
- Uterine Swabs: These are usually sterile, double-guarded swabs that are inserted through the cervix into the uterine body to collect samples of uterine lining or fluids.

After the sample is collected, each swab is carefully labelled with the mare's identification and the date and time of collection. Samples are placed in sterile containers for transport to a laboratory or for immediate analysis. If required, the collected samples are then sent to a laboratory for analysis, which may include microbiological cultures, cytology, or other tests, depending on the purpose of the swabbing.

Samples Taken Post Abortion

Referral of samples post-abortion in mares is a crucial veterinary procedure aimed at diagnosing the cause of abortion, identifying potential pathogens and preventing further reproductive problems. The steps involved in referring samples post-abortion are as follows [25].

Recognition of Abortion

The process typically begins when a mare experiences an abortion, which is the premature expulsion of a foetus before it is capable of survival. The abortion may be observed by the mare's owner or detected by a vet during routine checks, such as rectal palpation or ultrasound.

Initial Assessment

When an abortion occurs, it is essential to promptly assess the mare's condition, as she may require immediate medical attention or supportive care. The foetus and placenta should be carefully examined to determine their condition, as this information may be vital for subsequent diagnostic testing.

Sample Collection

To determine the cause of the abortion, various samples should be collected from both the mare and the aborted foetus [25]:

- Mare samples: Swabs or other samples are collected from the mare's reproductive tract to check for the presence of infectious agents, such as bacteria, viruses, or fungi. These samples may include vaginal swabs, uterine swabs and blood samples.
- Foetal samples: Tissues and fluids are collected from the aborted foetus. These samples may include foetal organs, placental tissues, foetal fluids (amniotic fluid, foetal blood) and any abnormal structures or lesions.

All collected samples must be properly labelled with the mare's identification, date and a clear description of the sample type. Samples should be securely packaged to prevent contamination or damage during transportation. They may need to be kept cool, depending on the nature of the samples and the time it takes to reach the diagnostic laboratory. The samples are typically sent to a specialised veterinary diagnostic laboratory for analysis. It is important to choose a laboratory that is experienced in handling reproductive samples and diagnosing abortion cases in horses.

Diagnostic Testing

At the laboratory, the various samples undergo a range of diagnostic tests, including:

- Microbiological cultures: To identify any bacterial or fungal infections.
- Polymerase chain reaction (PCR) testing: To detect the presence of specific viral deoxyribonucleic acid (DNA) or ribonucleic acid (RNA).
- Histopathology: Examining tissue samples under a microscope to identify abnormalities or lesions.
- Serological testing: Blood samples may be tested for the presence of antibodies to specific pathogens.

Reporting Results

Once the laboratory completes the analysis, they provide a detailed report to the referring vet and the mare owner. The report includes information on the cause of the abortion if identified, as well as recommendations for treatment and future breeding management.

Treatment and Prevention

Based on the diagnostic findings, the referring vet may recommend appropriate treatment for the mare and provide guidance on preventing future abortions. This may include vaccination, biosecurity measures or management changes to reduce the risk of further reproductive problems. Referring to samples post-abortion is essential for understanding the underlying cause of the abortion and taking appropriate steps to ensure the mare's future reproductive health. It requires close collaboration between the mare owner, the referring vet and the diagnostic laboratory to achieve a successful diagnosis and treatment plan.

Histopathology

Tissue Biopsies

Tissue biopsies are collected for histopathological examination. They can be more useful than FNAs and smears as they often lead to a more definitive diagnosis. A biopsy is a sample of tissue which has been taken from a live animal. Various techniques can be used for this, but the most common ones used include excision, incision, punch, needle and endoscopic biopsies. There are a number of sites in the horse that are suitable for a biopsy.

Skin

Skin biopsies are often thought to be the most useful technique for investigating skin conditions. Sedation and local anaesthesia are usually required. The site of the biopsy should not be clipped or surgically scrubbed as this could negatively affect the results. The patient should be positioned so that the person carrying out the biopsy has full visualisation of the site and can stand in a safe place. Common skin biopsy techniques include punch biopsy, elliptical biopsy or an excisional biopsy. The method used would be decided by the case vet [3].

Liver and Lung

The patient should be sedated and suitable restrained. The sample site should be clipped and aseptically prepared. After the local anaesthetic has been infiltrated, the sample is taken by a vet using a Tru-cut technique [3]. Ultrasound may be used to identify the biopsy site beforehand.

Muscle

The patient should be sedated and suitable restrained. The sample site should be clipped and aseptically prepared. After the local anaesthetic has been infiltrated, the sample is taken by the vet using sharp dissection or a Bergstrom needle introduced through the skin.

Endometrium

Endometrial biopsies are indicated for the routine investigation of barren mares and for the investigation of specific endometrial pathology. Biopsies are obtained with specially designed forceps. The mare is restrained as for routine gynaecological examinations with her tail bandaged and rectum evacuated of faeces. The mare is scanned to confirm that she is not pregnant. The perineum is hygienically prepared, and sterile biopsy forceps are introduced into the mare's vagina by the vet, with a gloved hand, through the cervix and on into the uterine body where the biopsy is taken. Tissues are carefully removed from the forceps with a needle or fine forceps to avoid artefactual damage and are fixed immediately in Bouin's fluid (preferred to formalin fixation). A fine-tipped sterile swab may be used to sample the inside of the jaws of the biopsy instrument for bacterial culture [26].

Bone Marrow

The patient should be sedated and suitable restrained. The skin overlying the sternum should be clipped and aseptically prepared. After the local anaesthetic has been infiltrated, the sample is taken by the vet using a Jamshidi needle [3]. The iliac crest can also be used as an alternative sample site.

Tissue samples or biopsies should ideally be preserved in 10% formal saline as this will inhibit the process of autolysis, which is the digestion and breakdown of all or part of a cell by its own enzymes. The thinner the tissue samples, the quicker 10% formal saline will fix the sample. Depending on the sample size, it can take 12–24 hours to fix completely. Muscle biopsies should be placed in an empty sterile container and ideally transported on ice. If there is any doubt as to how samples should be fixed or transported, the laboratory assessing the samples should be contacted for advice. Care needs to be taken when carrying out tissue biopsies; the sample itself would be classed as hazardous, and the formal saline used to preserve it is toxic and irritant, so PPE should be worn at all times [1–3].

Skin and Hair

Patient Preparation and Sample Collection

Horses commonly suffer from dermatological conditions. The testing of skin and hair aids in identifying ectoparasites and conditions such as dermatophytosis (ringworm). Various techniques can be used to obtain skin and hair samples, for example hair plucks, skin scrapes and adhesive tape impressions.

When collecting skin and hair samples, it is unlikely the patient will need any form of chemical restraint unless the area is painful. Physical restraint will include a headcollar and leadrope or a bridle. A set of stocks can also be used for extra restraint. Hair plucks, hair brushings and acetate tape preparation require no skin preparation; in fact, preparing the area, clipping and cleaning could be detrimental to the sample being collected. The affected area would need to be clipped for skin scrapes, as this will allow for a more accurate scrape, and a better visualisation of the affected area.

Hair Plucks

Hair plucks are often used for dermatophyte culture. As dermatophytosis is a zoonotic disease, extra care should be taken when taking samples from horses suspected of having this infection. Gloves should be worn and disposed of safely after use. Any equipment used should be thoroughly disinfected afterwards. The horse should be adequately restrained as a small number of hairs are plucked from the margins of the affected area. Often, artery forceps are used for this as there is more chance of including the roots with the pluck. The hairs are then placed onto a microscope slide with a drop of mineral oil, and a cover slip. The slide is labelled and then examined under a microscope

[2, 3]. A dermatophyte quantitative polymerase chain reaction (qPCR) test is now available in the United Kingdom.

Hair Brushings

These are rarely performed in horses but may be used to investigate dermatophytosis [3].

Acetate Tape Preparations

These are mostly used for identifying Oxyuris eggs from around the perineal and tail area. Gloves should always be worn prior to carrying out this sampling technique. Once the horse is restrained, clear adhesive tape is applied to the skin surface to collect any epidermal debris or eggs. The tape is then removed from the area and placed directly onto a microscope slide, ready for examination. If required, the tape can be stained with Diff-Quick [1, 2].

Skin Scrapings

These may be performed in order to identify mites such as Chorioptes. Coat hair should be clipped away, and mineral oil should be applied to the sample site. A scalpel blade should be held between the thumb and forefinger. The skin to be scraped should be stretched with the other hand. The sample site should then be gently scraped with the scalpel blade until capillary ooze is identified. The depth of scraping will vary according to the parasite in question. The sample should be collected into a sterile container or applied directly to a microscope slide [1, 3].

Impression Smears

Two types of impression smears can be carried out on lesions. If the lesion is producing exudate, such as an ulcer or from the underside of a crust, a direct impression smear will be carried out. With the patient restrained and the sampler wearing gloves, a microscope slide is gently pressed onto the lesion to collect the exudate. The sample is then air-dried and can be stained. For an indirect impression smear, often used due to a difficult location, a cotton swab could be used to collect any exudate, which is then rolled onto a microscope slide, dried and stained [1].

Swab Samples

Skin swabs can be used to identify bacterial, fungal and yeast skin conditions. The swab is rolled over the surface of the affected area for example the skin or the surface of a wound. In some circumstances, gross contamination may need to be removed from the sample site before the sample is taken. If this is required, sterile saline should be used. Swabs that use charcoal as a transport medium, are ideal for this type of sampling as the charcoal prolongs the viability of pathogenic organisms [1–3].

The technique for obtaining a wound swab sample is as follows [1]:

1) Ensure the patient is correctly restrained by a competent handler wearing PPE.
2) Assemble the required equipment: gloves, appropriate swabs and a pen for labelling.
3) Wear gloves.
4) Select an appropriate swab, e.g. charcoal swab for bacteriology.
5) Collect sufficient material for analysis by gently rotating the swab to cover the surfaces without traumatising the wound or causing discomfort to the patient. Contamination should be avoided.
6) Replace the swab into the cover tube avoiding any further contamination and secure the lid.
7) Remove gloves and dispose of them correctly.
8) Label the swab with the location the sample was taken from, e.g. left carpus.
9) Label the swab with the animal's name, owner's name and the date.

If the swab is being sent to an external laboratory, it should be packaged following current packaging guidelines (see Section 8.6). Alternatively, the swab can be rolled or smeared onto a microscope slide, stained and viewed with a microscope.

Bacteriology

Bacterial Culture

Although many bacteria are crucial to health, some are harmful and can cause disease. Therefore, it is important to culture bacteria and allow them to multiply in laboratory conditions to observe their growth and facilitate the identification of species. This will aid the formulation of more specific and effective treatment programmes.

Bacteria are microorganisms which will only grow when the environment is suitable. Important environmental factors include:

- The correct temperature.
- The correct pH.
- The availability of water.
- The availability of essential nutrients.

These environmental factors need to be provided when growing bacteria under laboratory conditions. This is achieved by using various culture mediums specific to the type of bacteria being grown.

Bacterial Culture Media

In a laboratory, bacteria are grown within a culture media. There are two types of media used in veterinary practice: liquid media (also commonly known as a broth) and solid media. Liquid broth supplies all the nutrients needed for bacteria to grow successfully, such as an enrichment broth, which will be selective for a particular bacterium. Solid media is made up of gelatine and agar (a derivative of seaweed). Agar can be bought ready to use in sterile Petri dishes. Agar plates must be kept in the fridge and stored upside down when unused. This is because the reduced temperature in the fridge can cause a film of condensation to develop on the agar plate; if this drips onto the unused agar, it will render it useless. Solid media can be classified as displayed in Table 8.9.

Table 8.9 Different types of bacterial growth media and their uses.

Type	Uses	Examples of medium
Simple or basal media	This media is a general-purpose media and provides all nutrients required for basic growth, such as *Escherichia coli*. They are generally used for the primary isolation of microorganisms	Nutrient agar
Enriched media	This media is used to culture bacteria that needs extra nutrients. For example, blood, serum or egg yolk can be added to a simple media to make them an enriched media	Blood agar – often used to detect haemolysis Chocolate agar – contains heated blood
Selective media	This media is designed to allow the growth of a particular bacterium, while suppressing the growth of another bacterium	MacConkey agar – contains bile salts which inhibit most gram-positive bacteria Deoxycholate citrate agar – used for growing salmonella Sabouraud agar – used to grown fungi such as (ringworm)
Transport media	This media is used when specimens need to be transported immediately after collection. It helps to maintain the viability of the specimen	Stuarts transport medium – used for aerobic bacteria

Source: Vicky Milne.

Method for Inoculating an Agar Plate

To produce a bacterial culture, careful handling of both the sample and the agar plate is imperative; any artefacts could create unreliable results.

The method for inoculating an agar plate is as follows:

1) PPE should be worn.
2) The Petri dish should be clearly labelled; often, client name, case number and date are used as a minimum.
3) An inoculation loop should be heated in the flame of a Bunsen burner to sterilise it. The loop should then be left to cool for a few seconds in the air before being used. If the inoculating loop is too hot, it will destroy the bacteria in the sample.
4) The cooled, sterilised loop should be dipped into the sample.
5) The lid of the Petri dish should be removed, and the side containing the agar should be picked up. The sample should be smeared into a small well; care should be taken to keep the inoculating loop almost parallel to the surface of the agar to stop the loop from digging into the agar.
6) The inoculating loop should be heated again, using the same method as in step 3.
7) The inoculating loop should be placed on the edge of the well and used to make a set of short streaks, all going in the same direction, right angles from the initial well (Figure 8.24).
8) The inoculating loop should be heated again, using the same method as in step 3.
9) The inoculating loop should be placed on the edge of the first set of short streaks, and further streaks should be created at right angles.
10) The inoculating loop should be heated again, using the same method as in step 3.
11) The inoculating loop should be placed on the edge of the second set of streaks, and a third and final set of streaks should be created at right angles from the second streaks.
12) The lid should be replaced on the agar plate, and it should be put into an incubator upside down (agar side on top) at 37 °C.
13) The plate can be examined between 18 and 24 hours for bacterial growth (Figure 8.25). If there is no growth, it may need to be re-incubated for a further 18 hours.

Microscopic Analysis of Bacteria

Bacteriological examination of samples can be performed in practice or samples may also be sent away to an external laboratory.

There are three ways in which a bacterial smear can be prepared:

1) Directly from a swab, by rolling the swab directly onto a microscope slide.
2) From a liquid that is either pipetted onto the slide or put there using a sterile wire loop.
3) Directly from an agar plate, by removing a portion of the bacterial culture and mixing it with sterile saline.

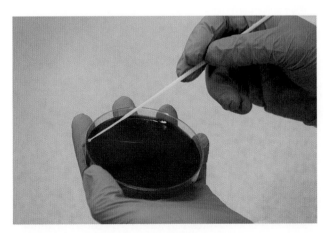

Figure 8.24 Inoculation of an agar plate with a bacterial sample. *Source:* Rosina Lillywhite with permission from Liphook Equine Hospital.

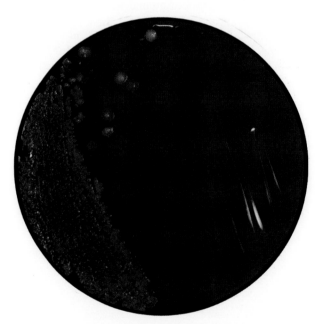

Figure 8.25 Bacterial growth on an agar plate. *Source:* Rosina Lillywhite with permission from Liphook Equine Hospital.

Examining the colony that has grown on the agar will firstly require a gross analysis, as different species of bacteria have their own characteristics. To further identify the bacteria, a smear should be made on a microscope slide. This should then be stained and examined with a microscope.

The method for producing a bacterial smear is as follows:

- Wear appropriate PPE (for bacteriology, this should include as a minimum: gloves, an apron, goggles and a facemask).
- Clean a microscope slide with a lint-free tissue and label it with the patient's details.
- Using a Bunsen burner, pass the slide through the flame.
- Using a sterile inoculating loop (using the same method as when plating onto agar), place one drop of water onto the slide.
- Using the same inoculating loop, collect a small portion of the bacterial culture that has been grown on the agar and place it onto the water drop on the slide.
- Mix the water and sample on the slide until it has been spread evenly.
- Allow the smear to air dry thoroughly.
- Once dried, the sample should be fixed by passing the slide through the flame of a Bunsen burner three times.

The slide can then be stained, which will aid in the identification of the type of bacteria cultured. Common stains to be used for bacteriology include methylene blue, and gram stain (see Tables 8.10 and 8.11). Methylene blue stain will colour the cells or the background so that the cells' size, shape and arrangement can be visualised. Gram-stained smears will highlight a difference between cells as follows:

- Gram-positive bacteria will stain blue/purple.
- Gram-negative bacteria will stain pink/red.

Table 8.10 Method for using Methylene blue stain on a bacterial smear.

Methylene blue stain
1) Wear suitable PPE
2) Place the microscope slide onto a staining rack
3) Cover the slide with 1% methylene blue stain
4) Leave for a minimum of two minutes
5) Hold over a sink at a 45% angle and rinse the smear with distilled water, then leave to dry standing vertically
6) The smear is now ready for examination using X100 objective with oil immersion

Source: Vicky Milne.

Table 8.11 Method for using Gram stain on a bacterial smear.

Gram stain
1) Wear suitable PPE
2) Place the bacterial smear onto a staining rack
3) Flood the smear with crystal violet for 30 seconds – 1 minute
4) Rinse the smear using tap water
5) Flood the smear with Gram's iodine for 30 seconds – 1 minute
6) Rinse the smear using tap water
7) Decolourise the smear using acetone for five seconds
8) Rinse the smear using tap water
9) Flood the smear with carbol fuchsin (or safranin) for 30 seconds – 1 minute
10) Rinse the smear using tap water
11) Air dry the smear
12) The smear is now ready for examination using X100 objective with oil immersion

Source: Vicky Milne.

See Chapter 6 for more information regarding gram-positive and gram-negative bacteria [1–3].

Antibiotic Sensitivity

Many bacteria are now resistant to some commonly used antibiotics, which means the drug is unable to destroy the bacteria. Therefore, if a bacterial infection is not responding as expected to a course of antibiotics, it is important to establish an effective treatment quickly, and antibiotic sensitivity testing can be performed to assist with this. For more information regarding antibiotic resistance, see Chapter 6.

To conduct antibiotic sensitivity testing, specialised discs impregnated with antibiotics are placed on the surface of an agar plate previously inoculated with a pure bacterial culture. This sample is then incubated for 18–24 hours before being removed and examined. If the bacteria are susceptible to the antibiotic, there will be a lack of bacterial growth near the disc, which indicates the antibiotic will be effective. If the bacteria are resistant to the antibiotic, bacteria will grow directly around the disc, which indicates the antibiotic would be ineffective (Figure 8.26). The vet can use the results of this test to prescribe an effective course of antibiotics and this in turn, helps to reduce the risk of antibiotic resistance developing [1–3].

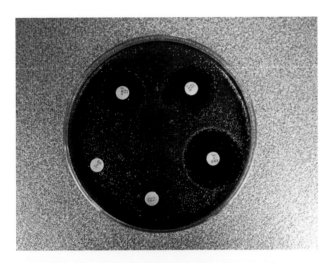

Figure 8.26 Antibacterial sensitivity plate. The organism was sensitive to three of the antibiotics (no growth zone around the disc) but resistant to the other two antibiotics (no zone of inhibition). *Source:* With permission from BSAVA Textbook of Veterinary Nursing 5th Edition. © BSAVA.

8.3 Commercial Test Kits

Deoxyribonucleic Acid (DNA) Testing

DNA profiling is carried out by breed registration authorities and is most commonly used to verify the pedigree of an animal. Each breed registration authority will have specific kits that they will send out to practice to facilitate sample collection. A number of different samples may be required including hair, blood, semen and buccal swabs [27].

Weatherby provides a range of genetic testing for both Thoroughbred and non-Thoroughbred horses. Genetic testing that can be carried out includes [28]:

- Coat colour screening: This can help to determine coat colour information from the genetic profile.
- Genetic trait testing: Helps to identify genes which can assist with making decisions around mating and breeding.
- Genomic testing: Helps to facilitate the breeding of healthier and more successful animals.
- Jaundice foal syndrome screening: This can help to diagnose and prevent this syndrome by checking the mare's blood and colostrum for the presence of dangerous antibodies to ensure the delivery of a healthy foal.
- Karyotyping: It helps to detect chromosomal abnormalities that may cause reproductive problems and prevent a successful pregnancy.
- Parentage verification: Used for Thoroughbreds and non-Thoroughbreds. This helps to obtain accurate parentage information.

- Pedigree allocation: Assists in the allocation of unknown parentage.

Weatherbys and other breed societies have clear guidelines that need to be followed carefully in order for the submission form and samples to be accepted. All guidelines should be read and followed carefully before the samples are collected.

SNAP© Tests

'SNAP' testing refers to a group of quick and convenient tests that can be performed anywhere, for example, out in a yard or at a veterinary practice (Figure 8.27). The most commonly used SNAP test in equine practice would be the SNAP∗Foal IgG. This is an enzyme immunoassay (EIA) for detecting immunoglobulin G (IgG). EIAs use an enzyme linked to an antibody to detect the antibody–antigen compound via enzymatic reactions. These tests are important when dealing with neonatal foals suspected of having a failure of passive transfer (see Chapter 15 for further information). On average, test results take seven minutes and are easy to interpret, meaning treatment can start immediately if required. SNAP kits must be stored at 2–8 °C before use. They can be used with whole blood, serum, or plasma. Contents of a kit include sample diluent, anti-equine IgG conjugate, SNAP foal IgG devices and sample loops [29].

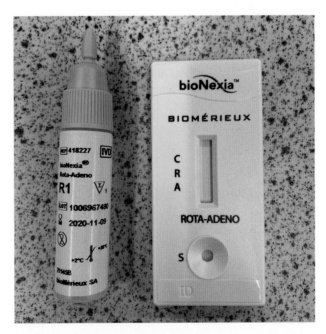

Figure 8.27 SNAP tests can be used anywhere for a quick and convenient diagnosis. *Source:* Vicky Milne. with permission from B&W Equine Hospital.

StableLab EQ-1 Handheld Reader

This handheld reader detects serum amyloid A (SAA), a protein produced by the liver and will rapidly increase in response to inflammation caused by infection. SAA readings can provide information relating to the severity of infection and these can be assessed quickly, often before any clinical signs develop and the horse's response to treatment can be monitored. The reader takes around 10 minutes to record a result, and it can be used on yards as well as in a hospital setting. This test can be run on whole blood, serum or plasma samples. The equipment needed to run the test includes an EQ-1 Reader and a Stablelab SAA cartridge, a pipette pack (used for serum samples) and BloodCaptor bulbs (used for whole blood) [30].

8.4 Causes of Sample Deterioration or Loss

Damage to samples, contamination to samples or incorrect paperwork can cause potential errors and inaccuracies in laboratory results. Within the veterinary laboratory, errors can occur at any stage of the process, including the pre-analytical, analytical and post-analytical stages. Most laboratory errors occur during the processing of samples, which is found in the pre-analytical stage.

Pre-analytical

- Incorrect test chosen.
- Incorrect preparation of the patient.
- Poor handling of the sample.
- Delay in running the laboratory test.
- Incorrect paperwork, including mislabelling of samples and incorrect sample location.

Analytical

- Spillage of samples.
- Contamination of the sample during testing.
- Errors with the laboratory equipment.

Post-analytical

- Incorrect recording of the laboratory results.
- Incorrect reporting/interpretation of the laboratory results.
- Delay in reporting the results.

This helps to emphasise how important attention to detail and adherence to correct storage and packing protocols is to obtaining the correct test results, which then facilitates correct and timely treatment for the patient in the first instance [1–3].

8.5 Packaging of Samples

It is common to send samples to external laboratories for analysis. It is important that samples are correctly packaged before being sent externally, as this will ensure that they arrive in an acceptable condition. Legal packing requirements for samples must be complied with [1].

Legal Packaging Requirements

Packaging regulations are in place to protect postal workers, transportation and laboratory staff. The sender is responsible for ensuring that samples are packaged correctly. The World Health Organisation (WHO) provides guidance for the transportation of pathological samples. Air transport regulations are the most restrictive; therefore, all packaging and shipping should comply with the international air transport association (IATA) regulations [1]. Most samples sent from veterinary practices to laboratories are classified as 'diagnostic substances' and fall under classification UN3373 (Category B infectious substances) [1]. Samples that fall under this classification must be packaged for transport according to the P650 or Packing Instruction 650 guidelines. According to P650 guidance, packaging must have the following components [1]:

- A primary receptacle containing the specimen.
- A secondary container or receptacle.
- Outer packaging with suitable cushioning or sturdy protective outer material for the sample being sent.

The packaging must also have the following qualities [1]:

- Capable to withstand a 1.2 m drop test.
- Capable to withstand internal pressure of 95 kilopascal (kPA).
- Be leakproof.
- Have enough absorbent material to absorb any leakages.
- Clearly show the words 'Diagnostic Specimen Licence no. UN3373' with a diamond-shaped mark (Figures 8.28 and 8.29).

External laboratories may provide practices with supplies, containers and packaging to use when sending samples for analysis. These may include [1]:

- Containers, including blood collection tubes and universal containers.
- Forms and paperwork.
- Absorbent material.

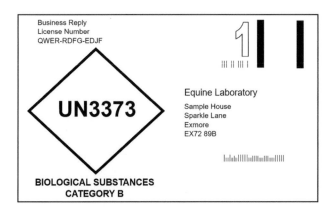

Figure 8.28 Example of address label on packaging for UN3373 (Category B infectious substances). *Source:* Rosina Lillywhite.

- Secondary layers such as a plastic biohazard bag and/or a polystyrene box.
- Tertiary layer, such as a padded bag or envelope.
- Labels for the tertiary layer including 'UN3373 Category B Infectious Material' together with a UN3373 symbol, laboratory address and space for the practice address.

Samples should be packaged carefully in a clean environment.

The suggested method for packing and posting samples is as follows [1]:

1) PPE should be worn to avoid contamination and exposure to potential zoonoses
2) The sample is to be checked to ensure it has been preserved correctly.
3) Ensure the container has been labelled with the animal's name, breed, age, sex, owner's name and date.
4) Ensure the container is airtight, moisture proof and robust.
5) Ensure the total volume or mass of the sample in one package does not exceed 50 ml or 50 g.
6) Wrap the container in sufficient absorbent material to absorb the total volume of fluid in the sample should there be a leak.
7) It is good practice to wrap the container in bubble wrap for extra protection.
8) Place the sample in the secondary bag and expel any excess air before sealing it.

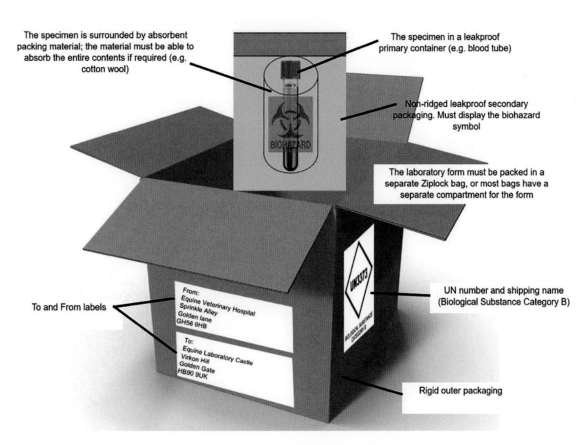

Figure 8.29 Example of packing and marking for Category B infectious substances. *Source:* Rosina Lillywhite.

9) Ensure that the laboratory paperwork and any additional forms have been fully completed. Place the paperwork in a plastic bag that is separate from the sample.

10) Place all items into the tertiary layer, such as a pre-paid padded bag supplied by the laboratory. Ensure that it is sealed securely.

11) Ensure the outer packaging contains the name and address of the sender.

12) Ensure the outer packaging states the nature of the sample and any special instructions such as 'handle with care', 'fragile' or 'pathological specimen'.

13) Ensure that the sample is sent by first-class post or via a courier.

When labelling samples and postage bags, a permeant, waterproof marker should be used.

8.6 Laboratory Sample Paperwork

Most external laboratories will supply paperwork for the completion and dispatch of samples being sent from different veterinary practices. Forms should include as standard [1]:

- Practice details and name of the case vet.
- Owner's name and address.
- Animal's name.
- Age and sex of animal.
- Test required.
- Date sample collected.
- Date sample despatched.
- Sample type.
- Sample site.
- Relevant history, clinical findings and therapy or treatment given.

Internal records of all samples processed 'in-house' or sent externally should be kept as a matter of good practice. Most veterinary practices either keep an online record or have a laboratory book where all samples that are to be sent to an external laboratory are recorded. Details to be recorded include:

- Date sample taken.
- Date sample posted.
- Patient identification (case number, owner and animal).
- Type of sample.
- Tests required.
- Name of case vet.
- Name of staff member who packaged the sample.

These details are important to be able to track samples and chase results if needed.

8.7 Laboratory Results

Results should be recorded on the clinical notes of a patient, carefully and accurately. Results should also be entered into the laboratory record book. Often, results from an external laboratory will be sent via email and can be downloaded to the patients' clinical records. Results from external laboratories may also include an interpretation of the results. The results should also be reported to the case vet, who requested the tests. Communication skills are important here, and test results should be reported quickly and efficiently to the appropriate vet. Senior RVNs should seek to assist newly qualified RVNs and student veterinary nurses (SVNs) with this to ensure that the process is standardised and successful across the nursing team.

Laboratory test results form part of the data upon which the case vet will make a clinical diagnosis or treatment decision [1]. Therefore, their clinical significance should be considered alongside any errors that may have occurred. All laboratory tests are subject to errors, and, if these occur, they should be identified and communicated to the case vet at the first possible instance [1]. It may be that the test will need to be repeated, and any unnecessary delay may affect the welfare of the patient being treated. It is important that RVNs have the knowledge to identify an inaccurate result or error so that the veterinary team can work together to rectify the error and amend the treatment programme for the patient in question.

References

1 Mullineaux, E. (2020). Veterinary laboratory equipment and techniques. In: *BSAVA Textbook of Veterinary Nursing*, 6e (ed. B. Cooper, E. Mullineaux, and L. Turner), 492–530. British Small Animal Veterinary Association: Gloucester.

2 Allan, L. and Ackerman, N. (2016). Laboratory diagnostic aids. In: *The Complete Textbook of Veterinary Nursing*, 3e (ed. V. Aspinall), 637–664. London: Elsevier.

3 Naylor, R.J., Hillyer, L.L., and Hillyer, M.H. (2012). Laboratory diagnostics. In: *Equine Veterinary Nursing Manual*, 2e (ed. K. Coumbe), 201–225. Oxford: Blackwell Science.

4 Health and Safety Executive. (2003). Safe working and prevention of infection in clinical laboratories and similar facilities [Online]. Available at: www.hse.gov.uk/pubns/clinical-laboratories.pdf (accessed 10 September 2022).

5 Health and Safety Executive. (2023) Health and Safety at Work Act 1974 [Online]. Available at: www.hse.gov.uk/index.htm (accessed 12 September 2022).

6 Health and Safety Executive. (2023). Control of substances hazardous to health (COSHH) [Online]. Available at: www.hse.gov.uk/coshh (accessed 10 September 2022).

7 DeltaNet. (2023). What is the Environmental Protection Act 1990? [Online]. Available at: https://www.delta-net.com/knowledge-base/health-and-safety/environmental-awareness/what-is-the-environmental-protection-act-1990 (accessed 1 September 2022).

8 http://Legislation.gov. (2023). The Hazardous Waste (England and Wales) Regulations 2005 [Online]. Available at: www.legislation.gov.uk/en/uksi/2005/894/made (accessed 1 September 2023).

9 Health and Safety Executive. (2023). Legislation – first aid at work [Online]. Available at: www.hse.gov.uk/firstaid/legislation.htm (accessed 10 September 2022).

10 Innovative Cleaning Services. (2023). Laboratory cleaning checklist [Online]. Available at: https://www.ics-oc.com/blog/laboratory-cleaning-checklist (accessed 10 September 2022).

11 University of Bristol. (2017) Using a microscope [Online]. Available at: www.bristol.ac.uk/media-library/sites/vetscience/documents/clinical-skills/Using%20a%20Microscope.pdf (accessed 12 September 2022).

12 Barrelet, A. and Ricketts, S. (2002). Haematology and blood biochemistry in the horse: a guide to interpretation. *In Practice* 24: 318–327.

13 Rossdales Veterinary Surgeons (2023). Haematology [Online]. Available at: https://www.rossdales.com/laboratories/tests-and-diseases/haematology (accessed 20 August 2023).

14 Liphook Equine Hospital. (2023). Haematology and biochemistry [Online]. Available at: https://liphookequinehospital.co.uk/equine-laboratory/laboratory-services/haematology-and-biochemistry (accessed 20 August 2023).

15 Corley, K. & Stephen. J. (2008). Chapter 19: Appendix. In: *The Equine Hospital Manual* (eds. K. Corley and J. Stephen), 670–684. West Sussex: Wiley-Blackwell.

16 Irwin Porter, G. (2012). Laboratory diagnostic aids. In: *BSAVA Textbook of Veterinary Nursing*, 5e (ed. B. Cooper, E. Mullineaux, L. Turner, and T. Greet), 508–535. BSAVA: Gloucester.

17 Rossdales Veterinary Surgeons. (2023). PPID diagnosis [Online]. Available at: https://www.rossdales.com/laboratories/guides/ppiddiagnosis#:∼:text=Pituitary%20Pars%20Intermedia%20Dysfunction%20(PPID)%20remains%20the%20most%20commonly%20diagnosed,inhibition%20of%20the%20pars%20intermedia (accessed 24 September 2023).

18 Rossdales Veterinary Surgeons. (2023). Diagnosing insulin dysregulation and equine metabolic syndrome [Online]. Available at: https://www.rossdales.com/laboratories/guides/diagnosing-insulin-dysregulation-equine-metabolic-syndrome (accessed 24 September 2023).

19 Rossdales Veterinary Surgeons. (2023). Urinalysis [Online]. Available at: https://www.rossdales.com/laboratories/tests-and-diseases/urinalysis (accessed 20 August 2023).

20 Rossdales Veterinary Surgeons. (2023). Pleural fluid [Online]. Available at: https://www.rossdales.com/laboratories/tests-and-diseases/pleural-fluid (accessed 31 January 2023).

21 Rossdales Veterinary Surgeons. (2023). Cerebrospinal (CSF) fluid [Online]. Available at: https://www.rossdales.com/laboratories/tests-and-diseases/cerebrospinal-csf-fluid (accessed 31 January 2023).

22 Rossdales Veterinary Surgeons. (2023). Skin disease: sampling [Online]. Available at: https://www.rossdales.com/laboratories/guides/skin-disease-sampling (accessed 24 September 2023).

23 Adams, W., England, G., Hanks, M., and Girling, S. (2012). Reproduction, and obstetric and paediatric nursing. In: *BSAVA Textbook of Veterinary Nursing*, 5e (ed. B. Cooper, E. Mullineaux, L. Turner, and T. Greet), 831. BSAVA: Gloucester.

24 Mair, T.S., Love, S., Schumacher, J. et al. (ed.) (n.d.). *Equine Medicine, Surgery and Reproduction*, 2e. London: Saunders Elsevier.

25 Davies Morel, M. (2021). *Equine Reproductive Physiology, Breeding and Stud Management*, 5e. Oxfordshire: CAIB.

26 Rossdales Veterinary Surgeons. (2023). Endometrial biopsy [Online]. Available at: https://www.rossdales.com/laboratories/tests-and-diseases/endometrial-biopsy (accessed 24 September 2023).

27 Munroe, G. (2012). Genetics. In: *Equine Veterinary Nursing Manual*, 2e (ed. K. Coumbe), 77. Oxford: Blackwell Science.

28 Weatherbys. (2023). Equine services [Online]. Available at: https://www.weatherbysscientific.com/our-services/equine#breeding-consultancy (accessed 10 May 2023).

29 IDEXX. (2023). SNAP foal IgG test [Online]. Available at: https://www.idexx.com/en/equine/in-house-diagnostics/snap-foal-igg-test (accessed 10 May 2023).

30 Zoetis. (2023). Zoetis adds Stablelab® handheld diagnostic test to its equine portfolio [Online]. Available at: https://news.zoetis.com/press-releases/press-release-details/2019/Zoetis-Adds-Stablelab-Hand-held-Diagnostic-Test-to-its-Equine-Portfolio (accessed 10 May 2023).

Further Reading

For further information on PPID and EMS visit: https://sites.tufts.edu/equineendogroup.

9

Pharmacology and Dispensary Management

Phillippa Pritchard[1], Rosina Lillywhite[2], and Marie Rippingale[3]

[1] *Liphook Equine Hospital, Liphook, Hampshire, UK*
[2] *VetPartners Nursing School, Greenforde Business Park, Petersfield, UK*
[3] *Bottle Green Training Ltd, Derby, UK*

Pharmacy Terminology and Abbreviations

Generic name – This is the active ingredient within the medicinal product, for example, phenylbutazone [1].

IM – Intramuscular: An injection of a medicinal product into a muscle.

IV – Intravenous: An injection of a medicinal product directly into the vein.

IVFT – Intravenous fluid therapy: Administering fluids via the intravenous route.

PO – Per os: This is Latin meaning 'by mouth' therefore, PO refers to the administration of a medicinal product by mouth.

PR – Per rectum: Administration of a medicinal product via the rectum for absorption via the mucous membranes.

Proprietary name – This is also known as the brand or trade name for the medicinal product. This is a name given by the drug company for marketing purposes, for example, Equipalazone [1].

q – Every: For example, q4 hours = every 4 hours.

S/C – Subcutaneous: An injection of a medicinal product into the subcutaneous layer of the skin.

SID – Once daily.

BID – Twice daily.

TID – Three times daily.

QID – Four times daily [1].

9.1 Legal Requirements for Storing and Supplying Veterinary Medicines

Three main pieces of legislation are relevant within the veterinary industry and play a pivotal role in ensuring the safe and responsible supply of veterinary medicines.

The Medicines Act 1968

This piece of legislation was the first comprehensive licensing system for medicines in the United Kingdom (UK); the law governs the manufacture and supply of drugs [2, 3]. Since the Medicines Act came into effect in 1968, multiple amendments have been made to ensure that the legislation is kept up to date [3].

The Medicines Act provides a system of licensing for manufacturing and dealing in medicines; the act also classifies medications into three categories:

- Prescription Only Medicines
- Pharmacy medicines
- General sales list [2–4]

Medicines controlled under the misuse of drugs legislation fall into prescription-only medications or pharmacy-only medications. Pharmacy arrangements are covered under this act, including pharmacy premises registration and protection of the terms 'Pharmacist' and 'Pharmacy' [5].

Veterinary medicines were removed from the scope of the Medicines Act when the Veterinary Medicines Regulations were introduced in 2013 [6]; enforcement of this Act rarely affects the general public [3].

Veterinary Surgeons Act 1966

The administration of medications by registered veterinary nurses (RVNs) is regulated under the Veterinary Surgeons Act 1966 (Schedule 3 Amendment) Order 2002. This states that only veterinary nurses registered with the Royal College of Veterinary Surgeons (RCVS) can administer medicines under the direction of a veterinary surgeon (vet). Student veterinary nurses (SVNs) enrolled with the RCVS for training can administer medication under the direct supervision of a vet or RVN [7, 8]. See Chapter 3 for more information on Schedule 3.

Veterinary Medicines Regulations 2013

In October 2013, the Veterinary Medicines Regulations were developed to regulate the manufacture, marketing, supply, advertising and classification of veterinary medicines and medicated feedstuffs [6]. In May 2024, significant changes to the Veterinary Medicines Regulations in the United Kingdom came into force, primarily through the Veterinary Medicines (Amendment etc.) Regulations 2024. These amendments updated the existing Veterinary Medicines Regulations 2013 to better align with current needs and practices, with a focus on improving regulatory oversight, reducing administrative burdens, and addressing antimicrobial resistance. Details of the Veterinary Medicines (Amendment etc.) Regulations 2024 can be found in the Further Reading section.

Legal Categories of Veterinary Medicines
Prescription-only-medicines: Veterinarian (POM-V) [5]
Only a vet can prescribe medications from this category. On 1st September 2023, the RCVS under care guidance changed. This meant that vets no longer had to carry out a physical assessment of an animal to take them 'under their care'. Under the new guidance published by the RCVS, a vet can accept an animal as 'under their care' when they are given and accept responsibility for it. Before prescribing a POM-V medication for an animal, the vet must carry out a clinical assessment. According to the new under care guidance, it is now up to the vet to decide whether this clinical assessment needs to include a physical examination or not, except for a number of circumstances which are as follows:

- Where a notifiable disease is suspected
- When prescribing controlled drugs (unless there are exceptional circumstances)
- When prescribing antibiotics, antifungals, antiparasitics or antivirals (unless there are exceptional circumstances*)

*NB The proximity of physical examination to prescribing will be slightly different depending on the species being treated)

Please see the Further Reading section for more information.

A written prescription is NOT required if the vet supplies the medication; however, clients with animals on long-term medications may request a written prescription to enable them to buy the medicines on the internet. Before prescribing the medication, the vet must be satisfied that the client or the person administering the medication (yard owner, for example) is going to administer the medication correctly. Therefore, they must assess the competency of the client before prescribing the medication.

- Updated lists of POM-V medications can be found on the veterinary medicines directorate (VMD) website at https://www.gov.uk/government/organisations/veterinary-medicines-directorate.

Veterinary medicinal products (VMPs) categorised as a POM-V often have one or more of the following:

- A new active ingredient
- Safety concerns
- It is deemed that veterinary knowledge is required for the use of the product
- The drug has a narrow safety margin
- Government policy

Medicated feedstuffs tend to now sit in the POM-V category [9].

Prescription-only Medicine – Veterinarian, Pharmacist or Suitably Qualified Person – (POM-VPS) [7]
- These medications can only be supplied by a Veterinarian, Pharmacist or a Suitably Qualified Person (SQP). The animal medicines training regulations authority (AMTRA) now use the term; registered animal medicines advisor (RAMA).
- The prescription can be in writing or oral, and a clinical assessment is not necessary.

A VMP is generally classified as a POM-VPS when it has the following characteristics:

- It is used to prevent endemic disease in herds, flocks or individual animals.
- There is some risk for the user, consumer, animal or environment. However, users can be advised of this by verbal or written instructions.
- Adequate training can be given for the regular use.

Non-food Animal Medicine – Veterinarian, Pharmacist, Suitable Qualified Person (NFA-VPS) [7]
- These medications can only be supplied by a Veterinarian, Pharmacist or a Suitably Qualified Person (SQP).
- The prescription can be in writing or oral, and a clinical assessment is not necessary.
- It must be a non-food-producing animal.

Authorised Veterinary Medicine – General Sales List (AVM-GSL)
- Any retailer may supply it; there is no restriction on their supply.

Table 9.1 Legal drug categories for veterinary medicines in the United Kingdom [9].

Classification	Meaning	Types of medicines	Examples
CD	Controlled drugs	Prescription-only medicines that are also classified under the Misuse of Drugs Regulations 2001	Opioid analgesics
POM-V	Prescription-only Medicines – Veterinarian	Medicines can be supplied with a valid prescription from a Veterinarian	Analgesics, antimicrobials
POM-VPS	Prescription-only medicines – Veterinarian, Pharmacist, Suitably Qualified Person	Medicines can be supplied with a valid prescription from a Veterinarian, Pharmacist or Suitably Qualified Person	Anthelmintics
NFA-VPS	Non-Food Animal – Veterinarian, Pharmacist, Suitably Qualified Person	Medicines can be supplied without a valid prescription from a Veterinarian, Pharmacist or Suitably Qualified Person	This category is not applicable to horses as they are considered to be a food-producing species. For cats and dogs, some topical ectoparasite treatments fit into this category
AVM-GSL	Animal Veterinary Medicine – General Sales List	Can be supplied by most retailers such as supermarkets and pet shops	Dietary supplements and insect repellents
SAES	Small Animal Exemption Schemes	Allows certain medicines to be sold without marketing authorisation for certain animals not intended for human consumption	Some anthelmintics for small animals

Source: Phillippa Pritchard.

- VMPs are placed in this category when:
  - There is a wide safety margin
  - They are used for common ailments
  - Special advice on their use is not required.

Table 9.1 summarises the legal categories of drugs in the United Kingdom.

Veterinary Medicines

Each medicine authorised for use within the United Kingdom has a marketing authorisation number (MAN); some animal medicines do not need market authorisation (MA), and some products are not considered animal medicines under the small animal exemption scheme (SAES), for example, animals that are exclusively pets. Poultry and equines are considered to be food-producing animals, so all medications would require a MAN even if the equine is considered to be a pet by the owner, and not intended for human consumption. If a product requires an MAN, then the producer would need to apply to the vto be a marketing authorisation holder (MAH). There are specific criteria that must be met to become a MAH. Products can be classified as either pharmaceutical or biological. Biological products contain substances from a biological source, for example, immunological medicines or medicines derived from blood or plasma. Pharmaceuticals, however, are chemically synthesised, and their structure is known.

MAH veterinarians can import medications licensed in other countries to treat their patients using the special import scheme (SIS). The imported medications are used on the prescribing cascade system described below using the SIS page on the VMD website [10, 11].

The Prescribing Cascade System

The cascade system provides guidance for vets on the authorised use of medications for treating animals. Each veterinary medicine is authorised for use to treat a specific condition or indication in a particular species or several species [12]. Details can be found on the datasheet provided with the product packaging, within the national office of animal health (NOAH) compendium or on the NOAH website.

The cascade system allows vets to use unlicensed medications required to prevent unnecessary suffering to their patients [7]. The cascade system displayed in Figure 9.1 must be followed. In this case, the term 'unlicenced' does not mean that the medication does not have a license but that it is not licensed for the condition that the vet is attempting to treat.

Vets are responsible for the choice of the product, and consent from the owner must be sought prior to the administration of treatment. The vet or a person acting under their direction must administer the medication. When using medications under the cascade system, the vet should

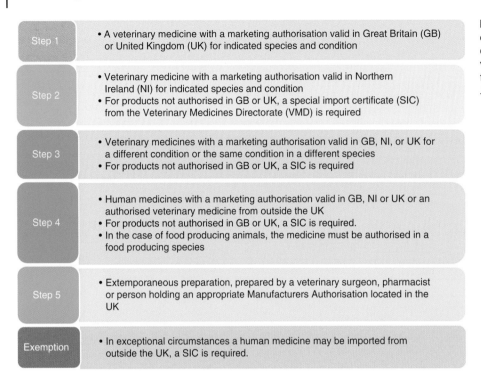

Step 1	• A veterinary medicine with a marketing authorisation valid in Great Britain (GB) or United Kingdom (UK) for indicated species and condition
Step 2	• Veterinary medicine with a marketing authorisation valid in Northern Ireland (NI) for indicated species and condition • For products not authorised in GB or UK, a special import certificate (SIC) from the Veterinary Medicines Directorate (VMD) is required
Step 3	• Veterinary medicines with a marketing authorisation valid in GB, NI, or UK for a different condition or the same condition in a different species • For products not authorised in GB or UK, a SIC is required
Step 4	• Human medicines with a marketing authorisation valid in GB, NI or UK or an authorised veterinary medicine from outside the UK • For products not authorised in GB or UK, a SIC is required. • In the case of food producing animals, the medicine must be authorised in a food producing species
Step 5	• Extemporaneous preparation, prepared by a veterinary surgeon, pharmacist or person holding an appropriate Manufacturers Authorisation located in the UK
Exemption	• In exceptional circumstances a human medicine may be imported from outside the UK, a SIC is required.

Figure 9.1 The steps in descending order of suitability for dispensing medications for veterinary surgeons in Great Britain following the cascade system [12]. *Source:* Phillippa Pritchard.

balance out the expected benefits to the animal with the risks of using medications under the cascade.

These should include risks to the following [12]:

- The animal
- The owner
- The person administering the medications
- To consumers of products from the treated animals, which may contain residues
- The environment
- The wider public health, such as increased antimicrobial resistance

Food-producing Animals

As a general rule in the United Kingdom, most horse owners consider their horses to be pets, but the Law sees them as food-producing animals; therefore, any medications that have no minimum inhibitory concentration (MIC) published must not be used in a horse intended for human consumption. Part II of Section IX of the equine passport allows the owner to permanently sign the horse out of the human food chain. This allows vets to administer unlicensed medications during illness. If a horse has already been signed out of the human food chain in their passport, a new owner cannot change this and decide the horse is then intended for human consumption. However, if a horse is designated for human consumption, a new owner can sign it out of the human food chain in the passport [13].

Regulatory Bodies

A regulatory body is a public organisation or government agency responsible for legally regulating aspects of human activity.

The role of the regulatory body is to establish and strengthen standards and ensure consistent compliance with them. Various regulatory bodies oversee the different sectors of veterinary medicine.

Department for environment, food and rural affairs (DEFRA) – is responsible for improving and protecting the environment, aiming to grow a green economy and supporting world-leading food farming and fishing industries. Their work contributes to sustainability, productivity and resilience in agriculture and also enhances biosecurity and raises standards of animal welfare. DEFRA also work alongside the food standards agency (FSA) to protect and improve human food safety [14].

The VMD – is an executive agency of DEFRA who contributes to the protection of public health and meeting high standards of animal welfare. The VMD also work closely with the FSA to protect and improve human food safety. The VMD are responsible for:

- Monitoring and taking action on reports of adverse events from veterinary medicines.
- Testing for residues of veterinary medicines or illegal substances in animals and animal products.
- Assessing applications for and authorising companies to sell veterinary medicines.

- Controlling how veterinary medicines are made and distributed.
- Advising the government ministers on developing veterinary medicines policy and putting it into action.
- Making, updating and enforcing UK legislation on veterinary medicines.

Other VMD priorities include influencing the development of revised legislation for veterinary medicines, medicated feedstuffs and residue surveillance and playing a leading role on antibiotic resistance in the United Kingdom and internationally [15].

Animal and plant health agency (APHA) – the APHA (APHA), formerly known as the animal health and veterinary laboratories agency (AHVLA), is an executive agency of DEFRA. The agency's main task is to protect the health and welfare of animals and the general public from disease. It conducts work across Great Britain on behalf of DEFRA, the Scottish Government and the Welsh Government. APHA provides vets with Vet Gateway, an online portal for vets to access APHA's services, systems, operating instructions, guidance, news and intelligence on new and re-emerging animal health threats [14].

RCVS – the statutory regulator under the Veterinary Surgeons Act 1966 responsible for keeping a register of vets and RVNs eligible to practice in the United Kingdom, setting standards for veterinary education and regulating the professional conduct of vets and RVNs and produce the professional codes of conduct that all vets and RVNs must follow. Their Royal Charter allows them to award fellowships and certificates [16].

RCVS Knowledge is a separate charity that was established to promote and advance the study of veterinary medicine by providing grants to support educational and research activities [16].

AMTRA – is a non-profit organisation that is appointed by the secretary of state to keep its register of RAMAs also known as SQPs. As well as keeping the register, AMTRA can instigate disciplinary processes should anyone fail to follow the code of practice and keep records of a mandatory system of continuing professional development (CPD). AMTRA work with Harper Adams University to develop and maintain a qualification syllabus that meets the requirements of the Secretary of State [7]. To remain on the AMTRA list of RAMAs CPD must be undertaken; this is logged-in points through AMTRA-accredited CPD options. If the equine-only pathway is completed, the post-nominals J-SQP can be used. People registered as J-SQPs are required to accumulate 30 CPD points and also pay an annual fee to remain on the register [7].

Vetpol Ltd – offers online training for SQPs via the awarding body LANTRA; the VMD has appointed Vetpol as an independent regulator of SQPs [6]. An SQP who is registered with Vetpol must carry out 3 hours of CPD per year. If qualified as an equine-only SQP, an annual fee must also be paid to remain on the register [17, 18].

VetSkill Ltd – is part of The office of qualifications and examinations regulation (Ofqual) and the council for the curriculum, examinations & assessment (CCEA) approved awarding organisation providing a variety of courses for the veterinary industry [20]. SQPs registered with VetSkill must carry out 5 hours of CPD per year if qualified as an equine-only SQP and pay an annual fee to remain registered [19].

Table 9.2 Summarises the CPD requirements for registered SQPs under the different awarding organisations.

Storage Requirements and Dispensary Management

All medications have a data sheet or a summary of product characteristics (SPCs) sheet. These documents contain details of storage for the medication. When searching for a data sheet for a medication, either the NOAH website, app or printed text can be used [20]. NOAH provides the following information for all medications listed within the compendium:

Qualitative and quantitative composition:

- Pharmaceutical form
- Clinical particulars
- Pharmacological particulars
- Pharmaceutical particulars
- Marketing Authorisation Holder (if different from distributor)
- Marketing Authorisation Number
- Significant changes
- Date of the first authorisation or date of renewal
- Date of revision of the text
- Any other information
- Legal category
- Global trade item number (GTIN)

Medication Storage

Proper medication storage is critical when working within a pharmacy. It is essential to know the temperature ranges specified within the data sheets, which can be found under pharmaceutical particulars. Correct storage prevents damage or inactivation of the products.

Considerations for temperature ranges are as follows:

- Some medicines require storage between 2 and 8 °C. Products can be irreversibly degraded if the temperature goes outside of this range, even briefly, so monitoring storage temperature is vital.
- The temperature of any refrigerators being used to store veterinary medicines should be monitored daily.

Table 9.2 Summary of CPD requirements for SQPs [5, 17–19].

Species	SQP code	AMTRA	VetSkill	Vetpol
Companion, Equine + Farm	R	80 points in 2 years	15 h (10 h CPD/5 h personal study)	6 h per year (3 for RVNs)
Farm + equine	G	60 points in 2 years	10 h (5 h CPD/5 h personal study)	5 h per year (2.5 for RVNs)
Farm + companion	K	60 points in 2 years	10 h (5 h CPD/5 h personal study)	5 h per year (2.5 for RVNs)
Equine + companion	E	50 points in 2 years	10 h (5 h CPD/5 h personal study)	5 h per year (2.5 for RVNs)
Farm only	L	50 points in 2 years	5 h per year	3 h per year (1.5 for RVNs)
Equine only	J	30 points in 2 years	5 h per year	3 h per year (1.5 for RVNs)
Companion only	C	30 points in 2 years	5 h per year	3 h per year (1.5 for RVNs)
Avian only	A	30 points in 2 years	5 h per year	3 h per year (1.5 for RVNs)
Companion + avian	CA	40 points in 2 years	10 h (5 h CPD/5 h personal study)	5 h per year (2.5 for RVNs)
Equine + avian	JA	40 points in 2 years	10 h (5 h CPD/5 h personal study)	5 h per year (2.5 for RVNs)
Equine, companion + avian	EA	60 points in 2 years	15 h (10 h CPD/5 h personal study)	6 h per year (3 for RVNs)
Avian and farm	AL	Not applicable (N/A)	10 h (5 h CPD/5 h personal study)	5 h per year (2.5 for RVNs)
Companion, avian + Farm	CAL	N/A	15 h (10 h CPD/5 h personal study)	6 h per year (3 for RVNs)
Avian Equine + farm	S	N/A	15 h (10 h CPD/5 h personal study)	6 h per year (3 for RVNs)
Companion, equine, avian + farm	XA	N/A	15 h (10 h CPD/5 h personal study)	7 h per year (3.5 for RVNs)

Source: Phillippa Pritchard.

A maximum/minimum thermometer should be used and this should be read and reset daily. All temperatures should be recorded. Continuous data loggers to monitor the temperature are now widely used as these are convenient. However, these should only be used if an audible alarm or flashing light alarm alerts the user to temperatures deviating from the required range. Weekly downloading of the temperatures into graph format is helpful to determine trends in temperature fluctuations. The problem with this is that without an alarm system, deviations from the required ranges will not be noticed until the data is downloaded. Data from these systems should be downloaded at least weekly [5].

- Some medicines require storage at temperatures below 15 °C. Since most practices do not have a cool room, a refrigerator would provide appropriate storage for such products, provided storage below 8 °C does not affect the medicine.
- Medicines that require storage at 25 °C or below can usually be stored at room temperature. Depending on the location of the pharmacy within the practice and the environmental temperatures reached, air conditioning may be required to maintain a stable ambient temperature. The ambient temperature must be monitored and recorded to ensure that the pharmacy meets the RCVS practice standards scheme (PSS) requirements [16].

- Excessive heat (greater than 40 °C) may be a cause for concern for ambulatory vets as temperatures within the car are often much higher than the ambient temperature [16]. Steps must be taken to ensure that the storage requirements are maintained even when stored in vehicles. Each vehicle must have a working fridge complete with temperature monitors. Insulated medication storage boxes should be used to minimise the temperature increase in extremely hot weather, and minimum and maximum thermometers should be used to monitor the temperature of vehicles and the medications kept within them.
- Light-sensitive medications should be stored in coloured bottles, and if dispensed in smaller quantities, they should be dispensed in coloured bottles [21].

Controlled Drugs

The Misuse of Drugs Regulations (2001) is associated with medications classified as controlled drugs (CD). These drugs have a high chance of misuse, abuse or addiction. There are five schedules within the controlled drug classifications; each has specific requirements for requisition, storage, record keeping, prescribing and disposal. CDs are available for use in veterinary medicine but may only be prescribed by a vet and supplied by a vet or a pharmacist [7, 22].

Schedule 1

- These drugs have little or no therapeutic value and are under the strictest control.
- These are the drugs that are most likely to be abused, and they include lysergic acid diethylamide (LSD), heroin and cannabis.
- Vets have no authority to possess or prescribe these drugs.
- The Home Office may agree to a vet using these medicines for research purposes; however, appropriate permissions must be obtained in the first instance [22].

Schedule 2

- These drugs have much therapeutic value but are highly addictive and, therefore, subject to abuse.
- These drugs are subject to strict prescription, dispensing, destruction and record-keeping requirements.
- These include morphine, pethidine, fentanyl, ketamine and quinalbarbitone.
- The requisition must be made in writing to the supplier and signed by a vet. The requisition itself can be typed, but the vet's signature must be signed in ink, and their RCVS number will also be required.
- These drugs must be stored in a locked, permanently secured cabinet which can only be opened by vets or personnel authorised by them. A communal key in one draw is NOT acceptable.
- A CD register must be maintained, recording all purchases and each individual supply within 24 hours.
- Destruction must take place in the presence of a person authorised by the Secretary of State, such as a vet from another practice or a police officer (for more information, see below on disposal of drugs).
- All invoices must be kept for two years [22].

Schedule 3

- These drugs also have therapeutic value, but the potential for abuse is reduced. They are, therefore, subject to fewer strict requirements compared with Schedule 2 drugs.
- Includes pentobarbital, phenobarbital, buprenorphine and midazolam.
- Subject to the same prescription and requisition requirements as Schedule 2.
- These drugs do not need to kept in a register as with Schedule 2.
- Buprenorphine MUST be kept in a locked cabinet; however, it is advised that all Schedule 3 drugs are locked away.
- All invoices must be kept for two years [7].

Schedule 4

- These drugs are not subject to safe custody or recording requirements and include diazepam, clenbuterol and anabolic steroids.
- These drugs are exempt from most restrictions of CDs.
- All invoices must be kept for two years [5].

Schedule 5

- These drugs are exempt from all requirements other than all invoices must be kept for two years.
- They include some preparations containing codeine or morphine in small amounts [7, 22].

Special Cases

Quinalbarbitone

- This drug is currently classified as a Schedule 2 CD, but it does not require safe custody (i.e. it does not need to be kept in the CD cabinet). However, it is good practice to keep it secure.
- It does need to be recorded in a CD Register [5].

Buprenorphine

- This drug is classified as a Schedule 3 CD, and its use does not need to be recorded in the CD Register, but safe custody does apply (i.e. it does need to be kept locked in a CD cabinet) [5].

Midazolam

- Midazolam has been moved from Schedule 4 to Schedule 3, and therefore, prescription requirements apply.
- It does not need to be kept in the CD cabinet although the RCVS recommends that all Schedule 3 CDs are kept in the CD cabinet. Recording in a CD register is not required [5].

Dispensary Management

Management of the dispensary may fall under the remit of RVNs, although larger practices may have a dedicated pharmacy manager. Managing the dispensary involves ensuring that the correct drug is available in the correct strength, and in sufficient quantities, to cater for the practice caseload. Pharmacy duties and stock levels will vary from practice to practice. It can be a balancing act when deciding on stock levels within the pharmacy. Enough stock should be available without having too much capital tied up in that stock. This will ensure there is minimal wastage from having out-of-date stock within the practice [23].

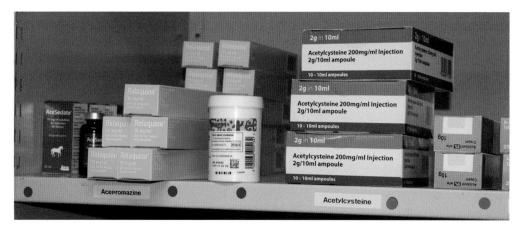

Figure 9.2 Appropriately labelled shelves in pharmacy. *Source:* Rosina Lillywhite.

Best practice for pharmacy management includes the following:

- Set stock levels to allow accurate stock holding.
- Have a named person responsible for stock control.
- Storing medicines in a logical order in the original packaging; it is ideal to organise the pharmacy alphabetically. It makes the most sense to use the active ingredient for this as then, when the trade name changes due to a change in supplier, it does not upset the order of the shelves [22] (see Figure 9.2).
- Supplying a product leaflet or SPC with all dispensed medicines; these can also be supplied in electronic form.
- Dispense medicines with the shortest expiry date first and rotate the stock at the point of every delivery. For example, put the new stock behind the old stock to ensure that medicines do not go out of date.
- Store medicines with the same batch number and expiry date together.
- Record batch numbers and expiry dates of dispensed medications on the animal/client records [23].

Vetsafe

The Veterinary Defence Society (VDS) has launched Vetsafe. This is a confidential significant event reporting service that is used for quality improvement purposes and to aid in risk management in veterinary practice. This involves a log of incidences of patient harm or other losses and also near misses in practice. It is essential to understand that even highly trained and motivated professionals make mistakes. The aim of VetSafe is to help practices learn from mistakes without allocating blame or judgement on co-workers [24]. VetSafe can:

1) Help clinicians to understand why mistakes happen
2) Help practices develop solutions to improve the quality of care

3) Share learning
4) Help practices track significant events and comply with the RCVS PSS
5) Support second victims – clinicians involved in mistakes [24]

Pharmacovigilance

According to the World Health Organisation (WHO), pharmacovigilance is the science relating to detecting, assessing, understanding and preventing adverse effects or any other medicine/vaccine-related problem [25].

The VMD are responsible for obtaining information from veterinary professionals, members of the public and pharmaceutical companies on adverse reactions. The information received is vital in monitoring the safety of veterinary medicines and identifying previously unknown hazards or side effects [24].

For a product to remain authorised for use, the benefits of administering the product must outweigh the risk of suffering reactions; if the risks outweigh the benefits, the product will be removed from the market. The adverse reaction reports allow the VMD to assess the risks and act appropriately, including updating the product literature with potential side effects [24].

Record Keeping

The CD section above covers record keeping for CDs. Plenty of other records are to be kept within veterinary practice.

POM-V and POM-VPS drugs: records must be kept, including incoming and outgoing transactions to include:

- Date of receipt and supply, which includes administration by the vet.
- Name and quantity of the VMP.
- Name and address of the supplier or recipient.

- If there is a written prescription, the name and address of the person who wrote the prescription and a copy of the prescription.
- Batch number (for products used for non-food producing animals, the batch number only needs to be recorded either on the date of receipt of the batch or the date the batch is first supplied or used).
- The purpose of recording batch numbers is to provide traceability of specific batches of products. This is intended to provide a basis for effective recall of a batch or batches of a product should this become necessary and provide traceability of the use of medicines in food-producing animals.
- Whether or not the cascade has been used [5].

All the above records should be kept for a minimum of five years [7].

Drug Use and Dispensing

When supplying POM-V medicines, they should be dispensed with an appropriate label with the following information:

- Name and address of the owner
- Name and address of the approved premises
- Date of supply
- Keep out of reach of children
- For animal treatment only
- For external use only
- Name, quantity, strength and directions for the use of the product [7]

Broached Vials

The broach date for vials should adhere to the information found on the datasheet. Most vials are to be used within 28 days of first broaching; however, some time periods are shorter. For example, reconstituted Excenel should be used within 7 days of first being broached and should be kept in the fridge thereafter [7, 20].

Out-of-date Stock

It is illegal to supply or administer a medicine after the expiry date detailed on the packet or to obscure the expiry date on the packaging of any medicine. Requirements in the European Union (EU) and national legislation to ensure the stability and safety of the products, mean that some products, such as injectables, have an in-use shelf-life. This is the timeframe in which a drug must be used after it has been broached, and this must remain within the expiry date of the drug. The following points should be followed in relation to out-of-date stock [26]:

- For most multidose injectables, the in-use shelf-life is usually, but not always, 28 days, thus making it an offence to administer the product 28 days after the first day of broaching. Multidose vials should be marked with the date of broaching and use-by date.
- Bright-coloured stickers can be helpful to draw attention, but all multidose vials with an in-use shelf-life now have a space to write this information on the bottle.
- Any medicine left in the vial after the specified time must be discarded. The required dose should be withdrawn immediately, and the remainder disposed of for single-use ampoules.
- Oral liquids should generally be disposed of six months after opening.
- When date checking, the short-dated stock should be marked and brought to the front of the shelf to be used first.
- Any stock that has gone out of date should be separated and details should be recorded before disposal.

CDs

All CDs must be destroyed by denaturing to render them irretrievable, but only the destruction of Schedule 2 CDs requires independent witnessing. There are commercially available denaturing kits used to destroy out-of-date stock CDs and returned CDs. These kits contain granules that react with liquids to form a solid gel. Drugs in liquid form should be removed from ampoules and vials and poured into the denaturing kit. Fentanyl patches can be folded upon themselves and placed in the gel with everything else, and tablets should be crushed, mixed with water and added to the gel [22].

The container should then be stored in a locked cabinet for 24 hours to allow the gel to solidify. The container is then sent as pharmaceutical waste through the practice waste contractor. Residual CDs are not usually denatured in this way because their destruction is required daily, which would prove too costly. Instead, residual drugs can be rendered irretrievable by collection into cat litter. Periodically, this cat litter is sent to the waste contractor as pharmaceutical waste [5, 22].

CDs may be presented for destruction in three different circumstances:

- Residual or waste drug – a whole ampoule of a CD (e.g. 10 mg morphine) is dispensed to a patient, but only 5 mg is administered to the patient, and the remainder is denatured. The amounts administered and denatured are recorded on the same line of the CD register to ensure the whole vial is accounted for. Double signing is good practice. This does not have to be witnessed by an independent person.
- Out-of-date drug stock. Destruction of out-of-date stock falls under the Misuse of Drugs Regulations (2001) and must be witnessed. This includes expired 'in-use

shelf-life' (e.g. a part-used bottle of methadone which has been open for more than 28 days). The expired stock should be kept in the cabinet, labelled appropriately and separated from in-date drugs. It should not be marked out of the running balance in the CD register until it is destroyed.

- For Schedule 2 CDs, the destruction must be witnessed by an RCVS Assessor or VMD inspector, a controlled drug liaison officer (CDLO) from the police force (a list of CDLOs can be found on the Association's website) or an independent vet.
- In order to be considered independent of the practice, another vet must have no personal, professional or financial interest in the practice where the drug is destroyed (i.e. locum team members or family members cannot do this).
- The independent vet must not be paid to witness the denaturing, apart from reasonable travel expenses. The RCVS number of the independent vet should be recorded in the CD register.
- For Schedule 3, 4 and 5 CDs, destruction does not need to be witnessed by an independent witness, but it is good practice to have it witnessed by another team member [5].
- Returned drug: The drug has been dispensed to a patient; there is no requirement to have the destruction of this drug witnessed or recorded. However, it is good practice to witness it with another staff member [22].

9.2 The Role of the Suitably Qualified Person – SQP

What is an SQP/RAMA?

An SQP or RAMA has undergone training to advise and prescribe some veterinary medicines under the Veterinary Medicines Regulations (2013). SQPs are commonly employed in pet shops, feed merchants and veterinary practices to allow non-veterinarians to prescribe selected products [27]. Each SQP must complete a base module and exam for each species that they want to prescribe for, the exams that must be passed as well as an oral exam [27]. Each awarding body allocates a code to denote what area of study the SQP has carried out; for example, an AMTRA SQP who has studied equine only is a J-SQP if they have undertaken equine and small animal they would be an E-SQP [7]. Typically, RVNs can just take the species-specific written and oral exam to avoid duplication of previous training. The current categories of SQP are:

- R-SQP: All animals
- C-SQP: Companion animals only
- J-SQP: Equines only
- L-SQP: Farm animals only
- A-SQP: Avian only
- E-SQP: Companion & Equines only
- K-SQP: Companion & Farm only
- CA-SQP: Companion & Avians only
- G-SQP: Equines & Farm only
- JA-SQP: Equines & Avians only
- EA-SQP: Companion, Equines & Avians only

The SQP qualification is now part of some RVN qualifications. If this is the case, specific SQP practical examinations will need to be passed to gain the qualification [27].

Duties and Responsibilities of an SQP

A SQP can dispense POM-VPS, NFA-VPS and AVM-GSL medications; they must follow the SQP code of conduct produced by the VMD [24]. SQPs like RVNs are not permitted to diagnose conditions. They are, however, permitted to identify a parasite and prescribe appropriate treatment. SQPs are not permitted to prescribe POM-V medications but can dispense them under the direction of a vet. An SQP must not split packaging; for example, they are not allowed to dispense loose tablets or a split a container of liquid (unless under the direction of a vet). A SQP can dispense part boxes of blister packs as the inner packaging is not broached, and a data sheet or leaflet is placed in with the part pack [20].

In order to dispense a medication, an SQP must [19, 34]:

- Ensure that the person giving the treatment is competent.
- Check the age, sex, weight, lifestyle and temperament of the patient as well as previous treatments.
- Make sure that medications are prescribed on a patient-by-patient basis.
- Ensure that owners are made aware of contraindications and/or warnings
- Provide a written prescription on request that contains the following information:
- Record the name, address and telephone number of the person prescribing the product
- Record the qualifications and registration enabling the person to prescribe the product
- Record the name and address of the owner/keeper of the animal(s)
- Record the identification of the animal, including species being treated
- Record the details of the premises that the animal is kept at if different from the owner/keeper
- Record the date of prescription

- Provide a signature if they are prescribing the product or check the signature of the prescriber if they are dispensing the product
- Record the name and amount of the product prescribed
- Record the dosage and administration instructions
- Record the any necessary warnings
- Record the withdrawal period (for food-producing animals) even if this is nil
- Record the batch number of the product
- Record the the reason for prescribing the product

A vet providing a written prescription should include all of the information above and a statement if it is being prescribed under the cascade. SQPs cannot prescribe medicines off license in this way. Prescriptions are valid for six months from the date of prescription unless the prescriber specifies a shorter period [19].

Anyone altering a written prescription without authorisation to do so is committing an offence. If a supplier doubts the validity of a prescription, they should contact the prescriber to check [10].

The VMRs apply to online pharmacies as well as over-the-counter sales, and internet retailers should be accredited with the VMD accredited internet retailer scheme (AIRS). Retailers are then able to display the VMD logo on their website [28].

The RCVS states that a vet may make a reasonable charge for written prescriptions. However, the client should be given sufficient information on medicine prices and informed of any significant changes to the prescription charges at the earliest opportunity. Vets are advised to direct their clients to online retailers under AIRS for the supply of veterinary medicines [12].

Supplying Medicines Prescribed by Other Registered Qualified Persons (RQP), Including Non-SQPs

When supplying medicines that a different RQP has prescribed from separate premises, an SQP must:

- Only supply the product specified on the prescription.
- Ensure that the RQP who wrote the prescription has the correct qualifications to prescribe it.
- Check that the prescription is suitable for the condition; if there is any doubt, then the prescriber should be contacted before the supply.
- Ensure that the medicine is supplied to the person named on the prescription.

An SQP cannot supply a substitute product to the one on the prescription. If the SQP cannot honour the prescription with the exact medication or disagrees with the prescription, they can refuse the supply request [19].

If the RQP is within the same premises, they can delegate the supply of the medicines to a colleague so long as [19]:

- They have the prescribed or supplied medicine.
- They have checked that the medicine has been correctly selected from stock.
- They have set the medicine aside for the customer.
- They are satisfied that the person dispatching the product is competent to do so.

Code of Practice

The SQP code of practice developed by the VMD is updated periodically. It details legislation that must be followed by SQPs as well as registration bodies. The code also details the requirements for prescriptions and supply of medicines, prescription details and record keeping for SQPs [19].

Requirements of Registered Premises

The VMD has produced a set of criteria for registered premises that can supply veterinary medicines. These are as follows:

- The premises must be approved and registered with the VMD.
- SQPs listed must be listed on the current SQP register.
- The qualifications of the SQPs present must be appropriate for the product range to be supplied.
- The premises must be a permanent building with a fixed address.
- It must be secure from unauthorised access.
- Must have facilities to enable veterinary medicines storage requirements to be met.
- Have measures in place to prevent pests from entering.
- Have veterinary medicines storage areas separated from food/drink areas for human consumption and from toilet and washroom areas.
- Clients must not be able to self-serve veterinary medicines except those under the AVM-GSL category, homeopathic remedies and those under the SAES [29].

Requirements for Packaging and Labelling of Veterinary Medicines

According to the RCVS, the phrase 'under their care' is interpreted as:

- The vet has the responsibility for the health of the animal by the owner or agent.
- The responsibility must be real and not nominal.
- The animal must have been seen immediately before prescription or recently enough for the vet to have personal knowledge of the animal's condition or its current health

status to enable a diagnosis. What amounts to recent enough must be a matter for the professional judgement of the vet.

- The vet must maintain clinical records for that herd/individual [29].

As per the cascade system described previously, the vet should prescribe a medicine for use in the target species, for the condition being treated and used at the dosage recommended by the manufacturer. Where no such medicine is available and to avoid unnecessary suffering, the vet can treat the animal with other medicines following the cascade [29].

If there is not an appropriate product for food-producing animals, the cascade is still able to be used with the following conditions:

- The treatment in any particular case is restricted to animals on a single holding.
- Any medicine imported from another country must be authorised for use in a food-producing species in that country.
- The active substance contained must be listed in the register as part of the VMDs product database.
- The vet responsible for prescribing the medicine must specify a withdrawal period and keep specified records [29].

Recommended Containers for Veterinary Medicines

Vets can only supply veterinary medicines from a premises that is registered with the RCVS as a 'veterinary practice premises', in accordance with the VMR. The VMD is responsible for ensuring compliance with the VMR, including registering, and inspecting veterinary practice premises. Newly registered premises will be inspected within six months of registering. The frequency of further inspections is determined using a risk-based approach, with the most compliant premises inspected every four years. However, less compliant premises may be inspected more frequently. If a practice is a member of the PSS, then a practice standards inspector will be responsible for ensuring that the practice is compliant with the VMR during the PSS inspection [16]. Inspectors will check that medications are stored and dispensed correctly. Some medicines are adversely affected by light, temperature, humidity and rough handling [5].

- Tablets should be dispensed in original packaging if possible. If loose tablets or capsules are repackaged from a bulk container, then they should be dispensed in child-resistant containers, and a package insert should be supplied. Tablets in blister packs can be dispensed in original

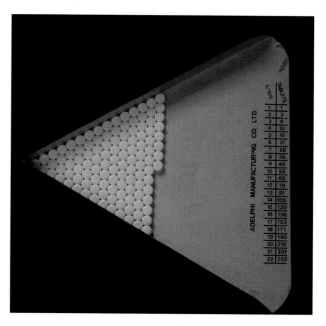

Figure 9.3 Pill counter in use. *Source:* Rosina Lillywhite.

packaging or a similar cardboard box. If bulk packages are to be broached, the tablets should be dispensed in a suitable container with a child-proof lid, a tablet counter should be used, and the tablets should not be handled without gloves.

Figure 9.3 shows a pill counter being used. 14 full rows is 105 tablets + 8 single tablets = 113 tablets altogether.

- Preparations for external application should be dispensed in coloured fluted bottles.
- Oral preparations should be dispensed in glass bottles with child-resistant closures; medications that are adversely affected by light should be dispensed in amber bottles instead [5].

Precautions When Handling Medicines

Cytotoxic Drugs

Cytotoxic drugs or antineoplastics are widely used in treating cancers; they contain toxic chemicals to cells, preventing replication or growth. The toxicity of these drugs means they present a significant risk to those who handle them; exposure can occur through the following:

- Skin contact or absorption
- Inhalation of aerosols and drug particle
- Ingestion
- Needle stick injuries [2, 5]

Under the Control of Substances Hazardous to Health (COSHH) regulations (2002), employers must create a risk assessment for cytotoxic drugs evaluating the risks and decide on appropriate measures to control employee exposure to these substances [2].

Control measures to reduce exposure can include:

- Reducing the number of employees that may be exposed as well as keeping their exposure to a minimum.
- Safe handling and storage of medicines and disposal of equipment used into appropriate containers (purple-lidded containers), good hygiene and appropriate training.
- Personal protective equipment (PPE) should be provided appropriately for the medications being used.
- A risk assessment is carried out in practice [22].

In equine practice, the most commonly used cytotoxic medication is mitomycin C eye drops. This medication slows down the division of cells and destroys cells that are rapidly dividing [42].

Product Labelling

A veterinary medicine label used by an SQP should include the following information:

- The owner's name and address
- Identification of the animal
- Date of supply and the expiry date
- Product name and strength
- Total quantity of the product supplied in the container
- Instructions for dosage
- Name of prescribing veterinary surgeon
- Specific pharmacy precautions, including storage, disposal and handling
- The wording 'Keep out of reach of children' and 'For animal treatment only'
- Withdrawal period
- And other necessary warnings
- 'For external use only' should be included on products for topical use [27]

All labels should be typed. If the information will not fit on one label, then an extra information sheet is permissible. To comply with the current VMR, records of all products supplied on prescription must be kept for five years. Batch numbers should be recorded on purchase and delivery to the practice, but it is not necessary to record the batch number of each medication supplied to an animal [7].

Information that Should be Provided to a Client Concerning the Administration of Medicines

Storge requirements for clients should be present on the dispensing label, such as 'keep out of reach of children' and 'for animal use only'. Other storage requirements are present on the data sheets that should be dispensed with the medication, and the owner is encouraged to read about the medication before administering it to the patient. Also,

present on the datasheet are precautions to take when handling the medication under the heading 'clinical particulars' and disposal of residual medications found under the heading 'pharmaceutical particulars'. These should be verbally communicated to the client and informed that the information is on the data sheet provided [7].

Demonstrating Techniques for Clients

The most common medications clients would be expected to administer are PO or oral medications. These can come in the form of tablets, capsules, liquids, suspensions, granules or powders. Often, these are administered directly into feeds, but some medications are less palatable than others, so it is not uncommon to need to administer this via a dosing syringe or catheter-tipped syringe (CTS). Details of suitable solutions to mix medications with should be explained to the client. If the patient has metabolic disorders, high-sugar solutions such as molasses should be avoided. The technique for correctly mixing the medication should also be explained to the client to facilitate effective administration. Some tablets may be placed in a piece of apple or carrot. It is important to make the administration of medication a positive one for the patient, especially if it is part of a long-term treatment programme [5].

It is unlikely that a client would be expected to IV injections but asking a client to administer IM injections is not uncommon. Usually, this would involve administering hormones (oxytocin) or some antibiotics. It is important to ensure that the client receives training relating to the correct injection site/sites for the medication. Photos can provide a visual reference for clients to refer to. However, the first injection should be in the presence of a RVN or a vet to ensure that the client is confident in administering the medication safely. The disposal of needles and syringes should be discussed, and a plan should be put into place to make sure that they are disposed of correctly [7]. For further information regarding correct injection sites and techniques, please see Chapter 17.

Calculations for Drug Doses

RVNs may be required to calculate drug doses. Drug calculations must be worked out carefully to ensure that the correct dose is administered to the patient. The formula required to work out doses for medications is as follows [30]:

$$\text{Dose} = \frac{\text{Bodyweight (kg)} \times \text{Doserate (mg/kg)}}{\text{Concentration}\left(\frac{\text{mg}}{\text{ml}} \text{ or mg/tab}\right)}$$

Example 1   Oral medication [31]

The vet has prescribed a 14-day course of meloxicam in the form of Metacam oral suspension for horses at a concentration of 15 mg/ml. The horse weighs 650 kg, and the dose rate is 0.6 mg/kg as stated in the datasheet [26].

$$650 \, \text{kg (bodyweight)} \times 0.6 \, \text{mg/kg (dose rate)}$$
$$= 390 \, \text{mg}$$

$$390 \, \text{mg} \div 15 \, \text{mg/ml (drug concentration)}$$
$$= \textbf{26 ml of Metacam oral once daily}$$

For a 14-day course:

$$26 \, \text{ml (daily dose)} \times 14 \, \text{(days required)}$$
$$= \textbf{364 ml required in total for 14 days}$$

Metacam oral for horses comes in 2 sizes of 100 and 250 ml, so this patient would require 2 × 250 ml or 4 × 100 ml to allow enough for a 14-day course.

Example 2   Tablets

The vet has prescribed a six-month supply of 1mg pergolide in the form of Prascend for a 125 kg donkey. Using the dose rate of 2 μg/kg stated in the datasheet [21].

$$125 \, \text{kg (bodyweight)} \times 2 \, \mu\text{g/kg (dose rate)}$$
$$= 250 \, \mu\text{g}$$

$$250 \, \mu\text{g} \div 1 \, \text{mg (drug concentration)}$$
$$= 250 \, \mu\text{g of 1 mg tablets}$$

In this case, the dose rate units, and the units for the strength of the tablet are different. For the dose to be accurate, the units must be the same, so need to be converted to μg (micrograms). There are 1000 μg in 1 mg.

Therefore, the calculation would be:

$$\text{Dose} = 250 \, \mu\text{g} \div 1000 \, \mu\text{g}$$
$$= \textbf{0.25 of a tablet per day.}$$

For a 6-month supply, there are approximately 30 days a month, so 30 × 6 = 180 days

180 days × 0.25 tablets = **45 tablets** for a 6-month course.

Example 3   Injectable medication [31]

The vet has prescribed procaine penicillin as Depocillin 300 mg/ml and gentamycin as Genta Equine 100 mg/ml injection for a 450 kg horse. Dose rates, as per the datasheets, are 12 mg/ml for Depocillin and 6.6 mg/ml for Genta Equine [32].

Depocillin

$$450 \, \text{kg (bodyweight)} \times 12 \, \text{mg/kg (dose rate)}$$
$$= 5400 \, \text{mg}$$

$$5400 \, \text{mg} \div 300 \, \text{mg/ml (drug concentration)}$$
$$= \textbf{18 ml}$$

Genta Equine

$$450 \, \text{kg (bodyweight)} \times 6.6 \, \text{mg (dose rate)} = 2970 \, \text{mg}$$

$$2970 \, \text{mg} \div 100 \, \text{mg/ml} = 29.7 \, \text{ml.}$$

If the vet agrees, this can be rounded up to 30 ml.

Calculating the correct dose of medication is imperative to prevent under or overdosing. A calculator can be used, and the resulting dose should be checked by another qualified staff member (RVN or vet) to reduce the chance of human error occurring [30].

Calculating the Percentage of a Solution

Some medications are recorded as a % of a solution for the concentration instead of milligrams per ml. In these cases, to understand how many mg/ml are in a solution, the calculation below should be followed. The data sheet should specify the mg/ml; however, it is good practice to be able to convert a % solution to mg/ml [30].

The % solution is described as the number of grams of a drug per 100 ml of medium. Using oxytetracycline as Engemycin for reference [21], the concentration of the solution is 10%. A 10% solution is 10 g of the drug per 100 ml of the liquid in the bottle, so **10 g** of the drug to **100 ml** of liquid [31].

To find out how many mg/ml that is [48]:

$$1 \, \text{ml solution} = 10 \, \text{g drug}/100 \, \text{ml solute}$$
$$= 0.1 \, \text{g within the solute}$$

To convert the grams to milligrams, simply multiply by 1000

$$0.1 \, \text{g} \times 1000 = 100 \, \text{mg/ml of solution}$$

Therefore **10% solution is equal to 100 mg/ml**

Let's try another one:

$$0.5\% \text{ solution contains } 0.5 \, \text{g of drug to every}$$
$$100 \, \text{ml of solution so :}$$
$$0.5 \, \text{g} \div 100 \, \text{ml} = 0.005 \, \text{g within the solute}$$

To convert this to mg multiply by 1000

$$0.005 \times 1000 = 5 \, \text{mg/ml of solution}$$

Therefore, **0.5% solution is equal to 5 mg/ml.**

Standard Units and International Units

International units (IU) are assigned to international standards according to the WHO guidelines; they are calibrated

Table 9.3 Conversion of basic units used for drug calculations [30].

Quantity	Units	Symbol	Relationship
Mass (Weight)	Kilogram	kg	
	Gram	g	1 kg = 1000 g
	Milligram	mg	1 g = 1000 mg
	Microgram	mcg or μg	1 mg = 1000 mcg
Volume	Litres	l	
	Millilitres	ml	1 l = 1000 ml
	Cubic centimetre	cc	1 ml = 1 cc

Source: Phillippa Pritchard.

into units of biological activity following extensive studies. This allows the assessment of biologicals in a consistent and internationally agreed manner; IU are used when determination of mass is not possible or appropriate. There may also be no agreed reference methods available, or a simple mass unit does not adequately define the measure of activity. In equine practice, the most commonly seen substances that are measured in IU are heparin and insulin [14].

Standard Units

Most commonly in relation to drug calculations, standard units are more commonly known as the metric system. This includes kilograms (kg) and litres (L) [20]. It is essential to understand the relationship between these and the smaller units as situations may arise where one measurement may need to be converted from one unit to another, such as milligrams to micrograms [20].

Table 9.3 shows the common conversions of basic units used in drug calculations.

9.3 Pharmacology

Pharmacology is a scientific discipline focused on studying the properties, interactions, and mechanisms of action of drugs and their effects on living organisms. This field encompasses a broad range of research areas, including drug composition, synthesis, and the molecular and cellular mechanisms by which drugs exert their therapeutic or toxic effects. Clinical pharmacotherapeutics is a specialised branch of pharmacology dedicated to understanding how drugs can be used to treat various diseases and medical conditions. It involves evaluating medication efficacy, safety, and optimal use in clinical settings to improve patient outcomes through tailored drug therapies. This sub-discipline integrates pharmacology and clinical medicine principles to develop and refine therapeutic strategies for individual patients and populations.[33].

Pharmacokinetics

Pharmacokinetics in veterinary medicine is the study of how drugs move through the bodies of an animal and is essential for understanding how to administer and manage medications across various species. This field involves the same four processes as in human medicine: absorption, distribution, metabolism, and excretion. Each of these have unique considerations for different animals. The four processes are defined as follows in the context of veterinary pharmacokinetics:

- Absorption: how the drug enters the bloodstream from the administration site, such as the stomach or skin.
- Distribution: how the drug spreads through the body's fluids and tissues.
- Metabolism: how the body chemically alters the drug, usually in the liver, to facilitate its elimination.
- Excretion: how the drug or its metabolites are removed from the body, mainly through urine or faeces.

Drug Absorption

Drug Absorption is affected by the route of administration, the disease status of the patient and the formulation of the drug [33].

Route of Administration

There are many routes of drug administration, but the most commonly used in equine medicine are oral, topical, S/C, IM and IV. Generally, for a drug to reach its site of action and have an effect, it must enter the systemic blood circulation; the route of administration will affect how long this takes. The only exceptions are drugs that act locally, i.e. they are applied directly to the area they work on. Mepivacaine hydrochloride is an example of a locally acting drug that does not need to enter circulation to reach its site of action [33].

Bioavailability refers to the amount of a drug that reaches the circulation intact. Medications given via the IV route have 100% bioavailability due to no absorption phase; this means the body can utilise 100% of the drug. This is also known as the bioavailability of one. Medications given by all other routes are said to have a bioavailability of less than one, as less than 100% of the dose will reach the circulation intact. Bioavailability is affected by the rate at which the drug is absorbed and the ease of absorption. Generally, the better the blood supply to an area, the quicker the absorption rate. Drugs administered intramuscularly are usually absorbed quickly. S/C injections have the lowest bioavailability due to the skin having a poor blood supply and some of the medication will be lost in the S/C fat [33].

Orally administered drugs travel through the gastrointestinal tract, which leads to large quantities being absorbed by the small intestine. Liquid preparations are generally absorbed more quickly than tablets, capsules and granules, as these need to undergo a dissolving process known as dissolution before absorption can occur. Some oral drugs are formulated as a 'sustained release' preparation, where dissolution and subsequent absorption are slowed. Sustained release is not the same as a tablet that is enteric coated; these tablets have been developed to protect the medication from the acid within the stomach. After an oral drug is absorbed across the intestinal wall, it enters the hepatic portal circulation, which directly transports it to the liver. One of the roles of the liver is to remove potentially toxic substances before they reach systemic blood circulation. Drugs may be partially or wholly broken down because of this mechanism, known as the first-pass effect. The first-pass effect is one reason that some medications cannot be administered orally or that the dose rate of an oral preparation is much higher when compared with a parenteral preparation of the same drug. Due to the need for dissolution, the time taken to reach the absorption site, and the first-pass effect, orally administered drugs tend to have a comparatively low bioavailability [33].

Other factors also affect the rate of absorption:

- Tissue perfusion directly affects the absorption rate; for example, a drug injected into an active, well-perfused muscle is absorbed more quickly than one injected into an inactive muscle due to a limited blood supply [33].
- Vasoconstriction or vasodilation will cause reduced or enhanced blood flow to an area, so exposing the patient to cold or hot environmental temperatures will affect the absorption rate when injecting via the S/C route.
- Disease conditions that affect the perfusion of the horse, shock and peripheral vasoconstriction both affect the absorption [33].
- The formulation of a drug can significantly influence its absorption. Hydrophilic drugs dissolve more easily in water, while lipophilic drugs dissolve more easily in fat. When drugs are administered via the IV or IM route, they enter the extracellular fluid. For IM administration, the drug must diffuse through this fluid to reach the circulation, making hydrophilic drugs more readily absorbed via these routes.
- In contrast, medications administered orally or via the S/C route must diffuse through cell membranes to reach the bloodstream. Since cell membranes are composed of phospholipids, lipophilic drugs can pass through them more easily, facilitating their absorption. Understanding these characteristics helps in selecting the appropriate route of administration for optimal drug efficacy. The pH of the drug and the environment can affect absorption because it can affect the drug's hydrophilic or lipophilic tendencies. Manufacturers sometimes advise that orally administered drugs should be given with food to improve absorption [33].

Drug Distribution

The movement of drugs from the systemic circulation into the body tissues is known as distribution. Most pharmaceuticals must reach a target area for their desired effect, known as the therapeutic effect. When a drug enters the systemic circulation, drug molecules attach themselves to a specific site on plasma proteins (notably to albumin); this is known as protein binding. Once bound to a plasma protein, a drug molecule becomes inactive and unable to move into body tissues. For a drug to be active, it must detach from the plasma protein, becoming unbound or 'free.' The balance between bound and unbound drug molecules in the circulation is maintained constantly. As free drug molecules move into the tissues, more bound drug molecules are released to preserve this equilibrium. Similarly, the concentration of unbound drugs in circulation and within tissues will always balance along a concentration gradient. It's crucial to understand that plasma proteins are not the target tissues, and drug binding to these proteins produces no physiological effect. Instead, drug-plasma protein binding creates a 'reservoir' of the drug, but only the free (unbound) drug is available to tissues to exert a therapeutic effect. [33].

Factors Affecting Drug Distribution

Some drugs bind more strongly to plasma proteins than others – these are termed highly protein-bound. The more highly protein-bound a drug is, the less free drug is available to distribute into the body tissues. The administration of large doses of highly protein-bound drugs is often necessary to achieve a therapeutic effect. Some drugs bind to the same site on plasma proteins; if these drugs are given together, this may result in the less bound drug not having binding sites leaving elevated amounts of the free drug leading to toxicity; this means that certain medications should not be administered together [33].

The body has natural circulatory barriers these include:

- The blood–brain barrier – the capillary walls in the brain have a different structure from others, which means that only highly lipophilic drugs are able to cross into the brain tissue. Drugs that must reach the brain to have an effect, for example, general anaesthetics, must be sufficiently lipophilic to cross the blood–brain barrier [33, 34].

- The placental barrier – the placenta acts as a natural barrier to the foal; the placental barrier, however, is not as efficient at preventing drugs from passing into the foetal circulation, so caution must be exercised when treating pregnant animals.
- The testicular barrier – the blood–testis barrier [35, 36], which is created by adjacent Sertoli cells near the basement membrane, serves as a 'gatekeeper' to prohibit harmful substances from reaching developing germ cells, most notably post-meiotic spermatids [34–36]. Like the placental barrier, the blood-testis barrier is not as effective as the blood–brain barrier, and most drugs can enter if the concentration is high enough [36].

These barriers exist to protect the body from circulatory toxins that may cause the body harm [37].

Tissue perfusion has an effect on absorption rate and speed of distribution. Organ/organs with high perfusion will be able to distribute drugs quickly. In contrast, organ/organs with poor perfusion, although they will receive the drug, will be in a lower concentration and take longer to disperse there due to the drop in the blood plasma. Distribution of a drug follows a concentration gradient; this causes a drug to leave a well-perfused area, enter back into circulation and enter less well-perfused areas; this is known as re-distribution. An example of this is the anaesthetic agent thiopental, which is lipophilic and redistributes to the adipose tissues, causing the animal to regain consciousness. If a horse is suffering from circulatory issues or ischaemia, this should be considered when planning and monitoring medications. Figure 9.4 displays the concentrations of the different routes of administration and how quickly they reach therapeutic levels [33].

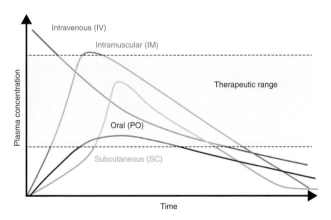

Figure 9.4 Plasma concentration levels after drug administration via different routes. *Source:* Rosina Lillywhite.

Drug Metabolism

The horse's circulation will metabolise or biotransform drugs as it would with any foreign substance within the circulation. This process of metabolism leaves a resultant product known as a metabolite. As a general rule, this transformation happens within the liver; however, other organs, such as the kidneys and the lungs, can be involved. Biotransformation is not a process that transforms a substance into a less harmful substance. The process is just making the substance more excretable [33].

In some cases, the metabolite can be more active in the body than the original drug molecule. This can be an advantage if it is impossible to give the active form of the drug in the first place; this is known as giving a prodrug; for example, the corticosteroid prednisone is metabolised into prednisolone. Alternatively, the metabolite can be as active as the original drug or even more toxic than the original drug [33].

The Metabolic Process

All drug eliminations need to be excreted via body fluids. Therefore, all metabolites must be hydrophilic to be eliminated. This happens in two phases [33]:

Phase I Metabolism can involve reduction or hydrolysis of the drug, but the most common biochemical process that occurs is oxidation. Oxidation is the chemical reaction that occurs when apples turn brown when exposed to the oxygen in the air [37].

Phase II This phase involves conjugation (joining) – this is where an attachment of an ionised group attaches to the drug. These groups can include glutathione, methyl or acetyl groups. These metabolic processes usually occur in the liver. The attachment of an ionised group makes the metabolite more water-soluble, facilitating excretion activity [37].

Example
Using aspirin as an example of a drug being metabolised - Aspirin undergoes phase I hydrolysis to salicylic acid. - In phase II, it is conjugated with either glycine or glucuronic acid forming a range of ionised metabolites that can then be excreted in the urine [37].

Factors affecting drug metabolism:

- Metabolic systems – a key metabolic system found in the liver is known as the mixed-function oxidase system. This system uses an enzyme known as cytochrome P450. This is introduced if one or more drugs it metabolises is present. This means continual use of drugs metabolised by P450 will need an ever-increasing dose rate to achieve a therapeutic dose. Phenobarbital uses this method, which is a drug used to control seizures, meaning that the dose would need to be adjusted to meet the seizure needs of the patient [33].

- Drug interaction – some enzymes are realised by the presence of the drug they metabolise; instead, they are always present, meaning a fixed number of enzymes are circulating. If two or more drug types that use the same enzymes are given simultaneously, a delay in metabolism and the possibility of toxicity occurs. Some drugs cause the inhibition of certain enzymes, which may result in the metabolism of that drug, or another drug, being slow. Inadequate liver function can also affect drug metabolism, as the production of the necessary enzymes may be impaired. This could be due to disease, but it should be kept in mind that neonatal and geriatric animals may also have reduced liver function [33].

Drug Elimination

Drugs are eliminated from the body via many routes such as the liver and kidneys through faeces and urine. Other methods of elimination include:

- Respiratory secretions
- Saliva
- Sebum
- Milk

The rate at which a volume of fluids can be completely cleared of a drug is known as the drug clearance rate and is measured in litres/hour (l/hr). The rate at which a drug is eliminated from the body, known as the elimination rate, and is measured in milligrams/hour (mg/hr). Both of these work together, and if there is high clearance, the elimination is also high [38].

Elimination Half-life and the Therapeutic Range

The term elimination half-life is used to describe the amount of time it takes for the concentration of a drug to drop by 50% in the circulation by metabolism and elimination. However, this does not mean that given the same length of time again, the drug will be eliminated entirely, as this is not the case, as the elimination rate does not always continue at the same pace, although this can also be the case [33].

The elimination half-life is crucial because it can determine when a drug's repeat doses are required to maintain the drug concentration in the blood sufficiently high to ensure that enough is available for distribution to the tissues and for a therapeutic effect. If this is not understood, several things could arise [33]:

- Giving repeat doses too frequently will result in drug levels climbing too high, causing toxicity.
- Leaving too long a time interval between repeat doses means that the blood concentration levels will drop too low to have a therapeutic effect in the tissues.

Maintaining optimal amounts of drug concentration in the blood so that neither toxicity nor ineffectiveness is created is known as keeping the levels within the therapeutic range or margin. Some drugs have a wide therapeutic range, meaning a large overdose must be administered before toxicity occurs. An example of a drug with a wide therapeutic range is pyrantel. Drugs with a narrow therapeutic range cause toxicity with even the slightest overdose, such as quinidine. For more information regarding adverse reactions, see Section 9.6 [33].

Pharmacodynamics

Pharmacodynamics play a pivotal role in drug development. This is the study of how drugs affect the body, focusing on the mechanisms of drug action and the resulting physiological and biochemical responses. It explores what the drug 'does' to the body, including interactions with cellular receptors, enzymes, and other molecular targets. By understanding these interactions, pharmacodynamics helps to determine the efficacy, potency, and safety of a drug, which is essential for optimising therapeutic use and guiding the development of new medications. [33].

Receptor-mediated Pharmacodynamics

Drug action is achieved by specific receptor sites within protein molecules attached to the cell membrane. Cell receptor sites are differentiated by their size or shape; cells will not have all receptor sites, and each cell will have a different range and number of sites [33].

Agonists and Antagonists

Agonists and antagonists are two types of drugs that interact with cellular receptors to influence physiological responses:

- Agonists: These drugs bind to receptors and activate them, mimicking the action of the body's natural chemicals. When an agonist binds to a receptor, it produces a similar response to the endogenous (naturally occurring) substance, effectively enhancing or triggering the same biological effect.
- Antagonists: In contrast, antagonists bind to receptors but do not activate them. Instead, they block the receptor, preventing the natural chemicals or agonists from

binding and producing a response. Antagonists can bind to the primary active site or to a different site (allosteric site) on the receptor, inhibiting its action and thereby stopping or reducing the intended physiological response. [38].

The main difference between these two drugs is that one simulates the intended reaction, whereas an antagonist binds to the receptor and stops/slows responses. Agonists essentially mimic the activities of normal neurotransmitters such as acetylcholine and emulate a similar reaction from the receptors they bind to. A great analogy to think of is a vending machine. Usually, to buy a drink, you would insert a coin into the machine, and the response is for it to dispense your favourite drink. An agonist in this scenario would be to use a metal disc of the same size as a coin to insert into the machine, thus using the same coin slot with a mimic coin to obtain a drink. An antagonist does the

opposite of an agonist. It binds to receptors and stops the receptor from producing a desired response. Returning to the analogy, it's like jamming the machine's coin slot so that it cannot perform its function until the blockage is removed [38]. Figure 9.5 shows the different drug bindings in relation to regular cellular activity.

Some drugs known as partial agonists or antagonists only partly block a receptor site; these block the cell but do not necessarily have much effect themselves. There are also drugs that, depending on the receptor site, can be both antagonists and agonists [33, 38].

Affinity and Competitiveness

Most drugs bind temporarily to receptor sites, and when present in sufficient quantities, they outcompete endogenous ligands (natural substances) for these sites. As the drug concentration decreases, endogenous ligands can

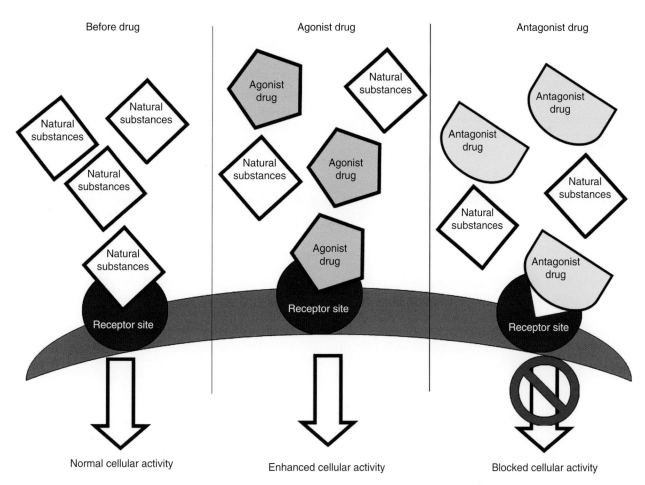

Figure 9.5 Drug binding in relation to typical cellular activity. *Source:* Rosina Lillywhite.

reclaim the receptor sites, causing the drug to dissociate. Due to this process, the effects of competitive drugsare reversible. In contrast, some drugs, known as non-competitive or irreversible drugs, remain bound to the receptor once attached. Their effects continue until the drug is metabolised and broken down, making them persistent in their action [33].

For a drug to connect with a receptor site, it must be attracted to that receptor. This attraction is known as affinity. Drugs with a strong affinity for the receptor site are usually highly effective and produce an excellent therapeutic response. Because they may remain in situ for more extended periods, the chances of toxicity are higher. The opposite is true for drugs with a weak affinity as they will leave receptors quicker and cause a lower case of toxicity [33, 37, 38].

Some drugs have the same receptor binding sites; if they were administered simultaneously, the drug with the weaker affinity would have no chance of binding to a receptor site because they would be full with the more potent affinity drug. An example of this would be morphine and butorphanol tartrate. This is an excellent example to remember: if a horse is likely to have surgery and require morphine, sedation with butorphanol tartrate should be avoided [33].

Down-regulation and Up-regulation

Long-term use of drugs requires careful management due to potential effects on receptor sites, which can lead to either down-regulation or up-regulation:

- Down-regulation is the prolonged use of a drug can cause a decrease in the number of receptor sites available for binding. This reduction results in a diminished therapeutic response over time, meaning the horse will require higher doses to achieve the same effect.
- Up-regulation occurs during extended drug use which can lead to an increase in the number of receptor sites. If the drug is suddenly discontinued, the previously blocked endogenous ligand can now bind to the increased number of receptors, potentially causing an enhanced and possibly harmful effect on the body. [33].

Specificity, Potency and Efficacy

- Drug Specificity (also known as selectivity) refers to the ability of the drug to act on a limited number of receptor sites. This is generally desirable because it allows for targeted treatment of the affected tissue or organ, minimising the potential for side effects by not affecting receptors in other parts of the body [33].

- Potency is the amount of drug needed to produce a therapeutic effect. A more potent drug requires a smaller dose to achieve the desired therapeutic outcome [33].
- Efficacy is the ability of a drug to produce a therapeutic effect. It is important not to confuse efficacy with potency. Potency compares two drugs of the same type, with the more potent drug requiring a smaller dose. Efficacy, on the other hand, compares two different types of drugs that produce a similar response; the drug that elicits a more satisfactory response is considered more efficacious [33].

Non-Receptor-Mediated Pharmacodynamics

Not all drugs exert their effects via receptors. There are several other pharmacodynamic mechanisms. These include:

- Antimicrobial drugs: these drugs directly target and act on pathogenic microorganisms in the body. Unfortunately, they can also affect commensal (beneficial) microorganisms.
- Chelating agents: these are used to remove toxic metals from the body, chelating agents bind with these metals to form less harmful substances. For example, ethylenediaminetetraacetic acid (EDTA) is often administered to treat lead poisoning by chelating the lead, thereby reducing its toxicity.
- Chemical action: this involves drugs that work through physical action, such as activated charcoal, which absorbs toxins to treat poisonings.

9.4 Common Classifications of Medications

Analgesics

Analgesics are drugs that prevent or relieve pain without loss of sensation. There are two main types of analgesics used in veterinary medicine and these are known as narcotic analgesics and non-steroidal anti-inflammatory drugs (NSAIDs) [33]:

- **Narcotic analgesics** – these medications get the name narcotic from their ability to cause 'sleepiness' in the patient. They can also be known as opiate analgesics derived from poppy seeds; however, medical opioids are synthetically produced. All opioids bind to opioid receptors in the central nervous system (CNS) to produce their analgesic effect; opioids are commonly used in preanaesthetic protocols to reduce the required general anaesthetic agents. They are also regularly used for patients who are already experiencing pain or for those who are about to undergo a painful procedure. Pre-emptive analgesia helps to reduce wind-up, which is a term used to describe sensitisation of the nervous system to further stimuli which can amplify pain, and lead to chronic pain states [21, 39, 40].

The three primary opioid receptors are Mu (only use lowercase μ for μ), Kappa (K uppercase or lowercase k) and Delta (upper case Δ and lowercase δ) the main emphasis in veterinary literature are with regards to μ and Kappa receptors.

Opioids are described as one of the following:
- An agonist: produces a noticeable effect
- A partial agonist: has a partial effect
- An antagonist: produces no effect.

μ receptors are primarily responsible for the analgesic effects that opioids produce. Full μ agonists include morphine and fentanyl, and butorphanol is a partial μ agonist and an antagonist, but it can still provide a moderate analgesic effect. Naloxone is a μ antagonist, so it can be used as a reversal agent for opioid analgesics.

Side effects can include respiratory depression, decreased gastrointestinal (GI) motility, euphoria, pupillary miosis (constriction) or mydriasis (dilation) [21, 39].

- **NSAIDs:** these medications decrease inflammation and work by blocking the activity of cyclooxygenase (COX) enzymes, which also inhibit the production of prostaglandins. Research in the 1990s shows that there are two forms of COX enzyme [33, 41]:
  - COX-1 is constantly present in a number of organs and produces prostaglandins, which are involved in the physiological regulation of organs such as the kidney and stomach. In the kidney, prostaglandins cause vasodilation in conditions requiring increased blood flow. In the stomach, they maintain mucosal perfusion, stimulate gastric mucus production and inhibit acid production.
  - COX-2 is only created when there is an insult to the tissue. It produces prostaglandins, which initiate the inflammatory response. NSAIDs that selectively inhibit COX-2 without significantly inhibiting COX-1 would, in theory, decrease inflammation without decreasing the production of normal prostaglandins; some NSAIDs are COX-2 selective [33].

By definition, NSAIDs reduce inflammation but also reduce fever (antipyretic) and pain perception (analgesic). When an injury occurs, the initial trauma and pain signals cause COX-2 enzymes to be produced in the spinal cord, leading to 'wind-up', the process of increasing ease with which pain signals can be sent up the spinal cord to the brain. When NSAIDs are used before surgery, they block COX production of these prostaglandins, reducing the number of pain signals being sent and lessening the perception of pain [21]. Most side effects of NSAIDs involve the GI tract in horses; right dorsal colitis (leading to protein-losing enteropathy) may occur, with accompanying signs of colic and diarrhoea. Hypoalbuminemia (low levels of albumin in the blood) may be evident on clinical pathologic evaluation, and there is potential for progression to ulceration and perforation. Theoretically, COX-2 selective (COX-1 sparing) NSAIDs should cause few or no GI adverse effects. However, in animals, COX-2 selective NSAIDs have been shown to cause gastritis, erosion, ulceration and enteropathy. COX-2 is also involved in protective mechanisms of the gastric mucosa; COX-2 selectivity confers relative GI safety [42].

GI blood loss may be further complicated by impaired platelet function. NSAIDs, by inhibiting COX-1, prevent platelets from forming thromboxane A2 (TXA2), a potent aggregating agent. Delayed clotting time would therefore be expected, and this occurs with aspirin but much less so with COX-2 selective NSAIDs. Aspirin irreversibly binds to platelet COX-1; however, with other NSAIDs, the binding is competitive. After long-term treatment with NSAIDs other than aspirin, blood dyscrasias (blood-related health conditions or hematologic diseases) have been reported in cats, dogs and horses [42]. COX-2 prostaglandins mediate protective renal vasodilation during hypotension. Animals with underlying renal compromise receiving NSAIDs could experience exacerbation or decompensation of their disease. Maintaining hydration and renal perfusion is essential in animals receiving NSAIDs, especially those undergoing anaesthesia or surgery, and in horses with colic. COX-2 selective NSAIDs are not safer regarding the potential for nephropathies, including papillary necrosis and interstitial nephritis [42].

Opioid Analgesics

Opioid analgesics are critical for managing pain in equine patients. They work by binding to opioid receptors in the CNS, providing effective relief from both visceral (organ) and somatic (skin and superficial tissue) pain. However, their use requires careful consideration due to potential side effects and variations in efficacy.

Morphine
Mechanism of action: morphine is a pure μ opioid agonist that provides effective pain relief by binding to μ receptors in the CNS. It is particularly effective for visceral pain, but its effectiveness for superficial pain can be limited [21].

Administration: morphine can be administered via the IV, IM or epidural routes.

- **IV administration**: rapid onset but short duration of action. A 0.66 mg/kg IV dose produces approximately 30 minutes of analgesia for superficial pain and 1 hour for mild visceral pain [21].
- **IM administration**: variable results in analgesia, often not significantly effective for noxious stimuli [21].
- **Epidural administration**: provides regional analgesia for procedures involving the hindlimbs or perianal area when combined with other drugs [21].

Side effects: morphine can cause CNS excitement, increased locomotor activity, and decreased GI function, increasing the risk of intestinal impaction. It also has the potential to cause histamine release, leading to urticaria and severe vasodilation if administered too quickly IV [40].

Fentanyl

Mechanism of action: fentanyl is a potent μ agonist with greater potency than morphine but a shorter duration of action [21].

Administration:

- **IV infusion**: requires constant rate infusion (CRI) due to its short half-life [21].
- **Transdermal patches**: commonly used, especially in long-term pain management. Patches are placed on clipped and cleaned areas of the skin and should not be cut to maintain the correct release rate of the drug [21].

Factors affecting absorption:

- **Skin thickness**:
  - **Impact**: the thickness of a horse's skin can significantly impact the rate and extent of fentanyl absorption. Thicker skin may slow down the absorption process, while thinner skin might allow for quicker and more efficient drug penetration.
  - **Anatomical differences**: different areas of a horse's body have varying skin thicknesses. For example, the skin on the neck is generally thicker compared to the skin on the flank or groin areas. Selecting a site with appropriate skin thickness is essential to ensure consistent drug delivery.
  - **Considerations**: regular monitoring of the horse's response to the patch will be required. It may be necessary to adjust the location or application method based on individual skin characteristics.
- **Skin perfusion**:
  - **Impact**: skin perfusion, or the amount of blood flow to the skin, plays a critical role in drug absorption. Areas

with higher blood flow enhance the absorption of fentanyl, while areas with poor perfusion may result in slower and less predictable drug uptake. Temperature, humidity, and the horse's overall health can influence skin perfusion. Warmer temperatures and physical activity can increase blood flow, potentially enhancing absorption, whereas cold environments might reduce perfusion.
  - **Considerations**: choosing areas with consistent and reliable blood flow can improve the efficacy of fentanyl patches. Sites such as the inner thigh or lower abdomen, where blood flow is generally more stable, may be preferred. Keeping the horse in a stable environment with controlled temperature and humidity can help maintain consistent drug absorption rates.
- **Patch location**:
  - **Impact**: the location of the patch is crucial for effective drug delivery. Sites that are less prone to movement and abrasion will maintain better contact with the skin, ensuring continuous drug release. Placing patches on areas that experience frequent movement or friction, such as near joints or areas that rub against tack or other equipment, can disrupt the adhesion of the patch and the consistency of drug delivery.
  - **Onset and duration**: therapeutic levels are typically reached between 12 to 24 hours after application, with effects lasting between 24 to 72 hours. Due to variability in absorption, additional injectable analgesia is often required until the full effect is achieved.

Side effects: similar to morphine, including the risk of misuse and incorrect disposal [43].

Buprenorphine

Mechanism of action: buprenorphine is a partial μ agonist and kappa (κ) antagonist, providing moderate analgesia with a ceiling effect, meaning increasing the dose does not increase analgesia but prolongs its duration [40].

Administration:

- **Mucous membranes**: readily absorbed across mucous membranes [40].
- **IV administration**: slow onset of action, with a significant delay in effect (at least 45 minutes) but prolonged duration (up to 11 hours at a dose of 0.01 mg/kg IV) [40, 44].

Side effects: can cause excitement, increased spontaneous locomotor activity, and decreased gastrointestinal function [40, 44].

Butorphanol

Mechanism of action: butorphanol is a mixed agonist-antagonist opioid, acting as a κ agonist and a weak μ antagonist, providing a rapid onset of analgesia [40, 45].

Administration:

- **IV administration**: produces a rapid onset of effect with a dose-dependent duration, lasting between 15 to 90 minutes [40, 45].

  Advantages: butorphanol generally produces fewer gastrointestinal side effects compared to other opioids and is less likely to cause severe changes in gastrointestinal function and transit time [40, 45].

  Side effects: can cause CNS excitement, often seen as exaggerated responses to external stimuli and muscle twitching [40, 45].

  Clinical uses: commonly combined with other anaesthetic, sedative, or analgesic drugs due to its synergistic effects, particularly with alpha-2 agonists like detomidine. It also has a strong cough suppression effect and causes less respiratory depression than full μ agonists [33].

NSAIDs

NSAIDs are essential in equine medicine for managing pain, inflammation, and fever. These medications work by inhibiting the cyclooxygenase (COX) enzymes responsible for the production of prostaglandins, which are mediators of these symptoms. NSAIDs can be broadly classified into non-specific COX inhibitors and selective COX inhibitors. This section focuses on non-specific COX inhibitors commonly used in horses.

Acetylsalicylic Acid (Aspirin)

Mechanism of action: aspirin is a non-specific COX inhibitor that irreversibly inhibits the COX enzymes, reducing the formation of prostaglandins and thromboxanes which are are crucial for platelet aggregation and vasoconstriction. By inhibiting thromboxane production, aspirin decreases platelet aggregation, lowering the risk of thrombus formation [39, 40].

Clinical uses:

- **Antiplatelet effects**: aspirin is a potent antiplatelet effects make it valuable in preventing thrombus formation in conditions where blood clot prevention is crucial, such as certain vascular disorders or post-surgical care [39, 40].
- **Pain and inflammation**: while aspirin can reduce pain and inflammation, its use in horses is limited due to the potential for GI side effects [39, 40].

Administration and dosage:

- **Dosage**: the dosage of aspirin for horses varies based on the intended therapeutic effect. It is essential to use veterinary-specific aspirin formulations, as human formulations can lead to severe side effects or death in horses [39, 40].

Side effects:

- **GI side effects**: aspirin can cause gastrointestinal ulcers and bleeding, limiting its use as a routine NSAID in equine practice [39, 40].
- **Renal effects**: long-term use or high doses may adversely affect renal function, necessitating caution in horses with compromised kidney function [39, 40].

Phenylbutazone

Mechanism of action: phenylbutazone, commonly known as "bute," is a non-specific COX inhibitor that alleviates pain and inflammation, primarily in musculoskeletal conditions [39, 40].

Clinical uses:

- **Musculoskeletal pain**: widely used for treating musculoskeletal inflammation, including conditions such as laminitis, arthritis, and other joint issues [39, 40].
- **Colic pain**: Less effective for visceral pain associated with colic compared to other NSAIDs or opioids [39, 40].

Administration and dosage:

- **Dosage**: administered orally or IV. The dosage is adjusted based on the severity of the condition and the horse's response to treatment [39, 40].

Side effects:

- **GI ulceration**: Increases the risk of gastric ulcers [39, 40].
- **Renal issues**: Can cause renal papillary necrosis if renal perfusion is decreased, leading to water retention and sodium imbalance [46].
- **Tissue necrosis**: Extravasation (injection outside the vein) can cause tissue necrosis. Although rare, bone marrow suppression is a potential side effect [46].

Special considerations:

- **Protein binding**: highly protein-bound (over 99% in horses). Caution is required in horses with hypoalbuminemia as this may increase the risk of adverse effects [46].

Flunixin Meglumine

Mechanism of action: flunixin meglumine is a potent non-specific COX inhibitor with significant anti-inflammatory, analgesic, and antipyretic effects [40].

Clinical uses:

- **Musculoskeletal injuries**: effective for managing pain and inflammation associated with musculoskeletal injuries [40].
- **Colic pain**: used to alleviate pain from colic and other abdominal issues [40].
- **Respiratory and systemic conditions**: also used for respiratory diseases, endotoxemia, and mastitis. It has shown effectiveness in mitigating some adverse effects of bacterial endotoxins, increasing survivability from endotoxemia [39, 40].

Administration and dosage:

- **Dosage**: administered orally or IV. Dosage varies based on the condition being treated [40].

Side effects:

- **GI Issues**: Similar to other NSAIDs, it can cause GI irritation or ulceration [40].
- **Renal effects**: caution is required in cases of compromised renal function [40].

Diclofenac

Mechanism of action: diclofenac is a non-specific COX inhibitor used primarily for topical treatment of localised inflammation [21, 40].

Clinical uses:

- **Topical application**: applied to the skin over distal limb joints to manage lameness and inflammation. Therapeutic concentrations are reached within 6 to 18 hours, making it effective for localised treatment without systemic side effects in many cases [21, 40].
- **Ophthalmic use**: available in ophthalmic formulations for treating uveitis in horses [21, 40].

Administration and dosage:

- **Topical**: applied directly to the affected area. Proper application is crucial to avoid systemic absorption and ensure effectiveness [21, 40].

Side effects:

- **Systemic absorption**: although the risk is low, systemic side effects may occur if diclofenac is used extensively over multiple sites [21, 40].

- **Precautions**: application should be carried out with gloves to prevent drug absorption through human skin, protecting the handler from potential side effects [21, 40].

COX-2 Inhibitors

COX-2 inhibitors are a subclass of NSAIDs that specifically target the COX-2 enzyme. This enzyme is primarily responsible for the production of prostaglandins that mediate inflammation and pain, unlike COX-1, which also produces prostaglandins involved in protecting the stomach lining and regulating kidney function. By selectively inhibiting COX-2, these drugs aim to reduce inflammation and pain while minimising GI and renal side effects commonly associated with non-specific NSAIDs.

Carprofen

Mechanism of action:

- **Carprofen**: carprofen is a COX-2 selective inhibitor with additional weak inhibition of the 5-lipoxygenase pathway, which also contributes to its anti-inflammatory effects. This dual action helps reduce inflammation and pain with potentially fewer side effects on the gastrointestinal tract compared to non-selective NSAIDs [47].

Clinical uses:

- **Licensing**: carprofen is licensed for use in horses in some countries but not in the UK. Therefore, in the UK, it must be used under the cascade system, which allows the use of unlicensed drugs when no suitable licensed alternatives are available [47].
- **Dose**: The recommended dose for horses is 0.7 mg/kg, either orally or given IV. This dosage has shown minimal accumulation in the plasma, indicating a favourable safety profile with proper use [47].

Administration and dosage:

- **Oral and IV use**: Carprofen can be administered orally or via the IV route at a dose rate of 0.7 mg/kg. There is no evidence of accumulation in plasma at this dose, suggesting it can be safely used over a treatment course [47].
- **IM injections**: have shown elevated plasma creatine kinase levels, indicating potential muscle cell damage, so caution is advised with this route [47].

Side effects:

- **Muscle cell damage**: elevated plasma creatine kinase levels suggest possible muscle damage with IM injections [47].

- **General safety**: carprofen is generally considered safe with minimal evidence of accumulation and a favourable margin of safety [47].

Meloxicam
Mechanism of action:

- **Meloxicam**: meloxicam selectively inhibits COX-2, reducing inflammation and pain with less impact on COX-1, which helps protect the stomach lining and renal function [48].

Clinical uses:

- **Licensing**: meloxicam is licensed in the UK for treating inflammation and pain in both acute and chronic musculoskeletal disorders in horses. It is also used for managing abdominal pain in equine patients [48].
- **Inflammatory conditions**: while licensed for musculoskeletal disorders, meloxicam may also be used off-license for other inflammatory conditions if justified under the cascade system [48].

Administration and dosage:

- **Oral and IV use**: administered at a dose of 0.6 mg/kg. The oral preparation has high bioavailability (around 98%), making it effective and convenient for oral administration [48].
- **Special populations**: its use is contraindicated in foals under six weeks of age, lactating mares, and pregnant horses [48].

Side effects:

- **GI Issues**: There have been reports of gastric ulceration and right dorsal colitis [48].
- **Renal effects**: Similar to other NSAIDs, caution is required with renal function, particularly in compromised animals [48].

Firocoxib
Mechanism of action:

- **Firocoxib**: firocoxib is a highly selective COX-2 inhibitor designed to alleviate pain and inflammation by targeting the COX-2 enzyme without significantly affecting COX-1, thereby reducing the risk of GI and renal side effects [49].

Clinical uses:

- **Licensing**: firocoxib is licensed in the UK for managing pain and inflammation associated with osteoarthritis (OA) and lameness in horses [49].

- **Additional uses**: it can be used off-license for other inflammatory conditions if justified under the cascade system. Studies suggest it may also be beneficial for ocular conditions and post-colic surgery pain management [49].

Administration and dosage:

- **Ocular penetration**: firocoxib has been found to have superior ocular penetration compared to flunixin meglumine, making it useful for eye conditions [49].
- **Visceral analgesia**: it has been shown to be an effective visceral analgesic and may be useful following colic surgery, although it is not licensed for this use [49].

Side effects:

- **Age restrictions**: contraindicated in animals under ten weeks of age. Its safety in horses under one year of age is not well established [49].
- **Pregnancy concerns**: laboratory studies indicate potential risks, such as embryological and foetal malformations, delayed parturition, and reduced survival, making it contraindicated during pregnancy [49].
- **General safety**: while it has a favourable safety profile, monitoring for any signs of GI or renal issues is recommended [49].

Other anti-inflammatory drugs.

Dimethyl Sulfoxide (DMSO)
Mechanism of action:

- **Free radical scavenging**: DMSO scavenges oxygen-free radicals, which are implicated in tissue damage following physical or chemical trauma. By neutralising these radicals, DMSO reduces oxidative stress, helping to mitigate inflammation and cellular damage. This mechanism is particularly beneficial in acute injury scenarios where oxidative stress plays a significant role in tissue damage [40].
- **Reduction of oedema**: DMSO effectively reduces oedema by decreasing fluid accumulation in tissues. This property is beneficial in conditions where inflammation causes significant swelling, such as soft tissue injuries, laminitis, and post-surgical recovery. Reducing oedema helps alleviate pain and restore normal function [40].
- **Analgesic properties**: DMSO provides analgesia, making it useful in managing pain associated with inflammation and trauma. It can be particularly effective in treating conditions like laminitis and other acute inflammatory conditions in horses [40].
- **Carrier for other medications**: due to its ability to penetrate biological membranes, DMSO is often used as a

carrier for other medications, such as corticosteroids and antibiotics. This enhances their absorption and effectiveness when applied topically, allowing for targeted therapy in conditions requiring multi-faceted treatment approaches [40].

Clinical uses:

- **Intracranial pressure**: DMSO can be used to decrease intracranial pressure, making it a valuable drug for managing head trauma in horses. This application can be critical in stabilising horses with severe head injuries [50].
- **Joint disease**: DMSO has been administered via the intra-articular route based on its anti-inflammatory and free radical scavenging properties, which may benefit inflammatory joint diseases like arthritis. However, administration via the intra-synovial route should be avoided as it can damage chondrocyte metabolism, potentially worsening joint health [40].
- **Topical and IV administration**: DMSO can be administered both topically and via the IV route. When applied topically, the area should be clipped to ensure better absorption, and when used IV, it should be administered slowly to avoid adverse effects [40].

Administration and Dosage:

- **Topical**: DMSO should be applied to a clipped and clean area of skin to enhance absorption. To maximise the efficacy of the drug, the skin should be free from dirt and debris [40].
- **IV**: DMSO should be administered slowly or via a CRI to avoid adverse effects such as muscle tremors, diarrhoea, colic, haemolysis, and haemoglobinuria. Clinical signs of adverse reactions typically abate within 10 minutes of discontinuing the infusion [50].

Side effects:

- **Adverse reactions**: rapid IV administration can cause muscle tremors, diarrhoea, colic, haemolysis, and haemoglobinuria. These side effects necessitate careful monitoring during administration [50].
- **Precautions**: PPE should be worn when handling DMSO to prevent contact with the skin, as it can be absorbed through human skin, causing systemic effects. This precaution helps prevent potential health risks to the handler [51].

Hyaluronic acid (HA)
Mechanism of action:

- **Synovial fluid component**: HA is a natural component of synovial fluid, contributing to its viscosity and lubricating properties, which are essential for the smooth movement of joints. This action helps protect cartilage surfaces from wear and tear during movement [40].
- **Anti-inflammatory effects**: HA has anti-inflammatory properties by suppressing prostaglandin production and scavenging free radicals that are destructive to joint cartilage and tissue. This dual action helps maintain joint health and function [40].

Clinical uses:

- **Joint lubrication**: HA increases the thickness or viscosity of joint fluid, acting as a lubricant between cartilage surfaces, which helps reduce friction and wear in joints. This property is particularly beneficial in managing OA and other degenerative joint diseases [40].
- **Inflammation relief**: HA is used to relieve inflammation of the synovium, the membrane lining the joint, providing relief from pain and improving joint mobility [40].

Administration and dosage:

- **Systemic IV and intra-articular injection**: HA can be administered either systemically via IV injection or directly via the intra-articular route to target specific areas of inflammation and provide lubrication. The route of administration depends on the condition being treated and the desired therapeutic effect [40].
- **Product variability**: many different equine injectable HA products are available. It is essential to read the package insert information on each product to understand the limitations and safe administration routes. This ensures the correct use of the product and maximises its therapeutic benefits [33].

Glucosamine and Chondroitin Sulphate
Mechanism of action:

- **Cartilage repair**: glucosamine aids in cartilage repair and maintenance by serving as a building block for the synthesis of glycosaminoglycans, essential components of joint cartilage. This helps to repair and maintain healthy cartilage, which is crucial for joint health [24].
- **Anti-inflammatory properties**: glucosamine has inherent anti-inflammatory properties that help reduce joint inflammation and associated pain. This property makes it beneficial in managing chronic joint conditions [24].
- **Water attraction and enzyme inhibition**: chondroitin sulphate attracts water to the cartilage matrix, maintaining its elasticity and resilience. It also inhibits cartilage-degrading enzymes, slowing cartilage degeneration and promoting joint health [24].

Clinical uses:

- **OA management**: these nutraceuticals are often used to manage OA in horses. They can reduce pain, improve joint function, and potentially slow the progression of cartilage degeneration. This makes them valuable in managing chronic joint diseases [24].
- **NSAID alternative**: by reducing the need for NSAIDs, glucosamine and chondroitin sulphate offer a safer long-term management option for chronic joint conditions. This can help mitigate the side effects associated with prolonged NSAID use [24].

Administration and dosage:

- **Oral administration**: glucosamine and chondroitin sulphate are typically administered orally in the form of supplements. The dosage varies depending on the product and the severity of the condition being treated. Consistent administration is key to achieving and maintaining therapeutic levels [24].
- **Veterinary guidance**: these supplements should be administered under veterinary guidance to ensure appropriate dosing and monitoring for efficacy and safety. Regular veterinary check-ups are essential to adjust the treatment plan as needed [24].

Side effects:

- **General safety**: these compounds are generally safe, but more research is needed to fully understand their long-term benefits and optimal use in different animal species. This ongoing research helps to optimise treatment protocols [24].
- **Veterinary supervision**: regular monitoring and adjustments may be necessary to ensure the best outcomes for the horse. Veterinary supervision helps to catch any potential issues early and adjust the treatment plan for maximum benefit [24].

Antiarrhythmic Drugs

Antiarrhythmic drugs are crucial in treating arrhythmias, which are irregular patterns of electrical activity in the heart. These abnormalities can result in either a faster-than-normal heart rate (tachyarrhythmias) or a slower-than-normal heart rate (bradyarrhythmias). The causes of arrhythmias are varied, ranging from electrolyte imbalances and structural heart diseases to systemic conditions and drug reactions. The choice of antiarrhythmic drug depends on the specific type of arrhythmia, the underlying cause, and the overall health of the horse. These drugs can be categorised into three main classes: beta-blockers, calcium channel blockers, and sodium channel blockers.

Categories of Antiarrhythmic Drugs

Beta-Blockers (β-Blockers): beta-blockers work by blocking the stimulation of β1 receptors in the heart, leading to a decrease in heart rate and strength of contraction. These drugs are also known as negative inotropes.

Mechanism of action:

- **Beta-blockers**: beta-blockers reduce the effects of endogenous catecholamines (like adrenaline) on the heart. This results in decreased heart rate (chronotropic effect) and reduced force of cardiac contractions (inotropic effect) [33].
- **Considerations**: horses treated with beta-blockers often need increasing dosages to maintain the therapeutic effect due to up-regulation of β receptors. Abrupt cessation of treatment should be avoided to prevent sudden availability of β1 receptors to endogenous stimulators, which could exacerbate arrhythmias [33].

Calcium channel blockers: calcium channel blockers reduce the rate of impulse generation and conduction across the heart by preventing calcium from entering the cells of the heart and arteries.

Mechanism of action:

- **Calcium channel blockers**: these drugs relax and open blood vessels by blocking calcium entry, which reduces the contractility of the heart muscle and slows down the heart rate [33].
- **Use in equine medicine**: they are not commonly used in equine medicine but can be employed in specific cases where control of arrhythmia through other means is not effective [33].

Sodium channel blockers: sodium channel blockers have a local anaesthetic action and reduce ectopic beats or extrasystoles, which are contractions occurring outside of the normal heartbeat.

Mechanism of action:

- **Sodium channel blockers**: these drugs inhibit the sodium channels during depolarisation, reducing the excitability of the heart muscle and helping to stabilise the cardiac rhythm [33].

Specific Antiarrhythmic Drugs used in Equine Medicine
Lidocaine
Lidocaine is a sodium channel blocker that is commonly used to treat premature ventricular contractions and ventricular arrhythmias in horses. It is particularly effective in stabilising the heart's electrical activity by inhibiting the rapid influx of sodium ions during the depolarisation

phase of the cardiac action potential. This action helps to reduce the excitability of the heart muscle and prevent abnormal heart rhythms [52].

Mechanism of action:

- **Lidocaine:** lidocaine works by binding to sodium channels in the cardiac cell membrane, blocking the rapid influx of sodium ions that occurs during the initial phase of the cardiac action potential. This inhibition slows down the rate of depolarisation, thereby stabilising the myocardial cell membrane and reducing the likelihood of ectopic beats or extrasystoles. Lidocaine is most effective against ventricular arrhythmias and is less effective against atrial fibrillation or atrial flutter due to its specific action on sodium channels primarily active during ventricular depolarisation [52].

Administration:

- **IV administration:**
  - **CRI:** due to its rapid metabolism and short half-life, lidocaine is often administered as a CRI to maintain therapeutic blood levels. The CRI method ensures a steady and continuous delivery of the drug, providing consistent antiarrhythmic effects [52].
  - **Bolus dosing:** in situations where CRI is not feasible, multiple small bolus doses can be administered. However, this approach requires careful monitoring to avoid fluctuations in blood drug levels that can lead to subtherapeutic effects or toxicity [52].
- **Local anaesthetic use:**
  - **Topical and injectable:** Lidocaine is also widely used as a local anaesthetic in equine practice. It can be applied topically to mucous membranes or injected into tissues to provide localised pain relief [21].
  - **Combination with epinephrine:** when used as a local anaesthetic, lidocaine is sometimes combined with epinephrine. Epinephrine causes vasoconstriction, which slows the absorption of lidocaine, prolonging its anaesthetic effect. However, caution is needed if lidocaine with epinephrine is used IV, as the vasoconstrictive properties of epinephrine can exacerbate arrhythmias [21].

Side effects:
CNS:

- **Sedation:** horses may exhibit sedation, characterised by lethargy and reduced alertness [52].
- **Ataxia:** loss of coordination and balance can occur, making the horse appear unsteady on its feet [52].
- **Drowsiness:** the sedative effects of lidocaine can lead to drowsiness, affecting the horse's overall activity levels [52].

Cardiovascular system:

- **Hypotension:** rapid administration of lidocaine can cause a drop in blood pressure due to its vasodilatory effects [52].
- **Cardiac depression:** high doses or rapid administration can depress myocardial contractility and lead to decreased cardiac output [52].

GI side effects:

- **GI disturbances:** although rare, some horses may experience colic symptoms following the administration of this drug [52].

Local anaesthetic use:

- **Injection site reactions:** localised reactions at the site of injection can include swelling, pain, and redness [52].
- **Caution with epinephrine:** when lidocaine is combined with epinephrine, care must be taken to avoid exacerbating arrhythmias due to the vasoconstrictive effects of epinephrine [52].

Monitoring and precautions:

- **Close monitoring:** horses receiving lidocaine, especially via CRI, should be closely monitored for signs of toxicity and adverse reactions. Continuous electrocardiogram (ECG) monitoring is recommended to detect any changes in heart rhythm [52].
- **Adjusting dosages:** dosages may need to be adjusted based on the horse's response and any observed side effects. Vets should be prepared to modify the treatment regimen to ensure safety and efficacy [52].
- **Pre-existing conditions:** caution is warranted in horses with pre-existing liver or kidney disease, as these conditions can affect the metabolism and excretion of lidocaine, increasing the risk of toxicity [52].
- **Gradual discontinuation:** when discontinuing lidocaine therapy, it should be tapered off gradually to prevent rebound arrhythmias or other adverse effects [52].

Quinidine

Quinidine is a sodium channel blocker used to treat various types of arrhythmias, particularly atrial flutter and fibrillation in horses. As an antiarrhythmic agent, quinidine works by slowing the conduction of electrical impulses through the heart, thereby stabilising the cardiac rhythm [40, 53].

Mechanism of action:

- **Quinidine:** quinidine functions by inhibiting the fast sodium channels in the myocardial cells. This action slows the rate of depolarisation and conduction velocity in the heart, thereby prolonging the action potential and refractory period. As a result, quinidine helps to restore normal sinus rhythm in horses experiencing atrial fibrillation or flutter by preventing the rapid, irregular electrical signals that cause these arrhythmias [40, 53].

Clinical uses:

- **Conversion of atrial fibrillation**:
  - **Atrial fibrillation**: quinidine is primarily used to convert atrial fibrillation to normal sinus rhythm in horses. Atrial fibrillation is a common arrhythmia in horses, especially in larger breeds and those with underlying heart conditions [40].
  - **Administration**: quinidine is typically administered orally in the form of quinidine sulphate or quinidine gluconate. The dosage and administration schedule can vary depending on the severity of the arrhythmia and the individual response of the horse. IV preparations are available in some regions but are less commonly used due to their potential for severe side effects [40].
- **Close monitoring**:
  - **ECG**: Due to the risk of severe side effects, horses receiving quinidine should be closely monitored using ECG to track heart rhythm and detect any adverse reactions early [40].
  - **Clinical observation**: regular observation for clinical signs of toxicity, such as changes in heart rate, respiratory distress, and gastrointestinal symptoms, is crucial [40].

Side effects: quinidine has a narrow therapeutic index, meaning the range between an effective dose and a toxic dose is small. Consequently, close monitoring is essential to avoid adverse reactions [40].

Common side effects:

- **Lethargy**: reduced energy levels and general fatigue are common, likely due to the drug's effect on cardiac output and overall circulation [40].
- **Mucosal swelling**: swelling of mucous membranes, such as those in the mouth and nasal passages, can occur, potentially leading to respiratory complications [40].

Respiratory side effects:

- **Nasal oedema**: swelling in the nasal passages can cause laboured or noisy breathing, making it difficult for the horse to breathe normally [40].
- **Laboured or noisy respiratory sounds**: Respiratory distress may manifest as laboured breathing or abnormal respiratory noises, indicating potential complications [40].

GI side effects:

- **Colic**: GI upset, including excessive gas and colic, can be a side effect, likely due to changes in gut motility and circulation [40].
- **Diarrhoea**: diarrhoea is a frequent side effect, which can lead to dehydration and electrolyte imbalances if not managed promptly [40].

Cardiovascular side effects:

- **Ventricular arrhythmia**: quinidine can paradoxically cause new arrhythmias, including ventricular arrhythmias, which can be life-threatening [40].
- **Ventricular fibrillation**: this severe arrhythmia can lead to sudden cardiac death if not treated immediately [40].

Severe side effects:

- **Sudden death**: due to the risk of ventricular fibrillation and other severe arrhythmias, there is a potential for sudden death, especially if the horse is not closely monitored during treatment [40].

Precautions and contraindications:

- **Pre-existing conditions**:
  - **Horses with underlying heart disease or electrolyte imbalances**: these horses should be evaluated carefully before administering quinidine, as they are at higher risk for adverse reactions [40].
  - **Electrolyte monitoring**: regular monitoring of electrolyte levels, particularly potassium and calcium, is essential during treatment to prevent exacerbation of arrhythmias [40].
- **Alternative treatments**:
  - Due to the potential for severe side effects, alternative antiarrhythmic treatments or supportive care may be considered, particularly for horses that do not tolerate quinidine well [40].
- **Preparation for emergency procedures**:
  - **Emergency drugs and equipment**: facilities treating horses with quinidine should be equipped with emergency drugs and equipment, such as defibrillators (where possible) and IV fluids, to manage potential complications promptly [40].

Propranolol

Propranolol is a non-selective beta-blocker that acts on both β1 and β2 adrenoceptors, making it useful in managing various cardiac conditions by modulating heart rate and myocardial contractility [54].

Mechanism of action:

- **Beta-adrenergic blockade**: propranolol blocks the effects of catecholamines (adrenaline and noradrenaline) on β1 and β2 receptors [54].
- **Heart rate reduction**: it decreases the heart rate (negative chronotropic effect) by reducing the rate of sinoatrial (SA) node discharge [54].
- **AV node conduction**: it slows atrioventricular (AV) node conduction velocity, prolonging the refractory period of the AV node [54].
- **Decreased contractility**: propranolol reduces myocardial contractility (negative inotropic effect), which can help manage arrhythmias and reduce the oxygen demand of the heart [54].

Clinical uses:

- **Supraventricular and ventricular tachycardia**: propranolol is used to treat both supraventricular and ventricular tachycardias, especially when other therapeutic agents have failed [54].
- **Quinidine-induced arrhythmias**: it can be used to manage ventricular tachyarrhythmias induced by quinidine, a sodium channel blocker [54].
- **Administration routes**: propranolol can be administered orally or via the IV route, depending on the urgency and specific needs of the treatment [54].

Sotalol

Sotalol is a non-selective β-adrenergic blocking drug with additional potassium channel-blocking effects, making it a versatile antiarrhythmic agent [21, 55].

Mechanism of action:

- **Beta-blockade**: decreases myocardial contractility and heart rate by blocking β1 and β2 receptors [21, 55].
- **Potassium channel blockade**: prolongs the action potential and refractory period by inhibiting potassium channels, stabilising cardiac rhythm [21, 55].

Clinical uses:

- **Atrial fibrillation**: used to treat atrial fibrillation by stabilising electrical activity in the atria [21, 55].
- **Ventricular and supraventricular tachycardia**: effective for both types of tachycardia, as well as premature complexes [21, 55].
- **Oral administration**: typically administered orally, preferably on an empty stomach to enhance absorption [21, 55].

Side effects:

- **Overdose risks**: overdose can lead to severe side effects such as [21, 55]:

– Aggravation of existing arrhythmias
– Polymorphic ventricular tachycardia
– Hypokalaemia (low potassium levels)
– Hypotension (low blood pressure)
– Exacerbation of congestive heart failure
– Bradyarrhythmias (slow heart rate)

Digoxin

Digoxin is a cardiac glycoside used to manage certain heart conditions by increasing myocardial contractility and controlling heart rate [40].

Mechanism of action:

- **Increased calcium availability**: diagoxin enhances the amount of calcium available for myocardial contraction, thus increasing the force of each contraction (positive inotropic effect) [40].
- **Vagal effects**: diagoxin exerts parasympathomimetic effects, which help slow the heart rate and reduce AV node conduction (negative chronotropic and dromotropic effects) [40].

Administration:

- **Oral and IV forms**: can be administered orally or via the IV route. The oral form has variable bioavailability, necessitating careful monitoring and dose adjustments [40].
- **Therapeutic monitoring**: regular monitoring of plasma levels is essential to ensure therapeutic effectiveness and avoid toxicity [40].

Side effects:

- **Cardiac dysrhythmias**: includes various types of arrhythmias, which require careful monitoring [40].
- **Non-cardiac effects**: depression, ataxia (loss of coordination), and GI disturbances like diarrhoea [40].
- **Toxicity**: signs of toxicity need to be monitored closely, especially in horses with renal impairment, as digoxin is excreted via the kidneys [40].

Dobutamine

Dobutamine is a beta-adrenergic agonist primarily used for its inotropic effects on the heart [40, 56].

Mechanism of action:

- **β1 receptor agonism**: stimulates β1 receptors in cardiac muscle, enhancing myocardial contractility with minimal effects on heart rate or systemic vascular resistance [40, 56].
- **Higher dose effects**: at higher doses, it also has some β2 and alpha (α)1 effects, which can influence vascular tone and resistance [40, 56].

Clinical uses:

- **Hypotension during anaesthesia**: commonly used to treat hypotension during anaesthesia, improving cardiac output and tissue perfusion [40, 56].
- **Cardiogenic shock**: effective in managing cardiogenic shock by increasing cardiac output [40, 56].

Administration:

- **IV administration**: administered IV, often as a continuous infusion to maintain stable plasma levels and therapeutic effects [40, 56].

Side effects:

- **Tachyarrhythmia**: this is the primary side effect, especially at high doses or in critically ill horses. Monitoring and dose adjustments are necessary to avoid complications [40, 56].

Anticonvulsant drugs

Anticonvulsant medications are crucial in controlling seizures, which result from excessive electrical activity in the brain. Seizures in horses can be life-threatening due to their size and the risk of injury to the horse and handlers. There are two main types of seizures: generalised and focal. Generalised seizures affect the entire brain, leading to convulsions and loss of consciousness, while focal seizures involve only part of the brain, causing localised muscle tremors or movements without loss of consciousness. Foals are more commonly treated for seizures than adult horses [21, 33].

Phenobarbital

Mechanism of action: phenobarbital is a barbiturate that acts as a CNS depressant. It enhances the inhibitory effects of gamma-aminobutyric acid (GABA) at the GABA-A receptor, reducing neuronal excitability and the likelihood of spontaneous depolarisation. This suppression of electrical activity helps decrease the frequency and severity of seizures [40, 57].

Therapeutic monitoring:

- **Plasma concentrations**: regular monitoring of plasma levels is critical to ensure therapeutic efficacy and prevent toxicity. The therapeutic range for phenobarbital in horses is generally 15-45 µg/mL [40, 57].
- **Dosage adjustments**: dosages may need to be adjusted based on plasma concentration results, clinical response, and any side effects observed [40, 57].

Adverse effects:

- **Sedation and ataxia**: common initial side effects that usually decrease as the horse acclimates to the medication [40, 57].

- **Increased intake**: horses may experience polyphagia (increased food intake), polydipsia (increased water intake), and polyuria (increased urination) when first starting treatment [40, 57].
- **Hepatotoxicity**: phenobarbital can cause liver damage, often unpredictable and idiopathic. Regular liver function tests are recommended to detect early signs of hepatotoxicity [40, 57].

Benzodiazepines

Benzodiazepines are effective anticonvulsants and muscle relaxants, commonly used for their rapid onset of action in emergency seizure control. They enhance the effect of GABA, the primary inhibitory neurotransmitter in the brain [40].

Mechanism of action: benzodiazepines bind to specific sites on the GABA-A receptor, increasing GABA's affinity for the receptor and enhancing its inhibitory effect. This results in CNS depression, muscle relaxation, and reduced seizure activity [40].

Commonly used benzodiazepines:

Midazolam:

- **Use in horses**: licensed for use in horses, particularly useful in premature or neonatal foals for controlling seizures and as a muscle relaxant [33, 58].
- **Mechanism**: increases GABAergic inhibition at multiple brain sites, including the brainstem, limbic system, amygdala, hippocampus, and hypothalamus [33, 58].
- **Administration**: can be administered via the IV or IM routes. It has a rapid onset and short duration, making it suitable for acute seizure control [33, 58].

Diazepam:

- **Use in horses**: not officially licensed for equine use but widely used due to its effectiveness [33, 59].
- **Mechanism**: enhances GABA-mediated inhibition quickly penetrating the blood-brain barrier [33, 59].
- **Clinical applications**: often used as the first line of treatment for seizure activity before midazolam was licensed for equine use. It is also used as a sedative in foals [33, 59].
- **Administration**: typically administered IV. Its effects are rapid but short-lived [33, 59].
- **Side Effects**: Minimal side effects include ataxia and muscle weakness due to its muscle relaxant properties. Tolerance can develop with long-term use, limiting its effectiveness over time [33, 59].

Antihistamines

Histamine is an endogenous compound found in high concentrations in the gastrointestinal tract, lungs, and skin. It plays a significant role in immune responses and allergic reactions. In humans, histamine is a primary mediator of allergic reactions. However, in animals, the role of histamine in allergies is less pronounced, except in specific respiratory conditions where histamine-induced bronchoconstriction can be significant. Antihistamines in equine medicine are primarily used to counteract this bronchoconstriction by antagonising H1 receptors in the smooth muscle of the bronchioles [33].

Clenbuterol Hydrochloride

Mechanism of action: clenbuterol hydrochloride is a β2 adrenergic agonist that stimulates β2 adrenoceptors, leading to bronchodilation. It also enhances ciliary movement within the respiratory mucosal cells and has a mucolytic effect, which helps to thin and reduce the viscosity of mucus [60].

Clinical uses:

- **Allergic respiratory disease**: clenbuterol is used to treat conditions where allergic reactions cause bronchoconstriction [60].
- **Respiratory infections**: helps in managing respiratory infections by improving airway patency [60].
- **Severe equine asthma (formerly known as recurrent airway obstruction or RAO)**: commonly used in horses with severe equine asthma to alleviate symptoms by reducing bronchoconstriction and mucus viscosity [60].

Administration and dosage:

- Available in oral granules, oral syrup, or injectable formulations [60].
- Dosage and administration routes may vary based on the severity of the condition and the discretion of the prescribing vet [60].

Contraindications:

- **Cardiac disease**: not recommended for horses with cardiac disease due to the risk of exacerbating heart conditions [60].
- **Pregnant mares**: should not be used in late pregnancy as it can reduce uterine contractions, potentially affecting labour [60].

Side effects:

- **Transient vasodilation**: temporary widening of blood vessels [60].
- **Tachycardia**: increased heart rate [60].
- **Sweating and muscle tremors**: commonly observed side effects which typically subside after discontinuation [60].

Dembrexine Hydrochloride

Mechanism of action: dembrexine hydrochloride acts as a mucolytic agent, thinning and reducing the viscosity of mucus in the respiratory tract [40].

Clinical uses:

- **Respiratory diseases**: indicated for the symptomatic treatment of acute, sub-acute, and chronic respiratory diseases affecting both the upper and lower respiratory tract, particularly where excessive or thickened mucus is present [40].

Administration and dosage:

- Administered according to the specific product guidelines, usually orally or via injection [40].

Side effects:

- No reported side effects in horses, even at doses up to 15 times the therapeutic range [40, 61].

Ciclesonide

Mechanism of action: ciclesonide is a corticosteroid used to alleviate inflammation in the respiratory tract. It is particularly effective for severe equine asthma and other related conditions [20].

Clinical uses:

- Used to manage the symptoms of severe equine asthma [20].

Administration and dosage [20]:

- Designed to be used with an inhaler, requiring the horse to be cooperative for effective administration
- Commonly prescribed as a 10-day course

Contraindications [20]:

- Pregnant women should not handle this medication due to potential risks

Side effects [20]:

- Mild nasal discharge can occur as a side effect but is generally not severe

Antimicrobials

Antimicrobials are agents used to kill or inhibit the growth of microorganisms, including bacteria, fungi, and viruses. In equine medicine, antimicrobials are critical for treating various infections and maintaining the health of horses. This chapter section will focus primarily on antibacterial agents, their mechanisms, spectrum of activity, and considerations for their use.

Antibacterial Agents

Antibacterial agents are classified based on their mechanism of action and their effect on bacteria. They can be either bactericidal, meaning they kill bacteria, or bacteriostatic, meaning they prevent the replication of bacteria, allowing the immune system of the host to manage the bacterial population effectively [33, 62].

Antibacterial Selection

It is up to the prescribing vet to choose and prescribe the correct antibacterial medication. Factors to consider are as follows:

1) **Spectrum of activity**: the range of pathogens an antibacterial is effective against. This includes whether the drug is effective against gram-positive, gram-negative, aerobic, or anaerobic organisms [40].
2) **Site of infection**: the ability of the drug to reach the site of infection in effective concentrations, considering factors like tissue penetration, ability to cross the blood-brain barrier, and presence in body fluids.
3) **Concentration requirements**: the necessary concentration of the drug to inhibit or kill bacteria, influenced by the minimum inhibitory concentration (MIC) for specific pathogens.
4) **Host factors**: consideration of the patient's age, weight, organ function (particularly liver and kidneys), immune status, and any known allergies or intolerances to medications [21].
5) **Side effects and drug interactions**: potential adverse effects and interactions with other medications being administered to the horse. Monitoring for signs of toxicity is crucial to ensure the chosen antibiotic does not exacerbate any existing conditions.

Key principle: the use of narrow-spectrum antibiotics is preferred to minimise resistance. Broad-spectrum antibiotics should be reserved for cases where narrow-spectrum drugs are ineffective [21].

The main classes of antibacterial drugs availible in veterinary medicine are summarised in Table 9.4.

Beta-lactams

Beta-lactam antibiotics, including penicillins, cephalosporins, and related compounds, are fundamental in antimicrobial therapy in equine medicine due to their broad-spectrum activity against many gram-positive, gram-negative, and anaerobic organisms. The selection of an appropriate beta-actam antibiotic involves understanding the drug's mechanism of action, spectrum of activity, pharmacokinetics, and potential adverse effects.

Penicillins

Mechanism of action: penicillins exert their bactericidal effect by inhibiting the synthesis of bacterial cell walls. They specifically target penicillin-binding proteins (PBPs) involved in the cross-linking of the peptidoglycan layer of the bacterial cell wall. This inhibition leads to the weakening of the cell wall, causing it to rupture and ultimately leading to cell death. Because cell wall synthesis occurs during cell division, penicillins are most effective against actively dividing bacteria. The combination of penicillins with bacteriostatic antibiotics is contraindicated, as these require bacterial growth for optimal activity [33].

Clinical uses:

- **Methicillin-resistant staphylococcus aureus (MRSA)**: MRSA has acquired resistance to all beta-lactam antibiotics, including penicillins, making infections with this organism particularly challenging to treat. Treatment typically requires alternative classes of antibiotics [21].
- **Absorption and distribution**: penicillins are generally well absorbed when administered via injection or orally. They are widely distributed in the body but do not penetrate well into the eye, brain, or prostate due to their hydrophilic nature [40].
- **Excretion**: most penicillins are excreted unchanged by the kidneys. They are actively transported by renal tubules into the urine, achieving high urinary concentrations, which makes them effective for treating urinary tract infections [40].

Adverse reactions:

- **Hypersensitivity reactions**: the most common adverse effect of penicillins is hypersensitivity, which can range from mild urticaria to severe anaphylaxis. Anaphylaxis is more common with injectable formulations and requires immediate treatment with adrenaline and corticosteroids. Close monitoring is essential following administration to detect early signs of hypersensitivity [21].
- **GI disturbances**: while less common, GI side effects such as diarrhoea can occur, particularly with oral formulations.

Cephalosporins

Mechanism of action: cephalosporins, similar to penicillins, inhibit bacterial cell wall synthesis by binding to PBPs.

Table 9.4 The main classes of antibacterial drugs available in veterinary medicine [21, 33].

Class	Mechanism of action	Subdivision	Spectrum of activity	Examples of drug	Example of conditions where the antibiotic is used as a first-line defence
Aminoglycosides	Interfere with bacteria synthesis Bactericidal		Primarily gram-negative anaerobes	Gentamycin, neomycin, amikacin	Contaminated wounds with synovial sepsis, contaminated wounds with open fractures, peritonitis, contaminated surgery, high-risk surgery, neutropenia, endocarditis
Tetracyclines	Interfere with protein synthesis Bacteriostatic		Broad spectrum Gram positive, gram negative, Chlamydophila Rickettsia	Oxytetracycline, Doxycycline	Cellulitis, solar abscess with P3 involvement, secondary pneumonia, severe equine asthma, periapical abscessation
Potentiated Sulphonamides	Inhibit metabolic pathway involved in folic acid synthesis Generally, bactericidal	Combination of two classes of agent / Diaminopyrimidine and a sulphonamide	Broad spectrum Gram positive / Gram negative and some protozoa	Trimethoprim / Sulfadiazine	Cystitis, pyelonephritis, mastitis, neutropenia, patent urachus, umbilical infections, premature/dysmature foal, meningitis, pyoderma, upper respiratory infection, periodontal disease, bacterial cholangiohepatitis, dermatophilosis congolensis (mud fever)
Macrolides	Inhibit bacterial protein synthesis Bacteriostatic and bactericidal		Gram positive and anaerobes	Erythromycin, azithromycin, clarithromycin	*Rhodococcus Equi*, Pneumonia
Nitroimidazoles	Damage bacterial deoxyribonucleic acid (DNA) bactericidal		Anaerobes	Metronidazole	Severe sepsis, contaminated wounds with open fracture, peritonitis, pleuropneumonia, abdominal abscesses, canker
Chloramphenicol	Inhibit bacterial protein synthesis Bacteriostatic		Broad spectrum	Chloramphenicol	Mild corneal ulceration, severe corneal ulceration
Beta-lactams	Interfere with the synthesis of the bacterial cell wall Bactericidal	Narrow spectrum penicillins	Gram-positive anaerobes	Penicillin	Contaminated wounds with synovial sepsis, contaminated wounds with open fractures, *Streptococcus equi* (Strangles), primary sinusitis, guttural pouch empyema, primary pneumonia, peritonitis, clean surgery, contaminated surgery, high-risk surgery
		Aminopenicillins	Gram-negative organisms Beta-lactamase-producing gram-positive organisms Pseudomonas spp.	Ampicillin and amoxicillin / Methicillin, cloxacillin	Severe respiratory infections but may cause severe diarrhoea and subsequent colic or death
		Beta lactamase-resistant penicillins	First generation – broad spectrum others Gram positive and gram negative and anaerobes	Ticarcillin, piperacillin	Intrauterine treatment of endometritis caused by beta-haemolytic streptococci
Protected DO NOT USE as a first defence →		Antipseudomonal penicillins Cephalosporins first to fourth generations	From first to fourth oral bioavailability decreases and gram-negative spectrum increases	First – Cefalexin Second – Cefuroxime Third – Ceftiofur, cefovecin Fourth – Cefquinome	Sepsis, severe sepsis, neonatal pneumonia, meningitis Use after culture and sensitivity as a last resort
Fluroquinolones Protected DO NOT USE as a first defence →	Damage bacterial DNA Bactericidal		Broad spectrum, especially gram-negatives and gram-positives	Enrofloxacin Marbofloxacin	Can be used to treat bacterial infections of the eye, lungs and abdomen after culture and sensitivity Avoid use in foals as they may damage the articular cartilage

Source: Phillippa Pritchard and Rosina Lillywhite.

This action disrupts the formation of the peptidoglycan layer, leading to bacterial cell lysis and death. Cephalosporins are classified into generations based on their spectrum of activity and resistance to beta-lactamases, with each successive generation generally having a broader spectrum and greater beta-lactamase resistance.

Clinical uses:

- **Renal or urinary tract infections**: due to high urinary concentrations, cephalosporins are effective for treating urinary tract infections [33].
- **Hypersensitivity reactions**: cephalosporins have a lower incidence of hypersensitivity compared to penicillins. However, they can still cause allergic reactions, including fever, rashes, and eosinophilia [21, 33].

Adverse reactions:

- **GI upset**: Similar to penicillins, GI disturbances such as diarrhoea can occur, particularly with oral cephalosporins.
- **Renal implications**: high doses or prolonged use can impact renal function, necessitating monitoring of renal parameters during treatment.

Aminoglycosides

Mechanism of action: aminoglycosides bind to the bacterial ribosomal ribonuecleic acid (RNA), specifically the 30S subunit, disrupting protein synthesis and leading to the production of defective proteins, which ultimately kills the bacteria. They require active transport into bacterial cells, which is oxygen-dependent, rendering them ineffective against anaerobic bacteria. The efficacy of aminoglycosides is enhanced when combined with cell wall-inhibiting antibiotics like penicillins, which facilitate their entry into bacterial cells [21, 33, 40].

Administration and distribution:

- **Parenteral administration**: aminoglycosides are usually administered via the IV or IM route due to poor GI absorption. They are well absorbed through abraded skin, making them useful for irrigating surgical sites [33, 40].
- **Distribution**: these drugs do not cross the blood-brain barrier and are not effectively secreted into the respiratory tract when nebulised. However, they achieve high concentrations in the lining of the respiratory tract and urine due to renal excretion [40].

Clinical uses:

- **Contaminated wounds and synovial sepsis**: effective for treating joint infections and contaminated wounds [21, 33].

- **Open fractures**: used to prevent osteomyelitis.
- **Peritonitis**: effective in treating abdominal infections [40].
- **High-risk surgeries**: prophylactic use to prevent postoperative infections.

Adverse reactions:

- **Nephrotoxicity**: aminoglycosides can cause kidney damage, necessitating close monitoring of renal function, especially in dehydrated or geriatric horses [21, 33, 40].
- **Ototoxicity**: potentially toxic to the inner ear, causing hearing damage.
- **Early toxicity signs**: signs include the appearance of casts or increased protein in the urine. Elevated blood urea nitrogen (BUN) and creatinine levels indicate significant renal impairment [21].

Tetracyclines

Tetracyclines are bacteriostatic antibiotics that inhibit bacterial growth and reproduction rather than killing them outright. This mode of action requires a functional immune system in the horse to help overcome the infection. Two commonly used tetracyclines in equine medicine are doxycycline and oxytetracycline, each with distinct properties and applications [21].

Doxycycline

- **Lipophilicity**: doxycycline is lipophilic, allowing it to be readily absorbed through the GI wall when administered orally. This property makes it particularly useful for treating systemic infections where oral administration is preferred.
- **Clinical uses**: doxycycline is often the drug of choice for treating infections involving the CNS and for managing Lyme disease which is caused by the spirochete bacterium Borrelia burgdorferi. Lyme disease is transmitted by ticks and can lead to symptoms including lameness, fever, and neurological signs in horses. The ability of doxycycline to effectively penetrate the blood-brain barrier makes it an ideal choice for CNS infections.
- **Excretion**: doxycycline is primarily excreted via the liver into the intestine, influencing its dosing and potential side effects. This excretion route can benefit horses with renal issues, as it places less burden on the kidneys when compared to other antibiotics.

Oxytetracycline

- **Injectable formulation**: oxytetracycline is commonly used as an injectable formulation in equine practice. It is well absorbed from IM injection sites, making it suitable for treating various infections in horses, particularly those where oral administration is not feasible or effective.

- **Clinical uses**: oxytetracycline is often used to treat respiratory, joint, and other systemic bacterial infections. One notable use of oxytetracycline is treating contracted foal tendons. Administering oxytetracycline helps to relax and elongate the tendons, aiding in correcting this condition [21].
- **Excretion**: oxytetracycline is excreted by the kidneys, making monitoring renal function during treatment important, especially in dehydrated or older horses.

Binding with calcium: a significant issue with tetracyclines, including doxycycline and oxytetracycline, is their strong affinity for binding with calcium. This can lead to the yellowing of teeth, particularly in young horses whose teeth are still developing. The binding of tetracyclines to calcium can also reduce their bioavailability, meaning their absorption and effectiveness can be decreased if administered with calcium-rich feeds [21].

Administration considerations: when administering tetracyclines, particularly oxytetracycline, via IV injection, it is crucial to adhere to proper administration protocols to avoid severe adverse reactions. Rapid IV injection of oxytetracycline can result in cardiac arrhythmia, collapse, and even death due to its effects on cardiac muscle. Therefore, it should be administered slowly, typically over one minute, as recommended in the datasheet. This slow administration helps mitigate the risk of sudden cardiovascular complications [21].

Sulphonamides and Potentiated Sulphonamides

Sulphonamides were among the first widely used antimicrobials, leading to high levels of bacterial resistance over time. These bacteriostatic agents inhibit bacterial growth by disrupting folic acid synthesis. In equine medicine, sulphonamides are frequently combined with trimethoprim, a potentiating agent that enhances their antibacterial effects, creating potentiated sulphonamides [21].

Mechanism of action: Sulphonamides interfere with bacterial metabolism by inhibiting the enzyme dihydropteroate synthase, which is crucial for synthesising folic acid. Folic acid is necessary for bacteria's DNA, RNA, and protein synthesis. When combined with trimethoprim, which inhibits dihydrofolate reductase (another enzyme in the folic acid pathway), the combination results in a synergistic effect, effectively blocking two sequential steps in the bacterial folic acid pathway. This dual blockade provides a broader spectrum of activity and reduces the likelihood of resistance developing compared to using sulphonamides alone [21, 36].

Spectrum of activity: potentiated sulphonamides exhibit a broad spectrum of activity against a wide range of gram-positive and gram-negative bacteria and some protozoa. Despite widespread resistance among many bacteria, common protozoal infections encountered in equine practice remain susceptible. These include Eimeria species and other protozoa that may cause gastrointestinal disturbances in horses (these are not commonly found in UK populations).

Pharmacokinetics: sulphonamides and potentiated sulphonamides are well absorbed from the GI tract in monogastric animals, including horses. Once absorbed, they are widely distributed throughout the body, reaching therapeutic concentrations in various tissues and fluids, including crossing the blood-prostate barrier, placenta, milk, and the blood-brain barrier to reach the cerebral spinal fluid (CSF). This extensive distribution makes them effective for treating various respiratory, urinary tract, and CNS infections. Excretion of sulphonamides varies; some are excreted unchanged in the urine, while others are metabolised by the liver before renal excretion. In the case of potentiated sulphonamides, both components must be present in the tissues simultaneously to achieve the desired antibacterial effect. This requirement often leads clinicians to administer these drugs twice daily, even though once-daily dosing might be recommended, to maintain effective tissue concentrations.

Clinical uses: sulphonamides are commonly used for their broad-spectrum antibacterial properties. They are frequently employed in treating respiratory infections, such as bacterial pneumonia and urinary tract infections. Additionally, they are used for wound infections and gastrointestinal infections caused by susceptible organisms. Specific formulations used in equine practice include Trimethoprim-sulphonamide (TMPS) combinations available in oral forms. These formulations are convenient for horse owners to administer and ensure consistent dosing [21].

Adverse reactions: while sulphonamides and their potentiated forms are generally safe, they can cause adverse reactions in horses. Common side effects include pruritus (itching), facial swelling, and hives (urticaria). More severe reactions, though less common, can include liver necrosis and liver failure. Horses may also experience GI disturbances such as diarrhoea or colic [21]. Following recommended dosing guidelines and monitoring horses closely during treatment is crucial to minimise the risk of adverse reactions. In cases of hypersensitivity or severe reactions, discontinuation of the drug and supportive care may be necessary.

Fluoroquinolones

Fluoroquinolones are a class of broad-spectrum antibiotics effective against various bacterial infections. They are particularly useful for treating skin, respiratory, and urinary tract infections caused by gram-negative bacteria such as *pseudomonas, klebsiella, escherichia coli,* and *salmonella.* Both aminoglycosides and fluoroquinolones require high peak concentrations for their bactericidal activity, which is crucial for their effectiveness [21, 33].

Pharmacokinetics and absorption: oral absorption of fluoroquinolones is generally good in small animals like cats and dogs, but it is more variable in horses and ruminants. In adult horses, fluoroquinolones are absorbed relatively well when administered orally, which allows for their use in systemic infections. However, foals do not absorb these drugs as efficiently, making oral administration less effective in younger animals. Fluoroquinolones are highly lipophilic, enabling them to accumulate in high concentrations in various tissues and bodily fluids. This includes the kidneys, liver, lungs, bone, joint fluid, aqueous humour of the eye, and respiratory tissues. This extensive tissue penetration makes fluoroquinolones particularly effective for treating infections in these areas.

Metabolism and excretion: enrofloxacin is the primary fluoroquinolone used in equine medicine. After administration, the kidneys excrete enrofloxacin, but a significant portion (up to one-fourth) is metabolised into ciprofloxacin. Ciprofloxacin is metabolised and excreted via both the liver and kidneys, contributing to the effectiveness of the drug in treating systemic infections [21, 33].

Clinical uses: fluoroquinolones are employed to manage several types of bacterial infections in horses:

1) **Respiratory infections**: fluoroquinolones treat bacterial pneumonia and other lower respiratory tract infections due to their excellent penetration into respiratory tissues.
2) **Urinary tract infections**: their high concentration in the kidneys makes them suitable for treating urinary tract infections caused by susceptible bacteria.
3) **Skin and soft tissue infections**: fluoroquinolones are effective for treating skin infections and soft tissue infections, particularly those involving resistant gram-negative bacteria. Enrofloxacin is available in both oral and injectable forms, allowing flexibility in administration based on the specific needs of the patient [21, 33].

Safety and adverse effects: fluoroquinolones are generally considered safe for adult horses; however, their use must be carefully managed due to potential adverse effects. Possible side effects in adult horses include GI disturbances such as diarrhoea (colitis), colic and hypersensitivity reactions. Therefore, it is essential to monitor horses closely during treatment with fluoroquinolones and to use these antibiotics judiciously to avoid unnecessary adverse effects and to preserve their efficacy by preventing the development of resistance. Another potential concern with fluoroquinolones is their potential to affect joint cartilage development adversely. This has been well-documented in rapidly growing dogs, where it can lead to joint cartilage lesions and other developmental issues. Although similar studies have not been conducted in horses, avoiding fluoroquinolones in young horses, especially those still undergoing rapid growth phases, is prudent to mitigate any potential risk [21, 33].

Macrolides

Macrolides, including erythromycin and azithromycin, are significant in treating various bacterial infections in horses, particularly those affecting the respiratory system. These antibiotics are particularly valuable for their efficacy against gram-positive bacteria and certain other pathogens, their ability to penetrate tissues, and their relative safety in horses with penicillin allergies [21].

Mechanism of action: macrolides inhibit bacterial protein synthesis by binding to the 50S ribosomal subunit, thereby preventing the translocation step of protein elongation. This action is bacteriostatic, which inhibits the growth and reproduction of bacteria, allowing the immune system of the horse to combat the infection effectively.

Erythromycin

Erythromycin is widely used for its effectiveness against gram-positive bacterial respiratory infections. This antibiotic accumulates in respiratory secretions, making it particularly effective for treating infections such as bronchitis, pneumonia, and other lower respiratory tract infections [21]. One notable application of erythromycin in equine medicine is treating *rhodococcus equi* infections in foals. *Rhodococcus equi* causes severe pneumonia in foals, which can be life-threatening if not treated promptly. Erythromycin, often combined with rifampicin, is a standard treatment for this condition [21]. However, erythromycin administration can lead to GI side effects in horses, most notably diarrhoea. This adverse reaction usually resolves once the medication is discontinued, but it necessitates careful monitoring and supportive care during treatment.

Azithromycin

Azithromycin, an erythromycin derivative, offers a broader spectrum of activity and is particularly effective against certain pathogens, such as Mycoplasma species, which can be involved in equine pneumonia. The pharmacokinetics of azithromycin include a longer half-life and better tissue penetration, make it a valuable alternative when first-line antibiotics fail or when dealing with resistant infections [21]. Azithromycin is commonly used to treat *rhodococcus equi* infections in foals, similar to erythromycin. Its broader spectrum also makes it effective against various other bacterial infections, including those involving mixed flora or atypical pathogens.

Considerations in treatment: when using macrolides, particularly in foals, it is essential to ensure that the medication does not inadvertently come into contact with the mare. Macrolides, especially erythromycin, can cause severe and potentially fatal colitis in adult horses if ingested. This risk underscores the importance of proper handling and administration techniques. For instance, rinsing the foal's mouth thoroughly after administering the medication can help prevent accidental transfer to the mare during nursing [21].

Nitroimidazoles

Nitroimidazoles, with metronidazole being the most commonly used agent in equine medicine, are crucial for treating infections involving anaerobic bacteria. Metronidazole is particularly effective for infections where anaerobes are suspected or confirmed due to its unique mechanism of action under low oxygen conditions.

Mechanism of action: metronidazole is metabolised into an active form within the bacterial cell under anaerobic conditions. This active form disrupts DNA and nucleic acid synthesis, leading to bacterial cell death. This mechanism makes metronidazole particularly effective against anaerobic bacteria, which thrive in low-oxygen environments. It is ineffective against aerobic bacteria, which require oxygen for growth [21].

Clinical uses:

1) **Pleuropneumonia**: this is a severe infection involving the lungs and pleural cavity, often caused by a mix of aerobic and anaerobic bacteria. Metronidazole is used in conjunction with other antibiotics to ensure broad-spectrum coverage and effectively target the anaerobic component of the infection.
2) **Peritonitis**: inflammation of the peritoneum, often following GI rupture or surgery, can involve anaerobic bacteria. Metronidazole is included in the antibiotic regimen to combat these anaerobes and reduce the risk of severe infection and complications.
3) **Abdominal abscesses**: intra-abdominal abscesses often harbour anaerobic bacteria. The ability of metronidazole to penetrate the walls of abscesses and reach the anaerobic bacteria makes it a valuable treatment option.
4) **Post-surgical prophylaxis**: the risk of anaerobic bacterial infection is high after colic surgery or other abdominal procedures. Metronidazole is used prophylactically to prevent such infections, contributing to better surgical outcomes and reducing postoperative complications [21].

Forms of administration: metronidazole is available in several forms, providing flexibility in administration based on the condition of the patient and the clinical scenario [21]:

- **Oral preparations**: these are commonly used for long-term treatment or when IV administration is not feasible. However, the bitter taste of metronidazole can make oral administration challenging, requiring flavoured pastes or mixing with feed.
- **IV preparations**: IV administration ensures rapid drug delivery to the bloodstream, making it ideal for acute infections and situations where quick therapeutic levels are necessary.
- **Rectal preparations**: these are occasionally used when oral or IV routes are unsuitable, such as severe oral ulcers or oesophageal strictures.

Adverse effects and considerations: while metronidazole is generally well-tolerated, it can cause adverse effects, particularly at higher doses or with prolonged use. Notable side effects include the following [21]:

- **Neurological effects**: reversible, transient neurological side effects can occur, including loss of balance, disorientation, and nystagmus. These effects are more common with higher doses and long-term administration.
- **GI disturbances**: metronidazole can cause anorexia and diarrhoea, although these side effects are less common in horses than in small animals.
- **Hypersensitivity reactions**: although rare, hypersensitivity reactions can occur, necessitating discontinuation of the drug and appropriate supportive care.

Monitoring and management: due to potential neurological side effects, horses receiving metronidazole should be closely monitored, especially at higher doses or for extended periods. If signs of neurological impairment are observed, the drug should be discontinued, and supportive treatment provided. Most neurological side effects are reversible upon discontinuation of the drug [21].

Chloramphenicol

Chloramphenicol is a broad-spectrum antibiotic used for its efficacy in treating infections caused by various bacteria. Its mechanism of action and ability to penetrate various tissues makes it a valuable tool, particularly in treating eye infections [21].

Mechanism of action: chloramphenicol exerts its antibacterial effects by binding to the 50S ribosomal subunit of bacteria, inhibiting peptide bond formation and thus disrupting protein synthesis. This action is bacteriostatic at lower concentrations, preventing bacterial growth and reproduction. At higher concentrations, it can be bactericidal, directly killing the bacteria. This dual action allows for dosing flexibility based on the infection's severity and the response needed [21].

Safety and toxicity concerns: chloramphenicol can affect mitochondrial protein synthesis in mammalian cells, leading to bone marrow suppression. This suppression is usually reversible upon discontinuation of the drug, but it poses a significant risk when used for extended periods or at high doses. In humans, chloramphenicol has been linked to fatal aplastic anaemia, a rare but serious condition where the bone marrow fails to produce sufficient blood cells. Because of this severe risk, chloramphenicol use in animals intended for the human food chain is strictly prohibited [63]. While the risk of aplastic anaemia in horses is not as documented as it is in humans, the potential for bone marrow suppression warrants cautious use. Regular monitoring of blood parameters during prolonged therapy is advisable to detect any early signs of bone marrow suppression [21].

Pharmacokinetics and tissue penetration: one of the most valuable attributes of chloramphenicol is its excellent tissue penetration. It effectively crosses various barriers, including the blood-brain barrier, making it suitable for treating CNS infections. Additionally, it penetrates well into the prostate gland and ocular tissues, which are often challenging sites for antibiotic delivery [21].

Clinical uses:

1) **Ophthalmic infections**: chloramphenicol is most commonly used in the form of eye drops or ointments to treat bacterial corneal ulceration. Corneal ulcers in horses can be caused by trauma or bacterial infections, and timely treatment is crucial to prevent severe complications or vision loss. The ability of chloramphenicol to penetrate the corneal tissue effectively makes it an excellent choice for these infections.

2) **Respiratory and CNS infections**: given its ability to cross the blood-brain barrier, chloramphenicol can be used to treat bacterial meningitis or other CNS infections in horses, although its use for such conditions is less common and typically reserved for cases where other antibiotics have failed or are unsuitable.

Administration and dosage: chloramphenicol is available in various forms, including oral, injectable, and topical preparations. The choice of administration route depends on the location and the severity of the infection. Topical preparations such as eye drops or ointments are preferred for ophthalmic use. Systemic infections may require oral or injectable forms, although these are used less frequently due to the risk of adverse effects and the need for careful monitoring [21].

Adverse effects and monitoring: while chloramphenicol is generally well-tolerated in horses, adverse effects can occur. These can include the following [63]:

- **Bone marrow suppression**: during prolonged treatment, regular blood tests are recommended to monitor for any signs of bone marrow suppression.
- **GI disturbances**: horses may experience diarrhoea or colic, particularly with oral administration.
- **Hypersensitivity reactions**: although rare, allergic reactions can occur and should be monitored.

Rifampicin

Rifampicin, a member of the rifamycin class, is a potent antimicrobial with both bactericidal and bacteriostatic properties. Its unique mechanism of action and ability to penetrate tissues make it particularly useful in treating certain infections in horses, especially foals. Due to the risk of developing resistance when used alone, rifampicin is often combined with other antibiotics, enhancing its efficacy and broadening its spectrum of action [21, 33].

Mechanism of action: rifampicin works by inhibiting the DNA-dependent RNA polymerase enzyme in bacteria, thereby blocking RNA synthesis. This inhibition prevents bacterial replication and protein synthesis, leading to bacterial cell death (bactericidal effect) or halting growth (bacteriostatic effect) depending on the concentration and susceptibility of the bacteria. Rifampicin selectively targets bacterial RNA polymerase, leaving mammalian cells unaffected, contributing to its safety profile in therapeutic use [21].

Clinical uses:

1) ***Rhodococcus equi* infections**: rifampicin is widely used with erythromycin or azithromycin to treat *rhodococcus equi* infections in foals. *Rhodococcus equi* is a significant pathogen causing pneumonia in foals, characterised by lung abscesses and severe respiratory distress. The combination therapy is effective because rifampicin penetrates intracellularly, where *rhodococcus equi* resides, and works synergistically with macrolides to enhance bacterial destruction.

2) **Other bacterial infections**: rifampicin is also used to treat various bacterial infections in horses when combined with other antibiotics like aminoglycosides, beta-lactams, or doxycycline. This combination therapy is crucial for managing infections caused by resistant bacteria and preventing the emergence of rifampicin-resistant strains.

3) **Fungal infections**: although primarily an antibacterial, rifampicin has been noted to enhance the effects of antifungal agents like amphotericin B. This combination can be effective against fungal infections such as those caused by aspergillus species. While less common, aspergillus infections can be severe and require aggressive treatment.

Pharmacokinetics and tissue penetration: rifampicin is well-absorbed following oral administration and widely distributed throughout the body. It penetrates well into various tissues, including the lungs, liver, and intracellular compartments, which is critical for treating infections like *rhodococcus equi* pneumonia in foals. Its ability to reach intracellular sites of infection makes it particularly effective in treating intracellular pathogens.

Side effects and considerations: while rifampicin is generally well-tolerated in horses, it has some notable side effects which are as follows [21]:

- **Discolouration of body fluids**: One of the most distinctive side effects of rifampicin is the reddish-orange discolouration of urine, sweat, tears, and saliva. This harmless but noticeable effect results from the pigmentation of the drug and can also cause plasma to appear reddish, resembling haemolysis. Owners should be informed about this discolouration to prevent unnecessary alarm.
- **Hepatotoxicity**: rifampicin can cause the elevation of liver enzymes, indicating potential liver stress or damage. Regular monitoring of liver function tests is advisable during prolonged therapy, especially in foals or horses with pre-existing liver conditions.
- **Drug interactions**: rifampicin is a potent inducer of cytochrome P450 enzymes, which can affect the metabolism of other concurrently administered drugs. This interaction necessitates careful consideration and possible adjustment of dosages for drugs metabolised by the liver.
- **GI disturbances**: as with many antibiotics, rifampicin can cause GI side effects, including diarrhoea and colic. These side effects are usually transient and resolve upon discontinuation of the drug.

Antiviral Medications

Antiviral medications are designed to target specific viruses and are generally safe for the host. Unlike broad-spectrum antibiotics that can target multiple types of bacteria, most antiviral drugs are selective for specific viruses. Although less common, broad-spectrum antivirals can treat a wider range of viral infections. These medications differ from viricides, which are chemical agents that inactivate or destroy virus particles on surfaces or in the body [21].

In equine medicine, the use of antiviral medications is relatively limited compared to other therapeutic categories. However, they are critical in managing specific viral infections that can significantly impact equine health and performance [21].

Aciclovir

This is one of the few antiviral medications used in equine practice. It is a synthetic nucleoside analogue that inhibits viral DNA polymerase, an enzyme essential for viral DNA replication. By interfering with this enzyme, aciclovir effectively halts the replication of herpesviruses, reducing the severity and spread of the infection.

Clinical uses:

1) **Equine herpesvirus (EHV) infections**: EHV, particularly EHV-1 and EHV-4, can cause respiratory disease, neurological disorders, and reproductive issues in horses. Aciclovir is used to manage these infections, especially during outbreaks, to control the spread and mitigate symptoms. While not always curative, it can significantly reduce viral shedding and disease severity.
2) **Equine superficial punctate keratitis**: this condition, caused by EHV, results in corneal inflammation and lesions. Aciclovir is applied topically as an ointment to treat the viral component of this eye disease, promoting healing and reducing discomfort.
3) **Sarcoids**: although primarily caused by bovine papillomavirus, some evidence suggests that antiviral treatments can be beneficial in managing equine sarcoids. In topical form, Aciclovir is sometimes used to treat these skin tumours, particularly when they exhibit aggressive behaviour or resist other treatments.

Formulation and administration: aciclovir is primarily available as a topical ointment for equine use. This formulation is suitable for direct application to affected areas, such as the eyes or skin lesions, ensuring high local concentrations of the drug where it is needed most [21].

Considerations and side effects: while aciclovir is generally well-tolerated, some considerations must be kept in mind [21]:

- **Topical application**: care must be taken to apply the ointment correctly to avoid contamination and ensure effective dosing. Proper hygiene and the correct technique are essential to prevent further infection or irritation.
- **Side effects**: adverse effects are rare, including mild local irritation at the application site. Monitoring for any signs of allergic reaction or increased irritation is essential.

Other antiviral agents: while aciclovir is the most commonly used antiviral in equine medicine, research and development continue to explore other antiviral agents that could benefit horses. These might include:

- **Valacyclovir**: a prodrug of aciclovir, which has better oral bioavailability. It could potentially be used for systemic treatment of EHV infections.
- **Famciclovir**: another nucleoside analogue with potential applications in treating viral infections in horses, particularly for systemic or severe cases.

Emerging research and applications: recent advances in veterinary virology and pharmacology are exploring new antiviral treatments for equine use. Research focuses on improving existing drugs' efficacy, discovering novel antiviral compounds, and developing vaccines that can help prevent viral infections [21].

Gene therapy and immunomodulators: gene therapy and immunomodulatory treatments are also being investigated to enhance the horse's immune response to viral infections. These therapies aim to boost the horse's natural defences, making it more resistant to infections and reducing the reliance on antiviral medications [21].

Vaccination: vaccination remains a cornerstone of viral infection control in equine medicine. While not an antiviral medication per se, vaccines prepare the horse's immune system to fight off specific viruses, reducing the incidence and severity of outbreaks [21].

Antifungal Medications

Antifungal medications are critical in treating various fungal infections in horses. Dermatophytosis (ringworm) is the most common fungal condition in equine patients, but antifungals are also used to treat fungal eye conditions and guttural pouch mycosis, which are often caused by aspergillus species. Understanding the different classes of antifungal medications, their modes of action, and their specific usesis essential for effective treatment [21, 33].

Table 9.5 summarises examples of commonly encountered antifungal medications.

Overview of Antifungal Medications

Griseofulvin

Mode of action: griseofulvin disrupts mitotic spindle fibres, inhibiting cell division in dermatophytes and fungi that cause skin infections like ringworm [21].

Clinical uses: Griseofulvin is primarily used to treat dermatophytosis in horses. It is absorbed orally through the digestive tract, though absorption is enhanced when administered with a fatty meal.

Administration and dosage: since it is poorly absorbed topically, griseofulvin is administered orally.

Contraindications: griseofulvin is contraindicated in pregnant animals due to the risk of congenital disabilities developing in the foetus.

Side effects: side effects may include anorexia and diarrhoea. The liver metabolises the drug, so liver function should be monitored during treatment.

Azoles

Mode of action: azoles inhibit the synthesis of ergosterol, a crucial component of the fungal cell membrane, leading to increased membrane permeability and cell death [21].

Table 9.5 Table of commonly encountered antifungal medications [21, 33].

Class	Examples	Mode of action	Spectrum of activity	Additional information
Griseofulvin	Griseofulvin	Disrupts mitotic spindle fibres Fungistatic	Dermatophytes (ringworm)	Given orally
Azoles	Ketoconazole Miconazole (Malaseb) Itraconazole Enilconazole (imaverol)	Inhibits formation of fungal cell membrane Fungistatic	Broad spectrum	Mostly topical use
Polyenes	Nystatin, Natamycin Amphotericin B	Interferes with fungal cell membrane Fungicidal	Broad spectrum	Amphotericin B highly toxic for systemic use. Others used topically
Systemic iodine therapy	Potassium iodide	Unknown	Broad spectrum	Given orally. Toxicity and resistance can occur. Administration of iodine in the diet of pregnant mares may cause congenital hypothyroidism in foals

Source: Phillippa Pritchard.

Examples and uses:

- **Ketoconazole and miconazole (Malaseb®)** are primarily used topically to treat fungal skin infections.
- **Itraconazole**: used to treat dermatophytes and guttural pouch mycosis in horses. It is often preferred due to its relatively low toxicity and effectiveness.
- **Voriconazole**: sometimes used to treat fungal keratitis in the equine eye, given its ability to penetrate ocular tissues effectively.

Administration and dosage: azoles can be administered topically or systemically, depending on the infection's location and severity [21].

Side effects: generally take 5-10 days to take effect. The most common side effects are associated with the GI tract such as anorexia and diarrhoea.

Polyenes

Mode of action: polyenes bind to ergosterol in the fungal cell membrane, creating pores that cause cell contents to leak, leading to cell death [21].

Examples and uses:

- **Nystatin and natamycin**: these are typically used topically for superficial fungal infections.
- **Amphotericin B**: used for treating deep or systemic mycoses. It is highly effective but also highly toxic, particularly to the kidneys.

Administration and dosage: amphotericin B is administered primarily via IV injection due to poor GI absorption.

Side effects: the most significant side effect is kidney toxicity, which requires close monitoring. Other side effects include fever and anorexia.

Systemic Iodine

Mode of action: the exact mode of action is unknown, but systemic iodine therapy is believed to disrupt various metabolic processes in fungi.

Examples and uses: potassium iodide is given orally to treat broad-spectrum fungal infections.

Administration and dosage: administered orally, potassium iodide is effective but must be used cautiously due to potential toxicity and the risk of resistance.

Contraindications: administration in pregnant mares may cause congenital hypothyroidism in foals.

Specific Antifungal Medications

Amphotericin B

Mode of action: it binds to ergosterol in fungal cell membranes, creating pores that cause critical materials to leak out, leading to cell death.

Administration: given primarily via IV injection due to poor GI absorption.

Clinical uses: amphotericin B is a potent antifungal for treating deep or systemic mycoses, such as aspergillosis in horses [21].

Side effects: significant side effects include kidney toxicity, fever, and anorexia, with kidney damage being the most critical concern.

Antineoplastic Medications

Antineoplastic medications, also known as chemotherapy or cytotoxic drugs, treat various cancers in equine patients. These medications target and kill rapidly dividing cancer cells, which can help manage and reduce tumour growth. In horses, the primary cancers treated with antineoplastic drugs include squamous cell carcinomas (SSCs), sarcoids, and melanomas [64].

Types of antineoplastic medications and their uses
Mitomycin C

Mechanism of action: mitomycin C works by cross-linking DNA, inhibiting DNA synthesis and ultimately leading to cell death. This makes it effective against rapidly dividing cancer cells.

Clinical uses: mitomycin C is an antimicrobial with cytotoxic properties, primarily used to treat SCCs of the third eyelid following surgical excision. SCCs are common in horses and can be aggressive, often requiring a combination of surgical and medical treatments [4, 65].

Side effects: potential side effects include damage to red blood cells and kidneys and immune system suppression.

Safety precautions: due to its cytotoxic nature, proper PPE should be worn when handling mitomycin C, and syringes and other administration materials should be disposed of in designated cytotoxic waste containers [4, 66].

AW-3-LUDES

Mechanism of action: fluorouracil interferes with DNA and RNA synthesis, inhibiting cancer cell growth and proliferation.

Clinical uses: AW-3-LUDES contains fluorouracil, used to treat human skin cancers and equine sarcoids, which are one of the most common skin tumours in horses and can be challenging to treat due to their recurrent nature.

Application: it should only be applied to affected areas, and precautions must be taken to avoid sun exposure on treated skin, as it can increase sensitivity and risk of severe sunburn.

Notes: AW-3-LUDES - this cream, which used to be known as 'Liverpool cream', was created by Derek Knottenbelt to treat equine sarcoids. It can only be brought by vets and applied by vets due to its ability to harm the surrounding tissue if used incorrectly [66, 67].

Cisplatin

Mechanism of action: cisplatin forms cross-links in DNA, preventing replication and transcription, leading to cell death.

Clinical uses: cisplatin is used intralesionally for treating equine skin tumours, including sarcoids, spindle-cell tumours, squamous cell carcinomas, and melanomas.

Administration: the drug is injected directly into the tumour under general anaesthesia, often using an electrical current to increase drug uptake, a procedure known as electrochemotherapy. This treatment is typically repeated three times at two-week intervals.

Considerations: electrochemotherapy with cisplatin is performed under general anaesthesia to ensure the horse remains still and to maximise the efficacy of the treatment [67, 68].

Oncept® vaccine

Mechanism of action: this vaccine stimulates the immune system of the horse to recognise and attack melanoma cells, reducing tumour size and limiting its ability to spread.

Clinical uses: developed by Merial/Boehringer Ingelheim, the Oncept® vaccine is designed to help the immune system target an enzyme concentrated in melanoma cells. Although initially developed for dogs, some horses have responded well to this treatment [68].

Administration: horses receive an initial series of four vaccinations, followed by boosters every six months. This treatment is currently off-licence for horses, meaning it is not officially approved for use in equines, but it may be used under veterinary discretion.

Cost and accessibility: the Oncept® vaccine procedure is costly and typically available only through veterinary internal medicine specialists [68].

Bacillus Calmette-guerin (BCG)

Mechanism of action: BCG induces a strong local immune response, destroying tumour cells. It is one of the oldest forms of cancer immunotherapy and has shown efficacy in treating equine sarcoids.

Clinical uses: BCG, an attenuated vaccine derived from *Mycobacterium bovis*, is used to treat sarcoids, especially those around the eye, through intralesional injection [69].

Administration: BCG is injected directly into the tumour, stimulating an immune response that helps to shrink and eliminate the tumour. This treatment is particularly useful for sarcoids in sensitive areas, such as around the eyes, where surgical removal might be challenging [69].

Antiparasiticide Medications

Antiparasiticidal medications play a crucial role in maintaining horses' health and wellbeing by controlling internal and external parasites. The ideal antiparasiticide should possess several key characteristics to ensure efficacy and safety [33]:

1) Selective toxicity: the drug should be highly toxic to the parasite but not harmful to the host animal.
2) Economic viability: the treatment should be cost-effective, particularly important for owners managing multiple horses.
3) Broad spectrum: effective against all stages of the parasite lifecycle with one application, minimising the need for repeated treatments.
4) Safety: safe for use in elderly horses, youngstock, pregnant, lactating, and debilitated animals.
5) Resistance management: does not promote the development of resistance in parasite populations.

Modern Worming Programmes

Modern worming programmes focus on breaking the parasite life cycle to control parasite populations effectively. These programmes often include a combination of strategic deworming and pasture management practices. Various antiparasiticides are used to control endoparasites (internal parasites), ectoparasites (external parasites), or both (endectocides) [33].

Classes of Antiparasiticides

Macrocyclic Lactones

Examples: ivermectin (Eqvalan™), doramectin (Dectomax™), moxidectin (Equest™).

Mechanism of Action: these drugs cause paralysis in parasites by enhancing the release of GABA, an inhibitory neurotransmitter, leading to starvation and death of the parasites [21].

Clinical uses:

- Effective against a broad range of nematodes and arthropods.
- It is commonly used for controlling gastrointestinal roundworms, lungworms, and bots.

Safety and side effects: signs of overdose include hypersalivation, ataxia, depression, coma, and seizures. There is no antidote, so careful dosing is essential [21].

Benzimidazoles

Examples: fenbendazole (Panacur Equine Guard™).

Mechanism of action: disrupts the normal function of parasitic cells by binding to β-tubulin, inhibiting the formation of microtubules, and eventually killing the parasite over 24 hours [21].

Clinical uses:

- Widely used to treat nematode infections.
- Effective against adult and larval stages of various roundworms.

Safety and side effects: generally safe with a broad margin of safety. Some resistance has been noted in parasite populations, emphasising the need for strategic use [21].

Tetrahydropyrimidines
Pyrantel (Strongid P™) **Mechanism of action**: acts as a depolarising neuromuscular blocking agent, causing parasite paralysis.

Clinical uses:

- Effective against roundworms and tapeworms (in double doses).
- Commonly used as part of a rotational deworming programme.

Safety and side effects: well-tolerated with minimal side effects. Overdose is rare but can cause signs of toxicity similar to cholinergic crisis [21].

Praziquantel
Mechanism of action: disrupts the integument of the parasite, leading to paralysis and death [21, 70].

Clinical uses:

- Effective against a wide range of tapeworms.
- Often combined with other antiparasiticides, such as ivermectin, to extend the spectrum of activity.

Safety and side effects: generally well-tolerated. Transient GI disturbances may occur.

Pyrethrins and pyrethroids **Mechanism of action**: disrupts the nervous system of insects, leading to paralysis and death [7].

Clinical uses:

- Control of external parasites like flies, lice, and mites.

Examples and specific uses:

- **Permethrin**: found in household fly sprays and cattle ear tags, also used in equine practice as Switch®. It acts as both an insecticide and a repellent. Toxic to cats, caution is needed in areas where cats are present.

- **Cypermethrin**: approved for use in livestock and equines, commonly used in products like Deosect® for controlling lice and as a fly repellent.

Safety and side effects: generally safe for use in horses, but care should be taken to avoid overexposure and potential toxicity in other animals, especially cats [7].

For a more information about worming programmes and anthelmintics, please see Chapter 5.

Corticosteroids

Corticosteroids are a class of steroid hormones produced by the adrenal gland cortex, divided into two main categories: mineralocorticoids and glucocorticoids. These drugs are crucial in managing inflammation, immune responses, and various physiological processes in horses [33].

Mineralocorticoids
Function: mineralocorticoids, such as aldosterone, are primarily involved in regulating water and electrolyte balance. They control sodium and potassium levels in the body, affecting fluid balance and blood pressure. In equine medicine, their use is limited due to their minimal anti-inflammatory effects [33].

Glucocorticoids
Function: glucocorticoids, such as cortisol and cortisone, have potent anti-inflammatory and immunosuppressive properties. They inhibit phospholipase A2, an enzyme involved in the arachidonic acid pathway, thereby reducing the production of inflammatory mediators like prostaglandins and leukotrienes. This inhibition helps manage inflammation, allergic reactions, and autoimmune conditions [33].

Common Glucocorticoids used in Equine Practice
Hydrocortisone
Clinical uses: hydrocortisone is a short-acting glucocorticoid used topically to treat inflammation from stings, insect bites, and skin irritation. Its effects are relatively mild compared to other glucocorticoids, making it suitable for localised inflammatory conditions [33].
Administration: available in creams, ointments, and lotions for topical application.
Side Effects: minimal when used topically as directed. Overuse can lead to skin thinning and delayed wound healing.

Cortisone
Clinical uses: cortisone is a short-acting glucocorticoid that must be converted to hydrocortisone in the liver to become active. It is found in some topical preparations

and used similarly to hydrocortisone for localised inflammation [33].

Administration: available in topical preparations, sometimes in combination with other medications.

Side Effects: similar to hydrocortisone, it has minimal systemic effects when used topically.

Prednisolone

Clinical uses: prednisolone is an intermediate-acting glucocorticoid with effects lasting 12–36 hours. It is suitable for alternate-day dosing and ideal for managing long-term allergic or inflammatory conditions. Prednisolone is also used in intra-articular injections to treat arthritis and other joint inflammations in horses [33, 40].

Administration: available in oral tablets, injectable forms, and as a component in intra-articular injections.

Side effects: potential side effects include immune suppression, increased risk of infection, gastric ulcers, and changes in glucose metabolism. Long-term use requires careful monitoring to prevent complications [33, 40].

Dexamethasone

Clinical uses: dexamethasone is a long-acting glucocorticoid with effects lasting 48 hours or more. It is used for its potent anti-inflammatory effects in treating many conditions, including severe allergies, inflammatory diseases, and autoimmune disorders.

Administration: available in injectable forms, oral tablets, and topical preparations.

Side effects: due to its potency and prolonged action, dexamethasone has a higher risk of side effects compared to other glucocorticoids. These can include immune suppression, increased susceptibility to infections, gastric ulcers, muscle wasting, and delayed wound healing. Recent studies indicate no significant risk of laminitis in healthy horses when used appropriately, although the risk should always be weighed against the potential benefits of treatment [21, 71, 72].

Considerations for use

1) **Monitoring and dosage**: careful monitoring and appropriate dosing are critical to minimise the risk of side effects, especially with long-term use. Regular veterinary check-ups and blood tests can help detect early signs of adverse effects.
2) **Alternating day dosing**: for long-term conditions, alternate-day dosing of intermediate-acting glucocorticoids like prednisolone can help reduce the risk of side effects while maintaining therapeutic efficacy.
3) **Combination therapy**: combining glucocorticoids with other treatments, such as NSAIDs or disease-modifying drugs, can enhance treatment efficacy and reduce the required glucocorticoid dose.

4) **Laminitis risk**: although recent studies suggest a low risk of laminitis in healthy horses, glucocorticoid use in horses with underlying systemic conditions or predispositions should be carefully considered and monitored.
5) **Withdrawal and tapering**: gradual tapering is essential when discontinuing long-term glucocorticoid therapy to prevent adrenal insufficiency and allow the horse's adrenal glands to resume normal cortisol production [72].

Diuretics

Diuretics are medications that promote urine production and fluid removal and are often used to manage various conditions such as heart disease, pulmonary issues, and cerebral oedema. Diuretics help reduce fluid overload and alleviate symptoms associated with these conditions by enhancing the excretion of water and electrolytes [33].

Frusemide (Furosemide)

Mechanism of action: frusemide, also known as furosemide, is a potent loop diuretic that acts on the ascending loop of Henle in the kidneys. It inhibits the reabsorption of sodium and chloride, leading to increased excretion of these electrolytes and water. This results in a significant increase in urine production [33, 73].

Clinical uses:

1) **Heart disease**: in horses with congestive heart failure, frusemide helps reduce fluid accumulation in the lungs and body tissues, improving breathing and reducing swelling.
2) **Exercise-Induced pulmonary haemorrhage (EIPH)**: frusemide is occasionally used to control EIPH, where horses bleed from the lungs during intense exercise. Using frusemide for this purpose is controversial and regulated in competitive equine sports due to concerns about its performance-enhancing effects and potential side effects [33, 73].

Administration: frusemide can be administered via the IV, IM or oral routes, depending on the clinical situation and urgency.

Side effects and considerations:

- **Hypokalaemia**: long-term use of frusemide can lead to potassium depletion (hypokalaemia), necessitating potassium supplementation or dietary adjustments.
- **Dehydration and electrolyte imbalance**: excessive diuresis can cause dehydration and imbalances in other electrolytes, such as magnesium and calcium.

- **Monitoring**: regular electrolyte levels and kidney function monitoring are essential, especially during prolonged treatment.

Mannitol

Mechanism of action: mannitol is an osmotic diuretic that increases the osmolarity of the blood, drawing water out of tissues and into the bloodstream, which is then excreted by the kidneys. It does not get reabsorbed by the renal tubules, ensuring the continued excretion of water [21].

Clinical uses:

1) **Cerebral oedema**: mannitol is used to reduce intracranial pressure and cerebral oedema following head trauma. Drawing fluid out of the brain tissue helps alleviate pressure and prevent further damage.
2) **Kidney damage and poisoning**: mannitol aids in the management of acute kidney injury and poisoning by increasing urine flow and promoting the elimination of toxins.

  Administration: mannitol is typically administered via the IV route due to its rapid onset of action [21].

Side effects and considerations:

- **Fluid and electrolyte imbalances**: mannitol can cause imbalances in fluid and electrolytes, so careful monitoring is required.
- **Dehydration**: excessive diuresis may lead to dehydration, necessitating the careful management of fluid therapy.
- **Contraindications**: mannitol should be used with caution in horses with pre-existing heart disease or severe dehydration.

General considerations for diuretic use in horses

1) **Indications and contraindications**: diuretics should be based on a thorough clinical assessment, considering the horse's overall health status and specific medical conditions. Contraindications, such as dehydration or electrolyte imbalances, must be addressed before initiating diuretic therapy.
2) **Monitoring**: regular fluid balance, electrolytes, and kidney function monitoring is critical during diuretic therapy. Blood tests and clinical evaluations help ensure that the horse maintains a stable internal environment and that any adverse effects are promptly managed.
3) **Adjustments and supportive care**: depending on the horse's response, adjustments to the diuretic dose or additional supportive care, such as electrolyte supplementation or fluid therapy, may be necessary. This helps

to mitigate the risk of adverse effects and ensures the efficacy of the treatment.
4) **Veterinary supervision**: diuretic use in horses should always be supervised by a vet, ensuring that the benefits of the treatment outweigh the risks and that the therapy is tailored to the individual needs of the horse.

Tranquillisers and Sedatives

Tranquillisers and sedatives are essential tools in equine medicine for managing anxiety, facilitating handling and examination, and providing pre-anaesthetic calming effects. While both classes of drugs aim to calm horses, their mechanisms and effects differ slightly [21, 33].

Tranquillisers

Function: tranquillisers primarily reduce anxiety and induce a state of tranquillity without causing significant sedation or drowsiness. They are particularly useful for horses that must remain calm and cooperative during transport, routine examinations, or minor procedures [21, 33].

Acepromazine   Class: phenothiazine
Clinical uses: acepromazine is commonly used to calm horses for transport examinations and as a pre-anaesthetic agent. It works by blocking dopamine receptors in the brain, reducing anxiety and inducing a state of calm [74].

  Administration: acepromazine can be administered in injectable and oral forms depending on the horse's specific needs and the situation.

Side effects and considerations:

- **Vasodilation and hypotension**: acepromazine can cause significant vasodilation, leading to hypotension. This is of particular concern in hypotensive patients, such as those with blood loss or dehydration.
- **Penile prolapse**: in stallions, acepromazine has been linked to penile prolapse, which may be transient or, in rare cases, permanent. Although the risk is small, this necessitates cautious use in entire males to avoid complications [74].
- **Dose adjustment**: careful dose adjustment is needed based on the horse's size, health status, and intended use to minimise risks and ensure effective calming.

Sedatives

Function: sedatives produce a deeper state of calm, often leading to drowsiness or light sleep, without significant analgesic effects. They are useful for more invasive procedures, prolonged examinations, or requiring a higher degree of immobility [21].

Alpha-2 agonists

Class: alpha-2 adrenergic agonists

Mechanism of action: these drugs work by binding to alpha-2 adrenergic receptors in the CNS, decreasing the release of norepinephrine and reducing alertness. This produces sedation, muscle relaxation, and some degree of analgesia [21].

General considerations:

- **Cardiovascular effects**: alpha-2 agonists can cause bradycardia (slow heart rate) and hypotension (low blood pressure), necessitating careful monitoring during use.
- **Potentiated sulphonamides**: these drugs should not be used in combination with potentiated sulphonamides due to the risk of fatal arrhythmias.

Specific alpha-2 Agonists

Romifidine

Duration of action: romifidine has a longer action duration than other alpha-2 agonists, making it suitable for procedures requiring extended sedation [75].

Clinical uses: commonly used for dental procedures, minor surgeries, and other prolonged sedation interventions.

Side effects: similar to other alpha-2 agonists, including bradycardia and hypotension.

Xylazine

Onset and duration: xylazine has a rapid onset of effects, typically within 5 minutes, and a relatively short duration of around 20 minutes [76].

Clinical uses: ideal for quick procedures such as minor wound treatments, diagnostic imaging, and short-term restraint.

Side effects: includes bradycardia, hypotension, and transient hyperglycaemia.

Detomidine hydrochloride

Combination use: often combined with butorphanol to enhance sedation and provide better analgesia [21, 77].

Clinical uses: suitable for deep sedation procedures, such as standing surgeries or intensive diagnostic workups.

Contraindications: should not be used with potentiated sulphonamides due to the risk of fatal arrhythmias.

For more information regarding drugs used during anaesthesia, see Chapter 10.

9.5 Routes of Administration for Medications

The administration route significantly affects the duration of action and bioavailability of a specific drug. The choice of route depends on several factors, including the disease being treated, the available drug formulations, the patient's condition and temperament, and the owner's ability to administer the medication [78].

Factors to consider:

- **The disease being treated**: some conditions may require systemic treatment, while others might be effectively managed with localised therapy.
- **Drug formulations**: the physical and chemical properties of the drug, such as solubility and stability, influence the choice of administration route.
- **Patient condition and temperament**: the horse's health status, behaviour, and ease of handling affect the feasibility of certain routes.
- **Owner's ability**: the practicality of the owner's administration, especially for long-term treatments, is a critical consideration [7, 79].

Table 9.6 displays the main routes of administration for medication, including the advantages and disadvantages of each [3].

Other Routes of Administration

Oral, topical, IV, IM and S/C routes of drug administration are discussed in more detail in Chapter 17. Other routes of drug administration are discussed below.

Nebulisation/inhalation

Nebulisation and inhalation therapies effectively deliver medications directly to the respiratory tract, which is particularly beneficial for treating airway diseases [79–81].

Key considerations for nebulisation/inhalation

1) **Mechanism and equipment**:
   - **Nebulisers**: these devices convert liquid medications into a fine mist that can be inhaled. They are commonly used for equine asthma and acute respiratory infections.
   - **Inhalers and masks**: inhalers with spacers or masks can deliver aerosolised medications, ensuring that the horse inhales the full dose.
2) **Applications**:
   - **Equine asthma**: nebulisation is particularly useful for chronic airway diseases, where anti-inflammatory medications, bronchodilators, and mucolytics can be administered directly to the lungs, improving respiratory function and reducing symptoms.
   - **Anaesthesia**: during anaesthesia, a vaporiser is used to mix volatile anaesthetic agents with oxygen. This mixture is then delivered via an endotracheal tube to maintain anaesthesia. Accurate control of the

Table 9.6 Advantages and disadvantages of different routes of medication administration [3].

Route	Advantages	Disadvantages	Notes
Oral	• Convenient and easy for the owner to medicate at home, especially convenient for long term medications	• Difficult to identify if the full dose has been consumed in some situations • Absorption and distribution of the drug is relatively slow compared to injectable medications • Food in the stomach can affect the absorption • Not suitable if the patient is unconscious or difficult to dose • Some drugs cause stomach irritation and diarrhoea • Gastric acid can denature some drugs • Liver enzymes may break down a drug before it reaches the systemic circulation	Once absorbed through the intestine the drugs pass to the liver before reaching the circulation and the site of action
IV	• Direct delivery to the systemic circulation 100% bioavailability • Drugs that are irritant to tissues can be given via this route	• Aseptic technique essential to avoid reduce the risk of infection • Commonly requires IV catheter placement for repeated dosing to prevent repeated venepuncture • Risk of thrombus formation at catheter site • Drug must be in a solution formulation • Extravascular injection can cause severe tissue damage	Some level of skill is required to administer the medicines correctly to avoid damage to the vessels or intra articular administration of medicines
IM	• Drugs in suspension can be given IM • Absorbed more quickly than the S/C route	• Guidance should be followed regarding the amount of medication to be injected per injection site to reduce incidence of localised reactions (see Chapter 17) • Accidental IV injection can occur unless the operator aspirates the syringe to check for venepuncture • Patient compliance plays a large part in the ability to complete a course of IM injections	Commonly used is the gluteal muscle, pectorals and the trapezius. Large volumes are tolerated better in the gluteal muscles
S/C	• Generally, pain free but this is drug dependent	• Absorption can take 30 minutes • Local reactions can occur	Requires an injection to be administered into the bottom of a skin tent where loose skin is available These areas lack large blood vessels and have a poor nerve supply Fluids should be non-irritant to prevent tissue necrosis
Epidural	• Provides standing analgesia to the perianal area to allow for surgery to be performed • Can provide analgesia for up to 8 h	• Strict aseptic technique required	Catheters can be placed into the epidural space to facilitate treatment

Table 9.6 (Continued)

Route	Advantages	Disadvantages	Notes
Intradermal	• Involves injecting a panel of allergens into a small, clipped area on the neck of the horse. Sedation is required • Any skin reaction is measured over 24 h • Allergens that have caused a reaction can then be administered in a vaccine to reduce the individual horses' allergic response	• Well tolerated	Commonly used for allergy testing
Intraarticular	• Commonly carried out in equine practice for identifying areas of discomfort during lameness examinations	• Strict aseptic technique	Corticosteroids and local anaesthetic commonly injected under standing sedation
Intraperitoneal	• Facilitates flushing of the peritoneal cavity without the need for a general anaesthetic • Large volumes of fluids can be flushed into and out of the cavity	• Aseptic technique required • Risk of puncturing abdominal organs	Rarely used in equine practice

Source: Phillippa Pritchard.

anaesthetic depth is essential for the safety and efficacy of the procedure.

3) **Acute conditions**:
   - **Emergency treatment**: nebulisers can be used in acute respiratory distress situations to quickly deliver bronchodilators and other medications, providing rapid relief of symptoms.
   - **Infection management**: antibiotics and antifungal agents can be nebulised to treat respiratory infections, ensuring high local concentrations at the site of infection with minimal systemic exposure.
4) **Advantages and disadvantages**:
   - **Advantages**: direct delivery to the respiratory tract allows for high local medication concentrations, rapid onset of action, and reduced systemic side effects.
   - **Disadvantages**: requires specific equipment and proper technique to ensure effective delivery. Horses may need to be acclimated to the use of masks or nebulisers to reduce stress and ensure compliance.

Figure 9.6 shows a horse with a nebuliser in place ready for the administration of medication.

Rectal Administration

Rectal administration is unsuitable for patients with diarrhoea or severe dehydration. Most commonly, enemas are given rectally to relieve impactions in foals and adult

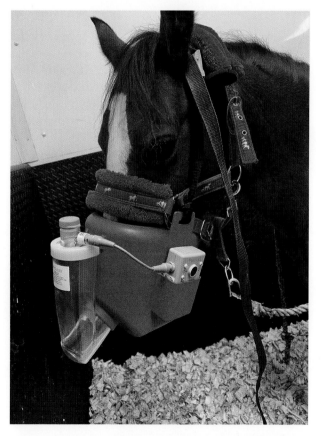

Figure 9.6 A patient wearing a nebuliser. *Source:* Cassie Woods.

patients. If patients are refluxing and require oral medications, these may be suitable to administer via the rectal route, for example, metronidazole tablets [80, 82].

Antibiotic Resistance

The British Equine Veterinary Association (BEVA) has produced a toolkit to help to protect the antibiotics used in practice and provide guidelines to ensure that they are used appropriately. It is of critical importance that antibiotics are used sparingly to ensure their efficacy in the future. The toolkit that BEVA has produced allows each practice to audit and use antibiotics responsibly, to limit the development of resistance and to protect the antibiotics that are available for the future [83]. Please see Chapter 6 for more information.

Recently, in the United Kingdom, the VMD has found that there was a 55% reduction in antibiotic use in food-producing animals between 2014 and 2021; this includes an 83% reduction in critically important antibiotics for human medicines. This shows a good understanding of protecting antibiotics and reducing the unnecessary use of antibiotics within veterinary practice [84].

Records of Administration

A medication administration record should be filled out for every patient. Details recorded should include the patient's name, owner's surname and, ideally, a case number. Medication administration information to be recorded includes:

- The name of the medication
- The strength of the medication
- The amount of medication given
- The time the medication was given
- The site of administration (including the side if applicable)
- The initials of the person who administered the medication
- Any adverse reactions that were observed at the time of administration [7, 19].

9.6 Adverse Reactions

Knowledge of adverse reactions in patients is important. The following terms are essential when referring to adverse reactions:

- Side effect: a documented problem in addition to the desired effect (not necessarily harmful).
- Special precaution: a measure taken in advance to prevent dangerous or unpleasant effects.
- Contra-indication: a specific situation meaning it should not be used.

Adverse reactions can be classified according to the suspected cause [33]:

- A: Augmented – enhanced drug effect. These are predictable reactions and tend to be dose dependent. They are associated with low mortality. Examples of this would include: opioids causing respiratory depression or gentamycin causing nephrotoxicity. There is more risk associated with higher doses or short-interval dosing.
- B: Bizarre – allergic or unusual reactions. These tend to be unpredictable and not dose dependent. They are associated with high mortality. An example would be a penicillin reaction.
- C: Continuing/chronic – occurs due to continuous therapy. These reactions persist for a long period of time. An example of this would be gastric ulceration for long-term NSAID use.
- D: Delayed. These reactions occur a long time after treatment. An example would be the teratogenicity of griseofulvin, carcinomas.
- E: End of treatment. These reactions occur upon withdrawal of therapy. These reactions are uncommon in horses.

The chances of a patient having an adverse reaction increase with the number of medications used. Generally, polypharmacy is a term used if five or more drugs are used. However, some sources suggest that any multiple medications administered can increase the chances of a reaction. In some cases, a known drug interaction is deliberately used as it has a therapeutic value. Drug interactions used in this way are as follows [33]:

- Summation: the response seen is equal to the combined responses of the individual drugs. Numerical explanation: $1 + 1 = 2$.
- Synergism: the response is greater than the combined responses of the individual drug. Numerical explanation: $1 + 1 = 3$.
- Potentiation: this is where one ineffective drug enhances the effect of another drug. Numerical explanation: $0 + 1 = 2$.
- Antagonism: this is where one drug inhibits the effects of another drug. Numerical explanation: $1 + 1 = 0$.

Understanding what issues need to be reported in the event of a patient suffering an adverse reaction is essential. The following responses should be reported:

- Adverse reaction
- Lack of efficacy
- Reactions affecting humans and animals of all species

Any reactions that fall into the above categories must be reported to the VMD through the suspected adverse reaction surveillance scheme (SARSS). Reports should be made to the VMD online via their website. Anyone may report to the scheme, including pet owners. In practice, RVNs may take on this responsibility. Any reactions, even if only suspected, should be reported. Details required include the animal details, the product, the batch number and the signs observed. All findings are shared with the drug manufacturer, who may contact the vet if more details are required [33].

References

1 Lane, D.R., Guthrie, S., and Griffith, S. (2016). *Dictionary of Veterinary Nursing*, 4e. Edinburgh: Elsevier.

2 Legislation Covering Medicines | Department of Health [Internet]. Health 2015. [cited 2023 Mar 14]. Available from https://www.health-ni.gov.uk/articles/legislation-covering-medicines.

3 Participation E. Medicines Act 1968 [Internet]. Statute Law Database [cited 2023 Mar 14]. Available from https://www.legislation.gov.uk/ukpga/1968/67/contents.

4 What are the UK drug laws? [Internet]. DrugWise. 2015 [cited 2023 Mar 14]. Available from https://www.drugwise.org.uk/what-are-the-uk-drug-laws/.

5 Nind, F. and Mosedale, P. (2022). BSAVA Guide to the Use of Veterinary Medicines. BSAVA Guide to the Use of Veterinary Medicines [Internet]. [cited 2023 Feb 27]; Available from https://www.bsavalibrary.com/content/chapter/10.22233/9781905319862.app2.

6 The Veterinary Medicines Regulations 2013 [Internet]. Queen's Printer of Acts of Parliament; [cited 2023 Mar 14]. Available from https://www.legislation.gov.uk/uksi/2013/2033/made.

7 Cooper, B., Mullineaux, E., and Turner, L. (ed.) (2018). *BSAVA Textbook of Veterinary Nursing*, 5e, 738–774. Gloucester: British Small Animal Veterinary Association.

8 18. Delegation to veterinary nurses [Internet]. Professionals. [cited 2023 Mar 14]. Available from https://www.rcvs.org.uk/setting-standards/advice-and-guidance/code-of-professional-conduct-for-veterinary-surgeons/supporting-guidance/delegation-to-veterinary-nurses/.

9 Legal category [Internet]. [cited 2023 Mar 14]. Available from https://www.noahcompendium.co.uk/home/legal-category.

10 Marketing authorisations for veterinary medicines [Internet]. GOV.UK. 2022 [cited 2023 Mar 14]. Available from https://www.gov.uk/guidance/marketing-authorisations-for-veterinary-medicines.

11 Import a medicine for veterinary use into the UK [Internet]. GOV.UK. 2021 [cited 2023 Mar 14]. Available from https://www.gov.uk/guidance/apply-for-a-certificate-to-import-a-veterinary-medicine-into-the-uk.

12 The cascade: prescribing unauthorised medicines [Internet]. GOV.UK. 2021 [cited 2023 Mar 14]. Available from https://www.gov.uk/guidance/the-cascade-prescribing-unauthorised-medicines.

13 The Horse Passports Regulations 2009 [Internet]. Queen's Printer of Acts of Parliament; [cited 2023 Mar 14]. Available from https://www.legislation.gov.uk/uksi/2009/1611/made.

14 APHA regulatory and compliance policy [Internet]. GOV.UK. 2018 [cited 2023 Mar 14]. Available from https://www.gov.uk/government/publications/ahvla-regulatory-and-compliance-policy.

15 About us [Internet]. GOV.UK. [cited 2023 Mar 14]. Available from https://www.gov.uk/government/organisations/department-for-environment-food-rural-affairs/about.

16 The role of the RCVS [Internet]. Professionals. [cited 2023 Mar 14]. Available from https://www.rcvs.org.uk/how-we-work/the-role-of-the-rcvs/.

17 Vetpol SQP Training and Registration [Internet]. Vetpol. [cited 2023 Mar 14]. Available from: https://vetpol.uk/.

18 CPD Policy [Internet]. Vetpol. [cited 2023 Mar 14]. Available from: https://vetpol.uk/vetpol-policies/cpd-policy/.

19 Veterinary Medicines Directorate (2017). Suitably Qualified Persons [SQPs] Code of Practice [Internet]. Secretary of State for the Department for Environment, Food and Rural Affairs. Available from chrome-extension://efaidnbmnnnibpcajpcglclefindmkaj/https://assets.publishing.service.gov.uk/government/uploads/system/uploads/attachment_data/file/895802/PCDOCS-_1060282-v11-Revised_SQP_Code_of_Practice_-_April_2017.pdf.

20 Home [Internet]. [cited 2023 Mar 14]. Available from https://www.noahcompendium.co.uk/home.

21 Bill, R.L. (2017). *Clinical Pharmacology and Therapeutics for Veterinary Technicians*, 4e. Missouri: Elsevier.

22 Controlled drugs: recording, using, storing and disposal [Internet]. GOV.UK. 2022 [cited 2023 Mar 14]. Available from https://www.gov.uk/guidance/controlled-drugs-recording-using-storing-and-disposal.

23 How to manage the practice dispensary [Internet]. The Veterinary Nurse. [cited 2023 Mar 14]. Available from https://www.theveterinarynurse.com/review/article/how-to-manage-the-practice-dispensary.

24 Society TVD. Home [Internet]. The Veterinary Defence Society. [cited 2023 Mar 14]. Available from https://www.thevds.co.uk/.

25 Pharmacovigilance [Internet]. [cited 2023 Mar 14]. Available from https://www.who.int/teams/regulation-prequalification/regulation-and-safety/pharmacovigilance.

26 Clinical particulars – Genta-Equine® 100 mg/ml Solution for Injection for Horses [Internet]. [cited 2023 Mar 14]. Available from https://www.noahcompendium.co.uk/.

27 The role of the SQP and their use in practice by Hollie Jane Millington [Internet]. British Veterinary Nursing Association. 2022 [cited 2023 Mar 14]. Available from https://bvna.org.uk/blog/the-role-of-the-sqp-and-their-use-in-practice-by-hollie-jane-millington/.

28 9. Practice information, fees and animal insurance [Internet]. Professionals. [cited 2023 Mar 14]. Available from https://www.rcvs.org.uk/setting-standards/advice-and-guidance/code-of-professional-conduct-for-veterinary-surgeons/supporting-guidance/practice-information-and-fees/.

29 Retail of veterinary medicines [Internet]. GOV.UK. 2018 [cited 2023 Mar 14]. Available from https://www.gov.uk/guidance/retail-of-veterinary-medicines.

30 Moore, M.C. and Palmer, N.G. (2001). *Calculations for Veterinary Nurses*, 1e, 129–139. Oxford: Blackwell Science Ltd.

31 Lake, T. and Green, N. (2017). *Essential Calculation for Veterinary Nurses and Technicians*, 3e. Missouri: Elsevier.

32 Clinical particulars – Depocillin® 300 mg/ml suspension for injection [Internet]. [cited 2023 Mar 14]. Available from https://www.noahcompendium.co.uk/

33 Ackerman, N. and Aspinall, V. (2016). *Aspinall's Complete Textbook of Veterinary Nursing*, 3e, 427–475. Edinburgh: Elsevier Ltd.

34 Rosa, B. (2020). Equine drug transporters: a mini-review and veterinary perspective. *Pharmaceutics [Internet]* 12: 1–19. Available from www.mdpi.com/journal/pharmaceutics.

35 Linlin, S., Mruk, D.D., Yan, C. et al. (2011). Drug transporters, the blood–testis barrier, and spermatogenesis. *Society for Endocrinology [Internet]* 208 (3): 207–223. Available from https://joe.bioscientifica.com/view/journals/joe/208/3/207.xml.

36 Pardridge, W.M. (2012). Drug transport across the blood–brain barrier. *Journal of Cerebral Blood Flow & Metabolism* 32 (11): 1959–1972.

37 RLO: The Liver and Drug Metabolism [Internet]. [cited 2023 Feb 28]. Available from https://www.nottingham.ac.uk/nmp/sonet/rlos/bioproc/liverdrug/page_three.html.

38 Agonists and Antagonists [Internet]. UTS Pharmacology. 2022 [cited 2023 Feb 28]. Available from https://lx.uts.edu.au/pharmacology/article/agonists-and-antagonists/.

39 Bertone, J., Linda, J., and Horsepool, I. (2004). *Equine Clinical Pharmacology*, 1e. London: Saunders.

40 Cole, C., Bentz, B., and Maxwell, L. (2015). *Equine Pharmacology*, 1e. Iowa: John Wiley and Sons Inc.

41 Ziegler, A.L. and Blikslager, A.T. (2020). Sparing the gut: COX-2 inhibitors herald a new era for treatment of horses with surgical colic. *Equine Veterinary Education* 32 (11): 611–616.

42 Nonsteroidal Anti-inflammatory Drugs in Animals – Pharmacology [Internet]. MSD Veterinary Manual. [cited 2023 Feb 27]. Available from https://www.msdvetmanual.com/pharmacology/inflammation/nonsteroidal-anti-inflammatory-drugs-in-animals

43 Fentanyl use in horses | Vetlexicon Equis from Vetlexicon | Definitive Veterinary Intelligence [Internet]. [cited 2023 Mar 15]. Available from https://www.vetlexicon.com/treat/equis/generics/fentanyl.

44 Buprenorphine use in horses | Vetlexicon Equis from Vetlexicon | Definitive Veterinary Intelligence [Internet]. [cited 2023 Mar 15]. Available from https://www.vetlexicon.com/treat/equis/generics/buprenorphine.

45 Butorphanol use in horses | Vetlexicon Equis from Vetlexicon | Definitive Veterinary Intelligence [Internet]. [cited 2023 Mar 15]. Available from https://www.vetlexicon.com/treat/equis/generics/butorphanol.

46 Phenylbutazone use in horses | Vetlexicon Equis from Vetlexicon | Definitive Veterinary Intelligence [Internet]. [cited 2023 Mar 15]. Available from https://www.vetlexicon.com/treat/equis/generics/phenylbutazone.

47 Carprofen use in horses | Vetlexicon Equis from Vetlexicon | Definitive Veterinary Intelligence [Internet]. [cited 2023 Mar 15]. Available from https://www.vetlexicon.com/treat/equis/generics/carprofen.

48 Meloxicam use in horses | Vetlexicon Equis from Vetlexicon | Definitive Veterinary Intelligence [Internet]. [cited 2023 Mar 15]. Available from https://www.vetlexicon.com/treat/equis/generics/meloxicam.

49 Frisbie, D. and Donnell, J. (2014). Use of firocoxib for the treatment of equine osteoarthritis. *Veterinary Medicine: Research and Reports* 2014: 159.

50 Schleining, J.A. and Reinertson, E.L. (2007). Evidence for dimethyl sulphoxide [DMSO] use in horses. Part 2: DMSO as a parenteral anti-inflammatory agent and as a pharmacological carrier. *Equine Veterinary Education [Internet]* 19 (11): 598–599. [cited 2023 Mar 15]. Available from https://doi.org/10.2746/095777307X255869.

51 Schleining, J.A. and Reinertson, E.L. (2007). Evidence for dimethyl sulphoxide [DMSO] use in horses. Part 1: DMSO as a topical and intra-articular anti-inflammatory agent. *Equine Veterinary Education [Internet]* 19 (10): 545–546. [cited 2023 Mar 15]. Available from https://doi.org/10.2746/095777307X248641.

52 Lidocaine use in horses | Vetlexicon Equis from Vetlexicon | Definitive Veterinary Intelligence [Internet]. [cited 2023 Mar 15]. Available from https://www.vetlexicon.com/treat/equis/generics/lidocaine.

53 Quinidine use in horses | Vetlexicon Equis from Vetlexicon | Definitive Veterinary Intelligence [Internet]. [cited 2023

Mar 15]. Available from https://www.vetlexicon.com/treat/equis/generics/quinidine.

54 Propanolol use in horses | Vetlexicon Equis from Vetlexicon | Definitive Veterinary Intelligence [Internet]. [cited 2023 Mar 1]. Available from https://www.vetlexicon.com/treat/equis/generics/propanolol.

55 Sotalol use in horses | Vetlexicon Equis from Vetlexicon | Definitive Veterinary Intelligence [Internet]. [cited 2023 Mar 15]. Available from https://www.vetlexicon.com/treat/equis/generics/sotalol.

56 Dobutamine use in horses | Vetlexicon Equis from Vetlexicon | Definitive Veterinary Intelligence [Internet]. [cited 2023 Mar 15]. Available from https://www.vetlexicon.com/treat/equis/generics/dobutamine.

57 Phenobarbital use in horses | Vetlexicon Equis from Vetlexicon | Definitive Veterinary Intelligence [Internet]. [cited 2023 Mar 15]. Available from https://www.vetlexicon.com/treat/equis/generics/phenobarbital

58 Midazolam use in horses | Vetlexicon Equis from Vetlexicon | Definitive Veterinary Intelligence [Internet]. [cited 2023 Mar 15]. Available from https://www.vetlexicon.com/treat/equis/generics/midazolam.

59 Diazepam use in horses | Vetlexicon Equis from Vetlexicon | Definitive Veterinary Intelligence [Internet]. [cited 2023 Mar 15]. Available from https://www.vetlexicon.com/treat/equis/generics/diazepam.

60 Clenbuterol hydrochloride use in horses | Vetlexicon Equis from Vetlexicon | Definitive Veterinary Intelligence [Internet]. [cited 2023 Mar 15]. Available from https://www.vetlexicon.com/treat/equis/generics/clenbuterol-hydrochloride.

61 Dembrexine hydrochloride use in horses | Vetlexicon Equis from Vetlexicon | Definitive Veterinary Intelligence [Internet]. [cited 2023 Mar 15]. Available from https://www.vetlexicon.com/treat/equis/generics/dembrexine-hydrochloride.

62 Haggett, E.F. and Wilson, W.D. (2008). Overview of the use of antimicrobials for the treatment of bacterial infections in horses. *Equine Veterinary Education* 20 (8): 433–448.

63 Chloramphenicol use in horses | Vetlexicon Equis from Vetlexicon | Definitive Veterinary Intelligence [Internet]. [cited 2023 Mar 15]. Available from https://www.vetlexicon.com/treat/equis/generics/chloramphenicol.

64 Antineoplastic [Chemotherapy] Drugs – Reproductive Health | NIOSH | CDC [Internet]. 2022 [cited 2023 Mar 14]. Available from https://www.cdc.gov/niosh/topics/repro/antineoplastic.html.

65 Taylor, S. and Haldorson, G. (2013). A review of equine mucocutaneous squamous cell carcinoma. *Equine Veterinary Education [Internet]* 25 (7): 374–378. Available from https://doi.org/10.1111/j.2042-3292.2012.00457.x.

66 Equine Cancer and Sarcoids – Equine Hospital – University of Liverpool [Internet]. [cited 2023 Mar 15]. Available from https://www.liverpool.ac.uk/equine/common-conditions/sarcoids/.

67 Fluorouracil [Topical Route] Precautions – Mayo Clinic [Internet]. [cited 2023 Mar 15]. Available from https://www.mayoclinic.org/drugs-supplements/fluorouracil-topical-route/precautions/drg-20063877.

68 EMA (2018). Oncept IL-2 [Internet]. European Medicines Agency. [cited 2023 Mar 14]. Available from https://www.ema.europa.eu/en/medicines/veterinary/EPAR/oncept-il-2.

69 Newton, S.A. (2010). Periocular sarcoids in the horse: three cases of successful treatment. *Equine Veterinary Education [Internet]* 12 (3): 114–167. Available from https://doi.org/10.1111/j.2042-3292.2000.tb00030.x.

70 Tapeworm infection – Diagnosis and treatment – Mayo Clinic [Internet]. [cited 2023 Mar 15]. Available from https://www.mayoclinic.org/diseases-conditions/tapeworm/diagnosis-treatment/drc-20378178.

71 Cornelisse, C.J. and Robinson, N.E. (2012). Glucocorticoid therapy and the risk of equine laminitis. *Equine Veterinary Education [Internet]* 25 (1): 39–46. Available from https://doi.org/10.1111/j.2042-3292.2011.00320.x.

72 McGowan, C., Cooper, D., and Ireland, J. (2016). No evidence that therapeutic systemic corticosteroid administration is associated with laminitis in adult horses without underlying endocrine or severe systemic disease. *RCVS Knowledge Veterinary Evidence [Online]* 1 (1): 1–17.

73 Diuretics: Types, Uses and Side Effects [Internet]. Cleveland Clinic. [cited 2023 Mar 14]. Available from https://my.clevelandclinic.org/health/treatments/21826-diuretics.

74 Bettschart, R. and Johnston, M. (2011). Confidential enquiry into perioperative equine fatalities:CEPEF4-achance to gain new evidence about the risks of equine general anaesthesia. *Equine Veterinary Journal [Internet]* 44 (1): 7. Available from https://doi.org/10.1111/j.2042-3306.2011.00483.x.

75 Romifidine use in horses | Vetlexicon Equis from Vetlexicon | Definitive Veterinary Intelligence [Internet]. [cited 2023 Mar 15]. Available from: https://www.vetlexicon.com/treat/equis/generics/romifidine.

76 Xylazine use in horses | Vetlexicon Equis from Vetlexicon | Definitive Veterinary Intelligence [Internet]. [cited 2023 Mar 15]. Available from: https://www.vetlexicon.com/treat/equis/generics/xylazine.

77 Detomidine hydrochloride use in horses | Vetlexicon Equis from Vetlexicon | Definitive Veterinary Intelligence [Internet]. [cited 2023 Mar 15]. Available from https://www.vetlexicon.com/treat/equis/generics/detomidine-hydrochloride.

78 Valverde, A., Rickey, E., Sinclair, M. et al. (2010). Comparison of cardiovascular function and quality of

recovery in isoflurane-anaesthetised horses administereda constant rate infusion of lidocaine or lidocaine andmedetomidine during elective surgery. *Equine Veterinary Journal [Internet]* 42 (3): 192–199. Available from https://doi.org/10.1111/j.2042-3306.2010.00027.x.

79 Coumbe, K. (2012). *Equine Veterinary Nursing*, 2e, 385–431. Oxford: Blackwell Science Ltd.

80 Corley, K. and Stephen, J. (2008). *The Equine Hospital Manual*, 1e. Oxford: Blackwell Publishing Ltd.

81 DeNotta, S., Mallicote, M., Miller, S. et al. (2023). *AAEVT's Equine Manual for Veterinary Technicians*, 2e, 305–323. Hoboken: John Wiley and Sons Inc.

82 Auer, J., Stick, J., Kummerle, J. et al. (2019). *Equine Surgery*, 5e, 143–198. Missouri: Elsevier.

83 Protect Me Toolkit | BEVA [Internet]. [cited 2023 Feb 27]. Available from https://www.beva.org.uk/Protect-Me.

84 Reducing antibiotic use in pets – Veterinary Medicines Directorate [Internet]. 2022 [cited 2023 Mar 15]. Available from https://vmd.blog.gov.uk/2022/11/23/reducing-antibiotic-use-in-pets/.

Further Reading

Davis, E.W. and Legendre, A.M. (1994). Successful treatment of guttural pouch mycosis with itraconazole and topical enilconazole in a horse. *Journal of Veterinary Internal Medicine [Internet]* 8 (4): 304–305. Available from https://doi.org/10.1111/j.1939-1676.1994.tb03239.x.

Electrochemotherapy for Sarcoids [Internet]. [cited 2023 Mar 15]. Available from https://www.rvc.ac.uk/equinevet/information-and-advice/fact-files/electrochemotherapy-for-sarcoids

Legislation.gov.uk. (2024). The Veterinary Medicines (Amendment etc) Regulations 2024 [Online]. Available at: https://www.legislation.gov.uk/uksi/2024/567/contents/made (accessed 13 July 2024).

RCVS. (2023). Under care – new guidance [Online]. Available at: https://www.rcvs.org.uk/setting-standards/advice-and-guidance/under-care-new-guidance/ (accessed 13 July 2024).

10

Anaesthesia and Analgesia

Alison Bennell[1], Kate Loomes[2], and Marie Rippingale[3]

[1] *Philip Leverhulme Equine Hospital, University of Liverpool, Wirral, UK*
[2] *Rainbow Equine Hospital, Malton, UK*
[3] *Bottle Green Training Ltd, Derby, UK*

Glossary

Analgesia drugs which act to relieve the sensation of pain, which are needed to provide basic welfare standards during painful procedures.

Barotrauma in the lung, refers to alveolar rupture due to elevated transalveolar pressure.

Cardiac output (CO) the volume of blood ejected from the heart in 1 minute.

General anaesthesia (GA) a state of controlled unconsciousness.

Heart rate (beats/minute) the number of heart beats counted per minute.

Minute volume minute volume (MV) is the volume of gas exhaled by the patient in 1 minute.

Neuroleptanalgesia deep sedation and analgesia.

Premedication a drug/combination of drugs given pre-operatively to cause a mental calming effect which facilitates handling and the entire anaesthesia process.

Respiratory rate (RR) or respiratory frequency (R_f) number of breaths per minute.

Sedation mental calming and reduced reactiveness to external stimuli. This facilitates the performance of a range of procedures, from imaging through to surgery

Stroke volume the volume (mlL) of blood ejected by each heart beat.

Tidal volume (V_T) the amount of gas that is moved during inspiration and expiration in one respiratory cycle. Approximately 10--15 ml/kgs.

Ventilation Ventilation-perfusion (V/Q) mismatch when ventilation does not match perfusion within one lung unit . Two extremes of mismatch are: No ventilation but good perfusion, and good ventilation but no perfusion [1, 2].

10.1 The Principles of Anaesthesia

Introduction

Anaesthesia is defined as: 'the loss of sensation in a part or the whole body by controlled, reversible suppression of the central nervous system'. Anaesthesia and analgesia are essential for modern-day veterinary practice, ensuring patient welfare, providing chemical restraint or immobility, and ensuring that required legal responsibilities are met. Equine anaesthesia is challenging and rewarding however, morbidity and mortality rates still remain high when compared to many other domesticated species [3].

Types of Anaesthesia and Analgesia

Anaesthesia can be provided or facilitated in equine patients in a variety of ways which include:

GA: a state of controlled unconsciousness caused by reversible suppression of the central nervous system (CNS)

- Immobilises the patient and allows positioning of the horse for optimal surgical access, for example, dorsal recumbency.
- Carries considerable risk of morbidity and mortality, particularly during the recovery period.

Epidural (extradural) anaesthesia: a drug is injected into the extradural space of the spinal canal (this is the space outside the dura mater, which is the outermost layer of the meninges). This is different from a spinal injection, where the injection is performed into the subarachnoid space (this is the space inside of the arachnoid mater, which is the middle layer of the meninges and contains the cerebrospinal fluid which bathes the spinal cord). Spinal

Textbook of Equine Veterinary Nursing, First Edition. Edited by Rosina Lillywhite and Marie Rippingale.
© 2025 John Wiley & Sons Ltd. Published 2025 by John Wiley & Sons Ltd.
Companion website: www.wiley.com/go/equineveterinarynursing

injections are performed very uncommonly in horses. For further information, see Chapter 12.

Noteworthy points about epidural anaesthesia are:

- Analgesic drugs, mainly local anaesthetics, alpha-2 adrenoceptor agonists and opioids can be used.
- Local anaesthetics can only be used in small doses in the sacro-coccygeal/inter-coccygeal spaces to desensitise the tail/perianal/perineal area to avoid motor blockade of the hind limbs and inadvertent recumbency, which can have fatal consequences.
- Particularly useful for dystocia or perineal surgery, under-standing sedation.
- It can also be used for analgesia (alpha-2 agonists and opioids) for standing surgery or for surgery under GA.

Local anaesthesia: reversible block of neural transmission (sensory and/or motor function).

Many methods to administer local anaesthetics are available:

- Topical: the application of local anaesthetic (sprays, creams, solutions) to the surface of the target tissue, commonly skin, mucous membranes and the eye, for example, the cornea, larynx and nasopharynx. Topical application has limited clinical uses other than for specific conditions/procedures, but is easy and minimally invasive to perform.
- Infiltration: a local anaesthetic is injected into subcutaneous tissues. Commonly and easily performed for surgical procedures, but desensitising large areas can be difficult and large volumes of local anaesthetic may be required, for example, a local bleb at the site of an intravenous (IV) catheter or a line block at an incision site.
- Regional: specific nerves supplying the area concerned are blocked. Examples include perineural anaesthesia of limbs and the head. This minimises the volume of local anaesthetic required and avoids the need for injection directly into/near the target area.
- Perineural: injection of local anaesthetic around a nerve or nerves, which supply the target area.
- Intra-synovial: injection of local anaesthetic into a joint (intra-articular), bursa or tendon sheath. This must be performed aseptically to avoid introducing infection.
- IV regional local anaesthesia: a local anaesthetic is injected into a vein (usually in a limb) where a tourniquet has been applied, to prevent the circulation of the drug. The area distal to the tourniquet will then be anaesthetised. This is easy to perform, but the application of a tourniquet can be resented in conscious horses.

Other points to consider are as follows:

- Local anaesthesia allows standing surgeries to be carried out as the patient cannot feel pain in the surgical area.

- Local anaesthetics can also be used for surgeries under GA as part of the analgesic protocol.
- Local anaesthetics have toxic effects at large doses, so care should be taken to monitor the total doses used.

Dissociative anaesthesia: a type of anaesthesia characterised by catalepsy, catatonia, analgesia and amnesia. The drug interferes with the transmission of sensory information into the cerebral cortex. Ketamine is the main dissociative drug used in equine anaesthesia.

Sedative Drugs

As horses are a prey species with a strong fight or flight response, it can be dangerous for them and personnel when trying to perform certain procedures, even if those procedures are non-painful. Sedative agents can be used, and these decrease the response to external stimuli to allow a range of procedures to be undertaken safely, from diagnostic imaging to invasive surgeries, when adequate pain relief is also administered. It is worth always remembering that sedated horses are not always entirely predictable or safe, and they can still move suddenly and quickly, with minimal warning, and this can cause injury to personnel, the patients and damage to equipment.

Common sedative drugs used in horses for standing sedation include the phenothiazine acepromazine, alpha-2 adrenoceptor agonists and opioids. Additional analgesic drugs and the administration of local anaesthetics are also required to desensitise areas for surgery and ensure that pain is abolished or minimised. For short procedures, horses are often sedated with a single bolus of sedation, a one-off IV injection, for example, which will allow sufficient time for the procedure to be completed. For longer procedures, additional boluses, or 'top-up doses', usually a smaller dose than the initial one, may be required. This will inevitably cause peaks and troughs in the level of sedation, when the horse will be most deeply sedated shortly after drug administration, and as the sedative drugs 'wears off' (via drug redistribution, metabolism and excretion discussed later), the horse becomes more lightly sedated. Another method to maintain a steadier plane of sedation for longer procedures is to administer drugs as a constant rate infusion (CRI) via an ongoing IV drip or by fluid pump, or syringe driver, to continually administer low doses of drug to the patient, to avoid periods of excessively deep or light sedation.

The Physiology of GA

Various routes of administration exist for sedation and anaesthetic agents. These include:

- Oral
- Transmucosal

- Subcutaneous
- Intramuscular (IM)
- IV
- Inhaled

Different routes of administration will cause variability in the rate of drug uptake and the amount of drug delivered to target tissues. Many complex factors will influence drug availability, such as concentration at the site of administration, local blood flow, drug pK_a, drug molecule size, pH of the surrounding fluid and surface area of the absorptive site. IV administration of drugs means the whole dose is administered directly into the circulation immediately, so it is often the route of choice for many drugs (see Chapter 9 for further information).

The altered CNS function is the cornerstone of anaesthesia, and anaesthetic agents reduce consciousness and perception. Drugs can do this in two ways:

- Inhibition of excitatory pathways
- Potentiation of inhibitory pathways

For drugs to reach their target organ, they must first gain entry to the systemic circulation, where they will then be delivered around the body. As the main desired effect of most anaesthetic agents is action within the CNS, these drugs must first traverse the blood–brain barrier, which is present along the microvasculature of the CNS and presents a diffusion barrier which impedes the influx of many compounds from blood to the brain.

The Effect of Anaesthetics on the Respiratory and Cardiovascular Systems

The respiratory system functions to supply oxygen to the body and eliminate the waste produced as carbon dioxide. Oxygen is needed for cellular respiration, the process of energy production through metabolic reactions which takes place in cells. Energy from nutrients and oxygen combine to make adenosine triphosphate (ATP), which is used on a cellular level as an energy source. Water and carbon dioxide are the waste products made during aerobic metabolism. The critical oxygen tension is the level that is required for metabolic consumption to prevent tissue hypoxia. When oxygen levels in the body fall below a certain level, such as during intense exercise, the body also relies on anaerobic metabolism to produce energy from carbohydrates. This process requires different cellular processes and produces lactic acid as a waste product.

Oxygen is therefore vital to life, and respiratory function, including gas exchange in the alveoli, must continually occur to provide oxygen to the body. Some anaesthetic agents can be delivered to the respiratory system, and are inhaled to get into the bloodstream. These volatile anaesthetic agents are vital as a method of maintaining GA. In terms of respiratory function, anaesthesia depresses the ventilatory response to hypercapnia, has effects on pulmonary gas exchange, can change bronchial muscle tone (bronchoconstrict or bronchodilate) and in combination with a large animal being placed in lateral or dorsal recumbency, will reduce functional residual capacity and can cause significant hypercapnia and hypoxaemia.

As Guedel documented in the early 1900s, with increasing anaesthetic depth, cardiorespiratory function decreases [4]. One of the aims of anaesthesia is to maintain the functions of the autonomic nervous system, in a state of relative normality, but many anaesthetic drugs have profound effects on cardiovascular and respiratory function. Anaesthesia can affect cardiac output, heart rate, systemic vascular resistance (vasodilation or vasoconstriction), myocardial contractility and cardiac conduction.

Effect of Anaesthetic Agents on the Autonomic Nervous System

There are three components of the Nervous System:

- CNS: brain and spinal cord
- Autonomic nervous system (ANS)
- Peripheral nervous system (PNS)

Anaesthetic drugs have wide-ranging effects, not only the effects aimed at the CNS. The ANS regulates involuntary physiological processes such as heart rate, respiration, blood pressure, digestion, reproduction and this will also be affected by many of the anaesthetic drugs used. Generally, anaesthetic agents used for induction of anaesthesia and anaesthetic maintenance will depress these systems, especially at higher doses. When performing any anaesthetic, it is worth remembering the common complications associated with anaesthesia and depression of homeostatic mechanisms, particularly the three H's which are defined as:

- Hypotension
- Hypoventilation
- Hypothermia

Effect of Anaesthetic Agents on the Hepatic and Renal Systems

Anaesthesia can also affect other organs, with the liver and kidneys also being worthy of consideration. Both these organs require significant blood flow to maintain normal function, so changes in blood pressure can affect their function greatly, especially renal function. Conversely, renal and hepatic functions are also vital for the metabolism and excretion of many of the drugs used, and any dysfunction can cause an accumulation of drugs, which can be problematic for a smooth and swift recovery.

Pain

Pain is defined by the International Association for the Study of Pain as 'an unpleasant sensory and emotional experience associated with actual or potential tissue damage, or described in terms of such damage' [5]. Recognition and treatment of pain are pivotal to optimise the welfare of our patients, particularly in the peri-operative period. The pain pathway is complex and acute pain, which can be beneficial to protect against further injury, and it occurs when there is tissue damage in the body. Persistent pain, on the contrary, is deleterious to health and can result in distress. Nociceptors (pain receptors) are located in many tissues such as skin, muscle, joints, periosteum and other soft tissues. Tissue damage can be physical (pressure, ischaemia), thermal (hot, cold) or chemical (when pain-producing/inflammatory substances are released around nerve fibres).

Once nociceptors receive input in peripheral tissues, the signal is then converted into an electrical signal (**transduction**), which is then transmitted along nerves to the spinal cord (**transmission**). **Modulation** of this information occurs at various sites within the CNS, and this step is responsible for hypoalgesia (reduced sensation when it is protective, e.g. allowing an animal to run away from a predator) but is also involved in the development of persistent pain states, including hyperalgesia (abnormally heightened sensitivity to pain) and allodynia (pain due to a stimulus that does not normally provoke pain). This information is finally passed to higher centres, and pain is **perceived** at a conscious level (see Figure 10.1).

Many drugs exert their effect on part of the pain pathway, to alter the signals produced and aim to decrease the level of pain perceived by the animal. It is important to remember that in an animal under GA, although pain cannot be perceived by the unconscious brain, the rest of the pain pathway is still 'in action', so when that animal recovers, pain is then perceived and can be distressing. This emphasises the need for adequate pain control in all patients. Pain scoring systems have gained popularity over the past few years [2] and are a useful tool to help improve pain recognition, especially in horses, who as a prey species, do not always demonstrate pain behaviours in the same way other companion species do. See Chapter 14 for more information on pain scoring.

Analgesics can work on several different parts of the pain pathway, including nociceptors, the spinal pathways and the brain (Figure 10.2).

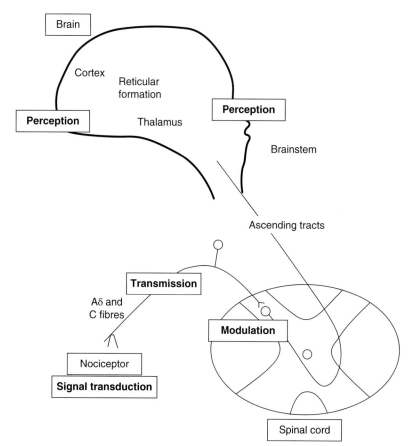

Figure 10.1 Simplified pain pathway. *Source:* Adapted from Wiley.

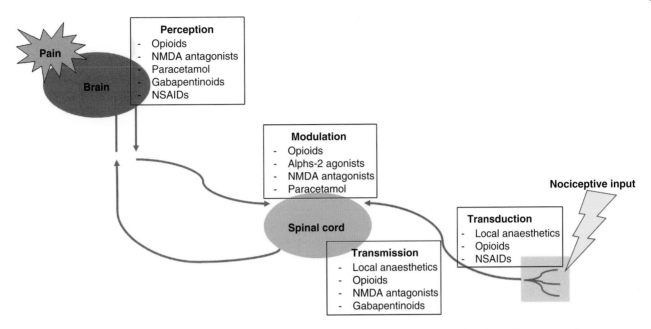

Figure 10.2 Action of different analgesics at different parts of the pain pathway. *Source:* Dr Alison Bennell.

Local anaesthetics prevent nociceptor activation and stop pain at sites of signal transmission. Non-steroidal anti-inflammatory drugs (NSAIDs) reduce nociceptor stimulation, by reducing inflammatory mediators. Many agents act at the modulation stage, impacting transmission to the brain. These include *N*-methyl-ᴅ-aspartate (NMDA) antagonists, opioids, alpha-2 agonists and gabapentin [6].

Pre-emptive Analgesia

Pre-emptive analgesia is a concept where antinociceptive/analgesic drugs/techniques are administered prior to the painful stimulus/surgery. The aim is to prevent 'wind up', which is the sensitisation of the nervous system to further stimuli that can amplify pain. Persistent pain is well-recognised and problematic to treat, and the aim of timely and effective analgesia is to minimise the risk of animals developing chronic pain states.

Multimodal Analgesia

Multimodal analgesia is the use of two or more pharmacological classes of analgesic drugs, to target different receptors/areas of the pain pathway to lead to improved efficacy of analgesia, while minimising side-effects of individual drugs. NSAIDs, opioids and alpha-2 agonists are commonly used, alongside drugs such as ketamine [7].

Recovery from Anaesthesia

Recovery from anaesthesia is dependent on many factors, and is determined by the speed of drug redistribution and clearance. Initial recovery from the effect of drugs can be seen when the drug is removed from the circulation and redistributed to other body tissues, including lean muscle and fat. The drug is then eliminated from the body, via excretion, metabolism or both. Emergence from volatile anaesthesia is dependent upon pulmonary elimination of the inhalational agent, which is determined by alveolar ventilation, pulmonary blood flow, the solubility of the volatile agent and the duration of administration. Volatile agents undergo minimal metabolism, and metabolism occurs in the liver and kidneys. Injectable agents need to be cleared from the systemic circulation, and their redistribution and elimination will be influenced by their drug properties (protein binding and lipid solubility), patient pathophysiological states (obesity, pregnancy, age), perfusion to organs responsible for metabolism and excretion and the functional status of clearance organs (metabolism may be delayed in patients with hepatic dysfunction).

Balanced Anaesthesia

The term balanced anaesthesia is a term given to a drug protocol addressing the needs of the patient throughout the perianaesthetic period. The use of several different classes of drug give rise to a multimodal approach, reaping the benefits of multiple drugs, while aiming to reduce the likelihood of negative side effects of each drug, as smaller doses can be used for each.

Triad of Anaesthesia

GA consists of a triad of:

- Unconsciousness
- Analgesia
- Muscle relaxation

The ideal anaesthetic agent produces all three of the above, with no side effects, but this is almost impossible to achieve without causing undesirable adverse effects. This means instead, multiple drugs with specific actions are often used, to provide effective and safe anaesthesia, while aiming to minimise the risk of unwanted side effects.

Objectives of Premedication

Premedication, the pre-operative administration of drugs to decrease patient stress levels and improve ease of patient handling, can also decrease the requirements for other anaesthetic agents and provide analgesia, depending on the agent(s) used. A range of medications are commonly used, including phenothiazines (acepromazine), alpha-2 agonists, opioids and NSAIDs. As a result, the entire peri-anaesthetic period from induction through to recovery should be smoother. Usually, after premedication, horses are moderately to profoundly sedated before anaesthesia is induced.

Methods Used for Maintaining GA

GA can be maintained via two main techniques:

- Inhalational/volatile anaesthetic agent, delivered in a carrier gas.
- IV anaesthesia is administered either via boluses or an infusion.

Inhalational/Volatile Anaesthetic

Volatile agents are the mainstay of anaesthetic maintenance during hospital anaesthesia, and are administered by inhalation via a breathing system.

Carrier Gases

A carrier gas is a gas which passes through the vaporiser to deliver an inhalational anaesthetic agent to the patient. Oxygen is an indispensable carrier gas, as it is required for vital metabolic processes to keep the patient alive. Additive carrier gases included medical air, nitrous oxide and even gases such as xenon, although they were seldom used outside research settings due to expense.

Total Intravenous Anaesthesia (TIVA)

TIVA is the mainstay of field anaesthesia, as minimal equipment is needed and procedures are usually of short duration, which makes them well suited to anaesthesia being maintained with injectable agents. Several agents are available for TIVA, either alone or in combination, with ketamine, alpha-2 agonists and guaiphenesin (GGE – a muscle relaxant), which are commonly used.

When TIVA is undertaken, premedication and induction are often the same or very similar to that used with volatile maintenance.

Top-up Doses

GA is then maintained with 'top up' doses, which means giving pre-calculated doses of an anaesthetic drug, usually ketamine, every 10–15 minutes. This aims to achieve a suitable plasma level of the drug to maintain anaesthesia. Alpha-2 agonists can also be administered with some top-up doses of ketamine to help maintain sedation and smooth anaesthesia.

Infusion Maintenance

Anaesthesia can also be maintained with an IV infusion of drugs, usually ketamine, GGE and alpha-2 adrenoceptor agonists, a mixture commonly referred to as a 'triple drip'. This is then administered, by a giving set, to maintain a sufficient depth of anaesthesia.

The choice between methods of TIVA is largely down to personal preference, familiarity with each protocol, drugs available and length of procedure. For example, a short field anaesthetic (20 minutes) would probably lead to the wastage of a 'triple drip' solution after it has been made and the expense associated with said wastage. However, for longer anaesthetics, it may be more straightforward to use an infusion as it will maintain a steadier plasma level of agents and ideally a smoother plane of anaesthesia, with fewer peaks and troughs, which are associated with repeated boluses. An overview of IV verses inhalational maintenance can be found in Table 10.1.

Neuromuscular Blockade

Moderate muscle relaxation is commonly achieved using various drugs in a standard anaesthetic protocol when adequate anaesthetic depth is achieved, but to enhance the degree of muscle relaxation due to anaesthetic drugs, excessive doses of these agents would need to be given. Additional muscle relaxation may be required for certain types of surgical procedures, such as ophthalmic procedures where the eye needs to be immobile and central or some orthopaedic and soft tissue procedures. Neuromuscular blocking agents (NMBAs), also known as relaxants or paralytic agents, are unique agents which cause relaxation of skeletal muscle by interfering with normal neuromuscular transmission. They do not provide

Table 10.1 IV versus inhalational maintenance overview.

IV – bolus administration or infusion	Inhalational administration
Minimal equipment needed, so less initial outlay of cost	Expensive/specialist equipment required for delivery
Elimination depends on organ function	Can change depth of anaesthesia quickly
Upper limit to duration of anaesthesia, without causing drug accumulation and adversely affecting recovery	Can maintain anaesthesia for a longer time period
Generally quicker recoveries (but accumulation of drugs and poorer quality recoveries if GA > 60 minutes)	May have slower recoveries
Reduced stress response	Risk of exposure to waste anaesthetic gases
Better cardiovascular function	Easier to deliver oxygen as trachea is always intubated

Source: Dr Alison Bennell.

analgesia, sedation or anaesthesia. Examples include atracurium and rocuronium.

Stages and Levels of Anaesthesia

CNS Function

In 1937, Guedel described a well-defined system pertaining to assessment of anaesthetic depth [4], with the anaesthetic agent, ether, after premedication with morphine and atropine.

Stage 1: Analgesia and amnesia. From induction of GA to loss of consciousness.

Stage 2: Delirium and unconsciousness. From loss of consciousness to onset of automatic breathing.

Stage 3: Surgical anaesthesia. From automatic respiration to respiratory paralysis

Stage 4: From apnoea (stoppage of breathing) to death. Anaesthetic overdose-caused medullary paralysis.

This system allows a basic understanding of the continuum of depth of anaesthesia, from consciousness to overdose and potential death. The introduction of newer drugs, and the use of balanced anaesthetic techniques, make the description seem rather basic, but still a useful reference to allow understanding of the consequences of using increasing dosages of an anaesthetic agent.

Phases of Anaesthesia

Before a general anaesthetic is administered to a patient, pre-anaesthetic checks and patient preparation need to be undertaken, including placing an IV catheter for further drug administration.

Following this, the process of GA can be divided up into four phases:

- **Premedication:** the animal is given drugs to calm it. Analgesic drugs are often also given for pre-emptive analgesia (±antimicrobials if indicated).

- **Induction:** the initiation of unconsciousness, muscle relaxation and analgesia (the triad of anaesthesia). This is usually by IV injection of induction agent(s).

- **Maintenance:** the animal remains anaesthetised so that the procedure can be carried out. This can be by inhalational agents or total IV methods.

- **Recovery:** anaesthesia is stopped, and the animal is allowed to recover and regain consciousness. This is the most dangerous phase of anaesthesia, supported by strong evidence in the literature [8]. Horses need to be able to stand during the recovery period, and go from a state of being closely monitored, with cardio-respiratory support, to minimal physiological support. Catastrophic injury can also occur during attempts to stand.

Anaesthetic Depth

Depth of anaesthesia is a commonly used term to describe the level of CNS and autonomic depression caused by administration of anaesthetic agents. As the dose of anaesthetic agent administered increases, the depth of anaesthesia increases and level of CNS depression also increases. Monitoring CNS function by assessing reflexes, such as palpebral reflexes and anal tone, allow the anaesthetist to titrate the anaesthetic agents to the lowest possible level, while maintaining an adequate depth of anaesthesia to ensure patient welfare. There is a fine line between achieving a plane of anaesthesia required to perform procedures, and overdose, with associated adverse outcomes. Table 10.2 provides a summary of methods used to subjectively assess anaesthetic depth.

Anaesthetic Calculations

Calculations are an essential everyday component of anaesthesia, from calculating drug dosages and fluid rates to calculating how much oxygen the patient needs while under

Table 10.2 Summary of methods used to subjectively assess anaesthetic depth.

Indicator	Plane of anaesthetic depth		
	Light	Adequate	Deep
Eye position	Rapid nystagmus[a]	Wandering	Central, dilated pupils
Palpebral reflex	Brisk	Slow	Absent
Corneal reflex	Present	Present	Present, may be slow
Lacrimation	Tear overflow	Some	None
Anal tone	Present	Present	Absent
Spontaneous movement/increase in muscle tone	Present	Absent	Absent
Respiratory rate/pattern	Can all vary and are influenced by drug protocol and physiological state of animal		
Blood pressure			
Heart rate			

[a] Nystagmus is also present during ketamine induction and maintenance (TIVA).
Palpebral reflexes are best performed in horses by gently stroking the eyelashes. Corneal reflexes are not checked due to risk of damaging the corneal surface.
Source: Dr Alison Bennell.

anaesthesia. Calculations can be intimidating, but with practice, confidence soon follows.

Use of Calculators

Calculators are helpful whenever drug calculations are required. However, if the numbers do not seem correct, calculations should be double-checked to ensure accuracy.

Gross Error Checks

Calculation errors can have problematic outcomes, ranging from situations such as a mild overdose to potentially fatal overdose or significant safety issues for personnel. Gross error checks aim to minimise the potential for errors to be made.

There are several ways to reduce possible errors, and these include:

- Ensuring familiarity with drugs and their dosages (including actual volumes administered)
- Working in mg/kg rather than volume when discussing doses with colleagues
- Using tables/written dosages
- Ensuring familiarity with the drugs used (there are different concentrations of xylazine available meaning it can be easy to give a large overdose by accident if the anaesthetist believes they are using the less concentrated solution)
- Ensuring drugs are clearly and legibly labelled
- Ensuring that information and calculations are double-checked with a colleague

Calculation of Minute Volume and Tidal Volume

This calculation is needed when using non-rebreathing breathing systems and is useful to know when considering positive pressure ventilation settings.

Minute volume = tidal volume (ml) × respiratory rate (breaths per minute)

The average tidal volume for a horse is 10–15 ml/kg.

Respiratory rate is between 6 and 8 breaths/minute.

Minute volume for a horse is approximately: $10 \times 6 = 60$ ml/kg bodyweight.

Fresh Gas Flow Rates

In equine anaesthesia, rebreathing systems, such as a large animal circle, are the mainstay of administering oxygen and volatile anaesthetic agents. Occasionally, in smaller animals, or foals, a small animal circle or non-rebreathing system may be used.

Rebreathing systems require lower oxygen flow rates due to the removal of exhaled CO_2 via soda lime in the circle, whereas non-rebreathing circuits rely on a higher fresh gas flow (FGF) to remove the CO_2 (and expired gases) from the circuit and into the scavenging. Using non-rebreathing systems in horses would be impossible due to the high oxygen flow rates needed.

When the patient is first placed on a rebreathing system, an initial higher FGF is used for two reasons:

- To denitrogenate the breathing system, as it was full of room air prior to starting anaesthesia that gas needs to be replaced with oxygen.
- As oxygen carries the volatile agent, it must be ensured that an adequate amount of volatile agent is being

administered to maintain anaesthesia, so an initial high FGF ensures that the concentration of inhalant in the system is increased.

After the initial high FGF for approximately five minutes, the FGF can be reduced to maintenance rates as the patient only requires enough oxygen to meet the metabolic demand. Metabolic oxygen demand is 4–10 ml/kg. When the lower end of this rate is used, a leak-proof breathing system must be used, and any losses from the circuit are added on (a side-stream capnograph will draw approximately 200 ml/min into the monitor). Higher FGF will be needed when vaporiser settings are changed, or if just oxygen is to be administered to the patient, as this will speed up the change of volatile concentration in the breathing system.

Another note to remember, only applicable to miniature horses and foals, is that flowmeters are poorly calibrated at <1 l/min, so it is wise to use this as a minimum, even if the FGF is calculated as <1 l/min.

Calculation Formulae
Drug Dosages
Converting units:

1000 mg = 1 g, so

- To convert mg to g, divide by 1000.
- To convert g to mg, multiply by 1000.

1000 mcg = 1 mg, so

- To convert mcg to mg, divide by 1000.
- To convert mg to mcg, multiply by 1000

% to mg/ml:

A percentage solution is defined as the weight of the solute (in grams) per 100 ml volume of drug (also known as weight divided by volume or w/v).

For example, a 2% lidocaine injection is made up of 2 g of lidocaine dissolved in 100 ml of carrier solution. and 50% glucose contains 50 g of glucose in 100 ml of carrier solution.

To calculate a dose of medication:

Dose (mg/kg) × patient bodyweight (kgs), then divide by drug concentration (mg/ml).

For further information on calculating drug doses, see Chapter 9.

Infusions

IV infusions make it possible to administer medications at a low rate, continually. They are commonly used for drugs such as sedatives and analgesics and can be very useful, as they eliminate the peaks and troughs associated with intermittent dosing. There are two ways to administer IV infusions – either via a syringe driver/pump or in a small volume of IV fluids with a standard giving set.

Using a Pump/Syringe Driver

Infusion doses may be in mg/kg/minute, mg/kg/hour or mcg/kg/minute. It is often easier to work in mg/kg/hour, so it is worthwhile to calculate this first. Then take the dose (in mg/kg/hour) and multiply it by patient weight (in kg). Then, divide this by the drug concentration (in mg/ml) to get the infusion rate in ml/hour.

When administering infusions via fluids and a giving set, a sensible drip rate needs to be calculated, so often a small volume of fluid is used (e.g. 500 ml/hour).

To calculate the volume of the drug to add to a small volume of fluids:

- Calculate the rate of the drug needed in ml/hour (dose × weight/concentration, remembering to convert the units as necessary)
- Add the drug to a reasonable amount of fluid to last the estimated procedure length (500 ml/1 l) – this is purely to work out a reasonable drip rate, not for IV fluid administration
- Work out the drip rate.

e.g. if 500 ml is to last 60 minutes, and a giving set is 20 drops/ml

- 500 ml/3600 seconds = 0.14 ml/second
- at 20 drops/ml = 0.14 × 20 = approximately 3 drops/second

Many infusions, particularly of sedative drugs, need to be titrated to effect, but sensible starting doses are available in many texts [9].

10.2 Anaesthetic Drugs

An effective anaesthetic protocol often contains a number of different classes of drugs. As mentioned previously, the use of several different classes of drugs gives rise to a multimodal approach, where the benefits of using multiple drugs are reaped against a reduced likelihood of negative side effects occurring, as smaller doses of each drug can be used. The main properties of commonly used sedative and anaesthetic drugs are summarised in Table 10.3.

Sedatives

Achieving Effective Sedation

It is the role of the veterinary surgeon (vet) in charge of the anaesthetic to prescribe the medication required. The administration of these medications may be delegated to

Table 10.3 Summary of the main properties of commonly used sedative and anaesthetic drugs.

Drug class	Clinical effect	Mechanism of action	Side effects
Phenothiazines	Mental calming: mild–moderate	Dopamine antagonist	Hypotension No analgesia
Alpha-2 agonists	Sedation: dose-dependent, can be profound Analgesia Some muscle relaxation	Alpha-2 adrenoceptor agonist in CNS (sedation) and periphery. Analgesic effects due to actions at both sites	Vascular tone changes and bradycardia (reduced CO) Diuresis Sweating
Opioids	Analgesia	Opioid receptors in CNS. Action at receptor will depend on drug (agonist/antagonist)	Can reduce gastrointestinal motility Can increase locomotor activity
Benzodiazepines	Muscle relaxation Used for co-induction with ketamine	γ-Aminobutyric acid type A (GABA$_A$) agonist	No analgesia Cause ataxia so not used for sedation in adult horses. Used commonly for sedation in neonatal foals
Volatile agents	Anaesthetic maintenance	Unknown	Hypotension Hypoventilation
Ketamine	Anaesthetic induction Analgesia	NMDA antagonist Dissociative anaesthetic	Can cause excitation Sympathomimetic effects
Thiopental (ultra-short acting barbiturate)	Anaesthetic induction Also useful peri-operatively if unexpected movement to deepen plane of anaesthesia quickly	GABA$_A$ agonist	No analgesia Irritant if injected perivascularly/extravascularly Can cause prolonged/ataxic recovery, especially if repeated doses used

Source: Dr Alison Bennell.

a registered veterinary nurse (RVN). If 'top up' doses of medication are required, these should be prescribed by the vet. Top up doses can be prescribed by the vet and discussed with the RVN prior to the start of the procedure. See The British Equine Veterinary Association (BEVA) Schedule 3 guidelines for further information (details in the 'Further reading' section the end of this chapter). Effective sedation can be achieved with several drugs, delivered by various routes. The vet will give consideration to the horse's temperament and the likely level of sedation required when deciding what drug and dose to choose. The external environment is a hugely important factor in achieving successful sedation, so a calm, quiet environment is optimal, with minimal interruptions. It is also worth remembering individual response to sedatives can be extremely variable. It is often easier to give more drugs if the desired effect is not achieved, as an over-sedated horse can be a challenge to deal with.

Phenothiazines (Acepromazine)

Acepromazine, a phenothiazine, exerts its mental calming effect by its actions of dopamine-antagonism and subsequent depression of the reticular activating system of the CNS. It can be administered orally, or via the IV or the IM route. The sedation caused by acepromazine is mild, and can be unpredictable, especially when given to horses who are very stimulated or 'wound-up'. Acepromazine causes hypotension, so it should be avoided in horses where there is pre-existing hypotension/hypovolaemia, for example, sick colics or patients who have suffered a significant haemorrhage. It is also contraindicated on the data sheet in breeding stallions due to the risk of priapism/paraphimosis, but as with many theoretical contraindications, it can be used after gaining informed consent from the owner if it is felt the potential benefits outweigh the potential risks of its use. The onset of action of mental calming is slow, around 30–45 minutes and it lasts for approximately 4–6 hours, but can last longer with higher doses. Acepromazine is often used in combination with other drugs, or as an initial pre-medicant, as it will not cause profound sedation when given alone. It provides no analgesia. Acepromazine undergoes hepatic metabolism and renal excretion.

Alpha-2 Adrenoceptor Agonists

Alpha-2 agonists are the mainstay of equine sedation. They provide predictable and dose-dependent sedation and also have analgesic and muscle relaxant properties. Alpha-2 adrenoceptors are found in the CNS and periphery giving rise to the clinical effects seen. Xylazine, romifidine and detomidine are licensed in the United Kingdom. All are licensed to be given by the IV route and detomidine is also licensed for IM and transmucosal administration, which is particularly useful in fractious or poorly handled horses. Xylazine has the quickest onset of action, about 2–3 minutes, compared to 5 minutes for romifidine and detomidine when given IV. Xylazine also has the shortest duration of action, about 20 minutes. Detomidine has a duration of action of around 40–60 minutes, and romifidine has around 60 minutes. After alpha-2 agonist administration, vasoconstriction and a transient increase in blood pressure causes reflex bradycardia. Vascular tone then relaxes and blood pressure returns to near normal. Respiratory effects are largely unimportant as although animals may show a slight decrease in respiratory rate, tidal volume may increase. The muscle relaxation caused by alpha-2 agonists in horses leads to ataxia, with romifidine generally causing the least ataxia when effective doses of alpha-2 agonists are used. Other important side effects of alpha-2 agonist administration include diuresis, sweating and decreased gastrointestinal motility. Alpha-2 agonists undergo hepatic metabolism and renal excretion.

Opioids

Opioids are often used in sedative protocols, but are discussed in detail in the analgesia section.

Benzodiazepines

Benzodiazepines are discussed later as they are used as sedative drugs in foals but not in adult horses.

Injectable Induction Agents

Ketamine and thiopental are induction agents that can be used for induction of anaesthesia in horses in the United Kingdom. These drugs are often used alongside co-induction agents, such as benzodiazepines and GGE, used for their muscle relaxant properties.

Ketamine

Ketamine is a dissociative anaesthetic agent and is an NMDA antagonist. It is the most commonly used induction agent in horses. Dissociative anaesthesia is characterised by catalepsy, and is accompanied by nystagmus. Due to the effect of ketamine on receptors, it is also an excellent analgesic, providing analgesia at sub-anaesthetic doses, although this only lasts for a short period of time. Horses need to be adequately sedated with alpha-2 agonists prior to induction of anaesthesia with ketamine, or excitation can occur, which can be dangerous for both the patient and any personnel involved. In healthy animals, ketamine causes indirect stimulation of the cardiovascular system (via the sympathetic nervous system), but in unhealthy animals, myocardial depression can be seen. Respiration and respiratory reflexes are maintained after ketamine administration, with horses often demonstrating an apneustic breathing pattern (deep inspiration and inspiratory pauses). Another effect of ketamine is that muscle hypertonus is seen at/immediately after induction. Co-administration of benzodiazepines helps to offset the muscle rigidity, smoothing the process of induction and inducing recumbency. This makes placing a mouth gag and subsequent tracheal intubation easier. This effect also facilitates the hoisting and transportation of horses into the theatre. Ketamine has a relatively short onset of action, of approximately 60–90 seconds and duration of action is 10–20 minutes. Ketamine is rapidly redistributed to tissues from the CNS, so recovery can be rapid. It undergoes hepatic metabolism and renal excretion, and when prolonged infusions are used, the production of an active metabolite, norketamine, can accumulate and cause poor-quality recoveries. For this reason, TIVA protocols with ketamine are kept under 60 minutes duration.

Thiopentone/Thiopental

Thiopentone is an ultra-short-acting barbiturate, and a GABA$_A$ agonist, which is still used in equine anaesthesia. It can be used as an IV induction agent, and is also useful when unexpected movement/a light plane of anaesthesia is encountered as it is quick acting and will deepen anaesthetic depth promptly. It has an onset of action of around 20–30 seconds and a duration of action of 10–20 minutes. Thiopentone causes a good level of muscle relaxation, and although ideally used after alpha-2 agonist premedication, it can be used without prior sedative administration, to induce GA. Thiopentone is an extremely alkaline medication (pH 10.5), and if injected perivascularly, it can cause significant irritation and tissue sloughing, so a patent IV catheter must always be used for administration. Thiopentone will cause a reduction in myocardial contractility, can cause mild vasodilation and mild respiratory depression. Thiopentone is redistributed to tissues, and this can be limited in animals with low body fat and neonates, which can cause slower recoveries. It has no analgesic properties. Thiopentone undergoes hepatic metabolism and renal excretion. Due to slow metabolism, and its propensity to redistribute to fat, recovery can become prolonged when multiple doses or infusions are used, so it is not suitable for TIVA maintenance. There is no current UK-licensed thiopentone for veterinary use, although there are veterinary-licensed products available to import.

Benzodiazepines

Benzodiazepines are often used for co-induction of GA as they are centrally-acting muscle relaxants, useful in offsetting the muscle hypertonus caused by ketamine. Midazolam and diazepam are most commonly used; Midazolam is currently licensed for co-induction of anaesthesia in the United Kingdom. Benzodiazepines also cause sedation in some species, but they are not administered as sedative agents to horses as the muscle weakness they cause produces panic, which is difficult to manage safely. They can be used in neonates, however, as they tend to lie down voluntarily after administration. Benzodiazepines have few side effects, with minimal cardiovascular or respiratory depression at clinically useful doses. They have no analgesic effects. Benzodiazepines undergo hepatic metabolism and renal excretion.

Guaiphenesin/Glyceryl Guaiacolate Ether (GGE)

GGE is another centrally acting muscle relaxant, acting on spinal cord and brainstem pathways to reduce postural muscle tone. It is commercially available as a 10% solution, which can be used for co-induction of anaesthesia, or as part of a TIVA protocol. GGE must be administered via the IV route and is combined with anaesthetic drugs as it provides minimal sedation and no analgesia. GGE can also be a vascular irritant, so care must be taken when administering, and it is advisable to flush IV catheters well before removing them after GGE has been used, to ensure no traces are drawn through the perivascular tissues. GGE undergoes hepatic metabolism and renal excretion.

Other Induction Agents

Propofol and alfaxalone are anaesthetic induction agents licensed in small animal species. Although they can be used off-license in horses, ketamine is the mainstay of equine induction agents. The volumes required of propofol and alfaxalone make them more suited to miniature horses and foals, when they can be used via the cascade. See Chapter 9 for further information regarding the cascade.

Inhalation Anaesthetics

Volatile Agents

In the United Kingdom, isoflurane is licensed for use in horses and is the mainstay of inhalational maintenance, but sevoflurane and desflurane can be used, when justified via the cascade. The exact mechanisms of action of volatile anaesthetic agents still remain elusive, although this is likely due to receptor-based mechanisms. Inhalational anaesthetic agents are administered, carried in oxygen, into the respiratory tract, where they passively diffuse via the lungs into the bloodstream. Both respiratory and physical factors will determine the speed of uptake, and the amount of drug taken into the bloodstream. Once dissolved in the blood, the inhalational agent is then distributed to the organs, including the target organ, the brain, where they have to cross the blood–brain barrier to be effective.

Anaesthetic potency is described by a concept known as minimum alveolar concentration (MAC). MAC describes the amount of anaesthetic agents where 50% of the sample population does not respond to noxious stimuli (e.g. skin incision) with purposeful movement. This gives a guide as to how much anaesthetic agent is required to achieve a level of anaesthetic depth where surgery can be humanely performed. MAC is inversely related to potency; therefore, a high MAC relates to an agent with a low potency. MAC values vary depending on the source; however, MAC values for commonly used inhalation agents are as follows:

- Isoflurane: 1.3%
- Sevoflurane: 2.3%
- Desflurane: 7.6%

Volatile agents cause vasodilation and myocardial depression, leading to dose-dependent hypotension. They are also respiratory depressants, especially in horses, so dose-dependent hypoventilation is seen [10]. Volatile agents possess no analgesic properties.

Carrier Gases

Nitrous Oxide

Nitrous oxide, a colourless gas which is an NMDA-antagonist, is well recognised for its analgesic properties when inhaled. Other volatile anaesthetic agents work through different receptors and channels, so they work synergistically to cause a volatile-sparing effect. Nitrous oxide has low anaesthetic potency, meaning a concentration of over 100% is required to achieve MAC anaesthesia, which is clearly impossible to achieve at atmospheric pressure. However, the physiochemical properties mean its use alongside volatile anaesthetic agents can speed up the onset of inhalational agents due to its 'second gas effect'. This means as nitrous oxide diffuses rapidly across the alveolus, it concentrates the remaining alveolar gases (volatile agent, oxygen), which increases the driving pressure of volatile agent into the bloodstream. Another sequelae of nitrous oxide's physiochemical properties is its propensity to diffuse into gas-filled spaces. This can be particularly problematic in horses, due to the considerable amounts of gas found in a normal gastrointestinal tract, and in abnormal ones, such as commonly found in horses with colic. Diffusion hypoxia occurs when delivery of nitrous oxide ends and the direction of diffusion reverses (from blood into the alveolar space); this means that alveolar oxygen may be diluted, and therefore the animal requires pure oxygen (100%) rather than room air (20%) for at least 3 minutes after termination of nitrous oxide delivery to prevent hypoxia.

Nitrous oxide has significant global warming potential and is a significant contributor to the greenhouse effect in the United Kingdom, as well as having ozone-depleting potential. The negative environmental impact is a major reason for a recent decline in use. Nitrous oxide has also been implicated in reduced fertility and negatively impacts pregnancies in female theatre workers, so it is regulated under the Control of Substances Hazardous to Health (COSHH) regulations in the United Kingdom.

As mentioned previously, oxygen is an indispensable carrier gas. Additive carrier gases include medical air, and even gases such as xenon, although they are seldom used outside research settings due to expense.

Analgesics

Opioid Analgesics

Opioids, one of the oldest forms of analgesia, exert their effects by binding to opioid receptors, which are largely found in the CNS, but also peripherally in areas such as joints. Different classes of opioids are used in veterinary medicine, based on the subset of opioid receptors on which they exert their effects. Pure mu-agonists, such as methadone, pethidine and morphine are efficacious analgesics. Partial mu-agonists such as buprenorphine are also useful analgesics. Mu-antagonists/kappa agonists, such as butorphanol, provide little analgesia, but are often combined with alpha-2 agonists to aid sedation. When selecting an appropriate opioid, several factors need to be considered: legalities/licensing/the cascade, the level of analgesia desired, the drug onset and duration of action, route of administration and potential side effects. Cost and availability are also practical factors worth consideration. Opioids can be administered via several routes with IV (not pethidine), IM, intra-articular and extradural routes all well described in the literature.

At clinically used doses, cardiovascular side effects are minimal, as are respiratory effects. Opioids can cause a reduction in propulsive gastrointestinal motility and ileus, particularly with repeated dosing. Many texts discuss the possibility of opioid-induced excitation, although this is seldom seen clinically for various reasons [11]. Painful animals are far less likely to experience opioid-induced excitation, and in non-painful animals the administration of sedation, such as alpha-2 agonists, prior to opioid administration will also decrease the likelihood of this side effect.

NSAIDs

NSAIDs are the most commonly prescribed class of drugs used to treat pain in horses. Their mode of action is to block specific enzymes, cyclooxygenase or COX, which is a vital part of the arachidonic acid pathway leading to the production of prostaglandins, which are involved in inflammation. Many licensed NSAIDs are available in the United Kingdom, including phenylbutazone, flunixin, meloxicam, suxibuzone and firocoxib, to name a few. NSAIDs have recognised negative side effects, including gastrointestinal injury (gastric ulceration and right dorsal colitis) and renal injury. Gastrointestinal side effects are usually seen when high doses are used, when NSAIDs are used for long periods of time, or in foals.

The choice of NSAID needs to take into consideration licensing (e.g. phenylbutazone is not to be administered to food-producing horses), cost, route of administration, availability and palatability. NSAIDs are commonly used due to their relatively cheap cost, ease of owner administration and relatively good safety profile, particularly in healthy animals.

Local Anaesthetics

Local anaesthetics are true analgesics as they block the transmission part of the pain pathway, so no action potential is produced in nociceptive fibres when nociceptors are stimulated. Local anaesthetics exert their actions by blocking voltage-gated sodium channels. Many different local anaesthetics exist, with procaine, lidocaine and mepivacaine being licensed in horses, although bupivacaine is commonly used due to its longer duration of action (Table 10.4). Local anaesthetics can be used in many ways, including topical application, splash blocks, local infiltration, peripheral nerve blocks, intrathecal administration, epidural injection and IV infusion.

Local anaesthetics can cause local tissue irritation and when used in high doses, can cause toxicity. This is most likely seen when IV infusion is used, or when supramaximal doses are used for local infiltration. Toxicity is seen in the CNS, and at higher doses cardiotoxicity is also seen.

Other Agents with Analgesic Properties
Paracetamol

The use of paracetamol in the veterinary world has gained momentum over the past few years, but its analgesic mechanisms are not completely understood, and its metabolism is complex. It is largely believed that paracetamol exerts its actions via an active metabolite, AM404, which acts on vanilloid and cannabinoid receptors in the CNS. Although no equine-licensed product is available, and there is limited literature available on its use in the horse, it can

Table 10.4 Main properties of commonly used local anaesthetics.

Drug	Onset of action	Duration of action	Notes
Procaine	5–10 minutes	45–60 minutes	Licensed preparation includes adrenaline
Lidocaine	Fewer than 120 seconds	Up to 2 hours without adrenaline, up to 3 hours with adrenaline	Licensed preparation includes adrenaline
Mepivacaine	30–120 seconds	2–3 hours	Most commonly used for nerve blocks for lameness investigation
Bupivacaine	5–10 minutes	4–8 hours	Unlicensed

Source: Dr Alison Bennell.

be a useful additional drug when dealing with painful equine patients.

Gabapentin

Gabapentin produces its analgesic actions through ion channel effects, and can be useful in persistent pain states. It can cause sedation/mental calming and ataxia.

Others

As has been discussed previously, alpha-2 agonists [12] and ketamine also have analgesic actions.

Neuromuscular Blocking Agents

Neuromuscular blocking agents (NMBAs) are agents which paralyse skeletal muscle movement, including respiratory muscles and ocular muscles, by blocking the movement of neurotransmitters at neuromuscular junctions. They do not provide any analgesia or anaesthesia, so they must always be used in combination with anaesthetic and analgesic drugs, or the patient will be awake and aware, but unable to move. NMBAs are not commonly used in equine anaesthesia, but are indicated in some types of surgery, such as ophthalmic procedures where the eye needs to be in a central position. Horses who have had NMBAs administered will require mechanical ventilation. The effectiveness of neuromuscular blockade requires monitoring with a peripheral nerve stimulator. Some subjective components of monitoring anaesthetic depth, such as eye position, nystagmus and reflexes, are abolished when NMBAs have been administered.

NMBAs are classified into depolarising and non-depolarising agents, according to their mechanism of action:

- Depolarising agents such as Succinylcholine/suxamethonium are rarely indicated for use in horses. Succinylcholine/suxamethonium causes depolarisation at the neuromuscular junction, initially producing intense muscle contractions followed by relaxation. Its clinical usefulness is limited by its short duration of action and side effects such as cardiac dysrhythmias, tachycardia and the effects of intense muscle contraction (increased potassium levels, metabolic acidosis).
- Non-depolarising agents such as atracurium and rocuronium act as antagonists at the postsynaptic receptor, meaning muscle contraction cannot be initiated as acetylcholine cannot bind to this receptor.

Monitoring neuromuscular function is important when NMBAs are used as it allows the assessment of the effectiveness of blockade and if repeat dosing with the NMBA is required. It will also reduce the incidence of complications associated with residual blockade in recovery, allowing the anaesthetist to decide if the block has worn off, or needs to be antagonised or reversed to ensure it is safe to attempt to recover the patient. There are several techniques used to monitor neuromuscular function, all based on the fact that NMBAs stop transmission at the neuromuscular junction and therefore muscle function. A peripheral nerve stimulator, placed with an electrode over an accessible peripheral nerve, will evoke a response in the corresponding muscle. This can then be quantified and monitored throughout the anaesthetic to monitor the effectiveness of blockade.

Because NMBAs block skeletal muscle function, it is vital to ensure normal muscle function is restored prior to recovery and tracheal extubation. Ideally, the length of time the NMBA agent is active for should be matched to the specific drug chosen. However, there are times when the residual blockade is still present at the end of the procedure. In the case of non-depolarising NMBAs, as they are competitive agonists, reversal of the drug is possible by increasing the amount of acetylcholine at the neuromuscular junction. This can be achieved by using drugs such as neostigmine or edrophonium, although commonly seen side effects include bradycardia and bronchospasm. Sugammadex, a reversal agent, is also available, which encapsulates some NMBAs, such as rocuronium, rendering it ineffective.

10.3 Anaesthetic Equipment

Function and Maintenance of the Anaesthetic Machine

An anaesthetic machine comprises several components (Figure 10.3). The design and arrangement of the machine and its components may influence the individual appearance of the anaesthetic machine. However, the overall functional aim of the anaesthetic machine is a common one: to deliver oxygen and inhalational anaesthetic agents to the patient in a controlled manner and to remove exhaled gases.

Components of the Large Animal Anaesthetic Machine

The main components of a large animal anaesthetic machine include:

- Gas supply
- Common gas outlet (CGO)
- Flowmeter
- Vaporiser
- Breathing system
- Carbon dioxide absorbent canister
- Rebreathing bag
- Adjustable pressure limiting (APL) valve or pressure relief valve
- Oxygen alarm
- Oxygen emergency flush
- Mechanical ventilator (may be an additional component).

Gas Supply

Cylinders Cylinders are made of thin-walled seamless molybdenum steel, in which gases and vapours are stored under high pressure [13]. Compressed gas cylinders can be used to store and supply medical gases. They have several features which facilitate their safe use (Figure 10.4). Smaller size cylinders, such as size E, may be mounted on the anaesthetic machine for use in small animal patients. If cylinders are machine-mounted, they must be clamped onto the machine by a yoke arrangement and secured tightly using a wing nut [14]. Larger cylinders, such as size J, are commonly used in large animal anaesthesia. Large-size cylinders are not usually machine-mounted due to their size and weight. Larger cylinders are usually stored in a location that is easy to access for delivery and safe for storage. Cylinders may be used individually or linked together to form a manifold. Cylinders forming a manifold may be divided into two groups, to allow a swift changeover from one supply to the other when one manifold is exhausted. The number of cylinders on the manifold depends on the expected demand [13].

Cylinder Safety Cylinders should be housed in a well-ventilated room, built using fire-proof material and located away from the main buildings of the hospital [13]. The cylinder housing should provide shelter from the extremes of temperature associated with hot and cold weather. Cylinders should not be stored near flammable materials such as oil or grease or near any source of heat [13]. The manifold room should not be used as a general cylinder store,

Figure 10.3 Example of a large animal anaesthetic machine with a large animal circle breathing system and mechanical ventilator. *Source:* Dr Kate Loomes.

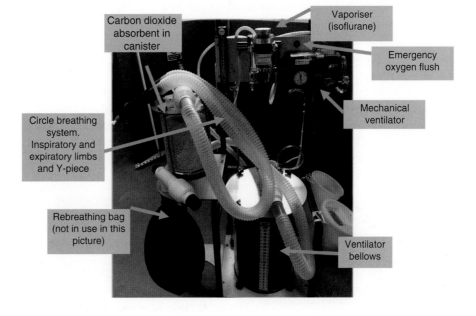

Carbon dioxide absorbent in canister

Vaporiser (isoflurane)

Emergency oxygen flush

Mechanical ventilator

Circle breathing system. Inspiratory and expiratory limbs and Y-piece

Rebreathing bag (not in use in this picture)

Ventilator bellows

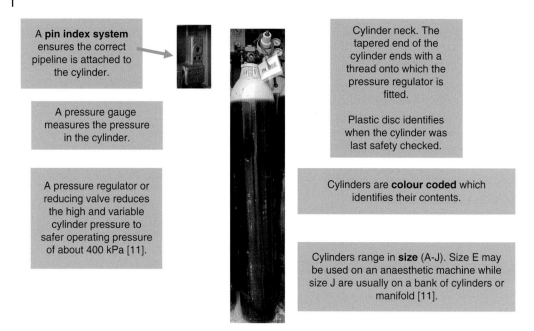

A **pin index system** ensures the correct pipeline is attached to the cylinder.

A pressure gauge measures the pressure in the cylinder.

A pressure regulator or reducing valve reduces the high and variable cylinder pressure to safer operating pressure of about 400 kPa [11].

Cylinder neck. The tapered end of the cylinder ends with a thread onto which the pressure regulator is fitted.

Plastic disc identifies when the cylinder was last safety checked.

Cylinders are **colour coded** which identifies their contents.

Cylinders range in **size** (A-J). Size E may be used on an anaesthetic machine while size J are usually on a bank of cylinders or manifold [11].

Figure 10.4 Compressed gas cylinders have several features which facilitate their safe use. *Source:* Dr Kate Loomes.

and empty cylinders should be removed to avoid confusion [13].

Piped Gases Copper alloy pipes are used to form a conduit for gas from a central supply point to regions of the hospital where medical gases are required. The gas outlets or sockets are colour and shape coded to accept the matching Schrader probes [13] (Figure 10.5). Flexible colour-coded pipelines are used to connect the anaesthetic machine to the gas outlets [13]. The gas outlets or sockets may be wall or ceiling mounted. The probe for each gas supply has a protruding indexing collar with a unique diameter, which fits the Schrader socket assembly for the same gas only [15]. If the connection is faulty, or the wrong hose is connected to the wall Schrader valve, the hose will disconnect from the wall when pulled during the 'tug test' [16].

Pressure Regulators or Pressure Reducing Valves Pressure regulators are unique for each gas and are required to be fitted to all cylinders. They provide a constant low pressure suitable for delivery to the anaesthetic machine from the

variable high-pressure cylinders. The pressure delivered from a cylinder is far too high to be used safely with apparatus where a sudden surge of pressure may accidentally be delivered to the patient [14]. Pressure regulators protect the components of the anaesthetic machine against pressure surges [13]. They ensure that a constant flow rate is maintained from a cylinder irrespective of the cylinder contents [14].

Common Gas Outlet (CGO)

The CGO delivers gas from the flowmeter and vaporiser to the anaesthetic breathing system [17]. There is usually one CGO per machine. Machines must have no more than one CGO unless there is an integral circle breathing system; in this case, the gas flow may be switched between this and the CGO [14]. The CGO may be fixed or swivelled through 90° (Cardiff Swivel) and should be robust enough to withstand the attachment of heavy equipment [14]. The swivel design of the CGO reduces the risk of disconnection or kinked tubing when either the patient or the anaesthetic machine is moved. The CGO is a standard size (22 mm

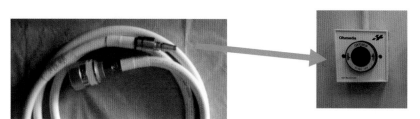

Figure 10.5 The Schrader probes and gas outlets or sockets for an individual gas have a unique shape and colour to avoid errors in connection. *Source:* Dr Kate Loomes.

male/15 mm female) allowing for connection of breathing apparatus [18].

Flowmeter (Rotameter)

Flowmeters are variable orifice, fixed-pressure devices [16] which control the fresh gas flow (FGF). The FGF is the gas which enters the breathing system from the common gas outlet on the anaesthetic machine. The gas contains oxygen and an inhalational anaesthetic agent if the gas has passed through a vaporiser. Flowmeters accurately control the flow of gas through the anaesthetic machine [14]. One flowmeter is provided on the anaesthetic machine for each gas and are individually calibrated [13]. The flowmeter tubes are a specific length and diameter for each gas. The control knob is colour-coded for each gas and is a safety feature. The tubes have an anti-static coating on both surfaces, preventing the bobbin from sticking [15]. The tube is leak-proofed at the top and bottom by 'O' rings, neoprene sockets or washers [14]. The bobbin will rise as gas flows increase and stop where gravity equals the pressure of upwards gas flow [16]. The bobbin is visible throughout the length of the tube [15]. The bobbin may have a white dot to allow observation that the bobbin is freely spinning and not lodged in the tube. The reading is taken from the top of the bobbin or if a ball is used (Figure 10.6), then the reading is usually taken from the midpoint of the ball [13]. To minimise risk of hypoxic gas mixtures being delivered to the patient, some machines will mechanically link flow-control valves to ensure that a minimal ratio of oxygen to other gases is provided [18].

Flowmeter Mechanism of Action The control knob opens a needle valve which allows gas to flow in and enter the tapered tube. The gas flowing up the tube holds the bobbin in a floating position. The higher the flow rate, the higher the bobbin position [13]. The bobbin floats and rotates inside the sight tube, without touching the sides, giving an accurate measurement of the gas flow [14].

Vaporiser

Many inhalational agents are liquids under normal storage conditions and need to be in a vapour form before they can be administered to a patient [19]. A vaporiser adds a controlled amount of inhalational agent, after changing it from liquid to vapour, to the fresh gas flow [13]. Vaporisers can be classified according to their location 'inside' or 'outside' the breathing system:

Inside the Breathing System

- Gases pass through a very low-resistance, draw-over vaporiser according to the patient's respiratory efforts. Examples are; Goldman, Oxford Miniature Vaporiser.
- Draw-over vaporisers are subjected to very variable flow rates as they rely on a patient's respiratory effort to draw gas over the vaporising surface [19].
- As air flows into the vaporiser, it is directed into either the vaporising chamber to collect vapour or into a bypass

Figure 10.6 An oxygen flowmeter.
Source: Dr Kate Loomes.

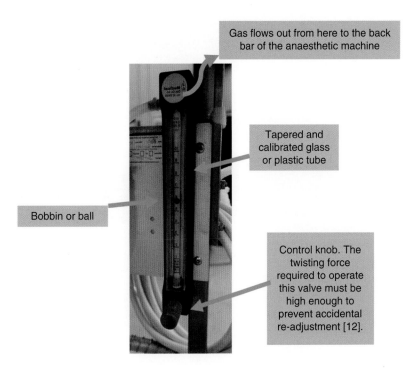

Gas flows out from here to the back bar of the anaesthetic machine

Tapered and calibrated glass or plastic tube

Bobbin or ball

Control knob. The twisting force required to operate this valve must be high enough to prevent accidental re-adjustment [12].

chamber. Wicks increase the surface area for vaporisation in some models.

- Draw-over vaporisers use fresh gas flow at atmospheric pressure, driven by the patient's respiratory efforts [20].
- Draw-over vaporisers may be used in portable systems or when compressed gas is not available [20].
- Gas pathways must offer minimal resistance to flow so as not to compromise the patient's ventilation. This requirement for low resistance may restrict the design of the vaporiser components [19].

Outside the Breathing System

- Gases are driven through a **plenum** (high resistance, unidirectional) vaporiser due to gas supply pressure [13] (Figure 10.7).
- Plenum is the term which describes a 'pressurised' chamber [19].
- The gas is split into two streams. One passes into the bypass channel; the other goes into the vaporising channel. Gas in the vaporising channel becomes saturated with vapour, which then mixes with the bypass channel to dilute it to the % on the dial before leaving the vaporiser.
- They have features to compensate for temperature change – a metal jacket that keeps temperature constant and a bimetallic strip that allows more gas into the chamber as it cools.
- Plenum vaporisers have high internal resistance, requiring fresh gas at above atmospheric pressure [20].

- Plenum vaporisers are more accurate due to design features which overcome the challenges of variable gas flow rates.
- Vaporiser accuracy increases if the carrier gas is pressurised to make it as dense as the vapour, allowing it to readily mix rather than pass over the vaporising chamber [19].

Vaporiser Safety Features

- **Push (release) button:** Most vaporisers have a push button, which must be activated before the dial can be turned. This push button cannot be used until the vaporiser is seated firmly on the back bar, ensuring that the vapour is not delivered if installation is incorrect [15].
- **Interlock mechanism:** All modern vaporisers come equipped with an interlock mechanism, which prevents more than one vaporiser from being used at the same time, thus causing an accidental overdose [15]. If two vaporisers are mounted side by side on the back bar, when the control dial of one vaporiser is turned on, a rod is released on either side of the vaporiser, which then engages the control dial of the adjacent vaporiser and immobilises the dial [15].
- **Transport setting:** Modern vaporisers may have a separate transport setting, which prevents spillage of the liquid agent into the bypass channel, which may risk potential overdosing when the vaporisers are used [15].
- **Keyed filling:** All newer vaporisers have keyed/funnel filling systems with unique sizing that are agent specific.

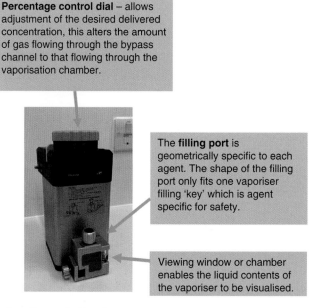

Percentage control dial – allows adjustment of the desired delivered concentration, this alters the amount of gas flowing through the bypass channel to that flowing through the vaporisation chamber.

Temperature compensation 'tec'.

Bimetallic strips. Two metals strips with different coefficients of thermal expansion. As temperature decreases the strips bend allowing more fresh gas flow to enter the vaporisation chamber.

Wicks and baffles in the vaporising chamber increase the surface area available for vaporisation.

The **filling port** is geometrically specific to each agent. The shape of the filling port only fits one vaporiser filling 'key' which is agent specific for safety.

Viewing window or chamber enables the liquid contents of the vaporiser to be visualised.

Figure 10.7 Example of a plenum vaporiser. *Source:* Dr Kate Loomes.

The bottles of inhalational anaesthetic agents are either fitted with specific nozzles or have filling adaptors which match the vaporiser filling port.

- **Colour coding:** Vaporisers are colour-coded to match the colour of the bottles of inhalational agents for which they are specific. For example, isoflurane is purple, sevoflurane is yellow and desflurane is blue.

Care and Maintenance

- Each hospital must ensure that all equipment including vaporisers are serviced at the regular intervals designated by the manufacturer and that a service record is maintained [21].
- The calibration of each vaporiser is agent-specific [13].
- Vaporisers must always be stored upright to prevent leakage of anaesthetic agents into the bypass channel.
- Vaporisers should never be tipped up or severely tilted as spillage of anaesthetic agent into the bypass channel results in dangerously high concentrations of agent leaving the vaporiser [18].

The Anaesthetic Breathing System

The breathing system conducts oxygen and anaesthetic gases from the common gas outlet to the patient and removes exhaled gases from the patient [17]. In the equine hospital setting, a large animal circle breathing system is most commonly used for the delivery of inhalational anaesthetic agents and oxygen to maintain GA. Circle breathing systems use one-way valves to unidirectionally route gases through the carbon dioxide absorbent material and back to the horse [17]. The optimal functioning of one-way valves is crucial to prevent rebreathing of exhaled gases. The Waters'

to-and-fro system is valveless and gases are exhaled through the carbon dioxide absorbent into a rebreathing bag and drawn back through the absorbent during inhalation [17]. Advantages and disadvantages of the circle breathing system and the Waters' to-and-fro system are presented in Tables 10.5 and 10.6.

Carbon Dioxide Absorbent and Canister

Various carbon-dioxide absorbent materials are available. Soda lime can be used to absorb exhaled carbon dioxide when a circular breathing system is used. Carbon dioxide is absorbed by chemical reactions [17]. Soda lime granules are placed in an appropriately sized canister for the size of patient and the circle breathing system in use. Soda lime consists of 94% calcium hydroxide and 5% sodium hydroxide with a small amount (<0.1%) of potassium hydroxide [13]. Exhaled gases pass through the soda lime granules in the canister allowing carbon dioxide absorption to take place. An exothermic reaction occurs and water and heat are produced. The warmed and humified gas then joins the fresh gas flow to be delivered to the patient [13]. Soda lime granules undergo a pH change in response to carbon dioxide absorption, which allows the use of indicator dyes to show when the absorption capacity is exhausted [22]. The colour change is specific to each brand of soda lime and should be verified before use to avoid confusion. 1 kg of soda lime on average can absorb 250 l of carbon dioxide [22]. A canister containing 5 kg of absorbent material typically remains active for a period of 6–8 hours of GA (assuming a 450 kg horse and 5 l/min oxygen flow rate) [17]. However, the duration that carbon dioxide absorbent material is effective before it must be changed varies with the size of the horse, the individual CO_2 production

Table 10.5 Advantages and disadvantages of the circle breathing system.

Advantages	Disadvantages
Low fresh gas flows can be used resulting in greater economy	Increased resistance created by the carbon dioxide absorbent canister and one-way valves
Dead space remains constant [15]	Long inspiratory and expiratory limbs can create equipment dead space particularly in smaller horses
Inspired gas is warmed and moistened	The Y-piece may be heavy which creates drag on the endotracheal tube
Low flow systems result in less environmental pollution	Anaesthetic agent concentration may be slow to change if low fresh gas flows are used
Mechanical ventilation can be easily used with a circle breathing system	The equipment can be expensive to buy and can be complicated to repair
Temperature is relatively uniform throughout the system [15]	Equipment is not easily transported
Minimum chance of inhaling alkaline dust from the absorbent material [15]	

Source: Dr Kate Loomes.

Table 10.6 Advantages and disadvantages of the to-and-fro system.

Advantages	Disadvantages
Simple to use	The horizontal position of the carbon dioxide absorbent canister can lead to 'channelling' of gases which reduces carbon dioxide absorption efficiency
Portable	The carbon dioxide absorbent becomes exhausted on the surface closest to the patient first and then as anaesthesia progresses, this area of exhausted absorbent extends which results in increased equipment dead space over time [20]
Easy to assemble/dissemble	The close proximity of the canister to the patient connector also creates some drag on the endotracheal tube as the canister can be quite heavy
Straightforward to clean	The close positioning of the canister to the patient connector can lead to inhalation of irritant dust from the carbon dioxide absorbent [20]
Relatively rapid change in anaesthetic concentration for a given fresh gas flow [15]	The close positioning of the canister to the patient connector can lead to heat being produced near to the endotracheal tube attachment [15]

Source: Dr Kate Loomes.

(metabolic rate) of the horse, the fresh gas flow and the size and location of the canister [17]. The best method of monitoring when to change carbon dioxide absorbent material is to monitor inspired gas for CO_2 using a capnograph [17].

Rebreathing/Reservoir Bag

The terminology used for the bag depends on the breathing system in which it is used [21]:

- **Rebreathing bag:** the bag in any breathing system where the patient's exhaled gases can/do pass into the bag (e.g. Bain, circle and Waters' to-and-fro breathing systems) [23].
- **Reservoir bag:** the bag in any breathing system where the patient's exhaled gases do not pass into the bag (e.g. Magill and Lack breathing systems) [23].

The reservoir or rebreathing bag is the rubber bag that is situated in the breathing system. It allows the accumulation of gas during exhalation and creates a 'reservoir' of gas for inhalation. Patient breathing can be visualised as the reservoir/rebreathing bag deflates and inflates in time with the patient's respiratory pattern. The reservoir/rebreathing bag should be of such a size that the capacity to which it may be easily distended must exceed the patient's tidal volume [23] (tidal volume (V_T) = 10–15 ml/kg bodyweight). The reservoir/rebreathing bag needs to be at least 2–6 times the patient's tidal volume. The maximum volume of the bag should be 5–10 times the tidal volume [17].

Adjustable Pressure Limiting (APL) Valve or Pressure Relief Valve

The APL valve allows the escape of exhaled and surplus gases from a breathing system but does not allow entry of the outside air [22]. The pressure required to open the valve

is low to minimise resistance to expiration [22]. The valve can be manually opened and closed. The 'open' or 'closed' position of the APL valve can be adjusted, which determines when the 'escape' pressure is reached.

Oxygen Supply Failure Alarm

Ideal characteristics of an oxygen alarm include:

- Activation of the alarm depends on the pressure of oxygen itself [13]
- The alarm requires no batteries or mains power [13]
- The energy required to operate a gas-powered alarm signal can be derived from the oxygen supply pressure [14]
- The alarm gives an audible signal which is distinct in character and of sufficient duration and volume to attract attention [13]
- The alarm should warn of impending failure and then alarm again when failure has occurred [13]
- The alarm should have pressure-linked controls that interrupt the flow of other gases when the alarm comes into operation. It should be impossible to resume anaesthesia until the oxygen supply is re-established [13].

Ritchie Whistle

The Ritchie Whistle was introduced in the 1960s, and forms the basis for most modern oxygen failure devices [14]. The Ritchie Whistle uses the failing oxygen supply for power and requires no other power supply [14]. The alarm is powered by an oxygen supply at a pressure of 420 kPa. When the oxygen pressure drops, the pathway of oxygen through the valve changes causing a whistle sound. This whistling sounds continuous until oxygen pressure falls to 40.5 kPa. When oxygen pressure falls to 200 kPa, the valve cuts off the supply of anaesthetic gases to the patient and allows the patient to inspire room air [14].

Emergency Oxygen Flush

An emergency oxygen flush is located upstream from the back bar and flowmeters. The oxygen delivered is at high pressure and does not pass through the vaporiser [16]. It directs a high-pressure flow of oxygen directly to the common gas outlet from the source, either pipeline or cylinder, bypassing all intermediate meters and vaporisers [15]. Barotrauma may result from accidental deployment of the emergency oxygen flush, particularly in smaller patients. Use of the emergency oxygen flush is contraindicated when a patient is connected to the machine because oxygen will be delivered at flows of 30–40 l/min and at a pressure of 400 kPa thereby putting the patient's airways at severe risk of barotrauma. Use of the emergency oxygen flush should be restricted to the flushing of breathing systems when not connected to a patient [18]. To prevent accidental activation, the emergency oxygen flush button is usually placed in a recessed setting and will deactivate as soon as the finger activating the switch is removed [15].

Scavenging

The COSHH regulations sets out the legal requirements for protecting the health of people in the workplace from hazardous substances: anaesthetic gases and volatile agents are covered by COSHH. The regulations apply to people who are exposed to anaesthetic gases and volatile agents during the course of their work [24].

In order to estimate exposure in the operating theatre, the following items should be considered [24]:

- For what period of time are staff exposed?
- Is there a gas scavenging system in place?
- How effective is the ventilation?
- Is there any leakage from the anaesthetic equipment, breathing system or scavenging system into the operating theatre?
- Is the gas flow turned off when not in use?
- Are vaporisers filled in ventilated areas or filled and drained with 'keyed filling devices'?

Monitoring Exposure Levels of Anaesthetic Gases

To ensure that the methods in place to reduce workplace exposure to anaesthetic gases are effective, regular personal exposure limits should be measured. Personal exposure levels can be measured by taking time-weighted air samples in the breathing zone of those potentially most exposed (usually the anaesthetist). Personal diffusive sampling techniques are suitable for measuring exposure to anaesthetic agents, and the diffusive samplers are small and easily attached to clothing [24].

Minimising Anaesthetic Gas Exposure

Minimising exposure to waste anaesthetic gases involves maintenance of equipment, training of personnel and regular routine exposure monitoring [13]. Routine leak testing of equipment should be carried out, and active scavenging should be available in locations where inhalational agents are used. Effective ventilation in operating theatres can help to control infection and also help to control exposure to anaesthetic gases. Air movement should ensure that any leakage of the anaesthetic agent is diluted and removed from the theatre environment [24]. In the United Kingdom, current recommended maximum accepted concentrations over an 8-hour time period are: 50 particles per million (ppm) for isoflurane.

Methods to reduce theatre pollution of waste anaesthetic gases include:

- Adequate ventilation and air conditioning with frequent and rapid changing of the theatre air. Fifteen air changes per hour is the minimum suggested [24].
- Use of cuffed endotracheal tubes [23].
- Use of circle breathing systems.
- Consider the use of TIVA.
- Utilise regional anaesthesia where appropriate.
- Use partial intravenous anaesthesia (PIVA) to reduce inhalational agent requirements.
- Avoiding spillage by using a fume cupboard during vaporiser filling.
- Fill vaporisers with their key-fill devices to reduce spillages [23].
- Ensure the recovery room is well ventilated. Recovery areas are at high risk for environmental anaesthetic gas pollution due to the levels of anaesthetic gas in the exhaled air from recovering patients.
- Connection of the endotracheal tube to the anaesthetic breathing system before delivering anaesthetic gases. The oxygen should be turned on first, before connection of the endotracheal tube to the breathing system. Once the endotracheal tube is securely connected to the breathing system, the vaporiser can be turned on [23].
- Regular monitoring of personal anaesthetic gas exposure levels.
- Implementation of an effective scavenging system [13].

Scavenging Systems

A scavenging system is capable of collecting waste gases from the breathing system and discarding them safely [13]. They consist of several components: a collecting system, a transfer system, a receiving system and a disposal system [25]. Passive scavenging is now not recommended, but both types of systems are described to highlight the differences between systems [25].

Passive Scavenging

- Simple and low cost.
- The collecting system connects to the patient's breathing circuit or ventilator via a 30 mm conical connection [16].
- The disposal conduit is usually a wide bore pipe which leads from the anaesthetic machine to the atmosphere directly or via the theatre ventilation system [13].
- The exhaled gases are driven by the patient's expiratory effort or by mechanical ventilation.
- Recirculation or reversal of the gas flow may occur [13].
- Compression or occlusion of the housing could result in leakage of gases into the room, so tubing should be made of non-compressible material and should not be placed on the floor [13].
- Passive and semi-passive scavenging systems may not control exposure to the occupational exposure standards. Therefore, monitoring personal exposure is important to check the performance of the scavenging equipment [24].

Active Scavenging

- The collecting and transfer system is similar to that of passive scavenging [13].
- Collecting systems in active scavenging systems have an 'air brake' to prevent pressure damage to the patient's lungs [16].
- The air brake is a large bore opening, such as slits in the collecting system casing, that allows room air to enter the system if excess negative pressure develops or scavenged gas to exit the system if positive pressure develops in the scavenging. Waste gases then travel through wide-bore tubing, known as the transfer system, to a reservoir referred to as the receiving system [16].
- The disposal system requires sub-atmospheric pressure to create a vacuum [25].
- A vacuum pump applies gentle suction to the APL valve so that waste gases are sucked away [23].
- An air brake unit (Figure 10.8) is used in the system to isolate the patient from the negative pressures created by the pump in the disposal system.

Absorption Systems (Activated Charcoal)

- Absorption systems consist of a canister, charcoal particles and transfer tubing connecting the canister to the APL valve of the breathing system or expiratory valve of the ventilator [13].
- Absorption systems can remove vapours of volatile anaesthetic agents but not nitrous oxide [25].
- They may be used when scavenging is not available.
- The weight of the canister indicates the degree of exhaustion [13].

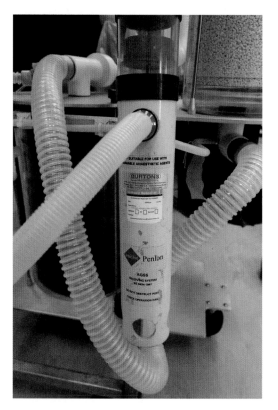

Figure 10.8 Barnsley receiver air-brake. *Source:* Marie Rippingale.

Anaesthetic Breathing Systems

Anaesthetic breathing systems function to deliver oxygen and an inhalational anaesthetic agent to the patient and remove carbon dioxide. Breathing systems can also be used to deliver controlled mechanical ventilation (CMV) to the patient.

Useful Terminology

- Tidal volume (V_T). The volume of gas exhaled in one breath and is between 10 and 15 ml/kg.
- Respiratory rate (RR) or respiratory frequency (R_f). Number of breaths per minute.
- Minute volume or minute ventilation (MV). The volume of gas exhaled by the patient in 1 minute. This is calculated using tidal volume (V_T) × respiratory frequency (R_f) and is approximately 200 ml/kg/minute.
- Dead space: this is the volume of inhaled gas that never takes part in gas exchange as it does not reach the alveolar level and is therefore 'wasted' ventilation. The total dead space volume is all the gas that is inhaled but does not take up any CO_2 or give off any O_2, which is known as physiological dead space (V_{Dphys}) [14].
- Physiological dead space = airway dead space + alveolar dead space [14].

Figure 10.9 Diagram of a large animal circle breathing system showing the component parts labelled: fresh gas flow inlet (F), vaporiser (V), inspiratory (I) and expiratory (E) limbs, Y-piece (Y), one-way valves (O), carbon-dioxide absorbent canister (C), rebreathing bag (B) and an adjustable pressure limiting (APL) valve. *Source:* Dr Kate Loomes.

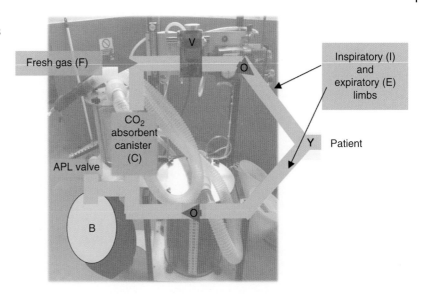

- Equipment dead space: this is the volume of gas inside equipment that extends the airway dead space in front of the lips (e.g. a face mask or endotracheal tube that extends in front of the lips) [14, 15].
- Ventilation: perfusion (V/Q) mismatch: when ventilation does not match perfusion within one lung unit. The two extremes of mismatch are:
- No ventilation but good perfusion. Blood passes through the lung without participating in gas exchange and contributes to 'shunt volume'.
- Good ventilation but no perfusion. Gas moves in and out of the lungs units but no blood is present so gas exchange does not occur. This volume is alveolar dead space [1, 2].
- Between these two extremes, there is a spectrum of varying degrees of V/Q mismatch, which can occur in each lung unit.

Anaesthetic breathing systems are broadly classified into rebreathing and non-rebreathing systems.

Rebreathing Systems

Equine anaesthetic breathing systems are the most commonly rebreathing systems. The two main types of rebreathing systems include the **circle** and the **to-and-fro** system.

Circle System

The circle breathing system is a very popular choice of equine anaesthetic breathing system. The circle breathing system consists of a fresh gas flow inlet, inspiratory and expiratory limbs, Y-piece, one-way valves, a carbon-dioxide absorbent canister, a rebreathing bag and an APL valve.

Circle systems come in different sizes: large circles (Figure 10.9) and small circles (Figure 10.10).

Pathway of Gas Around a Circle Breathing System

- Fresh gas flow enters the inspiratory limb, which is connected via a 'Y-piece' to the patient's endotracheal tube.
- The inspiratory limb may contain a one-way valve which ensures unidirectional gas flow.
- The patient then exhales the gases via the expiratory limb, which contains a one-way valve ensuring unidirectional flow of exhaled gas to the rebreathing bag and carbon dioxide absorbent canister.
- Once the gas has passed through the canister, it re-enters the inspiratory limb and mixes with fresh gas before being inhaled by the patient.
- The advantages and disadvantages of the circle breathing system are displayed in Table 10.5.
- **To-and-fro (Waters' canister) system**
- The Waters' to-and-fro breathing system is portable, simple to use and straightforward to assemble, disassemble and clean.
- The system consists of a fresh gas inlet, carbon-dioxide absorbent canister, rebreathing bag and an APL valve (Figure 10.11).
- Pathway of gas around a Waters' to-and-fro breathing system.
- Fresh gas enters the system near the patient connector; the patient inhales this gas and then exhales through the carbon dioxide absorbent canister. The gas then enters the closed rebreathing bag situated next to the canister before returning to the patient via the same route.

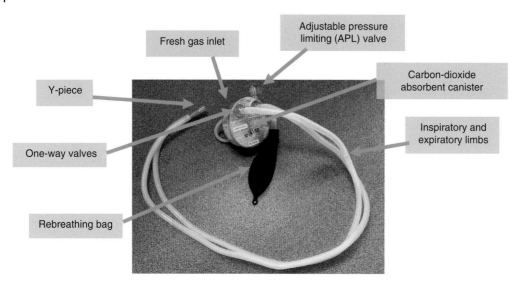

Figure 10.10 Diagram of a small animal circle breathing system the component parts labelled: fresh gas flow inlet, inspiratory and expiratory limbs, Y-piece, one-way valves, carbon-dioxide absorbent canister, rebreathing bag and an adjustable pressure limiting (APL) valve. *Source:* Dr Kate Loomes.

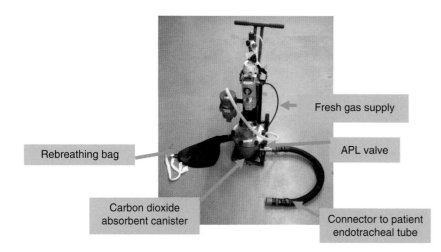

Figure 10.11 Example of the Waters' to-and-fro rebreathing system with the following parts labelled: connector to the patient's endotracheal tube, fresh gas supply, adjustable pressure limiting (APL) valve, carbon dioxide absorbent canister and rebreathing bag. *Source:* Dr Catriona Mackenzie.

- The advantages and disadvantages of the to-and-fro system are displayed in Table 10.6

Non-rebreathing Systems

Non-rebreathing systems are mainly used in small animal anaesthesia but can be used in foals. Their use is limited to foals <25 kg bodyweight. Non-rebreathing systems rely on fresh gas flow to maintain a one-way flow of gases and avoid rebreathing of exhaled carbon dioxide. They do not contain carbon dioxide absorbent canisters or one-way valves. There are several types of non-rebreathing systems available, which are named according to Mapleson's classifications (Tables 10.7 and 10.8). The advantages and disadvantages of non-rebreathing systems are displayed in Table 10.9.

Controlled Mechanical Ventilation

Controlled mechanical ventilation (CMV) is routinely used in equine anaesthesia, with many different options available to facilitate the delivery of mechanical breaths [26]. In anaesthetised horses, the dose-dependent respiratory depression produced by isoflurane [27] and the effect of recumbency may necessitate CMV to improve pulmonary function [28]. The ventilators available for use in horses may vary in design and appearance. However, they are all based on the same physical principle: the application of an inspiratory flow of gas to inflate the lungs,

Table 10.7 Mapleson D (Ayre's T-piece and the Bain system).

Breathing system	Ayre's T piece	Bain
Fresh gas flow (ml/kg/minute)	500–600	200–400
Maximum bodyweight (kg)	10	15–20
Use with controlled mechanical ventilation?	Yes	Yes
Image		

Source: Dr Kate Loomes. Images used with kind permission from Dr Victoria Phillips.

Table 10.8 Mapleson A (Lack and Magill system).

Breathing system	Magill	Lack
Fresh gas flow (ml/kg/minute)	160–200	160–200
Maximum bodyweight (kg)	25–30	25–30
Use with controlled mechanical ventilation?	No	No
Image		

Source: Dr Kate Loomes. Images used with kind permission from Dr Victoria Phillips and Marie Rippingale.

Table 10.9 The advantages and disadvantages of non-rebreathing systems.

Advantages	Disadvantages
Low resistance to breathing. No carbon dioxide absorbent canister or one-way valves in the system	High fresh gas flows are required which makes use uneconomical for patients >25 kg bodyweight
Changing delivered anaesthetic agent concentration is rapid	High fresh gas flows can lead to increased expense and environmental pollution
Cheaper to purchase compared to rebreathing systems	Narrow inspiratory and expiratory limbs may cause increased resistance to breathing in larger foals
	Inspired gas can be cold and dry which can lead to hypothermia in small foals

Source: Dr Kate Loomes.

Table 10.10 The advantages and disadvantages of implementing controlled mechanical ventilation in healthy adult horses.

Advantages	Disadvantages
CMV results in a reduction in the work of breathing [30]	CMV results in negative cardiovascular effects including a reduction in venous return and cardiac output [30]
CMV can effectively treat hypoventilation	CMV may have the potential to cause lung injury
CMV may be used to reduce atelectasis by using techniques such as continuous positive airway pressure (CPAP) and positive end-expiratory pressure (PEEP) [31]	CMV may cause increases in proinflammatory cytokines, which have been associated with inflammatory lung diseases [22]
CMV can be used with techniques such as a recruitment manoeuvre (RM) to re-inflate collapsed alveoli [31]	The provision of CMV requires expensive equipment which must be maintained

Source: Dr Kate Loomes.

thereby overcoming the forces that resist thoracic expansion and the flow itself [26]. Techniques to provide ventilatory support in horses exclusively use positive pressure to expand the lungs [29]. The provision of CMV may also be referred to as intermittent positive pressure ventilation (IPPV). While CMV is a common technique employed in equine anaesthesia, there can be negative effects. During 'normal' spontaneous respiration, intra-thoracic pressure is sub-atmospheric, which favours venous return to the heart. When CMV is employed, intra-thoracic pressure becomes positive, which reduces venous return to the heart and therefore has a negative cardiovascular effect. This effect may be particularly noticeable in hypovolaemic horses. The advantages and disadvantages of implementing CMV in healthy adult horses are displayed in Table 10.10.

Ventilator Types

There are three main types of ventilators: direct blowers, bellow-squeezers and piston-driven ventilators [26].

Direct Blower – Demand Valve

- For use during the recovery period.
- Delivers a high flow of oxygen (approx. 60–160 l/min) via attachment to the endotracheal tube.
- Provides assisted ventilation if a horse is apnoeic in the recovery box after disconnection from the mechanical ventilation.
- A demand valve can be used to assist horses during spontaneous breathing as the horse's respiratory effort should open the valve. However, this generates resistance to inspiration and expiration causing an increase in negative airway pressure which can result in lung injury or pulmonary oedema [32]. Therefore, once spontaneous breathing has resumed in the recovery box, the endotracheal tube cuff should be deflated.

- The tidal volume (V_T) delivered depends on the inspiratory time for which the demand valve is actioned.
- V_T = Inspiratory flow (L/s) × inspiratory time (s) [26].

Bellow Squeezer – Bellows in a Box

- This is the most common type of ventilator used in equine practice.
- Large animal ventilators usually have a bag-in-box design whereby a gas flow introduced in the box compresses the rebreathing bag or bellows and forces gas from the anaesthesia machine into the horse's lung [29].
- Pressurised gas is delivered into the box, which results in the squeezing of the bellows, which delivers a breath to the horse [26].
- The bellows contain the respiratory gas mixture from the patient and are separated from the driving gas in the surrounding box [29].
- Bellows may be standing (ascending) or hanging (descending) depending on which direction they move from the stationary position [26].
- If a leak develops in the bellows, then the system may underperform.
- The driving gas can in principle be oxygen, but usually for economic reasons compressed air is used [29].
- Bellows may use compressed gas as the source of both the power and driving force [26].

Piston Driven – Tafonius®

- A piston moves up and down, regulated by a motor to compress or decompress the gas in the cylinder, which is directly connected to the anaesthetic circuit [26].
- No bellows or reservoir bags.
- Within the piston cylinder, there is a 'virtual bag' [26].
- Requires an electrical power source.

Ventilator Settings

Ventilator settings can be adjusted to deliver CMV, which is tailored to each horse. The variables that can be adjusted differ between ventilators. In the volume-controlled mode, the adjustable variable is tidal volume, whereas in the pressure-controlled mode, it is peak inspiratory pressure [29]. Other adjustable variables may include respiratory frequency (R_f), inspiratory flow rate and time, inspiratory to expiratory ratio (I : E ratio), and expiratory time [29]. The ventilator can be set to deliver a certain volume or peak inspiratory pressure at a pre-set frequency independent of the patient's spontaneous efforts [30]. It is important to recognise that changes in the compliance of the thoracic compartment will influence ventilator performance differently [29]. Large animal ventilators display airway pressure, but they do not measure effective tidal volume. A rough visual estimation of the tidal volume can be made using graduations on concertina-type bellows [29].

The following formulas explain how the variables can be adjusted to tailor CMV:

- Tidal volume (V_T) = Inspiratory flow (L/s) × inspiratory time (s) [26].
- Respiratory frequency (bpm) = 60 seconds/(inspiratory time (s) + expiratory time (s)).

As a general rule, these are recommended settings for delivering CMV to an adult horse:

> **Tidal volume = 10–15 ml/kg**
> **Respiratory frequency = 6–8 breaths per minute**
> **Peak inspiratory pressure = 20–30 cmH₂O [29]**
> **I:E ratio 1 : 2 to 1 : 3 [33]**

Ventilator settings can be tailored to target arterial carbon dioxide tension ($PaCO_2$) values of 45–60 mmHg [33]. If blood gas analysis is not available, ventilation tailored to achieve an end-tidal carbon dioxide tension ($ETCO_2$) of 35–45 mmHg should maintain the $PaCO_2$ within a normal range. However, blood gas analysis is preferable to ensure that normal $PaCO_2$ values are achieved, particularly in compromised horses [34].

Monitoring the Effect of Controlled Mechanical Ventilation

CMV has significant effects on the cardiorespiratory systems and also has negative cardiovascular effects, including hypotension. A ventilator-induced reduction in venous return may occur and is consistent with a cyclical depression in systolic arterial pressure synchronised with the ventilator cycle. This variation between pressure waves is known as pulse pressure variation and is more pronounced during CMV in hypovolaemic horses. CMV may have an unpredictable effect on arterial oxygen tension (PaO_2). CMV is usually effective in correcting hypoventilation and hypercapnia. However, it is important not to cause hypocapnia.

Endotracheal Tubes

Endotracheal intubation during inhalation anaesthesia is routine in veterinary medicine.

Endotracheal intubation:

- Maintains airway patency
- Efficiently delivers inhalational anaesthetic agents
- Minimises personnel exposure to waste anaesthetic gases [37]

Endotracheal intubation is usually performed blind in horses. If assistance is required, endoscopic guidance can be used to visualise the larynx during endotracheal intubation in difficult cases.

Intubation Procedure: How to Intubate a Horse

- The horse's mouth should be thoroughly rinsed with water prior to anaesthetic induction. Even horses muzzled for several hours prior to anaesthesia can retain food in the cheek pouch area [35].
- A large dosing syringe or garden hose is inserted lateral to the cheek teeth, and a stream of water is directed into the cheek pouch area. Both sides of the mouth are flushed until no food material is observed in the effluence [35].
- After induction of GA, it is important to assess the depth of anaesthesia and degree of muscle relaxation prior to attempting endotracheal or nasotracheal intubation.
- The largest-diameter tube that can be inserted without excessive force should be selected [35].
- It is important to use minimal force when performing endotracheal intubation [39], as the force applied to pass an inappropriately large endotracheal tube (ETT) through the glottis may result in laryngeal injury.
- The tube cuff should be inflated before insertion and observed for leaks and then deflated [35].

Endotracheal Intubation [35]

- A most common method for horses undergoing inhalational agent anaesthesia.
- The anaesthetic technique should provide a depth of anaesthesia sufficient to relax the masseter muscles and permit insertion of the mouth speculum or gag.

- Extend the head and neck to align the oral cavity with the larynx and trachea.
- Gently retract the tongue through the interdental space.
- The lubricated ETT is then inserted into the mouth in the midline and advanced to the pharynx, carefully avoiding the cheek teeth. Advance the tube with the concave surface of the tube directed towards the palate. Rotate through 180 degrees as the tip of the tube enters the pharynx and gently advance it through the larynx.
- If resistance is met during this procedure, then the tube may be directed towards the pharyngeal wall or oesophagus. Retract the tube by 10 cm and rotate before gently re-advancing. Several attempts may be required for successful intubation. It is important to use minimal force during re-directing and advancing of the tube to avoid laryngeal and pharyngeal trauma.
- If the tube is correctly inserted, then airflow can be detected at the end of the tube when the horse breathes spontaneously or when the chest is compressed.

*Note: During endo/nasotracheal intubation, spontaneous respiration should be present. Horses do not typically show a period of apnoea after the induction of GA, which may be experienced in small animals where the agents used for anaesthetic induction are different.

Nasotracheal Intubation [35]
- A smaller-diameter tube is used for nasotracheal intubation compared to endotracheal intubation.
- Method: the tip of the nasotracheal tube should be well lubricated and inserted through the nostril in a ventral-medial direction, directing the tube tip into the ventral nasal meatus. Advance the tube gently and slowly into the pharynx. Gently advance through the larynx. Slow rotation of the tube may facilitate passage through the larynx.
- If resistance is met in the nasal cavity, this may indicate the tube is too large or that the tube is not in the ventral meatus.
- Verification of correct nasotracheal tube placement and the process for detecting leaks are the same as described for ETT placement.

*Note: the relatively smaller airway produced by nasotracheal intubation increases the resistance to breathing. The nasal tube should be exchanged for an ETT if increased airway resistance compromises adequate ventilation or causes respiratory distress [35].

Types of ETT
Silicone
- Poor resistance to kinking/bending.
- Non-reactive and can withstand heat sterilisation [35].

Red Rubber
- Poor resistance to kinking.
- Can cause tissue reaction.
- Breakdown with heat sterilisation [35].

Tube Selection
An appropriately sized ETT helps to prevent leakage of air, minimises laryngeal and/or tracheal injury and limits airway resistance [37]. Increased airway resistance can occur through the use of narrow ETT [32]. Airway resistance decreases as the ETT diameter increases. Endotracheal intubation can decrease work of breathing by bypassing the upper airway [38]. However, using an ETT with too narrow internal diameters results in an increase in resistance and work of breathing [38]. Using too large an ETT and/or excessive force to place the ETT should be avoided and this can cause tracheal/laryngeal damage [35]. Intubation using a 30 mm internal diameter ETT in an average-sized horse (500 kg) has been documented to have a high rate of tracheal injury [36]. Selection of an appropriate ETT size develops with experience. A 20–25 mm internal diameter tube is suitable for most adult horses. Ultrasound measurements of the trachea have been used in humans to predict ETT size [39]. Further studies are needed to develop a technique to accurately measure the tracheal size in horses [37].

Checking for Patency
Correct placement of the ETT can be confirmed by the presence of airflow consistent with expiration. Horses should breathe spontaneously after induction of GA and ETT placement, so there should be no need to compress the chest to check for ETT patency. Apnoea after induction of GA and/or ETT intubation may be a cause for concern, and the reason for apnoea should be investigated immediately. Once the ETT is attached to an anaesthetic breathing system, correct ETT placement can be confirmed by visualising movement of the rebreathing bag synchronous with the horse's inspiratory and expiratory respiratory pattern. Correct ETT placement can also be verified using capnography. If a capnograph trace of relatively normal appearance is present after connection of the breathing system to the ETT, then tracheal intubation can be confirmed. A leak around the cuff may be diagnosed using the capnograph trace. The rectangular shape of the capnograph trace will not be present as CO_2 escapes around the cuff and is therefore not sampled at the Y-piece. It is important to confirm correct ETT placement prior to connection of the ETT to the breathing system when CMV is used. This is because there is potential for gastric distension and rupture if the ETT is incorrectly placed (into the oesophagus) and CMV delivers positive pressure ventilation to the stomach via the oesophagus.

Cuff Inflation

The cuff on the tube should be inflated in order to prevent air leakage around the ETT, thereby avoiding room contamination with anaesthetic gas [37]. The cuff on the ETT should be inflated in order to prevent pulmonary aspiration of fluids such as gastric contents, blood or surgical lavage fluids [35]. The cuff should be inflated until no leak is discernible, and the cuff pressure should be checked using a pressure gauge to minimise tracheal epithelial damage [40]. To manually check for escape of air around the cuff, place a hand or stethoscope on the horse's neck in the region of the cuff during a forced inspiration. If vibration is detected as air escapes around the ETT, it is likely that a leak is present [41]. The cuff is inflated with air to seal the airway when the lung is pressurised to 20–25 cmH$_2$O. This is accomplished by connecting the patient end of the ETT to the Y-piece of the breathing system and squeezing the rebreathing bag or compressing the ventilator bellows to develop pressure within the breathing system of 20–25 cmH$_2$O.

A leak may be present if:

- There is a rush of air from the nostrils.
- There is an odour of inhalational agent present in the room.
- There is an inability to maintain positive airway pressure [35].
- Airflow around the ETT is palpable using a hand placed externally on the larynx, or the leaking airflow may be audible as a low-grade rumbling sound.

Complications Associated with ETTs

Reported complications of tracheal intubation in the horse include laryngeal haematomas on the epiglottis and arytenoids, swollen tongue, pharyngeal perforation, epiglottic trauma and retroversion, laryngeal mucosal damage, laryngeal paralysis/paresis [35].

Injury to the larynx and/or trachea associated with endotracheal intubation, may be caused by:

- Excessive force used during intubation.
- Use of a relatively large ETT.
- Over-inflation of the ETT cuff.
- Positioning of the ETT cuff near the thoracic inlet.
- Changes in position of the neck of the horse with the ETT cuff inflated [42].
- Chemical-induced injuries can occur due to failure to rinse off disinfectants [36].
- Incorrect placement. Inadvertent oesophageal intubation and connection to the anaesthetic machine may result in dangerous gastric distension. Verification of tube placement must be performed before connection of the ETT to the breathing system and delivery of gases.

ETT Obstruction

Defects or weakness in the cuff can lead to asymmetric inflation and may result in cuff herniation and obstruction of the lumen of the ETT [43].

Nasotracheal Tubes

Nasotracheal intubation can cause haemorrhage in the ventral or middle meatus, with the potential for airway obstruction by blood clots as well as aspiration [40].

Cuff-related Complications

- It is important to avoid over-inflating the cuff as there is a risk of tracheal or laryngeal injury due to pressure exerted on the tracheal wall.
- Tracheal injury may also occur due to cuff movement if the neck is flexed or extended while the cuff is inflated [44].
- Ensure that the ETT is disconnected from the anaesthetic breathing system when moving the horse [41].
- To achieve optimal cuff inflation, intra-cuff pressure monitoring is recommended in human and veterinary species, although this is not routine [37, 45].
- Consider auscultating the trachea during inflation of the ETT cuff and CMV, to detect the minimum occlusive volume to ensure a seal around the cuff [36].
- Palpation of the larynx or auscultation using a stethoscope during ETT cuff inflation may detect turbulent airflow around the ETT cuff, which is indicative of a leak. Laryngeal palpation/auscultation can also be used to estimate the minimum occlusive volume to achieve a seal.
- Pilot balloon palpation is an inaccurate way of assessing the ETT cuff inflation in dogs, and monitoring cuff pressures with a manometer is recommended [36]. It is likely that the same principle applies to horses.

Maintenance of Endotracheal Tubes

ETTS should be regularly inspected for signs of wear or damage. Particular attention should be paid to the cuff. Check cuff integrity prior to using an ETT on every occasion.

Cleaning, Sterilisation and Storage

ETTs and nasotracheal tubes (NTTs) should be cleaned as soon as possible after extubation. ETTs and NTTs for horses are expensive and not disposable [36]. Clean all tubes thoroughly inside and out. The presence of organic material impedes chemical disinfection. After being cleaned or gross contamination, tracheal tubes can be soaked in an appropriate disinfectant solution to further reduce the chance of nosocomial infection [36]. Ensure thorough rinsing of the tracheal tubes prior to storage/use. Chemical injury to the airway can be caused by residual disinfectant on the ETT or NTT. Silicone is the only material that can withstand steam autoclaving. Manufacturer recommendations for temperature and contact time should be followed [36]. Store ETTs and NTTs carefully and ensure that they are not in contact with anything. Custom-made racks can be used to hang ETTs and NTTs. It is useful to store ETTs and NTTs in size order to facilitate rapid selection of a particular size.

Safety Checks

The performance of pre-anaesthetic safety checks are a crucial part of pre-anaesthetic preparation.

Endotracheal Tubes   Prior to use, ETTs and NTTs must be checked for patency and closely inspected for signs of damage. The integrity of the cuff must be verified before use on every occasion.

Anaesthetic Machine Check

- Performing a 'pre-use' check to ensure the correct functioning of anaesthetic equipment is essential to patient safety [18].
- The anaesthetist has a primary responsibility to understand the function of the anaesthetic equipment and to check it before use [18].
- The correct steps to follow to carry out an anaesthetic machine safety check are displayed in Table 10.11.

A note should made in the patient's anaesthetic record that the anaesthetic machine check has been performed, that appropriate monitoring is in place and functional, and that the integrity, patency and safety of the whole breathing system has been assured [18]. This verification of machine checks may be incorporated into the surgical safety checklist and performed for each patient.

Checking Equipment Used for TIVA

When TIVA is used, there must be a continuous IV infusion of anaesthetic agent or agents; interruption may result in awareness [18]. In equine anaesthesia, awareness may result in sudden movement, which can be dangerous to the horse and to personnel. Anaesthetists using TIVA must be familiar with the drugs, the technique and all equipment and disposables being used [18]. If an infusion pump is used, its function and calibration must be checked before use. Infusion lines must be correctly placed in infusion pumps and free of obstruction or points of compression. Infusion lines must be patent and primed with a solution ready for use. The drugs required for the procedure and consumables should be readily available. During TIVA sites of IV infusions should be visible so that they may be monitored for disconnection, leaks or infusion into subcutaneous tissues [18].

Equipment Fault Reporting

A responsible person or persons should be appointed to organise repair and servicing of anaesthetic equipment. Faulty equipment including the nature of the fault may be recorded in a log book or reported directly to the responsible person. Where there are multiple pieces of the same type of equipment such as infusion pumps; each individual infusion pump should be identifiable so that recurring faults affecting a single piece of equipment can be identified.

Servicing of Equipment

Each hospital must ensure that all machines are fully serviced at the regular intervals designated by the manufacturer and that a service record is maintained [18]. As it is possible for errors to occur when reassembling an anaesthetic machine, it is essential to confirm that the machine is correctly configured for use after each service.

Emergency Power Supply

Anaesthetists should be aware of the options available in the event of mains power failure. A backup generator should be available, and backup batteries for monitors should be available and charged. Alternative methods of ventilating a patient (for example, a rebreathing bag) should be available in the event of mechanical ventilator failure.

Anaesthetic Monitoring Equipment

The Association of Veterinary Anaesthetists (AVA) recommends that a dedicated anaesthetist should be available to monitor each case. The dedicated anaesthetist should be a qualified member of veterinary staff who has received anaesthesia training [46]. Basic 'hands-on' monitoring of anaesthesia requires no equipment and is a core skill for every anaesthetist. Basic monitoring techniques that require no equipment, including ocular and mucous membrane assessment and pulse palpation, are recommended for every general anaesthetic procedure [47]. As technology advances, many more electronic monitoring options have become available [47]. Electronic monitoring equipment should not replace the 'hands-on' approach to monitoring but may be used to complement it. An understanding of the function and limitations of monitoring equipment is crucial to enable its effective use and correct interpretation. For each case, a minimum panel

Table 10.11 The correct steps to follow to carry out an anaesthetic machine safety checks.

Ensure all flow control valves and vaporisers are turned off

Oxygen/Medical Air Supply
For individual cylinder supply: Check that each cylinder is secured in place. Open each cylinder in turn and check the pressure, label each cylinder 'full' or 'in-use' accordingly. Replace any cylinders that are empty
For pipeline gases: Open the cylinders or the manifold as applicable. Check that the contents of the cylinders are adequate for the intended anaesthetic duration. Label cylinders 'full' or 'in-use' accordingly and replace any empty cylinders
Check the connection between the gas pipelines and the supply ports using the 'tug test' [19]

Oxygen Flowmeter
Slowly turn the oxygen flowmeter control valve on and then back off again. Watch the bobbin as you do so; the function should be smooth with the bobbin rising as you open the valve and then falling back to zero as you close the valve. The bobbin should be spinning and free of resistance. Repeat with the other gases

Vaporiser
Check that the vaporiser is securely fastened to the back bar and that the locking mechanism is fully engaged [19]. Check that the vaporiser is full of agents but not overfilled and that the filling port is tightly closed [9]. Turn the percentage control dial all the way on and then off again. The function should be smooth

Oxygen Supply Failure Alarm
Turn the oxygen flow meter control valve on and then disconnect the oxygen supply. The oxygen supply failure alarm should be audible and continuous until supply is restored

Soda Lime
Check canister contents (colour change and indicated level of use) [19]

Scavenging
Passive scavenging: Check the connection of the scavenging tubing to the adjustable APL valve. Check the length of the scavenging tubing from the anaesthetic machine connection to the external exit point and ensure that the tubing is not obstructed at any point and that there are no signs of wear or damage
Active scavenging: Turn on the scavenging and ensure that the float inside the Barnsley receiver or similar receiving device is elevated and spinning

Mechanical Ventilator
Ensure that the tubing associated with the ventilator is correctly configured. Check that pressures/volumes/times are appropriately set for the size of the patient. Check that alarms are functioning if present. Prepare an alternative method of ventilation in the event of ventilator malfunction

Leak Test for a Circle Breathing System
For a circle breathing system and reservoir bag:
Plug the patient's end of the breathing system, close the APL valve and turn on the fresh gas flow to inflate the reservoir bag. Inflate bag to a set pressure or so that it is moderately distended. Turn off the fresh gas flow and observe for any loss of pressure or volume within the system
After performing the leak test, **ALWAYS** remember to re-open the APL valve
Using the two-bag test: Attach the patient end of the breathing system to a reservoir bag or 'test-lung'. Set the fresh gas flow to 5 l/min and ventilate manually. Check that the whole breathing system is patent, and the unidirectional valves are moving. Check the function of the APL valve by squeezing both bags [19]
For a circle breathing system and mechanical ventilator:
Using the two-bag test: Attach the patient end of the breathing system to a reservoir bag or 'test-lung'. It may be useful to place the 'test lung' in a box or bin to simulate the thorax. Turn on the ventilator and check that the ventilator cycles correctly according to pre-set pressures and/or volumes

Monitors
Check monitors are working and configured correctly. Check alarm limits and volumes [19]

Source: Dr Kate Loomes.

of electronic monitoring, including capnography, pulse oximetry, electrocardiography (ECG) and blood pressure monitoring devices has been recommended [48]. It is recognised that anaesthesia in horses is performed in a variety of places with different facilities and using various drug combinations [47]. Table 10.12 provides a summary of electronic monitoring devices used in equine practice. Anaesthetic monitoring is covered in more detail in Section 10.5.

10.4 Anaesthetic Risks and Induction

Anaesthetic Risks

The preliminary results of The Confidential Enquiry into Perioperative Equine Fatalities 4 (CEPEF 4) study suggested that horses still carry a high risk of mortality associated with GA [3]. The total mortality from perioperative complications was found to be 1%. This is still high

Table 10.12 Summary of electronic monitoring devices used in equine practice.

Monitoring equipment	When to use	Reason for use	How to use	Comments
Capnography	Capnography should be employed during the GA of all intubated patients	Capnography measures the amount of carbon dioxide (CO_2) that is expired (end tidal CO_2 ($ETCO_2$) [50] and inspired (fractional inspired CO_2 ($FiCO_2$) in one breath	CO_2 absorbs infra-red light. A sensor detects how much infrared light is absorbed and this is directly comparable to the level of CO_2 expired in one breath [51]. The CO_2 tension during the respiratory cycle is displayed as a number and also as a trace, or capnograph. Capnography may use mainstream or side stream analysers. Side stream analysers are the common type in practice	Capnography provides an insight into ventilation, anaesthetic depth, cardiac output as well as any equipment malfunction [50]. It can be used to diagnose rebreathing, airway obstruction or leaks in the breathing system or anaesthetic machine [50]
Pulse oximetry	Pulse oximetry can be employed in all patients under GA	Pulse oximetry provides a non-invasive, continuous and inexpensive method to assess the cardiovascular and respiratory functions of horses under anaesthesia [52]	Pulse oximetry uses red and infra-red light to detect the saturation of haemoglobin with oxygen (SpO_2). The principles of measurement are based on the different light absorption spectra of oxyhaemoglobin and deoxyhaemoglobin, and the detection of a pulsatile signal [53, 54]	Limitations include interference due to light, movement, poor perfusion and the absence of a commercially available pulse oximeter calibrated for horse blood [53]
Electrocardiography (ECG)	ECG can be used to identify abnormal cardiac rhythm before or during anaesthesia [53]	Electrical activity in the heart is detected by skin electrodes and can be transformed into a characteristic trace, the morphology of which corresponds to events in the cardiac cycle	Conduction of electrical activity in the heart follows a fairly fixed pathway: from the sinus node, across the atrial myocardium, through the atrioventricular node, His bundle, bundle branches, and Purkinje system to the ventricular myocardium [55]. This electrical activity generates a characteristic ECG waveform which can be used to assess heart rate and rhythm. Recognition of the normal P-QRS-T morphology is required in order to accurately assess an ECG recording and the timing intervals [55]	Good electrical contact is required between the clips and the skin, and this can be facilitated using alcohol or electrode gel [53]
Arterial blood pressure measurement (ABP)	ABP should be measured in all horses under GA	ABP measurement provides important information relating to the cardiovascular system [58]. ABP monitoring is particularly important in haemodynamically compromised horses, for example, those undergoing colic surgery	There are two ways to measure ABP: **Direct (invasive) arterial blood pressure (IBP) measurement:** In horses, IBP is considered the gold standard ABP measurement technique [59]	In situations where IBP monitoring is not available/viable, then NIBP measurement can be performed however, this is not as accurate in adult horses compared to foals

Table 10.12 (Continued)

Monitoring equipment	When to use	Reason for use	How to use	Comments
			Indirect or non-invasive blood pressure (NIBP) measurement: Inaccuracy and poor reliability of NIBP devices compared with IBP mean they remain underused in horses [60]. NIBP measurement may be useful in foals, where placement of an arterial catheter may be more challenging	
Central Venous Pressure (CVP)	CVP is not routinely monitored in horses but may be measured for experimental reasons	CVP provides information relating to blood volume and cardiac preload. It may be used in states of hypo and hypervolaemia and used to assess the response to treatment	Measuring CVP is complex and includes placing an IV catheter through the jugular vein into the right atrium and observing the characteristic pressure waveforms and values on an oscilloscope or IBP monitor.	This technique is invasive, challenging and requires trained personnel. The technique itself and the catheter can cause arrhythmia, infection and trauma [61].
Blood gas analysis	Arterial blood gas analysis is useful in all horses undergoing GA to assess adequacy of ventilation and acid base balance [62]	Blood gas analysis provides information about respiratory and cardiovascular function and metabolic status [53, 63, 64]. The level of accuracy and the information gained cannot be replaced by any non-invasive method [65, 66] such as pulse oximetry or capnography	Arterial blood samples are usually drawn from a pre-placed peripheral arterial catheter used for direct blood pressure measurement. Peripheral catheters used for this purpose are most commonly placed in the facial, transverse facial or metatarsal artery. Venous blood samples are usually drawn from the jugular vein	Blood gas analysis is limited by the number of samples taken and the time needed to obtain the results; therefore, the samples are collected as needed, most often at intervals of 30 or 60 minutes but more frequently if the patient's condition requires it
Thermometers	Monitoring body temperature is important during GA, and particularly important in foals	Maintenance of normothermia is required to preserve normal physiological function [66]. GA inhibits vasoconstriction which allows generalised redistribution of body heat. A decrease in body temperature occurs as heat is lost to the environment [53]	The end of the thermometer should be lubricated. The lubricated end of the thermometer should be inserted about 2 inches into the rectum and held against the rectal wall to avoid faecal material, which may cause an inaccurate reading. Once the thermometer alarm sounds, the thermometer should be carefully removed, the reading noted, and the thermometer should be turned off and cleaned	Rectal temperature should be monitored at 15 minutes intervals during inhalational anaesthesia [53]

Source: Dr Kate Loomes.

compared to mortality rates reported for cats and dogs. However, the preliminary data from CEPEF 4 suggested that the current mortality rate for horses is lower than 20 years ago [3]. Even though risks seem to be getting lower, consideration must be given to the fact that equine patients still carry a high risk for GA. Vets and RVNs involved with equine anaesthesia must do everything possible to reduce risk in elective and emergency patients.

American Society of Anaesthesiologists (ASA) Anaesthetic Risk Score

Once the history has been taken, and a physical examination has been carried out (see Chapter 12), the patient should be assigned to one of the ASA physical status classes [67]. Allocation of an ASA score can help the anaesthetist to decide whether anaesthesia can proceed or whether further investigations and/or stabilisation are required first [67]. The basic ASA descriptors are given below; however, a recent veterinary version has been devised. Please see the further reading for more information.

ASA physical status classes [67]:

1) Normal healthy animal. No delectable underlying disease (cannot be an emergency).
2) Mild systemic disease but causing no obvious clinical signs or incapacity (animal compensating well).
3) Severe systemic disease-causing clinical signs (animal not compensating fully, substantial functional limitations).
4) Severe systemic disease that is a constant threat to life.
5) Moribund is not expected to survive without the procedure.

E. An 'E' should be added to any class to identify the patient as an emergency (where a delay in treatment will significantly increase the threat to life or limb).

If pre-operative support or stabilisation is required, this may include [68]:

- Anxiolysis/sedation
- Analgesia
- Oxygen supplementation
- Fluid therapy
- Blood transfusion
- Assistance with thermoregulation, for example, rugs, bandages and heat lamps
- Medical support
- Surgical procedures, for example, tracheostomy

The patient should be monitored carefully; all treatments and observations should be recorded. If the patient is deemed fit for anaesthesia, pre-anaesthetic preparations can proceed.

Risks for Specific Patients

It is beyond the scope of this section to discuss every specific risk and management protocol for high-risk patients. However, the most important considerations are summarised below. Readers are directed to the texts in the reference list for further information.

Colic Patients

Horses with colic are often considered to be one of the most high risk patients to anaesthetise. The results of CEPEF 4 suggest that mortality for horses undergoing colic surgery is around 3.4%, which is high when compared to non-colic patients at 0.6% [3]. The positive news is that fatal outcomes for colic, and non-colic patients are less frequent than 20 years ago when the previous CEPEF study was conducted [3]. The reason colic patients are such a high risk to anaesthetise is that they often present with a wide range of physiological states, which can vary depending on the type of obstruction present. There are two types of gastrointestinal tract (GIT) obstructions: non-strangulating and strangulating [68].

Non-strangulating GIT Obstructions

With non-strangulating obstructions, secretions tend to accumulate in the gut lumen, leading to extracellular fluid loss, which promotes the development of hypovolaemia [68]. Bacterial fermentation of gut contents may cause a build-up of gas. This, along with the accumulation of fluid in the gut lumen, leads to distension of the gut, and this causes pain. Distension and displacement of the gut can also put traction on the mesentery causing further pain [68]. The stretch caused to the gut wall compromises its perfusion, and it becomes ischemic, hypoxic and oedematous, compromising perfusion further. This system of events leads to the mucosa becoming 'leaky' and endotoxaemia and systemic inflammatory response syndrome (SIRS) occurs, which serves to complicate the initial hypovolemia further [68].

Strangulating GIT Obstructions

With strangulating lesions, the mucosal barrier becomes compromised more quickly, and this allows bacteria and toxins to enter the bloodstream [68]. In this case, endotoxaemia and hypovolaemia co-exist from the start. Ischaemic bowel becomes necrotic, and peritonitis can develop as a result of this, which adds to pain levels.

Clinical Signs

Hypovolaemia is initially characterised by tachycardia and weak peripheral pulses. Later on, cold, pale extremities and tachypnoea will develop. Tachypnoea helps to produce a respiratory alkalosis to compensate for the metabolic acidosis that commonly occurs. Eventually, the animal reaches a point where it can no longer compensate, and the periphery demands more perfusion. Significant vasodilation occurs, which then causes a drop in blood pressure. This loads the blood with acidic metabolites and causes the patient to deteriorate rapidly [68].

An endotoxaemic patient will present with a dull and depressed demeanour. Disseminated intravascular coagulation (DIC) may be present, and this develops secondary to the primary disease. DIC is characterised by the activation of the coagulation cascade. The disease process is dynamic with early thrombosis being followed by perfuse bleeding. Haemorrhagic diathesis (a tendency to bleed easily) is often seen, which manifests as petechiae (pinpoint spots) on mucous membranes. Congested mucous membranes and a prolonged capillary refill time may also be observed.

Clinical Examination and Preparation

A quick but thorough examination is required. Human safety should be a primary consideration when dealing with painful colic patients. Handlers should wear sufficient personal protective equipment (PPE) such as a hard hat, gloves and steel toe-capped boots. The need for sedation and or analgesia should be assessed quickly. Any medication required should be prescribed by the case vet. Following this, the RVN can administer the medication. Once it is safe to do so, the following procedures can commence [68]:

- A full assessment of all clinical parameters (see Chapter 17).
- A blood sample may be taken to assess packed cell volume (PCV) and total solids.
- Vascular access should be secured by placing an IV catheter.
- Blood and peritoneal fluid lactate concentration should be assessed.
- A nasogastric tube should be passed to check for accumulation of reflux in the stomach.
- An ultrasound examination of the abdomen.
- Abdominocentesis could be carried out by the treating vet. Fluid should be tested for cellularity, protein and lactate.
- The vet will carry out a rectal examination to further assist with a diagnosis.

Considerations for Anaesthesia

It is beyond the scope of this section to discuss all considerations for anaesthesia in colic patients; however, the most important considerations are summarised below. Readers are directed to the texts in the reference list for further information.

- **Medication:** As stated previously, analgesia and sedation must be administered in the first instance. Medications used will include alpha-2 agonists, NSAIDs and opioids. Readers are referred to Section 10.2 for further information. Gastric decompression should also be considered as this can help to relieve pain [68]. For the anaesthetic, drugs that are minimally cardio-respiratory depressants should be selected.
- **Fluid therapy:** May be required pre-operatively. If significant hypovolaemia is present, hypertonic saline or colloids may be required to improve the intravascular volume prior to anaesthetic induction and early maintenance of anaesthesia. Both of these treatments should be followed by isotonic crystalloids. For more information about fluid therapy, see Section 10.5.
- **Monitoring:** Colic cases require close observation, and the use of multiparameter monitoring equipment is essential [68].
- **Patient positioning:** In hypovolaemic patients, dorsal recumbency further compromises venous return and cardiac output. This may cause the patient to decompensate acutely and die in the period when it is hoisted from induction to the operating theatre [68]. If body position changes are required, they should be performed relatively slowly and gently. The patient should be closely monitored at all times.
- **Ventilatory support:** May be required, especially if significant abdominal distension is present. IPPV used in hypovolaemic patients may significantly reduce thoracic vena cava blood flow and venous return to the heart. This will reduce cardiac output and blood pressure [68].
- **Reperfusion/re-oxygenation injury:** This can happen when blood flow to previously compromised gut is re-established. Products of anaerobic metabolism subsequently enter the main circulation [68]. Reactive oxygen species can be produced in previously ischaemic and/or damaged tissue. For these reasons, patients can crash shortly after the affected gut is un-twisted [68]. For information on cardiopulmonary cerebral resuscitation (CPCR) procedures, see Section 10.6.

Post-operative Care

Colic cases will require close monitoring and ongoing support in the first few days following surgery. Analgesia and fluid therapy are paramount to a successful recovery [68]. Acid–base and electrolyte imbalances may require attention. The patient will also require nutritional support and intensive nursing care. See Chapter 13 for further information.

Limb Fractures

Horses with limb fractures pose a significant risk when presented for GA. The most significant concerns relate to guiding the horse safely into recumbency, and then successfully recovering it from recumbency to a standing position without further catastrophic injury occurring. Good analgesia will be required as these patients are often painful and agitated [68]. Slings can be used for assisted induction to safely lower the horse into recumbency. Not all horses will tolerate being put in a sling, so the temperament of the patient should be considered before this is attempted. Rope recovery should be considered for these patients to facilitate a safe transition from recumbency to standing following the anaesthetic.

Neonates (<4 Weeks)

Neonatal foals carry specific considerations for GA. An accurate weight is essential for these patients to ensure correct drug dosing. In the first two weeks of life, cardiac output is largely dependent upon heart rate as the ventricles are less compliant. For this reason, alpha-2 agonists should be avoided where possible, as they cause a marked reduction in heart rate and cardiac output [68]. Midazolam or diazepam may be used to provide sedation and encourage recumbency. Pulmonary hypertension should be avoided, especially in the first week of life, as a transitional circulation exists at this time. The foetal ductus arteriosus and foramen ovale are only functionally closed. Marked pulmonary hypertension can cause these structures to re-open, creating a shift back to a foetal circulation that leads to a vicious cycle of worsening hypoxaemia [68]. Causes of pulmonary hypertension include hypovolemia, hypothermia, hypoxaemia, acidosis and pain [68]. An appropriate anaesthetic breathing circuit should be selected for example a non-rebreathing circuit for very small foals, or a small circle for larger foals [68].

Neonatal foals are prone to hypothermia due to their large surface area to volume ratio. Heat should be conserved as much as possible, and the following should be considered [68]:

- Clipping and wetting of the surgical site should be minimised.
- Heat should be retained by using insulative blankets, heated mattresses and warm air devices, for example a Bair hugger, if appropriate for the surgery being carried out.
- IV fluids and fluids used for lavage should be warmed before use.
- The ambient temperature in the theatre should be maintained between 15 and 20 °C.

Neonates are prone to hypoglycaemia as the neonatal liver has a limited ability to store glycogen and therefore has a poorly developed ability for glucogenesis. In neonatal foals, there is a high metabolic rate, which leads to a high demand for glucose [67]. For this reason, foals are rarely starved before GA. Neonatal foals are prone to gastric ulceration, and gastroprotectants should be considered in high-risk patients. Stringent monitoring should be carried out during the anaesthetic (see Section 10.5 for details). The foal should be kept warm and dry in recovery. Oxygen administration can continue until the foal is in sternal recumbency. Foals that are 100–150 kg can be assisted to stand [69]. Once the foal is steady on its feet, it should be reunited with the dam as quickly as possible and allowed to feed.

Older Foals (>4 Weeks)

Healthy older foals can be considered more like mature horses. Alpha-2 agonists can be used for sedation. Premedication may still result in recumbency, which can make the induction process smoother and safer for all involved [68].

Geriatric Patients

Geriatric patients may have significant age-related co-morbidities which require consideration for anaesthetic management [69].

Pituitary Pars Intermedia Dysfunction (PPID)

PPID also known as equine Cushing's disease (ECD) (see Chapter 13 for further information) may be a consideration in a geriatric horse. Hyperglycaemia associated with PPID may cause abnormalities leading to alternations in body fluid and electrolyte imbalances. Therefore, the hydration and electrolyte status of the patient should be checked before GA, where possible [69]. PPID can cause muscle wasting and weakness in geriatric patients; therefore, careful positioning and padding should be considered under GA to reduce the chances of post-anaesthetic myopathy (PAM) or post-anaesthetic neuropathy (PAN) developing [69]. Some horses with PPID can develop chronic hypercortisolism, and this can lead to osteoporosis. This is a consideration for patients during recovery as the risk of developing complicating pathological fractures could be higher [69]. Assisted recovery could be used to help to address this risk.

Musculoskeletal Considerations

Musculoskeletal disease and lameness, specifically osteoarthritis, represent the second most frequent reason for referral and a major reason for euthanasia in geriatric horses [70]. As stated above, careful positioning and padding should be used along with rope-assisted recovery in these cases. Multimodal analgesia should also be considered to ensure adequate comfort levels in these patients [69].

Respiratory Considerations

Equine asthma is the most prevalent respiratory disease seen in geriatric horses [70]. The primary anaesthetic concerns associated with equine asthma are bronchoconstriction and hypoxaemia. If a horse is presented for an elective procedure with poorly controlled asthma, the procedure should be postponed until the condition is under control [71]. In urgent or emergency cases, pre-anaesthetic optimisation can be achieved with short-term dose escalation of medications such as bronchodilators and steroids. Administration of inhaled salbutamol just prior to anaesthesia could be considered, which has been shown to improve oxygenation in anaesthetised horses [71]. Subsequent administration of salbutamol at the end of anaesthesia may help to reduce hypoxaemia during recovery [71].

Cardiovascular Considerations

Cardiac murmurs are detected in more than 20% of horses aged 15 years or older [69]. Geriatric horses should have a full pre-anaesthetic clinical examination to help to identify any murmurs or arrhythmias before anaesthesia is induced. If abnormalities are detected, and it has been deemed safe to continue with the anaesthetic, particular attention should be paid to maintaining fluid balance and blood pressure. Stringent monitoring of the cardiovascular system should occur, as detailed in Section 10.5.

Obesity

Obesity is a growing problem in equine populations and is a serious health concern. Obesity asserts negative effects on the cardiovascular system; therefore, an important first step when considering an anaesthetic in an obese equine patient is to identify any cardiac or cardiovascular abnormalities if they exist [69]. A thorough clinical examination should be carried out. In addition, indirect blood pressure monitoring could be used to identify hypertension, and an ECG could be used to assist in identifying cardiac dysrhythmias [69]. Both ventilation and oxygenation are affected by obesity. Hypoxaemia and hypoventilation in obese equine patients could be addressed using the following strategies [69]:

- Pre-oxygenation: administration of oxygen via a nasal catheter at 151 l/min for 3 minutes between sedation and induction. This is well tolerated and can help to increase the mean partial pressure of oxygen (PaO_2) during anaesthetic induction.
- Positive pressure ventilation: positive pressure ventilation can be administered, with an increased fraction of inspired oxygen (FiO_2) via a demand valve after intubation, during transportation from induction to the operating theatre and while positioning the horse on the operating table.
- Mechanical ventilation: IPPV should be initiated at the beginning of the GA.
- Evaluate arterial blood gas status: an arterial blood gas reading should be obtained within the first 20 minutes following induction, to acquire a baseline reading. This can be used to compare further values throughout the anaesthetic.
- Alveolar recruitment manoeuvres (ARMs): temporarily, airway pressure is increased during mechanical ventilation in order to open up any collapsed alveoli and improve oxygenation.
- Positive end-expiratory pressure (PEEP): administration of a higher PEEP via a mechanical ventilator is often combined with ARM to further improve oxygenation.
- Aerosolised salbutamol: can be administered via the ETT.
- Increase cardiac output: This can be achieved using IV fluids and/or inotropes such as dobutamine.

The risk of an obese the patient developing a PAM must be considered. Adequate padding and careful positioning must be carried out. The anaesthetic time should be kept to an absolute minimum. Blood pressure should be monitored throughout the procedure, and hypotension should be prevented with the use of IV fluids and dobutamine if necessary. If the proposed procedure is an elective one, the patient could be sent away to follow a weight loss management program and come back for the surgery when appropriate weight loss has been achieved.

Caesarean Section

A parturient mare presented for a caesarean section will have similar needs to those of any acute case. There are two additional considerations one being the effect of the gravid uterus on the mare and the other being the effect of anaesthetic drugs on the foal [72]. Risk factors include exhaustion and marginal dehydration in the mare. Anaesthetic drugs should be considered carefully, and barbiturates should be avoided. The major risk for caesarean sections in mares is the compression of the vena cava when the mare is placed in dorsal recumbency [72]. Serious or fatal hypotension can occur if the mare is placed symmetrically in dorsal recumbency. For this reason, recommendations are to tilt the mare off midline as much as possible (Figure 10.12) and monitor for hypotension with direct blood pressure monitoring [72]. Caution should be taken not to overload the dependent gluteal muscle when tilting the patient, as this could contribute to the risk of developing a post anaesthetic myopathy. A separate team with

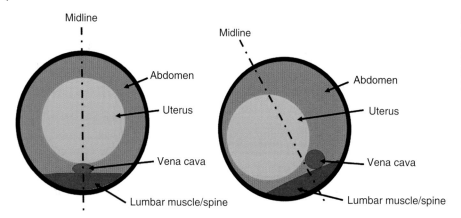

Figure 10.12 A mare undergoing a caesarean section should be tilted off midline as much as possible to reduce the pressure from the gravid uterus on the vena cava [6]. *Source:* Rosina Lillywhite.

equipment and medication should be prepared to perform resuscitation on the foal.

Trauma

The acute trauma case will often present as distressed and painful. If the horse has been injured during an athletic endeavour, it may also be restless and excitable, which can make these patients dangerous to handle. Personnel should wear PPE when handling these horses. Sedatives and analgesics should be considered in the first instance. Other risk factors for these patients are dehydration, blood loss and hypovolaemia. If the horse has lost a substantial amount of blood, the circulating volume should be restored prior to anaesthesia. The exception to this is if anaesthesia is required to stem the source of bleeding [72].

If hypovolemia is suspected, phenothiazines should be avoided as the resulting hypotension may cause the horse to lose consciousness. Colloids such as gelofusine or plasma may be given to help to restore circulating volume. Isotonic crystalloids should also be given to address dehydration. If a large amount of blood has been lost, a blood transfusion should be considered. Hypertonic saline may also be administered if circulatory collapse is suspected. This must always be followed up with isotonic crystalloids [68]. The vet in charge of the case will prescribe the fluids required for the stabilisation protocol. The RVN can then administer these fluids as directed. The patient should be monitored constantly throughout this procedure. Once the patient has been stabilised, anaesthesia can commence.

Anaesthetic Induction

Before anaesthesia is induced, the patient should be carefully assessed and prepared. Patient preparation is covered in detail in Chapter 12. Induction is a potentially dangerous time for the patient, and any veterinary personnel involved. PPE should be worn, and induction protocols should be adhered to. As discussed in Section 10.2, anaesthesia is most commonly induced in horses using IV agents. It is

important that the patient has been adequately premedicated before induction is attempted.

Premedication

Premedication is the administration of an appropriate medication prior to anaesthesia to facilitate induction, maintenance and recovery. Premedication often involves using many different types of medication together to give a balanced overall effect. This is known as multi-modal anaesthesia. Medications used for premedication include phenothiazines, alpha-2 agonists, NSAIDs and opioids. These medications and their uses are discussed in Section 10.2. Antibiotics may need to be administered prior to anaesthesia. The vet in charge of the anaesthetic and the surgeon should discuss and agree on the antibiotics required prior to surgery, and these should be given pre-operatively. Antibiotic protocols should be in place and based on the BEVA 'Protect ME' campaign, aimed at promoting responsible antimicrobial use and any emerging evidence-based practice. See Chapter 6 for more information. The RVN should liaise closely with the case vet to develop an anaesthetic protocol that is appropriate for each individual patient. Once the has prescribed the required medication, the RVN can calculate drug doses and administer the medication for the premed.

The Induction Process

The RVN must have all equipment and medication prepared before induction takes place. This also involves checking and preparing ETTs, as described in Section 10.3. In a practice setting, horses are usually induced in a padded induction box (see Chapter 11 for further information). The patient must be sedated with an alpha-2 agonist prior to induction. To optimise sedation, alpha-2 agonists are often combined with an opioid. This sedative must be given enough time to take effect and will work much better if given in a quiet, calm environment. Once the patient is deemed ready, anaesthesia can be induced by the anaesthetist. Induction agents used in horses are discussed in Section 10.2. The most common medications used are ketamine and midazolam or diazepam.

During induction, the RVN should assist the anaesthetist with patient restraint and positioning. There are different methods for trying to control anaesthetic induction for equine patients.

- Free fall: the patient is left alone in the induction box after the induction medication is given. This method is generally not recommended as the horse is not controlled during induction and can land awkwardly. This method is sometimes used if the horse is very large and there is not sufficient room for handlers to stay in the induction box safely.
- Support from handlers: generally, two handlers will hold the horse, ensuring that the head is kept down to prevent the horse from falling over backwards as it loses consciousness.
- Swing door: some induction boxes incorporate a crush door that forms part of the wall of the induction box and can be folded out. During induction, the horse is positioned between the door and the wall of the box (Figure 10.13). This provides control as the horse

assumes recumbency. The door is then folded back into the wall of the induction box during recovery [73].
- Tilt tables: few equine hospitals use tilt tables for induction. The horse is sedated and positioned adjacent and parallel to the table, orientated vertically. Bellybands are placed under the horse and are tightened to provide support as anaesthesia is induced. When the horse is anaesthetised, the table is rotated to a horizontal position [73].
- Sling induction: the horse is sedated and put into a sling before anaesthesia is induced. During induction, the sling takes the weight of the horse, and it is lowered into recumbency in a controlled manner. This method is useful for the induction of fracture patients, to prevent possible displacement of the fracture as recumbency is achieved. The use of this method also depends on the temperament of the patient, as not all horses will tolerate being put into a sling. This method requires experienced personnel.

There are advantages and disadvantages to each induction method. The RVN should discuss the most appropriate method to use with the anaesthetist, considering the facilities and trained personnel available, as well as the temperament of the patient.

Following induction, monitoring of vital signs should begin as soon as possible [68]. The patient will be intubated as described in Section 10.3 (Figure 10.14). As this is happening, the horses' hooves will be covered (Figure 10.15), hobbles will be applied, and the patient will be attached to the hoist in readiness to be transported into the operating theatre. Health and safety must be considered at all times during this process, and appropriate PPE worn by personnel. In some practices, the horse is attached to the anaesthetic circuit in the induction box before being transported into the theatre. In other practices, the horse is attached to the anaesthetic circuit once it has been

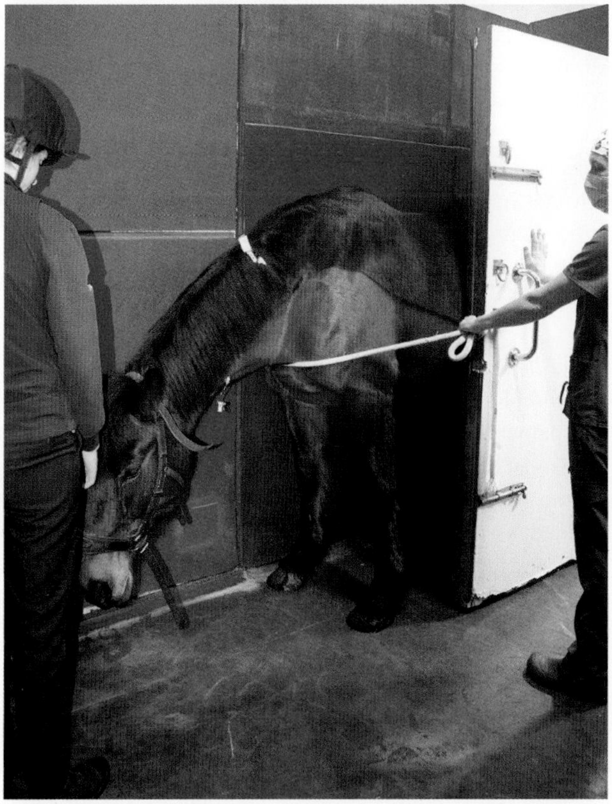

Figure 10.13 Swing door induction. *Source:* Rosina Lillywhite.

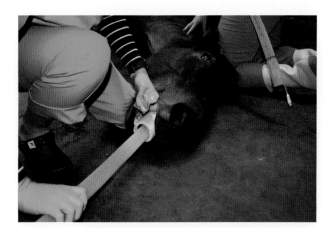

Figure 10.14 A horse being intubated. *Source:* Rosina Lillywhite.

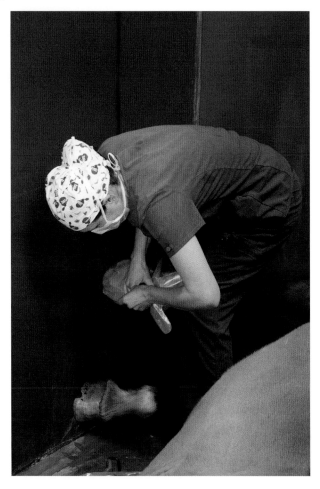

Figure 10.15 Horses hooves are covered before they are attached to the hoist. *Source:* Rosina Lillywhite.

transported into the theatre. In either situation, the anaesthetic circuit should be set up ready, having been leak tested previously. Once the patient is deemed ready by the anaesthetist, it can be transported into the theatre on the hoist and carefully positioned ready for the surgical procedure. Anaesthetic monitoring equipment should be set up ready so it can be attached at the earliest possible moment. For more information regarding monitoring equipment, see Section 10.5.

10.5 Monitoring Techniques for Anaesthetised Equine Patients

Introduction

During equine anaesthesia, the anaesthetist aims to balance the preservation of normal equine physiology while providing an adequate plane of anaesthesia and analgesia to enable the procedure to be performed.

To achieve this, the following must be considered:

- The patient must be continuously assessed.
- Parameters should be documented every 5 minutes.
- The anaesthetist must have knowledge of which parameters to monitor, how to accurately monitor them and how to interpret the findings [47].

Anaesthetic Monitoring Observations

All basic monitoring techniques that require no equipment, such as ocular and mucous membrane assessment and pulse palpation, are recommended for every general anaesthetic procedure [47].

Level of Consciousness

Guedel [74] described the stages and planes of anaesthesia in humans after the administration of ether. Guedel's classification of anaesthetic depth remains in use today [74] (see Section 10.1 for further details). The maintenance of an adequate plane of anaesthesia is very important in horses due to the potential for injury to personnel and/or the patient in the event of movement. Furthermore, an inappropriately deep plane of anaesthesia may significantly compromise physiological function.

Reflexes and Observations Indicative of Anaesthetic Depth

Monitoring reflexes and patient characteristics using a 'hand-on' approach is a crucial and fundamental skill for the equine anaesthetist in both field and hospital settings [47].

Anaesthetic depth as determined by eye position, ocular reflexes, presence of nystagmus and muscle or anal tone helps the anaesthetist avoid too light or too deep a plane of anaesthesia [75].

Ocular Reflexes and Movement
Palpebral Reflex
The palpebral reflex is triggered by stroking the cilia [47]. Care must be taken not to test this reflex repeatedly as it will fatigue [47]. Contact with the corneal surface should be avoided, as this will produce a false result and may cause corneal injury. A very rapid blink or spontaneous blinking may indicate a light plane of anaesthesia. The palpebral reflex is progressively depressed as anaesthetic drug effects intensify [66]. In most horses under inhalational agent anaesthesia, the palpebral reflex should always be present. An absent palpebral reflex may indicate a deep plane of anaesthesia. However, since the palpebral response can be significantly depressed by inhalational agents, in some horses, it may become absent during surgical levels of

inhalational agent anaesthesia [66]. After induction of GA with ketamine, an active palpebral reflex is maintained during the transition from injectable to inhalational agent anaesthesia [66]. During TIVA, the palpebral reflex is often more brisk during a surgical plane of anaesthesia, particularly when agents such as ketamine are used.

Corneal Reflex

Touching the cornea may cause corneal injury, so routine evaluation of the corneal reflex is not recommended [47]. Touching the cornea should always provoke a blink response. The absence of a corneal reflex with any anaesthetic drug protocol should raise concern of an anaesthetic overdose [66].

Nystagmus

Nystagmus describes a repetitive, rhythmic and involuntary oscillation or movement of the eyeball. The rate of nystagmus is variable. During volatile agent anaesthesia, nystagmus can indicate an inadequate or light plane of anaesthesia. The development of a brisk palpebral reflex and the appearance of nystagmus are associated with the lightening of anaesthesia, and the eye may also rotate dorsocaudally [53]. TIVA involving the administration of ketamine, causes the eye to be either centrally placed or directed slightly rostroventral, the palpebral reflex is brisk and small amplitude nystagmus is often present [53].

Anal Reflex

A reduction in anal contraction on stimulation is associated with increasing anaesthetic plane [66].

Muscle Tone
Neck

Palpation of the neck muscles is a useful way to assess muscle relaxation and depth of anaesthesia. Increased tension or tightening of the muscles in the neck and shoulders may indicate a light plane of anaesthesia [66].

Limbs

Palpation of limb muscle tone is a useful method to assess anaesthetic depth. Muscle tone should be relaxed, and the distal limb should be easily moved with no resistance to manual flexion/extension. A response to surgery or 'lightening of the plane of anaesthesia' is usually signalled by an increased tone or slow movement of the forelimbs [76]. Shivering and increased muscle tension (particularly in the neck and legs) are often useful indicators of an inadequate plane of anaesthesia for surgical stimulus, although impending conscious or unconscious movement remains challenging to predict [47].

Swallowing
During inhalational agent anaesthesia, swallowing may indicate a light or inadequate plane of anaesthesia. TIVA may not be appropriate for airway surgery, as swallowing can occur throughout surgery [76].

Reflexes and Patient Observations During TIVA

During TIVA, horses may appear lightly anaesthetised, often with a brisk palpebral reflex, occasional nystagmus, swallowing, and lacrimation, good muscle tone, and yet little response to surgery [76].

Anaesthetic Monitoring Observations of the Cardiovascular System

Most anaesthetic and sedative agents have effects on the cardiovascular system. Therefore, during sedation and GA, it is important to monitor the cardiovascular system. Injectable and inhalant anaesthetic drugs used in horses may decrease cardiac output and reduce arterial blood pressure [77]. The detrimental effects that anaesthetic agents may have on cardiovascular function necessitate that anaesthetic drugs are titrated to effect.

Useful Terminology

- Heart rate (beats/minute): The number of beats counted per minute. The normal heart rate in an anaesthetised adult horse is 30–45 beats per minute [77].
- Stroke volume: The volume (ml) of blood ejected by each heartbeat [78].
- Cardiac output (CO): The volume of blood ejected from the heart in 1 minute [79] CO = heart rate (HR) × stroke volume (SV) (ml/min).
- Systole: The period of ventricular contraction [78].
- Diastole: The period of ventricular relaxation [78].
- Systemic vascular resistance: Resistance of the circulation = mean arterial pressure (MAP)/CO [79].
- Systemic arterial blood pressure: Systemic vascular resistance (SVR) × CO [80].
- Systolic arterial pressure: The maximum pressure generated [78].
- Diastolic arterial pressure: The minimum pressure generated [78].
- Pulse pressure: The difference between the systolic and diastolic arterial pressure [78].
- Mean arterial pressure: The average over each complete cardiac cycle. This can be approximated to diastolic pressure plus one-third of the pulse pressure [78].
- Systemic vascular resistance (SVR): Is used to describe how well the blood flows around the circulation. The tone of the vessels directly affects resistance to blood flow. Vasoconstriction results in increased SVR, while vasodilation results in decreased SVR.
- Central venous pressure (CVP): Is the intraluminal blood pressure within the intrathoracic cranial vena cava [59].

- Oxygen delivery: This is the product of arterial oxygen content (CaO_2) and CO [81].

During GA, it is important to monitor the cardiovascular system continuously and assess the effects of anaesthetic drugs on cardiovascular function. An appropriate level of anaesthesia needs to be maintained while minimising the negative effects of the drugs on the cardiorespiratory system.

Manual Palpation of Pulse Rate and Quality

A rapid and effective method of making a subjective assessment of cardiac output is by palpating a peripheral pulse. Heart rate can be counted, and the strength of the pulse can be estimated as subjective [82]. The normal heart rate for anaesthetised horses is 30–45 beats per minute [83]. The pulse rate should match the heart rate. Gentle pressure on a peripheral artery using a finger enables palpation of the expansion of the artery as pressure builds. The rise in pressure (pulse pressure) equates to the systolic pressure minus the diastolic pressure [82]. A strong pulse indicates a large stroke volume, and a weak pulse indicates a low stroke volume [82].

Mucous Membrane Colour

Subjective indication of peripheral tissue perfusion. Normal mucous membrane colour is pink in most horses. Pale pink or greyish mucous membranes may indicate poor perfusion due to either reduced CO or vasoconstriction, which is common after alpha-2 agonist administration [56]. Congested or bright red mucous membranes can be secondary to vasodilation. This is occasionally seen with hypercapnia but, more commonly, in cases of septic shock [47]. Mucous membrane colour should not be relied upon for assessment of oxygenation status and rather, used as a prompt for further investigation [47].

Capillary Refill Time (CRT)

CRT offers a subjective indication of peripheral perfusion. In healthy horses, CRT is less than 2 seconds. Slow or sluggish capillary refill times (>2 seconds) and pale pink or greyish colouration may indicate poor perfusion [56].

Monitoring the Cardiorespiratory Systems with Equipment

Electronic monitoring methods should not replace the anaesthetist's 'hand-on' core skills in monitoring anaesthesia but should complement them. During equine anaesthesia, cardiovascular monitoring usually consists of an ECG and IBP measurement [84]. Supporting MAP is important in the prevention of severe complications, such as myopathies [84].

ECG

An ECG is used to monitor heart rate and rhythm. A surface ECG records the electrical activity of depolarisation and repolarisation of myocardial tissue, using electrodes placed at the skin [57]. While the consistent placement of the electrodes may aid in producing a familiar trace, any orientation of pairs of electrodes will produce a waveform if they span the heart [56]. The ECG trace represents events in the cardiac cycle (Figure 10.16):

- P wave = atrial depolarisation.
- PR interval = conduction through the atrioventricular (AV) node.
- QRS complex = ventricular depolarisation.
- T wave = ventricular repolarisation [57].

The base-apex lead is the most common lead system used for ECG analysis in horses [59]. Electrical impulses which spread across the heart muscle can be detected and amplified at the skin surface using electrodes [47, 55]. A minimum of three electrode contact points with crocodile

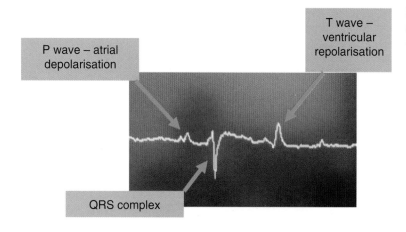

Figure 10.16 Example of an electrocardiograph: showing the P-wave, QRS complex and T-wave. *Source:* Dr Kate Loomes.

clips or adhesive gel electrodes can be configured in a 'base–apex orientation' [55]:

- The red right arm electrode (−) is clipped on the neck in the right jugular furrow.
- The yellow left arm electrode (+) is clipped at the apex of the heart over the left fifth intercostal space several inches from the midline [85].
- The left leg electrode is clipped on the neck or shoulder. Recognition of the normal P-QRS-T morphology is required in order to accurately assess an ECG recording and the timing intervals [55].

The normal HR for anaesthetised horses is 30–45 beats per minute [83]. The normal HR for anaesthetised foals maybe 35–60 beats per minute, as their resting heart rate is 100 beats per minute at birth [83, 86]. In horses, heart rate may not vary significantly with anaesthetic depth or surgical stimulation. Heart rate is not a reliable indicator of appropriate anaesthetic depth in horses. Bradycardia <25 beats per minute and may occur in response to increased vagal tone or the administration of agents such as alpha-2 agonists or dobutamine [87]. Tachycardia >50 beats per minute [20] and may be associated with sympathetic stimulation, pain, hypoxaemia, dobutamine administration or tourniquet use [87, 88]. An ECG enables further investigation of rhythm disturbances, for example, second-degree (AV) block (Figure 10.17), atrial premature contractions, ventricular premature contractions and atrial fibrillation (Figure 10.18).

Arterial Blood Pressure (ABP) Measurement

ABP is a marker of circulatory status and is the product of CO and SVR [59]. Blood flow rather than blood pressure is the driving force for tissue perfusion. However, while the direct measurement of flow is currently impractical, blood pressure is used as an estimate of flow [59]. ABP can be measured using direct (invasive) or indirect (non-invasive) methods.

Invasive Arterial Blood Pressure (IBP) Monitoring

ABP measured directly or invasively (IBP) is considered the gold standard ABP measurement technique [58]. The technique requires an intra-arterial catheter connected to a transducer via a non-compliant fluid-filled extension set [59] (Figure 10.19). The lateral dorsal metatarsal artery, the transverse facial artery and the facial artery are most commonly used for arterial catheterisation [59] (Figure 10.20). The fluid extension set should be visually inspected for air bubbles, kinks, fluid leaks, obstructions, or clots, which can lead to damping the system response and erroneous ABP measurements [59].

Measurement of arterial pressure using a peripheral arterial catheter is commonly practised in equine anaesthesia because hypotension has adverse consequences in horses,

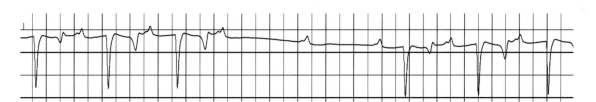

Figure 10.17 Second-degree AV block. This is a regularly irregular rhythm where the heart misses a beat in a regular rhythm. It is the most common intraoperative rhythm disturbance seen. Second-degree AV blocks rarely require treatment and usually resolve spontaneously. See Chapter 13 for further information. *Source:* Dr Mark Bowen.

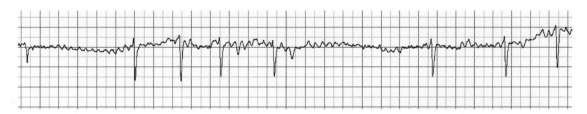

Figure 10.18 Atrial fibrillation. This is an irregularly irregular rhythm which occasionally develops during anaesthesia. The atria contract randomly causing an irregular and sometimes extreme tachycardia. Treatment may not be required if blood pressure remains normal. If treatment is required, electrolyte infusion, reduction of the volatile agent and dobutamine can be initiated depending on the circumstances [73]. A horse found to be in atrial fibrillation prior to GA should be treated and converted prior to anaesthesia [73]. See Chapter 13 for further information. *Source:* Dr Mark Bowen.

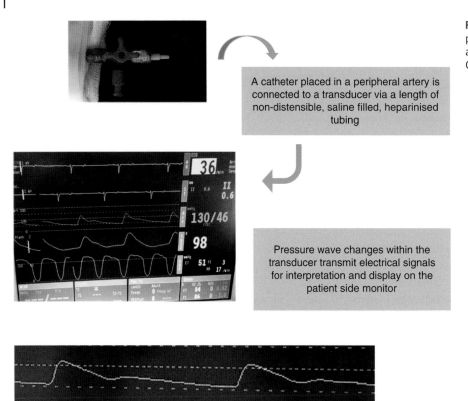

A catheter placed in a peripheral artery is connected to a transducer via a length of non-distensible, saline filled, heparinised tubing

Pressure wave changes within the transducer transmit electrical signals for interpretation and display on the patient side monitor

Figure 10.19 A catheter placed in a peripheral artery is used to measure arterial blood pressure directly during GA in horses. *Source:* Dr Kate Loomes.

Figure 10.20 Arterial trace generated from catheterisation of the dorsal metatarsal artery in a horse in lateral recumbency. *Source:* Dr Kate Loomes.

and the arterial catheter facilitates sampling for blood-gas analysis [89]. Direct ABP monitoring provides a continuous display of pressure waveforms and values for systolic arterial pressure (SAP), mean arterial pressure (MAP) and diastolic arterial pressure (DAP) [59]. (Figure 10.21). Catheterisation of a peripheral artery is required in order to measure arterial blood pressure directly.

Arterial catheterisation must be performed using an aseptic technique and requires skill and practice to perform effectively.

Potential complications of arterial catheterisation include:

- Haemorrhage from the site
- Haematoma formation
- Tissue damage/necrosis
- Infection

Saline-filled, heparinised, non-distensible tubing is used to connect the arterial catheter to an electrical transducer, which is connected to a monitor. Pressure wave changes within the transducer transmit electrical signals for

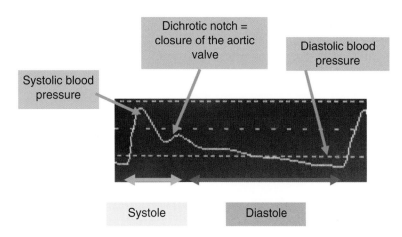

Dichrotic notch = closure of the aortic valve

Diastolic blood pressure

Systolic blood pressure

Systole

Diastole

Figure 10.21 Arterial trace generated from catheterisation of the mandibular branch of the facial artery. Features of the arterial waveform reflect the distension and behaviour of the vasculature. *Source:* Dr Kate Loomes.

interpretation and display on the patient-side monitor [58]. The electrical transducer is placed at the level of the heart. The measurement and display of systolic, diastolic and mean arterial blood pressure values and the arterial pressure waveform provide important information regarding cardiovascular function and status [83]. Equine anaesthetists normally aim to maintain MAP above 70 mmHg [81]. Since intra-compartmental pressure in the dependent muscles of adult horses, on an adequately padded surface, reaches values of 30–40 mmHg [90] and a vascular transmural pressure needs to be greater than 30 mmHg for adequate microcirculation [91], a MAP >70 mmHg should support adequate tissue perfusion in healthy horses. Normal DAP in healthy adult anaesthetised horses is >45 mmHg. Low DAP (<45 mmHg) may indicate relative (due to vasodilation) or absolute (due to haemorrhage or dehydration) hypovolaema [87].

Hypotension is usually defined as MAP <70 mmHg [92]. Causes may include:

- Anaesthetic overdose
- Reduced circulating volume
- Administration of drugs causing vasodilation (acepromazine, isoflurane, sevoflurane).

When hypotension occurs, contributing factors such as decreases in circulating volume (for example, blood loss), cardiac output or systemic vascular resistance should be considered [81]. Hypotension is commonly corrected with dobutamine during GA.

Hypertension occurs when MAP > 100 mmHg. Causes may include:

- Pain
- Sympathetic stimulation
- An inadequate plane of anaesthesia
- ± surgical stimulus
- Hypercapnia
- Hypoxaemia
- Hyperthermia
- Administration of drugs causing vasoconstriction (alpha-2 adrenoreceptor agonists) [87, 88].

Both severe hypotension and hypertension should be prevented to avoid the negative effect of abnormal tissue perfusion [60].

Non-invasive Blood Pressure (NIBP) Monitoring

NIBP or indirect methods of measuring blood pressure include manometric measurements (Korotkoff sounds) as well as oscillometric and Doppler methods [59]. Oscillometric NIBP devices utilise a peripherally placed arterial bladder cuff to record pressure wave oscillations induced by blood flow turbulence during vascular release. The monitor measures MAP at maximal oscillation amplitude and then uses proprietary algorithms to calculate SAP and DAP [58].

Cuff placement sites include:

- Proximal tail base
- Metacarpus [58].
- Median
- Palmar digital arteries [80].

In situations where IBP measurement is not possible, oscillometric NIBP measurement may be used, but the limitations of the technique should be considered. Poor agreement between NIBP measured by an oscillometric device and IBP has been reported in horses [58, 93]. Devices that measure ABP non-invasively are routinely used in human and small domestic animal patients; however, inaccuracy and poor reliability compared with IBP mean they remain underused in horses [58].

Central Venous Pressure (CVP)

CVP is an estimate of preload and right ventricular filling pressure (right atrial pressure) and is an approximation of the ratio of blood volume to blood volume or vessel capacity [59]. Complex techniques and trained personnel are required to measure CVP; therefore, measurement of CVP is usually reserved for experimental procedures or specialist centres. There is evidence that jugular venous pressure has an adequate correlation with CVP in healthy, euvolemic, laterally recumbent anaesthetized adult horses [61]. One study showed that while jugular venous pressure cannot replace CVP measurement, but it may be used clinically to estimate CVP [61].

CO Monitoring

The measurement of CO can be used to indicate tissue perfusion and to assess the effects of drugs on circulation [77]. Techniques described for the measurement of CO include:

- Fick principle
- Electromagnetic flowmetry
- Indicator dilution methods
- Doppler echocardiography
- Thoracic electrical bioimpedance
- Pulse contour analysis
- Thermodilution method
- Transoesophageal echocardiography

Measurement of CO requires specific equipment and trained personnel and is usually reserved for experimental procedures or specialist centres.

Anaesthetic Monitoring Observations of the Respiratory System

Respiration should be observed carefully. Visualising the rate and degree of chest wall or rebreathing bag movement is a basic but important method of assessing respiratory rate and pattern. Tidal volume (V_T) may be roughly estimated by observing the degree of collapse of the rebreathing bag when using inhalational agent anaesthesia [83]. More sophisticated mechanical ventilators may have the facility to measure tidal volume using spirometry. Thoracic auscultation may be difficult in the recumbent horse due to positioning and extraneous background noise [83].

Useful Terminology

- Respiratory rate (RR) or respiratory frequency (R_f): the number of breaths per minute. The normal respiratory rate in a spontaneously breathing adult anaesthetised horse is 6–20 breaths per minute [83].
- Tidal volume (V_T): is the volume of air exhaled in a single breath (ml/kg)
- Minute volume (M_V): is the volume of gas exhaled by the patient in 1 minute (ml/kg/min). $M_V = RR \times V_T$.
- End-tidal carbon dioxide tension (ETCO$_2$): is the maximal partial pressure or concentration of CO$_2$ in the respiratory gases at the end of an exhaled breath [94].

- Dead space: is the part of a ventilated volume that does not participate in gas exchange [95].

Anaesthetic Monitoring of the Respiratory System with Equipment
Capnography

Capnometry is the measurement of carbon dioxide (CO$_2$) in a sample of gas [94]. Capnography provides information relating to ventilation, gas exchange and metabolism. During anaesthesia, end-tidal CO$_2$ partial pressure (ETCO$_2$) from the gases in the breathing circuit are sampled close to the patient [47]. Capnography is the continuous monitoring of the concentration or partial pressure of CO$_2$ in respiratory gases [94]. Capnography produces a continuous waveform of CO$_2$ partial pressure [47] (Figure 10.22). The characteristic shape of the capnograph corresponds to events in the respiratory cycle (Figure 10.23).

Infra-red spectroscopy is used to measure the CO$_2$ content of gas [94]. A beam of infrared light is passed across

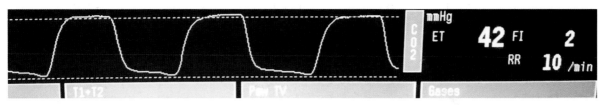

Figure 10.22 Carbon dioxide in expired gas is represented in a graphical form, with time on the *X*-axis and expired partial pressure of CO$_2$ on the *Y*-axis: the result is a capnography trace or waveform. *Source:* Dr Kate Loomes.

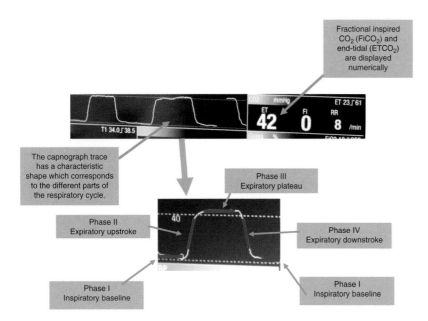

Figure 10.23 The capnograph trace has a characteristic shape which corresponds to the different parts of the respiratory cycle. Phase I (inspiratory baseline) represents inspiration and therefore, no CO$_2$ is detected. Phase II (expiratory upstroke) represents expiration of both dead space gas and alveoli gas from the respiratory bronchioles and alveoli. Phase III (alveolar plateau) represents expiration of alveolar gases. At the end of phase III, the maximal value of CO$_2$ measured is equivalent to the ETCO$_2$. Phase IV (expiratory downstroke) represents the beginning of the next breath, with the CO$_2$ content returning rapidly to zero. The continuous waveform allows a visual breath-by-breath assessment of a patient's airway and ventilation, with the contour of the waveform giving considerably more information than the ETCO$_2$ value alone [94]. *Source:* Dr Kate Loomes and Rosina Lillywhite.

the gas sample and directed to a sensor. The presence of CO_2 in the gas leads to a reduction in the amount of light which is transmitted to the sensor and a change in the circuit voltage [94]. This information is interpreted by the monitor, and a real-time continuous waveform is produced.

- **Normal ETCO$_2$ (normocapnia)** in a spontaneously breathing anaesthetised horse is 30–50 mmHg [83]. Mechanical ventilation can be tailored to achieve ideal ETCO$_2$ values between 35 and 55 mmHg in anaesthetised horses.
- **Decreased ETCO$_2$ (<30 mmHg) (hypocapnia)** indicates hyperventilation, which may be due to pain, excitement, light plane of anaesthesia or over-zealous use of mechanical ventilation.

A sudden drop in ETCO$_2$ may be a result of extubation, equipment failure, for example, a leak from the ETT cuff, massive pulmonary embolism or cardiopulmonary arrest [96] (Figure 10.24). Stepwise reductions in ETCO$_2$ (Figure 10.25) may be indicative of falling CO and is a cause for concern.

Capnography can provide evidence that the circulatory system is capable of CO_2 transport as a fall in cardiac output results in a reduction in ETCO$_2$ when ventilation is constant [47].

Increased ETCO$_2$ (>60 mmHg) (hypercapnia) may indicate hypoventilation due to anaesthetic agent-associated respiratory depression caused by CNS depression and respiratory muscle weakness [63]. Increased ETCO$_2$ may be seen in states of malignant hyperthermia, fever or sepsis [96]. There may be cardiovascular benefits of mild

hypoventilation, with some studies advocating maintaining PaCO$_2$ between 50–70 mmHg [33] or below 70–75 mmHg [97]. Note this reference is to PaCO$_2$ and not ETCO$_2$. Measurement of arterial carbon dioxide tension (PaCO$_2$) requires blood gas analysis. The difference between ETCO$_2$ and PaCO$_2$ can be used to estimate how effectively CO_2 is being transferred from the blood to the alveoli before being exhaled. Increased ETCO$_2$–PaCO$_2$ difference (>20 mmHg) indicates increased alveolar dead space ventilation, incomplete alveolar emptying, ventilation-perfusion mismatch or a leak in the sampling system [83]. ETCO$_2$–PaCO$_2$ difference tends to increase with increased anaesthetic time and is affected by body position and mode of ventilation. ETCO$_2$ gives a relatively poor indication of PaCO$_2$ in both healthy and compromised horses, especially during CMV [98]. For this reason, it is important to use blood gas analysis to provide an accurate PaCO$_2$. Capnography monitoring is key when performing CPCR, as the return of the waveform highlights the return of spontaneous circulation, indicating that the procedure has been successful [50].

Pulse Oximetry

Pulse oximetry displays heart rate and estimates the percentage of arterial blood haemoglobin which is saturated with oxygen (SpO$_2$) [83] (Figure 10.26). It indicates the presence of pulsatile flow to tissues and displays the pulse rate [47, 54] and a beat-to-beat value for arterial haemoglobin saturation (SpO$_2$) [52]. It can detect hypoxaemia without the need to measure arterial blood gas [52]. Pulse oximetry is non-invasive and offers immediate and continuous measurements of SpO$_2$ [47, 59]. The portable nature of

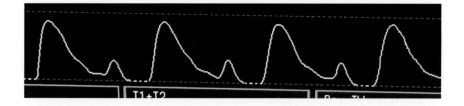

Figure 10.24 Decreased ETCO$_2$ and a loss of the normal capnograph shape may be seen when there is a leak around the endotracheal tube cuff. *Source:* Dr Kate Loomes.

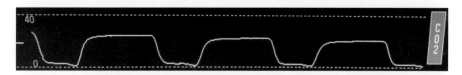

Figure 10.25 Stepwise reductions in ETCO$_2$ may be indicative of falling cardiac output and is a cause for concern. *Source:* Dr Kate Loomes.

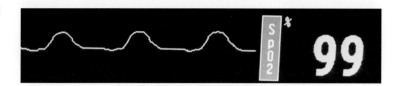

Figure 10.26 Pulse oximetry provides a digital and audible display of pulse rate [59]. *Source:* Dr Kate Loomes.

the pulse oximeter makes it useful for field anaesthesia [47]. A pulse oximeter uses two light-emitting diodes and a photodetector. Red and infrared light is transmitted through superficial tissue such as the tongue. A photodetector measures the relative absorption of light by arterial blood in the tissue. Pulse oximeters estimate SpO_2 by evaluating the relative absorption of light of two different frequencies, red (660 nm) and infrared (940 nm), by oxyhaemoglobin and the reduced form of Hb (deoxyhaemoglobin) [99].

Normal SpO_2 during GA in an adult horse receiving 100% oxygen is >95%. Oxygen is routinely used in veterinary anaesthesia as the sole carrier gas and therefore patients are commonly exposed to nearly 100% oxygen [100]. Hypoxaemia (SpO_2 < 95%) may be due to an inadequate oxygen supply, respiratory obstruction, ETT obstruction, ventilation-perfusion mismatch. Ventilation-perfusion inequality is the most common reason for the development of hypoxaemia in horses. Poor signal quality is the major reason for inaccuracy of pulse oximeters [98]. Inaccuracies may arise due to ambient light, movement and vasoconstriction. Inaccuracy of a pulse oximeter to obtain the exact correct heart rate correlates with the inaccuracy of SpO_2 readings [98]. Pulse oximetry and arterial blood analysis complement one another. Continuous monitoring of SpO_2 via oximetry can be coupled with intermittent arterial blood gas analysis as required [59].

The shape of the sensor, thickness of tissue placed within the sensor, presence of pigment and hair and movement of the patient can be responsible for the pulse oximeter failing to measure arterial oxygen saturation [53]. The pulse rate displayed on the oximeter must correspond to the rate obtained by palpation or ECG before the measurement can be assumed to be accurate. During GA, when 100% oxygen is being delivered: normal SpO_2 > 95%. Hypoxaemia (SpO_2 < 95%) mainly occurs due to ventilation-perfusion inequality but may also be caused by hypoventilation [54].

Arterial Blood Gas Analysis

Arterial blood gas analysis provides information relating to oxygenation, ventilation and acid–base balance [66]. Venous blood analysis provides information relating to assess ventilation and acid–base balance [63]. It is indicated in horses undergoing colic surgery or under GA with other causes of critical illness. Samples must be drawn anaerobically for accurate analysis of oxygenation parameters. Blood is introduced into a blood gas analyser, which contains a series of electrodes that measure pH, oxygen tension (PO_2) and carbon dioxide tension (PCO_2). The other information provided by the analyser is calculated from these measured parameters. Machines used to measure blood gas values may also offer the facility to measure electrolytes

(sodium, calcium, glucose and potassium), PCV, haemoglobin, lactate, urea and creatinine.

Arterial blood samples can be drawn from a peripheral arterial catheter placed for IBP measurement. If needle puncture is used, the site for arterial puncture should be prepared with an antiseptic. Clipping or shaving the hair may facilitate visualisation or palpation of the artery [59]. The blood should be collected in a syringe coated with heparin and kept anaerobic and on ice [59]. Blood gas analysis is not continuous, so its use is limited by the number of samples taken and the time taken to obtain the results. Samples should be collected as needed, most commonly every 30–60 minutes or more frequently if the horse's condition requires it [63]. Blood gas analysers use small electrodes which measure pH, arterial and venous tension of carbon dioxide ($PaCO_2$, $PvCO_2$) and oxygen (PaO_2, PvO_2). During GA in an adult horse, normal $PaCO_2$ is 40–60 mmHg and normal PaO_2 is 100–500 mmHg [83]. Increased $PaCO_2$ (>65–70 mmHg) (hypercapnia) indicates hypoventilation, which may be due to anaesthetic agent-associated respiratory depression or inadequate mechanical ventilation. Decreased $PaCO_2$ (<40 mmHg) (hypocapnia) indicates hyperventilation, which may be due to pain, excitement, light plane of anaesthesia or over-zealous use of mechanical ventilation. Severe hyperventilation resulting in hypocapnia may cause respiratory alkalosis and a reduction in cerebral blood flow [59].

Hypoxemia is defined as a state of reduced oxygen tension in arterial blood (PaO_2 < 60 mmHg) that can lead to reduced oxygen levels in the tissues (hypoxia) [63]. PaO_2 values <80 mmHg indicate hypoxemia and correlate with an SaO_2 < 95% [59]. Values below 60 mmHg (SaO_2 of approximately 90%) indicate severe hypoxemia [59]. Rapid desaturation of haemoglobin occurs below this level [98].

Spirometry

During clinical large animal anaesthesia, the use of spirometry to monitor ventilation is not routine because of the lack of a reliable and practical method adapted to large animals [101]. Purpose-made equipment does exist allowing the routine use of spirometry in horses in some centres. Spirometry measures tidal volume (V_T), minute ventilation (MV), dynamic compliance and resistance. Spirometry allowed continuous measurement of tidal and minute volume on a breath-to-breath basis and quick detection of any changes [101]. The information measured using spirometry can be used to create a pressure-volume (PV) loop, which provides information about compliance and a flow-volume (FV) loop, which determines the resistance [63]. Spirometers may use a pitot tube-based flow sensor with an integrated respiratory gas sample port and a dedicated host monitor. The pressure difference generated is converted to flow and volume.

The flow sensor is placed between the ETT and the breathing circuit [101].

Temperature

Temperature monitoring is important in all equine patients peri-operatively but particularly important in foals. All horses are susceptible to heat loss due to the vasodilatory effects of sedative and anaesthetic agents, which promote heat loss to the periphery. Perioperative hypothermia may be associated with an increased incidence of surgical-wound infection, weakness and ataxia during recovery [53]. Foals are particularly susceptible to hypothermia, owing to a large body surface area to mass ratio, minimal fat stores, depressed thermoregulatory centres in the brain and poor vasomotor tone [75]. Adverse effects of hypothermia include decreased anaesthetic requirements, prolonged recovery, bradycardia and hypotension unresponsive to catecholamine administration [75]. Methods to prevent and treat hypothermia should be instituted immediately at or before the onset of anaesthesia in foals [75]. Blankets, limb wraps and/or forced air warmers may be used to maintain normothermia depending on requirements and the ambient theatre temperature.

Equipment Observations

Oxygen analysers are incorporated into most anaesthesia monitors. Oxygen analysis can be performed in inhaled and exhaled gases and usually takes the form of a paramagnetic cell [102]. Volatile agent analysis can be carried out by some monitors. End-tidal and fractional-inspired volatile agent concentrations are displayed as a percentage. Oxygen cylinders should be checked before use to ensure that they contain enough oxygen for the anticipated anaesthetic duration. Spare cylinders should always be available and clearly labelled. A spare vaporiser should be available in case of equipment failure. Breathing systems and ETTs must be checked for leaks or imperfections prior to use. Leak testing is an important part of the pre-anaesthetic machine check and should be carried out prior to use in every patient.

Care Requirements of an Anaesthetised Equine Patient

Blood Loss

If a surgical procedure is anticipated to cause significant blood loss, the horse should be cross-matched before surgery to identify an appropriate blood donor or donor [87]. The blood volume of a horse is approximately 8% of its body weight (kg) [103]. Therefore, a 500-kg horse normally has about 40–50 l of blood [87]. Blood loss of less than 15% (<12 ml/kg) of total blood volume is often insignificant and may not be clinically detected [104]. It can often be fully compensated by physiological mechanisms and generally does not require fluid or blood-product therapy [105]. More severe haemorrhage, >25% of blood volume (>20 ml/kg), often requires crystalloid or blood product replacement. Acute blood loss of greater than 30% (>24 ml/kg) may result in haemorrhagic shock requiring resuscitation treatments [106, 107]. Blood loss of greater than 40% is characterised by marked clinical abnormalities, severe shock and imminent death [104].

Haemorrhage may also be classified as:

- Controlled haemorrhage (the haemorrhage has stopped).
- Uncontrolled haemorrhage, as often occurs with internal bleeding [108].
- Uncontrolled haemorrhage associated with internal bleeding (i.e. intracranial, thoracic, abdominal, or compartmental) or severe external haemorrhage (i.e. severe epistaxis associated with guttural pouch mycosis), which results in clinical signs of shock may yield a grave prognosis for survival in spite of appropriate attempts to resuscitate the patient [109].

The accurate quantification of blood loss can be difficult in the anaesthetised horse [107].

Changes in Physiological Parameters in Response to Haemorrhage

- **Haematocrit** (HCT) or PCV may not change significantly during acute severe blood loss in anaesthetised horses [107]. The PCV is typically unchanged during the first 12 hours in cases of mild or even moderate to severe blood volume loss [109].
- This is due to a delay in transcellular fluid shifts following acute blood loss, as well as splenic contraction and erythrocyte release in response to haemorrhage [104].
- **Total plasma protein (TPP)** follows a similar pattern to PCV alterations and may remain normal until fluid redistributes from the interstitial spaces. Hypoproteinaemia may be seen once transcellular fluid shifts have occurred [103, 109].
- **Heart rate:** if haemorrhage progresses to cause poor perfusion and poor delivery of oxygen, then low PCV and tachycardia may be seen [104].
- **Arterial blood pressure:** decreases in arterial blood pressure and pulse pressure can indicate acute blood loss [44]. Mean arterial pressure <60 mmHg is indicative of poor perfusion and poor oxygen delivery [104].
- **Oxygenation:** decreased PaO_2, SpO_2, venous oxygen saturation <50% can occur after severe acute haemorrhage in horses and may be indicative of poor tissue perfusion and oxygen delivery [104, 107]. As circulating red cell mass decreases, the oxygen-carrying capacity of the blood to deliver oxygen to the tissues wanes [109].

- **Peripheral tissue perfusion:** pallor, cold extremities and prolonged capillary refill time may occur in response to acute severe haemorrhage and can be indicative of poor tissue perfusion and oxygen delivery [104, 107].
- **Lactate:** elevated lactate (hyperlactaemia) >3–4 mmol/L after fluid resuscitation, metabolic acidosis and negative base excess can indicate poor perfusion and oxygen delivery after acute haemorrhage [104].

In cases of acute haemorrhage, changes in heart rate, respiratory rate, capillary refill time, and anxiety level are appreciated after approximately 15–20% of total blood volume is lost [104]. However, during GA, additional factors such as pre-haemorrhage arterial blood pressure and heart rate, surgical stimulation, body position, anaesthesia duration and administration of agents to support blood pressure may affect the physiological response to haemorrhage.

Methods used to quantify blood loss include:

- Weight differential of dry and used swabs.
- Suction bottle contents.
- Visual observation.
- Blood analysis.
- Changes in cardiovascular function associated with acute blood loss.

Urine Output

Urine output is an indicator of renal blood flow [59]. It may be used as an indirect marker of end-organ perfusion and fluid balance [59]. During GA, IV fluid therapy and the administration of drugs, including alpha-2 adrenoreceptor agonists may influence urine output [47]. Urine-specific gravity provides useful information in differentiating pre-renal azotaemia from renal failure [59]. Adult horses vary in terms of urine-specific gravity; however, dehydration should also result in concentrated urine, whereas renal failure yields isosthenuria [59, 110]. Urinalysis, with cytologic evaluation of sediment, complements the monitoring of renal function [59].

Treatment of Haemorrhage

One goal of routine IV fluid administration during inhalation anaesthesia is to maintain sufficient vascular volume and venous return to the heart despite anaesthetic-related vasodilation [87]. In the event of a haemorrhage, the administration of IV fluids and blood products should be tailored to the severity of the blood loss and the individual patient's physiological response.

Aim to support cardiac output and blood flow to vital organs and try to stop the bleeding [108]. If the haemorrhage can be controlled (for example, the vessel can be ligated), then initial efforts to resuscitate the horse should focus on increasing perfusion pressure and blood flow to organs as quickly as possible with crystalloids or colloids while assessing the need for whole blood transfusion [108]. IV fluids are needed to restore intravascular volume in cases of haemorrhagic shock. Unfortunately, these fluids can also dilute platelets and clotting factors and negatively affect clot formation [103]. The approach to fluid resuscitation requires consideration of the severity of the haemorrhage and the volume of blood lost together with the physiological response shown by the horse.

Crystalloids

Crystalloids can be defined based on their tonicity, use and/or electrolyte composition. Most crystalloids are isotonic, meaning that they have similar tonicity to fluid within the body, both intra- and extra-cellularly [111]. A variety of crystalloid fluids are available, but few are available in volumes large enough for the practical administration of horses. Most practices stock a single type of fluid. In general, it is a replacement fluid, as these are available in large sizes, are most commonly used, and can be given rapidly to patients in need of resuscitation [111]. Hartmann's solution or lactated ringers solution is commonly stocked by equine practices as a replacement fluid. These fluids have a composition that is similar to extracellular fluid but are not exactly the same. Therefore, given the electrochemical makeup of these fluids, maintaining patients on this type of fluids, beyond the initial replacement period, inevitably results in sodium loading and inadequate replacement of other electrolytes [111].

Isotonic Fluids

One of the most common reasons for fluid administration is the resuscitation of a critically ill patient with insufficient preload due to hypovolemic, distributive, or obstructive shock. These patients require rapid, significant intravascular volume expansion [111]. Rapid intravascular volume expansion is best achieved by administering fluids directly into the vascular space [111]. In order to achieve rapid administration of large volumes of fluid: a large (10–14) gauge catheter, wide-bore administration set, and the ability to suspend the fluids from a sufficient height above the horse are required [112]. Balanced crystalloid solutions such as Hartmann's solution can be used in relatively large volumes to improve circulating volume; however, the effect is relatively short-lived (20–30 minutes). After acute controlled haemorrhage, perfusion pressure and blood flow can be quickly improved by rapid (over 20–30 minutes) IV infusion of high volume (10 ml/kg) crystalloid solution (Hartmann's solution) [108]. The current approach is typically to administer a 10–20 ml/kg bolus of crystalloid followed by a reassessment of indicators of perfusion (e.g. heart rate, capillary refill time, pulse quality, extremity temperature, systemic lactate, urination, blood pressure) and intravascular volume (jugular fill) [113]. An additional infusion of 10–20 ml/kg may be needed to replace the blood volume lost from severe haemorrhage (>30% blood volume) [108]. Large-volume crystalloid replacement that allows the HCT to fall to an extremely low concentration could theoretically have a negative effect on microcirculatory flow by decreasing blood viscosity [114].

Hypertonic Saline

Available as a 7.2% solution with a high sodium content and a tonicity almost nine times that of plasma. Hypertonic saline has the potential of increasing both blood volume and blood pressure with low-volume administration due to the rapid shifts of the fluid between the cellular and interstitial spaces into the intravascular compartment following administration [108]. Administration of hypertonic solution results in significant and rapid fluid shifts into the intravascular space, initially from the other extracellular compartments (i.e. interstitial space) and will continue from the intracellular space [111]. After acute controlled haemorrhage, perfusion pressure and blood flow can be quickly improved by IV infusion of low volume (1–4 ml/kg) IV infusion of hypertonic saline. Hypertonic saline as a resuscitation fluid in haemorrhagic shock has been shown to have an immediate and favourable hemodynamic effect, decrease secondary inflammation via attenuating the leukocyte-activated endothelial damage, decrease the incidence of organ failure, and improve survival in some animal models of haemorrhagic shock [115]. In a model of induced haemorrhagic shock, administration of hypertonic saline resulted in rapid plasma volume expansion and urine output, along with sustained elevations in numerous cardiovascular parameters, including cardiac output, stroke volume, MAP and contractility [106].

Be aware that hypertonic solutions draw fluid from the interstitial space into the vascular space, therefore effectively depleting the interstitial space. Balanced isotonic crystalloid fluids (Hartmann's solution) can be used to replenish the interstitial space. For a sustained effect and to avoid ill effects of intracellular dehydration, hypertonic saline administration should be followed by larger quantities of IV isotonic replacement crystalloids [111]. Avoid the use of hypertonic solutions in foals due to the high sodium content. Despite such a rapid initial expansion, this effect is relatively short-lived, due to the redistribution of electrolytes and water across the vessel wall as expected with all IV crystalloid administration [111]. As a result of these fluid shifts, the effective expansion of circulating volume is in the order of 3.5 times the administered volume [113].

Colloids

Colloid administration generally has two goals: improving colloid oncotic pressure (COP) or inducing more rapid and sustained volume expansion than crystalloids during fluid resuscitation of critically ill patients [116]. Combining hypertonic saline and a synthetic colloid as an initial low-infusion volume treatment may be superior to hypertonic saline alone [117]. Although some synthetic colloids have been shown to be associated with acute kidney injury in people receiving resuscitation therapy, this undesirable effect in horses has not been reported [108]. Large volumes >10–20 ml/kg of colloids may impede coagulation. Statistically significant changes in coagulation testing. It should be recognised that most changes were mild, with values often remaining in the normal range and unlikely to be clinically significant [116]. Additional work is needed to evaluate these effects in clinical patients, particularly those more likely to be at risk for pre-existing thrombocytopenia, thrombocytopathies or coagulopathy [111], such as horses suffering from the effects of haemorrhage. Similar to a hypertonic saline infusion, colloid treatment may increase plasma volume 4 times compared to a similar volume treatment with a balanced isotonic crystalloid.

Natural Colloids

Natural colloids such as whole blood or plasma are often administered for a particular purpose in certain cases – such as replenishing red cells, plasma proteins and coagulation factors in the case of whole blood or for anti-endotoxic or coagulation benefits in the case of plasma [111].

Blood Products

If the horse has lost >30% blood volume and is suffering from haemorrhagic shock, it is likely that a whole blood transfusion will be needed as re-establishment of normal perfusion alone may not enable adequate oxygen delivery [108]. After the initial crystalloid treatments, whole blood transfusion should be strongly considered if clinical signs are not improving, HCT decreases to <18%, heart and respiratory rates remain above normal, blood lactate is not decreasing, or pulmonary venous oxygen tension remains <30 mmHg. These findings suggest the need for haemoglobin replacement [108].

Blood

Blood transfusion is a life-saving treatment for horses with acute haemorrhage [104]. Blood transfusions improve oxygen delivery to the tissues via increased blood volume and haemoglobin concentration [104]. Indications for blood transfusion may not be clear cut and an individual patient approach is warranted. The following factors may be indications for blood transfusion in cases of acute haemorrhage:

- Estimated blood loss greater than 30%.
- PCV less than 20% during an acute bleeding episode.
- Inadequate delivery of oxygen (DO_2) to the tissues, resulting from low haemoglobin (Hb) concentration [104].
- Blood lactate level of 4 mmol/L or more after fluid therapy.
- Oxygen extraction ratio 50% or greater [103].
- The delivery of oxygen to tissues (DO_2) is an important factor when considering the requirement for blood transfusion.
- DO_2 is determined by the oxygen content of the blood (CaO_2) and the cardiac output (Q) and can be calculated using the following formula [104]:

$$\text{Oxygen delivery} (DO_2) (mlO_2/100\,mL\,blood) = \text{Cardiac output (Q)} \times \text{Oxygen content of blood} (CaO_2)$$

where $CaO_2 = 1.36 \times [Hb] \times SaO_2 + (0.003 \times PaO_2)$; $[Hb]$ = haemoglobin concentration; SaO_2 = arterial oxygen saturation; PaO_2 = arterial oxygen tension and Q = (cardiac output = heart rate (HR) × stroke volume (SV)).

Fresh Whole Blood

Fresh whole blood is the blood product most commonly used to replenish red blood cell mass in horses [103]. There are over 400,000 possible equine RBC phenotypes, and no universal donor exists. Therefore, some blood type incompatibilities are likely between any donor and recipient. Therefore, prior to any blood transfusion, donor and recipient blood should be cross-matched [104]. However, in an emergency situation, a large, healthy gelding, can be used as a donor without prior testing, provided that both the donor and recipient are at a low risk of previous sensitisation to blood type alloantigens [104]. The ideal equine blood donor is a healthy, large (>500 kg), well-behaved gelding. No true universal donor exists, because there are 8 equine blood groups and 30 different factors [103].

Volume calculation [108]:

Litres of blood to transfuse =

$$[(\text{desired HCT} - \text{recipient HCT})/\text{donor HCT}] \times (0.08 \times \text{bodyweight (kg)})$$

The amount of blood required for transfusion can be estimated from the amount of blood lost during acute haemorrhage [103]. The entire blood volume lost does not need to be replaced, because volume has already increased through mobilisation of interstitial fluid, voluntary intake of water and administration of IV fluids. Approximately 25–50% of blood lost should be replaced, and packed red blood cells

(RBCs) may be used if concern exists about volume overload [103].

Administering the Transfusion

Pre-transfusion vital parameters should be recorded. The transfusion rate should not exceed 1 ml/kg for the first 15–30 minutes (0.25–0.5 ml/kg/hour), and the recipient's vital parameters should be closely monitored throughout the transfusion [104]. The infusion rate can be increased if no reactions are appreciated [104]. Transfusions should be completed in <4 hours to minimise potential bacterial growth [104]. Blood transfusions can be continued after recovery until the desired volume has been administered [104]. Fresh whole blood includes viable platelets and coagulation factors in plasma [103]. See Chapter 14 for more information regarding blood transfusions.

Packed RBCs

Packed RBCs are indicated for horses with chronic anaemia or those with acute blood loss and normovolaemia, such as when the volume has been replaced by crystalloid fluids [103]. However, stored blood can be affected by changes in pH, glucose, ATP and osmotic stability during storage, known as the 'storage lesion' [103]. Stored blood should be examined for storage lesions before use, and recommended maximum storage times should not be exceeded.

Plasma

Plasma transfusions are not useful for restoring oxygen-carrying capacity but may be used as an adjunctive treatment when colloid and clotting factors are desired [103].

Drainage and Collection of Fluids During Procedures
Urine Collection

Urinary bladder catheterisation is recommended in horses during GA to prevent contamination of the surgical site with urine. Urine collection also allows volume and urine-specific gravity to be monitored. Urinary catheters can be placed during GA in a theatre setting to minimise urine contamination in the operating theatre. They also enable monitoring of urine production and avoid excessive urination in the recovery box resulting in a wet, slippery floor [47]. See Chapter 17 for more information regarding urinary catheters.

Blood

Blood may be collected in a suction canister allowing volume and PCV to be measured. Swabs can be weighed to estimate the blood volume contained within the swabs.

Tourniquet Placement

Tourniquet placement has been associated with hypertension, and tourniquet deflation was associated with a decrease in blood pressure in anaesthetised horses [118]. Arterial hypertension and tachycardia developed within 15 minutes after a pneumatic tourniquet was placed 8–10 cm proximal to the right carpus and inflated to 800 mm of Hg [88]. Heart rate and mean arterial pressure decreased after the tourniquet cuff was deflated [88]. See Chapter 11 for more information.

Anaesthetic Records

In veterinary medicine, the vast majority of anaesthetic records are handwritten [56]. Maintaining an accurate and complete anaesthetic record is important in every case.

- Anaesthetic records are designed to allow entry of physiological data at 5-minute intervals throughout the anaesthetic duration.
- A free text column allows events to be recorded.
- Traditionally in human anaesthesia, records were handwritten. However, there is now a trend towards anaesthetic information management systems (AIMSs) [119].

Maintaining an Anaesthetic Record

The anaesthetic record is a medico-legal document [119]. The anaesthetic record is also useful for clinical communication, audit, education and research purposes [119].

Anaesthetic records require the insertion of different types of data:

- Quantifiable numerical value (e.g. heart rate, mean arterial blood pressure).
- Discrete elements comprised from predefined categories (e.g. pulse quality; good/moderate/poor) [119].
- Descriptive data (e.g. events which occurred).

The anaesthetic record:

- Provides a visual summary of the patient details, signalment, risk factors and an assessment of anaesthetic risk using the ASA physical classification score.
- Enables the anaesthetist to observe changing trends over time.
- Provides a snapshot of a range of physiological data which can be rapidly interpreted at any point during the anaesthetic period.
- Enables events to be recorded, which may facilitate discussion of a case retrospectively.

Positioning of the Anaesthetised Horse on the Operating Table

The responsibilities of the anaesthetist include the provision of a safe environment for the patient from the start of anaesthesia until after the animal has returned to standing in recovery [120].

- Conscious animals avoid uncomfortable postures, but with anaesthesia this protective mechanism is abolished [120] making it the responsibility of the theatre team to ensure optimal positioning and effective padding.
- In horses, the size of the body means that it is subjected to large forces during dorsal or lateral recumbency, and therefore small deviations from ideal positioning can have disastrous consequences [120].
- Poor positioning can result in trauma, neuropathy and/or myopathy [120].

Eye Protection

GA reduces or abolishes the protective palpebral reflex and decreases tear production in horses [121]. During GA and recovery, horses are at risk for corneal abrasions, so extra care should be taken to protect the eyes from drying or trauma during surgery or movement of the head [87]. Horses have laterally situated, prominent eyes, which may render them susceptible to trauma from physical contact with surfaces due to poor positioning, proximity of surgical drapes, contamination with surgical solutions or sweat during GA [122, 123]. Horses may be particularly susceptible to mechanical corneal trauma due to the position and prominence of their eyes, particularly during the anaesthetic induction and recovery periods, when direct corneal contact with the floor and walls of the recovery box is difficult to prevent [123].

In lateral recumbency:

- Lateral recumbency on the operating table was recognised as a risk factor for corneal abrasion in one prospective observation study [123].
- Ensure the eyelids of the dependent eye are closed.
- Ensure the non-dependent eye is lubricated. Use a single-use lubricant to avoid the potential for microbial contamination associated with multi-use vials.

In dorsal recumbency:

- Apply corneal lubrication.
- Use a single-use lubricant to avoid the potential for microbial contamination associated with multi-use vials.
- Ensure that both eyes are protected from mechanical trauma from drapes/equipment.
- Ensure that both eyes are protected from chemical trauma (e.g. solutions, particularly scrub solutions or sweat that may run down the face/cheek under the drapes).

Body Position and Padding

It is important that the whole of the horse's body is supported in the operating table [124]. Limb supports, inflatable cushions and foam wedges can be used to provide cushioning and support on the operating table. Fluid bags can also be useful, as these help to fill the small gaps that some cushions cannot [124]. The type of padding used on the operating table will vary according to the available facilities and preferences [120]. Foam mattresses should be firm and at least 30 cm thick. Mattresses should be covered with waterproof material to prevent contamination and slow its compression by reducing air leakage [120]. Air mattresses allow adjustment of the 'softness' of the surface depending on how much air is used to distend the mattress. Once the horse is positioned on the table, it is important that sufficient air is let out of the mattress to prevent the horse from lying on a hard surface [124]. Superficial nerves, such as the facial and radial nerves may be vulnerable to pressure damage during anaesthesia and recumbency. Special attention should be paid to padding and protecting these nerves from such pressure damage [87].

Dorsal Recumbency

- Ensure adequate padding under the animal to protect the back muscles [120].
- The padding should extend beyond the quarters of the horse and care must be taken not to allow the croup to overhang the table as this may result in damage to the cauda equina [120].
- The horse must be well supported at the shoulders. This will ensure that it is well-balanced and lies in a central position on the mattress [124].
- When hoisting the horse into the theatre, someone can be assigned to guiding the withers of the horse into the centre of the bed and positioning the shoulder cushions accordingly, depending on the size of the horse [124].
- The head should be carefully positioned in line with the body and padded to prevent the formation of pressure points. In particular, the poll should be well padded [124].
- Limbs should be supported so that they are not under tension.
- Avoid concurrent extension of both hindlimbs. This position places stress on the femoral nerves and possibly also the gluteal muscles [124]. Hyperextension of the pelvic limbs can cause femoral nerve paralysis [125, 126].

Lateral Recumbency

- Ensure that the entire body of the horse is supported by the padding.
- The head should be padded and positioned in as natural a position as possible [120].
- Remove the headcollar for the duration of anaesthesia to prevent the buckles or straps from exerting pressure on the facial nerve.

- The lower (dependent) forelimb should always be pulled forward to relieve pressure on the lower triceps muscle mass [120].
- The upper (non-dependent) forelimb should be supported but never pulled backward, as this disrupts venous drainage [127].
- Avoid forced extension of either forelimb as increased tension of the radial nerve may lead to overstretching [128] and the development of neuropathy.
- Be aware of and try to avoid abduction and/or endo-rotation of the scapula if the upper (non-dependent limb) is suspended in a semi-flexed position using a hoist. Abduction/endo-rotation of the scapula, consequent damage to the brachial plexus with possible vascular occlusion and ischaemia was hypothesised to be one possible cause of myopathy developing in the non-dependent limb in one case report [128].
- The hindlimbs should be supported slightly raised and parallel to each other. They should be supported sufficiently to allow a flat hand to be placed between the adductor muscles without difficulty [120].
- Ensure that the lower/dependent eye is protected when the horse is being moved.

Recovery Positioning

Horses should be allowed to recover from GA in an area that is safe and free from sharp objects, with a surface that provides sufficient padding to avoid muscle or nerve damage during recumbency, and good, non-slip footing when the horse attempts to stand [87]. Care should be taken over positioning for recovery. A box with a padded floor is ideal, but animals can be placed on a large pad in recovery if this is not available [120]. Mechanical trauma to the cornea may occur in recovery due to the position and prominence of horse's eyes and the difficulty in preventing physical contact between the eye and the floors and walls during recovery [123].

Anaesthetic Recovery

Recovery is a high-risk period during equine anaesthesia with studies indicating that most peri-anaesthetic complications occur during the recovery period [129–131]. Horses must be closely observed throughout the recovery process from a safe distance. While prompt intervention is important in the event of a recovery complication, it is imperative to ensure personnel safety during this potentially dangerous time. The recovery period commences when the horse is disconnected from the anaesthetic breathing system, or the administration of IV anaesthetic agents is ceased.

Monitoring horses during transfer to the recovery box is important since complications can arise during this process.

Disconnecting the Patient from the Anaesthetic Equipment and Materials

Horses that have received CMV during anaesthesia may experience a period of apnoea in recovery when the CMV is ceased. The apnoeic period may be of variable duration before spontaneous ventilation resumes [132]. Controlled ventilation during GA resulted in better oxygenation in the early recovery period but was associated with a period of apnoea [133]. Permissive hypercapnia during GA reduced the time to spontaneous ventilation during recovery and time to standing [134, 135].

Provision of Oxygen During Recovery

Oxygenation may be reduced during GA due to ventilation-perfusion inequality. The intrapulmonary shunt produced during GA persists in recovery while the horses remain in lateral recumbency, but oxygenation improves once they move to the sternal [136].

Methods to administer oxygen during recovery include:

Nasal Oxygen Insufflation

- Administration of nasal oxygen using flexible tubing.

Demand Valve

- Demand valves may be used to supplement oxygen during recovery. Demand valves increase the inspired oxygen fraction and supplement inspiration, which can improve hypoxaemia caused by hypoventilation in recovery [137].
- Oxygen delivered at 15 l/min via a demand valve or by insufflation into the trachea can help prevent hypoxaemia during recovery [137].
- The demand valve can be attached to the ETT and is able to deploy a flow rate of 60 l/min allowing a manual breath to be given to an adult horse.
- The valve mechanism allows a horse to activate the valve during spontaneous respiration, although deflating the ETT cuff is recommended during spontaneous respiration to reduce the airway resistance generated through the valve.
- Once the horse is breathing spontaneously and regularly, the demand valve is usually withdrawn.
- The flow rate of the demand valve must be appropriate for the size of a horse. Adult demand valves are not safe for use in ponies or foals.
- Demand valves must be used carefully to avoid increased dangerously high airway pressure [40].

Extubation

Once spontaneous respiration has returned and is regular, the ETT may be removed. It is very important to remember to deflate the ETT cuff prior to extubation. The timing of extubation may vary between anaesthetists and between patients. In some instances, the ETT may be left in place and secured until the horse returns to standing. If the ETT is removed, a nasopharyngeal or nasotracheal tube is often used to dilate the upper airway and maintain airway patency [138]. Nasal phenylephrine can be used to reduce the risk of upper airway obstruction [138]. Horses that have been positioned in dorsal recumbency intra-operatively can be at greater risk of post-anaesthetic partial upper airway obstruction due to increased nasal mucosal oedema [139].

Effects of Patient Positioning on Respiratory and Cardiovascular Function

The recumbency position of the horse during GA can have effects on every body system, the consequences of which must be considered by the anaesthetist. Dorsal recumbency was deemed to attract twice the anaesthetic risk compared to lateral recumbency in a survey of experienced equine anaesthetists [140]. If horses have been on the operating table in lateral recumbency, they should remain in the same recumbency during recovery unless there is a specified reason to change.

Respiratory Function

Recumbency greatly impacts ventilation because the diaphragm is dome-shaped in the horse and the pressure exerted by abdominal viscera forces air out of lung units causing collapse and the compression atelectasis to develop [101, 141].

Dorsal recumbency is associated with:

- Lower PaO_2 values compared to lateral recumbency [28].
- Greater gas exchange impairment compared to lateral recumbency [28].
- More compromised pulmonary function during GA compared with lateral recumbency, irrespective of the concentration of oxygen provided [100].
- A greater reduction in functional residual capacity and atelectasis formation as abdominal organs shift cranially to push against the diaphragm and thus compress a larger portion of both lungs leading to an increase in collapsing alveolar units [142].
- More severe ventilation–perfusion ratio (V/Q) abnormalities than horses placed in lateral recumbency [143].
- Lateral recumbency:
- Changing lateral recumbency (from one side to the other) should be avoided as it will worsen hypoxaemia [137].

Cardiovascular Function

Changing position from lateral to dorsal recumbency during hoisting may initially exacerbate hypotension secondary to shifting the weight of abdominal organs onto the caudal vena cava, thereby decreasing venous return to the heart [144].

Dorsal recumbency has been associated with more pronounced decreases in arterial blood pressure and cardiac output in spontaneously breathing anaesthetised ponies compared to lateral recumbency [145].

Effect of Hoisting on Cardiorespiratory Parameters

Mean arterial pressure temporarily decreases when horses are hoisted after isoflurane anaesthesia [144]. Arterial oxygenation decreases during hoisting and may remain below baseline when horses are returned back to left lateral recumbency [144]. Arterial carbon dioxide tension (PaCO$_2$) decreases during hoisting and may be associated with a mild increase in respiratory rate, which suggests adequate ventilation [144]. In systemically healthy horses, the observed functional impairments are not likely to be life-threatening, but the effects of hoisting may be more severe and longer lasting in systemically compromised horses and therefore much attention must be paid to monitoring blood pressures and oxygenation when hoisting sick equine patients [144].

Effects of Patient Positioning on Musculoskeletal System

Owing to the sheer weight of horses, the key to success is supporting all parts of the horse's body as well as possible [124]. In either lateral or dorsal recumbency, attention should be paid to good padding and positioning to avoid the development of pressure spots. In either lateral or dorsal recumbency, MAP should be maintained >70 mmHg to facilitate adequate microcirculation to muscles since the intra-compartmental pressure in the dependent muscles of adult horses, on an adequately padded surface can reach 30–40 mmHg [90].

Sedation During Recovery

Administration of an alpha-2 adrenoreceptor agonist immediately prior to recovery improves the quality of recovery compared to a control group receiving either saline or no drug administration [146]. Alpha-2 adrenoreceptor agonists provide analgesia but also increase the time available for the effects of the inhalational agents to wear off. If the horse attempts to rise while anaesthetics remains in the tissues following a long administration period, it may lead to repeated and unsuccessful attempts to stand, leading to a greater risk of injury [125].

Different alpha-2 adrenoreceptor agonists have been described for sedation recovery in horses:

- Xylazine (0.2 mg/kg IV) or romifidine (0.02 mg/kg IV) administered in the recovery box resulted in a better quality of recovery, fewer attempts to stand and better coordination compared to horses not receiving recovery sedation [147].
- Romifidine 0.02 mg/kg IV [148].
- Xylazine (0.1 mg/kg IV), detomidine (2 µg/kg IV) or romifidine (8 µg/kg IV) prior to recovery improved quality of recovery, prolonged times and decreased the number of attempts to stand compared to saline [149].
- Dexmedetomidine* 0.875 µg/kg [150].

*****Note:** dexmedetomidine is not currently licensed for use in horses in the United Kingdom.

Methods of Recovery

Unassisted

'Free' or unassisted recovery may be selected for horses whose temperaments preclude rope assistance. Unassisted recovery poses the minimum risk to personnel, but there may be a greater risk of injury to the horse or airway obstruction [83]. Horses usually rise from sternal recumbency by placing their front feet forward and contracting the extensor muscles of the hindlimbs to generate the force required to stand [83]. During this motion, the horse will move forward, so careful consideration should be given when positioning the horse for recovery. The environment should be quiet, calm and non-stressful [83]. The recovery room floor should be a dry, non-slip, compressible surface which provides traction even when set [83].

Methods of Assisted Recovery

Head and Tail Rope Assisted Recovery

Rope assistance may improve recovery time and quality in some horses. The decision to perform a rope-assisted recovery must be made considering individual patient, team and practice factors. Rope assistance cannot prevent fatalities in recovery [152]. Head and tail rope recovery aims to provide stability and direction to a horse during attempts to stand in recovery. One rope attaches to the halter and aims to control the direction of the horse's attempts to stand, while the second rope attached to the tail aims to assist and stabilise the horse during rising [152]. Research to date has shown conflicting results regarding rope-assisted recoveries. While some studies showed no benefit [153, 154], others have shown fewer attempts to stand, better recovery quality and fewer injuries in healthy horses assisted with ropes [155]. Rope-assisted recovery reduced fatal recovery complications and improved recovery quality in horses recovering from emergency colic surgery [131, 156].

Technical difficulties with ropes may include:

- Tangling of ropes around the legs
- Tail hair breakage
- Slipping of the knots
- Sudden release of head rope
- Loss of headcollar
- Tail fracture
- Facial nerve paralysis [152, 154, 155, 157]

A 'blanket' policy of rope recovery is not recommended due to the inherent variability in the temperament of horses and capabilities and experience of personnel [151]. At this time, insufficient evidence is available to permit a full recommendation regarding rope assistance during recovery from GA in horses [151]. The decision to use rope-assisted recovery must be made on an individual patient basis.

Sling Recovery

Sling recoveries have been described and seem to reduce the risk of injury in recovery, particularly in horses with existing musculoskeletal injuries [87]. Successful use of a sling requires more personnel, as well as experience in placing and fitting the sling on a recumbent horse [87]. Sedation is typically required, and some horses may fight the sling or refuse to cooperate [87].

Pool Recovery

Using a pool for recovery can be useful for recovering horses from GA when difficult recoveries are anticipated due to the horse's injury, size, demeanour, duration of anaesthesia, or risk of further injury [158]. The technique can be more time and labour-intensive than a standard stall recovery 169]. One study reported that 17% of horses developed pulmonary oedema after submersion in water [158]. Post-operative incisional infections may occur as a result of water submersion, and particular attention needs to be paid to surgical site closure and bandaging [158].

Pool-Raft System [159]

- During a pool recovery, a large animal sling is fitted to the anaesthetised horse, which is then hoisted up and placed into a rubber recovery raft. The raft is then lowered into a heated pool.
- The pool raft system avoids submersion of the horse in water as the horse is put into a rubber recovery raft.
- The technique allows the horse to float, which avoids the negative pulmonary effects which may be encountered with submersion in water.
- Once the horse begins to wake up, they are hoisted out of the pool and the raft and placed in a recovery box.

- Studies have shown the pool-raft system is a safe option for recovery from GA.
- Although the pool-raft system is not a fail-safe system, it appears to decrease the complications of recovering horses in a high-risk category.
- Potential disadvantages of this system are added expense and manpower necessary in building, maintenance, and usage, as well as size limitations of the raft itself.
- See Further Reading for more information.

Field Recovery Techniques

It is advised that a second vet or an RVN accompanies the primary veterinary surgeon when a field anaesthesic is planned [160]. Additional sedation is not usually required for recovery after short periods of anaesthesia [160]. However, the duration of anaesthesia and the temperament of the horse should be taken into consideration. If the horse does attempt to stand too soon, it may be ataxic. If it is safe to do so, administering sedation may prolong the period of recumbency [160]. After positioning the horse in lateral recumbency for recovery, a leadrope can be attached to the halter to control the horse once it stands [161]. Headcollars should be padded, and care should be taken to reduce pressure on the facial nerve from buckles and restraint techniques since facial nerve paralysis is a potential complication [160]. The horse's eye should be covered to reduce the amount of light stimulation. Ensure a quiet environment for recovery to reduce premature recovery and attempts to stand. Most horses will roll to sternal recumbency within 45 minutes and then stand shortly thereafter [162]. Most horses will stand within 20–40 minutes of the end of field anaesthesia. Enough time should be allowed for the veterinarian to stay for the entire recovery period [160]. Do not closely restrain the head of the horse as it attempts to stand [162]. The handler holding the rope should wear protective gloves and a hat. Ensure the immediate environment is free of obstacles/hazards and people.

The area selected for performing GA in a horse, should be at least 4 × 4 metres in size and should be free from obstruction [162]. Horses tend to place their front feet forward and then push themselves to a standing position with the use of the rear legs [162].

Assessment of When Patient Can Safely Return to Stable

Horses should remain in the recovery suite until ataxia and incoordination associated with recovery from GA have resolved. Full muscle strength should be present before attempts are made to return the horse to the stable. Stumbling or limb knuckling is a sign of muscle weakness and an indication that the horse is not ready to return to the stable. No signs of nystagmus or evidence of visual disturbances should be present.

Post-anaesthetic Complications

The recovery period after GA is a time of high risk in horses. The vast majority of fatalities occur in recovery [129–131]. In horses, the recovery phase of anaesthesia is the least controllable component of the horse's overall anaesthetic experience [163], making this phase potentially dangerous for intervention by personnel.

Limb Fracture

Fractures that occur during recovery, while not common, are one of the most devastating complications of equine anaesthesia [87]. Limb fracture was the most common reason for recovery fatality in the preliminary findings of a recent, large, multi-centre study where limb fractures accounted for 28% of all peri-anaesthetic fatalities in horses ASA I-II [3]. Horses undergoing fracture repair are also at increased risk of repeat fractures at the surgery site. This was the most common cause of recovery fatality in horses ASA III in a recent large multi-centre study [3]. In the event of a horse sustaining a suspected fracture during recovery, imaging may be required to clarify the site and nature of the injury. Sedation or re-induction of GA may also be required to enable safe examination.

Cardiorespiratory Abnormalities

Hypotension, hypoventilation, hypoxaemia, hypothermia and dysrhythmias may occur both during maintenance of anaesthesia and also in recovery [138]. Monitoring of horses from a safe distance during the recovery phase facilitates early identification of these abnormalities and allows prompt intervention. Horses should be continuously observed during the recovery phase to facilitate early identification of a complication.

Post-anaesthetic Myopathy Neuropathy Syndrome (PAMNS)

In clinical cases, the neurogenic and myogenic components of PAMNS may occur separately, concurrently or in subsequent order [128]. Post-anaesthetic myopathy usually occurs in muscles of the trunk or legs but smaller muscles, such as the masseter may be affected [164]. Nerves affected, which have been reported, include facial, radial, obturator, peroneal and facial [40]. Neuropathy and myopathy may be hard to distinguish, which may lead to under-reporting of neuropathy. The aetiology of PAMNS is complex. Contributing factors are thought to include:

- Lateral body position [126, 165]
- Bodyweight [126]
- Intra-compartmental muscle pressure (ICMP)
- Hypotension with associated inadequate tissue perfusion [166, 167]
- Venous stasis [128]
- Length of procedure [165–167]

Post-anaesthetic myopathy and/or neuropathy has a reported incidence of between 0.02% and 0.9% [129, 130, 165, 168–170]. In lateral recumbency, PAMNS can occur in the dependent [171], or the non-dependent limb [128], indicating that care must be taken with the positioning and padding of all limbs. ICMP is greater in the triceps and extensor carpi radialis muscle masses of the dependent forelimb compared to the non-dependent limb in lateral recumbency [171]. An increase in ICMP and a reduction in muscle perfusion can occur if the venous return is obstructed by limb positioning [127]. This can lead to compartmental syndrome developing, where a decrease in muscle perfusion can cause severe myopathy [73].

This syndrome can occur in any group of muscles that are contained within an inextensible envelope or compartment, usually made up of muscle fascia and adjacent periosteum [73] (Figure 10.27). Within such a compartment, there is no outlet for the relief of applied pressure and a reduced ability to expand in volume. This leads to an increased internal pressure. In the compartmental syndrome, the cycle of events is set up as follows [73]:

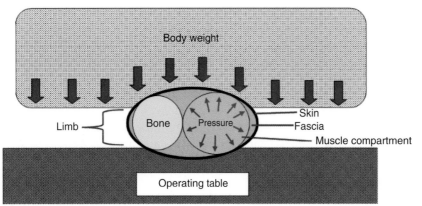

Figure 10.27 Compartmental syndrome. An osteofascial compartment that cannot expand in volume is prone to the development of compartmental syndrome if the pressure within the compartment rises. On the operating table, the horses' body weight pressing on the dependent limb muscles causes pressure in such osteofascial compartments to increase [73]. *Source:* Rosina Lillywhite.

- Pressure in the compartment rises either due to external pressure or trauma-induced damage, causing cellular swelling.
- The increased pressure prevents capillary perfusion and causes ischaemia (blood supply restriction).
- Ischaemia causes hypoxia, which causes further cell damage and swelling.
- Swelling increases the pressure and the cycle continues.

Maintaining a MAP greater than 70 mmHg is recommended during GA since the ICMP in the dependent muscles of adult horses, on an adequately padded surface, reaches 30–40 mmHg [90] and vascular transmural pressure needs to be greater than 30 mmHg to support adequate microcirculation [91]. PAMNS has also been reported to affect the non-dependent limb, indicating that positioning of the non-dependent forelimb should be done judiciously [128]. Clinical signs of PAMNS are first seen in the recovery period and include pain or discomfort resulting in box walking and sweating [40]. Hard, swollen, painful muscles are seen and in severe cases the horse will be unable to stand. Myoglobin released into the circulation from damaged muscles may lead to the production of myoglobinuria or dark red/brown urine [73]. Large quantities of myoglobin may block and cause damage to the renal tubules, which can cause pain and, in some cases, fatal renal failure [73]. PAMNS has a direct influence on recovery and may increase the probability of catastrophic injury [128]. Treatment for PAMNS is largely supportive and patient-specific but may include:

- Administration of IV fluids: This can help to prevent myoglobin accumulation in the renal tubules. Large volumes (20–40 l) of IV crystalloids should be given [73]. Any acid–base imbalances should be corrected.
- Administration of analgesia: Pain can be severe in some cases, so analgesia is required on welfare grounds and to improve safety for the personnel handling the horse [73].
- Administration of sedation: May help to calm the horse and ease discomfort [73].
- Administration of acepromazine: To promote vasodilation and therefore muscle perfusion.
- Application of a sling or support bandages [163]: Maintaining the horse in a sling is ideal if they will tolerate it. However, this will specialist equipment and experienced personnel.
- In the absence of a sling, the horse should not be forced to keep attempting to stand, as this may cause further damage [73].
- If the patient is recumbent they should be maintained in sternal recumbency to reduce the risk of hypostatic pneumonia developing. If this is not possible, they should be turned every four hours if it is practical and safe to do so.

- Food and water should be provided close by if the patient is recumbent.
- The horse should be kept warm and comfortable. The application of grooming, massage and tender loving care (TLC) will improve the horses' demeanour and can contribute to their recovery [73].
- Clinical improvement in PAMNS is usually seen within 12–24 hours [163].

Colic

Post-anaesthetic colic (PAC) is the most common peri-anaesthetic complication in horses [170–172]. The cause of PAC may be multifactorial. Factors which may contribute to the development of PAC may include:

- The effect of sedative or anaesthetic agents on gastrointestinal motility [173, 174].
- Management changes associated with hospitalisation including altered dietary intake, disturbed or altered water intake.
- Administration of opioids [172].
- Peri-operative pain [175].
- The surgical procedure [176].
- Increasing anaesthetic duration [177].

When PAC occurs, it is most likely to occur on the day of or the day after surgery [170] or within 72 hours of surgery [172]. In many cases, a specific cause of colic may not be identified. Pelvic flexure impaction, large colon displacement, caecal impaction, caecal distension, ileus and peritonitis have been reported as types of PAC [170]. Diarrhoea/colitis was seen in 4.6% of PAC cases in one large single-centre study [170]. The treatment required depends on the specific cause of the colic.

Post-anaesthetic Ileus

The diagnosis is based on small intestinal dysmotility and/or distension with reflux of large volumes of intestinal content, tachycardia, abdominal discomfort, reduced faecal output or absent borborygmi [178]. After colic surgery, post-operative ileus was estimated to occur in up to 20% of cases [178]. Medical therapy may include fluid therapy, parenteral nutrition, flunixin and/or prokinetic agents, including lidocaine or metoclopramide. Fluid therapy and/or parenteral nutrition may also be required [178].

Spinal Cord Malacia

A rare complication, however, is the occurrence of spinal cord malacia almost always necessitating euthanasia. Most cases are in young male horses (<2 years of age) undergoing anaesthesia of less than 1.5 hours duration [40]. While the precise aetiology remains unknown, the following mechanisms have been proposed:

- Reduced perfusion and ischaemia of the spinal cord in dorsal recumbency [179].
- Reduced venous return due to compression of the vena cava by abdominal contents [180–182].
- Vitamin E deficiency destabilising spinal cord membranes [183].
- Stretch ischaemia of the spinal cord, verminous arteritis and embolism [184].

In recovery, affected horses struggle to stand and show progressive paraparesis or paraplegia of the hindlimbs [40]. This often means that the horse presents in a dog-sitting position. Over time, clinical signs progress and the forelimbs may also become affected. Reports have indicated that euthanasia is required in all cases [40]. Histopathological findings depended on the duration and severity of clinical signs [40].

Airway Obstruction

Airway obstruction during recovery can cause pulmonary oedema, which is often fatal if airway patency is not restored extremely quickly [40].

Airway obstruction may occur as a result of:

- Bilateral laryngeal paralysis.
- Nasal mucosa hyperaemia and obstruction of the external nares in the recovery box [32].

Pulmonary oedema resulting from upper airway obstruction has been referred to as negative pressure pulmonary oedema (NPPO), as the development of large negative intra-thoracic pressures is probably involved [32]. Clinical signs include tachypnoea, dyspnoea, presence of pink frothy fluid at the nares and mouth, distress and abnormal lung sounds [185–187]. When the airway is obstructed, the priority is to restore patency, for example, by performing endotracheal intubation or tracheostomy [32]. Oxygen insufflation can be achieved via the ETT or tracheostomy site using suitably sized tubing [32]. Acepromazine may be useful as it decreases anxiety and lowers systemic and pulmonary blood pressures [32]. Endobronchial suction may be needed to remove fluid in the proximal airway [187], while terminal airways may require diuretic therapy, such as furosemide. Other treatments may include bronchodilators, NSAIDs or glucocorticoids [32].

10.6 Anaesthetic Emergencies

This section will discuss the anaesthetic emergencies which may occur during GA in equine patients. As far as possible, these emergencies should be prevented; however, if they do

occur, they must be recognised and treated promptly to avoid potentially life-threatening consequences.

Hypoxaemia

Hypoxaemia is reduced arterial oxygen concentration and is best diagnosed using arterial blood gas analysis [188]. Cyanotic mucous membranes may be seen if the hypoxaemia is severe.

Causes of intraoperative hypoxaemia include:

- Respiratory depression leads to hypoventilation due to anaesthetic agents used.
- Ventilation-perfusion mismatch: This is where blood flowing through the compressed lungs of an anaesthetised horse does not become fully oxygenated because the compressed lung is poorly ventilated [73]. This problem is exacerbated in large horses positioned in dorsal recumbency [188].
- Ventilation perfusion mismatch also occurs when normally ventilated areas of the lung are not perfused.
- Lung atelectasis (collapse): The two primary causes of atelectasis are compression of lung tissue and absorption. Absorption atelectasis occurs when gases in an expanded alveolus are absorbed rapidly across the alveolar membrane into the bloodstream, and this leads to alveolar collapse [49]. Once alveolar collapse has occurred, it tends to stay collapsed. If this occurs in a large number of alveoli, it can result in a significant area of atelectasis, and this will significantly impair gas exchange [49].
- Reduced delivery or failed delivery of oxygen in the event of pipeline failure or an empty cylinder.

Treatment of intra-operative hypoxaemia includes [188]:

- Administering oxygen with an inspired concentration of 100%.
- Check for a respiratory obstruction and, if present, amend this immediately.
- Use PIVA techniques to enable a reduction in inhalational agent concentration.
- IPPV and other ventilation strategies, such as ARM or PEEP ventilation.
- Maximise cardiac output by administering fluid therapy and positive inotropes such as dobutamine if required.
- Administration of aerosolised salbutamol via the ETT [189].

Hypercapnia

Hypercapnia is increased arterial carbon dioxide concentration. It is usually diagnosed via blood gas analysis [188].

Causes of intraoperative hypercapnia include:

- Anaesthetic agents can cause central respiratory depression. This can lead to hypoventilation and carbon dioxide retention [73].
- A disease or a body condition that restricts thoracic movement and therefore tidal volume. This results in impaired ventilation and hypercapnia.
- Hypercapnia often leads to respiratory acidosis, which increases sympathetic stimulation, and this has the potential to increase the chance of cardiac dysrhythmias, in the presence of volatile anaesthetic agents [73].
- A degree of hypercapnia is acceptable and can have beneficial effects on arterial blood pressure; however, if readings rise above 60–70 mmHg treatment should be initiated.
- The decision to treat hypercapnia can also be based on blood gas analysis readings. The pH should not fall below 7.20 where possible [73].

Treatment of intra-operative hypercapnia includes [73]:

- Reducing the depth of anaesthesia. This may improve ventilation by reducing the level of respiratory depression. PIVA can be used to facilitate this process.
- Carbon dioxide retention can easily be treated by increasing ventilation. This can be achieved effectively with IPPV.

Hypotension

Hypotension is low blood pressure and is usually diagnosed through direct blood pressure monitoring. Hypotension is defined as a MAP reading below 70 mmHg. It is a major contributing factor in the development of post anaesthetic myopathy. Maintaining normal blood pressure is also vital to maintain blood flow to vital organs such as the kidneys.

Causes of intraoperative hypotension include [188]:

- Vasodilation is caused by volatile agents.
- Hypovolaemia. This can be relative due to vasodilation, or absolute due to a reduced circulating volume in a normal vascular space.
- Acid–base balance and electrolyte disturbances.
- Cardiac arrhythmias.
- Pre-existing conditions such as shock and diseases causing cardiovascular derangements such as colic.

Treatment of intraoperative hypotension [188]:

- Minimise cardiovascular depression caused by anaesthetic agents, including lightening the plane of anaesthesia where possible.
- Administration of IV fluid therapy to support the cardiovascular system.

- Administration of positive inotropes to increase the contractility of the heart and raise the blood pressure. Dobutamine is commonly used as it has a rapid onset and short duration of action. Dobutamine is carefully administered to effect by IV infusion. Overdose can cause tachycardia and cardiac arrhythmias. Therefore, careful monitoring is required during administration.

Respiratory Obstruction

Respiratory obstruction is covered in Section 10.5.

Respiratory Arrest

Respiratory arrest is the cessation of breathing, and this results in apnoea. This can easily be recognised by an absence of chest movements, an absence of breathing bag movements and an absence of expired CO_2 (if capnography is being used). If apnoea is left untreated, life-threatening hypoxaemia and hypercapnia will occur [190]. Apnoea can occur during induction and after placement of the ETT. Apnoea most commonly happens after a horse is moved from a ventilator and placed in recovery. There is often a period of apnoea before spontaneous breathing resumes after IPPV is ceased.

Causes of respiratory arrest:

- Respiratory obstruction. The ETT should be checking for kinks.
- Excessive resistance in the breathing circuit. The breathing circuit should be checked, and any problems rectified. For example, the APL valve is closed during spontaneous ventilation.
- Anaesthetic overdose leading to CNS depression and cardiac arrest. Anaesthetic depth should be checked and amended as required.
- Severe respiratory disease or the effect of endotoxaemic shock in colics. For example, this can cause cardiorespiratory arrest, which may present first as respiratory arrest.

Treatment of respiratory arrest:

- Manual stimulation of the larynx or a firm compression of the chest.
- Surgical stimulation may be successful in the restoration of breathing.
- IPPV should be initiated if spontaneous respiration does not resume.
- It is important to establish and manage the underlying cause of apnoea for the anaesthetic to proceed safely [190].

Cardiopulmonary Arrest (CPA)

Types of Arrest

Respiratory and cardiac arrest may occur together as these systems are intrinsically linked within the body, or one may follow the other. Whatever the initiating cause, or which system was affected first, a vicious cycle is entered into and eventually arrest of both systems occurs. This is known as a CPA [191].

There are two types of CPA: acute and chronic. Acute arrests are not expected [191]; for example, a healthy horse undergoing a castration who has been anaesthetised a bit too deeply and stops breathing. If the arrest was recognised and treated immediately, the prognosis would be better than for a chronic arrest. Chronic arrests are multifactorial [191]; for example, a geriatric horse with severe equine asthma (formally known as recurrent airway obstruction or RAO) who is already hypoxemic is undergoing colic surgery for a large colon torsion, which has caused dehydration, hypovolaemia and endotoxaemia. These conditions superimpose until the myocardium can no longer cope, arrhythmias develop and the heart stops. The prognosis for these cases is poor [191].

Recognising the Signs of CPA

Clinical signs of CPA are as follows [188]:

- No palpable pulse
- No heart sounds
- Absent palpebral and corneal reflexes
- Altered capillary refill
- Cyanotic or pale mucous membranes
- Central eye position
- Pupillary dilation
- Respiratory arrest seen as apnoea or terminal gasping
- No haemorrhage at the surgical site

Monitoring modalities such as an ECG, capnography, IBP monitoring and pulse oximetry can help to identify the signs of CPA quickly enough for treatment to be successful.

ECG abnormalities that may pre-empt CPA include [192]:

- Asystole
- Ventricular rhythm
- Ventricular fibrillation (Figure 10.28)
- Markedly irregular or slow ECG activity

Capnography can help to identify decreases in CO. A capnograph steps down during CPA as ETCO$_2$ decreases. This capnograph pattern is only associated with the development of CPA. IBP monitoring will show a loss of the arterial wave or a sudden reduction in mean arterial blood pressure. Pulse oximetry will show a reduction in oxygen saturation.

If an unusual ECG rhythm is noted, the pulse rhythm and quality should be checked immediately [192]. One of the difficulties with the identification of CPA is that the horse can appear to be becoming light [73]. Signs such as nystagmus, blinking, agonal breathing and jerking of the limbs often prompt the anaesthetist to increase the volatile agent. By the time these signs disappear the horse is brain dead, and resuscitation is unlikely to be successful [73]. The success of resuscitation attempts relies on the speed of detection [73]. CPA may occur for a variety of reasons, including hypoxia, hypercapnia, inhalation agent overdose and vagal stimulation leading to asystole [73].

Cardiopulmonary Cerebral Resuscitation (CPCR)

The immediate goals of resuscitation during CPA are to re-establish myocardial and cerebral perfusion and oxygenation; hence, 'cerebral' has been added to cardiopulmonary resuscitation, which is now known as CPCR [191].

Equine-specific evidence-based guidelines for CPCR are currently lacking, and there are substantial variabilities in techniques used in practice. This section will give an overview of current recommendations for equine CPCR; however, in the event of an emergency, practice protocol should be followed. The reader is also encouraged to refer to the Veterinary Emergency and Critical Care Society Reassessment Campaign on Veterinary Resuscitation (RECOVER) guidelines detailed in the Further Reading section.

Preparing for CPCR

Organised management of the CPCR procedure is essential to its success. Before every surgery, roles should be assigned to members of staff should CPCR be required. These include, as a minimum:

- One person to take charge and oversee the procedure. This should be the anaesthetist.

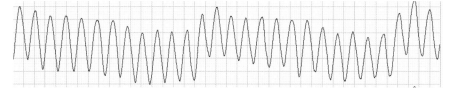

Figure 10.28 Ventricular fibrillation. This is a fatal dysrhythmia where there are no organised ventricular depolarisations. *Source:* Dr Gayle Hallowell.

- One person to take responsibility for IPPV and control of the anaesthetic circuit under the direction of the anaesthetist.
- One person to draw up medication as required and record any interventions carried out.
- At least two people to perform chest compressions. This is a mentally and physically exhausting procedure and should not be attempted by one person alone.
- One person to monitor the patient and attach any extra monitoring equipment required.

Regular resuscitation simulations should take place, as this allows staff to become familiar with what will happen and what their role will be in event of a CPA. Simulations will also facilitate the identification of broken or missing equipment [193].

A 'crash box' containing a selection of needles and syringes, IV catheters, fluid-giving sets, a tracheostomy tube and a stethoscope should always be close to hand. The crash box should also contain appropriate medication (see 'Advanced Life Support' section. The contents of the crash box should be checked and restocked regularly. The dates of any medications contained in the crash box should be noted and changed when they become close to exceeding the expiry date. A chart of drug doses for emergency situations should remain in the crash box permanently.

Immediate Action

Before any action is taken, the following must be considered:

- Is resuscitation appropriate? Is this an acute arrest or a chronic arrest, and what does this mean for the prognosis of the patient?
- Has informed consent has been obtained from the owner? The conversation surrounding resuscitation should have been had during the admission of the patient. Alternatively, details regarding resuscitation are often explained on the consent form.

If resuscitation is to go ahead, the time should be noted, and extra help should be requested. The horse must be immediately positioned in the right lateral recumbency. This can be difficult if the patient is undergoing abdominal surgery in dorsal recumbency. Depending on the circumstances, the abdomen can be packed quickly and secured with two or three sutures through all layers of the abdominal wall [192]. If the horse is undergoing an elective procedure such as an arthroscopy, it might be advisable to move the patient to the recovery box before initiating CPCR. The reason for this is that if the horse is successfully resuscitated, it will be awake and moving, and therefore more difficult and dangerous to hoist. This is situation-dependent and will be decided by the anaesthetist in charge of the case.

The volatile anaesthetic agent should be turned off, and 100% oxygen should be given at a flow rate of 10–15 l/min. The pressure relief valve on the anaesthetic circuit should be opened, and the emergency oxygen flush button pressed to flush out as much anaesthetic agent as possible [192]. If this is not possible, room air is now thought to be as just as effective [193].

Basic Life Support (BLS)

The order of BLS used to be Airway (A), Breathing (B) and Circulation (C); however, recent changes have seen the prioritisation of C in both human and now veterinary medicine [191]. A and B are still important, but starting C as soon as possible can lead to a more favourable outcome. It has been suggested that the original prioritisation of A, B and C may be more appropriate for foals [193]. This decision would remain with the anaesthetist in charge of the case at the time of the CPA.

Circulation
Cardiac Pump Chest Compressions

External chest compressions in horses used to focus on the 'cardiac pump' method, which was centred on chest compressions over the heart area. The cardiac pump method is based on the theory that alternate chest compressions squeeze and release the heart, establishing a forward flow through the chambers [191]. Practically, this involves a member of staff jumping onto the horse, landing with the knee and shin on the high point of the thorax, just behind the triceps muscle mass [192]. This poses a risk of injury to the person performing the compressions and to the horse, who could sustain rib fractures as part of the procedure.

Thoracic Pump Chest Compressions

The 'thoracic pump' method of chest compressions is now recommended to aid circulation in foals or adult horses [193]. In this method, the aim is to evoke pressure changes in the chest. Positive pressure occurs during the compression of the chest, and negative pressure occurs during release and chest wall recoil. This facilitates alternating cardiac output and venous return, which serves to establish a one-way blood flow [191]. With this method, the horse or foal is placed in lateral recumbency, and the hands of the person performing the chest compressions should be placed over the widest portion of the chest wall (caudodorsally). The chest should be depressed to approximately 30–50% of its width [194] with a 1 : 1 compression to relaxation rate at 100 compressions per minute [195].

Whichever method is used, performing chest compressions on horses and foals is exhausting. Recommendations are to change the person performing chest compressions every 2–3 minutes as they fatigue and will end up performing the compressions ineffectively [193]. The success of chest compression is most effectively monitored by measuring end-tidal carbon dioxide (ETCO$_2$). A reading of 12–18 mmHg is suggestive of adequate cardiac output [193]. If ETCO$_2$ is unavailable, pupil size can be monitored to assess the effectiveness of chest compressions. Marked dilation of the pupils occurs when blood flow to the brain is substandard. Pupils will be neutral in size if blood flow to the brain is adequate [193]. Chest compressions should be continuous. The ECG is an essential monitoring tool during CPCR as it provides information on heart rhythm, and this information can be used to inform interventions such as drug administration or defibrillation. Unfortunately, ECGs are suspectable to motion artefacts, and this means that meaningful rhythm analysis cannot be obtained during chest compressions [196]. Therefore, chest compressions must be paused for essential rhythm analysis to take place. Recommendations are the chest compressions should not be stopped for more than 10 seconds every 2 minutes for monitoring to occur [193].

Internal Cardiac Massage

Internal cardiac massage can be carried out in the horse, but this involves thoracotomy to allow direct access to the heart and is rarely performed.

Airway

If the patient is not already intubated, an ETT should be placed immediately. The ETT should be checked for patency, and the anaesthetic circuit and oxygen supply should be checked to ensure optimal function.

Breathing

IPPV should be initiated even if the horse or foal appears to be breathing for themselves [73]. A ventilator is the preferred method for IPPV. Manual techniques in adult horses can be effective but will be physically tiring for the operator. If foals are not intubated, and breaths are being given using a self-inflating bag valve device, some coordination between breaths and chest compressions will be required [193]. One fast breath should be given every 10 seconds [193]. Resuscitative measures can be continued for as long as there are still signs of brain activity [73]. However, if no response is seen after 15–20 minutes, resuscitation is unlikely to be successful [191].

Advanced Life Support (ALS)

Once BLS has been carried out, ALS can begin. ALS includes Drugs (D), Electrical defibrillation (E) and Follow-up (F). By this stage, any monitoring equipment available should be attached if this has not already been done so. Stages D, E and F can be carried out more or less at the same time, guided by monitoring devices, the ECG in particular [191].

Drugs

The evidence for value of the use of pharmacological agents in CPCR is either completely lacking or weak [193]. Nevertheless, if drugs are to be administered, they should be prescribed by the veterinary surgeon in charge of the anaesthetic. RVNs can work out drug doses, draw up medication and administer medication under the direction of the veterinary surgeon. Drugs used for resuscitation should be administered IV as absorption from sublingual and intratracheal administration is poor at best [193]. Administering drugs directly into the heart is no longer recommended.

Depending on the underlying arrest rhythm, the assumed cause of the arrest, the duration of CPCR, administration of vasopressors, anticholinergics and antiarrhythmics may be indicated as part of ALS [196]. Vasopressors can be beneficial during CPCR as they act to redistribute blood flow from peripheral vascular beds to the heart, brain and lungs via an increase in vascular tone [196]. The most commonly used vasopressor is adrenaline, which is used at low doses during CPCR. High doses have been associated with adverse effects in humans. One reason for this is that adrenaline causes an increase in myocardial oxygen consumption and therefore an increase in the incidence of ventricular tachyarrhythmias after the return of spontaneous circulation (ROSC) [196].

Vasopressin is becoming increasingly popular for use either instead of adrenaline or alongside it during CPCR. Vasopressin acts via a different receptor system from adrenaline and may convey a more reliable increase in vascular tone [196]. Vasopressin is less likely to increase myocardial oxygen consumption and therefore reduces the risk of post-ROSC cardiac tachyarrhythmias compared to adrenaline [196]. Clinical evidence to support the use of vasopressin over adrenaline is lacking in the horse; therefore, vasopressin administration may be considered interchangeably or in combination with adrenaline during CPCR.

Atropine is an anticholinergic drug and is no longer recommended for routine use during CPCR unless a vagal event has triggered the CPA [193]. This is more common during acute gastrointestinal, respiratory or ocular disease [196]. Antiarrhythmic drugs such as lidocaine or magnesium sulphate may be administered to treat ventricular fibrillation. In a situation where there is no defibrillator available and the patient is in ventricular fibrillation, the efficacy of these drugs is likely to be low [196]. Doxapram is a respiratory stimulant and is no longer recommended for use in CPCR. It increases cerebral and myocardial oxygen demand and can be detrimental when a patient is already hypoxaemic [191].

The use of other drugs such as corticosteroids, calcium and sodium bicarbonate are controversial and depends on the individual circumstances surrounding the CPA [191].

Electrical Defibrillation

Electrical defibrillation is the method of choice for the conversion of pulseless ventricular tachycardia or ventricular tachycardia to sinus rhythm [196]. Electrical defibrillation is not recommended for asystole [191]. Electrical defibrillators are rarely available in equine practice. Where they are available, they should be used with caution.

Follow-up

Aftercare and treatment will depend on the status of the patient as well as the original cause of the CPA. Heart rhythm abnormalities and hypotension may require treatment. If atropine has been used, small doses of dobutamine should be given to prevent severe tachycardia [73]. The cause of the original CPA should be investigated and treated.

CPCR Success

CPCR has a place in equine veterinary practice. Efforts in foals and ponies are more likely to be effective; however, success in adult horses has been reported [197]. A favourable outcome depends on prompt identification of the CPA, the type of arrest and therefore the prognosis for the patient, organised and well-trained staff and the instigation of an effective CPCR process.

Acknowledgement

With thanks to The Philip Leverhulme Equine Hospital for their assistance in gaining images for this chapter.

References

1 Moreno-Martinez, F., Mosing, M., and Senior, M. (2022). Controlled mechanical ventilation in equine anaesthesia: physiological background and basic considerations (part 1). *Equine Veterinary Education* 34: 320–329. https://doi.org/10.1111/eve.13476.

2 West, J.B. and Luks, A. (2016). Ventilation-perfusion relationships: how matching of gas and blood determines gas exchange. In: *West's Respiratory Physiology: The Essentials*, 10e (ed. J.B. West and A. Luks), 63–86. Alphen aan den Rijn: Wolters Kluwer.

3 Gozalo-Marcilla, M., Bettschart-Wolfensberger, R., Johnston, M. et al. (2021). Data collection for the fourth multicentre confidential enquiry into perioperative equine fatalities (CEPEF4) study: new technology and preliminary results. *Animals* 11: 2549. https://doi.org/10.3390/ani11092549 (accessed 29 November 2022).

4 Keys, T.E. (1975). Historical vignettes: Dr. Arthur Ernest Guedel 1883–1956. *Anesthesia & Analgesia* 54 (4): 442–443. https://doi.org/10.1213/00000539-197507000-00008 (accessed 29 November 2022).

5 Gleerup, K.B. and Lindegaard, C. (2016). Recognition and quantification of pain in horses: a tutorial review. *Equine Veterinary Education* 28: 47–57. https://doi.org/10.1111/eve.12383 (accessed 29 November 2022).

6 Dugdale, A. (2010). Pain. Chapter 3. In: *Veterinary Anaesthesia. Principles to Practice* (ed. A. Dugdale), 8–30. Wiley Blackwell.

7 Sanchez, L.C. and Robertson, S.A. (2014). Pain control. *Equine Veterinary Journal* 46: 517–523. https://doi.org/10.1111/evj.12265 (accessed 29 November 2022).

8 Gozalo-Marcilla, M. and Ringer, S.K. (2021). Recovery after general anaesthesia in adult horses: a structured summary of the literature. *Animals (Basel)* 11 (6): 1777. https://doi.org/10.3390/ani11061777 (accessed 29 November 2022).

9 Michou, J. and Leece, E. (2012). Sedation and analgesia in the standing horse 1. Drugs used for sedation and systemic analgesia. *In Practice* 34: 524–531. https://doi.org/10.1136/inp.e6423 (accessed 29 November 2022).

10 Brosnan, R.J. (2013). Inhaled anesthetics in horses. *Veterinary Clinics of North America: Equine Practice* 29 (1): 69–87. https://doi.org/10.1016/j.cveq.2012.11.006 (accessed 29 November 2022).

11 Clutton, R.E. (2010). Opioid analgesia in horses. *Veterinary Clinics of North America: Equine Practice* 26 (3): 493–514. https://doi.org/10.1016/j.cveq.2010.07.002 (accessed 29 November 2022).

12 Valverde, A. (2010). Alpha-2 agonists as pain therapy in horses. *Veterinary Clinics of North America: Equine Practice* 26 (3): 515–532. https://doi.org/10.1016/j.cveq.2010.07.003 (accessed 29 November 2022).

13 Al-Shaikh, B. and Stacey, S. (2007). *Essentials of Anaesthetic Equipment*, 3e. Elsevier: Churchill Livingstone.

14 Diba, A. (2012). Chapter 4. The anaesthetic workstation. In: *Ward's Anaesthetic Equipment*, 6e (ed. A.J. Davey and A. Diba), 65–105.

15 Subrahmanyam, M. and Mohan, S. (2013). Safety features in anaesthesia machine. *Indian Journal of Anaesthesia* 57: 472–480.

16 Record, N. and Beecroft, C. (2021). Principles of the anaesthetic machine. *Anaesthesia and Intensive Care Medicine* 23 (1): 1–5.

17 Bednarski, R.M. (2009). Anesthetic equipment. In: *Equine Anesthesia – Monitoring and Emergency Therapy* (ed. W.W. Muir and J.A.E. Hubbell), 315–331. USA: Elsevier.

18 Taylor, S. (2013). A whistle-stop tour of the anaesthetic machine. *Veterinary Nursing Journal* 28 (1): 8–36. https://doi.org/10.1111/j.2045-0648.2012.00255.x.

19 Davey, A.J. (2012). Chapter 3. Vaporizers. In: *Ward's Anaesthetic Equipment*, 6e (ed. A.J. Davey and A. Diba), 41–64.

20 Boumphrey, S. and Marshall, N. (2011). Understanding vaporizers. *Continuing Education in Anaesthesia, Critical Care and Pain* 11 (6): 199–203.

21 Hartle, A., Anderson, E., Bythell, V. et al. (2012). Checking anaesthetic equipment 2012. Guidelines of the Association of Anaesthetists of Great Britain and Ireland. *Anaesthesia* 67: 660–668.

22 Davey, A.J. (2012). Chapter 5. Breathing systems and their components. Chapter 5. In: *Ward's Anaesthetic Equipment*, 6e (ed. A.J. Davey and A. Diba), 107–138.

23 Dugdale, A. (2010). Anaesthetic breathing systems. Chapter 9. In: *Veterinary Anaesthesia. Principles to Practice* (ed. A. Dugdale), 76–92. Wiley Blackwell.

24 Health Services Advisory Committee (1995). *Anaesthetic Agents: Controlling Exposure Under COSHH*. Suffolk, UK: Health and Safety Commission. HSE Books.

25 Bailey, S. (2012). Chapter 18. Atmospheric pollution. In: *Ward's Anaesthetic Equipment*, 6e (ed. A.J. Davey and A. Diba), 385–398.

26 Moreno-Martinez, F., Senior, J.M., and Mosing, M. (2021). Controlled mechanical ventilation in equine anaesthesia: classification of ventilators and practical considerations (part 2). *Equine Veterinary Education* https://doi.org/10.1111/eve.13527.

27 Steffey, E.P., Hodgson, D.S., Dunlop, C.I. et al. (1987). Cardiopulmonary function during 5 hours of constant dose isoflurane in laterally recumbent spontaneously breathing horses. *Journal of Veterinary Pharmacology and Therapeutics* 10: 290–297.

28 Day, T.K., Gaynor, J.S., Muir, W.W. et al. (1995). Blood gas values during intermittent positive pressure ventilation and spontaneous ventilation in 160 anesthetized horses positioned in lateral or dorsal recumbency. *Veterinary Surgery* 24: 266–276.

29 Moens, Y. (2013). Mechanical ventilation and respiratory mechanics during equine anesthesia. *Veterinary Clinics of North America: Equine Practice* 29: 51–67. https://doi.org/10.1016/j.cveq.2012.12.002.

30 Mosing, M. and Senior, J.M. (2018). Maintenance of equine anaesthesia over the last 50 years: Controlled inhalation of volatile anaesthetics and pulmonary ventilation. *Equine Veterinary Journal* 50: 282–291.

31 Hopster, K., Jacobson, B., Hopster-Iversen, C. et al. (2016). Histopathological changes and mRNA expression in lungs of horses after inhalation anaesthesia with different ventilation strategies. *Research in Veterinary Science* 107: 8–15.

32 Senior, J.M. (2005). Post-anaesthetic pulmonary oedema in horses: a review. *Veterinary Anaesthesia and Analgesia* 32: 193–200. https://doi.org/10.1111/j.1467-2995.2005.00186.x.

33 Kerr, C.L. and McDonell, W.N. (2008). Oxygen supplementation and ventilatory support. In: *Equine Anaesthesia: Monitoring and Emergency Therapy*, 2e (ed. W.W. Muir and J.A.E. Hubbell), 332–352. Missouri: Elsevier.

34 Koenig, J., McDonell, W., and Valverde, A. (2003). Accuracy of pulse oximetry and capnography in healthy and compromised horse during spontaneous and controlled ventilation. *The Canadian Journal of Veterinary Research* 67: 169–174.

35 Bednarski, R.M. (2009). Tracheal and nasal intubation. In: *Equine Anesthesia – Monitoring and Emergency Therapy* (ed. W.W. Muir and J.A.E. Hubbell), 277–287. USA: Elsevier.

36 Burns, P.M. (2020). Orotracheal intubation in the horse – is bigger better? *Equine Veterinary Education* 32: 314–318.

37 Ferreira, T.H., Allen, M., De Gaseri, D. et al. (2021). Impact of endotracheal tube size and cuff pressure on tracheal and laryngeal mucosa of adult horses. *Veterinary Anaesthesia and Analgesia* 48: 891–899.

38 Tomasic, M., Mann, L., and Soma, L. (1997). Effects of sedation, anesthesia, and endotracheal intubation on respiratory mechanics in adult horses. *American Journal of Veterinary Research* 58: 641–646.

39 Altun, D., Orhan-Sungur, M., Ali, A. et al. (2017). The role of ultrasound in appropriate endotracheal tube size selection in pediatric patients. *Pediatric Anesthesia* 27: 1015–1020.

40 Deutsch, J. and Taylor, P.M. (2021). Mortality and morbidity in equine anaesthesia. *Equine Veterinary Education* 34: 152–168.

41 Trim, C.M. (2015). Endotracheal intubation in horses – are complications truly rare? *Equine Veterinary Education* 27: 176–178.

42 Miller, C. and Auckburally, A. (2020). Tracheal rupture following general anaesthesia in a horse. *Equine Veterinary Education* 32: 62–65. https://doi.org/10.1111/eve.13019.

43 Bergadano, A., Moens, Y., and Schatzmann, U. (2004). Two cases of intraoperative herniation of the endotracheal tube cuff. *Schweizer Archiv für Tierheilkunde* 146: 565–569.

44 Díaz, M.D.M., Hewetson, M., and Kaartinen, J. (2022). Tracheal trauma and pneumonia secondary to endotracheal intubation in a horse undergoing general anaesthesia, computerised tomography and myelography. *Equine Veterinary Education* 34 (3): 106–109.

45 Briganti, A., Portela, D.A., Barsotti, G. et al. (2012). Evaluation of the endotracheal tube cuff pressure resulting from four different methods of inflation in dogs. *Veterinary Anaesthesia and Analgesia* 39: 488–494.

46 Association of Veterinary Anaesthetists. Guidelines for Safer Anaesthesia. https://ava.eu.com/resources/anaesthesia-guidelines.

47 Dagnall, C., Khenissi, L., and Love, E. (2022). Monitoring techniques for equine anaesthesia. *Equine Veterinary Education* https://doi.org/10.1111/eve.13581.

48 Martinez, E.A., Wagner, A.E., Driessen, B. et al. (2008). American College of Veterinary Anesthesiologists guidelines for anesthesia in horses. Available online: https://acvaa.org/wp-content/uploads/2019/05/Guidelines-for-Anesthesia-in-Horses.pdf (accessed 30 January 2021).

49 Murrell, J. and Ford-Fennah, V. (2012). Anaesthesia and analgesia. In: *BSAVA Textbook of Veterinary Nursing* (ed. B. Cooper, E. Mullineaux, and L. Turner), 725–735. British Small Animal Veterinary Association.

50 Wallace, A. (2021). Capnography: the best anaesthetic monitoring tool? *Veterinary Nursing Journal* 36: 319–322.

51 Thomas, J.A. and Lerche, P. (2011). Chapter 5: Anaesthetic monitoring. In: *Anesthesia and Analgesia for Veterinary Technicians*, 164–167. Elsevier.

52 Zoff, A., Dugdale, A.H.A., Scarabelli, S. et al. (2019). Evaluation of pulse co-oximetry to determine haemoglobin saturation with oxygen and haemoglobin concentration in anaesthetized horses: a retrospective study. *Veterinary Anaesthesia and Analgesia* 46: 452–457.

53 Trim, C.M. (2005). Monitoring during anaesthesia: techniques and interpretation. *Equine Veterinary Education* 15: 30–40. https://doi.org/10.1111/j.2042-3292.2005.tb01825.x.

54 Sage, A.M., Ambrisko, T.D., and Martins, F.D.C. (2021). Evaluation of fingertip pulse oximeters for monitoring haemoglobin oxygen saturation in arterial blood and pulse rate in isoflurane-anaesthetised horses breathing greater than 90 percent oxygen. *Equine Veterinary Education* https://doi.org/10.1111/eve.13592.

55 Mitchell, K.J. (2019). Equine electrocardiography. *The Veterinary Clinics of North America. Equine Practice* 35: 65–83. https://doi.org/10.1016/j.cveq.2018.12.007.

56 Taylor, P. and Clarke, K.W. (2007). Chapter 5 – Monitoring. In: *Handbook of Equine Anaesthesia*, 2e, 87–104. Philadelphia, PA: Saunders Elsevier.

57 Jago, R. and Blissitt, K. (2022). How to record a good quality ECG in horses. *In Practice* 46–53.

58 Pratt, S., Barnes, T.S., Cowling, N. et al. (2022). Bias associated with peripheral non-invasive compared to invasive arterial blood pressure monitoring in healthy anaesthetised and standing horses using the bionet BM7V. *Veterinary Sciences* 9: 52. https://doi.org/10.3390/vetsci9020052.

59 Magdesian, K.G. (2004). Monitoring the critically ill equine patient. *Veterinary Clinics of North America: Equine Practice* 20: 11–39.

60 Shih, A.C. (2019). Cardiac monitoring in horses. *Veterinary Clinics of North America: Equine Practice* 35: 205–215. https://doi.org/10.1016/j.cveq.2018.12.003.

61 Tam, K., Rezende, M., and Boscan, P. (2011). Correlation between jugular and central venous pressures in laterally recumbent horses. *Veterinary Anaesthesia and Analgesia* 38: 580–583. https://doi.org/10.1111/j.1467-2995.2011.00667.x.

62 Jeawon, S.S., Katz, L.M., Galvin, N.P. et al. (2018). Determination of reference intervals for umbilical cord arterial and venous blood gas analysis of healthy Thoroughbred foals. *Theriogenology* 118: 1–6.

63 Stefanik, E., Drewnowska, O., Lisowska, B. et al. (2021). Causes, effects and methods of monitoring gas exchange disturbances during equine general anaesthesia. *Animals* 11: 2049.

64 Barton, L.J., Devey, J.J., Gorski, S. et al. (1996). Evaluation of transmittance and reflectance pulse oximetry in a canine model of hypotension and desaturation. *Journal of Veterinary Emergency and Critical Care* 6: 21–28.

65 Guedes, A. (2018). Blood gases. In: *Interpretation of Equine Laboratory Diagnostics*, 57–65. Hoboken, NJ, USA: John Wiley & Sons.

66 Hubbell, J.A.E. and Muir, W.W. (2009). Chapter 8 – Monitoring anaesthesia. In: *Equine Anaesthesia*, 2e, 149–170. Missouri, MO: Saunders Elsevier.

67 Dugdale, A.H.A., Beaumont, G., Bradbrook, C. et al. (ed.) (2020). Chapter 2: Patient safety. In: *Veterinary Anaesthesia Principles to Practice*, 9–10. Oxford: Blackwell Publishing.

68 Dugdale, A.H.A, Beaumont, G., Bradbrook, C. et al. (eds.) (2020). Chapter 30: equine anaesthesia. In: *Veterinary Anaesthesia Principles to Practice*, 447, 464–469. Blackwell Publishing: Oxford.

69 Hay Kraus, B. and Johnson, P. (2022). Anaesthetic management for endocrine diseases and geriatric horses. In: *Equine Anaesthesia and Co-existing Disease* (ed. S. Clark-Price and K. Mama), 232–236. Hoboken: Wiley-Blackwell.

70 Ireland, J.L. (2016). Demographics, management, preventative health care and disease in aged horses. *Veterinary Clinics of North America: Equine Practice* 32: 195–214.

71 Lascola, K. and Clark-Price, S. (2022). Anaesthetic management for inflammatory or infectious respiratory diseases. In: *Equine Anaesthesia and Co-existing Disease* (ed. S. Clark-Price and K. Mama), 56. Hoboken: Wiley-Blackwell.

72 Taylor, P.M. and Clarke, K.W. (2007). Chapter 8: Anaesthesia in special situations. In: *Handbook of Equine Anaesthesia*, 180–183, 189–191. London: Saunders.

73 Taylor, P.M. and Clarke, K.W. (2007). Chapter 7: Anaesthetic problems. In: *Handbook of Equine*

Anaesthesia, 123–129, 131–132, 137–139, 148. London: Saunders.

74 Guedel, A.E. (1927). Stages of anesthesia and a re-classification of the signs of anesthesia. *Current Researches in Anesthesia & Analgesia* 6 (4): 157–162.

75 Fischer, B. and Clark-Price, S. (2015). Anesthesia of the equine neonate in health and disease. *Veterinary Clinics of North America: Equine Practice* 31 (3): 567–585. https://doi.org/10.1016/j.cveq.2015.09.002.

76 White, K. (2015). Total and partial intravenous anaesthesia of horses. *In Practice* 37: 189–198.

77 Schwarzwald, C.C., Bonagura, J.D., and Muir, W.W. (2009). The cardiovascular system. Chapter 3. In: *Equine Anesthesia. Monitoring and Emergency Therapy*, 2e (ed. W.W. Muir and J.A.E. Hubbell), 37–100. Saunders Elsevier.

78 Elkington, T. and Gwinnutt, C. (2009). Introduction to cardiovascular physiology. *Anaesthesia Tutorial of the Week* 125: 1–128.

79 Mellema, M. (2009). Cardiac output monitoring. In: *Small Animal Critical Care Medicine* (ed. D. Silverstein and K. Hopper), 894–898. St Louis, MO: Saunders Elsevier.

80 Corley, K.T.T. (2002). Monitoring and treating haemodynamic disturbances in critically ill neonatal foals. Part 2: assessment and treatment. *Equine Veterinary Education* 14 (6): 328–336.

81 Schauvliege, S. and Gasthuys, F. (2013). Drugs for cardiovascular support in anesthetized horses. *Veterinary Clinics of North America: Equine Practice* 29: 19–49. https://doi.org/10.1016/j.cveq.2012.11.011.

82 Levick, J.R. (2010). Assessment of cardiac output and peripheral pulse. Chapter 7. In: *An Introduction to Cardiovascular Physiology*, 5e (ed. J.R. Levick), 108–115. Hodder Arnold.

83 Hubbell, J.A.E. and Muir, W.W. (2009). Chapter 21 – Considerations for induction, maintenance and recovery. In: *Equine Anaesthesia*, 2e, 381–396. Missouri, MO: Saunders Elsevier.

84 Schauvliege, S., Van den Eede, A., Duchateau, L. et al. (2009). Comparison between lithium dilution and pulse contour analysis techniques for cardiac output measurement in isoflurane anaesthetized ponies: influence of different inotropic drugs. *Veterinary Anaesthesia and Analgesia* 36: 197–208. https://doi.org/10.1111/j.1467-2995.2009.00446.x.

85 Durando, M.M. and Young, L.E. (2003). Cardiovascular examination and diagnostic techniques. In: *Current Therapy in Equine Medicine*, 5e (ed. N.E. Robinson), 572–585. Philadelphia: WB Saunders.

86 Robertson, S.A. (2005). Sedation and general anaesthesia of the foal. *Equine Veterinary Education* 15: 94–101.

87 Wagner, A.E. (2008). Complications in equine anesthesia. *Veterinary Clinics of North America: Equine Practice* 24: 735–752.

88 Abrahamsen, E., Hellyer, P.W., Bednarski, R.M. et al. (1989). Tourniquet-induced hypertension in a horse. *Journal of the American Veterinary Medical Association* 194: 386–388.

89 Rousseau-Blass, F., Pige, C., and Pang, D.S.J. (2020). Agreement between invasive and oscillometric arterial blood pressure measurements using the LifeWindow multiparameter monitor and two cuff sizes in anesthetized adult horses. *Veterinary Anaesthesia and Analgesia* 47: 315–322.

90 White, N.A. and Suarez, M. (1986). Change in triceps muscle intracompartmental pressure with repositioning and padding of the lowermost thoracic limb of the horse. *American Journal of Veterinary Research* 47: 2257–2260.

91 Young, S.S. (1993). Post-anesthetic myopathy. *Equine Veterinary Education* 5: 200–203.

92 Valverde, A., Giguere, S., Sanchez, L.C. et al. (2006). Effects of dobutamine, norepinephrine, and vasopressin on cardiovascular function in anesthetized neonatal foals with induced hypotension. *American Journal of Veterinary Research* 67: 1730–1737.

93 Tearney, C.C., Guedes, A.G.P., and Brosnan, R.J. (2016). Equivalence between invasive and oscillometric blood pressures at different anatomic locations in healthy normotensive anaesthetised horses. *Equine Veterinary Journal* 48: 357–361. https://doi.org/10.1111/evj.12443.

94 Kerslake, I. and Kelly, F. (2017). Uses of capnography in the critical care unit. *BJA Education* 17 (5): 178–183.

95 Drábková, Z., Schramel, J.P., and Kabeš, R. (2018). Determination of physiological dead space in anaesthetized horses: a method-comparison study. *Veterinary Anaesthesia and Analgesia* 45: 73–77.

96 Thawley, V. and Waddell, L.S. (2013). Pulse oximetry and capnometry. *Topics in Companion Animal Medicine* 28: 124–128.

97 Blissitt, K.J., Raisis, A.L., Adams, V.J. et al. (2008). The effects of halothane and isoflurane on cardiovascular function in dorsally recumbent horses undergoing surgery. *Veterinary Anaesthesia and Analgesia* 35: 208–219.

98 Koenig, J., McDonell, W., and Al-Shaikh, A. (2003). Accuracy of pulse oximetry and capnography in healthy and compromised horses during spontaneous and controlled ventilation. *Canadian Journal of Veterinary Research* 67 (3): 169–174.

99 Shoemaker, W.C. (2000). Invasive and noninvasive monitoring. In: *Textbook of Critical Care*, 4e (ed. W.C. Shoemaker, S.M. Ayres, A. Grenvik, et al.), 74–92. Philadelphia: WB Saunders.

100 Uquillas, E., Dart, C., Perkins, N. et al. (2018). Effect of reducing inspired oxygen concentration on oxygenation parameters during general anaesthesia in horses in lateral or dorsal recumbency. *Australian Veterinary Journal* 96: 46–53. https://doi.org/10.1111/avj.12662.

101 Moens, Y.P.S. (2010). Clinical application of continuous spirometry with a pitot-based flow meter during equine anaesthesia. *Equine Veterinary Education* 22: 354–360. https://doi.org/10.1111/j.2042-3292.2010.00066.x.

102 Langton, J.A. and Hutton, A. (2009). Respiratory gas analysis. *Continuing Education in Anaesthesia, Critical Care & Pain* 9 (1): 19–23.

103 Mudge, M.C. (2014). Acute hemorrhage and blood transfusions in horses. *Veterinary Clinics of North America: Equine Practice* 30 (2): 427–436.

104 Radcliffe, R.M., Bookbinder, L.C., Liu, S.Y. et al. (2022). Collection and administration of blood products in horses: transfusion indications, materials, methods, complications, donor selection, and blood testing. *Journal of Veterinary Emergency and Critical Care* 32: 108–122. https://doi.org/10.1111/vec.13119.

105 Magdesian, K.G., Fielding, C.L., Rhodes, D.M. et al. (2006). Changes in central venous pressure and blood lactate concentration in response to acute blood loss in horses. *Journal of the American Veterinary Medical Association* 229 (9): 1458–1462.

106 Schmall, L.M., Mulr, W.W., and Robertson, J.T. (1990). Haemodynamic effects of small volume hypertonic saline in experimentally induced haemorrhagic shock. *Equine Veterinary Journal* 22: 273–277. https://doi.org/10.1111/j.2042-3306.1990.tb04266.x.

107 Wilson, D.V., Rondenay, Y., and Shance, P.U. (2003). The cardiopulmonary effects of severe blood loss in anesthetized horses. *Veterinary Anaesthesia and Analgesia* 30: 80–86.

108 Divers, T.J., Radcliffe, R.M., Cook, V.L. et al. (2022). Calculating and selecting fluid therapy and blood product replacements for horses with acute hemorrhage. *Journal of Veterinary Emergency and Critical Care* 32: 97–107. https://doi.org/10.1111/vec.13127.

109 Hurcombe, S.D.A., Radcliffe, R.M., Cook, V.L. et al. (2022). The pathophysiology of uncontrolled hemorrhage in horses. *Journal of Veterinary Emergency and Critical Care* 32: 63–71. https://doi.org/10.1111/vec.13122.

110 Knottenbelt, D.C. (2003). Differential diagnosis of polyuria/polydipsia. In: *Current Therapy in Equine Medicine*, 5e (ed. N.E. Robinson), 828–831. Philadelphia: WB Saunders.

111 Crabtree, N.E. and Epstein, K.L. (2021). Current concepts in fluid therapy in horses. *Frontiers in Veterinary Science* 8: 648774. https://doi.org/10.3389/fvets.2021.648774.

112 Nolen-Walston, R.D. (2012). Flow rates of large animal fluid delivery systems used for high-volume crystalloid resuscitation. *Journal of Veterinary Emergency and Critical Care* 22: 661–665. https://doi.org/10.1111/j.1476-4431.2012.00817.x.

113 Magdesian, K. (2015). Replacement fluids therapy in horses. In: *Equine Fluid Therapy*, 1e (ed. C. Fielding and K. Magdesian), 161–174. Ames, IA: Wiley Blackwell https://doi.org/10.1002/9781118928189.ch12.

114 Naumann, D.N., Beaven, A., Dretzke, J. et al. (2016). Searching for the optimal fluid to restore microcirculatory flow dynamics after haemorrhagic shock: a systematic review of preclinical studies. *Shock (Augusta, Ga.)* 46 (6): 609–622.

115 Motaharinia, J., Etezadi, F., Moghaddas, A. et al. (2015). Immunomodulatory effect of hypertonic saline in hemorrhagic shock. *Daru* 23: 47–55.

116 Epstein, K., Bergren, A., Giguere, S. et al. (2014). Cardiovascular, colloid osmotic pressure, and hemostatic effects of 2 formulations of hydroxyethyl starch in healthy horses. *Journal of Veterinary Internal Medicine* 2: 223–233. https://doi.org/10.1111/jvim.12245.

117 Jernigan, P.L., Hoehn, R.S., Cox, D. et al. (2016). What if I don't have blood? Hextend is superior to 3% saline in an experimental model of far forward resuscitation after hemorrhage. *Shock (Augusta, Ga.)* 4 (3 Suppl 1): 148–153.

118 Copland, V.S., Hildebrand, S.V., Hill, T. et al. (1989). Blood pressure response to tourniquet use in anesthetized horses. *Journal of the American Veterinary Medical Association* 195 (8): 1097–1103.

119 Mair, A. and Mathis, A. (2018). Completeness of handwritten preanaesthetic records at two veterinary referral institutions. *Veterinary Anaesthesia and Analgesia* 45 (2): 129–134. https://doi.org/10.1016/j.vaa.2017.08.007.

120 Johnson, C.B. (2005). Positioning of the anaesthetised horse. *Equine Veterinary Education* 7 (41): 41–44.

121 Brightman, A.H., Manning, J.P., Benson, G.J. et al. (1983). Decreased tear production associated with general anaesthesia in the horse. *Journal of the American Veterinary Medical Association* 182: 182–243.

122 White, E. and Crosse, M.M. (1998). The aetiology and prevention of peri-operative corneal abrasions. *Anaesthesia* 53: 157–161.

123 Scarabelli, S., Timofte, D., Malalana, F. et al. (2018). Corneal abrasion and microbial contamination in horses following general anaesthesia for non-ocular surgery. *Veterinary Anaesthesia and Analgesia* 45 (3): 278–284. https://doi.org/10.1016/j.vaa.2017.12.002.

124 King, K.E. (2015). How to prepare and position a horse for theatre. *The Veterinary Nurse* 5 (10): 588–591.

125 Young, S.S. and Taylor, P.M. (1993). Factors influencing the outcome of equine anaesthesia: a review of 1,314 cases. *Equine Veterinary Journal* 25: 147–151.

126 Franci, P., Leece, E.A., and Brearley, J.C. (2006). Post anaesthetic myopathy/neuropathy in horses undergoing magnetic resonance imaging compared to horses undergoing surgery. *Equine Veterinary Journal* 38: 497–501.

127 Taylor, P.M. and Young, S.S. (1990). The effect of limb position on venous and compartmental pressure in the forelimb of ponies. *Journal of Veterinary Anaesthesia* 17: 35–37.

128 Oosterlinck, M., Schauvliege, S., Martens, A. et al. (2013). Postanesthetic neuropathy/myopathy in the nondependent forelimb in 4 horses. *Journal of Equine Veterinary Science* 33 11: 996–999. https://doi.org/10.1016/j.jevs.2013.03.181.

129 Dugdale, A.H., Obhrai, J., and Cripps, P.J. (2016). Twenty years later: a single-centre, repeat retrospective analysis of equine perioperative mortality and investigation of recovery quality. *Veterinary Anaesthesia and Analgesia* 43: 171–178.

130 Laurenza, C., Ansart, L., and Portier, K. (2020). Risk factors of anesthesia-related mortality and morbidity in one equine hospital: a retrospective study on 1,161 cases undergoing elective and emergency surgeries. *Frontiers in Veterinary Science* 6: 514.

131 Nicolaisen, A.-S.K., Bendix Nygaard, A., Christophersen, M.T. et al. (2020). Effect of head and tail rope-assisted recovery of horses after elective and emergency surgery under general anaesthesia. *Equine Veterinary Education* https://doi.org/10.1111/eve.13397.

132 Wright, B.D. and Hildebrand, S.V. (2001). An evaluation of apnea or spontaneous ventilation in early recovery following mechanical ventilation in the anesthetized horse. *Veterinary Anaesthesia and Analgesia* 28: 26–33.

133 Bardell, D.A., Mosing, M., and Cripps, P.J. (2020). Restoration of arterial oxygen tension in horses recovering from general anaesthesia. *Equine Veterinary Journal* 52: 187–193.

134 Thompson, K.R. and Bardell, D. (2006). The effect of two intra-operative end-tidal carbon dioxide tensions on apnoeic duration in the recovery period in horses. *Veterinary Anaesthesia and Analgesia* 43: 163–170.

135 Brosnan, R.J., Steffey, E.P., and Escobar, A. (2012). Effects of hypercapnic hyperpnea on recovery from isoflurane or sevoflurane anesthesia in horses. *Veterinary Anaesthesia and Analgesia* 39: 335–344.

136 Marntell, S., Nyman, G., and Hedenstierna, G. (2005). High inspired oxygen concentrations increase intrapulmonary shunt in anaesthetized horses. *Veterinary Anaesthesia and Analgesia* 32: 338–347.

137 Mason, D.E., Muir, W.W., and Wade, A. (1987). Arterial blood gas tensions in the horse during recovery from anesthesia. *Journal of the American Veterinary Medical Association* 190: 989–994.

138 Lukasik, V.M., Gleed, R.D., Scarlett, J.M. et al. (1997). Intranasal phenylephrine reduces post anesthetic upper airway obstruction in horses. *Equine Veterinary Journal* 29: 236–238.

139 Shawley, R.V. and Bednarski, R.M. (1991). Endotracheal intubation in the horse. In: *Equine Anesthesia Monitoring and Emergency Therapy* (ed. W.W. Muir and J.A. Hubbell), 310–324. St. Louis, MO: Mosby Year Book.

140 Hubbell, J.A.E., Muir, W.W. III, and Hopster, K. (2022). Hypothesis article rethinking equine anaesthetic risk: development of a novel Combined Horse Anaesthetic Risk Identification and Optimisation tool (CHARIOT). *Equine Veterinary Education* 34 (3): 134–140. https://doi.org/10.1111/eve.13563.

141 Hedenstierna, G. and Edmark, L. (2010). Mechanisms of atelectasis in the perioperative period. *Best Practice & Research: Clinical Anaesthesiology* 24: 157–169.

142 Mosing, M. and Senior, M. (2017). Maintenance of equine anaesthesia over the last 50 years: controlled inhalation of volatile anaesthetics and pulmonary ventilation. *Equine Veterinary Journal* 50: 282–291. https://doi.org/10.1111/evj.12793.

143 Nyman, G. and Hedenstierna, G. (1989). Ventilation-perfusion relationships in the anaesthetised horse. *Equine Veterinary Journal* 21 (4): 274–281.

144 Cerullo, M., Driessen, B., Douglas, H. et al. (2020). Changes in arterial blood pressure and oxygen tension as a result of hoisting in isoflurane anesthetized healthy adult horses. *Frontiers in Veterinary Science* 7: 601326. https://doi.org/10.3389/fvets.2020.601326.

145 Gasthuys, F., DeMoor, A., and Parmentier, D. (1991). Haemodynamic effects of change in position and respiration mode during a standard Halothane anesthesia in ponies. *Journal of Veterinary Medicine* 38: 203–211. https://doi.org/10.1111/j.1439-0442.1991.tb01003.x.

146 Loomes, K. and Louro, L.F. (2020). Recovery of horses from general anaesthesia: a systematic review (2000–2020) of risk factors and influence of interventions during the recovery period. *Equine Veterinary Journal* 54: 201–218.

147 Bienert, A., Bartmann, C.P., Von Oppen, T. et al. (2003). Recovery phase of horses after inhalant anaesthesia with isofluorane (Isoflo®) and postanaesthetic sedation with romifidine (Sedivet®) or xylazine (Rompun®). *Deutsche tierärztliche Wochenschrift* 110: 244–248.

148 Woodhouse, K.J., Brosnan, R.J., Nguyen, K.Q. et al. (2013). Effects of postanesthetic sedation with romifidine or xylazine on quality of recovery from isoflurane anesthesia in horses. *Journal of the American Veterinary Medical Association* 242: 533–539.

149 Santos, M., Fuente, M., Garcia-Iturralde, P. et al. (2003). Effects of alpha-2 adrenoceptor agonists during recovery from isoflurane anaesthesia in horses. *Equine Veterinary Journal* 35: 170–175.

150 Guedes, A.G.P., Tearney, C.C., Cenani, A. et al. (2017). Comparison between the effects of postanesthetic xylazine and dexmedetomidine on characteristics of recovery from sevoflurane anesthesia in horses. *Veterinary Anaesthesia and Analgesia* 44: 273–280.

151 Lloyd, F. and Murison, P. (2021). For horses undergoing general anaesthesia, are rope recoveries or free recoveries better? *The Veterinary Evidence Journal* 6 (3): 1–17.

152 Niimura Del Barrio, M.C., David, F., Hughes, J.M.L. et al. (2018). A retrospective report (2003–2013) of the complications associated with the use of a one-man (head and tail) rope recovery system in horses following general anaesthesia. *Irish Veterinary Journal* 71: 1–9.

153 Auer, U. and Huber, C. (2013). A comparison of head/tail rope-assisted versus unassisted recoveries of horses after patrial intravenous general anaesthesia. Abstracts presented at the Association of Veterinary Anaesthetists Spring meeting, 22nd–23rd March 2012, Davos, Switzerland. *Veterinary Anaesthesia Analgesia* 40 (1): 1–28. https://doi.org/10.1111/vaa.12001.

154 Rüegg, M., Bettschart-Wolfensberger, R., Hartnack, S. et al. (2016). Comparison of non-assisted versus head and tail rope-assisted recovery after emergency abdominal surgery in horses. *Pferdeheilkunde* 32 (5): 469–478. https://doi.org/10.21836/PEM20160508.

155 Arndt, S., Hopster, K., Sill, V. et al. (2019). Comparison between head-tail-rope assisted and unassisted recoveries in healthy horses undergoing general anesthesia for elective surgeries. *Veterinary Surgery* 49 (2): 329–338. https://doi.org/10.1111/vsu.13347.

156 Louro, L.F., Robson, K., Hughes, J. et al. (2021). Head and tail rope-assisted recovery improves quality of recovery from general anaesthesia in horses undergoing emergency exploratory laparotomy. *Equine Veterinary Education* 2021: https://doi.org/10.1111/evj.13516.

157 Bird, A.R., Morley, S.J., Sherlock, C.E. et al. (2019). The outcomes of epidural anaesthesia in horses with perineal and tail melanomas: complications associated with ataxia and the risks of rope recovery. *Equine Veterinary Education* 31: 567–574.

158 Tidwell, S.A., Schneider, R.K., Ragle, C.A. et al. (2002). Use of a hydro-pool system to recover horses after general anesthesia: 60 cases. *Veterinary Surgery* 31: 455–461. https://doi.org/10.1053/jvet.2002.34662.

159 Sullivan, E.K., Klein, L.V., Richardson, D.W. et al. (2002). Use of a pool-raft system for recovery of horses from general anesthesia: 393 horses (1984–2000). *Journal of the American Veterinary Medical Association* 221 (7): 1014–1018.

160 McFadzean, W. and Love, E. (2017). How to do equine anaesthesia in the field. *In Practice* 39: 452–461. https://doi.org/10.1136/inp.j4582.

161 Hubbell, J.A.E. (1999). Recovery from anesthesia in horses. *Equine Veterinary Education* 11: 160–167.

162 Hubbell, J.A.E. (2013). How to produce twenty minutes of equine anesthesia in the field. *AAEP Proceedings* 59: 469–471.

163 Muir, W.W. and Hubbell, J.A.E. Anesthetic-associated complications. Chapter 22. In: *Equine Anaesthesia. Monitoring and Emergency Therapy* (ed. W.W. Muir and J.A.E. Hubbell), 397–417. Saunders Elsevier. Equine.

164 Clark-Price, S.C., Gutierrez-Nibeyro, S.D., and Santos, M.P. (2012). Anesthesia case of the month. EPAM. *Journal of the American Veterinary Medical Association* 240: 40–44.

165 Johnston, G.M., Eastment, J.K., Taylor, P.M. et al. (2004). Is isoflurane safer than halothane in equine anaesthesia? Results from a prospective multicentre randomised controlled trial. *Equine Veterinary Journal* 36: 64–71.

166 Lindsay, W.A., McDonell, W., and Bignell, W. (1980). Equine postanesthetic forelimb lameness: intracompartmental muscle pressure changes and biochemical patterns. *American Journal of Veterinary Research* 41: 1919–1924.

167 Richey, M.T., Holland, M.S., McGrath, C.J. et al. (1990). Equine post-anesthetic lameness: a retrospective study. *Veterinary Surgery* 19: 392–397.

168 Johnston, G.M., Eastment, J.K., Wood, J.L.H. et al. (2002). The confidential enquiry into perioperative equine fatalities (CEPEF): mortality results of phases 1 and 2. *Veterinary Anaesthesia and Analgesia* 29: 159–170.

169 Bidwell, L.A., Bramlage, L.R., and Rood, W.A. (2007). Equine perioperative fatalities associated with general anaesthesia at a private practice – a retrospective case series. *Veterinary Anaesthesia and Analgesia* 34: 23–30.

170 Jago, R.C., Corletto, F., and Wright, I.M. (2015). Peri-anaesthetic complications in an equine referral hospital: risk factors for post anaesthetic colic. *Equine Veterinary Journal* 47: 635–640.

171 Lindsay, W.A., Pascoe, P.J., McDonell, W.N. et al. (1985). Effect of protective padding on forelimb intra-compartmental muscle pressures in anesthetized horses. *American Journal of Veterinary Research* 46: 688–691.

172 Senior, J.M., Pinchbeck, G., Dugdale, A.H.A. et al. (2004). A retrospective study into risk factors and prevalence of post-anaesthetic colic after orthopaedic surgery in horses. *Veterinary Record* 155: 321–325.

173 Lester, G.D., Bolton, J.R., Cullen, L.K. et al. (1992). Effects of general anesthesia on myoelectric activity of the intestine in horses. *American Journal of Veterinary Research* 53: 1553–1557.

174 Merritt, A.M., Burrow, J.A., and Hartless, C.S. (1998). Effect of xylazine, detomidine, and a combination of xylazine and butorphanol on equine duodenal motility. *American Journal of Veterinary Research* 59: 619–623.

175 Steinbrook, R.A. (1998). Epidural anesthesia and gastrointestinal motility. *Anesthesia & Analgesia* 86: 837–844.

176 Andersen, M.S., Clark, L., Dyson, S.J. et al. (2006). Effect of perianaesthetic morphine on the prevalence of colic in

horses after general anaesthesia for MRI or nonabdominal surgery. *Equine Veterinary Journal* 38: 368–374.

177 Borland, K.J., Shaw, D.J., and Clutton, R.E. (2017). Time-related changes in post-operative equine morbidity: a single-centre study. *Equine Veterinary Education* 29: 33–37.

178 Lefebvre, D., Pirie, R.S., Handel, I.G. et al. (2016). Clinical features and management of equine post operative ileus: survey of diplomates of the European Colleges of Equine Internal Medicine (ECEIM) and Veterinary Surgeons (ECVS). *Equine Veterinary Journal* 48: 182–187.

179 Schatzmann, U., Lang, J., Ueltschi, G. et al. (1981). Tracheal necrosis following intubation in the horse. *Deutsche tierärztliche Wochenschrift* 88: 102–103.

180 Blakemore, W.F., Jefferies, A., White, R.A.S. et al. (1984). Spinal cord malacia following general anaesthesia in the horse. *Veterinary Record* 114: 569–570.

181 Yovich, J.V., LeCouteur, R.A., Stashak, T.S. et al. (1986). Post anesthetic hemorrhagic myelopathy in a horse. *Journal of the American Veterinary Medical Association* 188: 300–301.

182 Wan, P.Y., Latimer, F.G., Silva-Krott, I. et al. (1994). Hematomyelia in a colt: a post anesthesia/surgery complication. *Journal of Equine Veterinary Science* 14: 495–497.

183 Stolk, P.W.T., van der Velden, M.A. and Binkhorst, G.J. (1991) Thoracolumbar myelomalacia following general anesthesia in horses. In: *Abstract in the Compendium on the 4th International Congress of Veterinary Anesthesia*. Utrecht, The Netherlands, 100.

184 Dugdale, A.H. and Taylor, P.M. (2016). Equine anaesthesia-associated mortality: where are we now? *Veterinary Anaesthesia and Analgesia* 43: 242–255.

185 Abrahamsen, E.J., Bohanon, T.C., Bednarski, R.M. et al. (1990). Bilateral arytenoid cartilage paralysis after inhalation anesthesia in a horse. *Journal of the American Veterinary Medical Association* 197: 1363–1365.

186 Dixon, P.M., Railton, D.I., and McGorum, B.C. (1993). Temporary bilateral laryngeal paralysis in a horse associated with general anaesthesia and post anaesthetic myositis. *Veterinary Record* 132: 29–32.

187 Tute, A.S., Wilkins, P.A., Gleed, R.D. et al. (1996). Negative pressure pulmonary edema as a post-anesthetic complication associated with upper airway obstruction in a horse. *Veterinary Surgery* 25: 519–523.

188 Murrell, J.C. and Ford-Fennah, V. (2012). Anaesthesia. In: *Equine Veterinary Nursing* (ed. K. Coumbe) 456, 458, 459. West Sussex: Wiley-Blackwell.

189 Robertson, S.A. and Bailey, J.E. (2002). Aerosolized salbutamol (albuterol) improves PaO_2 in hypoxaemic anaesthetized horses – a prospective clinical trial in 81 horses. *Veterinary Anaesthesia and Analgesia* 29 (4): 212–218.

190 Murrell, J.C. and Ford-Fennah, V. (2020). Anaesthesia and analgesia. In: *BSAVA Textbook of Veterinary Nursing*, 5e (ed. B. Cooper, E. Mullineaux, and L. Turner), 733. Gloucester: BSAVA.

191 Dugdale, A.H.A., Beaumont, G., Bradbrook, C. et al. (ed.) (2020). Chapter 51: Cardiopulmonary cerebral resuscitation (CPCR). In: *Veterinary Anaesthesia Principles to Practice*, 627–631. Blackwell Publishing, Oxford.

192 Corley, K. (2008). Cardiopulmonary resuscitation. In: *The Equine Hospital Manual*, 1e (ed. Corley, K. and Stephen, J.). 5–6. Blackwell Publishing: Oxford.

193 Hallowell, G.D. (2016). Cardiopulmonary resuscitation: a waste of time? *Equine Veterinary Education* 28 (5): 245–252.

194 Fletcher, D.J., Boller, M., Brainard, B.M. et al. (2012). RECOVER evidence and knowledge gap analysis on veterinary CPR. Part 7: clinical guidelines. *Journal of Veterinary Emergency and Critical Care (San Antonio)* 22 (Suppl. 1): S102–S131.

195 Palmer, J.E. (2007). Neonatal foal resuscitation. *Veterinary Clinics of North America: Equine Practice* 23: 159–182.

196 Cooper, E. and Boiler, M. (2018). Cardiopulmonary resuscitation. In: *BSAVA Manual of Canine and Feline Emergency and Critical Care*, 3e (ed. L.G. King and A. Boag), 324–326. Gloucester: BSAVA.

197 Duggan, M., Schofield, W., and Vermedal, H. (2022). Successful cardiopulmonary resuscitation in an adult horse following cardiovascular collapse on recovery from general anaesthesia in the Trendelenburg position. *Equine Veterinary Education* 34 (3): e98–e105.

Further Reading

BEVA, (2024), 'BEVA guidance for Schedule three procedures', [Online], Available at: https://www.beva.org.uk/Portals/0/Documents/Nurses/Guidance%20for%20Schedule%20Three%20Procedures.pdf, [Accessed 13th February 2024].

Chiavaccini, L. (2022). REassessment Campaign On VEterinary Resuscitation: has the time come for horses? *Equine Veterinary Education* 34 (3): 177–199.

Michou, J.N., Dugdale, A.H.A. and Cripwell, D. (2019). Achieving safer anaesthesia with ASA [Online]. Available at: www.alfaxan.co.uk/news/achieving-safer-anaesthesia-with-asa (accessed 27 February 2023).

Sweeney, C. (2015). Unique New Bolton Center Pool Advances Equine Orthopaedic Surgery [Online], Available at: https://www.vet.upenn.edu/about/news-room/bellwether/new-bolton-post/winter-2015/pool-recovery-story (accessed 13 April 2023).

11

Theatre Practice
Rosie Heath[1], Nicola Rose[2], and Rosina Lillywhite[3]

[1] *Mickleham, Dorking, Surrey, UK*
[2] *Ash Vale, Aldershot, Surrey, UK*
[3] *VetPartners Nursing School, Petersfield, UK*

Glossary

Antisepsis Prevention of sepsis by destruction or inhibition of microorganisms using an agent that may be safely applied to living tissue [1].

Asepsis The absence of bacteria, viruses, and other microorganisms [1].

Disinfectant An agent that destroys microorganisms – generally chemical agents applied to inanimate objects [1].

Disinfection The removal of microorganisms but not necessarily their spores [2].

Endogenous Microorganisms that originate from within the body of an animal [2].

Exogenous Microorganisms found on the skin and coat [2].

Sepsis The presence of pathogens or their toxic products in the blood or tissues of the patient, more commonly known as infection [1].

Sterilisation Total elimination of bacteria or other living microorganisms [2].

11.1 The Principles of Operating Theatre Design and Use

Registered veterinary nurses (RVNs), should aim to create and maintain a clean, safe and effective surgical environment to help to prevent microorganisms and spores from multiplying; this is achieved by using sterilisation and disinfection techniques to eliminate microorganisms and spores. These techniques include autoclaving, cold sterilisation, daily damp dusting, periodic deep cleaning and the use of appropriate disinfection protocols. All equipment, instruments and furnishings used in the theatre or operating suite should be maintained in an aseptic manner. A fresh set of instruments must be used for each patient [3].

The theatre suite must not be a thoroughfare; there should be one way in, and another separate way out. Clearly defined clean and dirty areas of the theatre suite ensure aseptic techniques are easier to manage and have a reduced risk of contamination. When considering design and use, it is also essential to consider the personnel present during surgery; an increased number of personnel will increase the chance of contamination from factors such as skin particles and increased air movement. Operating areas should contain adequate lighting, flooring and wall coverings that are easy to clean, durable and have hygienic protection. It should be possible to control the temperature in these rooms and have positive pressure air ventilation. There should be minimal furniture and no open shelving in the theatre as this will harbour dust; all equipment, including the operating table, should be easy to clean. Standard operating procedures (SOPs) are essential when considering theatre use [4]. Important points relating to SOPs include:

- Following written SOPs help to ensure all staff follow the same procedure when cleaning, disinfecting and sterilising to maintain theatre asepsis.
- SOPs should be clear and regularly audited to ensure validity.
- SOPs should be usable by all members of staff.
- SOPs should include the correct dilution rates for cleaning and disinfecting, although not all disinfectants will remove microorganisms and their spores. For this reason, careful consideration must be employed when selecting a disinfectant. It is important to remember that most disinfectants are inactivated by organic material such as blood and faeces, so it is best practice to clean areas before disinfection occurs. Correct dilution of disinfectant is essential in order to reduce disinfectant resistance; manufacturer guidelines should always form part of SOPs.
- SOPs detailing daily damp dusting should also be available explaining the importance of daily damp dusting and

weekly and monthly deep cleans. It is best practice if working in a busy hospital theatre to do monthly bacterial swabbing of a range of areas within the theatre to identify if cleaning protocols are effective or not. The growth of bacteria of any kind could be detrimental to patient health, and prevention is always preferable over cure [2].

Ideally, every hospital or practice would be purpose-built, but the buildings used have often been modified and adapted over time due to costs and space requirements. When developing the perfect layout and design, there are many factors to consider, such as the location and flow of patients, staff and materials. In addition to being isolated from the usual traffic of the hospital, communicating with the pharmacy, radiography and emergency access, the surgical area must have the best ambient and operating lighting, the right furniture and a strict and efficient air-conditioning system. The theatre suite can be broken down into different areas, from the outside spaces to the inner theatre. The objective is to avoid possible contamination and the development of surgical site infections, as the most significant source of infection in postoperative wounds is caused by incorrect handling of the spaces shared by medical staff and patients [5].

Different areas of the surgical suite can be broken up into zones and can even be colour-coded to ensure that all personnel entering can clearly see where they can and cannot go. An example of this system is as follows:

- Black area – this area is considered the most contaminated area and includes all the corridors around the theatre and the horse preparation area before induction. In this area, staff may be dressed in outdoor footwear and clean uniform, but theatre attire is not required.
- Grey area – includes the induction and recovery boxes and the anaesthetised patient prep area. In this area, clean clothing should be worn by those entering from the black area, and theatre scrubs with boiler suits over the top should be worn from the yellow area.
- Yellow area – this should only be entered through a clean changing room from a black area. Nobody should enter directly from a black area, i.e. from the patient preparation area to the grey area for induction into yellow. Similarly, nobody should exit a yellow area anywhere except via a changing room. Clean theatre scrub suits and theatre hats should be worn when within the yellow area. This area includes the storage areas and scrubbing-in areas.
- White zone – area of maximum restriction, where the operating theatre and sterile storage are located. This should be accessed via a sterile corridor, and a one-way system should be in place, so the dirty traffic does not go back through the white area. Doors must remain closed at all times, and full theatre attire is required [5].

Regardless of the individual set-up in a practice, theatres can be separated into different essential areas. These requirements will be specific to the area, including induction and recovery, preparation area, operating theatre, scrubbing-up area, decontamination and sterilisation area, sterile storage and changing rooms [5].

Induction and Recovery Boxes

Ideally, there would be a separate induction and recovery box; however, this may not be practical or necessary in a smaller practice. The requirements of this area include:

- The room size needs to be large enough for the horse but should not be oversized as this will allow the horse to gain momentum that will only increase the chance of injury – typically, the ideal size is between 12 and 16 ft./4–5 m^2 [6].
- Padded walls and doors at least 8–10 ft./2.5–3 m high using robust surface material that can withstand high impacts and can easily be cleaned; this is usually a polyvinyl chloride (PVC) or rubber-based material; this will also minimise the risk to the patient during induction and recovery [2].
- Soft, rubberised floor with a non-slip surface that provides sufficient traction even when wet, has a drainage system and can readily be cleaned and disinfected [3].
- Some practices may opt for a box that has rounded corners and curved borders, while others have a more traditional square room; whichever type is used, there must be no unpadded square edges or protrusions, as these will lead to injury [3].
- The doorways should be wide enough for the horse to be safely hoisted through from the theatre and taken back to its stable on the opposing side.
- Lockable doors that are secured by transverse bars and/or floor/ceiling bolts [3].
- A pulley system is in place to enable rope recovery; this may be used in all recoveries or occasional ones. All bolts, pulleys and mechanisms should be high enough on the walls not to cause injury to the patient during recovery [2, 3].
- Adjustable lighting that enables visualisation of the horse when required, but during recovery, it is sometimes preferable to have lighting dimmed [2].
- Heating/Air conditioning (AC) system – recovery should be separately temperature controlled so that heating and cooling can be achieved as required. Cooling may not be necessary, depending on the ambient temperature of the general environment [3].
- Hoist – this is a gantry-mounted hoist that is ideally electrically operated; however, even if an electric one is used, a manual hoist should always be available in case of

malfunction. The hoist is essential for moving the horse from the induction box to the operating table and then to the recovery box. In some practices, where there is no preparation room, or the table is not mobile, the hoist will go directly into the theatre. While this may be unavoidable, it is not ideal since the hoist will invariably be contaminated with, for example,. oil and dust. Due to the hoist possibly being over the surgical incision, it is preferable to have a system that avoids the need for the hoist to enter the theatre itself, using a post-induction preparation area and movable operating bed [2].

- There are several ways of monitoring the horse during recovery; the simplest is a spy hole in the door that the person watching the horse can look through; however, the use of closed circuit television (CCTV) that runs to a monitor is preferable as the whole room can be visualised without any blind spots.
- Practices with a high surgical caseload typically have two or more recovery boxes; this allows a second horse to be anaesthetised while the first horse is recovering. The practice should have a number of recovery and induction boxes that suit their caseload; if there are more than necessary, this increases the chance of microorganisms growing on surface areas as they are not used and cleaned as often.

Preparation Area

This area is where the horse can be prepared for surgery, and ideally, the area should include the following features [4]:

- Situated in close proximity to the theatre suite – ideally, this will be a room that adjoins the induction box, so that once the horse is suitably prepared, it can be taken straight into the induction box.
- It needs to be large enough to prepare the horse safely but not too large as this will increase the surface area and encourage further bacterial growth.
- Contain equipment required for preparing the horse; this will vary depending on the individual practice but could include the following:
  - Clippers
  - Shoe removal kit
  - Hoof pick, scrubbing brush and bucket
  - Intravenous (IV) catheter equipment
  - Hosepipe for cleaning the floor
  - Large syringe and bucket for rinsing the mouth out
  - Grooming brushes
  - Tail bandages
  - Induction headcollar (ideally made from leather and padded)
  - Pre-operative sedation
- Sterile gloves and examination gloves

Operating Theatre

Depending on the caseload of the practice, it may be necessary to have at least two operating theatres. This allows for best practice, ensuring that one theatre is kept for 'clean' surgeries, such as elective orthopaedic procedures and fracture repairs. In contrast, the other theatre is used for 'contaminated' procedures, such as colic surgery and dental procedures. This approach ensures that procedures already contaminated do not transmit contamination to non-contaminated, potentially high-risk surgeries. Many practices do not have the luxury of having multiple theatres; if this is the case, cleaning protocols must ensure effective cleaning has been taken place. The requirements for the operating theatre include:

- **Size** – The theatre needs to be large enough to accommodate a horse positioned in dorsal or lateral recumbency and allow enough room for surgical equipment and a surgical team. Generally, a horse in lateral recumbency will take up double the space of one positioned in the dorsal recumbency. A theatre that is too small will compromise working conditions and make it harder to maintain asepsis; however, in contrast, a theatre that is too large will be difficult to keep clean and has a higher surface area for bacterial growth [7].
- **Floors** – Should be made of smooth, impervious, non-staining material that is easy to clean, hard-wearing and non-slip. Industrial vinyl or rubberised floors can be used. However, they may be damaged by heavy equipment (especially the operating table) and cleaning materials. If this happens, it will allow bacterial colonisation under the surface, making it difficult to keep clean. Screeded concrete can also be used. It is hard-wearing, non-slip and easily cleaned; however, the surface can chip away and pit, allowing water to form pools [7].
- **Walls and ceiling** – Should be painted with light-coloured waterproof paint. Anti-bacterial coatings are available, but they are expensive and are not long-lasting, so a re-painting schedule should be implemented. Other options for walls within the operating theatre include:
  - Epoxy Resin Coatings: Durable and resistant to chemicals and stains.
  - Vinyl Wall Coverings: Seamless, hygienic, and easy to clean.
  - Ceramic Tiles: Smooth, non-porous, and easy to disinfect, though grout lines must be minimised.
  - Stainless Steel Panels: Highly durable, easy to clean, and resistant to microbial growth. [7].
- **Operating table** – This should be adjustable to facilitate the needs of the patient and the surgeon. It should ideally be able to be raised, lowered and tilted as necessary, and

this is typically achieved by using a hydraulic or electric pump system. The table may have wheels to allow it to be moved around easily in the room, or it could remain in a fixed position. It is essential to consider that the typical equine patient will be large, heavy and difficult to move. The choice of operating table will depend on the size of the operating theatre, the amount and type of surgeries performed, and financial and personal considerations. There are a range of equine operating tables available:

- **Mobile** – These are typically beds that are on wheels and can be manoeuvred around the theatre suite and into the preparation area as required. Some beds have to remain attached to a power supply to be able to adjust but can be disconnected while the horse is being prepped. Others have a chargeable battery system that allows for completely unrestricted movement.
- **Fixed hydraulics** – These tend not to be as commonly used; as the name suggests, they are fixed, and therefore, there is no way to change the position in the room. They often have a pit under them so the bed can go right to the floor without damaging the hydraulics underneath, but this also creates an area that can build with debris and harbour microorganisms.
- **Inflatable** – These are ideal in a smaller practice with a minimal theatre caseload. They have layers of inflatable mattresses that build up height and are adjustable by removing air from the valves. These do have limitations and can be unstable in certain surgeries [2].

Ideally, the operating theatre should have minimal equipment in it. It should not have any shelving or unnecessary furniture, as this will harbour dust and microorganisms. Any shelving should be behind doors or in a separate area, such as sterile storage. Other important points to consider are as follows:

- **Drains** – Although they are a potential source of bacteria, drains are essential in an equine operating theatre if a good standard of asepsis is to be maintained. A good SOP should be in place detailing how to clean the drains to minimise the risk of bacterial growth. Floors should be gently sloped towards the drains to facilitate drying and prevent the pooling of water [4].
- **Electrical sockets/network interfaces** – There should be a good supply around the room, either recessed into the wall or suspended from the ceiling, and they should have protective covers. Care must be taken that these are out of reach from water and that they do not get wet during the cleaning process [8].
- **Lighting** – This is essential in the operating theatre; ideally, lighting should be flush with the ceiling to prevent dust from building up on surfaces; strip lighting is a good source of light in a theatre. There should also be an adjustable ceiling-mounted spotlight to allow illumination of the surgical site; these can come with single or multiple heads and have removable autoclavable handles to enable the surgeon to have the correct placement of light during a procedure [8].
- **Ventilation** – There should be a positive pressure ventilation system that allows frequent air changes in the operating theatre to remove airborne microorganisms and help maintain asepsis. This, however, is expensive and may not be feasible in smaller practices [4].
- **Windows** – Operating theatres are generally windowless, although windows are becoming more prevalent in newly built theatres, to provide clinical teams with natural light and may improve surgeons' mental well-being and consequently improve surgeon occupational health [9]. However, they should be airtight and soundproof, and the use of tinted glass will mean that blinds are not necessary as they will allow dust to build up on them. Some procedures may require them to be blocked off, i.e. the use of a laser, as this may be detrimental to the health of others.
- **Heating** – The ambient temperature should be 15–20 °C, so some form of heating is required. Airconditioning units may be used as part of the ventilation system, but these should not include a fan; fan heaters must be avoided as they will cause movement of dust and debris. Panel heating within walls is desirable but expensive. Modern wall-mounted radiators are often the most practical method but must be easily cleanable to prevent dust and debris from accumulating [10].
- **Wall clock** – For anaesthetic monitoring and timing of the surgery; if possible, this should be behind a see-through panel to avoid dust accumulation.
- Other fixtures and equipment include:

  - **Anaesthetic machines**, scavenging systems, storage for emergency drugs, and items needed in case of a cardiopulmonary arrest are also required. See Chapter 10 for more details.
  - **A dry wipe board** – where details such as swab numbers and sutures used are recorded.
  - **Theatre trolley** – For holding instruments during surgery. This should be made of stainless steel and, ideally, have two shelves with a guard rim around the edge to prevent instruments from falling on the floor. The mayo trolley is a type of theatre trolley with a removable tray for cleaning. These are adjustable in height and designed to sit over the patient; some also feature a pivot system to assist with placement over the operating table. These are not regularly used in equine practice as they would not easily fit over the equine patient [10].

- **Fittings for piped gases** – oxygen and occasionally nitrous oxide, and medical air for power tools – and scavenging systems may be wall-mounted or dropped from the ceiling.
- **X-ray viewers** – Tend to be portable now that digital imaging systems are mainly used, but this could be built into the wall, so the panel is flush with the wall surface.
- **Wall fittings** - rings in the wall or hoist systems may be used for positioning limbs for surgery [4].

Scrubbing-up Area

Ideally, this should be an adjoining room to the operating theatre, which can be reached via swing doors. Desirable features are as follows:

- Stainless steel scrub sinks at an appropriate height for staff; these should have either elbow- or foot-operated taps.
- Storage for sterile gowns, gloves and hand towels.
- The room should be large enough for the trolley to be laid out and for staff to gown and glove without contamination [7].

Decontamination and Sterilisation Area

A designated area within the theatre suite should allow for the decontamination of used equipment and sterilisation. This should be separate from the sterile storage area to prevent cross-contamination from dirty instruments and include the following features:

- A double sink – this will allow contaminated instruments to be submerged in instrument cleaner and then a sink of clean water to rinse off residual cleaning products [5].
- A range of brushes and cleaning tools to ensure kits are cleaned effectively.
- An ultrasonic cleaner to ensure that all organic matter is removed from instruments before sterilisation.
- A washing machine and tumble dryer to launder all drapes and clothing used in surgery.
- Packing materials required for re-packing clean instruments ready for sterilisation.
- An autoclave for the sterilisation of packed and clean materials.
- An ethylene oxide steriliser to sterilise materials that cannot be processed using an autoclave [11].

Sterile Storage

The sterile storage area should be accessible from all operating theatres and is where all sterilised equipment should be located. It should have the following features:

- There should be limited access to sterile storage, and it should be a temperature-controlled environment – temperature should be 18–23 °C, and humidity should be maintained at between 30% and 60% and not exceed 70% [5].
- The floors, walls and surfaces should be made of materials that are non-porous and able to withstand chemical agents used in cleaning and disinfection [12].
- Shelves used for storage of clean and sterile equipment are at least:
    - 25 cm (10 in.) off the floor
    - 45 cm (18 in.) from the ceiling and sprinkler heads
    - 5 cm (2 in.) from an outside (exterior) wall [6].
- Containers used for clean and sterile storage are
    - Kept clean and free of visible dust or soiling
    - Enclosed or covered
    - Clearly and accurately labelled [11].

Changing Rooms

Changing rooms should be located at the entrance to the theatre and should be marked as sterile areas; they should include the following features:

- External hooks for outdoor coats and jumpers
- Exterior shelving for footwear worn outside of the theatre
- Suitable changing facilities to cater for the individual needs of staff and visitors
- Labelled shelving for staff scrubs and visitor scrubs
- Contain theatre-use boiler suits that are clearly labelled, so that staff can carry out daily jobs inside without getting entirely changed if there is no surgery happening
- Contain theatre footwear that is clearly labelled
- Contain hats and masks
- Contain a written SOP for appropriate theatre attire [2].

11.2 Maintenance and Cleaning of the Theatre Suite

Theatre suite cleaning protocols must be strictly adhered to in order to maintain a clean environment with a low risk of contamination. All areas within the theatre suite must be easy to clean, preferably made of hard plastic or stainless steel and be anti-static. RVNs must understand the importance of maintaining this environment, the schedule for which can be broken down into daily tasks and periodic deep cleans which should typically be carried out on a monthly basis [10].

Daily Care

At the beginning of each day, before the daily operating list commences, all surfaces must be damp dusted; this includes overhead lights, the top of the hoist and anaesthetic monitoring equipment. Damp dusting involves the use of clean or new cloths with a suitable cleaning agent for theatre, to remove all dust particles which may have built up. Traditional dusting moves the dust particles around; therefore the cloth used must be regularly changed to prevent a build-up of bacteria [3].

Between surgeries, all areas within the operating room, including the operating table, any mattresses or stands, equipment and adjoining rooms, must be cleaned and disinfected with an appropriate disinfectant designed to kill microorganisms and their spores. All surfaces and equipment must first be cleaned with water +/− a detergent to remove all organic material before disinfection. Failure to do this may mean that the disinfection process is not achieved due to inactivation or partial inactivation of the active ingredient in the disinfectant by organic materials.

The cleaning process for the theatre suite should begin in the operating room, where the walls should be washed first, working down to the floor and towards the drain. The room should slope slightly towards the drain to prevent water pooling, which may encourage the growth of bacteria. Then, a cleaner safe for all surfaces can be used, using a scrubbing brush marked for theatre use only. Once all areas have been scrubbed, they must be rinsed with clean water. Finally, a disinfectant used at the correct dilution rate, following the manufacturer's guidelines, can be used and left to dry for more prolonged residual activity. The rest of the theatre suite can be cleaned following this same protocol, working from back to front and top to bottom. All surfaces must be wiped down with a disinfectant at the correct dilution at the end of each day, and if using reusable cloths, have a regular rotation of clean ones. All bins must be emptied between each surgery, including general, offensive, clinical and anatomical waste [10].

Other daily tasks may include:

- Care of clippers – clippers should be cleaned and sprayed with a hygiene spray. This will ensure that they are not contaminated when used on other patients.
- If a hoover is used in the theatre to clean any loose hair before scrubbing takes place, this will need regular cleaning and emptying.
- Putting away sterile supplies and ensuring the sterilisation process is complete.
- Stocking consumables and used items required for operating.
- Ensuring all items are in date.
- Changing over any equipment that may be required for emergency surgery out of hours [2].

Periodic Deep Cleaning

Methicillin-resistant *Staphylococcus aureus* (MRSA) is a bacteria that is resistant to commonly used antimicrobials in both animals and humans. It is paramount that the effective use of disinfectants in practice is adhered to. Regular swabbing should be carried out to ensure correct usage. MRSA is a nosocomial (hospital-acquired) bacteria that is one of the top causes of post-operative complications in hospitalised patients. Because of this, regular deep cleans must be factored into the running of a theatre suite; this should ideally be carried out every month along with monthly swabbing of a range of areas to ensure no bacterial growth has occurred, and that the disinfectant solutions and cleaning protocols used are effective. Deep cleaning the theatre suite means all areas, including drains, windows and coving are thoroughly cleaned. A wet vacuum could help reduce the amount of standing water (with regular filter changes required) or an industrial floor scrubber could be used [13].

All cleaning utensils and equipment used in the theatre must be colour-coded or marked 'Theatre use only'. This prevents contamination from other parts of the practice, which would be classed as 'dirty'.

Electrical Equipment Cleaning and Maintenance

Modern operating theatres contain a range of electrical equipment that will require special considerations when it comes to maintenance; these include:

- **Clippers** – These are essential items in theatre; they will be used to touch up any surgical site clipping and clip areas for arterial lines and emergency catheter placement. Clippers used in theatre must be 'Theatre-only' clippers and serviced annually. New clipper blades are recommended for each surgery ensuring the blades sharp and free from contamination; if this is not possible, they should be appropriately cleaned and sprayed with hygiene spray to prevent cross-contamination. Clippers should undergo portable appliance testing (PAT) annually.
- **Lighting** – Strip lighting and spotlights require annual servicing.
- **Operating table** – Annual servicing and PAT testing if there are electrical components, so the table is safe for use; if using hydraulic arms on the table, having spares is essential to allow for them to be replaced if they break during surgery.
- **Hoists** – Electric/manual, annual service by the manufacturer, keep well-oiled unless not required by the manufacturer. PAT testing is required for electric hoists.
- **Stretchers** – These are made out of fabric or plastic with handles to lift a patient. Due to the size of the horse, they

are not commonly used but are helpful for foals; these need to be checked for cracks.

- **Hobbles** – These are required to go around the patient's pasterns to lift the horse onto and off the surgical table. These need a weight certificate to be issued annually to ensure they are safe to use.
- **Autoclave** – Depending on usage, this will require either bi-annual or annual servicing and also require a boiler test done annually – this will require the manufacturer and a boiler inspector to be present at the same time, and the autoclave must be cold to carry this out, it is advised that it is switched off overnight to ensure that this is the case.
- **Ethylene oxide steriliser** – Annual service by the manufacturer and PAT testing.
- **Suction unit** – This is an essential item in the operating theatre for many reasons. It can be used for removing blood and fluid from the surgical field and occasionally for the aspiration of fluids from the oropharynx and nasopharynx during or after surgery, or for suctioning fluids and blood during surgical procedures. Various suction machines are available, and size should be considered – units range from one to four canisters depending on usage required, with a preference being for two canisters, to allow one to be quickly emptied while the other is in use (Figure 11.1). Fluid accumulation should be disposed

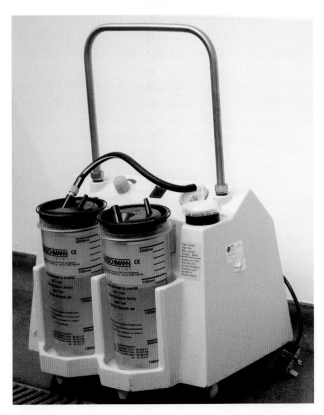

Figure 11.1 Double canister suction unit. *Source:* Rosina Lillywhite.

of appropriately, and some suction units have liners containing the fluid rather than pouring it down a sluice drain. Most suction units have manufacturers' guidelines for disposal and safe use and local and national waste disposal legislation. These must be thoroughly cleaned after use and disinfected, especially if a reusable canister is being used. These units must be sent off for servicing annually, so there is no drop in suction performance. They will also require an annual PAT test [4].

- **Diathermy unit** – This machine uses a high-frequency electrical current, which produces heat within the tissues at the point of application. The nature of the waveform of the applied current used in diathermy can vary in effect from continuous waveforms for cutting tissues and interrupted waveforms for coagulation. It is a valuable piece of equipment that allows rapid control of haemorrhages, minimising blood loss, and allows for clear visualisation of the surgical field. The electrical box should be damp dusted daily, ensuring that dust and debris do not build up. After each use of the diathermy, the earth plate should be cleaned and disinfected (if reusable). The cable and leads should be inspected for patency and then washed; the electrical ends should not be submerged in water unless the manufacturer's guidelines state that this is appropriate. The unit should be maintained according to 'the manufacturers guidelines and serviced and maintained regularly by a qualified engineer. PAT testing should be carried out annually. There are several types of diathermy machines available for surgical use. The two most common types are:
  - **Monopolar diathermy** – this typically uses a finger-switch pencil used for cutting and coagulation. This diathermy requires the patient to be 'earthed' or 'grounded' using a diathermy pad. In monopolar action, the electrical current oscillates between the surgeon's electrode through the patient's body until it meets the 'diathermy pad' (typically positioned on the patient's spine) to complete the circuit. If this is not present, the electricity will pass along the line of least resistance, which may be the patient or the surgeon leading to a severe electric shock or burning. The earth plate may be disposable or reusable.
  - **Bipolar diathermy** – does not require a ground or earth plate as the current passes through the tips of the forceps across the tissue. The current is usually activated using a foot pedal connected to the machine. Coagulation is achieved by applying the forceps directly to the source of the bleeding, by touching or clamping the vessel [4].
- **Cryosurgery equipment** – Uses extreme cold to destroy living tissue and aims to kill diseased cells in a target area, whilst causing minimal damage to the surrounding healthy tissue. Liquid nitrogen is most commonly used,

and after application to the area, the intracellular and extracellular water begins to freeze with its reduced temperature causing the formation of ice crystals, eventually leading to cell denaturation and death. Liquid nitrogen is a harmful substance, so many precautions are associated with its storage and use. To comply with Control of Substances Hazardous to Health (COSHH) regulations, a SOP should be in place to prevent accidents when storing and handling liquid nitrogen. All personnel involved in the use of liquid nitrogen should be trained and familiar with the SOP. Liquid nitrogen should be transported and stored only in containers supplied by the liquid nitrogen provider or a cryosurgical equipment manufacturer. These are insulated metal containers of varying sizes. The correct personal protective equipment (PPE) should always be worn when handling liquid nitrogen; this should include protective goggles, an apron and insulated gloves. Contact with the skin should be avoided as this will cause severe thermal burning. In veterinary practice, small specially developed thermos canisters are used as they are easy to handle and manipulate. The liquid nitrogen can be applied via a probe attachment that adheres to the tissue surface or from a more diffuse spray. Once the probe or spray attachment has been used, it will be frozen, so it should be left to thaw before being washed and disinfected. The remaining liquid nitrogen should be poured back into the main container [4].

- **Laser** – Laser stands for 'light amplification by stimulated emission of radiation' . Laser is used to seal small blood vessels and lymph vessels as it cuts, reducing bleeding and post-op swelling. It also allows the surgeon to be more precise in their actions since the tissues appear cleaner and more apparent. Laser seals off nerve endings as it cuts, reducing post-operative pain [14]. It kills bacteria instantly, effectively sterilising the operating area. It is helpful in minor procedures such as sarcoid removals and hobday surgeries. The laser machine requires an annual service by the manufacturer; the goggles must be regularly checked for defects to ensure they are safe for their intended use. It will also require PAT testing [4].

11.3 Roles in the Operating Theatre

The procedure for setting up the operating theatre varies slightly depending on the individual surgery and the patient. A foal will require a slightly higher ambient temperature than an adult horse, as foals cannot regulate their body temperature as efficiently. A colic surgery will require different equipment compared to a fracture repair. It is essential to be aware of the differences in surgical techniques, hospital or practice protocols and surgeon preferences. RVNs should be involved in the planning that goes into creating a surgical plan; a good plan should consider the needs of the patient, surgeon, anaesthetist and nursing team to minimise risk factors and increase the chances of success.

The correct order of surgeries is essential to reduce the risk of surgical site contamination. If space allows, two theatres are necessary for gold standard practice allowing for clean and dirty procedures to be separated into different theatres. However, if this is not possible, then the operating list should follow the stated order below from first to last:

- Clean – Elective orthopaedic procedure, implants may be used.
- Clean contaminated – Controlled entry into the gastrointestinal or respiratory tract.
- Contaminated – Open, fresh wound <6 hours old, small intestinal resections with no excess contamination.
- Dirty – Infected wounds >6 hours old, anal surgery, colon dump as these have an increased risk of MRSA due to the nature of the wound or area of the surgical site [10].

Theatre Attire

Good personal hygiene and general cleanliness are essential to maintaining asepsis within the theatre suite; before entering, all personnel should wash their hands; hand washing should occur regularly while working in the theatre suite. If clothing becomes contaminated at any stage, scrubs must also be changed, ideally personnel should shower before returning to the theatre. All jewellery, including watches, rings and earrings, must be removed before entering the theatre suite, as they harbour bacteria and risk contaminating the surgical site. If jewellery cannot be removed, it must be covered with tape. Finger nails must be kept short, and the use of nail varnish, including gel and acrylic, is much debated. The latest studies show that there is not an increase in the number of microorganisms if nail varnish is on and undamaged. However, if there is damage to the surface of the nail varnish, this can facilitate an increase in microorganisms. Therefore, current advice is to avoid wearing nail varnish or acrylics in the operating theatre.

No outdoor clothing or footwear should be worn inside the theatre suite. It is best practice for all personnel entering a theatre suite to either change into a two-piece scrub suit or cover their outerwear with a boiler suit. Theatre clothing should be made from cotton or polyester and worn inside the suite. It should be washed at the end of the day and changed between surgeries if necessary or thought to be contaminated; all laundering should be done within the theatre suite.

Footwear for theatre is typically croc-type shoes or wellingtons with non-slip, antistatic soles, which are easy to clean either in a washing machine or wiped over.

Scrub hats are required to ensure that hair and skin flakes do not contaminate the theatre; these can either be made from reusable cotton or be disposable. Using cotton hats has less environmental impact over disposable hats, especially in large practices that typically use large quantities of these items. Different designs cover long hair, short hair and beards [4].

There is currently mixed evidence on the use of surgical masks in the operating theatre and the reduction in postoperative site infections. There is not yet enough data to say that they should not be worn, so it is still believed to be best practice to wear a surgical mask during procedures; however, these should be changed between procedures or during if it is a lengthy procedure to minimise the chance of the mask losing efficacy [15].

Conduct

Effective and clear communication is critical to ensure the smooth, efficient running of the theatre suite; and minimise the chance of error due to human factors. Although all personnel within the operating theatre should understand where they can and cannot go, sometimes situations can occur where there is a break in sterility. If this situation occurs, an environment should be created that allows personnel to speak up without fear of retribution, allowing for immediate resolution.

As an RVN in theatre, there are three main roles, a circulating nurse, a scrubbed RVN, or an anaesthetist; these roles are equally crucial to the smooth running of an operating suite and have independent functions, but form part of the team that is crucial to enable surgery to happen [8]. The role of the RVN as an anaesthetist is covered in Chapter 10.

The Circulating Nurse

As the circulating nurse, it is essential to ensure that any ancillary and powered equipment is checked before the procedure starts and that any equipment relating to the procedure, including relevant gowns and gloves, are out and ready to open, maintaining sterility throughout.

The circulating nurse is responsible for positioning the patient correctly for surgery, preparing the patient and ensuring the correct site has been clipped and then prepared for surgery. Clipping, where possible, should be done before the patient enters the theatre to prevent contamination and reduce surgical time. In a gold-standard environment, clipping would be done in a preparation area outside the main theatre, so that the horse can be fully prepared on the theatre bed and then wheeled into the theatre. If this is not possible within the set-up, a hoover can be used to remove all hair and debris post-clipping, minimising the chance of contamination.

Applying a tourniquet or an Esmarch bandage may be a role for the circulating nurse and therefore needs to be understood. Esmarch bandage tourniquets are commonly used in theatre and are typically applied by the RVN before the surgical scrub has started. Esmarch tourniquets used during surgery can aid the surgeon in providing a bloodless surgical field which assists with the identification of anatomical structures. In turn, this helps to reduce operating time and therefore reduce surgical complications. Care is needed for prolonged use, as this could lead to ischemic damage or neuropathy of the limb depending on the location and time the tourniquet is in place. Tourniquets are commonly reusable and do not need to be sterile as the application occurs before the sterile scrub takes place, but will still need to be cleaned and disinfected between patients [4].

Esmarch bandage or Esmarch tourniquet is a typically 10 cm wide soft rubber bandage used to expel blood from a limb (exsanguinate). The bandage is applied to the distal end of the limb and extends proximally up the limb. The remaining bandage is used as a traditional tourniquet to cut off the blood supply. Once secured in place, the distal portion can be unravelled and tied around the tourniquet portion of the bandage. The limb is often elevated as the elastic pressure is applied. The exsanguination is necessary to enable some arthroscopic procedures to take place, as having blood in the surgical field would cause difficulty navigating the surgical area [16].

Once the horse has been correctly positioned and prepared for surgery, the circulating nurse can assist with dressing the surgeon, scrub nurse and opening sterile supplies. When passing sterile instruments to a scrubbed operator, it is essential to maintain asepsis at all times ensuring that the instrument handle is being passed first and directly into the hands or the surgeon or assistant. It is vital to know how to open all sterile packaging and to ensure that none comes in contact with the sterile field. Instruments should be opened in the order in which they will be used (e.g. trolley drape first followed by the surgical kit). It is also essential to stand in a position that avoids leaning over the sterile field and ensure that the surgeons' view is not obstructed. When passing sterile instruments, it is vital to take care and not damage any equipment when passing it to the surgeon [13].

The circulating nurse may be required to assist with draping the patient; it is essential to listen to the surgeon and act on their instructions to maintain sterility at all times.

During the surgery, the circulating nurse can clear away used materials, prepare cleaning products and pass any equipment or consumables that the surgeon may require during surgery. Recording of instruments and swab counts during surgery is essential for patient safety. Many practices will have kits made up of pre-counted swabs and a certain number of instruments included per kit. This should be the same number every time, but all equipment must be counted prior to the surgery start time. During surgery, the number of swabs or instruments removed from the sterile field must be accounted for; a whiteboard is helpful in theatre. A regular count during surgery is useful, with another count performed before closing. A final count of all instruments, needles and swabs should also be performed at the end of surgery. This is also an excellent time to invoice the materials used during the surgery to ensure the clients' billing is kept up to date and this prevent items from being forgotten.

Monitoring blood loss during equine surgery is complex, although swabs can be weighed and an estimate can be made if able to contain the blood in a bowl or bucket. If this is not possible, the circulating nurse should be vigilant with how often blood is washed away and communicate with the surgeon if at all concerned. However, a horse's large blood volume means that they seldom have a blood loss issue [4].

After the surgery, the circulating nurse may be required to place a bandage on the patient if they have had surgery on a limb and assist with transporting the horse to the recovery box. If not needed to assist with the recovery, the circulating nurse can clean the theatre and prepare for the next patient [2].

The Scrub Nurse

The role of the scrub nurse is to assist the surgeon with the sterile procedure by scrubbing into the surgery and passing instruments and consumables as required [4]. They must systematically scrub the skin on their arms and hands (see method below). Once they have achieved this, they can don a gown and gloves and assist with laying out the instruments on the trolley. Maintaining sterility is paramount, so an awareness of surroundings whilst acting as a scrubbed assistant is essential. When not required to pass instruments or assist, the scrub nurse should place their hands together or keep them on the trolly. This prevents the temptation of touching somewhere inadvertently.

As the scrubbed nurse, it is essential to have all instruments laid out on the instrument trolley and easily visible, making them easier to find when asked for them. The order

they are laid out in will be similar for all types of surgery, although there will be some key differences. Instruments on the trolley must be laid out in order of use and, depending on preference, left to right or right to left [10].

1) Towel clamps
2) Drape scissors
3) Scalpel blade

The instruments used next will depend on the surgery; the final instruments will always be the same

- Needle holders, also sometimes known as needle drivers
- Rat tooth forceps

Using the correct method to pass instruments to the surgeon is vital for ease, speed and safety; they must be given with the blade facing away from the surgeon and the handle placed into a finger grip. Ringed instruments must be passed into the surgeons' palms with points outwards and curves upwards. All instruments with ratchets must not have these engaged. A theatre nurse may open needles and syringes, and both the needle and cap must always be taken; the cap must remain in place until the syringe is ready for use.

When mounting and demounting a blade, the blade must face forward, down and away from the operator. This will help to prevent injury during the removal process.

Maintaining sterility of the trolley during procedures must be strictly adhered to; this is managed by an acute awareness of surroundings, ensuring all sharps are kept facing away with the blade laid on a clean, sterile swab so as not to pierce the trolley drape accidentally. Fluids must be kept to one end in case of strikethrough. All tissues removed should be placed onto a clean swab or metal dish to be dealt with at the end of surgery.

At the end of the surgery, the scrub nurse is responsible for performing a final count of swabs and instruments before closure; they can then take the surgical kit to be cleaned and decontaminated, ready for re-sterilisation [13].

Scrubbing into Surgery

The technique for scrubbing into surgery should follow a systematic method, starting with a skin antiseptic. This removes all organic material and microorganisms from the elbows down to the hands, as it is impossible to sterilise the skin. There are two typical scrub solutions commonly used in practice for traditional scrubbing techniques:

Chlorhexidine gluconate 4% – Has broad-spectrum antimicrobial qualities, is effective against organic matter, is virucidal and fungicidal, and has sporicidal properties. It has an improved residual effect compared to povidone-iodine. It is harmful to mucous membranes and has been proven to irritate tissues and be ulcerative to the eyes, so care should be taken in these areas [4].

Povidone-Iodine 10% – This also has broad-spectrum antimicrobial qualities, ineffective against organic matter, has virucidal and fungicidal properties and has a relatively short period of efficacy. Also found to be an irritant to tissues and should be used at the correct dilution if used around mucous membranes [10].

The Traditional Method of Hand Scrubbing

Research has shown that significant numbers of common skin bacteria continue to be removed after 5 minutes of scrubbing, but at 10 minutes, no more significant benefit ensues. Therefore, it is logical to adopt a scrubbing technique that takes 5–10 minutes, allowing time for rinsing between stages. The method for using both chlorhexidine gluconate and povidone iodine is as follows [17]:

1) Remove jewellery and watches, and ensure fingernails are short.
2) Adjust the water supply to a safe flow and temperature – this is usually elbow or foot operated, although no-touch sensors may also be used. Once the scrubbing has begun, the hands should not touch the taps, sink or soap dispenser; only use elbows or feet should be used. If they are inadvertently touched, repeat the last stage of the procedure.
3) Wash the hands thoroughly using a plain soap or surgical scrub solution and clean under the nails with a sterile nail pick – pre-prepared scrub brushes that contain a nail pick can be used.
4) After hand washing, the arms are washed up to and including the elbows. Always keep the hands above the elbows so that water drains down towards the unscrubbed arms to avoid recontamination – this phase aims to remove organic matter and grease from the skin.
5) Rinse both hands and arms by allowing water to wash away the soap from the hands to the elbows (avoid using the opposite hand to assist with the rinsing, which could lead to recontamination).
6) Repeat this procedure, beginning with the hands, using a surgical scrub solution such as chlorhexidine or povidone-iodine. Use minimal water to produce a lather so the scrub solution does not get diluted, reducing its bacterial properties. Correct contact times for the product used should be used.
7) Excessive amounts of water will rinse away the scrub solution before it has destroyed sufficient bacteria.
8) Rinse off the scrub solution from the hands but leave the arms coated.

9) Take a sterile scrubbing brush and scrub solution and systematically scrub the hands. Scrub the palms of the hand, wrist and four surfaces of each finger and thumb, nails and nailbed. Either rinse the brush, add more scrub solution and scrub the other hand, or discard it and take a second brush. It is advisable to avoid scrubbing the backs of the hands and arms as the skin here tends to be sensitive and scrubbing with a brush may damage the surface, increasing surface microorganisms. Some commercially available disposable scrub brushes have very soft bristles and a sponge back which may be less traumatic to this sensitive skin and allow scrubbing of this area without leading to excoriation. If a brush is used on the arms, then both hands and arms should be rinsed during stage 7.
10) Rinse the hands and arms as in stage 5.
11) Wash the hands and arms in surgical scrub solution, but this time finish just below the elbow, so there is no danger of contact with a previously unscrubbed area.
12) Rinse the hands and arms as before, and then turn off the tap using an elbow or foot.
13) Allow excess water to drip from the elbows before leaving the sink.
14) Take a sterile hand towel, holding it at arm's length, so it does not touch the scrub suit. Use a different section to dry each hand and arm. Discard the towel. It is a good idea to check the clock at the start and again before the final stage to ensure that the procedure has taken the allotted time [4].

Sterillium® Surgical Hand Preparation

This method is now widely replacing the traditional hand scrubbing technique in many practices. There are multiple benefits of using Sterillium®, which is fast-acting and has long-lasting efficacy with broad-spectrum antimicrobial qualities. It has virucidal, fungicidal and sporicidal properties with a long residual effect. Sterillium® is non irritating to tissues and can increase the skin's moisture levels with regular use [18].

The use of Sterillium® should start with a hand wash; any can be used; however, the manufacturer of Sterillium® makes a product called Baktolin®, which is a cleanser only and has no antimicrobial ingredients, it has a neutral pH, so it is much kinder to the skin. The hand wash only needs to occur before the first surgery of the day and does not need to be repeated, unless the hands get soiled between patients [18].

Once the hand wash has been completed, the following steps should be completed with Sterillium®; the process takes 90 seconds, using a timer and the hands must remain moist all this time. Immediately before starting, the Sterillium® timer is set and starts counting down [18].

1) A minimum of 1.2 ml of Sterillium® is dispensed into the palm of one hand.
2) The fingers of the opposite hand are dipped into the solution, working it under the nails.
3) The solution is spread onto the palm, fingers and back of the first hand.
4) This is repeated with the other hand, using another 1.2 ml Sterillium®.
5) Another 1.2 ml Sterillium® is dispensed into the palm of one hand and spread onto the forearm.
6) This step is repeated with the other forearm.
7) Finally, another 1.2 ml Sterillium® is dispensed into the hands, which are rubbed until the 90-second timer sounds and the hands are dry.
8) The hands are kept in a vertical position and are ready for gloving [17].

Closed Gloving

Most surgical gloves are made of latex, but it is now becoming more popular to have latex-free gloves available, as latex can cause a skin reaction in some people. Having non-powdered gloves is preferable for surgeries to prevent contamination from the powder when they are donned and during surgery. Still, powdered options, which tend to be cheaper, are suitable for minor procedures. All sterile gloves create an effective barrier and increase asepsis; depending on which technique is used, the asepsis is increased [3].

Disposable surgical gowns are commonly used and ensure asepsis is maintained; they are pre-packaged, pre-sterilised and water resistant. Reusable gowns are not as common in practice, but their use may increase due to their environmental benefits; however, they need to be washed, dried and packed, which some feel outweighs the cost of purchasing disposable gowns. Reusable gowns also lose their sterility rapidly when wet, as they are not typically water resistant, so 'strike-through' (fluid leaking through the gown) occurs. Most gowns come with side ties, providing better coverage and this means that the whole gown remains sterile.

The transition away from surgical gowns with ties at the back is driven by a focus on maintaining sterility and enhancing the safety of surgical procedures. Traditional gowns with back ties present several issues:

1) Sterility compromise: The back of the gown becomes non-sterile once the ties are fastened, as this process typically involves touching the gown's exterior, potentially introducing contaminants. This non-sterile area increases the risk of contamination during surgery.

2) Enhanced design features: Modern surgical gowns have front closures or wrap-around styles that ensure the entire gown remains sterile. These designs allow for a more straightforward and reliable process for maintaining sterility.
3) Infection control: The transition to gowns without back ties is crucial in reducing hospital-acquired infections (HAIs). This design shift helps minimise contamination, thereby protecting both patients and employees.
4) Ease of use: Gowns with front closures or Velcro straps are easier to secure and adjust, improving the surgical team's overall efficiency and effectiveness.[13].

The closed gloving technique should be used if preparing for surgery with a gown and gloves. Using this technique means the hands should not come out the end of the gown and contact the outside or the outside of the gloves. It is essential to realise that the hands can never truly be sterile, whereas the gown and gloves are [16]. The correct technique for closed gloving is as follows:

1) Ask the assistant to open the gown for you, take out the gown and place it on the sterile trolley (Figure 11.2); if using a disposable gown, carefully open the lining around the gown; care should be taken when opening not to touch your hands on the table surface and keep your hands on the inside of the lining.

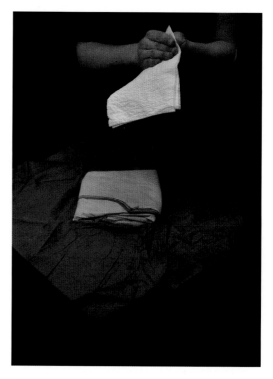

Figure 11.2 Opening a gown. *Source:* Rosina Lillywhite.

2) Pick the gown up and face the inside towards you with the arm holes visible, then gently slide arms into the arm holes while allowing the gown to drop towards the floor (Figures 11.3 and 11.4). *Make sure you are not standing near any surfaces that you may touch*

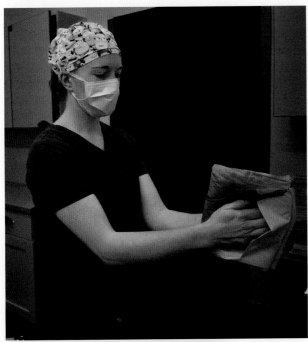

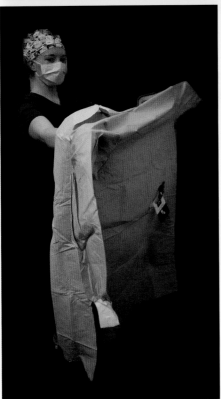

Figures 11.3 and 11.4 Putting on a gown. *Source:* Rosina Lillywhite.

3) You then need to ask your assistant to carefully, without touching the outside of the gown, fasten the top fastening at the neck and the tie in the back that has an external and internal tie that tie together, closing the back portion of the gown (Figures 11.5 and 11.6).
4) Ask the assistant to pass you a pair of gloves, take the inner packet without touching the outside packaging or allowing your fingers to leave the gown.
5) Place the glove packet on the trolley (Figure 11.7), ensuring that the fingers are pointing towards you, then open the glove packet, ensuring that you don't touch the surface, keeping your hands on the inside of the packet and within your gown at all times – the right glove is on the left, and the left glove is on the right (Figure 11.8).
6) Using the right hand, pick up the right glove by the rim of the glove's cuff. The hand is then turned upside down, so the fingers face the body and the glove is lying flat on the palm/wrist of the hand (Figures 11.9 and 11.10).
7) Next, with the left hand, grasp the rim of the glove on the right hand and pull the glove over the hand. At the same time, push your fingers out of the gown into the glove (Figures 11.11 and 11.12).

When the glove is on, repeat the process on the left hand and try to make final adjustments to the gown until both hands are in the gown.

8) Once both hands are safely inside the gloves, adjustments can be made; you should aim for the gown to be at knuckle height inside the gloves to ensure a good overlap between the two (Figure 11.13).
9) If using a side-tying gown, you now need to remove the cardboard tab from the short section of the tie and pass the tab to an assistant, informing them only to hold the end of the cardboard (most modern gowns are colour-coded to help with this). Figure 11.14.
10) Once they have hold of the tab, you need to spin around carefully. Once back to the front, pull out the tie from the tab and tie it to the side of the gown (Figure 11.15).
11) You are now sterile, provided your hands have not been on the outside of the gown at any point and have not touched any surfaces. Once gowned and gloved, stand with hands clasped in front of you to minimise the risk of contaminating yourself (Figure 11.16) [4].

Open Gloving

Open gloving is a technique used when a gown is not required; this would include minor procedures and sterile scrubbing [10].

1) The glove packet is opened so the fingers can point away from the body.

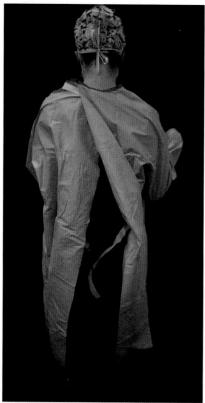

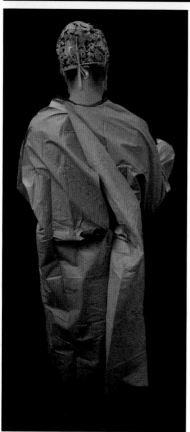

Figures 11.5 and 11.6 Tying the back of the gown. *Source:* Rosina Lillywhite.

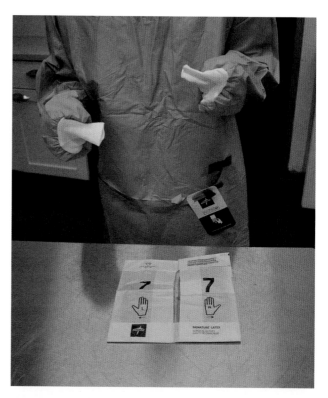

Figure 11.7 Put the glove packet on the trolley. *Source:* Rosina Lillywhite.

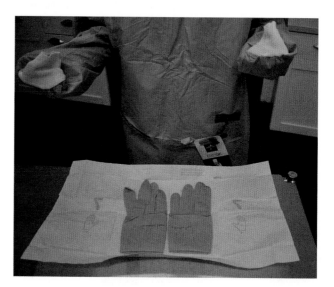

Figure 11.8 Opening the gloves. *Source:* Rosina Lillywhite.

2) Using the left hand, the right glove is picked up at the bottom of the folded back cuff and holding only the inner surface of the glove; it is pulled onto the right hand; the right thumb must hook under the cuff.

3) This is repeated on the left hand, but using the right hand, the free fingers tuck under the cuff to pull the

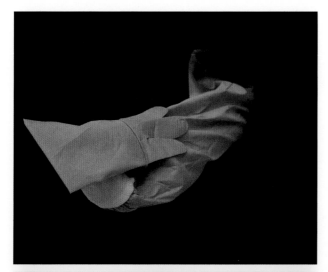

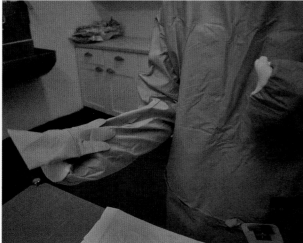

Figures 11.9 and 11.10 Picking up the glove. *Source:* Rosina Lillywhite.

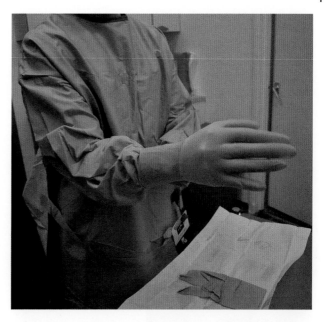

Figure 11.12 Putting the glove on. *Source:* Rosina Lillywhite.

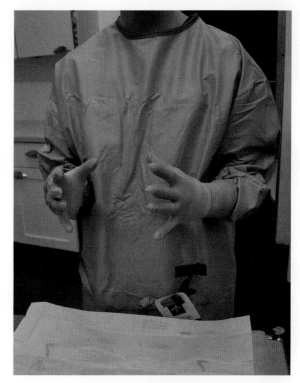

Figure 11.13 Both gloves are on. *Source:* Rosina Lillywhite.

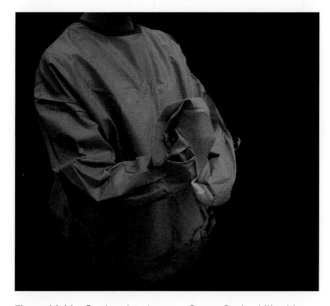

Figure 11.11 Putting the glove on. *Source:* Rosina Lillywhite.

glove onto the hand, only touching the glove's outer surface.

4) The left hand can finish gloving the right hand by taking the rim up to the wrist.

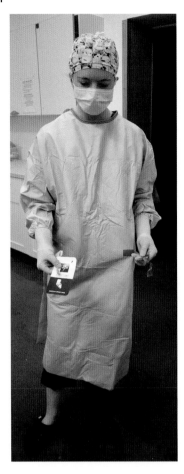

Figure 11.14 Passing the tab. *Source:* Rosina Lillywhite.

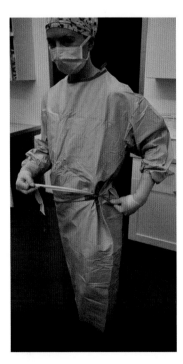

Figure 11.15 Tying the tab. *Source:* Rosina Lillywhite.

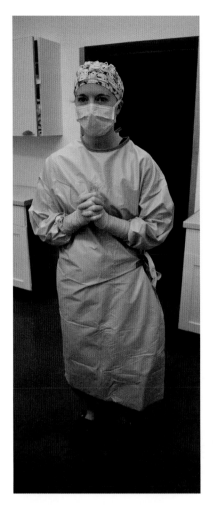

Figure 11.16 Completed closed gloving. *Source:* Rosina Lillywhite.

5) Now, the left hand can un-hook the glove of the right thumb and pull the rim up the wrist.
6) You have now finished gloving.

Once scrubbed, an acute awareness of surroundings must be adopted; maintaining good posture and only touching the sterile field are imperative for asepsis to be maintained. Keeping hands clasped together, above the waist and below the shoulders discourages touching of the non-sterile field [4].

Preparing an Instrument Trolley

Instrument trolleys should be laid up during the sterile scrub so surgery can start immediately. This can be done via an assistant handing the instruments and equipment to either the surgeon or the scrub nurse so they can lay them out; if the practice does not have enough staff for this, the scrub nurse may delay scrubbing in to assist the surgeon and then pass the kit to them to lay the trolley. Once the circulating nurse has completed the sterile scrub, the scrub nurse can scrub in and join the surgeon [8].

It is also possible to lay out the trolley before the surgery and then place a sterile drape over the top to prevent contamination before the surgery begins. This means that trolleys can be laid by a person wearing sterile gloves before the horse is anaesthetised; this can speed up the surgery time, especially when working in a smaller team. All equipment, instruments, drapes, suture materials, saline and other consumables required should be placed on the trolley. Lists with requirements for different procedures are helpful when several different RVNs work in the theatre. In some theatres, a checklist is used whereby the surgeon ticks or lists specific requirements for each surgery. Using the pre-laid trolley method may mean that there is a higher chance that instruments become contaminated; however, more research is required to understand this fully [4].

11.4 Instruments

RVNs should be familiar with the more commonly used surgical instruments and equipment. These can be expensive and should be well maintained and handled correctly.

Materials used for surgical instruments vary and will have an impact on the cost and lifespan of the equipment. Materials include:

Stainless Steel

- Stainless steel is the material of choice for most instruments.
- Stainless steel is a ferrous alloy with a minimum of 10.5% chromium content (ferrous metals contain iron and are magnetic. They are prone to rust and therefore require a protective finish, which is sometimes used to improve the aesthetics of the product).
- The name originates from the fact that stainless steel does not stain, corrode or rust as easily as ordinary steel.
- Steel is made stainless by adding nickel and chromium.
- The more chromium used in making stainless steel, the softer the alloy becomes, which is undesirable in manufacturing surgical instruments.
- Therefore, the mix required to make quality medical instruments is very specific and has well-defined parameters.
- It is expensive, but resists corrosion, is very strong and has a pleasing appearance [4].

Chromium-plated Carbon Steel

- Lower in price than stainless steal
- Will rust, pit and blister, especially when used with chemicals and saline
- Will blunt quickly [4]

Titanium

- Titanium is a very light, strong white metal, less than half the weight of steel.
- It has a desirable strength-to-weight ratio.
- Titanium is alloyed with 6% aluminium and 4% vanadium.
- One of titanium's most notable characteristics is that it is as strong as steel but is only 60% of its density, providing lightweight, flexible strength and decreases user fatigue.
- Excellent corrosion resistance in many environments, including oxidising acids and chlorides.
- This material can be heated up to 440 °C, making it suitable for heat sterilisation.
- Due to its complex machining and finishing processes, titanium instruments are more expensive [10].

Tungsten Carbide

- Tungsten carbide is among the hardest materials known and is sometimes referred to as a 'man-made diamond'.
- Is expensive.
- The primary advantage of tungsten carbide is its hardness, making it very resistant to wear and corrosion.
- To obtain its unique hardness, the unhardened tungsten carbide must be heat treated or 'sintered' at 1454–3200 °C.
- Tungsten carbide inserts are used in surgical instruments to enhance their performance and longevity.
- These inserts are micro-bonded to the working end of the device to provide years of increased performance.
- Tungsten carbide needle holders and forceps grasp more securely and are more durable than their stainless steel counterparts.
- Tungsten carbide scissors and bone rasps cut better and need much less sharpening than similar conventional instruments.
- Gold handles are used to identify instruments with tungsten carbide in the tips.; it is important to remember that it is only the tips that contain tungsten carbide, not the whole instrument [13].

Most practices will have specific instruments grouped together into kits. The contents of these kits will be based on the preference of the surgeon, and kits will be based on procedures or procedures common to specific practices. Each time these kits are packed, they must have precisely the same instruments so that everyone knows what should be in each kit, and it is easy to know if things are missing from it. Instrument sets can also be colour-coded using adhesive instrument tape that can come in various colours.

Common Instruments

Scalpel

This is the most common instrument for dividing tissue with minimal trauma. Most commonly used are scalpel handles with interchangeable single-use blades (Figure 11.17). The main advantage of interchangeable blades is consistent sharpness. A rounded (beaver) blade handle with a smaller interchangeable blade is mainly used for ophthalmic surgeries.

When trying to remember which size handle to use for which blade, it is helpful to remember the following:

- Blades with the numeric prefix of '1' (e.g. 10, 11, 12, 15) fit #3 or #7 blade handles.
- Blades with the numeric prefix of '2' (e.g. 20, 21, 22, 23, 24) fit #4 blade handles [4].

Towel Clips

They are used to attach drapes to the patient and instruments to the operating site. There are two types commonly used in equine practice (Figure 11.18):

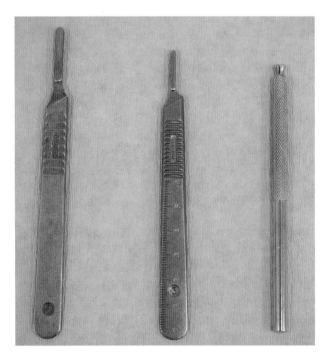

Figure 11.17 Scalpel blade handles – from left to right No. 4, No. 3, Beaver handle. *Source:* Rosina Lillywhite.

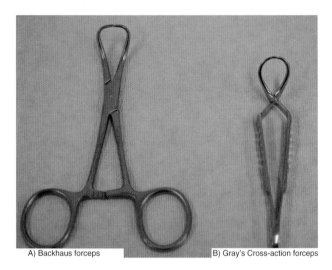

A) Backhaus forceps   B) Gray's Cross-action forceps

Figure 11.18 Towel clips – from left to right, Backhaus forceps, Grey's cross-action forceps. *Source:* Rosina Lillywhite.

- Backhaus forceps have ringed handles and curved, pointed, tongue-like tips.
- Gray's cross-action forceps are commonly used in small animal surgery; they have a strong spring-clip attachment, tend to have a smaller jaw and are more challenging to use in the equine patient [4].

Needle Holders

These are forceps designed explicitly for holding suture needles during stitching and knot tying. There are four main types in practice, and surgeons and RVNs will develop a personnel preference for one or more. Examples are as follows (Figure 11.19):

- **Olsen-Hegar needle holders** – have a cutting edge and a ratchet to hold the needle securely. These are common in practice due to not requiring scissors when suturing. This can, however, lead to unintentional suture cutting when learning to suture.
- **Mayo-Hegar needle holders** – resemble a pair of artery forceps. They have a ratchet but no scissor action; they are suitable for beginners.
- **McPhail needle holders** – handles have a spring ratchet, so the jaws open and close when squeezed to release or hold the needle.
- **Gillies needle holders** – have a scissor action for cutting suture ends but have no ratchet; this means the needle needs to be held in place by gripping the blades tightly, which can cause muscle fatigue for the user [2].

Figure 11.19 Needle holders – from left to right; Olsen Hegar, Mayo-Hegar, Mcphail, Gillies. *Source:* Rosina Lillywhite.

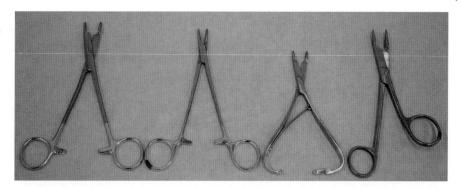

Dissecting Forceps

Also known as thumb forceps, they are designed to handle tissues and other materials and manipulate needles and other instruments while operating. They have a spring action, and the jaws are opposed by holding the metal blades together. They either have a plain or toothed end. Forceps with a plain end are used for handling delicate tissues such as viscera and are atraumatic, while toothed forceps are used for denser tissues and are traumatic. Forceps should be held in the pen grip, with the index finger running along one arm of the forceps and the thumb along the other to allow optimal fine motor control and access for ease of manipulation of tissue [10]. Examples are as follows (Figure 11.20):

- **Rat-toothed forceps** – Have a small rat-toothed grasping end and are used to hold (grip) skin/dense tissue. The teeth are designed to hold tissue without slipping.

They cause a degree of tissue damage, so they should not be used on delicate tissue.

- **Dressing forceps** – Originally designed for handling gauze. In addition to being used to hold gauze, dressing forceps can also be used during wound debridement to pull out pieces of infected or dead tissue, remove foreign material in a wound, or pull back the skin to visualise the area of an injury better. These forceps can also be used for handling sutures.
- **DeBakey forceps** – Have a plate with a ridge in the middle and have a distinct coarsely ribbed grip panel, as opposed to the finer ribbing on most other tissue forceps; this is designed to grip without tearing delicate tissue. They are atraumatic tissue forceps used on soft tissue and organs during surgery. They are typically large (some examples are upwards of 12 in. [36 cm] long) [4].
- **Adson-Brown** – Are used for holding dressing materials such as cotton and gauze during surgical procedures,

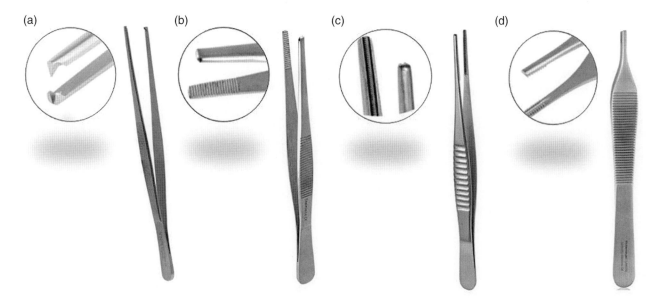

Figure 11.20 Dissecting forceps – from left to right Rat-toothed, Dressing, DeBakey, Adson-Brown. *Source:* Rosina Lillywhite.

holding and manipulating delicate tissues, etc. They have a broad thumb grasp for a firm grip, increased precision and control. Opposing surfaces are designed in the form of two longitudinal rows of fine [4].

Artery Forceps

They, also known as haemostatic forceps, are designed to clamp and occlude blood vessels and stop bleeding. They come in various shapes, sizes and lengths, but most have transverse striations to facilitate holding tissue; they should not be used as needle holders. Most types are available with both straight and curved heads. The most commonly used are as follows (Figure 11.21):

- **Halsted mosquito** – These are versatile, ratcheted, finger ring forceps used for clamping more delicate vessels and controlling blood flow and other clamping tasks in general surgical procedures.
- **Spencer wells** – One of the most commonly used artery forceps, is used to regulate blood flow in vessels. They have short, serrated jaws capable of totally sealing small blood vessels. When using them on larger vessels, they may temporarily limit blood flow. The handles of the Spencer Wells forceps are intended to be significantly closer together to prevent artery tangling inside them. Ratcheted versions often feature one or two locks. They are also available in a range of sizes with either curved or straight jaws.
- **Crile hemostatic** – Forceps are available in straight or curved. These forceps have a slightly lighter jaw than the Spencer Wells forceps. They are most commonly used for clamping blood vessels or tissue before cauterisation or ligation. They may also be used for soft tissue dissection, typically no deeper than 6–8 in. or in Laparotomy procedures. The lightweight modification provides the surgeon with greater control and a reduction in fatigue. Horizontal serrations of the entire length of the jaw and jaws half the length of the shank make this instrument unique.
- **Rochester Pean** – Are used for clamping more significant tissue and vessels for haemostasis and are typically longer than Spencer Wells with a larger head. The full horizontal serrations and availability in multiple lengths make these forceps a versatile instrument used in various procedures. They are available in curved or straight [19].
- **Kocher** – Is an instrument designed to aggressively grasp medium to heavy tissue or occlude heavy, dense vessels. They have horizontal serrations the entire length of the jaw and 1×2 teeth at the tip. The combination of full serrations plus teeth ensures a firm grip on the tissue or vessel. They are available either curved or straight and in multiple lengths [4].

Tissue Forceps

Tissue forceps are designed to grasp tissue with minimal trauma, but neither type should be used to hold viscera, for which more specialised forceps should be used. The most common types are as follows (Figure 11.22):

- **Babcocks** – These are finger ringed, ratcheted, non-perforating forceps used to grasp delicate tissue. They are frequently used with intestinal and laparotomy procedures. Babcock Tissue Forceps are similar to Allis forceps; however, they may be considered less traumatic due to their broader, rounded grasping surface. The jaws are circumferential, and the tips are triangular and fenestrated with horizontal serrations. They are beneficial for grasping tube-shaped structures.

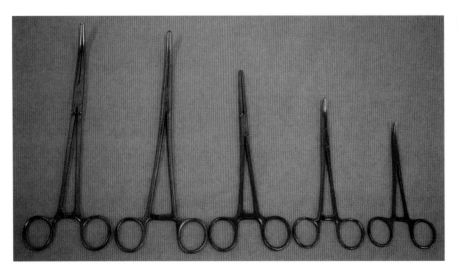

Figure 11.21 Artery forceps from left to right Kocher, Rochester Pean, Crile haemostatic, Spencer Wells, Halstead Mosquito. *Source:* Rosina Lillywhite.

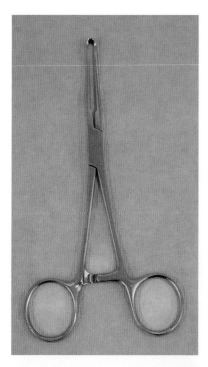

Figure 11.22 Allis tissue forceps. *Source:* Rosina Lillywhite.

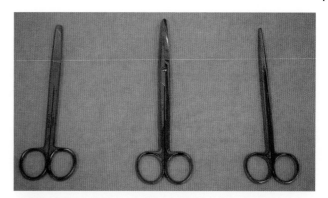

Figure 11.23 Scissors – from left to right Dressing, Mayo, Metzenbaum. *Source:* Rosina Lillywhite.

- **Allis tissue** – Is used to grab onto tissue or retract it. The forceps have serrated jaws and blades which curve towards the inside. The instrument comes with a ratcheted handle and is made to grab hold of tendons and fascia. Available straight or angled, this instrument also comes in a variety of lengths. The tip-end style varies to meet the procedure's needs or the surgeon's preferences.
- **Duval** – This is a general-purpose forceps that surgeons commonly use to grasp and statically retract tissues, especially during abdominal exploratory procedures. They have triangular jaws for clamping heavy tissues and a long-reaching shaft for deep surgical access with ring fingers and a rachet [4].

Scissors

Scissors are available in different sizes and lengths and can come with straight and curved blades. The tips may be blunt or short, and they should only ever be used for their intended purpose. Commonly used scissors include (Figure 11.23):

- **Mayo** – Wider and short with generally blunt ends, they come in various lengths; they are general-purpose scissors where the blade is approximately one-third of the overall instrument length. The straight version has a standard bevelled blade typically used for cutting surface tissue and muscle layers. Mayo's are versatile instruments that can be used in multiple procedures and settings [4].
- **Metzenbaum** – They are designed for cutting delicate tissue and blunt dissection and have a relatively long shank-to-blade ratio, similar to mayo scissors. The curved version can be used to reach deeper wounds allowing penetration into the wound, which cannot be easily achieved with the straight version [13].
- **Spencer stitch** – These are primarily used for suture removal. These scissors have a small hook-shaped tip on one blade that slides under sutures to lift them slightly before cutting for removal. This hook also holds the suture so it does not slip off the blade of the scissors before cutting. They typically have smaller, more delicate tips that are used for removing smaller sutures. They should not be used for cutting tissue.
- **Dressing or suture scissors** – Blunt/Blunt are the most commonly used as both tips have a blunt end, which means it is difficult to cause unwanted damage with blunt tips, i.e. when removing the dressing. Dressing Scissors, also known as Surgical or Operating Scissors, are versatile surgical instruments. They are often used for cutting materials such as drapes, sutures, tubing, or gauze. This product is straight with smooth, blunt/blunt tips [3].

Retractors

Retractors are used to aid exposure to the operating field or site and come in a range of shapes and sizes. Retractors can be segregated into two groups:

- Self-retaining
- Handheld

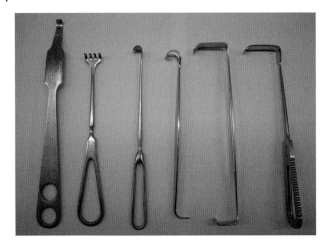

Figure 11.24 Handheld retractors – from left to right Hohmann, Volkmann, Koenig, Canny-Ryall, Army-Navy, Langenbeck. *Source:* Rosina Lillywhite.

Self-retaining retractors have a ratchet, and handheld retractors require an assistant to hold them in place. Examples of handheld retractors (Figure 11.24) [4]:

- **Hohmann** – Also known as Hohmann Muller Bone Lever or a Hohmann elevator. It is used to move tissue aside to allow for greater access to the surgical field. It has a slim flat long handle with two holes near the end and flares into a wide plate with a point-on end tip for ease of incision and contour. The Hohmann is available in several different lengths and tip widths. They are used during orthopaedic surgery.
- **Volkmann** – Allows surgeons to manipulate tissues during distal limb surgeries, especially those involving small incisions; they come with anywhere between one to six prongs, and these can be blunt, semi-sharp and sharp prongs for avoiding injury to nearby structures. They have a hollow tear-dropped handle for ease of use.
- **Koenig** – Allows the surgeons to mobilise, retract and grasp tissues to unveil the surgical field and its anatomical structures. They have a single concave blade for superior retraction.
- **Canny-Ryall** – Allows surgeons to grasp, mobilise and statically hold soft tissues to obtain maximum exposure to the surgical field and its cavities. It has a fenestrated blade to view the retracted tissues with an atraumatic terminal blade border to avoid haemorrhage. They have a solid handle for enhanced manoeuvrability.
- **Army-Navy** – The US military developed this retractor, hence the name. It is used for shallow, superficial wounds and is double ended, with both 90° angled blades facing towards one another. The handle is fenestrated for increased handling.

- **Langenbeck** – long handle teardrop-shaped with the centre of the handle cut out. It is a handheld instrument used to separate the edges of a surgical incision or wound actively; it can also hold back underlying organs and tissues so that body parts under the incision may be accessed.

Examples of self-retaining retractors (Figures 11.25–11.28) [4]:

- **Gelpi** – A specialist retractor often used for deep and superficial tissue retraction. Because of its distinctive form, it is suitable for retracting heavier tissues and

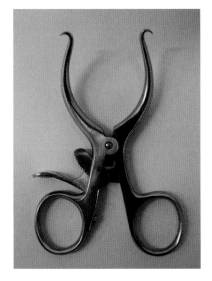

Figure 11.25 Gelpi retractor. *Source:* Rosina Lillywhite.

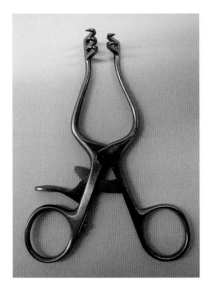

Figure 11.26 West retractor. *Source:* Rosina Lillywhite.

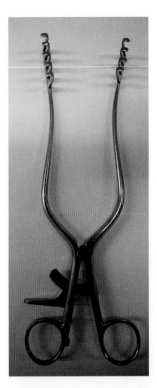

Figure 11.27 Travers retractor. *Source:* Rosina Lillywhite.

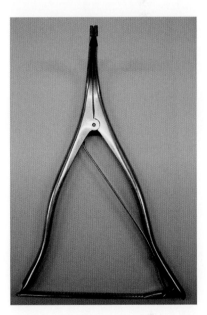

Figure 11.28 Inge retractor. *Source:* Rosina Lillywhite.

difficult-to-reach incision locations. Frequently used in equine practice, it comes in various sizes and has a single pointed end on each arm that points outwards. A locking mechanism allows the retractor to remain in place.

- **West** – A finger ring retractor with a cam ratchet lock, two into three or three into four sharp interlocking teeth. A popular instrument, most commonly used in large bone and joint procedures, it also helps with small, deep incisions and soft tissue dissection at a superficial level.
- **Travers** – An excellent alternative to the more commonly used Gelpi's, particularly for superficial soft tissue. It has four into five blunt hooks/prongs with a wide gap to retract the tissues. The length of the arms is typically longer than West's.
- **Inge** – Also known as the Inge Lamina Spreader, it is an orthopaedic instrument frequently used in human spinal procedures called a laminectomy or decompression surgery. However, they can be helpful in a dorsal spinous process resection in equines and other orthopaedic procedures. It features a double-spring plier handle with a bar ratchet used to spread apart or distract the lamina, bony fragments or joints.

Uncommon self-retaining retractors used and designed for retracting chests and abdominal walls are [10]:

- **Balfour** – Has three individually operable, outward-looking curved loops mounted on a bar. Inserting the blades into an incision and spreading them all allows full access to the tissue below. It is used for easily retracting bulky tissues. Due to most abdominal surgery not requiring retraction, it is not commonly used; however, there may occasionally be a use for it in less common thoracic or abdominal surgeries.
- **Gossett** – Are similar to Balfour retractors; however, they only have two curved loops mounted to a bar. They are used to actively separate the edges of a surgical incision in the abdomen; they hold back underlying organs and tissues so that body parts may be accessed.
- **Finochietto** – Similar to the Gossett/Balfour. Known as a rib spreader. It is a type of retractor specifically designed to separate ribs in thoracic surgery – rack-and-pinion-type stainless steel rib spreaders (with a thumb-screw to lock it in place). Figure 11.29.

Visceral Clamps, also known as bowel clamps, are designed to clamp the bowel in an atraumatic way. These are essential in abdominal surgery to minimise the risk of contamination by the intestinal content during a bowel resection, and several types are available [4]:

- **Doyen** – Has rounded ends that are suited for deep tissue manipulation (Figure 11.30). Grasps and secures sensitive tissues, including mucosal surfaces, intestinal walls and the omentum. It also functions as a haemostat, clamping blood arteries and preventing bleeding. This incorporates longitudinal striations that are used to clamp the bowel in an atraumatic manner.

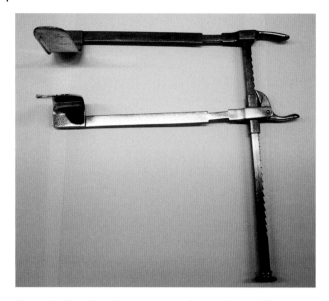

Figure 11.29 Finochietto retractor. *Source:* Rosina Lillywhite.

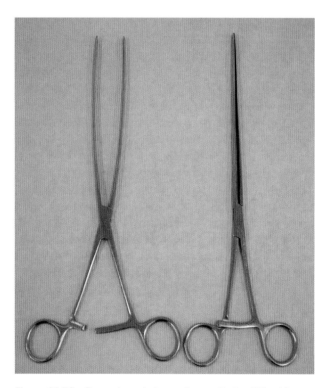

Figure 11.30 Doyen bowel clamp. *Source:* Rosina Lillywhite.

- **Parker-Kerr** – These are similar to the Doyen clamp but have smaller jaws making them less desirable for equine intestines; if they are used, it is predominantly on small intestinal resections, but they are less commonly used.

Orthopaedic Instruments

Orthopaedic instruments are used for surgeries where bone or cartilage is involved and are typically heavier and more durable than other instruments. The most common retractors used in orthopaedic surgeries are handheld Hohmann retractors, often used for retracting muscle, tendon or ligaments.

Some orthopaedic instruments are not widely used in smaller general practices, but a RVN needs to have an idea of the common instruments used (for more detail on fracture kits and instrumentation, see Chapter 12).

Common orthopaedic instruments include (Figures 11.31 and 11.32) [20]:

- **Osteotomes** – This instrument removes, divides and shapes bone and cartilage. It comes in various sizes and widths to suit the needs of the surgery. It can be used with a mallet and has a wooden or stainless-steel handle. Both sides of the blade have an evenly tapered edge.
- **Chisels** – Similar in appearance to the osteotome; however, this only has one tapered edge, and the other side is flat. This can also be used with a mallet and

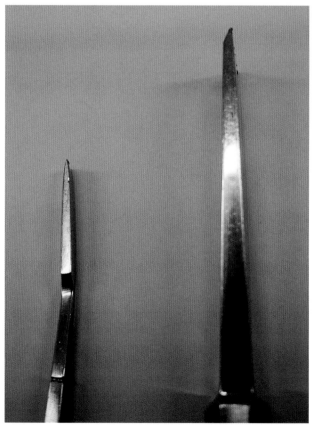

Figure 11.31 The ends of a chisel and osteotome – left osteotome, right chisel. *Source:* Rosina Lillywhite.

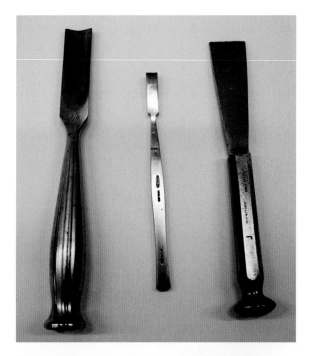

Figure 11.32 Left to right Gouge, Ostetome, Chisel.
Source: Rosina Lillywhite.

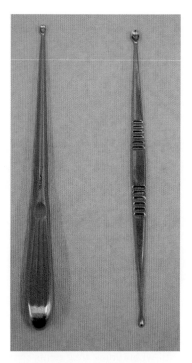

Figure 11.33 Left to right Bruns curette, Volkmann curette.
Source: Rosina Lillywhite.

comes in various sizes and widths to meet the user's needs [21].

– Tip: If you are struggling to remember the difference between an osteotome and a chisel, try to remember that the end of the word osteotome, 'tome' sounds similar to 'home'. If you can remember this, you can remember that, like a home, the osteotome has an end that looks like the roof of a house.

- **Gouges** – Easily distinguished by their concave shape. They are available in various widths and are used to remove large pieces of bone and cartilage.

Curettes

Curettes are easily recognised by their cuplike tip. They have sharp, oval, or round edges that help remove the diseased bone, cartilage, debris and damaged tissue from dense tissue surfaces. Their shape also makes them ideal for harvesting cancellous bone grafts, although this is not a common procedure in horses [22]. A wide variety of sizes and types of curettes are available (Figure 11.33):

- **Bruns** – Also called Spratt curettes or a Volkmann bone curette, have a straight or angled single oval cup at the end of a grooved handle. These are common in arthroscopic procedures and procedures that require a durable instrument for curetting.
- **Volkmann** – Also known as a Volkmann spoon, they are double-ended, having an oval cup on one end and an oval

or round cup on the other. These are used to scrape and debulk bone growths and fibrous tissues to perform fracture repair, and they are ideal for debriding soft tissue before wound repair.

Bone-holding forceps – Are designed to grip and hold bone fragments together to allow correct alignment during fixation.

Bone-reducing forceps – These, in some publications, are known as bone-holding forceps because they do a similar function. They position bone fragments and keep them in place during fracture repair and treatment. They usually have curved tips to avoid damage to the encompassing structure but are also available in straight tips (Figure 11.34). These can either have a ratchet closure mechanism or a screw lock [22].

Periosteal elevators – Are used to lift the periosteum and soft tissue from the surface of the bone before drilling or sawing; these are used in fracture repairs, sinus surgeries and some arthroscopies (Figure 11.35).

Bone Rongeurs

Rongeurs are strongly constructed instruments with a sharp-edged, scoop-shaped tip used to gouge bone. Rongeur is a French word that means rodent or 'gnawer'; in some practices, they are known as bone nibblers.

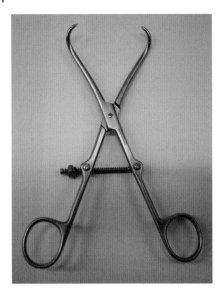

Figure 11.34 Bone-reducing forceps. *Source:* Rosina Lillywhite.

- **Ruskin** – These are useful when doing treatments that require bone contouring and cutting. It is equipped with a pair of sturdy jaws with sharp-edged opposing surfaces for this function. The rongeur also has a plier-style grip handle with horn finger resting projections. It is double hinged for more strength when cutting (Figure 11.36).
- **Ferris Smith** – Designed as intervertebral disk rongeurs in human and small animal surgery. It is an essential part of all arthroscopy kits. In equine practice, they are mainly used to remove fracture fragments and osteochondritis dissecans (OCD) chips. They are available in various sizes, working lengths, jaw strengths and a wide range of angles and designs (Figure 11.37) [4].
- **Bone cutters** – These are used in orthopaedic surgery to cut bone. They can grasp and manipulate and extract bones and are designed to cut out larger pieces of bone. They look similar to a large pair of nail clippers [20].
- **Bone rasps** – These are used to remove sharp edges following cutting, scraping, or curetting bone. They come in a variety of sizes and roughness.

Drills

These are hand held, can either be battery-operated or air-driven, and are commonly used in orthopaedic surgery [20].

- **Hand drills** are useful around delicate structures. When minimal drilling is required, such as the placement of orthopaedic wire in jaw fractures if the patient is weary of load noise and the surgeon is trying to place the wire in the standing patient; however, these are rarely used anymore with preference to the powered options.

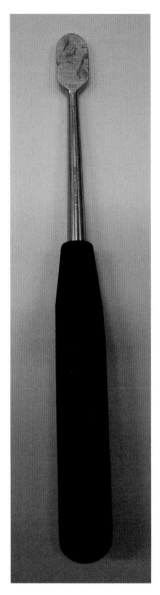

Figure 11.35 Periosteal elevator. *Source:* Rosina Lillywhite.

- **Battery-operated** – These can range from DIY store-brought to purpose-made surgical options; this will largely depend on case type and budget. These allow for more speed, energy and precision than hand drills. Care to follow manufacturer guidelines when sterilising. Batteries must be kept charged to prevent them from being flat when they are required. It is a good idea to have a charging schedule as even if not used, the battery will lose charge over time.
- **Air drills** – These are less expensive to buy and generally lighter in weight compared to battery-operated drills. These require attaching to an air hose and a supply of medical air to use them, meaning that they are now less

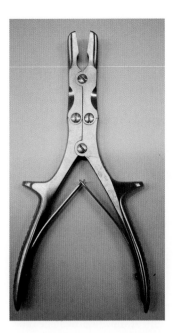

Figure 11.36 Ruskin Rongeur. *Source:* Rosina Lillywhite.

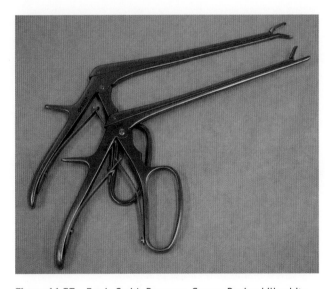

Figure 11.37 Ferris Smith Rongeur. *Source:* Rosina Lillywhite.

popular due to the limitation of having an air hose attached. Large practices that do multiple fracture repairs, will probably have one as a spare. Unlike battery-operated drills, these do not rely on being charged to work, so they are an excellent alternative if there is a battery failure mid-surgery.

- **Oscillating saws** – This is a surgical saw driven by electric or air power for cutting bones and other hard tissues. These saws are hand-held power tools with electric

motors to cause them to oscillate and can have either reciprocating or sagittal blades (reciprocating blades work with a 'push pull' motion like a manual hand saw). It's a very aggressive saw, which is not commonly used in equine practice. An oscillating saw makes tiny, rapid motion side-to-side and works well in confined spaces or for awkward cuts; this is widely used in equine surgery, for example, during sinus surgery [4].

Tip: If using any power tools that are air-driven, all couplings must be attached to the unit before the air supply is attached.

- **Wire forceps** and **wire cutters** – These are available in a selection of sizes. Wire cutters are predominately used for cutting the orthopaedic wire to length before and during surgery. Wire forceps are used for holding and twisting orthopaedic wire.
- **Gigli wire and handles** – These are used during a fetotomy (which means to dissect or to cut apart a dead foetus in utero [23]), to saw through bone with a cheese-wire effect to assist the surgeon in the removal of the foetus from the patient. These must be used with care as misuse could cause severe damage to the mare's uterus.
- **External fixators** – These are not extensively used in horses as they are typically not strong enough to be used on the limb of the horse; however, they have been successfully used in the repair of fractured mandibles. Generally, only hospitals will have the expertise and a team with the appropriate experience to carry out an eternal fixation (for more information, see Chapter 12).
- **Screws and plates** – Many sizes of plates and screws are required for fracture repair. This will include cortical and cancellous screws, locking compression plates (LCP) and screws. A variety will need to be kept in stock to ensure that a fracture repair can take place (for more detail on equipment, see Chapter 12).

Dental and Sinus Surgery Equipment

There is a vast array of dental equipment, including rasps and floats, which come in hand-operated and electrical. Battery-powered instruments have started to replace hand-held instruments due to better precision and ease of use; however, proper training must be given as they can cause complications with incorrect use.

- **Dental float** – These are used to smooth teeth that have rough edges or are overgrown. They are also known as rasps. They comprise a rectangular piece of metal affixed to a straight or angled handle. The blades have rough surfaces in fine, medium, or coarse grains. They can be made of carbide or tungsten carbide chips. The angled handles facilitate reaching the various sides of a tooth [12].

- **Equine molar cutter** – These are used to cut or trim molars. Heavy straight or angled jaws are situated on handles allowing the user to reach the back molar.
- **Wolf tooth elevator** – This is an essential instrument for removing wolf teeth. They are used to loosen the ligament attachment of a tooth. They have a tapered shaft affixed to a handle that can withstand a strike with a mallet. The shaft is designed to slide along the tooth's surface into the gum tissue [12].
- **Small tooth extracting forceps** – These are required to remove smaller teeth. They are curved, and resemble a pair of needle-nose pliers [21].
- **Cheek tooth extractors** – Have a wider jaw to grip more tooth area; some of these come with a ratchet to hold the instrument tightly to the tooth. One jaw of the forceps swivels, allowing several configurations so the user can choose the one that fits the tooth being extracted. A deciduous premolar-extraction forceps has blocky jaws that enable the user to maintain a good grip [21].
- **Dental tooth punch** – These are used to remove cheek teeth. Once a trephine has gained access to the sinus cavity, this instrument's shaft is inserted over the tooth so it can be struck out [21].
- **Periodontal dental probe** – These measure the depth of pulp chambers and pockets. These can come with colour bands known as banded probes or just plain. The banded probes allow for a better idea of measurement.
- **Equine dental mirrors** – These are circular mirrors fixed to a metal handle, allowing better visualisation within the oral cavity.
- **Horsley trephine** – These are used to create a hole in the sinus to allow sinusitis treatment. Trephines come in many different sizes; the size used will depend on the size of the horse, the surgeon and the sinus being accessed. The trephine is made up of sharp-angled blades arranged in a circle on the end of a long shaft with a T-shaped handle [21].

Equine Dental Speculum – Dental Gags

The equine dental speculum also called a gag, is used to visualise the teeth and enable safe palpation. There are many different types; the most common are [24]:

- **Millennium** – This is probably one of the most widely used dental gags in practice, comprised of an arched metal frame with an upper and lower bite plate and a side ratchet. The metal part of the speculum is attached to either a leather or synthetic strap. Once in place, the ratchet can be opened to allow for a safe oral cavity examination.

- **Offset Gunther** – This has a similar head strap to the millennium speculum. However, the bite plates are fixed to a straight metal bar that can position the upper jaw in different offset positions depending on the operator's needs. This gives better access to specific procedures such as minimally invasive transbuccal extraction (MTE). It uses a screw handle to open the jaw.
- **Schoupe** – This is a very simple gag and consists of a tightly coiled metal cylinder attached to an arm that is 'u' shaped. This holds the mouth open by inserting the coil between the cheek teeth, and it can be secured to the horse's headcollar. This is rarely used for dental procedures now as it has to keep moving to go between the sides of the mouth, but it can be helpful in gastroscopy and anaesthesia to keep the mouth open.
- **Butler** – This is similar to the Offset Gunther; however, it does not have a head strap, and you cannot offset the jaws. It is used predominately in anaesthesia to open the mouth for the placement of an endotracheal tube; it uses the same screw ratchet system as the Offset Gunther.

Ophthalmic Instrumentation

A vast array of instruments are used in ophthalmic surgeries. Still, the most common factor is that they are a lot smaller and more delicate than all the other instruments, especially compared with orthopaedic instruments. Common ophthalmic instruments include [4]:

- **Castroviejo corneal scissors** – These are double-spring ophthalmic scissors most commonly used during corneal procedures. It has jaws that are curved right with smooth edges and sharp/sharp tips. Different tips are used in different techniques:
  - Blunt tips for soft tissue protection
  - Angled blades for access to tight corners
  - Short blades to increase precision
- **Iris dissecting forceps** – These are multipurpose dissecting forceps commonly used for dissecting internal tissues. They are often used during ophthalmic procedures as they come with pointed tips that are ideal for sharp dissection of tissues. Used for dissecting delicate tissue, mucous membranes, blood vessels, skin and subcutaneous tissue. Serrated non-toothed with tweezers-like tips. They also have serrated thumb grips and a spring grip, which give optimum instrument control.
- **Capsule forceps** – Are used for holding the lens capsule during ophthalmic procedures with tips designed to avoid damage to the iris. They are oval shaped with a small cup and have a standard curve.

- **Castroviejo needle holders** – These are double spring instruments used for holding small, delicate needles in various microsurgical procedures. They feature a locking mechanism, a spring handle and a flat lock coupled with straight jaws.
- **Eyelid speculum** – This is a specialised device used in ophthalmic surgery to statically retract the eyelids to broaden the view of the surgical field; they use a screw ratchet to open and close the speculum [25].

Arthroscopy/Tenoscopy

Instruments required for both arthroscopy and tenoscopy tend to be the same and therefore are typically packed in one kit. For all key-hole surgery, an arthroscopy tower is required (Figure 11.38), which includes [26]:

- **Monitor** – This screen displays the images that the camera and scope get from within the surgical field. Ideally, this should be a high definition (HD) and have image capture software to allow photographs and videos to be taken through the procedure. The monitor, however, can only be in HD if the camera is also an HD camera.

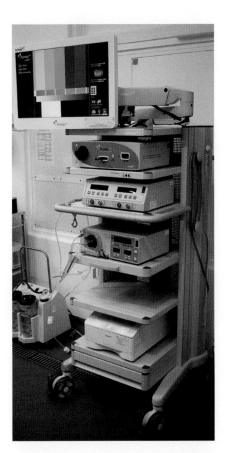

Figure 11.38 Arthroscopy tower. *Source:* Rosina Lillywhite.

In general, the whole system will be brought from the same manufacturer.

- **Light source** – A continuous high-intensity light source is necessary to illuminate structures within the joint or tendon space and acquire a good image. The light source provides light via the light cable to the arthroscope; most will emit 300W light power. With various types available, Xenon light sources are generally considered superior concerning image quality; however, they are expensive and have a relatively short lifespan of 350–500 hours. Therefore, many practices choose light-emitting diode (LED) light sources, as they are more economical and have a better lifespan of around 17,000 hours; another positive for LED is it generates very minimal heat and therefore does not require fan assistance. Most modern light sources automatically adjust the light, meaning the circulating nurse does not need to. It is essential that the correct light cable is attached to the light source and it is an appropriate length to meet the needs of the surgery [26].
- **Fluid irrigation system** – Also known as a fluid pump, this is used to distend and lavage during arthroscopic and tenoscopic procedures. This allows for visualisation during the procedure and flushes debris from the joint or tendon. These consist of a motorised pump providing fluid irrigation through pressurised roller systems. These pumps are available from a variety of manufacturers, and depending on the brand and model will depend on how it works. Some models now detect the pressure levels within the space and increase or decrease the fluid pressure to maintain the desired pressure; others rely on the circulating nurse to increase or decrease it as required throughout the procedure. Brand and model-specific sterile fluid irrigation tubing is needed; depending on the model, this can be a high cost as many are single-use [26].
- **Synovial resector** – Also known as 'shavers' or 'resector'. The handpiece contains an adjustable rotating blade within a sheath, to which a suction system can be attached, which is connected by a cable to an electrically-powered control unit that sits on the tower. The handpieces can be operated either by using buttons or a foot pedal attached to the control unit. Blade rotation can be adjusted either in oscillating or continuous unidirectional shearing modes. There are various blade attachments available, consisting of three basic categories: smooth-edged resectors (soft tissue), tooth-edged resectors (denser tissue) and bone burrs (bone exostosis). Blades are generally specific to the system, so care needs to be taken when ordering [25].
- **Gas insufflation system** – This is rarely used in arthroscopic or tenoscopic surgery; however, it is required for

laparoscopic surgery. Carbon dioxide gas is the most commonly used as it is deemed safest for the patient, having a lower risk of air embolus formation. However, some adverse effects do remain. Special systems must be used for gas insufflation, including a gas insufflation machine attached to a commercial gas cylinder and requiring a specialised sterile tubing set. If using gas insufflation for arthroscopic or tenoscopic surgery, it is essential to remember that without the fluid, the procedure will need to be followed with a flush, as debris will build up in the space [25].

The kit required to perform an arthroscopy, tenoscopy or laparoscopy is essentially the same. The laparoscopic instruments just have longer handles. The kit includes the following [25]:

- **Video camera** – This is required to project the image from the arthroscope or laparoscope's eyepiece, or lens, to the monitor. The video camera unit must be compatible with the scope's eyepiece in terms of HD quality, brand and model. Since camera cable 'plugs' can vary between different models of the same brand, it is essential to ensure that the camera head is compatible with the camera unit on the arthroscopy tower.
- **Ridged endoscopes** – Ridged endoscopes vary in diameter depending on where they are being used. The arthroscope is a delicate piece of equipment, as the lens and internal magnifying rod lens system can be easily damaged if not handled appropriately. Therefore, a protective sheath should be placed on the arthroscope when it is not in use.
- **Arthroscope cannula and obturator** – Arthroscopes are inserted into synovial structures encased in a protective sheath in the form of a stainless steel cannula; in a laparoscopy, these are often plastic and have slightly different attachments. These cannulae are available in a variety of self-locking mechanisms, which vary by brand, and are equipped with a variable number of stopcocks to allow fluid ingress and egress. The fluid irrigation system is attached to one of the stopcocks for ingress. An obturator is placed through the cannula lumen and is used to aid the insertion of the cannula into the joint, tendon sheath or abdominal cavity. Obturators are either sharp, blunt or conical (cone-shaped). Once in place, the obturator is removed and replaced by the arthroscope/laparoscope.
- **Egress cannula and obturator** – These are used for large-volume lavage to clear the visual field in the case of haemorrhage, or to remove debris. They are available in 3 and 4.5 mm diameters and require a blunt obturator for insertion into the joint.

- **Arthroscopic probe** – This is a blunt probe used to palpate and manipulate cartilage, fragments or lesions. Probes are available in various lengths, with different handles and tips, with variable angulation.
- **Magnetic probe** – Although not commonly listed as an essential instrument, magnetic probes are invaluable tools when they are required. Instrument breakages, although infrequent, can present a challenge, the most common breakage being the number 11 or 15 blades or needles or the shafts of small, angled spoon curettes, which occur due to excessive force. A magnetic probe can save a lot of time and stress by helping with retrieval within a joint [25].
- **Ferris Smith rongeurs** – Please see the above text under rongeurs.
- **Curettes** – Please see Bruns curette in the text above.

Laparoscopy

Most of the instruments in this kit would be extra-long handled and, like the arthroscopy kit, with the addition of a carbon dioxide insufflator (see above for more information).

Colic Surgery

Colic surgery would generally include standard instruments with the addition of bowel clamps (see standard instruments above for details of these).

The following instruments are specific to equine colic surgery:

- **Linear cutters** – These are used during anastomosis of the small and large intestines. There are two main types of staplers used in equine surgery these are:
  - Gastrointestinal anastomosis (GIA)
  - Intestinal linear anastomosis (ILA)

    These staplers are linear stapling instruments with two interlocking halves loaded with cartridges (single use loading units). Cartridge sizes for reusable stainless-steel GIA instruments are 50 or 90 mm long. Disposable reloadable GIA staplers are available in 60, 80 and 100 mm lengths. The reusable ILA stainless-steel stapler is available in 52 and 100 mm lengths.

    Gastrointestinal staplers apply four staggered rows of staples; cartridges contain cutting blades that divide tissues between the second and third rows of staples. The instrument separates into two halves, meaning each half can be placed into a bowel lumen or on either side of a hollow viscus. After closure, the push bar handle of the device is slid forward to fire the staples and the blade. The incision cut by the knife blade is 8 mm short of the last staple at the distal end. When used for side-to-side or functional end-to-end anastomoses, the result is a stoma with two rows of staples on either side. The instrument insertion site remains open and must be closed by suturing. The main indications for the use of GIA or ILA staplers in equine surgery are jejunocecostomy and jejunocolostomy [4].

- **Visceral retainer** (Figure 11.39) – Some also know these as a FISH®; this is the name given by a manufacturer. It is designed to effectively retain the omentum and viscera during the closure of the peritoneal cavity. It provides added anchorage and retentive power to speed closure and significantly reduces the risk of nicks and punctures. That means less trauma for patients [27].

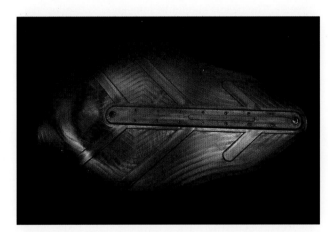

Figure 11.39 Visceral retainer. *Source:* Rosina Lillywhite.

Castrations

During castration, the veterinary surgeon will require a standard kit and some long-handles artery forceps. The extra instrument that most veterinary surgeons use is a pair of emasculators. The function of the emasculators is to simultaneously crush and cut the spermatic cord, preventing haemorrhaging while still detaching the testis from the animal. These must be cleaned and assembled correctly after every use and are always used nut to 'nut' [21].

11.5 Suture Materials

When looking for suture, it is essential to understand several terms; for common terms for suture (see Table 11.1).

Sutures can be broken down into different categories:

- Absorbable – A suture generally loses most of its tensile strength in 1–3 weeks and is fully absorbed within 3 months.
- Non-absorbable – A suture that is not absorbed by the body and must be removed.
- Natural – A suture that is made from natural substances.
- Synthetic – A suture made from an artificial product.
- Multifilament – A suture with multiple strands twisted together (braided) and sometimes coated.
- Monofilament – A suture made from a single strand [4].

Table 11.1 Common suture terminology [4].

Term	Meaning
Tensile strength	Initial tensile strength is a measure of the amount of tension applied in a horizontal plane necessary to break the suturing material Tensile strength is a measure of the time it takes for a suture material to lose 70–80% of its initial strength
Knot security	Knot security, defined as the ability of a knot to resist slippage and breakage as the load is applied, is a critical factor in maintaining the integrity of a tied suture Often the strongest suture has the poorest knot security
Tissue reaction	Low tissue reactivity means that the suture material should exhibit a minimal inflammatory response, which will not delay wound healing nor increase the infection rate. Tissue reaction is reflected through an inflammatory response, which develops during the first 2–7 days after suturing the tissue
Tissue drag	The degree of frictional force developed as the material is pulled through the tissue
Capillarity	Capillarity is the process by which fluid and bacteria are carried into the spaces of multifilament fibres. Capillary suture materials should not be used in contaminated or infected sites. Coating the suture reduces the capillarity of some sutures
Memory	The inherent capability of suture to return to or maintain its original gross shape. A material with high memory tends to unkink during knot tying, therefore, having poor knot security
Chatter	'Chatter' and tissue drag are the lack of smoothness or amount of friction while passing through tissue It is also the lack of smoothness when knot tying
Stiffness and elongation	The less force required to stretch a suture, the more it will elongate before it ruptures

Source: Rosina Lillywhite.

These terms can be used individually or in conjunction with one another to describe the properties and characteristics of an individual suture. The type of suture required is generally decided on by the person doing the suturing.

Most suture materials on the market can now be coated in triclosan; these sutures are known as 'Plus Sutures'. Triclosan is a broad-spectrum antibacterial agent. It helps reduce biofilm formation and bacterial colonisation, preventing the growth of the most common organisms associated with surgical site infection for at least seven days. The National Institute for Health and Care Excellence (NICE) has recommended to human health care that all suture materials used in human medicine should have this coating [28].

Absorbable Suture

An absorbable suture is used for closing internal tissue layers or organs that do not require longer-term support, as these suture materials lose their tensile strength within 60 days.

Synthetic suture material causes less tissue reaction than natural suture and is broken down by hydrolysis (in the presence of water).

Natural sutures cause more tissue reactions than synthetic sutures due to them being broken down by enzymatic degradation and subsequent phagocytosis [29].

For common absorbable suture and their properties, see Table 11.2.

Non-absorbable Suture

When permanent ligation or prolonged mechanical support is required, a non-absorbable suture is used for closures within slow-healing tissues. Non-absorbable suture materials maintain their tensile strength for longer than 60 days [4].

Table 11.3 shows the properties of common non-absorbable suture-used materials.

Suture Needles

As well as understanding the properties of a suture, it is essential to understand the type of needle required for the kind of suturing being performed. There are three basic components of a surgical needle [4]:

- **The suture attachment:**
  - Swaged needles – These are pre-connected to the suture; they are preferred in practice due to the enormous variations. Synthetic absorbable suture materials are only available individually pre-packaged with a swaged needle; this guarantees a needle is in perfect condition with the correct size needle-to-suture size ratio.
  - Eyed needles – These are reusable needles that are threaded with suture material. They are rarely used in practice due to their increased tissue trauma; this is caused by double the amount of suture material being passed through the tissue. Loss of shape, corrosion and blunting of the needle tip occurs relatively quickly due to repeated use and regular sterilisation.
- **The body** – The needle body is the central part of the needle between the point and the suture attachment. Length should be considered when choosing a suture needle. The needle should be long enough to allow penetration of both wound margins. The curvature of the body also affects its behaviour, and needles come in various shapes: straight, half-curved, or curved with 1/4-, 3/8-, 1/2-, or 5/8-circle shapes [4].
- **The point** – the point of a needle is the end used to penetrate the tissue. There are various different types available, and they have uses in different tissues.
  - **Cutting** – These are designed to suture dense or tough tissue. The cross-sectional appearance of the needle is usually a triangular cutting edge, which extends at least halfway along the shaft. The cutting edge is on the inside of the needle curve.
  - **Reverse cutting** – These have the cutting edge on the outside of the needle curve to improve strength and resistance to bending.
  - **Tapercut** – these are designed for dense tissues. The trochar point has a strong cutting tip on the needle's point with a robust round body. This reduces tissue trauma while increasing the penetration of the needle.
  - **Round-bodied** – These are designed to separate soft tissues rather than cut them. They are designed to be atraumatic but have limited penetration.
  - **Spatulated** – these are designed for thin, flat tissues. The cutting surfaces are on the lateral sides, with smooth sides on the inner and outer curvature of the needle. Used to pass through thin, flat tissue [8].

All of the required suture information can be found on the suture packet; see Figure 11.40 for an example.

Suture Technique

Once the suture has been selected, it is essential to understand the principles of the suture technique and which suture patterns should be used for the different procedures. Suture techniques can be categorised depending on the type of tissue apposition required; these categories include:

Table 11.2 Absorbable suture materials and their properties [4].

Suture type and trade name	Properties and structure	Advantages	Disadvantages
Type Surgical gut Trade names Catgut Plain gut Chromic gut	• Multifilament • Absorbed by phagocytosis and enzymatic degradation over 90 days • Tensile strength: 7–10 days untreated • Made from the submucosa of ovine (sheep) intestine or the serosa of bovine (cow) intestine • Chromic gut gets treated with a chromic salt solution which extends the holding strength to around 18–21 days	• Cheap • Good handling	• Generally superseded by synthetic materials as it can cause tissue reaction • Chromic gut is challenging to handle and has poor knot security when wet
Type Polyglactin 910 Trade names Vicryl Polysorb Unisynth Fast Hinglact	• Braided multifilament – generally always coated • Synthetic • Tensile strength reduction by 25% at day 14, 50% at day 21, and by 100% at day 35 • Resorption time: 56–70 days • Absorbed by hydrolysis • Coated to improve handling • Low memory • Tissue drag	• Good size-to-strength ratio • minimal tissue reaction • excellent handling properties • Stable in contaminated wounds. • High tensile/knot strength	• Considerable tissue drag if uncoated
Type Polyglycolic acid Trade Names Dexon Dexon II Safil	• Multifilament, braided • A polymer of glycolic acid. Dexon II is coated with polycaprolate • Absorbed by hydrolysis • Tensile strength reduction by 35% at day 14 and by 65% at day 21 • Absorption time: 60–90 days	• Good handling characteristics • Wide range of uses including in a contaminated environment	• Very rapid absorption in the oral cavity and in the presence of urine • Tends to drag through tissues • Less knot-breaking strength than polyglactin 910
Type Glycomer 631 Trade names Biosyn V-Loc	• Monofilament • Combined polymer of glycolide, dioxanore and trimethylene carbonate • Resorption time: 90–110 days • Tensile strength is 75% of at day 14 and 40% at day 21	• Monofilament suture with only minimal memory and excellent handling properties; minimal tissue reaction	• None known

(Continued)

Table 11.2 (Continued)

Suture type and trade name	Properties and structure	Advantages	Disadvantages
Type Polyglytone 6211 Trade name Caprosyn	• Monofilament • Copolymer of glycolide, caprolactone, trimethylene carbonate and lactide • Resorption complete within 56 days • Loses almost all tensile strength within 21 days	• It provides short-term tensile strength combined with very rapid absorption	• Rapid absorption
Type Polydioxanone Trade name PDS II	• Monofilament • Polymer of poly-*p*-dioxanone • Resorption time: 180 days • Tensile strength reduction by 25% at day 14, 30% at day 28, 50% at day 42	• Absorbable suture material that maintains tensile strength over a prolonged period • Less memory effect than polyglyconate	• Moderate knot security, moderate handling characteristics
Type Polyglyconate Trade name Maxon	• Monofilament • Copolymer of glycolide and trimethylene carbonate • Resorption time: 180 days • Tensile strength reduction by 25% at day 14, 50% at day 28, 75% at day 42	• Slow resorption and loss of tensile strength; three times stronger than polyglactin 910 at day 21 of wound healing; good knot security	• High memory effect, limited flexibility and moderate handling properties
Type Poliglecaprone 25 Trade name Monocryl Petcryl Mono	• Monofilament • Copolymer of glycolide and caprolactone • Absorption time: 90–120 days • Tensile strength reduction by 50% at day 7 and 80% at day 14; complete loss of tensile strength within 21 days	• Very low tissue drag owing to the smooth surface; good handling characteristics; high initial tensile strength; minimal tissue reaction	• Rapid loss of tensile strength but moderate resorption time

Source: Rosina Lillywhite.

Table 11.3 Non-absorbable suture materials and their properties [13].

Suture type and trade name	Properties and structure	Advantages	Disadvantages
Type Silk Trade name Sofsilk Silkam	• Braided multifilament; coated or uncoated • Raw silk, spun by the silkworm • Does not maintain tensile strength for more than six months loses 80% of tensile strength within 8 days • Slow absorption and persistence up to several years	• Excellent handling characteristics • Useful for ligatures • Cheap	• May potentiate infection – should be avoided in contaminated sites; has significant capillarity; incites some inflammatory reaction • Poor tensile strength
Type Surgical steel Trade name Surgical steel Steelex	• Monofilament or as a multifilament twisted wire • Alloy of iron • Biologically inert. • High tensile strength, which is maintained indefinitely • Non-capillary	• Greatest tensile strength of all sutures • Greatest knot security of all sutures; no inflammatory reaction	• Tissue movements against the inflexible ends may cause inflammation and necrosis • Poor handling properties • Cannot withstand repeated bending without breaking • Multifilament wire can fragment and migrate, leading to sinus tract formation
Type Nylon Trade name Dafilon Monosof Orlon	• Monofilament or multifilament • Polymer of polyamide • Intermediate tensile strength; monofilament nylon loses about 30% of its original tensile strength by two years because of chemical degradation • Multifilament nylon retains no tensile strength after six months	• Suitable for use in contaminated wounds; degradation products act as antibacterial agents	• Poor handling characteristics and poor knot security • Not recommended for use within serous or synovial cavities because buried sharp ends may cause frictional irritation
Type Polycaprolactam Trade name Supramid, Braunamid	• Multifilament with a polyamide coating • Polymerised caprolactam • Biologically inert • No tensile strength after six months • Capillarity	• Better tensile strength than nylon • Excellent handling properties, high knot security	• Intermediate tissue reactivity • It tends to form sinuses on implantation in tissues and is, therefore, best suited for use in the skin • Difficult to handle • Poor knot security
Type Polyester Trade name Mersilene Synthofil Dagrofil Ethibond Ticron	• Monofilament or multifilament • Uncoated or coated with polybutilate or silicone or polyethylene/vinyl acetate • Polyethylene terephthalate • Very high and sustained tensile strength • Biologically inert	• High tensile strength • Good handling characteristics. • Prolonged support	• Noncoated polyester fibres have a high coefficient of friction • Knot security is poor and is further reduced by coating • Causes marked tissue reaction and fibrous encapsulation • Should not be used in contaminated wounds
Type Polypropylene Trade name Premilene Prolene Surgipro	• Monofilament • Polyolefin plastic • Moderate tensile strength • Biologically inert	• Greatest knot security of all synthetic monofilament sutures; least thrombogenic suture material; minimal tissue reactivity and least likely to potentiate infection; high elasticity	• Slippery handling and tying characteristics

Source: Rosina Lillywhite.

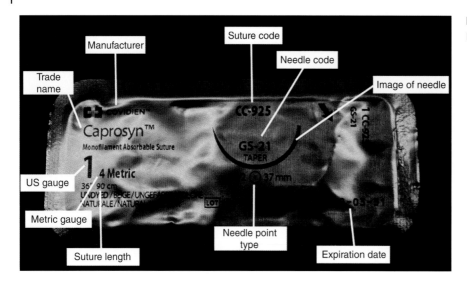

Figure 11.40 Understanding suture packaging. *Source:* Rosina Lillywhite.

- **Apposing sutures** – Bring the tissues together in direct apposition.
- **Everting sutures** – Bring the edges of the wound outwards.
- **Inverting sutures** – Bring the edges of the tissues inwards [4].

Surgical Knots

A critical part of suturing is the knowledge and understanding of knot tying; knots are essential to ensure that a suture line does not fail due to human error.

There are three critical components to a surgical knot:

- The loop – the part of suture material within the opposed or ligated tissue.
- The knot – made from several throws or a locking suture knot.
- The ears – the cut end of the suture, prevent the knot from being untied.

Knots can be hand-tied or instrument-tied. The basic surgical knot is known as the reef knot or square knot [8]. Figure 11.41 shows the step-by-step process of tying a square knot.

The other knot regularly used in equine surgery due to the thickness and tension of equine skin is the surgeon's knot; this has an initial double throw, not a single throw (Figure 11.42). Doing a double throw reduces the risk of losing the first throw's tension while the second throw is being placed. Hand tying can be used when suturing, but this

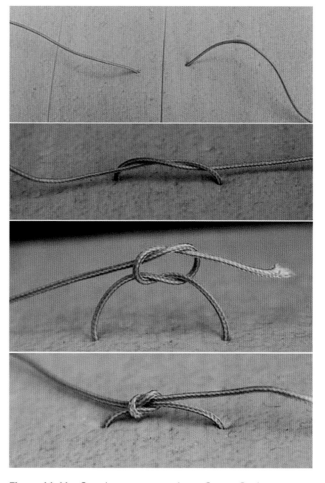

Figure 11.41 Step-by-step square knot. *Source:* Rosina Lillywhite.

will fail if there is a break in the suture or a knot slippage. To remove the suture, it must be pulled through the entire incision, meaning that the suture on the outside is pulled through the whole incision line, and this carries a significant risk of incisional contamination.

Ford interlocking – This is an appositional suture pattern. A simple interrupted suture is placed and knotted it, only the end of the suture material that is not attached to the needle is cut. The needle is brought up through the loop of the suture and then crossed the incision and inserted into the tissue on the opposite side as for a simple continuous pattern. The needle is taken across the incision and brought up through the tissue on the opposite side. As the needle exits the tissue, it is brought up through the loop of the previous suture. This is repeated along the incision. To finish the line, the needle is inserted back down into the tissue on the same side as it has just been brought out from and then passed across the incision to exit on the other side. The single end of the suture material on the first side is retained. The loop of material close to the needle to the single end is then tied [16].

Interrupted sutures – This is an appositional suture pattern; it is more time-consuming and uses more suture material than continuous sutures, as each suture is individually cut and tied. This could have cost implications but has the advantage of maintaining strength and tissue apposition should one suture break down [2].

Vertical mattress sutures – This is an everting suture pattern. It is helpful for poorly supported or mobile skin. The needle is inserted as per the simple interrupted suture approximately 5 mm from the wound edge and brought out the opposite side; in the same way, the needle is then reinserted closer to the wound edge on the emergent side (approximately 1–3 mm). A shallow bite is taken across the wound from the emergent side to the original side, coming out of the skin closer to the wound edge than the initial insertion point ('Far Far Near Near'). The knot is then tied on the original insertion side. Although it can be time-consuming to place, these sutures give an excellent cosmetic result and are good at tension relief. They have a minimal impact on the blood supply to the skin edges, although the margins of the wound must be healthy [1].

Horizontal mattress sutures – This is an everting suture pattern and can be time-consuming to place. They give a poor cosmetic result due to the eversion and gapping of the skin. They do, however, give good tension relief and therefore are helpful in wounds under tension. There is an increased risk of tissue hypoxia with these sutures compared to other suture types. The needle is inserted as per the simple interrupted suture and brought out the opposite

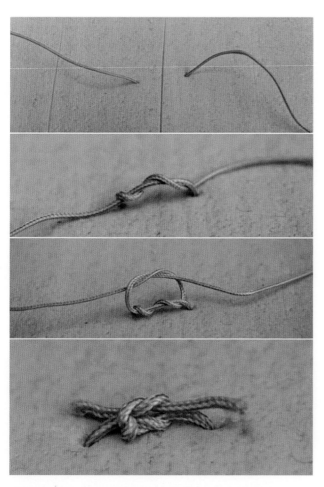

Figure 11.42 Step-by-step surgeons knot. *Source:* Rosina Lillywhite.

wastes a significant amount of suture material compared to using instruments. The knots of skin sutures should be pulled to one side of the incision. The suture loop should be loose; sutures placed too tightly will compromise the vascular supply and delay healing; there is also a chance that they may cause discomfort to the patient and cause patient interference [8].

Suture Patterns

There are multiple different suture techniques that are used in veterinary practice, but it is essential to understand the most commonly used techniques [4].

Continuous sutures – This is an appositional suture pattern; it is quick and easy to place as the sutures only have knots at either end of the wound; this also means less suture material is used, reducing the overall cost. The main disadvantage of this suture pattern is that the whole suture line side; in the same way, the needle is then reinserted adjacent to the emergence point on the far side of the wound and brought out on the near side i.e. like two simple interrupted sutures placed next to each other but traversing the wound in opposite directions; the path of the thread forms a rectangle. The knot is tied on the original side of the wound [4].

Cruciate sutures – This is an appositional suture pattern; however, if force is used, it can become inverting. Pass the needle through the skin on the far side of the incision. Pass the needle through the tissue on the near side of the incision. Then, pass the needle through the tissue again, approximately 1 cm away from the first part of the suture. Pull the suture through until the suture material lies flat over the top of the incision. The knot can then be tied, making sure when finished; the knot is not lying over the incision. The finished suture should look like a cross [4].

Purse string sutures – This is an inverting suture pattern. This suture may be used to reduce a rectal prolapse or temporarily close the anal sphincter before surgery of the rectum. It may also be used to close a hole in the thoracic wall after penetration by a foreign body (e.g. a stick). If the suture is placed after the tube is inserted, the tube lumen may become compromised. Placing a purse ring suture around the anal sphincter prevents the passage of faeces, which may prevent contamination of the surgical site. These sutures should always be removed following surgery. A line of sutures should by placed around the area that needs to be closed; so that the suture needle ends up at the same point as it started. A length of suture material should be left free from each end. The ends of the suture should be pulled up around the tube/hole and tied together. If the purse ring suture is around a penetrating foreign body, the foreign body should slowly be withdrawn as the suture is tightened [16].

Barbed sutures – Barbed sutures are becoming more popular in equine surgery. They work as knotless sutures as they have tiny barbs along the length of the material that act as anchors in the tissues. Using this type of suture allows for the convenience and speed of a continuous suture pattern but the security of an interrupted pattern. Depending on the manufacturer, the suture started using either a tab system or a loop system (it is essential that full training is sought before using these sutures). Once in place, the suture can be placed as a continuous suture; the other side of the incision is reached, and it can be tied off according to the manufacturer's recommendations; the suture can then be cut to be flush or at the same level as the skin. This is ideal for subdermal suturing as there will be no visible sutures. It is important to note that removal of this suture is difficult once placed, due to the barbs embedding into the tissue. To be removed, they must be taken through the tissue in the same direction as they were placed [30].

Other Methods of Closure

Staples – These are fabricated from surgical stainless steel. Before application, the skin staple is U-shaped. During application, the cross member is bent over an anvil, crimping it at two sites and bringing the legs together. This results in a rectangular shape of the closed staple, which is narrower than the original. Skin staples are suitable for the rapid closure of surgical incisions. They provide excellent wound edge eversion without strangulation of tissue. It was previously thought only to incite minimal tissue reaction; however, a large case series of horses undergoing exploratory celiotomy identified the use of staples for skin closure as a significant risk factor for developing a surgical site infection. This has led to a reduction in their use in equine practice. Staple removal is performed by a staple extractor, which compresses the cross member of the staple and straightens the legs, facilitating easy extraction [4].

Tissue adhesives (glue)

There are two types of tissue glue available:

- **2-Octylcyanoacrylate** – Tissue adhesives based on 2-octylcyanoacrylate are available as a dermal suture replacement. Advantages include faster closure, reduced cost, ease of application and no requirement for removal (unlike some sutures). They are considered equivalent to other methods of skin closure in terms of cosmetic outcome, infection rate and dehiscence rate. Tissue adhesives should not be applied to tissues within wounds; instead, they should be used on intact skin at the wound edges to hold the injured surfaces together. Adhesives are advantageous in superficial wounds or wounds in which the deep dermal layers have been closed with sutures [4].

- **Fibrin glues** – These are not commonly used in equine surgery yet, as further research is needed into their benefits. They are mainly composed of concentrated fibrinogen, thrombin and calcium chloride, thus duplicating the final stage of the coagulation process. Fibrin acts as a haemostatic barrier, adheres to surrounding tissue, and serves as a scaffold for migrating fibroblasts. The main advantages of fibrin glues are tissue compatibility, biodegradability and efficacy when applied to wet surfaces. Using fibrin glue as a carrier matrix for stem cells or bone marrow cells in a regenerative approach to treat musculoskeletal lesions is a more promising application in equine patients. Further potential applications include laparoscopic and endoscopic procedures and their use as a sealant in wound closure in combination with other techniques [4].

- **DERMABOND™ PRINEO™ Skin Closure System** – This is relatively new but has shown promise as an excellent closure product post laparotomy. The product comprises a self-adhering mesh and a 2-octyl cyanoacrylate liquid adhesive tube. The mesh is applied to one side of the skin incision and pulled across to approximate the skin edges. Once the mesh is placed, the adhesive is used around the edge, ensuring that the adhesive overlaps onto the skin edge all the way around. The adhesive is then thinly applied to the whole mesh. This then provides a proven strength, flexibility and microbial barrier to the skin incision, and it is hoped that this will minimise the occurrence of surgical site infections in these patients. A dressing is not required when using this product, as the mesh acts as a barrier [31].

Adhesive tapes – Modern cutaneous tapes play an essential role in wound closure in human surgery. Closure with microporous tape produces more resistance to infection than other closure techniques. Tapes maintain the integrity of the epidermis and thus result in less tension in the wound. These tapes can also be used over sutures to provide a partially closed environment and improve the overall cosmetic effect. Wound edge approximation is less precise with tape alone than with sutures. Wound oedema can lead to blistering at the tape margins and to the eversion of taped wound edges. Because of these disadvantages, tapes are not routinely used in equine surgery [4].

11.6 Instrument Care and Sterilisation

Instrument Care and Maintenance

Surgical instruments should always be carefully handled, especially ones with sharp edges and pointed ends. Most new instruments are supplied dry without lubrication. Before use, it is recommended that they are washed and dried carefully. Their moving parts (like a hinge or ratchet) should be lubricated with appropriate instrument lubricant or oil.

When cleaning instruments after use, correct PPE should be worn in line with the manufacturers' guidelines. Sharps (i.e. needles, glass vials and scalpel blades) should be disposed of safely. Specialised and delicate instruments should be cleaned separately from other general instruments.

After the cleaning process (see below), all instruments should be inspected for distortion, misalignment, sharpness and correct assembly. Pivot movements, ratchets and joints should also be checked for proper function [12].

The Cleaning Process

Once the surgery is complete, instruments should be cleaned as soon as possible to prevent blood, tissue debris or saline from drying onto them and potentially causing pitting or corrosion. The instruments should first be soaked or rinsed in cold water (ideally with an enzymatic cleaner). Hot water should be avoided as it causes blood coagulation, making cleaning more difficult and potentially damaging the surface of the instrument. Surgical instruments should be dismantled if possible, and ratchets or joints should be opened before submerging in cleaning fluid. Instruments should then be cleaned with a hand brush that has soft bristles and extra care should be taken for joints, ratchets and moving parts. Abrasive chemical agents should not be used as they may damage the surface of the instruments. Ordinary soap should also be avoided, as it causes an insoluble alkali film to form on the surface, trapping the bacteria and protecting them from sterilisation.

After the initial washing, instruments should be rinsed in clean, cold water to ensure no chemical cleaner remains and inspected for any damage. Instruments with a ratchet and moving parts should be lubricated using a water-soluble instrument lubricant. Oil-based lubricants should never be used as they interfere with the sterilisation process. The instruments should then be dried before being packed and sterilised [10].

Ultrasonic Cleaners

After initial washing, instruments can be placed in an ultrasonic cleaner. These are normally bench-top, suitable for veterinary use, relatively inexpensive and highly effective at removing debris from hard-to-reach areas where brushes cannot access. Ultrasonic cleaners use energy waves with a vibration frequency to produce tiny bubbles within the cleaning solution that form on the surface of the instruments. As the bubbles burst, energy is released, breaking the bonds that hold the debris to the surface.

Instruments are placed in a wire mesh basket in the ultrasonic cleaner, filling the unit as per the manufacturers' recommendation with an enzymatic cleaning product. The basket is placed within the solution, the lid is replaced and the unit is switched on (for about 5–10 minutes). The correct settings must be used; it should be noted that most ultrasonic cleaners have a heat function as well as the ultrasonic cleaning function. Because of this, it is important that the correct button is used so that the instruments are cleaned as opposed to heated [2].

Folding and Packing Materials

Many materials and containers are available for packing instruments for sterilisation, each having advantages and disadvantages. Selection will depend on several factors:

- Choice of sterilisation – steam or gas
- Size of autoclave/gasser
- Packaging being protective enough for the equipment

- Time taken to achieve sterility
- The ability for microorganisms to penetrate the inner layers
- Costs
- Personal preference [8]

Materials Used

Nylon film – Is designed specifically for use in the autoclave and is available in various sizes. It has the advantage of being reusable and is transparent so the contents can easily be identified. Its primary disadvantage is that it becomes brittle after use, resulting in the development of tiny holes that may not be seen and, therefore, contamination of the pack may occur. It is also difficult to remove sterile items from the pack without contaminating its contents and edges. These packs are often sealed with bowie-dickie tape [4].

Disposable seal-and-peel pouches – These bags are paperbacked with a clear plasticised front. They have a fold-over seal are available in various sizes; they may be used in an ethylene oxide (EO) steriliser or an autoclave. Seal-and-peel bags have also been made especially for hydrogen peroxide sterilisation. The risk of contamination when opening is small; double wrapping decreases the risk of damage to the instrument or contamination during storage or when opening the pack. These pouches are most suitable for single instruments, although large bags are available for small kits [10].

Paper-based sheets – These are used for packing long instruments. The most suitable type consists of a crepe-like paper that is slightly elastic and water-repellent. It is, therefore, ideal as an outer dust layer for packs with an inner drape layer. It is also acceptable to use an inner and outer layer of paper. Two sheets are generally used for kits; the two layers are typically different colours minimising the chance of contamination when opening, as the person opening and the person taking the contents can easily identify what can and cannot be touched. It is intended to be disposable but could be re-used if opened carefully and thoroughly checked for damage. These sheets come in a variety of sizes, and can also be cut to size [8].

Textile (drape) sheets – These are usually made from linen or a cotton/polyester combination and can be used for wrapping surgical equipment for sterilisation. They are conforming, strong and reusable but have the major disadvantage of being permeable to moisture. Usually, a double layer of linen is covered by a waterproof paper-based wrap for surgical packs; this also helps to identify which layer is sterile [4].

Drums – These are made from metal and contain vents on the side, which are closed after sterilisation. These can be used for instruments, drapes and gowns. Their main disadvantage is that they are frequently multi-used, so there is a degree of environmental contamination each time the lid is opened, and there is a chance of human error if the vents are left open [8].

Boxes and cartons – These are available in different shapes and sizes and can be sterilised in the autoclave. They are manufactured from non-toxic ethylene/propylene anti-static material to prevent dust attraction; they are also designed to withstand temperatures up to 137 °C and irradiation. They can be used for grouped instruments (specialised packs such as orthopaedic) and gown or drape packs. They are reusable and relatively inexpensive [2].

Metal boxes – These are commercially available sterilisation boxes made from stainless steel; they can have different coloured lids and engraved labels to indicate the contents (Figure 11.43). These boxes offer extra protection

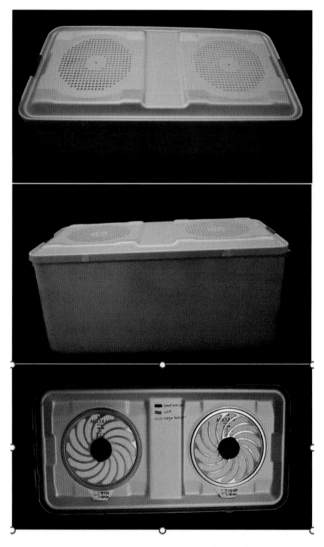

Figure 11.43 Bbraun sterilisation boxes. *Source:* Rosina Lillywhite.

against dust, fluids and transport damage. They have an inner tray that is removed by the surgeon and a removable outer lid, which the non-sterile person removes. All boxes contain filters in the lid, which means that the contents of the box will remain sterile for up to 12 months; the containers can be sterilised either in the autoclave or using ethylene oxide [32].

Sterilisation Indicators

External sterilisation indicators should be used in all cases when sterilising equipment; however, internal indicators should also be used when packaging bulky items so that heat, steam or chemical penetration can be checked. Indicators should be correctly used depending on the type of sterilisation as they have different requirements for correct temperature and pounds per square inch (PSI) values [4].

- **Chemical indicator strips** – Time, steam and temperature (TST) control strips show colour changes when the correct temperature, pressure and time have been reached. A strip is placed inside each package of instruments, and a new one must be used each time to prevent any false results. The correct strip must be used for the temperature of the autoclave used in practice, as this may also cause false readings [2].
- **Browne's tubes** – These work on the same principle, i.e. a colour change. Small glass tubes are partly filled with an orange-brown liquid that changes to green when certain temperatures have been maintained for a required period. Tubes are available to change at 121 °C, 126 °C or 134 °C. The correct tube must be selected for the correct cycle of the autoclave [16].
- **Bowie-Dick tape** – This is commonly used to seal instruments and drape packs. It is a beige-coloured tape with chemical strips that change to dark brown when certain temperatures are reached (121 °C). The disadvantage of these is they do not give information regarding time and pressure reached and, therefore, cannot be a reliable indicator of sterility [12].
- **Ethylene oxide indicator tape** – This is similar to Bowie-Dick tape; however, it is blue/green and has yellow strips that turn red when exposed to ethylene oxide. As with the Bowie-Dick tape, the main disadvantage is that it does indicate if the exposure has been for the correct length of time [8].
- **Indicator stickers** – These are provided by the manufacturer and have a yellow dot that turns blue following prolonged exposure to ethylene oxide. These are not 100% reliable as the colour change will also occur in prolonged light exposure and must be kept in the dark [4].
- **Dosemeter strips** – Are used for ethylene oxide sterilisation and undergo a colour change when exposed to

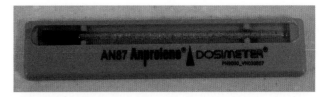

Figure 11.44 Ethylene oxide dosimeter strip. *Source:* Rosina Lillywhite.

ethylene oxide for the correct time (Figure 11.44). These must be placed in the centre of a load; this prevents change from occurring before the centre of the load is sterilised [33].

- **Spore tests** – These are strips of paper impregnated with dried spores and included in the load. On completion of the cycle, they are placed in the culture medium provided and incubated for up to 72 hours. If sterilisation is successful, there will be no growth seen. Spore systems are more accurate than chemical indicators, but the delay in obtaining the results is a significant disadvantage. A combination of both methods is recommended: a chemical indicator should be included in each load, and spore strips should be used at regular intervals. Vacuum-assisted autoclaves usually have visible temperature and pressure gauges on the front, and some systems have a paper recording chart indicating sterilisation efficiency [4].

How to Pack for Sterilisation

Gowns and Drapes

Reusable gowns and drapes should be washed, dried and inspected for damage prior to sterilisation. Gowns should then be folded correctly so that the outside surface of the gown is on the inside, allowing the user to don the gown in an aseptic manner. Plain drapes can be folded concertina style or so that two corners are on the top surface for easy opening when sterile and to allow free steam flow during sterilisation. Both gowns and drapes can also be sterilised with ethylene oxide or autoclaved. Generally, the autoclave is more widely used due to the quick cycle time. A hot air oven cannot be used as it will burn the material. Gowns and drapes can be sterilised in bags or packs. Hand towels can be placed with the gowns and drapes in the instrument pack if required [16].

Swabs

Swabs may be purchased sterile or non-sterile. When packed to sterilise, all staff should know how many have been packed (normally multiples of 2, 5 or 10). Swabs may be incorporated into instrument packs, supplied in drums or packed individually and should be sterilised the same way as drapes and gowns [4].

Urinary Catheters

These should not be reused as it would be impossible to be sure they are free from debris. They may be sterilised if they are opened in error but not used. Many brands of catheters may be sterilised by autoclaving, but the heat may damage some types. Some manufacturers do not sell sterilised catheters; if this is the case, the stylet can be removed, and the use of silicone spray down the lumen of the catheter can facilitate the removal of the stylet once in situ. If silicone spray is not used, the stylet may be challenging to remove once the catheter is in the patient, especially in male catheterisation. If using ethylene oxide for sterilisation, they must be thoroughly dry before sterilising [34].

Syringes

Some practices may choose to sterilise 30 or 50 ml syringes as part of a surgical kit. If so, they should be dissembled. Ethylene oxide is the best for sterilising plastic syringes, as temperatures in the autoclave will damage the plastic and rubber [10].

Liquids

These can be purchased pre-sterilised but can be sterilised in some modern autoclaves, as they have the appropriate cycle settings. It is crucial to choose the appropriate container for this, so that the container does not melt during the cycle. Liquid cycles have to be run without the drying part of the cycle so that the liquid does not evaporate during the sterilisation process. It is also worth remembering that the lids will require loosening on the bottles slightly to stop the pressure from building up and imploding the bottle [2].

Power Tools

These include air drills, saws and mechanical burrs; they are usually autoclavable, but the individual manufacturers' guidelines should be checked beforehand. Autoclaving can sometimes lead to the jamming of the motor and cause damage to the batteries. Ethylene oxide is often safer for all air-driven and battery-operated tools, but the manufacturer's guidelines should be followed at all times [13].

Packing a Surgical Kit

Instruments are usually packed together based on surgical preference and can have swabs and drapes packed in as well. The surgical kit may have a trolley drape form part of the wrapping so that when it is unfolded, the trolley gets covered at the same time. A trolley drape or paper-based sheets are essential when packing items for sterilisation in a box or carton. Unlike seal and peel packs, boxes and cartons do not have the necessary outer wrapping to maintain sterility during transport and storage. The trolley drape or paper-based sheets act as an additional barrier, protecting the contents from contamination and ensuring they remain sterile until they are ready to be used.

A metal or plastic tray is lined with a towel or linen drape sheet (these may have instrument pockets). The instruments should then be laid out in a specific order, and swabs, and other consumables can be added. A water-resistant wrap is laid over the top of the instrument trolley, followed by two layers of linen sheet. The tray is placed on top and then wrapped and sealed with bowie-dick tape. It should then be labelled to include the contents, date packed and by whom before sterilisation. Autoclavable plastic tips can be used to protect sharp or pointed instruments [13].

The Sterilisation Process

Sterilisation is achieved when microorganisms (including spores) are eliminated. Sterilisation can be divided into heat and cold sterilisation [10].

Heat Sterilisation

- Autoclave (steam under pressure)
  – Vertical, Horizontal, Vacuum-assisted
- Dry Heat
  – Hot-air oven, high-vacuum oven, convection oven

How Autoclaves Work

Although autoclaves vary in size and type, the basic principle stays the same. When water boils at 100 °C, some bacteria, spores and viruses are resistant to the heat and remain unchanged, even when exposed to higher temperatures for a long time. Increasing the pressure and steam temperature allows the autoclave to reach much higher temperatures; therefore, resistant microorganisms and spores will be destroyed by the coagulation of cell proteins. The increased temperature, not the pressure, leads to cell destruction. Table 11.4 displays the temperature,

Table 11.4 Temperature, pressure and time requirements for sterilisation [10].

Temperature (°C)	Pressure (psi)	Pressure (kg/cm^2)	Time (minutes)
121	15	1.2	15
126	20	1.4	10
134	30	2	3½

Source: Rosina Lillywhite.

pressure and time required to achieve sterilisation; and shows that the higher the temperature, the shorter the time needed for sterilisation [10].

A qualified engineer should service all autoclaves annually to ensure they remain in good working order and electrically safe. Vacuum-assisted autoclaves with a separate boiler should be serviced every six months to comply with health and safety regulations. The thermocouple is the probe that ensures that the temperature is reached during each sterilisation cycle. Thermocouple testing is recommended annually to ensure effective sterilisation.

The Autoclaving Process

A steam jacket surrounds the central chamber of the autoclave, where the pressure is raised (depending on the cycle). Steam enters the chamber, and as this happens, the air is displaced downwards because steam is lighter. When all the air is evacuated, vents are closed and steam continues to enter until the desired pressure is achieved. Once the air has been evacuated, steam entering the chamber condenses on the colder surfaces, i.e. instruments. The steam produces heat, penetrating the pack's innermost layer. The moisture increases the penetrability of the heat; as the temperature drops, the pressure returns to normal. The instruments are heat-dried in vacuum-assisted autoclaves, with filtered air replacing the exhausted steam. In modern systems, the door cannot be opened during this stage of the cycle [4].

Effective sterilisation also depends on the correct loading of packed instruments into the autoclave, as there should be adequate space between them to allow steam to circulate freely. Care should be taken to avoid overloading and blocking the inlet and exhaust valves. Before instruments are placed into the autoclave, they should be free of protein material to allow for effective steam penetration [2].

Steam under pressure (autoclave system) is the most widely used and efficient sterilisation method. It requires a considerable initial expense but is economical in the long run. Most items can be sterilised in the autoclave. Some plastic goods will need to be checked before autoclaving as these will be heat-sensitive. Manufacturer's guidelines should always be followed when sterilising items such as delicates, batteries and arthroscopes [10].

A vertical pressure cooker operates by boiling water in a closed container. It usually has an air vent at the top, which is closed, once the air is evacuated and pressure has built up. A disadvantage to this system is that air can get trapped underneath the steam, which would drop the temperature, and sterility is not guaranteed. It is also manually operated, so human error may also occasionally interrupt the cycle.

A horizontal or vertical downward-pressure autoclave is fully automatic and usually larger. It has an electrically operated boiler incorporated into the autoclave as a steam source. The air is then driven out more efficiently by the downward placement where there is an air outlet at the bottom (steam can escape by a vent at the top). These machines are generally designed for loose instruments rather than packs as they have poor penetrating ability and drying cycles. Packs would seem to be sterile but damp in places allowing entry of microorganisms during the storage period. Temperatures for this type of autoclave would range from 112 to 134 °C [4].

Vacuum-assisted autoclaves (porous load) (Figure 11.45) work on the same principle as the other two stated above but use a high-powered vacuum pump to help evacuate the air rapidly from the chamber at the beginning of the cycle. Steam penetration is instant after evacuation, and sterilisation takes place very quickly. A second vacuum also removes moisture after sterilisation and dries the load. This system is suitable for instruments, drapes and other surgical equipment as there is a choice of different

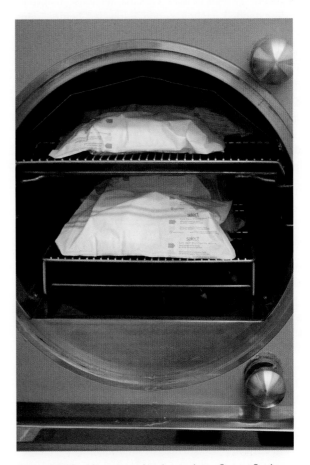

Figure 11.45 Vacuum-assisted autoclave. *Source:* Rosina Lillywhite.

cycles using different temperatures and pressures. Vacuum-assisted autoclaves are fully automatic with a failsafe mechanism that includes warning lights and alarms that indicate when a load is non-sterile or has not been sterilised effectively. They are much larger and more efficient than other types of autoclaves. The initial purchase cost is usually higher, but sterilisation efficiency and reliability outweigh this compared to the smaller types [4].

Dry Heat kills microorganisms by causing oxidative destruction of bacterial protoplasm. Microorganisms are much more resistant to dry heat than heat in the presence of moisture, so a higher temperature is required (150–180 °C). Dry heat below this temperature cannot destroy bacterial spores in <4/5 hours. With such high temperatures needed, it is also restricts the type of equipment which can be sterilised; fabrics, rubber and plastic cannot withstand these temperatures and damage will occur. Dry heat sterilisation is ideal for glass instruments, ophthalmic instruments, drill bits, powders and oils [12].

Hot Air Ovens are generally heated by electrical elements and are usually small in size, economical to run and less expensive. They have been mainly superseded by the autoclave, which is more effective for most materials. A more extended cooling period is needed before items may be used as a hotter temperature is necessary for sterilising (150–180 °C). They should be fitted with a safety door that cannot be opened until the load has cooled. It is essential not to overload hot air ovens to allow air to flow freely. Spore strip tests and 'Browne's tubes are available specially designed for hot air ovens [3].

Cold Sterilisation

Cold sterilisation can be achieved by use of the following:

- Ethylene oxide
- Commercial solutions
- Chemical, alcohol-based
- Gamma Radiation

Ethylene Oxide is an effective and penetrative method of sterilisation. Although concerns have been raised in the past about the level of toxicity if personnel are exposed. It is irritant to tissues and highly flammable, so the manufacturers' guidelines must be followed regarding operating, and COSHH regulations may make its use impractical in some veterinary practices.

Ethylene oxide deactivates the deoxyribonucleic acid (DNA) in cells and consequently prevents cell reproduction. This technique is effective against vegetative bacteria, fungi, viruses and spores. Many factors can influence the ability of ethylene oxide to destroy microorganisms, including temperature, pressure, concentration, humidity and exposure time. As the temperature increases, the ethylene oxide penetration power increases and the cycle duration

decreases. The only system available in the United Kingdom that operates at room temperature has a cycle of 12 hours or 24 hours + 2 hours of venting at the end of the process. Now, newer machines have a heating element, which speeds the cycle up to three and a half hours + venting [33].

Ethylene oxide is an effective method of sterilising different types of equipment. It can be limited due to the size of the container, duration of the cycle and concerns about toxicity. However, if the correct sterilisation chambers are used, this is not a valid concern. It is then mainly used for items that may be damaged by heat, such as fibre optic equipment, plastic equipment, ophthalmic or delicate equipment and battery-operated equipment. Equipment made from PVC should not be sterilised by this method as the material may react with the gas. Items previously sterilised by gamma-irradiation should not then be re-sterilised by this method [33].

The steriliser consists of a chamber fitted with a ventilation system to prevent gas from entering the work area (Figure 11.46). It should be located in a clean,

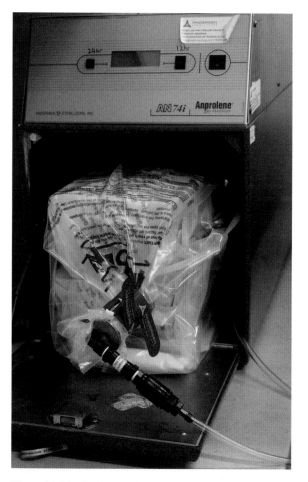

Figure 11.46 Andersens Anprolene steriliser. *Source:* Rosina Lillywhite.

well-ventilated area away from heavy foot traffic. The temperature of the room should be maintained at 20 °C during the cycle. Items for sterilising should be packaged and placed in a polythene liner bag. The plastic bag works as a gas diffusion membrane. Its function is to contain the gas from the ampoule and release it at a controlled rate during the sterilisation cycle. A gas ampoule containing the ethylene oxide liquid surrounded by a plastic shield is placed inside the plastic membrane (bag). The mouth of the bag is then closed and sealed around a plastic purge tube, which purges excess air out and allows for gas ventilation at the end of the cycle. The machine should then be set to purge so that all air is removed from the polythene liner bag. Once purged, the ampoule should be snapped at the tip from the outside of the bag, realising Anprolene gas. The door to the unit should be closed and locked, and the hours set (usually 12 but can be 24). The cycle is generally done overnight, and at the end of this period, extra time is required for ventilation before the unit is unlocked. Items can then be unloaded and put away. The unit door is also alarmed to prevent premature opening by human error [33].

Materials to be sterilised by ethylene oxide must be cleaned and dried thoroughly before being packaged as water on instruments at the time of exposure, may react with the gas and reduce its effectiveness. Any caps, bungs or stylets must be removed from instruments so that the gas can penetrate freely, and syringes should be packaged dissembled [8].

Commercial Solutions

Hydrogen peroxide sterilisation uses hydrogen peroxide gas plasma at a low temperature to sterilise efficiently. It has a very short cycle time (between 30 and 60 minutes), allowing quick sterilisation, so instruments can be returned to use quickly. It does not require high temperatures, and oxygen and water vapour are the only by-products, so it is less toxic than ethylene oxide. The system can be used for endoscopes, arthroscopes, light cables, plastic instruments, batteries and power drills. It cannot be used to sterilise paper or wood due to absorption [4].

Chemical disinfectant solutions are produced commercially, and some are ready for use; some will need diluting (usually with purified water) before use. Chemical solutions should ideally be used for disinfection, although some manufacturers guarantee sterilisation following a prolonged immersion (usually 24 hours). It is most commonly used for the cleaning of flexible endoscopes [4].

Manufacturers' guidelines regarding concentration, immersion and immersion times must be followed. Any cleaning, disinfectant or sterilisation product must be listed on the practice COSHH register; before immersion, check that the equipment can fully be submerged and will not be damaged by the solution. The chemical solution and the equipment for sterilising should be placed in a tray or bowl deep enough for the item to be fully submerged and preferably have a lid to prevent evaporation and contamination by airborne microorganisms. Following submersion, the item should be thoroughly rinsed in sterile water and dried before use. Chemical solutions should ideally be discarded after use, and a fresh solution should be made up each time [3].

Alcohol-based solutions such as ethanol and isopropyl alcohol work by denaturation and coagulating proteins; these are not commonly used to sterilise equipment and instruments [35].

Gamma irradiation can only be carried out under controlled conditions generally on an industrial level. Many pre-packed items, such as suture material and surgical gloves, are sterilised using this method. Due to the nature of the process, it is not commonly used for the day-to-day sterilising of instruments in practice [4].

Storage After Sterilisation

There should be a separate area in the theatre suite for storing sterile instruments and packs that should be kept dust-free, dry and well ventilated. Ideally, all packs should be kept in cupboards. They should be handled as little as possible to minimise the risk of damage and packed loosely on shelves. It is recommended that re-sterilisation takes place every 3–12 months, but some industries, such as human medicine, are moving to 'event-related' sterilisation. This means that depending on the material, storage conditions and amount of handling, if an item meets all of the above, it could remain sterile indefinitely. Due to generally poorer storage facilities in equine practice, it can be assumed that a re-sterilisation plan is the most effective way to maintain the sterility of surgical instruments [11].

References

1 Terms and definition [glossary] in nursing procedure – a simple learning for nurses [Internet]. Nursing articles, jobs, procedure, notes and question bank. [cited 30 January 2023]. Available from: http://www.canestar.com/terms-and-definition--glossary--in-nursing-procedure---a-simple-learning-for-nurses.html.

2 Coumbe, K. (2012). Equine Veterinary Nursing, 2e, 385–431. Oxford: Blackwell Science Ltd.

3 DeNotta, S., Mallicote, M., Miller, S. et al. (2023). AAEVT's Equine Manual for Veterinary Technicians, 2e, 305–323. Hoboken: John Wiley and Sons Inc.

4 Auer, J., Stick, J., Kummerle, J. et al. (2019). Equine Surgery, 5e, 143–198. Missouri: Elsevier.

5 etkho. (2022). All the keys to the correct design of an operating theatre [Internet]. ETKHO Hospital

Engineering. [cited 31 January 2023]. Available from: https://www.etkho.com/en/all-the-keys-to-the-correct-design-of-an-operating-theatre/.

6 Assisted recovery in horses awakening from general anesthesia | IVIS [Internet]. 2005 [cited 30 January 2023]. Available from: https://www.ivis.org/library/recent-advances-anesthetic-management-of-large-domestic-animals/assisted-recovery-horses.

7 AIA TLC (2018). Sizing rooms for equine hospitals [Internet]. EquiManagement. [cited 30 January 2023]. Available from: https://equimanagement.com/articles/sizing-rooms-for-equine-hospitals/.

8 Ackerman, N. and Aspinall, V. (2016). Aspinall's Complete Textbook of Veterinary Nursing, 3e, 427–475. Edinburgh: Elsevier Ltd.

9 Kiss, C. (2019). The Influence of Windows on Surgeons' Stress. Graduate School of Clemson University.

10 Cooper, B., Mullineaux, E., and Turner, L. (ed.) (2018). BSAVA Textbook of Veterinary Nursing, 5e, 738–774. Gloucester: British Small Animal Veterinary Association.

11 Storage of clean and sterile supplies in clinical areas [Internet]. Alberta Health Services. 2022 [cited 30 January 2023]. Available from: chrome-extension://efaidnbmnnnibpcajpcglclefindmkaj/https://www.publichealthontario.ca/-/media/documents/c/2017/cds-storage-sterility.pdf?la=en.

12 Sterilizing practices | Disinfection & sterilization guidelines | Guidelines library | Infection control | CDC [Internet]. 2019 [cited 30 January 2023]. Available from: https://www.cdc.gov/infectioncontrol/guidelines/disinfection/sterilization/sterilizing-practices.html.

13 Corley, K. and Stephen, J. (2008). The Equine Hospital Manual, 1e. Oxford: Blackwell Publishing Ltd.

14 Laser surgery [Internet]. Falkland Veterinary Clinic. [cited 06 February 2023]. Available from: https://falklandvets.co.uk/our-services/laser-surgery/.

15 Surgical face masks in the operating theatre: re-examining the evidence | Elsevier Enhanced Reader [Internet]. [cited 30 January 2023]. Available from: https://reader.elsevier.com/reader/sd/pii/S0195670100909125?token=0BBA741F12E665D83D131A7DD2E8D17FA2C381F09C29E3A4D3E97E8BA4F14FA3D9B981B52818B81B04CC4FEC75BC4212&originRegion=eu-west-1&originCreation=20230130221219.

16 Aspinall, V. (2014). Clinical Procedures in Veterinary Nursing, 3e, 128–174. Edinburgh: Elsevier Ltd.

17 Hand washing [Internet]. [cited 31 January 2023]. Available from: https://wvs.academy/learn/companion-animals/spay-neuter/preparation-and-principles/surgical-team-preparation/hand-washing

18 Sterillium – product range [Internet]. [cited 31 January 2023]. Available from: https://www.sterillium.info/en/product-range.

19 Rochester-pean artery forcep [Internet]. MAHR surgical. [cited 01 February 2023]. Available from: https://www.mahrsurgical.co.uk/products/instruments/general-surgery/artery-forceps/rochester-pean/.

20 Nixon, A.J. (2020). Equine Fracture Repair, 2e, 807–813. Hoboken: John Wiley and Sons Inc.

21 Sonsthagen, T.F. (2019). Veterinary Instruments and Equipment a Pocket Guide, 4e, 357–400. Missouri: Elsevier.

22 Themes UFO (2016). Orthopedic instruments [Internet]. Veterian key. [cited 02 February 2023]. Available from: https://veteriankey.com/orthopedic-instruments/.

23 VM224/VM224: how to perform a fetotomy in cattle: an illustrated guide [Internet]. [cited 02 February 2023]. Available from: https://edis.ifas.ufl.edu/publication/VM224.

24 Speculum & accessories archives [Internet]. Equine blades direct. [cited 07 February 2023]. Available from: https://equinebladesdirect.com/product-category/speculum-accessories/.

25 Corp, M.S. Eye surgical instruments and ophthalmic instruments [Internet]. [cited 07 February 2023]. Available from: https://www.surgicalinstruments.com/eye-instruments/eye-surgical-instruments.

26 Ryan, J. and Johnson, J. (2020). The equine nurse's approach to arthroscopic surgery: part 1 – equipment & instrumentation. *Veterinary Nursing Journal* 35 (9): 262–267.

27 FISH® glassman viscera retainer | Simple solution for abdominal closure | Adept-Med [Internet]. Adeptmed. [cited 07 February 2023]. Available from: https://adeptmed.com/the-fish/.

28 Plus sutures for preventing surgical site infection. NICE Guid [Internet]. 2021;1–18. Available from: https://www.nice.org.uk/guidance/mtg59.

29 Absorbable suture – an overview | ScienceDirect topics [Internet]. [cited 02 February 2023]. Available from: https://www.sciencedirect.com/topics/nursing-and-health-professions/absorbable-suture.

30 STRATAFIX™ spiral knotless tissue control devices | Ethicon [Internet]. J&J MedTech. [cited 06 February 2023]. Available from: https://www.jnjmedtech.com/en-US/product/stratafix-spiral-knotless-tissue-control-device/barbed-suture.

31 Dermabond prineo skin closure system | Ethicon UK & Ireland [Internet]. J&J MedTech. [cited 06 February 2023]. Available from: https://www.jnjmedtech.com/en-GB/product/dermabond-prineo-skin-closure-system.

32 Sterile container [Internet]. [cited 07 February 2023]. Available from: https://www.bbraun.co.uk/en/products-and-therapies/services/sterile-supply/sterile-container.html.

33 EOGas series 4 [Internet]. [cited 07 February 2023]. Available from: https://www.anderseneurope.com/view.php?id=5.

34 Themes UFO. (2016). Equine clinical procedures [Internet]. Veterian key. [cited 07 February 2023]. Available from: https://veteriankey.com/equine-clinical-procedures/.

35 Pop-Vicas, A.E., Keating, J.A., Heise, C. et al. (2021). Gaining momentum in colorectal surgical site infection reduction through a human factors engineering approach. *Infection Control & Hospital Epidemiology* [Internet] 42 (7): 893–895. Available from: https://www.cambridge.org/core/product/identifier/S0899823X20013227/type/journal_article [cited 05 October 2022].

12

Surgical Nursing and Patient Care

Natalie Karla Fisk¹, Lisa Harrison¹, Rosina Lillywhite², Marie Rippingale³, and Nicola Rose⁴

¹ *Rossdales Equine Hospital & Diagnostic Centre, Newmarket, Suffolk, UK*
² *VetPartners Nursing School, Greenforde Business Park, Petersfield, UK*
³ *Bottle Green Training Ltd, Derby, UK*
⁴ *Ash Vale, Guildford, Surrey, UK*

Glossary

General anaesthesic (GA) Medically induced loss of consciousness that renders the patient unarousable even with painful stimuli [1].

Local anaesthesia A local anaesthetic creates an absence of pain in a specific location of the body without a loss of consciousness [1].

Perioperative The period of a patient's surgical procedure; it commonly includes admission, anaesthesia, surgery and recovery [2].

Preoperative Occurring before a surgical operation [2].

Post-operative: The period following a surgical operation [2].

12.1 Admitting the Surgical Patient

The process involved in admitting the surgical patient will depend on individual practice policy. This policy will dictate who admits these patients and whether this is a registered veterinary nurse (RVN) or a veterinary surgeon (vet), the role is an important one. The admission period is a vital time to gather patient information, which can be used to enable the practice to deliver the best care possible to each individual patient. As part of this process, a preoperative check takes place to ensure that the horse is in a condition suitable for GA; this may include a physical examination and blood tests [3].

Before Admission

Before the horse is admitted to the hospital, the person responsible for the admission needs to consider:

- Admission time: booking a time slot for admissions may be wise. This ensures there are sufficient staff and time to admit the patient correctly and allow clients enough time to ask relevant questions [1].
- Medical history: make sure that all relevant medical history is attached to the admission documents so that all staff are aware of previous conditions that may affect the GA [4].
- Accommodation: ensure the horse has been allocated a suitable stable for their condition. There are many considerations to make when thinking about stabling:
  - Do they need to be near the recovery suite?
  - Will they require a stable in the intensive care unit (ICU)?
  - Are they stallions and therefore require a stable away from mares?
  - Do they need company?
- Admission documents: some practices now send out the basic documentation before the patient's arrival; if this is the case, the client's understanding should be checked thoroughly.
- Understanding the procedure: it is vital that the person responsible for the admission understands the procedure that is taking place so they can answer any questions the client may have [5].

Admission

Upon arrival, the client should be greeted in a friendly, welcoming way to ensure they feel comfortable. When admitting any patient, it is essential that the client does not feel rushed or unwelcome; this is especially relevant for surgical admission, as clients may be apprehensive about the procedure. The RVN must acknowledge why the client has come to the hospital, as the client will want to know that their horse will be cared for by the best team of people. When admitting horses, it is generally good practice to place the horse in a selected stable and then take the client to a quiet area away from the horse. This will reduce the chances of the client being distracted by the horse and will help them focus on the admission process. The admission process should include the following:

- Passport: The horse's passport should be checked for several things:
  - Part II of Section IX is signed, ensuring that the horse is not eligible to enter the human food chain [6]. This information should be recorded on the practice computer system.
  - The microchip: this should be scanned and compared with the number in the passport, ensuring the correct horse is admitted. There has also been an increase in the number of people using one horse's insurance against multiple horses meaning they only need one insurance policy for multiple horses that look the same. For this reason, all horses should have a microchip scanned at admission [7].
- Admission questionnaire: on admission, there should be some form of questioning to ensure that the horse is cared for in the best possible way. This questionnaire may have been sent to the owner before arrival; however, it should be checked with the owner to ensure no mistakes are made. The Ability Model assessment form is a good document to use for this. Please see Chapter 13 for further information.

Questions should include the following:

- The horse's usual diet: this can then be matched as closely as possible while the horse is at the practice. Some practices may require owners to bring food with them to ensure the horses' diet stays the same, and some clients may prefer to do this regardless of practice policy.
- The horse's typical routine: how is the horse kept at home? Is it used to being stabled?
- Current work level: finding out what type of work the horse is in and used for is essential to understanding the horse. If the horse is coming straight off the racecourse and is fit for racing, sudden changes to this could impact both its mental and physical well-being.
- Vaccination and worming status: the horse's vaccination status must be known. Some owners may not have kept their horse's vaccinations up to date. When admitting a surgical patient, the horse must be up to date with tetanus. If the horse is not up to date with tetanus, it should receive a dose of antitoxin and start a course of tetanus vaccinations. It is also important to know the worming history of the horse, as this may have an impact on the GA if they have a heavy worm burden [8].
- The horse's temperament: what is the typical character of the horse? Is the horse ordinarily quiet? Do they have behavioural problems? Does the horse get stressed in a stable? This is important, especially in the surgical patient, as if this is not known, it is hard to judge the horse post-operatively [9].
- Behaviour: what is the horse's behaviour like? Are they likely to bite, kick or rear? Could they cause harm to members of staff or other inpatients that get too close?
- Allergies: does the horse have any allergies that could cause issues while hospitalised? This is especially important if there are drug allergies, such as an allergy to penicillin.
- Relevant history: does the horse have any relevant history that is unknown to the practice?
- Concurrent illnesses that may affect the anaesthetic: for example, chronic lung infections, severe equine asthma (formally known as recurrent airway obstruction or RAO) or exertional rhabdomyolysis (see Chapters 10 and 13).
- Is the horse used to wearing a bit and a bridle?: it is good practice to handle unknown horses with a bridle, so identifying if a horse can wear a bridle is important.
- Contact details of the client: there must be correct contact details for the client so they can be contacted regarding their horse. It is also important to ensure the client has details about the practice and understands how to contact the practice out of hours.
- Consent – For full details on consent, see Chapter 3. It may be the responsibility of the RVN to gain consent for surgical procedures; this should come after the vet has had an in-depth conversation regarding the procedure and associated risks [10]. Although an RVN can gain consent from a client, the overall responsibility for informed consent lies with the vet. Consent for an anaesthetic must be obtained from the owner or someone acting on the owner's behalf [10]. Before the owner signs the consent form, they should be fully informed of the potential consequences of anaesthesia/surgery and its

potential risks. The surgical outcome should be discussed at length, so the owner is fully informed of the risks of the surgery and the risks that the anaesthetic may pose to the horse. The owner should have time to process whether they would like to proceed [10]. The vet should determine whether the client has processed the information and is fully informed of the potential risks.

- GA risks are covered in detail in Chapter 10; however, the primary considerations include the risk of myopathy, neuropathy and fracture following the GA. Myopathies and neuropathies are caused by long periods of recumbency, compression of the nerves and muscles and poor perfusion. The most common myopathy occurs when the triceps muscle is not pulled forward adequately when the horse is in lateral recumbency. Generally, myopathies are more painful for the patient due to ischaemic muscle damage. Neuropathies occur due to nerve compression, stretch, contusion, or transection, which can occur following surgical trauma or patient positioning compression of the nerve. This can happen if the patient is put into an abnormal position under GA, for example, over-extension of the limbs; neuropathies are not as obviously painful as a myopathy but can still cause lameness and an inability to move the affected limb [11].
- Labelling: once all paperwork is complete, the horse should have identity tags attached to its headcollar and put into the mane. This will ensure that the horse can be identified correctly. All items left with the horse should be clearly labelled to ensure that they are not misplaced.
- Weight: anaesthetic doses are calculated based on body weight. Therefore, obtaining an accurate weight for the patient before GA is important. The most accurate way to do this is to use an electronic weighbridge. If a weighbridge is unavailable, a weigh tape can be used, but these do not tend to be as accurate, so they are less ideal [12].

Post-Admission

After the client leaves, a complete clinical examination should occur; this may be done by an RVN or vet, depending on practice policy. All clinical parameters should be assessed (see Chapter 17). Emphasis should be put on the cardiovascular and respiratory systems. The musculoskeletal system should also be assessed to check for pre-existing lameness. If the initial assessment highlights any areas of concern, these should be investigated prior to anaesthesia. This may require further diagnostic tests to be performed, such as electrocardiography (ECG), radiography, ultrasonography, haematology and biochemistry. The decision to perform further diagnostic tests will be at the discretion of the case vet. Blood samples may

be taken for haematology to check for any underlying diseases and ensure the horse is fit for a GA.

Typically, equine patients being admitted for surgery are admitted the day before surgery; this allows the horse time to settle and adjust to the surroundings; some horses will have travelled long distances or maybe unsettled travellers. Admission, the day before surgery, also ensures that the practice has time to carry out the necessary preoperative checks. However, this may not be the case for several reasons:

- The horse is an emergency
- The client does not want the horse to stay or cannot afford for the horse to stay for extra time
- Practice policy
- A minor procedure that does not require the horse to be admitted to the practice for a more extended period

12.2 Preparing the Surgical Patient

Each surgery will require specific perioperative care; as an RVN, it is important to understand the requirements for the different procedures performed in practice [4].

Minor Surgery

Minor surgery generally includes minimally invasive surgeries with a low risk to the patient's health and welfare. This may be performed under standing sedation or GA [13].

Common minor surgeries may include:

- Sarcoid removal
- Standing splint bone removal
- Keratoma removal
- Pedal bone scrap

Standing Surgery

Standing surgery is a procedure that is performed under local anaesthesia and standing sedation. Procedures using this technique can be classified as minor, but some are also major surgeries [13].

Common standing surgeries include:

- Urogenital: cystotomy to remove uroliths
- Laparoscope: ovariectomy (removal of ovary/ovaries), nephrosplenic space closure, nephrectomy (removal of kidney), cryptorchidectomy (removal of a retained testicle – this can be performed standing or under GA via a laparoscopic technique if the testicle is in the abdomen)
- Upper airway and sinus surgery: tieback and or Hobday, sinus trephination, sinus flap

- Skin mass removal: melanoma removal, sarcoid removal, lumpectomy
- Orthopaedic: splint bone removal, lag screw placement, joint flush
- Dentistry: tooth removal, minimal invasive transbuccal extraction (MTE)

GA

A GA is carried out for any surgeries that require the horse to be fully unconscious for the procedure; for more information on GA, refer to Chapter 10. Horses carry a high mortality rate compared to humans and small animals; because of this, a GA must be used only when necessary to carry out a procedure [11].

Common surgeries completed under GA include [12]:

- Tenoscopy: keyhole surgery entering a tendon sheath
- Arthroscopy: keyhole surgery entering a joint space
- Fracture repair: bone repair using screws and/or plates
- Annular ligament desmotomy (ALD): the cutting of the ligament to create more room for the tendon to move
- Penile surgery: partial or complete resection
- Castration: removal of testicles

When preparing for any surgical procedures, it is important that the RVN is organised and understands the procedure that is due to happen; the following should be considered for all surgeries:

- Pain management: managing pain in horses can be difficult and varies from breed to breed. Certain breeds of horses and donkeys are more likely to mask signs of pain due to their nature as prey animals. It is useful to use multimodal analgesia for procedures. This usually involves the use of non-steroidal anti-inflammatory drugs (NSAIDs) and opioids, depending on the procedure. Pain scoring can be a valuable tool to use in the perioperative period. Each practice will have a specific pain scoring method to assess a patient's pain level; the pain scoring should be derived from a validated system; all staff members must use the same system. Pain scoring can ensure that a patient's pain level is managed sufficiently. If the pain score is high and the level of pain relief is insufficient, the RVN's job is to highlight this to the vet [11].
- Antibiotics: the use of antibiotics prior to surgery is a controversial subject; there are now many routine surgeries that may not require antibiotics, especially clean surgeries such as arthroscopies. The use of antibiotics for surgical cases will always be a practice-led discussion and should factor in the practice's infection rates and the best evidence base available; this should be reviewed regularly, as well as looking at protocols for patient preparation and

surgical cleaning, using resources such as The British Equine Veterinary Association (BEVA) ProtectMe toolkit, can also help with this decision-making process [14] (see Chapter 6 for more information).

- Equipment: all surgical instrumentation and equipment should be prepared in advance depending on the surgery and requirements of the vet (see Chapter 11 for more information). The RVN should check that any auxiliary equipment is working and that all surgical equipment is sterilised prior to the surgery commencing [4].
- Communication: with any surgery, good communication is essential. The RVN is part of a large surgery team, and all team members should have good lines of communication to prevent human errors from occurring [9] (see Chapter 2 for more information).

Once all these points have been discussed as a team and a surgical plan has been created, the horse can be prepared for surgery. This will include the following:

Starvation

The starvation of surgical patients is a much-debated topic, with some guidance set at starving for 6–12 hours prior to surgery. After the patient has metabolised the anaesthetic drugs, food is slowly introduced post-anaesthetic. Traditionally, starving equine patients before GA has been suggested to reduce diaphragmatic splinting and vena cava compression by an otherwise full gastrointestinal tract (GIT) [11]. This reduction during recumbency (particularly dorsal recumbency) is hoped to preserve pulmonary functional residual capacity (FRC), alveolar ventilation and venous return during GA [11]. However, there is a lack of evidence to support the starvation of equine patients prior to GA. Evidence suggests that starving horses increases circulating catecholamines (catecholamines are important in stress responses [15], and high levels can cause high blood pressure or hypertension). Another reason for not starving prior to GA is that it may increase the chance of postoperative ileus and/or caecal impactions. This has led to some hospitals now not having a starvation period. Specific, evidence-based guidelines for the starvation of equine patients prior to GA are not available at the time of writing. However, the following guidance can be considered when deciding on a starvation protocol [11]:

- Access to clean, fresh water should be allowed up until the time of premedication.
- Restricting access to concentrates and large meals of forage for around four to six hours prior to premedication might be prudent as a starting point to limit gut fill and the development of tympany. This may contribute to limiting increases in intra-abdominal pressure.

- It is difficult to justify restriction for patients who have true ab lib access to grazing or conserved or ensiled forages.
- Allowing access to food right up until the point of premedication would require a thorough mouthwash, especially if an endotracheal tube is to be placed.
- Alternatively, access to food could be restricted one to two hours prior to anaesthesia. This may help to address the problem of food in the oral cavity while mitigating against the detrimental effects of restricting food intake.

If access to food is to be restricted, the patient should be put in a stable containing nonedible bedding such as shavings or cardboard. Whichever starvation protocol is used within the practice, there are some instances where starvation is generally avoided regardless [12]:

- Foals: foals should not be starved as they could become dehydrated and hypoglycaemic, and this could cause complications during and after surgery.
- Donkeys and some native pony breeds: these patients carry a high risk of hyperlipemia. When these types stop eating, i.e. are starved, their body goes into a state of 'negative energy balance' (more energy is used up than is being taken in). When this happens, the body tries to use stored fat deposits as a source of energy [16]. This

results in free fatty acids circulating to the liver to be converted to glucose for use by the body. Control of this system is hormonal and should get shut down again. However, donkeys and small ponies cannot efficiently turn off this fat release, and fat levels soon build up in the circulation. Fat levels can be measured by testing the blood for triglycerides. Large amounts of fat cause the liver and kidneys to degenerate and fail, and eventually, all the organs in the body fail. The result is irreversible organ damage and death [17].

Table 12.1 identifies some possible advantages and disadvantages of starvation versus non-starvation of equine patients before a GA. As previously stated, there are arguments for either, which should be decided upon using the best evidence-based practice and statistics available [12].

Some surgeries require starvation to facilitate access to the surgical site, for example, a cystotomy. Under GA, the patient may need to be put into the Trendelenburg position (this is a term used to describe when the horse's head is lower than the body) to access the bladder. Other surgeries will require extended periods of starvation to enable a procedure to take place. Patients undergoing elective laparoscopy may be required to have a starvation period of between 24 and 48 hours [12]. This reduces the ingesta in

Table 12.1 Advantages and disadvantages of starvation versus non-starvation before surgery.

Starvation 6–12 h Advantages	Starvation 6–12 h Disadvantages	No starvation Advantages	No starvation Disadvantages
Reduces gut fill and, therefore, pressure on the diaphragm during anaesthesia	It can affect the horse's behaviour and increase stress levels which may mean that anaesthetic drugs are less effective	Horses are less stressed which means that the anaesthetic drugs are more likely to be effective	More intestinal gut fill and therefore more pressure on the diaphragm during anaesthesia
Reduces the weight of the abdomen on the lumbar musculature. Possibly reducing the chance of myopathy, especially in dorsal recumbency	Increase in stress hormones	Stress hormones are not as elevated	There may be a higher chance of myopathies and neuropathies due to the weight of the abdomen on lumbar musculature
It may decrease the chances of aspiration pneumonia due to reflux	Increased chances of hyperlipemia in some patients, e.g. donkeys	Reduced chances of hyperlipemia	There may be a higher chance of aspiration pneumonia
Reduced chance of rupturing the stomach on induction	It may cause equine gastric ulcer syndrome (EGUS)	Reduces the chance of EGUS developing	Increased chance of stomach rupturing on induction if full
Reduces the risk of aspiration of food material when the endotracheal tube is placed as there is no food material in the oral cavity (this risk can also be reduced with mouth cleansing prior to induction)	There may be an increase in post-operative ileus leading to pelvic flexure and caecal impactions	Increases the risk of aspiration of food material when the endotracheal tube is placed as there will food material in the oral cavity (this risk can also be reduced with mouth cleansing prior to induction)	There may be a reduction in post-operative ileus reducing the chances of pelvic flexure and caecal impactions

Source: Rosina Lillywhite.

the colon and cecum, allowing the surgeon access to the upper caudal abdomen.

It is vital to remember that horses do not require water removal before a GA.

Shoe Removal and Foot Preparation

Shoes should be removed before GA to reduce the risk of injury to the patient and to protect the floor of the knock-down box from damage. The feet must then be pared and thoroughly scrubbed clean and, after induction, covered with rectal sleeves prior to hoisting into the theatre to prevent contamination [3]. If shoe removal is not possible, the shoes can be taped up with adhesive tape before induction.

Scrupulous preparation is essential for surgery involving the foot or a structure close to the foot [3]. Bacterial numbers can be significantly reduced by removing the superficial hoof surface, for example, paring the feet with a hoof knife, applying a povidone-iodine scrub and using a 24-hour povidone-iodine soak. However, bacterial populations can persist after these disinfection techniques [4]. Chlorhexidine gluconate could be considered for pre-surgical foot preparation, as chlorhexidine has a residual activity against bacteria and is not inactivated by organic material, unlike povidone-iodine. This, along with paring the feet before surgery, could be a useful and effective cleaning technique, although there is currently no empirical evidence to support this. Regardless of the cleaning technique, a foot dressing should be applied after cleaning, then covered with an empty drip bag, and secured with an adhesive bandage to keep the area clean and dry [3].

Grooming

The horse should be groomed thoroughly to prevent contamination of the theatre. Some horses, especially those with long coats and feathers, may require bathing to facilitate asepsis [3]. The mane should be plaited if long, and the tail should be tied up and covered with a bandage or rectal sleeve.

Site Identification

The surgical site must be identified with the vet before surgery and documented in the relevant places according to practice policy. Best practice may include having standard operating procedures (SOPs) for routine procedures. Diagrams and explanations of the clipping and prepping process could be provided to ensure this is standardised throughout the hospital to minimise human error.

Clippers

When using clippers for surgical skin preparation and intravenous (IV) catheter placement, the recommended blade size is 40. Previously, it was thought that 50 blades were suitable as they clipped the hair closer to the skin. However, these blades can clip too closely to the skin, sometimes resulting in post-operative skin abrasions and acute dermatitis.

When clipping the patient, the blades must be flat to the skin and used gently. Clipping too vigorously can damage the skin, causing abrasions that increase the risk of bacterial colonisation from bacteria such as *Staphylococcus aureus*; this type of bacteria is commonly found in normal skin and only causes an issue if the skin becomes damaged [12].

Clipper blades must be cleaned between patients to prevent cross-contamination. Diseases such as dermatophytosis (ringworm) and lice are easily passed from patient to patient by inadequate cleaning and disinfection of clipper blades. The clipper blade cleaner used must be fungicidal, virucidal and bactericidal, and act as lubrication for the clipper blades. If the blades are not adequately lubricated, they can cause excess tissue drag and damage the patient's skin. Blades must be changed frequently, as blunt blades can cause skin trauma. Clipper blades should be sent off regularly for routine sharpening [1].

The surgical site should be clipped as much as possible before GA to minimise anaesthetic time. Equine patients are not ideal candidates for GA due to their large size. Clipping the day before surgery is considered controversial; some research suggests that the skin trauma caused by clipping causes residual skin bacteria to come to the surface and increases the risk of a surgical site infection (SSI). The hair protects the patient's skin surface, often shielding it from dirt [18]. Removing the hair the day before surgery and leaving the skin open to a contaminated, stable environment may lead to an increased risk of an SSI. However, it has also been suggested that clipping the night before and the minimal risk this poses to SSIs is outweighed by the benefits of reducing anaesthetic time. When the patient is clipped, will depend on individual practice policies, which should be linked to the best available evidence-based research [19].

When clipping for a surgical procedure, there should be a circumference of at least 5–10 cm around the patient's surgical site where possible. In some instances, such as young Thoroughbreds that are going to the horse sales, a smaller clip patch or none at all may be required to ensure that it is less visible when the horse is sold; this may be requested by the owners/trainers; this is a decision to be made by the vet.

IV Catheter Placement

Vascular access should be secured before any equine patient is anaesthetised [2]. This ensures that the anaesthetist has consistent IV access throughout the procedure, and this increases the safety of the patient and all theatre personnel. A wide-bore catheter is usually placed around the time of premedication. Please see Chapter 17 for further information on IV catheter placement. The catheter should be placed into the left jugular vein if the horse is positioned in dorsal recumbency or the uppermost vein if the horse is positioned in lateral recumbency [3].

Tail Bandaging

The application of a tail bandage aids in reducing microorganisms and contaminants entering the surgical theatre space; it also helps to ensure the tail does not contaminate the surgical site when moving the horse out of the theatre at the end of surgery and when recovering. Tail bandages come in a range of types. They can be a reusable, clean tail bandage, crepe bandage or self-adhesive bandage; whichever is chosen, it should be appropriately placed so that it does not interfere with the blood supply to the tail [2].

Mouth Cleansing

Rinsing the horse's mouth is vital to prevent the patient from aspirating food material during endotracheal tube placement [3]. A large dental syringe can be used for this, and the water should be warm. Mints or a small amount of mint oil can be added to the water to flavour it and make it more palatable to the patient. This will make the experience more positive for the patient.

Padded Headcollar

A leather padded headcollar should be applied to equine patients prior to induction. Leather is less likely to cause trauma, such as friction burns, when compared to nylon-webbing material [2]. The padding on the headcollar protects the superficial nerves near bony prominences from the metal rings on the headcollar. This helps to reduce the chance of the patient developing facial paralysis following anaesthesia. However, removal of the headcollar following induction is the only way to prevent this entirely.

Preparation of the Operating Theatre

Organisation and preparation of the operating theatre should take place the day before surgery where possible. It is important to be prepared and have all the necessary surgical instruments ready for the procedure. Sterilisation dates of all instruments and equipment to be used should be checked beforehand. Setting the room up before the patient and surgeon arrive helps to prepare prior to the procedure [4]. Preparations may include:

- Deciding the order of the day for procedures/discussion with surgeons
- Damp dusting surfaces
- Is the room clean and suitable for use?
- Checking equipment, drugs, anything broken or missing?
- Preparing sedation, analgesia, local anaesthetic, antibiotics and intravenous fluid therapy (IVFT) for prolonged procedures
- Checking surgical instruments
- Preparing and checking paperwork and a checklist

Surgical Safety Checklist (SSC)

The World Health Organization (WHO) has encouraged the use of SSCs to decrease errors and increase teamwork and communication in surgery [20]. Several human studies have shown a significant reduction in surgical-related morbidity and mortality (between 43% and 62%) following the implementation of and adherence to SSCs. These SSCs are designed to minimise/erase human factors (human factors are those things that affect an individual's performance). Research by Oxtoby et al. [21] suggests that 80% of adverse events are primarily related to human factors. Factors that the use of an SSC may eliminate include [22]:

- Operating on the incorrect horse or incorrect limb
- Having the horse positioned in an incorrect way
- Having the wrong surgical kit
- Not having a surgeon present
- Severe allergic reaction

The benefits of an SSC may arise from the opportunity for the team to pause for a moment and communicate in a busy setting, which encourages the sharing of collective responsibility within the surgical team. An SSC should be a simple checklist of instructions that are carried out at three intervals throughout the surgical period and should include the following considerations [20]:

Before the horse is induced:

- Has the identity been confirmed?
- Has consent for the procedure been obtained?
- Is the surgeon aware?
- Is the site clipped?
- Has the patient had its pre-op drugs?
- Has the patient been groomed?
- Have the feet been cleaned?

- Has the mouth been washed?
- Has the tail bandage been applied?
- Any allergies?
- Any expected issues with intubation?

Before skin incision:

- All staff members identify themselves with name and role
- Confirm the patient's name and procedure
- To the surgeon:
  - Are there any extras required?
  - How long will the procedure take?
  - Are there any concerns regarding blood loss?
- To the anaesthetist
  - Do you have any concerns with the anaesthetic?
- Nursing team
  - Has the equipment been sterilised?
  - Are there any known equipment issues?

Before the patient goes into recovery:

- Verbal communication of the procedure taking place
- Completion of the swab and instrument count verbalised
- For any samples taken during surgery, the patient details and test requirements should be read aloud
- Whether any equipment issues need addressing
- The verbalisation of the recovery and treatment plan [11]

A SSC should always be read aloud with the whole room pausing to listen and answer when appropriate; just using it as a tick list is not appropriate. If one person ticks these during the surgery, it will not prevent adverse events from happening. For more information on human factors or SSCs, please refer to VetLed and the WHO [22, 23].

Sedation Considerations

Sedation prior to GA is covered in detail in Chapter 10. Commonly used sedative drugs include the following:

- **Alpha 2 agonists:**
  - Xylazine
  - Romifidine
  - Detomidine
- **Opioids:**
  - Morphine
  - Butorphanol (counteracts morphine)
- **Phenothiazines:**
  - Acepromazine

A deeper level of sedation is usually required for standing surgery due to the horse being conscious. The surgeon may have to get themselves in dangerous positions to operate. Different sedation protocols are needed for different procedures,

and the right sedation for the right procedure must be selected. A sedation plan should be made when discussing the procedure with the surgeon [15]. A combination of IV, intramuscular and constant-rate infusions may be used. Xylazine is rarely used in standing surgery, as it is short-acting, so it does not give a good enough level and depth of sedation even for short procedures [15].

Constant-Rate Infusion (CRI)

For any procedures that are going on for some time or that use loud, noisy equipment, a CRI is typically a good method of administering sedation. It is created using a bag of saline spiked with a sedative (typically detomidine). It allows for a continuous delivery system of sedation to the patient to keep the patient on a level sedation plane without the patient transitioning between light and deep sedation, which can be a problem with 'top-up' sedation. CRIs are administered IV and require the following preparation [15]:

- IV catheter placement
- 500 ml bag of saline
- Giving set
- Detomidine 0.1–0.6 ug/kg (1.25 ml per bag) rate; 1 drop/s
- Xylazine 0.69 mg/kg, rate; 3 drops/s (if requested by the vet for use)

Local Anaesthesia

Local anaesthesia is essential for many surgeries; using anaesthesia locally in the area that is being operated on can reduce the amount of analgesia used, reduce the chance of wind-up or a chronic pain state developing and ensure that the horse has a more comfortable post-operative experience. It can also make a standing procedure safer for the surgeon as the horse cannot feel discomfort during the surgery. Types of local anaesthesia used include [15]:

- Nerve blocks: local anaesthetic is injected around a nerve or neurovascular bundle to remove the sensation to a particular area; the area should always be checked to make sure that desensitisation has occurred before the surgery starts [15].
- Line block: subcutaneous lidocaine is injected along the incision site. Relatively straightforward, it is often used when the surgical site is away from a nerve or nerve bundle. The block can be easier on the animal if a longer needle is inserted through the last injection site.
- Ring block: a specific type of field block. The entire limb is encircled with subcutaneous local anaesthetic to reach all nerves in the limb.
- Regional IV blocks: a tourniquet is placed on the limb, and local anaesthetic is injected into a vessel below

the tourniquet. The local anaesthetic is diluted to the level that it pushes out of the vasculature and into the tissues [15].

Types of Local Anaesthetic

The most common local anaesthetics used are as follows [15]:

- Mepivacaine hydrochloride (Intra-Epicaine)
- Bupivacaine hydrochloride (Marcaine)
- Prilocaine hydrochloride (Citanest)
- Lidocaine hydrochloride (Lignol)

Lidocaine with adrenaline is not for use in the skin as it has a vasoconstrictive effect and can cause tissue necrosis. Lidocaine with adrenaline increases the duration of anaesthesia; when used for local infiltration, its vasoconstrictive effect is an added benefit as it provides a bloodless operating field. Because of this, it is more commonly used in laparoscopic surgeries for desensitising internal structures and local infiltration during sinus surgery, throat surgery and perineal surgery [12].

When preparing local anaesthesia for a procedure, the correct type should be selected to prevent errors from developing. More information can be found in Chapter 10.

Epidural Anaesthesia

Epidural anaesthesia is most commonly used in standing procedures for rectovaginal fistula repairs in mares post-foaling and any procedures in the perianal area. The caudal epidural space is most frequently used; it is found by lifting the tail, creating a divot that can be palpated. Xylazine is the preferred drug for perineal analgesia; its analgesic effect lasts longer than detomidine and romifidine and is thought to last around 2.5 hours [24]. Morphine can be used for an epidural but is more commonly used to manage severe pain or painful long-term procedures. A long-term epidural can be achieved by placing an epidural catheter into the caudal epidural space. If using an epidural in horses, it is important not to overdose as this can affect the sensory and motor function of the hindlimbs [12]. It is important for RVNs to know the landmarks for this procedure when assisting the vet, as they will be involved with patient preparation. Figure 12.1 shows the different areas where an epidural can be placed; the first position is between the sixth lumbar vertebrae L6 and the first sacral dorsal spinous process S1; this is used for catheter placement for continuous caudal epidural anaesthesia (technically demanding, infrequently performed). The second position is between the first and second coccygeal vertebrae (C1 and C2). Needle placement

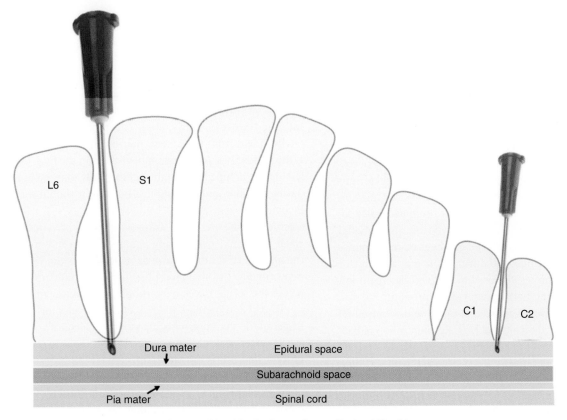

Figure 12.1 Needle placement for an epidural in the horse. *Source:* Rosina Lillywhite.

for caudal anaesthesia perpendicular direction. Once the needle is inserted, anaesthesia administration can occur, or a catheter can be introduced over 10–30 cm into the epidural space. After placement of the catheter, the needle can be removed and the catheter can be secured to the skin [24].

Surgical Site Skin Preparation

Surgical site preparation aims to remove debris and microorganisms from the dermal surface, reducing the risk of SSIs. The antimicrobial scrub used initiates this process aided by a validated scrubbing technique [25]. Complete sterilisation of the skin is impossible, and gradual recolonisation will occur.

Whether using chlorhexidine gluconate (CG) or povidone iodine (PI), the most crucial factor is that the two skin preparations are not mixed. The two products are considered incompatible and deactivate each other. CG is cationic (positively charged) and PI is anionic (negatively charged). The manufacturers recommend not using them together for this reason [1].

Both CG and PI are suitable for surgical skin preparation. Many studies have been conducted to determine which skin preparation is superior. CG is often considered superior due to its prolonged residual action [26]. PI has a short residual activity compared with CG. There is insufficient evidence to support the idea that PI is less of an irritant to the skin in comparison to CG. Some research papers have reported a higher incidence of acute contact dermatitis in dogs with the use of PI. In human medicine, strong ratios of PI have been known to cause chemical-type burns and contact dermatitis and strong solutions are also considered corrosive, so using the correct dilution rates is essential [26].

Alcohols such as ethyl alcohol and isopropyl alcohol are also used as disinfectants and antiseptics. Water is necessary to increase the microbial efficacy of alcohol and formulations of 60-90% are most effective [27]. The concentration of the product is more important that the type of alcohol used however, isopropyl alcohol has a greater bactericidal action than ethanol [27]. Alcohol can be used in combination with another antiseptic during skin preparation, for example CG. It can also be used to rinse off detergent left over from scrubbing with another skin antiseptic.

Some studies have suggested that CG should be rinsed off with saline rather than alcohol [27]. Recolonisation of bacteria on the surface of the skin has been shown to be more aggressive post-operatively when prepped with CG and rinsed with alcohol than if it had been prepped with CG and rinsed with saline. More research is needed into this area as the manufacturer recommends rinsing with

alcohol. In contrast, some studies looking at the effect of commercially available preparations of 2% chlorhexidine and 70% isopropyl alcohol found that alcohol enhanced the residual activity of CG [27]. Clearly, there is a need for more research in this area before a standardised skin preparation protocol can be produced for veterinary practice. Until more information is available, practices should continue to use skin protocols that are in place, if they are effective, but pay particular attention to correct dilution rates and contact times for skin antiseptic solutions.

CG should not be used in the skin preparation protocol for head and neck surgery, as it can cause ototoxicity (ear toxicity). This can induce hearing loss and balance problems. It is also very irritant to ocular surfaces and mucous membranes and can provoke ulcers, so PI is recommended for any surgery around these areas [12].

The scrubbing procedure may begin in the preparation room and be completed in the theatre, or the whole process may take place in the theatre. As there currently is no standardised skin preparation protocol for veterinary practice, the following steps should be treated as guidelines only [27]:

- Gloves should always be worn and changed with each step of the decontamination process. Patients should be clipped away from the operating theatre. If this is not possible, a hoover should be used in the operating theatre to remove the loose hair.
- When preparing patient limbs, the hair not included in the surgical site should be covered over where possible using a cohesive bandage to mark out the surgical site and cover the unclipped hair.
- Covering the patient's feet in rectal sleeves or bandaging material will help minimise the contamination brought into the theatre. A sterile sheet can protect the theatre environment from the horse's hair during surgery [2].
- If the patient has an operation near to or on the foot, this should be prepped the night before. This may include paring the foot and soaking in PI or CG; it should then be bandaged until surgery.
- Decontaminate the skin using a pre-skin preparation wash with mild neutralising shampoo. This minimises the amount of scrubbing and damage to the skin. It also saves time as the shampoo lifts much of the dirt/grease before the scrub. Excessive scrubbing can cause damage to the skin and increase the risk of SSIs developing [27].
- Rinse off the shampoo with 70% isopropyl alcohol or with sterile water, as the shampoo can inhibit the skin preparation agent if it is not rinsed off.
- CG is recommended for use at a 4% concentration. It is often challenging to create a lather and loosen grease with neat CG; therefore, a small amount of water is

sometimes added. Be aware that any concentration below 2%, i.e. 50:50, has been shown to be less effective against microorganisms, increasing the likelihood of SSIs developing post-operatively [28].

- Make up the skin preparation solution just before it is required; avoid making these up too far in advance, as this decreases the efficacy of the solution.
- The first stage of the skin prep should be carried out with non-sterile swabs using CG 4% or PI 7.5% (use as neat as possible on intact skin) [27]. The four corners of the swab should be held together, creating a middle surface area to scrub with keeping your hand behind the swab contact area and away from the patient.
- Lint-free swabs should be used to minimise the amount of gauze that is left behind on the patient. The first skin prep is finished once the swabs are visibly clean.
- Rinse with 70% isopropyl alcohol or sterile saline once the skin prep agent has had its contact time of 3–6 minutes (check manufacturer's guidelines) for CG and is thought to be slightly longer for PI at around 4–10 minutes (check manufacturer's guidelines) [27].
- The skin should be clean before the sterile skin preparation is initiated (second skin prep) with CG or PI – distilled or sterile water should be used (not tap water as the compounds react and reduce efficacy). This step is carried out with the operator wearing sterile gloves. If using CG, the contact time is around 3–6 minutes, and if using PI scrub 7.5% is 4–10 minutes, but always check the manufacturer's guidelines [27].
- Use isopropyl alcohol (70% dilution) spray or sterile saline swabs to remove detergent. Spray bottles should be wiped down after each use and routinely sterilised to prevent cross-contamination between patients. When using a spray bottle, the first spray should be aimed into a kick bucket or bin to prevent the spread of bacteria that may be harboured in the spray bottle nozzle [27].
- Allow the alcohol/saline to dry before the incision is made.
- Skin paint can be used as a final step. This is usually a mixture of CG 0.5% with industrial methylated spirits (which can be bought pre-made) [27]. Practice protocols may vary regarding the types and amounts of skin antiseptics used to create skin paint solutions.
- If using PI, then the solution must only be used as a skin paint and used neat. This can be applied using sterile swabs and sponge-holding forceps or by hand as long as sterile gloves are worn [12].
- Commercially available skin antiseptic solution applicators containing 2% CG and 70% isopropyl alcohol mixed together have been growing in popularity in human medicine and small animal practice. These could also be incorporated into skin preparation protocols in equine practice. As with any changes to a skin preparation

protocol, the efficacy of any changes should be monitored with a clinical audit.

Once the surgical site has been prepped, it should not be touched. The final surgical prep should be repeated if there's a break in asepsis.

The practice protocol for skin preparation should be followed in most cases. However, if an increase in SSIs is seen, a clinical audit should be carried out, and the skin preparation regime should be changed if considered appropriate. This should then be followed by another clinical audit to ensure that the changes have been effective.

Scrubbing patterns

'The Back-and-Forth Technique'

Gauze swabs should be folded into quarters by bringing the four corners together and holding by the corners. This produces a smaller contact area that is easier to control and limits the chance of fingers touching the patient. Move the gauze back and forth at the proposed incision site for approximately 15 seconds. It is the back-and-forth action that provides most of the cleaning. Discard the swab and select a new one. Gradually move out from the incision, keeping that back-and-forth action going, changing swabs regularly. Never return a dirty swab back to the incision site. A pattern of L and C shapes will keep the back-and-forth action going while enabling the swab to move away from the centre. This technique uses firm pressure as well as back-and-forth motion; evidence has shown that this method can penetrate the first five dermal layers [27].

The Circular Scrub Technique (Target or Bullseye)

Also known as the singular or concentrative pattern, historically, RVNs have used the circular scrub technique, which has often been favoured in the veterinary profession. Some evidence suggests the back-and-forth technique is superior to the circular scrub technique. This will vary on the particular area of the patient being prepared.

The circular motion technique starts with a centre point (where the incision is to be made) and moves outwards away from the centre point in a circular motion to the clipped edge. Once the edge is reached, or the swab is contaminated, it must be discarded [27].

Excessive pressure is unnecessary and will abrade the skin, causing inflammation and the incision may be more prone to healing complications if the dermal layer is compromised. It will also cause the native skin microbes to rise to the surface.

Figure 12.2 shows the two scrub patterns used in the equine patient when preparing for a surgical procedure [27].

(a)

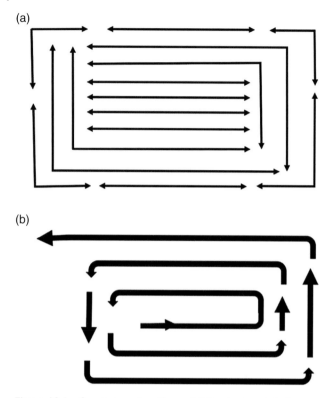

(b)

Figure 12.2 Surgical scrub patterns: (a) The back-and-forth technique for the surgical preparation of the patient and (b) the circular technique for the surgical preparation of the patient. *Source:* Rosina Lillywhite.

Skin Preparation for Ocular Surfaces

For ophthalmic surgery, a PI solution should always be used as CG has been shown to be more irritant to the surface of the cornea. Alcohol based solutions should not be used in this area [1]. PI should be used as follows [29]:

- Dilute in saline or distilled water
- Around eyelids and surrounding skin a 1:10 solution can be used (50 ml in 500 ml saline)
- Around corneal surfaces a 1:50 solution can be used (10 ml in 500 ml saline)

Some surgeons do not advocate clipping around the eye for intraocular surgery and opt to use adhesive drapes instead to protect the eye from hair and skin [1]. Other surgeons prefer to clip a minimal amount of hair around the eye. A water soluble gel can be applied to the hair and into the eye prior to clipping. The skin surrounding the eye is thin and sensitive, so a well functioning set of clippers and clean blades should always be used. The eye should be irrigated with saline several times following clipping to wash away any hair and remaining lubricant. The eye can then be irrigated with a dilute a 0.1-0.2% PI solution if required [1].

Skin Preparation for Wounds

This section will concentrate on preparing wounds for surgical procedures. For information on preparing wounds that do not require surgery, please see Chapter 13. Hydrogels are helpful to place into the wound to prevent further dirt, hair and contaminants from tracking deep into the wound when clipping and prepping around the area as it creates a barrier and rehydrates the wound. A hydrogel protects the wound, keeps it moist and aids wound healing [12]. PI can be used for preparing contaminated, chronic and acute wounds as it has a broad antimicrobial spectrum, lack of resistance, efficacy against biofilms and is tolerated well [30].

If appropriate, a PI solution can be used on contaminated wounds; iodine scrub should only be used on intact skin. This can be difficult when preparing a large area of skin with wounds and intact skin. The PI scrub is used to lift the dirt and grease from the skin; without its use, the preparation of the area can take longer. When preparing two separate areas due to intact skin and multiple wounds, the wound should be covered with sterile saline-soaked swabs, and then intact skin should be prepped with PI scrub [30]. This is then rinsed with sterile saline, and then the skin and wounds are prepared with a PI solution. PI has low cytotoxicity compared to CG, which has high cytotoxicity. The PI solution can be used to cleanse contaminated wounds before closure. A ratio for wound irrigation of PI solution (10%) should be applied in a 0.1–0.2% concentration. s. PI 7.5% scrub contains detergent and is unsuitable for cleansing wounds [31].

Saline is widely used for cleansing clean wounds and is often preferred due to its isotonic nature, which makes it non-toxic to tissues. This characteristic helps maintain cellular integrity and prevents additional tissue damage during wound care. Unlike tap water, saline does not contain various compounds that might irritate the wound or disrupt the osmotic balance.

In contrast, tap water can be beneficial for the initial cleaning phase of heavily contaminated wounds. Its abundance and cost-effectiveness make it a practical choice for flushing out debris and contaminants. However, tap water should be used cautiously because it is not isotonic and may contain minerals and other substances. After the initial decontamination with tap water, switching to an isotonic solution like saline is advisable to promote optimal healing conditions and avoid potential tissue irritation.

It's important to note that tap water should only be used when a constant supply of potable drinking water is available, ensuring it is free from harmful microorganisms. The primary advantage of tap water lies in its affordability and ready availability, making it a convenient option for the initial management of contaminated wounds [31].

Skin Marking

Sometimes, it is necessary to mark the surgery site with staples preoperatively. If this needs to be done, the skin should be clipped, shampooed rinsed and an initial skin prep should be carried out before staple insertion. The staples are then included in the skin preparation for surgical site preparation. Care should be taken when scrubbing, as it is easy to loosen the staples [12].

Bacterial Colonisation

Recolonisation of the surgical site will gradually occur after antiseptic preparation. The time this takes will depend on several factors, including, but not limited to, antiseptic preparation used, length of surgery time and type of drape. It is essential to know how these factors can affect the efficacy of the products used, as re-colonisation will increase the chance of SSIs. The occurrence of an SSI can cause major post-operative problems for a patient and can be caused by the patient, the surgical team, as well as the environment [30]. To minimise this risk, correct surgical attire must be worn when scrubbing a patient (see Chapter 11 for more information). RVNs should remain bare below the elbows, and hats and masks should be worn from the point of scrubbing to the end of closure to minimise airborne microorganisms from staff.

SSIs have various causes *staphylococcus aureus* is the most common bacteria associated with SSIs and is derived from the patients own skin flora.[12]. If the patient's skin is damaged from excessive scrubbing or clipping, this encourages bacteria to come to the surface, and increases the risk of a SSI developing. Plastic drapes are more likely to increase the risk of SSIs; however, iodophor-impregnated incise films are thought to reduce the risk, having shown fewer colonies of bacteria developing in the studies conducted [30]. Hair shafts and sweat glands go deep within the dermis; the longer a surgical site is left covered by a drape, the more likely the patient is to sweat and cause bacteria to resurface from the hair shaft or sweat gland. It is almost impossible to penetrate deep within the hair follicles. Prepping the surgical site just before the incision is made helps to prevent SSIs. If alcohol is used as a rinsing agent, it must be allowed to dry before the surgical incision is made. If diathermy or a laser is being used, alcohol should be avoided as it can cause burns [25].

12.3 Wounds

A wound is a disruption of the anatomical and cellular continuity of tissue. Wounds can be created accidentally or intentionally [1]. An example of an intentional wound is a surgical incision.

Physiology of Wound Healing

Wound healing is broken down into four stages: haemostasis, inflammatory, proliferation and maturation; these stages occur in an overlapping sequence of events that result in the repair of the damaged tissue. The healing process is initiated as soon as the injury occurs [12].

- Phase 1: haemostasis (cessation of bleeding): This phase happens immediately following the injury and is completed in hours. The first response of the body to the initial injury is to stop the flow of blood. The blood vessels constrict to help reduce the blood flow, and then platelets stick together to help seal the break in the wall of the blood vessel. Strands of fibrin adhere to the platelets and start to form a clot, and this clot helps to reduce blood loss.
- Phase 2: inflammatory: Occurs during the first 6–8 hours following injury [1]. The inflammatory phase begins shortly after the initial injury when the blood vessels leak transudate, which causes localised swelling. Activation of platelets and the presence of fibrin in the blood clot attracts neutrophils to the area [2]. The neutrophils function to clear up bacteria, necrotic tissue and foreign material. Neutrophils release inflammatory mediators that, in turn, attract macrophages into the tissue [2]. The macrophages perform the final stage of debridement before the next stage begins.
- Phase 3: proliferation: This phase normally occurs from day three following [1]. Granulation tissue develops at this stage to fill in the wound bed. Healthy granulation tissue is bright red in colour and even in appearance. Fibroblasts lay down a collagen matrix, and endothelial cells lay down new blood vessels (angiogenesis). Epithelial cells migrate over the top of the wound in a process known as epithelialisation. The wound starts to contract at this stage, and this process alone can close the wound by up to 30% [2]. Gradually, collagen fibres and scar tissue are laid down, and the wound progresses to the next stage.
- Phase 4: maturation: This phase occurs from 14 days after injury and can last for 12 months [1]. A collagen framework is laid down where a new dermal matrix is formed [3]. Fibroblasts help to improve tensile strength by remodelling the dermal tissues. Granulation tissue matures into scar tissue, and re-epithelisation occurs [3]. This scar tissue is the body's natural way of healing from an injury; however, it has only 80% of the original tissue tensile strength one-year post-injury [3].

Healing Times of Different Tissues

The basic physiology of wound healing remains the same for various tissue types: haemostasis, inflammation followed by proliferation and maturation. However, the length of time may differ considerably for the type of damaged tissue and the extent to which that tissue has been affected. Muscles and tendons generally take longer to heal due to the structural demands that are placed on them. These tissues require healing to a high level of strength and function. Muscle tissue should heal quickly, and immobilisation can help to allow strength to develop in the scar tissue [2]. The healing process for tendon and ligament injuries is slow, and rushing this process will only cause delays to the whole healing process. A tailored rehabilitation programme will often be needed for these types of injuries. Tissues in the GIT, urinary and reproductive tract heal more rapidly than the skin. The colon has the slowest healing time compared to the urinary bladder, which heals the fastest [2]. RVNs must understand the healing times of different tissues to ensure that rehabilitation plans and nursing care are tailored to the individual patient and are as effective as possible. Table 12.2 shows the average healing times for different tissue types; these times can be affected by external factors such as age, health status and SSIs [25].

Wound Healing Complications

RVNs should carefully monitor any wound, be it surgical or otherwise, for complications. Factors to look out for include [32]:

- Excessive amounts of purulent exudate.
- Erythema (reddening) of the skin edges and surrounding area
- Oedema (swelling) of the wound and the surrounding area
- Haematoma
- Pain on palpation

The wound should be assessed carefully and treated accordingly if any of these factors are identified.

Table 12.2 Tissue healing times.

Tissue type	Healing average healing time
Mucosa and skin	5–7 days
Subcutaneous and peritoneum	7–14 days
Fascia	14–28 days
Muscle	At least 60 days

Source: Rosina Lillywhite.

Types of Wounds

Wound types can be divided into open or closed wounds [12].

Open Wounds

- Incision: these are usually caused by a sharp object such as a scalpel (intentionally), glass or metal (accidentally). These injuries cause minor pain and the skin edges are cleanly cut with minor tissue damage [1].
- Laceration: this is a common type of wound. The skin edges are irregular, and there is extensive damage to underlying tissue. These wounds are painful. If the tissue has been lost, the laceration is termed an avulsion, for example, a degloving injury. A laceration extending into tendons, ligaments, synovial structures, or a body cavity is a complicated wound [1].
- Puncture: this is a wound caused by a sharp object that perforates tissue [1]. There is often a risk that these wounds penetrate a synovial structure. This should always be investigated thoroughly [1].

Closed Wounds

Closed wounds are injuries where the entire skin thickness has not been separated.

- Abrasion: these are friction injuries to the superficial surface of the skin or mucous membranes. These wounds are painful [1].
- Contusion: this results from bleeding and tissue destruction within and under intact skin. There is no division of the skin with these wounds [1].
- Burn: this is where the skin has been exposed to excessive heat, cold or a corrosive substance [1]. Please see Chapter 14 for more information regarding burns.

Classification of Wounds

A wound can be classified as follows:

- Clean wounds: these are the simplest of wounds, providing no complications occur. Clean wounds are created under aseptic conditions. For example, surgical incisions produced via scalpel blade causing minimal tissue damage. These 'clean' wounds do not enter body cavities such as the respiratory, gastrointestinal, or urogenital tracts.
- Clean-contaminated wounds: surgical incisions made into one of the body cavities mentioned previously are classified as 'clean-contaminated' wounds. Although these wounds are prepared under the same aseptic conditions as clean wounds, the entry into one of the tracts

introduces a level of contamination, making them fall into the 'clean-contaminated' category.

- Contaminated wounds: wounds obtained via accident, or a traumatic event are classed as 'contaminated'. These wounds often have a degree of environmental debris within them, for example, mud in a laceration wound on a tarsus.
- Dirty wounds: dirty wounds are those that are infected and exude purulent material. Traumatic 'contaminated' wounds can fall into this category if improper initial treatment is not sought.

Understanding the type and classification of the wound being dealt with is essential, as this has implications for the equipment and methods required for treatment.

Wound Closure Methods

The classification of the wound will impact the best management approach. There are different types of wound closure. These are as follows:

- Primary closure or first intention healing is the best choice of closure for clean wounds. Wounds closed by primary closure must be free from foreign material to give the wound the best chance of healing without complication [12].
- Delayed primary closure can be used for contaminated wounds which benefit from initial lavage and debris removal and then given a few days for any inflammation and swelling to reduce. The wound would then be closed after further lavage and possible debridement, generally done before the granulation process commences. Please see Chapter 13 for more information on wound lavage and debridement.
- Secondary closure can be used to surgically close wounds that have been left to develop a healthy granulation bed.
- Second intention healing is where wounds are not surgically closed but left to heal by granulation tissue formation and contraction. This method is often used for large wounds over areas of high movement, for example, the gluteal or pectoral muscles [3].

Many factors could cause a delay in wound healing; some of these complications can derive from the patient itself, for example, self-mutilation, systemic disease or other factors such as surgical complications, infection or poor wound management. The RVN plays a significant role in monitoring and assessing the progress of the wound during the healing process; it is essential to recognise complications as they arise to allow for a change in management as soon as possible, should it be required. Please see Chapter 13 for more information on the factors that delay healing [12].

Drains

Drains can be a helpful addition in wound management and healing in wounds where excess fluid accumulation is anticipated, predisposing the patient to seroma formation or where the infection is present, and drainage is beneficial. However, close monitoring and post-operative care are essential in ensuring the selected drain works correctly and, therefore, does not adversely affect the wound healing process [12]. Equine patients occasionally present with large, traumatic, open wounds, which can create large areas of dead space. Dead space develops between tissues after the disruption of subcutaneous connective tissues. This is undesirable because the fluid that typically fills this void provides a prime medium for bacterial growth [4]. Drains are often used in these situations to prophylactically reduce the chances of excess fluid accumulation. A drain should be sutured proximally, traverse the wound and exit through a small incision separate from the wound [3].

Types of Drains

Drains are classified by their action, which is either passive or active [5]. Passive drains use gravity and capillary action to allow fluid to drain freely from the wound. Active drains require 'active' suction to remove fluid or exudate. An active drain can be intermittently drained via a syringe or a chamber-like device for continuous drainage. Table 12.3 shows the different drains available for use in equine patients, the mechanisms by which they work and the advantages and disadvantages of each.

Figure 12.3 shows a Penrose drain on the left and a Jackson-Pratt drain on the right. Figure 12.4 shows a Jackson–Pratt drain placed in a large wound surgically repaired under GA.

Management of Drains

As mentioned previously, drains require careful post-operative monitoring and care. Things to monitor for are as follows [12]:

- Pain
- Increased exudate
- Swelling around the drain insertion
- Patient interference

Drains should be checked daily to ensure that they are still working correctly and are still patent. They should also be cleaned daily. During cleaning, the drain should be moved slightly to break any seal formed between the drain, the exudate and the surrounding skin [3].

Table 12.3 Types of surgical drain.

Passive drains

Type of drain	Material	Action and function	Advantage	Disadvantage
Gauze drains	Fine mesh gauze	Gravity Capillary action	Economical Step-by-step removal	Adherence of fibrin clots to gauze Risk of gauze fraying
Latex Penrose drain	Soft, pliable latex	Gravity Capillary action Mostly extraluminal drainage	Economical Many applications	Kinks easily Not applicable in body cavities No suction possible, collapse It may facilitate ascending infection
Silicone Penrose drain	Soft, pliable, nonreactive silicone	Capillary action Mainly extraluminal drainage	Minimal tissue irritation Use in latex-sensitive patients Radiodense marker	Not applicable in body cavities No suction possible
Rubber tube drains	Red Rubber	Gravity Capillary action	Because of relative stiffness, it is rarely compressed or occluded Suction possible	Increased foreign body reaction
Sheet drain (well [wave] drain')	Waved sheet of stiff red rubber	Gravity Capillary action	Because of relative stiffness, it is rarely compressed or occluded Can be cut to size	Increased foreign body reaction
Flexi-drain	12 parallel joined silicone tubes of 3-mm diameter	Gravity Capillary action	Good drainage along the tubes where they join Suction possible Can be cut to size	Mainly extraluminal drainage

Active drains

Type of drain	Material	Action and function	Advantage	Disadvantage
Redon drain	Round, multi-fenestrated polyvinyl chloride (PVC) with non-fenestrated extension tube	Intraluminal drainage	Excellent for evacuation of fluids from body cavities No collapse Used for lavage and drainage	Stiff Fenestrations may occlude
Jackson-Pratt drain	Flat silastic, multi-fenestrated drain with a non-fenestrated extension	Intraluminal drainage	Excellent for evacuation of fluids from body cavities Minimal tissue irritation	Expensive The suction function is only possible when implanted in an airtight space
Blake drain	Round or flat pliable silastic drain with longitudinal slits and protected spaces with a non-slit extension	Drainage through the longitudinal slits	Multifaceted slits reducing the risk of occlusion Minimal tissue irritation Radiodense marker No collapse possible	Expensive Voluminous The suction function is only possible when implanted in an airtight space
Trocar catheter	Round, multi-fenestrated tube Inserted with blunt trocar into body cavity	Drainage of body cavity Intraluminal drainage	Minimal tissue irritation Used for fluid drainage and lavage	Relatively easy dislodgement and interruption of adequate drainage Occlusion

Source: Rosina Lillywhite.

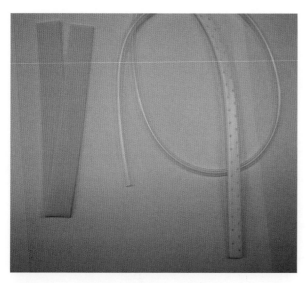

Figure 12.3 Left Penrose drain, right Jackson–Pratt drain. *Source:* Rosina Lillywhite.

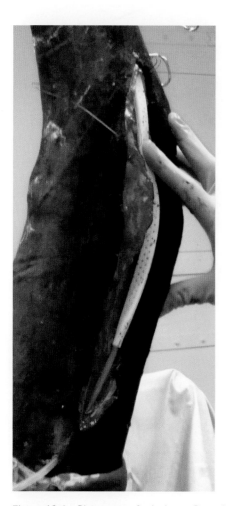

Figure 12.4 Placement of a Jackson–Pratt drain. *Source:* Rosina Lillywhite.

Drains, although often placed to prevent problems, may occasionally cause further complications such as:

- Some patients may react to some of the materials drains are made of, for example, latex.
- Bacteria may migrate up the drain lumen and contaminate the healing wound.
- Exudate draining freely from passive drains can cause skin scalding and irritation if the area below is not kept clean and dry. A barrier cream or emollient can be applied as necessary to help prevent this secondary complication.
- Where possible, the drain should be bandaged in place with a sterile dressing to absorb fluid from the end of the drain [2].

If complications of drains are not identified and addressed promptly, the outcome of the wound healing and, therefore, the patient's comfort and healing time can be significantly impacted.

Timing of drain removal is essential, as premature removal of the drain will be counterproductive unless complications have been encountered. Drains should not be left in situ for an excessive length of time. Drains are usually left in place for 24–48 hours but longer if drainage persists [3]. Active drains allow for a more precise assessment of drainage reduction. In comparison, passive drains rely on a subjective visual assessment of drainage reduction and improved exudate appearance. When the drain is removed, the skin suture is cut and the drain is pulled out swiftly [2]. It is important to pull the drain out in the correct direction, for example, with gravity, to avoid pulling the most contaminated end of the drain back through the wound.

Skin Grafts

Types of Skin Graft

A skin graft is the term used when a portion of skin is detached and relocated from one site to another. The aim is to significantly reduce the skin deficit, which should hasten wound healing [3]. Grafting is useful for distal limb wounds in horses when healing is delayed due to reduced blood supply and poor wound contraction [3].

There are different classifications of skin grafts. These are as follows:

Free Grafts:

1) Pinch Grafting:
   Pinch grafting is a commonly used technique in equine medicine due to its cost-effectiveness and relative ease of execution. It involves the removal of small pieces of skin (usually with a punch tool) from a healthy donor site and transferring them to the recipient wound bed. These

grafts are particularly useful for smaller wounds where a limited amount of skin is required for coverage.

2) Punch Grafts:

Punch grafting involves the use of a punch tool to extract circular sections of skin from the donor site. These grafts can vary in size depending on the diameter of the punch used. They are versatile and can be applied to wounds of different shapes and sizes, offering a tailored approach to equine wound management.

3) Tunnel Grafts:

Tunnel grafting involves creating tunnels beneath the recipient wound bed and inserting strips of donor skin into these tunnels. This technique is advantageous for wounds with irregular or undermined margins, as it allows for more extensive coverage and facilitates the establishment of a new blood supply.

4) Full-Thickness Sheet Grafts:

Full-thickness sheet grafts involve transplanting entire layers of skin from the donor site to the recipient wound bed. These grafts provide comprehensive coverage and are suitable for larger wounds or those requiring structural support. They can be further classified as meshed or unmeshed depending on whether the graft is expanded to cover a larger area by creating perforations.

5) Partial-Thickness Sheet Grafts:

Partial-thickness sheet grafts involve transplanting only the epidermis and a portion of the dermis from the donor site to the recipient wound bed. These grafts promote faster healing and minimise donor site morbidity compared to full-thickness grafts. Similar to full-thickness grafts, they can be meshed or unmeshed depending on the specific requirements of the wound.

6) Pedicle Grafts:

Pedicle grafts remain connected to the donor site by a vascular pedicle, which supplies blood to the graft during the initial stages of healing. However, in equine medicine, the use of pedicle grafts is limited due to the inelastic nature of equine skin, which makes it challenging to mobilise sufficient tissue for grafting without compromising vascular integrity. Additionally, the risk of vascular compromise and graft failure is higher with pedicle grafts in horses compared to other species.

Aftercare for Skin Grafts

Skins grafts should be dressed with a sterile, non-adherent dressing and bandaged to immobilise the graft site. This may sometimes require a Robert Jones Bandage (RJB) or a cast. If nosocomial infections associated with streptococci or pseudomonas are present in the hospital, the bandage should be changed daily for at least five or six days [1]. If nosocomial infections are not a concern, the bandage

should be left in place for four to five days to avoid unnecessary disruption to the delicate vascular attachments to the graft [1]. A bandage should be placed on the limb until the wound has completely epithelised. The patient should be carefully monitored for complications, and regular pain scoring should occur.

12.4 Fracture Repair

Bone Structure and the Response to Injury

Figure 12.5 shows the structure of an equine long bone; for more information on the structure and function of bone, see Chapter 4. However, this figure can be used as a reference point throughout this section.

Bone structure can renew and remodel to repair its surface; this is called bone activation. Bone can regenerate itself rather than healing through the production of scar

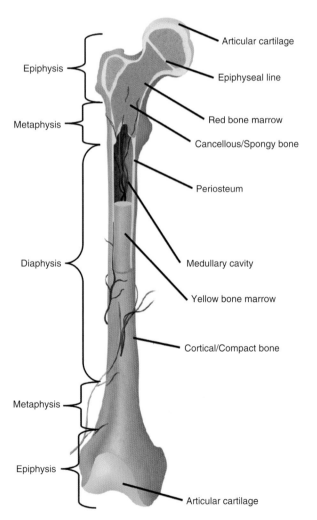

Figure 12.5 The structure of a long bone. *Source:* Rosina Lillywhite.

tissue like a tissue wound [1]. Once the bone structure has healed, it can resume 100% of its former strength again. The three main components of bone include:

- Bone osteogenic cells (osteoblasts, osteoclasts and osteocytes)
- Organic matrix (collagen)
- Minerals

Cortical bones are characterised by their compact structure and higher density levels, compared with cancellous bone, which is less dense and features a more porous composition[33].

Anatomical Orientation of a Fracture

Anatomical terms are often used to describe the location of a fracture:

- Articular: involves a joint
- Diaphyseal: a fracture in the midshaft or diaphysis of the bone
- Metaphyseal: a fracture of the area between the midshaft and at the end of the epiphysis
- Physeal: a fracture through the growth plate of a neonate
- Epiphyseal: a fracture of the epiphysis
- Condylar: a fracture of the epiphysis when the condyles are involved. For example, metacarpal or metatarsal III are the most common condylar fractures in horses [33].

Classifications of Fractures

Many terms can be used to classify fractures in equine patients. Table 12.4 shows the main fracture classifications seen in equine patients.

In the classification of fractures, terms such as "displaced" and "non-displaced" are used. "Displaced" indicates that the ends of the fractured bone are not aligned, potentially leading to improper healing without surgical intervention. Conversely, "non-displaced" describes fractures where the bone ends remain properly aligned, often not necessitating surgical fixation. Fractures can also be categorised as "open" or "closed". A "closed" fracture occurs when there is no breach in the skin, posing a lower risk of infection. On the other hand, an "open" fracture involves a break in the skin, significantly increasing the risk of infection and categorising it as contaminated. Repairing such fractures in horses can be particularly challenging. [33].

Fracture Healing

Direct fracture healing occurs when the fractured edges are so close together there is no callus formation. It is preferable to heal a fracture without callus formation as there is a direct union of the fractured edges; this is usually when the fracture has been fixed in the acute stage by surgical intervention. The surgeon can create a good union of the two edges, and the fracture cannot then be seen radiographically [33].

Indirect fracture healing is the natural process of bone recovery, typically observed when a fracture hasn't undergone surgical intervention. However, in certain instances, complex spiral fractures that have undergone surgical repair can exhibit bone remodelling and substantial callus formation [12].

In the acute phase, there is haemorrhage, clot formation and inflammation. This is to achieve haemostasis and to try to prevent infection. It then proceeds to the repair phase, which aims to recreate the previous function of the anatomy restoring vascular unity and repairing the structure of the bone back to load-bearing strength [12].

Inflammatory Phase

This occurs hours after injury and can last days. During this phase, the formation of blood clots and, in some cases, a haematoma can form. The inflammatory reaction stimulates the release of cytokines, growth factors and prostaglandins which are imperative for healing. Blood clots and haematomas become more organised, which are then infiltrated by fibrovascular tissue, forming a matrix for bone formation and primary callus [12].

Repair Phase

Depending on the fracture, this phase can last days to weeks. A callus forms around both fracture ends. Osteocytes are recruited to form new bone; this can be seen on radiographs from 7 to 14 days. Occasionally, fractures do not appear on radiographs until after 14 days. Because of this, if a fracture is suspected, it should be treated as one until after this time and has negative radiographs. The soft callus is formed into a hard callus over the next coming weeks [33].

Remodelling Phase

This is the longest phase and can continue for months, possibly years. The healed fracture and callus respond to external forces and functional demands during remodelling. Sometimes too much bone remodelling occurs and can be seen externally [12].

Depending on the severity of the fracture, healing can take 6–12 weeks. However, bone remodelling can continue for months and even years. Radiographs are taken at different intervals to assess callus formation and monitor the healing process [12].

Table 12.4 Fracture classification.

Type of fracture	Characteristics	Picture
Open or compound fracture	Any fracture where a bone has penetrated the skin surface	Fracture site; Bone fragment caused open wound; Skin edge
Closed fracture	Any fracture where the bone fragments have remained within the skin surface	Fracture site; Skin edge
Oblique fracture	Oblique fractures occur when the bone is broken at an angle. The fracture is a straight line that is angled across the width of the bone	Skin edge; Fracture site

Transverse fracture

Transverse fractures occur when the bone is broken perpendicular to its length.
The fracture pattern is a straight line that runs in the opposite direction of the bone

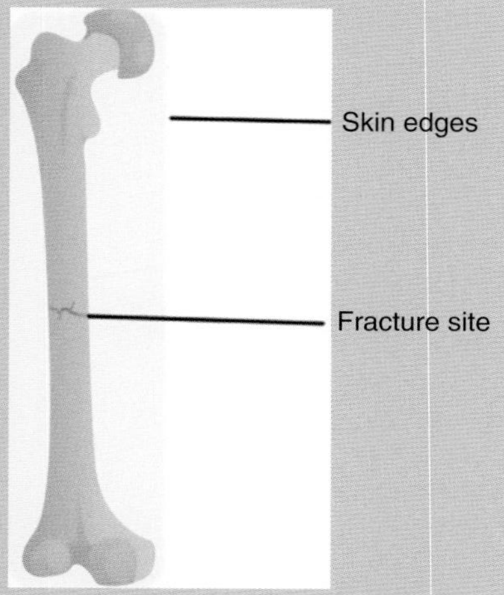

Skin edges

Fracture site

Spiral fracture

Spiral fractures happen when the bones are broken with a twisting motion.
They create a fracture line that wraps around the bone and looks like a corkscrew

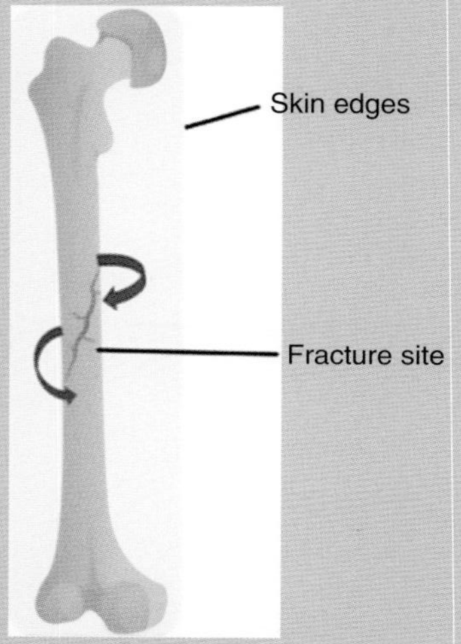

Skin edges

Fracture site

(Continued)

Table 12.4 (Continued)

Type of fracture	Characteristics	Picture
Comminuted/Multiple fractures	Comminuted or multiple fractures result in the bones' discontinuity, crumpling, or 'wrinkled' appearance. There are numerous breaks in one bone, often caused by sudden impact fractures are a type of broken bone. The term comminuted fracture refers to a bone that is broken in at least two places	Skin edges — Fracture site
Greenstick	A greenstick fracture is a partial thickness fracture where only the cortex and periosteum are interrupted on one side of the bone but remain uninterrupted on the other. They occur most often in long bones	Skin edges — Fracture site

Source: Rosina Lillywhite.

Considerations for Fracture Repair

Fracture fixation aims to restore the unity of the bone, so it is functional again while maintaining soft tissue function and essential stay apparatus.

- Reduction: it is essential to reduce the fracture for repair. If the fracture has not been adequately reduced, this will cause pain, callus bone formation and take longer to heal. This can also be completed by open or closed traction. Fracture-reducing forceps are used to align the bone and manipulate it back into position in a closed technique. In an open technique, this can be performed at surgery by visualising the fragments and manipulating them back into position [33].
- Fixation: fragments fixation is gained using the lag screw technique or plate and screw reduction; this reduces the fracture line and forcing clinical union [33].
- Blood supply: blood supply must be preserved as a fracture cannot heal without a blood supply [33].

If the fracture has been repaired or immobilised by conservative management, the primary goals are to [12]:

- Relieve pain.
- Keep the limb immobilised if necessary to prevent fracture displacement or delayed or non-union of the bone.
- Certain fractures cannot be immobilised, and restricted box rest and cross-tying may be necessary for these areas that are unlikely to be fixed surgically.
  - Pelvis
  - Humerus
  - Scapula
  - Sacrum

Surgical Equipment and Implantation

There are many different ways in which a fracture can be fixed; the main fixation techniques in equine surgery include [33]:

- Internal: using pins, plates and screws
- External: using external fixators (not very common in horses) are more often used for jaw fractures
- External coaptation: using splints and casts

Numerous factors can affect fracture healing; these factors include [33]:

- Age: foals heal much quicker than in adult patients because the bone is still growing, and the remodelling process will lead to complete bone healing. Older geriatric patients will take longer to heal due to thinning and weakening of the bones, which can make it harder for fractures to repair.
- Underlying disease: any underlying conditions will factor in on the time it takes to heal the bone; this can be a direct impact from the condition or the medication used to treat the condition.
- Infection/sequestrum: if there is an infection or a sequestrum present, the bone will be unable to heal until the infection is cleared and/or the sequestrum is removed; a sequestrum acts as a foreign body.
- Poor reduction at surgery will affect how the patient heals: more callus formation and bone remodelling will be present on radiographs.
- Good blood supply: adequate blood supply is essential for effective bone repair, requiring a good circulation to facilitate the healing process.
- Temperament: the horse's temperament will factor into bone healing and increased levels of stress may mean the horse is difficult to treat and manage. There is also some research that suggests there may be links to stress causing higher cortisol levels which may impact calcium uptake and, therefore, bone healing.
- Cost to the owner: the cost of fixation surgery may be too high for owners to afford, and elective euthanasia may be opted for.
- Prognosis: if the prognosis indicates a poor outcome, it's important to engage in thorough discussions with the owner, particularly regarding the potential inability of the horse to resume athletic activities, which may impact their interest in further treatment.

Complications of Fracture Healing

Complications that are seen with fracture healing include [12]:

- Non-union: describes the failure of the fracture to heal, often due to inadequate blood supply, excessive movement at the fracture site, or infection. This condition may necessitate additional interventions or surgical stabilisation to promote healing.
- Delayed union: this signifies a healing process that takes longer than expected and is often due to poor blood supply, inadequate immobilisation, or nutritional deficiencies. While the delayed union may eventually progress to complete healing, it may require prolonged monitoring and potentially additional interventions to support the healing process.
- Malunion: this condition occurs when the fracture heals in an abnormal position, impairing the function of the affected area. It is important to address this issue promptly, as it can result from inadequate fracture reduction, improper immobilisation, or complications during the healing process. Malunion in horses may require

corrective surgery to restore proper alignment and function, particularly if it causes pain or functional limitations, which can have significant long-term effects. Where possible, it is preferable for a fracture in the horse to be surgically repaired, as this stabilises the fracture. Casting and immobilising the fracture can be challenging and cause complications such as decubital ulcers and bandage sores from prolonged bandaging and casting. These complications can often become worse than the fracture itself [12].

Initial Treatment and Transportation

For the correct transportation methods for the fractured patient, please refer to Chapter 5. On arrival to the hospital, a suspected fracture should already have been assessed clinically by a referring vet, and appropriate RJB, cast or splint should have been placed either in full or half limb, depending on the location of the fracture. Any bandage, cast or support should immobilise the joint above and below the fracture to minimise movement and reduce the risk of displacing the fracture [8].

On initial examination, the vet examines the patient to assess where the fracture is before imaging. The fracture is manipulated to see if there is any crepitus (the sound or sensation produced when friction occurs between fractured parts of bone or bone and cartilage). A physical examination is carried out, taking the patient's vital signs and a blood sample for haematology may be taken [9]. The patient should be sedated (as directed by the vet) but not too heavily to avoid inducing ataxia. A sedation protocol suitable for GA or standing surgery should be used.

A set of four standard radiographic views depending on the location of the fracture should be taken; lateromedial, dorsopalmar/(plantar), dorsomedial palmar/(plantar) lateral oblique and dorsolateral medial oblique [2]. Depending on the nature of the fracture, initial examinations and radiographs may be taken with the dressing or cast in place. Analgesia should be given (as directed by the vet) if it has not already been, phenylbutazone, flunixin meglumine and morphine are suitable. Once the radiographs have been taken, the results and the prognosis should then be discussed with the owners. If the patient cannot return to athletic function, the owner may be unwilling to try treatment options; however, some horses will have owners who will want to explore all treatment options [34].

A RJB or standing cast bandage may be applied if the patient needs to wait for surgery until they are more stable. Some fractures may be managed conservatively, and a cast, RJB or cast bandage may be applied. There are various types of manufactured temporary splints on the market. These can be useful for the transportation of equine

patients to receive treatment for fractures; some examples of these include [33]:

- The Kimzey splint: This may be a suitable temporary solution before surgery or transportation in some fractures. However, they are unsuitable for spiralling condylar fractures or any fracture above the metatarsus or metacarpus as they only immobilise the distal limb. They are designed to take the weight off the patient's limb by placing the hoof into the metal foot capsule that acts as a dorsal splint, with the patient's toe perpendicular to the ground see Figure 12.6 for a Kimzey splint in situ. Figure 12.7a shows the forces and abnormal vectors generated by a sesamoid fracture. Figure 12.7b shows the neutralising effect of a dorsal splint applied to this fracture type. This is the effect that can be expected from a Kimzey splint, but it can also be achieved with a wooden splint taped to a bandage [12].
- Monkey splint: The concept behind the Monkey splint is identical to that of a dorsal splint and heel wedge. It comprises a concave plastic dorsal splint fixed to a flat bottom and a large, wedged footplate. The foot rests on the wedge, with the angle designed to align the metacarpophalangeal and interphalangeal joints in a neutral position. The splint is then secured to the limb by three broad Velcro straps. The Monkey splint's principal advantage is its ease of application; it can be used on the racetrack with no additional materials required [12]. This splint can allow transport off the track and

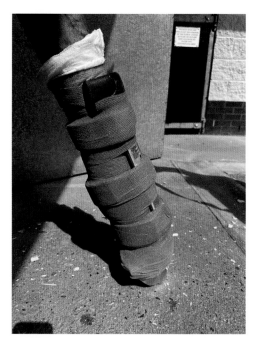

Figure 12.6 Kimzey leg saver splint. *Source:* Elaine Packer.

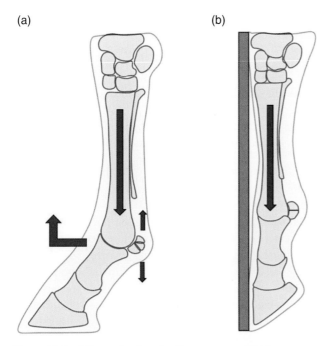

Figure 12.7 Effects of a dorsal splint on a sesamoid fracture. (a) shows the fracture displacement of the sesamoid without a dorsal splint in place. (b) shows the neutralising effect of a dorsal splint on a sesamoid fracture. *Source:* Rosina Lillywhite.

to a hospital with reasonable support of the third metacarpal bone and phalanges in dorsal alignment. It resists mediolateral foot rotation better than a dorsal splint. There are some disadvantages to the Monkey splint; the dorsal portion of the splint terminates in the proximal diaphysis (distal to the metacarpal tuberosity) of the third metacarpal bone, and therefore the construct is inadequate to resist extension of the fetlock joint. Additionally, the footplate produces significant limb lengthening and minimal mediolateral support; because of this, it is not suitable for long-term use [33].

- Compression boots: Commercial compression boots which offers circumferential distal limb support; these were initially marketed as the Farley compression boot (see Figure 17.68b in Chapter 17). They are shaped with a fetlock angle of approximately 135° to support the distal limb in a neutral (weight-bearing) position. They come in two different sizes and consist of an outer, rigid construct of copolymer plastic divided medially and laterally [33]. The dorsal portion has a sole plate to which the palmar portion is attached distally with a hinge. When the limb is placed into the dorsal half of the boot, the palmar half is raised and ski boot-type clips are secured. The boot has a medium-density polyurethane foam lining that provides comfort to the limb. The palmar component of the splint extends for less distance proximally than its dorsal counterpart to permit carpal flexion. The dorsal shell of

the splint should sit against the metacarpal tuberosity of the third metacarpal bone [33]. The original Farley compression boot was designed to fit most Thoroughbred forelimbs; however, they are not well tolerated in the hindlimbs due to the length and angle of the metacarpophalangeal joint. There have been alternatives made with the hindlimb in mind that are better tolerated. The only real disadvantage of compression boots is the expense of purchasing them; however, they are usually long-lasting and robust [33].

Open fractures are more difficult to manage and difficult to transport. They require adequate dressing and padding layers around the open fracture, and using a tourniquet may be necessary depending on the fracture's location. Some fractures, especially non-displaced fractures of the long bones, may take up to 14 days to appear on radiographs [33].

Methods for Treating Fractures

- External coaptation: this is often seen as the conservative approach to fracture repair, and owners sometimes perceive it as the cheaper option. However, this is not necessarily the case [12]. The bandage or cast materials can be expensive to purchase. Not being placed carefully can cause complications such as bandage bind and decubital ulcers, which can often be worse than the original problem. The fracture's location will depend on whether this method can be used, as the fracture needs to have immobilisation of the joint above and below the fracture, which cannot always be achieved. The placement of casts or RJBs requires someone experienced, or this can lead to failure of the treatment plan or complications. Sometimes, a bandage and cast can be used together to create a bandage cast [33]. These have the benefit of padding from the bandage and the support from the cast. These would not be a suitable treatment choice for displaced or comminuted fractures.
- Internal: this uses either the Association for the Study of Internal Fixation (ASIF) or Association for Osteosynthesis (AO) Lag screw fixation, pins, or plates [33].
- External: this is not a common method of fixation in an equine patient due to their size, as it uses external fixators to create a metal frame; these are often not strong enough to take the weight of the horse [33].

Placement of a RJB

A RJB is used to immobilise the limb and stabilise a fracture; this can be used in conservative treatment plans but can also be used to stabilise fractures that are not possible to fix with surgery, such as a fracture to the radius. If a wound is present, an appropriate dressing should be applied, which should be placed with orthopaedic padding. The bandage then consists of multiple layers of padding, such as cotton wool or gamgee, held in place and tightened by a densely knitted conforming bandage that allows for support and compression of the fracture [33]. Each layer is applied more tightly than the previous one, increasing the compression on the fracture. The outer layer of a RJB comprises a layer of a self-co-adhesive or self-adhesive bandage according to practice protocol. The finished RJB of the distal limb for a normal-size horse requires 10–15 rolls of cotton. Its diameter should be at least three times the diameter of the limb and should make the limb cylindrical in appearance. Figure 12.8 shows a patient with a distal limb RJB in place. This type of bandage cannot be used to stabilise a fractured limb for any length of time without adding splints due to compression of the padding layers [12].

On the other hand, if a splint is applied, the padding does not have to be so thick; however, the splint should be applied to a flat surface. Splinted full-limb RJBs can be reinforced further by applying an outer layer of fibreglass casting material, which should not be thick; two layers generally are adequate to provide support without making the bandage heavy and causing the patient to have problems ambulating around in the stable [33]. Figure 12.9

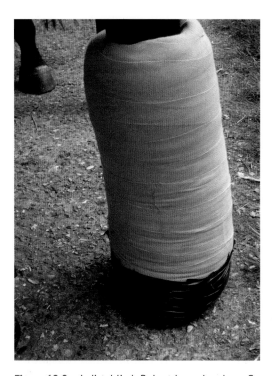

Figure 12.8 A distal limb Robert Jones bandage. *Source:* Rosina Lillywhite.

shows the correct splinting technique for a patient with a radial fracture.

Application of a Cast

Casts are used for a range of conditions as well as fracture repair; the correct application is vital as a cast can cause damage to the soft tissues. Three types of casts can be used in the equine patient; these include [33]:

- Standard casts: these consist of a thin padding layer under the cast tape, allowing the cast type to match the limb confirmation closely.
- Transfixation pin casts: transfixation pin casts are a type of external skeletal fixation used in equine medicine to stabilise fractures. This method involves the insertion of transfixation pins through the skin and into the bone above and below the fracture site. These pins are then connected externally to the casting material to create a rigid construct that reduced the weightbearing forces on the affected limb.
- Bandage casts: these have a large volume of padding material under the cast tape; this reduces the proximity of the cast to the limb, making the bandage cast inappropriate for rigid limb fixation. These are desirable when transitioning from a standard cast to a bandage or if cast sores have made it impossible to keep a standard cast in place.

Historically, casts were made from plaster of Paris (POP); however, this has largely been replaced by resin-impregnated fibreglass tapes. Although POP is largely unused, it does have some advantages over fibreglass tapes, including its low cost and superior conformability; however, there are more disadvantages to its use than advantages, including slow setting times, low strength, permeable to water, radio-opaque in comparison to fibreglass tape. Fibreglass tapes are available in 3.66 m lengths and widths ranging from 2 to 5 in. [33]. Fibreglass cast tapes are activated by submerging them into tepid water; this initiates a transformation of the resin to a rigid material within the fibreglass, which is irreversible. If the cast tape is hard before it has been activated by water, it should not be used as it will not work effectively. The equipment for the placement of a cast will depend on whether it is a bandage cast or a standard cast [33]:

Equipment Required for a Bandage Cast
- Suitable wound dressing
- Orthopaedic padding: This may not be required depending on how thick the bandage is on the limb
- Cotton wool
- Conforming, gauze bandage

(a) (b) (c)

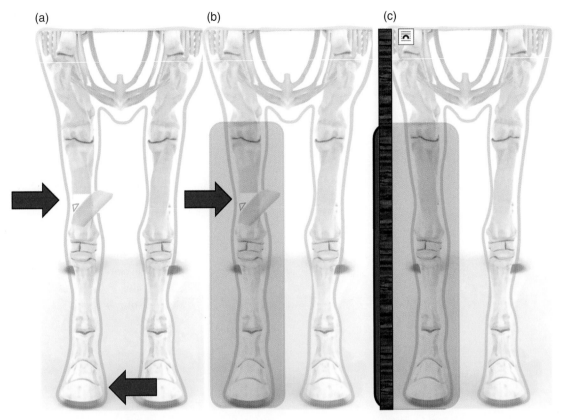

Figure 12.9 Splinting a radial fracture in the horse. Picture (a) shows a fracture of the proximal radius and the lateral and medial forces applied to the unsupported limb; this increases the chance that the distal bone fragment will penetrate the skin, causing a catastrophic displacement. Picture (b) shows immobilisation of the limb using an un-splinted RBJ; without a splint, there is still a lateral force and catastrophic medial displacement is still possible. Picture (c) shows a RBJ with a lateral splint extending to the shoulder; this combination eliminates the lateral force and minimises the chance of medial displacement of the fracture. Using this type of splint allows the patient to load the fractured limb [12]. If using a splint, it must be placed in the correct place depending on the fracture location. Table 12.5 displays the placement of splints for a range of fracture locations. *Source:* Rosina Lillywhite.

- Self-adhesive bandage material
- Cast material of the appropriate width
- Bucket with water
- Adhesive bandage material
- Cast saw: a bandage cast can sometimes be used as a removable cast allowing the dressing underneath to be changed and the cast to be reapplied over the top and taped together with a non-elastic bandage [33]

Equipment Required for a Standard Cast
- Tubigrip
- Dressing layer
- White tape
- Orthopaedic padding
- Scissors
- Cast material
- Hapla cast felt (helps to prevent cast sores)
- Vetlite cast to reinforce the bottom of the cast material (otherwise, the horse can wear through the bottom of

the cast). It is white and is thermoplastic mesh which is ventilated and very strong
- Tepid water for cast material
- Boiling water for the Vetlite cast layer
- Double gloves

After placement of the dressing, the cast can then be placed. Preparation before starting the casting is vital to ensure the process is smooth [33]:

- Ensure that there is a bucket with tepid water (20–25 °C) available; if Vetlite is being used, then a full kettle is required at the end of the process.
- Ensure that the correct width of cast tape is available and that it does not have any firm areas.
- Casting is made more efficient with one person applying the cast tape and another submerging the cast tape.
- All personnel that are handling the cast material should wear gloves as this will prevent cast material from adhering to the person's hands.

Table 12.5 Correct placement of splints for the equine patient.

Fracture type	Includes	Goal	Splinting technique
Distal forelimb fractures	Metacarpus, phalanges and sesamoids	• Achieve good alignment and soft tissue protection • The splint should include the foot and extend to the proximal metacarpus • There are commercially available splints	• Apply a medium-sized bandage from the coronary band to the proximal metacarpus • Place a wooden plank or other ridged material against the dorsal aspect of the limb and secure it in place with a non-elastic bandage or cast tape • The entire foot should be included in the splint to avoid further damage
Mid-forelimb fractures	Metacarpus, carpus and distal radius	• Achieve good alignment and prevent the lower limb from moving in all four directions • This is best achieved by using two splints positioned at right angles – a caudal splint placed from the ground to the top of the olecranon and a lateral splint from the floor to the elbow	• Apply a full limb RJB • Apply the caudal splint from the ground to the point of the elbow and secure it with a non-elastic bandage • Place the lateral splint extending from the ground to the elbow joint and secure it in place with non-elastic tape • The entire foot should be included in the bandage • Ensure that the splints are flat to the surface and cover the whole bandage and splints in a layer of non-elastic bandage
Upper forelimb fractures	Fractures above the carpus	• Achieve good alignment and prevent movement in all directions to prevent laceration to the medial aspect of the limb from sharp bone edges • Two splints should be applied at right angles – a caudal splint from the ground to the olecranon and a lateral splint from the floor to above the shoulder to prevent lateral movement of the limb	• Apply a full limb RJB • Place the caudal splint from the ground to the point of the elbow, securing it with non-elastic tape • Place the lateral splint from the ground to above the shoulder joint and secure it in place with non-elastic tape • The top of the splint can be secured with an elastic bandage in a figure of eight, including the neck, chest, through forelimbs and over the withers • Ensure that the splints are flat to the surface and cover the whole bandage and splints in a layer of non-elastic bandage
Proximal forelimb fractures	Fractures to the elbow and shoulder	• The goal is to fix the carpus, as this will mean the horse loses its triceps function • This is achieved by using one splint that extends from the ground to the elbow on the caudal aspect of the limb	• Place a medium-thickness bandage to the full forelimb • The caudal splint is then placed flat to the bandage and secured with a non-elastic bandage
Distal hindlimb fracture	Metatarsus, phalanges and sesamoids	• Achieve good alignment and soft tissue protection • The splint should include the foot and extend to the proximal metatarsus • There are commercially available splints	• Apply a medium-sized bandage from the coronary band to the proximal metatarsus • Place a wooden plank or other ridged material on the plantar aspect of the limb and secure it in place with a non-elastic bandage • The entire foot should be included in the splint to avoid further damage
Mid-hindlimb fractures	Metatarsus and tarsus	• The aim is to prevent movement in all four directions • This is accomplished by using two splints placed at right angles – the first placed on the caudal aspect of the limb from the ground to the highest point of the tarsus. The second is placed on the lateral aspect of the limb from the floor to the tarsus • For fractures involving the tarsal bones, the lateral splint should bend with the shape of the leg and extend higher	• Apply a full limb RJB from the coronary band to the stifle • Place the caudal splint extending from the ground to the highest point of the tarsus secure in place with a non-elastic bandage • Place the lateral splint extending from the ground to the highest point of the tarsus secure in place with a non-elastic bandage • The entire foot should be included in the splint
Proximal hindlimb fractures	Tarsus, tibia, fibula and stifle	• Immobilisation of these fractures prevents the fracture ends from damaging the surrounding tissues and penetrating the skin every time the limb is flexed or extended • The aim of alignment allows for the movement of the limb as well as the prevention of fracture collapse • A lateral splint should extend from the ground to the hip	• Apply a full limb RJB from the coronary band to the stifle • Place a lateral splint extending from the floor to the hip flat against the bandage to the hip. Secure in place with a non-elastic bandage • Secure the upper portion of the splint in place with an elastic bandage placed over the hip, through the legs, under the flank and over the lumber spine in a figure of eight • The entire foot needs to be incorporated into the splint

Source: Rosina Lillywhite.

- It may be advisable to put a drape or cover over the floor to protect the floor from cast material drips, which may be difficult to remove once dry.
- Once the person applying the cast is ready, the assistant can unwrap the first cast tape and submerge it into the tepid bucket of water.
- During immersion, the cast tape should be squeezed several times to ensure that the water activates the whole roll of cast tape.
- Whether excess water should be squeezed from the tape is specific to each manufacturer, and instructions are available on the package insert. As a rule, increasing water temperature and the number of squeezes while the roll is immersed and after the roll is removed from the water will decrease the setting time, as will an increase in the ambient temperature. A higher water temperature will also increase the exothermic reaction during cast curing – this may be seen as a negative as it will not allow for the cast to be placed entirely before it goes off.
- The cast tape should be placed immediately after being submerged and then wrapped around the limb, overlapping the cast material by half on each turn – it is important to remember that cast material cannot be made looser or tighter once in place, so the desired tension needs to be applied from the beginning.
- When the person who is applying the cast is halfway through a roll, the person assisting should be opening the next roll and submerge it in preparation; once a cast is started, it must be completed efficiently to prevent cast failure.
- Once the desired thickness is achieved, the cast should start to cure, which will cause the outside to heat up.
- If the cast goes under the foot, then there needs to be a reinforced toe and foot. This is achieved using Vetlite, a ventilated white thermoplastic mesh for splinting and casting. It is lightweight and very strong. When heated in hot water, it becomes a soft, malleable material that can be shaped into any configuration and hardens as it cools. If using this product, it needs to go into freshly boiled water; it is advisable to use tongs or another instrument to squeeze the material to ensure the water has softened the whole roll and avoid scalding the person handling it.
- Once the material becomes soft and malleable, it can be removed from the hot water and given to the person applying the cast. This material unwraps with the help of a plastic separator, which needs to be removed once unwrapped fully.
- A material known as Demotec 90 can be used instead of or as well as Vetlite. The aim is to improve the durability of the cast around the foot. Demotec 90 is a quick-setting resin supplied as a powder and liquid that forms a paste when mixed together (in a beaker provided with a spatula). The paste is then used on the bottom of the cast; it is essential to note that a texture needs to be added to this product to prevent the horse from slipping. This can be lines created by the spatula before the product sets.
- The last step of the process is to apply a self-adhesive bandage to the top of the cast to prevent any bedding material from going down the top of the cast, causing irritation and possible infection.

When a cast has been placed, it must be correctly monitored to ensure that complications arising from its placement are corrected promptly, ensuring no impact on the patient's recovery. Checks should include:

- At least once per day:
- Remove the self-adhesive bandage and ensure there are no signs of rubbing at the top of the cast, and check that it is not too tight on the dorsal, palmar/plantar aspects.
- At least twice per day:
- Assess temperature, respiration rate and heart rate (TPR) readings to help ensure early signs of pain or infection are identified.
- Check the underside of the cast to ensure that there is no damage to the toe/footplate; this could make the leg unstable and lead to bacteria infiltration.
- Feel the outside of the cast for 'hot spots' or areas of differing temperatures; this may indicate the development of a complication.
- Check that there is no damage to the visible areas of the cast and that there are no unpleasant odours coming from the cast.
- Carry out a pain assessment on the patient to ensure that there is no decrease in comfort level. See Chapter 14 for further information regarding pain scoring.

Surgical Equipment and Implantation

In horses, the simplest method of fracture repair is the lag screw fixation technique, which reduces and compresses the fracture site and stabilises it [33]. The fracture is reduced with bone-holding forceps (not always necessary), a gliding hole is drilled into the fragment (the exact width of the screw), and then the far cortex is drilled with a drill bit the same size as the core of the screw. The far cortex is tapped (unless a self-tapping screw is used), but the near cortex is not. When the screw is placed into the hole, it does not grip the fragment, just the far cortex. This technique compresses the fragment into place. The most common screw size used in equine surgery is 4.5 mm [33].

ASIF/AO systems

The term ASIF refers to internal fixation devices developed by the Association for the Study of Internal Fixation. In North America, these devices are classified under a system that is both patented and copyrighted by the association. In Europe, the equivalent classification is the AO system, developed by the Association for Osteosynthesis. Both associations have developed fracture fixation devices with four fundamental principles in mind; these are [33]:

- Restoration of anatomy
- Stable fracture fixation
- Preservation of blood supply
- Early mobilisation of the limb and patient

Instrumentation

As an RVN, it is crucial to understand the different instruments and how they function to aid in fracture fixation. Fracture fixation can be a stressful surgery, and familiarity with the equipment and how it is used is essential in ensuring the procedure runs smoothly [12].

Drills

The drill is an essential part of any fracture repair, which can be powered by either air or battery. Until recent years, the air-powered drill was always the preferred drill type as it had higher power and easier to handle. However, with

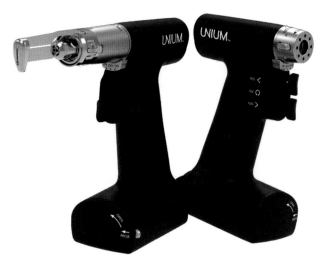

Figure 12.10 Battery-powered orthopaedic drill source. *Source:* From DePuy Synthes part of Johnson & Johnson.

higher-powered battery drills (Figure 12.10) and lighter batteries becoming available, most large practices will have battery-powered drills [1]. If battery drills are used, it is essential to remember that the batteries will need periodic charging to prevent them from becoming damaged and flat. It is typically good practice to have a backup drill if there is an issue mid-surgery that would mean the fracture repair could not be finished. Table 12.6 shows the advantages and disadvantages of both types of drills commonly used in equine practice. Some practices that do minor repairs,

Table 12.6 Advantages and disadvantages of orthopaedic drills.

	Advantages	Disadvantages
Battery	No airline required	Heavier use can cause user fatigue
	Batteries provide great freedom of movement	Batteries will require replacement and are expensive
	A double trigger feature allows for a change of direction when screwing and/or drilling with the simple pressure of a finger	Not all have autoclavable batteries
	More recent feature additions in battery surgical systems	It may require multiple batteries to ensure that battery failure does not impact surgery
		May have less power
Air powered	A reliable source of high power, with no requirement to replace batteries	Slightly more repairs than electric or battery if the air supply is dirty or humid
	High powered	Higher risk for fluid invasion that may cause the handpiece to get stuck
	Lighter and more balanced	The gas/air supply hose restricts movement as compared to a battery device
	The whole product is autoclavable	
	They are cheaper to repair, compared to battery and electric options	

Source: Rosina Lillywhite.

such as jaw wires, may have a standard electric drill designed for DIY; these are readily available and suitable for minor procedures; however, they pose an issue when cleaning and sterilising them [12].

Whichever drill is used in practice, the RVN must understand how it should be cleaned, maintained and sterilised to prevent damage during this process. The use of SOPs developed from the manufacturer's guidelines can aid with this.

Drill Bits

When using drill bits, the right drill bit is essential for the correct drill head being used. The AO (Figure 12.11) and ASIF drill bits require a quick coupling head (also known as a chuck), whereas rounded drill bits require a Jacobs chuck [33]. When placing lag screws, two sizes of double-fluted drill bits (the flute is the groove cut into the drill bit in a double-fluted drill bit; there are two cut opposite to each other, making it much stronger) are used for each size of screw to be inserted in lag fashion. There are larger sizes of 3.5, 4.5 and 5.5 mm bits used to prepare the glide hole for the respective sized screws. There are then the smaller sizes that represent the size of the core of the screw; these are 2.5, 3.2 and 4.0 mm bits. The size of each bit is marked on the quick coupler or the shaft. When using locking screws, the drill bit required is 4.3 mm and the screw is typically 5 mm in equine surgery [12].

Double Drill Guide

The double drill guide (Figure 12.12) is used with the drill bits and taps to apply the lag technique. A drill guide is essential to prevent further damage to the soft tissue from the instruments as they are used; it also helps to prevent the drill bit from bending during use. The purpose of it being double-ended means that one end supports the larger glide hole drill bit while the other supports the smaller lag hole. The 3.5, 4.5 and 5.5 mm drill guides are also used as the respective tap guides [12].

Universal Drill Guide

This type of drill guide is used for plate application and contains a 3.5, 4.5 or 5.5 mm drill sleeve on one end and a spring-loaded 2.5, 3.2 or 4.0 mm drill sleeve on the other. By applying pressure to the spring-loaded portion, the hole

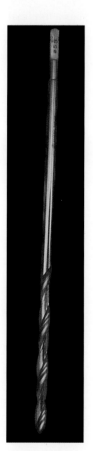

Figure 12.11 AO drill bit. *Source:* Rosina Lillywhite.

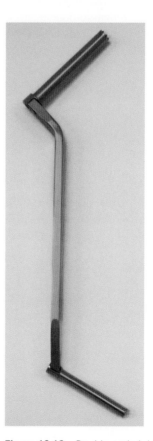

Figure 12.12 Double-ended drill guide. *Source:* Rosina Lillywhite.

is drilled in a neutral position, whereas when no force is used and the drill guide is positioned at the far end of the plate hole, the hole is drilled in a load position across the underlying bone [33].

Drill Guides for Plate Application

A 3.2 mm double-ended drill guide for the 4.5 mm dynamic compression plates (DCP) and limited contact dynamic compression plates (LC-DCP) with a 4.0 mm diameter hole at the other end. One end of the guide has a neutral drill barrel (green), which allows the drilling of a central hole through the oval plate hole, and the other end has an offset barrel (yellow), which results in a 1 mm offset hole to provide compression as the screws are tightened within the plate [33].

Drill Guides for Locking-head Screws

These drill guides are threaded perpendicularly into the plate hole (Figure 12.13). Care has to be taken to apply the drill guide to the plate precisely perpendicularly in all planes. It is best to initially turn the drill guide backwards when it makes contact with the plate to ensure it is lined up correctly; it can then be rotated clockwise to screw it into the plate appropriately [12]. It is prudent to double-check the orientation of the drill guide relative to the plate before

drilling is initiated. It is possible to place the drill guide cross-threaded into the plate, which locks it to the plate at an angle and allows the drilling of an inappropriately oriented hole for the locking-head screw. If these are placed incorrectly, the result could be a poorly seated screw and a plate with reduced performance [33].

Countersink

The countersink (Figure 12.14) is used to prepare a conical indentation in the cortical surface of the bone, to accept the curved underside of the screw head. It is 4.5 mm diameter tip fits into the glide hole. The countersink depression reduces the load at the screw head–shaft junction. A solitary contact point which develops when a screw is inserted obliquely or across a slanted surface, or a contact ring if the screw is inserted perpendicularly relative to the bone surface, is transformed into a broad contact area by the countersink depression [33]. The depression also reduces screw head protrusion on the bone surface, which is especially desirable with the 4.5 and 5.5 mm screws. Figure 12.15 shows the difference in a screw placed with and without a countersink. Not only is the screw placed without the countersink protruding has a minimal contact point in comparison to the one that has used a countersink [33].

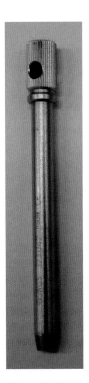

Figure 12.13 Drill guide for a locking plate. *Source:* Rosina Lillywhite.

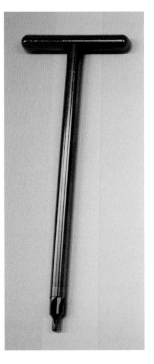

Figure 12.14 Countersink. *Source:* Rosina Lillywhite.

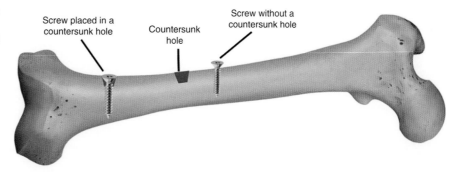

Figure 12.15 The difference between using and not using a countersink during screw placement. *Source:* Rosina Lillywhite.

Screw placed in a countersunk hole

Countersunk hole

Screw without a countersunk hole

Depth Gauge

The depth gauge (Figure 12.16) allows exact determination of the length of the prepared hole and therefore dictates the screw length. This device measures the screw length, including the screw head, and contains a conically shaped nose, which fits into the countersink depression in bone or the topside of the slot in the plate [12]. Therefore, the countersink hole, if one is being used, must be prepared before the depth gauge is used. The long thin probe of the depth gauge is inserted into the hole, and the opposite bone surface is engaged by the small hook on the probe end, followed by a direct measurement of screw length from the instrument's barrel. Direct measurement, including the plate's thickness, is obtained identically when the depth gauge is applied through the slot in the plate. When cleaning a depth gauge, it is essential to remember that it completely disassembles, allowing the centre lumen to be thoroughly cleaned and preventing debris from building up [12].

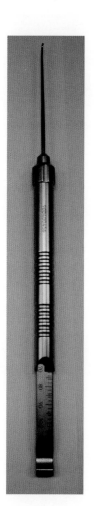

Figure 12.16 Depth gauge. *Source:* Rosina Lillywhite.

T-handle and Tap

The T-handle is used for manual tapping of the hole; as the name suggests, the handle is a T-shape with a quick-coupling end that the tap fits into, allowing the user to use it effectively. Taps (Figure 12.17) come in various sizes, corresponding to the drilled hole, and are used to precisely cut screw threads within the hole. When the lag technique is applied, threads are not cut in the over-drilled glide hole, which has the same diameter as the tap. The tap is inserted through the respective drill guide/tap sleeve to protect the soft tissues from additional trauma by the sharp cutting edges of the tap. The tap has three flutes along the cutting portion to accept bone debris formed during the cutting action. It is important to note that most screws now used in equine surgery are known as self-tapping; therefore, the use of a tap is not required [12].

Torque-limiting Devices

Because the locking-head screws secure into the threaded section of the combi holes within the locking compression plates (LCPs) rather than directly into the bone, using torque-limiting devices is essential, just as it is with regular screws. A torque-limiting device ensures that the correct amount of torque is applied to the screw, preventing over-tightening or under-tightening, which can compromise the stability and integrity of the fixation. Employing a torque-limiting attachment for the drill, or using

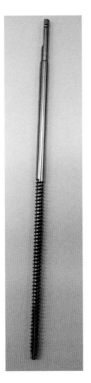

Figure 12.17 Tap. *Source:* Rosina Lillywhite.

screwdrivers equipped with torque control, ensures that the locking-head screws are fully inserted with the correct tension within the plate, thereby optimising the fixation and promoting proper healing [12].

Screwdriver

This can either be an attachment for the drill or a handheld, and a screwdriver with the correct coupling must be used; the most common screw heads in equine surgery are hexagonal and star drive heads, but Philips heads can also be used [12].

Figure 12.18 shows a large animal fragment system.

Screws

There are many different screw types available depending on the desired result, but all screws have the same structure, which includes [35]:

- Head: prevents sinking of the screw into the bone. Hemispherical in shape to increase the surface area for load transfer and to allow angulated insertion. Enables attachment of screwdriver, which may be star, hexagonal or Philips.
- Shaft: the length of the usable screw between the bottom of the head and the tip of the screw.
- Core: solid section from which the threads project outwards. The size of the core determines the strength of the screw and its fatigue resistance. The size of the drill bit used is equal to the core diameter.
- Thread: thread diameter is the maximum diameter of threads. Thread depth is half of the difference between thread diameter and core diameter. The thread depth determines the amount of contact with the bones, which determines the resistance to pull out. The size of the tap is equal to the thread diameter.

Figure 12.19 shows the location of these areas on the screw; knowing the type of screw and the different diameters (Ø) of these is essential when assisting with a fracture repair.

Screws can be manufactured from different materials, including [35]:

- Titanium
- Stainless steel
- Bioabsorbable

In equine surgery, stainless steel is still the most commonly used material for implants to be manufactured from. There is very little evidence to suggest that the increase in the cost of titanium implants would have enough of a

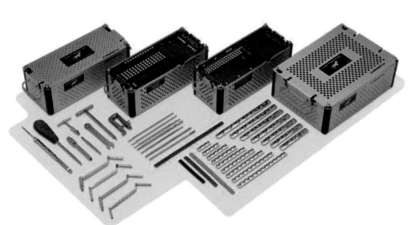

Figure 12.18 Large fragment system. *Source:* From DePuy Synthes part of Johnson & Johnson.

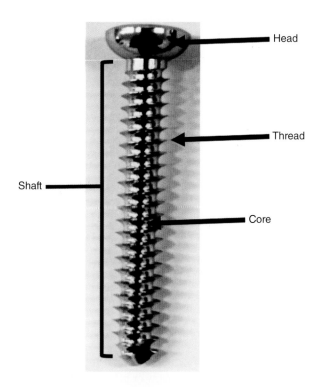

Figure 12.19 Labelled screw structure. *Source:* Rosina Lillywhite.

positive effect to justify the cost difference. Some evidence suggests that there may be a slight increase in the chance of implant failure with stainless steel; however, many suggest that they are of equal biomechanical properties. The use of bioabsorbable screws, while not widely used, has been used in some surgical repairs of incomplete unicortical condylar fractures of the metacarpal III (MCIII) in horses. While not common, this may reduce complications associated with implants as these are designed to absorb; however, this could also cause problems if absorption occurs before stabilisation [33].

Screws can be broken down into three main categories common to equine surgery; these are [33]:

- Cortical or cortex
- Cancellous
- Locking

Cannulated screws and headless screws are available; however, they are beyond the scope of this book as they are not commonplace in equine surgery.

Cortical or Cortex Screws

Cortical screws are used on cortical bone. They have a smaller diameter threading than cancellous screws, do not contain any regions of a bare shaft, and are the most widely

used screw type in equine fracture treatment. They vary in length depending on the size and manufacturer, but they all increase in length in 2 mm increments and can range from 10 to 100 mm in length [33].

Locking Screws

The locking screws have an increased core diameter with a finer diameter thread and pitch, creating a threaded bolt appearance and a greater strength ratio than cortical screws. The locking-head screw tips are either equipped with a self-tapping portion or, as occasionally used in human surgery, a self-drilling, self-tapping tip. The latter type of screw is only used as a unicortical screw, because protrusion of the sharp self-cutting tip into the surrounding soft tissues would result in significant damage and potential loss of function [33]. The 5.0 mm locking-head screw is preferred in equine fracture management. It is possible to use the smaller 4.0 mm locking-head screw in the same plate; however, these screws are weaker than the 5.0 mm screws and are rarely added to the fixation [33].

Cancellous Screws

These are designed for metaphyseal bone and are not commonly used in equine fracture repairs, thought to reduce tissue irritation at the base of the screw head. They are only used in the cancellous bone as the wider diameter thread helps to grip the spongier cancellous bone [35]. Cancellous screws have a wider thread height (1.45 mm) compared to cortex screws and a different pitch (angle of the threads relative to the long axis of the screw). These 6.5 mm diameter screws are available as partially threaded screws with either 16 or 32 mm of thread length or as fully threaded screws. 6.5 mm screws are available with lengths varying from 20 to 100 mm in 5 mm increments for fully threaded screws and 30–100 mm for 16 mm partially threaded screws. The 32 mm partially threaded cancellous screw is available in 45–100 mm lengths [33].

Figure 12.20 shows from left to right cortical, locking and cancellous screws.

Screws can also be allocated into self-tapping and non-self-tapping categories. Self-tapping screws create their thread path by cutting into the bone. Non-self-tapping screws require the use of a tap to create a thread path. Figure 12.21 shows the end of the screw tip; showing the screw on the left has a cutting notch in it, whereas the screw on the right has a rounded end [33].

Table 12.7 shows all the key characteristics of a screw that may be required when assisting in surgery or ordering replacements.

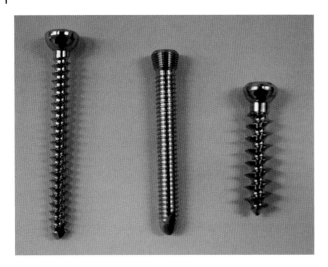

Figure 12.20 Types of screws: left, cortical, middle, locking and right, cancellous screws. *Source:* Rosina Lillywhite.

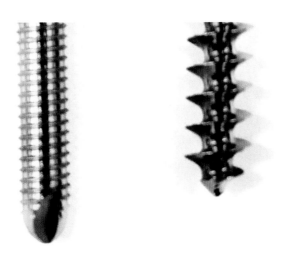

Figure 12.21 Screw ends: left, self-tapping tip; right, non-self-tapping tip. *Source:* Rosina Lillywhite.

Plates

There are many different plates used in veterinary surgery; however, the three main plates used in equine surgery are [33]:

- Dynamic compression plates (DCP)
- Limited contact dynamic compression plates (LC-DCP)
- Locking compression plates (LCP)

It is beyond the scope of this book to discuss other types of plates available as they are not commonplace in equine surgery.

Dynamic Compression Plates (DPCs)

The DCP is considered the basic plate in equine fracture treatment and is slowly becoming obsolete with the increased use of the LC-DCP or LCP systems. DCPs apply pressure to the two bone fragments so they can be trans-fixed [33]. They come in various sizes and are characterised by their width, this being narrow or broad and the number of holes, for example, a 9-hole narrow DCP plate. The plate has oval holes and can be used as a compression plate, neutralisation or buttress plate. Each technique is used for different fracture types [12].

- Compression plate: simple transverse fractures
- Neutralisation plate: oblique, spiral and comminuted fractures
- Buttress plate: stabilises a fracture site or is used as a bridge to stabilise a fracture that is not repairable. Bone grafts filled with cancellous bone are placed at the fracture to restore instability.

Table 12.7 Common orthopaedic screws and a summary of data.

Screw type	Size (mm)	Glide hole Ø	Thread hole Ø	Tap Ø	Core Ø	Head type
Cortical	3.5	3.5	2.5	3.5	2.4	⬣
	4.5	4.5	3.2	4.5	3.1	⬣
	5.5	5.5	4	5.5	4	⬣
Locking	4.0	Not used for lag fixation	3.2	Cannot buy non-self-tapping	3.4	★
	5.0	Not used for lag fixation	4.3	Cannot buy non-self-tapping	4.4	★
Cancellous	6.5	4.5	3.2	6.5	3	⬣

Source: Rosina Lillywhite.

Limited Contact Dynamic Compression Plate (LC-DCPs)

In humans and small animals, the application of DCPs has resulted in avascularity beneath the plate, which occasionally culminated in pathologic fracture following implant removal. The LC-DCP contains undercuts on the surface that contacts the bone, reducing the contact area between bone and plate, thereby improving bone vascularity maintenance [33]. A disadvantage of the LC-DCP in equine fracture repair has been soft tissue closure over the implants, which is complicated by the slightly wider plate stock in the LC-DCP, particularly when double plating. The top side of the LC-DCP is machined with oval holes of the dynamic compression unit (DCU) design. The DCU design contains an incline on either end of each hole, allowing compression to be applied on either side and, therefore, in either direction [33]. There is no designated middle of the plate, and the holes are arranged evenly along the entire length of the plate, in a staggered line for the broad plate and in a straight line for the narrow plate. When a screw is applied and tightened in load position through the thread hole, the screw head glides downward along the plate hole's incline towards the hole's centre. Therefore a fracture may be located anywhere along the plate and still be compressed by dynamic compression using adjacent screw holes [33].

Locking Compression Plates (LCPs)

The LCP (Figure 12.22) is a relatively new technique that allows locking screws and conventional screws in combination screw holes. Conventional screws are used if angulation is needed from the screw. These are placed into the hole without the threads. A locking plate does not have to precisely contact the underlying bone in all areas [33]. When the locking screws are tightened, they lock into the threaded screws of the plate. Stabilising parts of the bone without pulling the bone to the plate. Locking plate/screw systems do not disrupt the underlying cortical bone perfusion as much as conventional plates, which compress the plate to cortical bone. Locking plate/screw systems have been shown in human studies to provide more stable fixation than non-locking plate/screw fixations [33].

Figure 12.23 shows the narrow dynamic compression plate, broad dynamic compression plate and locking compression plate from left to right.

External Fixation

External fixation is sometimes required in horses, but this is relatively uncommon. External skeletal fixation (ESF) stabilises the fracture using pins inserted through a small stab incision in the skin and inserted into the bone via a Jacobs

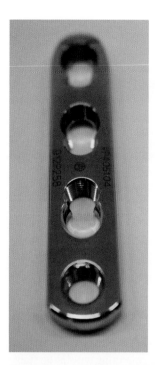

Figure 12.22 Locking compression plate. *Source:* Rosina Lillywhite.

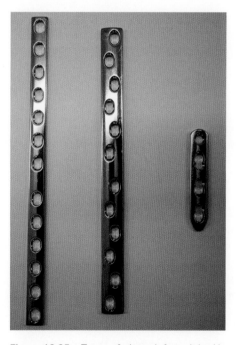

Figure 12.23 Types of plates left to right: Narrow dynamic compression plate, broad dynamic compression plate and a locking compression plate. *Source:* Rosina Lillywhite.

chuck or a power drill with Jacob's chuck attachment. If used on a limb, they are inserted through both cortical surfaces and fixed on the outside of the limb with bars, clamps and acrylic resin. The type of frame depends on the fracture

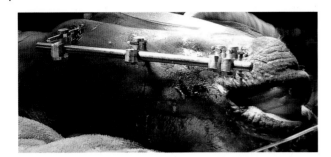

Figure 12.24 External fixator on a mandible. *Source:* Rosina Lillywhite.

itself. A simple frame would include three pins into a bar with clamps [33]. Due to the horse's size and weight, it is difficult to restrict them like a small animal, which, when used on the equine limb, can end in implant failure. They can be used more successfully in mandible fractures, especially if both mandibles are affected; however, care must be taken with the aftercare as the horse may cause further damage if the frame is caught on anything within the stable environment [12]. These types of devices, when used, tend to irritate the skin where the pins protrude, causing premature pin loosening and risk of infection. Application is complex and requires experience. Pins sizes range from 1.1 to 4 mm. Pins have a trocar end, and the opposite end is threaded. Figure 12.24 shows the placement of an external fixator on the mandible of a foal.

Acrylic Pin External Fixator (APEF) System

The APEF system is a slightly different method of external fixation with the same principles. Pins are inserted into the bone – which can be Steinman pins cut down to the appropriate size [33]. Corrugated tubing is placed around the pins that are protruding from the skin. This is then filled with polymethylmethacrylate, a type of bone cement. The ends of the corrugated tubing are blocked, filled with bone cement and supported until this hardens. A chemical process between the liquid and powder activates the bone cement. This generates heat, and the skin should be protected. Heat can also be conducted down the pins and cause necrosis of the bone. Soaked sterile saline swabs can be used for the skin and saline from a syringe or giving set lavaged gently onto the pins to reduce the heat [12].

Other Methods of Fracture Fixation

Intramedullary Pins
Intramedullary pins are also called Steinman pins (Figure 12.25), which are used for many different procedures. Initially, they were used for internal fixation. They come in a

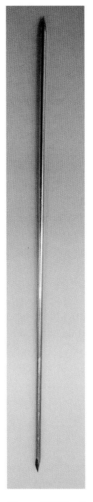

Figure 12.25 Steinmann pin. *Source:* Rosina Lillywhite.

range of widths from 1.6–8.0 m in diameter. They are placed into the medulla (central shaft of the bone) to secure a fracture and have a sharp end at both ends [33]. A power drill or a Jacobs chuck are used to insert them. This type of fracture fixation is not commonly used in equine practice due to the weight of the horse and the likelihood of implant failure.

Kirschner Wire
Also known as K-wires, these stiff, straight wires are sometimes necessary for repairing broken bones. They can be used with or without cannulated screws, which have a hollow central core allowing for wire placement. However, cannulated screws are not commonly used in equine patients due to the high risk of bending. When used, the wire can be threaded down the screw shaft and into the bone, providing additional stability during the healing process [12]. Figure 12.26 shows Kirschner wire and a Jacobs's chuck.

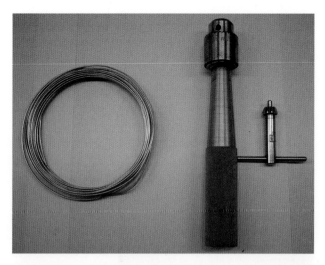

Figure 12.26 Kirshner wire and a Jacobs's chuck. *Source:* Rosina Lillywhite.

Broken Screw Extractor Sets

These are not used often, but they are helpful when needed. The extractor kit has a cannulated end that is placed over the top of the screw and clamps around the screw shaft for removal [33]. The set usually includes power screwdriver inserts and conical extractor sets – for stripped screw heads. Extraction bolts – for broken screws, drill or tap shafts. Hollow reamer tubes attach the centring pin and shaft to expose a broken portion of the screw and allow the extraction bolt to extract the screw. A T-handle with quick coupling is used for these attachments. Extraction pilers may also be in some extraction kits [12].

Placement of Lag Screws

- Reduce fracture with reduction forceps if necessary or manually.
- Drill the near cortex using a drill bit and a drill guide. The drill bit will need to be the same size as the cortical screw intended for use (for example 4.5 mm cortical screw will use a 4.5 mm drill bit).
- The far cortex is drilled using a 3.2 mm drill bit. This drill bit has the same diameter, which is similar to the inner part of the screw.
- A countersink is used to create a platform in the near cortex. If insufficient countersinking is carried out, it causes an eccentric loading and lessens the degree of compression. Too much countersinking can remove all the cortical bone around the circumference of the head of the bone. Once the screw is tightened, the screw can then enter the medullary canal and offers no resistance to the head of the screw.
- A depth gauge is then used to determine screw length.
- Tap the far cortex of the bone with a 4.5 mm tap.

- Insert a screw of the appropriate length measured. The near cortex of the screw should be observed when tightening to ensure cracking does not occur from over-tightening [36].

Standard Plate Technique in a Neutral Position

- First anatomical reduction – manual reduction or reduction forceps.
- Plate benders are used to shape the plate to fit the bone.
- Position the plate on the bone and primarily fix it.
- Select a drill guide position, Neutral – press the spring – loaded against the bone in the DC part of the LCP hole. The inner sleeve retracts. The rounded end of the outer sleeve slides along the hole angle into a neutral position. This allows neutral predrilling.
- Drill screw hole (3.2 mm for a large fragment set).
- Determine the screw length using a depth gauge of 4.5 mm measuring up to 110 mm.
- Tap the thread – if using self-tapping screws, then there is no need for this step.
- Insert a cortical screw using the screwdriver, and manually insert and tighten a standard screw with the measured length.
- The holes in LCP plates are larger at the two ends, allowing for cancellous screw insertion if needed.
- If a combination of the cortex and locking screws are used, then a cortex should be inserted first to generate interfragmentary compression [37].

12.5 Equine Dental Surgery

Common Dental Problems

Equine teeth continually erupt, and the natural process of wearing and grinding down teeth has become somewhat reduced due to domestication. Concentrates and short fibres such as chaff are commonly fed, reducing the time required for the horse to chew [2]. As a result, sharp edges develop on the cheek teeth, which can cause painful ulceration and laceration within the oral cavity. It is advised that a routine dental examination is performed at least annually, ideally six months, especially in geriatric patients, to enable these sharp tooth edges to be rasped before causing the horse discomfort. Equids can present with a variety of dental diseases. Some of these diseases include [9]:

- Tooth root infections/abscesses: This type of infection is a relatively common disorder within the equine mouth, occurring primarily in the cheek teeth. Both upper and lower cheek teeth are reported to become infected at similar rates. The terms tooth root abscess and tooth root infection are synonymous [38]. However, a more accurate term is apical infection (in dental anatomy, the apical foramen, literally translated as 'small opening of the apex', is the tooth's natural opening, found at the root's very tip) [39].

- Diastemata: Is a term that refers to the space between two teeth. Technically, there is no space between the cheek teeth, or there should not be. However, in some cases, a space develops as horses age; it is this space that causes an issue as food material gets packed into the gap [40].
- Periodontal disease: Usually starts with the impaction of food material, diastemata, gingival inflammation and formation of periodontal pockets. This process proceeds towards the dentoalveolar space, causing the detachment of tooth-supporting periodontal fibres.
- Fractured teeth: Traumatic fractures of equine teeth are uncommon; the incisors are more susceptible to damage from falls, kicks or mouth play behaviour. More commonly, cheek teeth fractures are identified, often found without a history of trauma. Loose fracture fragments or sharp edges may cause oral pain when eating, but these teeth are typically encountered when the smaller fragment has already been shed [38].

Some ongoing dental problems can cause secondary issues, such as sinusitis, due to the close proximity of the teeth to the sinuses.

Routine dental examinations require relatively minimal equipment; a gag will be required, ensuring the mouth is held open, allowing for a thorough examination in all areas of the mouth. A mirror, picks, probes, rasps and mouthwash syringe allow for an initial assessment [3].

Figures 12.27 and 12.28 show a commercially available dental bucket, hand rasps and dental mirror. It is important to keep the dental mirror in warm water, if possible, as this will prevent the mirror face from steaming up.

Various gags, also known as speculums, are available for equine dentistry. The procedure to be carried out will impact the one chosen, along with surgeon preference [12].

The Hausmann gag is a more commonly used gag for routine examinations and dental extractions. An incisor gag is used to gain visual access to the incisors, and the Gunther mouth gag, which can also be offset, are used for more complex procedures such as advanced extractions. Other gags, such as the swales and butler gag, are less commonly used nowadays. It can be helpful to have a range of gags available in practice to facilitate a wide range of dental procedures and patient sizes. Dental equipment such as mirrors, rasps and picks must be equine-specific due to the horse's large and long oral cavity. A mirror is an essential basic examination tool, allowing for inspecting all surfaces

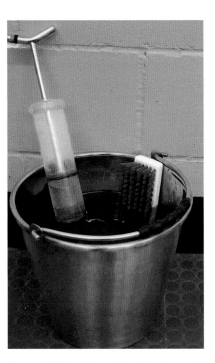

Figure 12.27 A dental bucket. *Source:* Lisa Harrison.

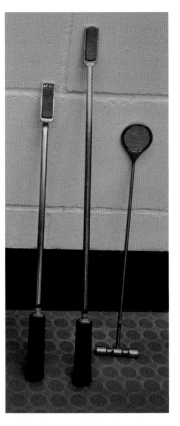

Figure 12.28 Selection of handheld dental rasps and a dental mirror. *Source:* Lisa Harrison.

within the oral cavity [12]. It is helpful to frequently dip the mirror in a bucket of warm water to minimise fogging. Various picks and probes are used to assess the surface of each tooth carefully. Manual rasps, alternatively known as hand floats, are available in various blades and angles. The material used to form the floating surface of the blade is the most important consideration for effective work. Various materials are used to compose the different blades of a rasp; the material used impacts the level of rasping. The most common blades are made of solid tungsten carbide; they have serrations cut into the surface, with various coarseness available.

The oral cavity of a horse is very long and dark, so a bright light source is essential to gain a good vision of what is going on in the horse's mouth. The surgeon commonly wears a battery-powered head torch so their hands remain free to use the necessary equipment to examine each tooth, often using both hands simultaneously. The light would ideally be situated at eye level for optimal illumination within the mouth. Some specialised lights can attach directly to the gag itself, eliminating the need to wear a head torch throughout the procedure. These lights are very much a surgeon's preference [9].

Some practices may be equipped with a video endoscopy system to which an oral endoscope is connected, giving a magnified image on a screen. These systems provide great visualisation into the back of the mouth and invaluable intraoperative guidance, for example, during extractions. Images and videos can be recorded on this system, enabling the surgeon to show and explain to clients their findings and dental work carried out [12].

The head of the patient needs to be in a comfortable, well-supported position throughout the procedure. Different styles of headstands facilitate different procedures; in the hospital setting, the horse's head is routinely placed in a head hoist allowing for ease of thorough examination. Other headstands are composed of a good sturdy base, the ability to adjust the height, some with a curved cradle for the chin to rest, and others with a flat headrest which can be angled to suit the needs of the procedure. Some of the newer headrests can be dismantled, enabling them to be easily transported to client facilities. There may be occasions when a combination of handstands may be required to complete a procedure, i.e. going from the head hoist onto a headstand for local anaesthesia administration prior to extraction [9].

Irrigation is important throughout dental procedures; an initial flush, quite often, a standard mouthwash syringe will wash away food material from the oral cavity. Flushing at intervals to remove dust and debris that accumulates is important to maintain good visibility throughout the procedure; it is suggested that an oral rinse solution can be prepared by mixing 10–20 ml of a 2% CG solution with one gallon of tap water. There are also various ready-made oral rinses available [12]. A general garden hose with a proprietary equine oral lavage attachment delivers a high-pressured flush that removes food material from diastemas; flushing sets are also commercially available; these are usually modified weed killer sprays. Some of the motorised units have irrigation systems built in to allow lavage throughout procedures, reducing dust, facilitating visualisation and reducing the risk of thermal damage during extensive overgrowth reductions.

Powered Tools

Hand rasps have been around for a long time, and while still proving beneficial in some circumstances, motorised units are fast becoming superior in the equine dental industry. This is due to the motorised units being more efficient and provided when used correctly, which can achieve a better result for the patient. The units come with various interchangeable handpieces and can also be used to widen interdental spaces during the treatment of diastemata [40].

Motorised rasps are driven by a motor with a cable connection to which varying handpieces connect. Ideally, the motor is small, lightweight, yet powerful while remaining quiet and durable. Some offer a foot pedal control, while others are controlled by hand. An important safety aspect of the motorised rasp should be the ability to start and stop quickly; this prevents trauma to the oral cavity should the patient move [9].

When used correctly, motorised tools provide greater precision and with less tissue trauma compared to hand instruments, reduction of large overgrowths is achieved more easily. In inexperienced hands, however, soft tissue damage, excessive removal of dentinal tissues and pulpar exposure can lead to significant trauma, pain and long-term consequences for the horse. Table 12.8 shows the advantages and disadvantages of using powered dental equipment.

12.6 Sinus Surgery

The equine head comprises a series of sinus compartments, divided into a caudal and a rostral group of sinuses. The sinus lining produces mucus that drains freely through the nasal passages in healthy horses. See Chapter 4 for more information on sinus anatomy [12].

Sinusitis, inflammation and/or infection of the sinuses can be primary or secondary, often resulting from a respiratory infection. At the same time, tooth root abscesses, tumours and sinus cysts can lead to the development of secondary sinusitis.

Table 12.8 The advantages and disadvantages of powered dental equipment.

Advantages	Disadvantages
Reduced procedure time, therefore sedation time and user fatigue	Some can be noisy, which may unsettle some patients
Some offer built-in irrigation	Expensive
Useful for advanced intricate procedures	High maintenance
Offer a more efficient reduction than hand rasping alone	Can fault. Undesirable once the horse is sedated and ready for the procedure
Usually improved patient compliance	Can cause over-reduction in the wrong hands. Also, irreversible damage if inadvertent comes into contact with neighbouring teeth
	Soft tissue damage
	Thermal trauma

Source: Lisa Harrison.

A nasal endoscopy can help identify the primary sinusitis signs. Further diagnostics such as radiography, computed tomography and, in some cases, scintigraphy may be required should the cause not be identified through endoscopy alone. However, the need for radiography or computed tomography to create a surgical plan is often required as using endoscopy alone cannot solely diagnose what is happening inside the sinus. Once diagnostics have been performed, sinus surgery may be indicated. There are several ways that a surgeon may enter the sinus; however, there is some key equipment that may be required to access the area [12].

Sinus Trephine

Access is gained, most commonly into the caudal group of sinuses via the frontal bone using a sinus trephine. Care must be taken not to introduce the instruments too far, causing trauma to underlying structures. A trephine removes a small circular piece of bone, allowing direct access into the sinus. Once access is gained, an endoscope can examine the affected sinus directly. Alternatively, a rigid arthroscope may also occasionally be used if this is the case, care must be taken as the bony protrusions and sharp edges can scratch the lens of the ridged endoscope as they are more delicate than a flexible endoscope. Care should be taken around the edges of the trephine hole, as this can damage the bending section of a flexible endoscope [12]. Access to the more commonly affected rostral group of sinuses is then achieved by sinoscopic fenestration of the maxillary septal bulla overlying these sinuses. It is essential to guide the scope around very carefully; the area is very vascular, and significant haemorrhage can occur. It is often beneficial to have packing material available in case of a severe bleed. Occasionally, a larger 'window' of bone may be removed to facilitate the removal of a mass or cyst lesion. This procedure is commonly known as a 'sinus flap' and, more precisely, a sinus osteotomy.

Further surgical instruments will be required; depending on surgeon preference, a hammer and chisels are often used. Alternatively, an air-driven or battery-operated oscillating saw may also be used. A foley catheter will be placed at the end of sinus surgery to facilitate 'flushing'. These catheters come in various sizes, the most commonly used for sinus flushing in the averaged size horse being 26–30 ft. The catheter is inserted into the trephine hole and kept in situ by the 'balloon', which is blown up with sterile water or air. The end of the catheter can be taped to the side of a leather headcollar, which then must stay on the horse or to the patient's forelock allowing the headcollar to be removed if necessary [9].

Flushing is often carried out using a saline solution; this can be made up by adding salt to water for an inexpensive, effective flushing solution. The dilute PI solution is another flushing solution often used in cases with severe infection; a 1% solution is tolerated well. A general garden weed killer pressure pump (bought new and unused) can be used to deliver the flush; this holds a substantial amount of flush at once, being both time efficient and effective. When flushing a horse using this method, it is essential to start slowly as horses can react to the sensation and mix the solution using warm water [12].

12.7 Requirements for Handover From the Operating Theatre

Handing over from the operating theatre, whether it is standing surgery or under GA, the principles are the same. The following details should be communicated with the patient exiting the theatre; most of these details are communicated on a SSC and into the patient's record [12]:

- Patient details
- Allergies
- Temperament
- Surgery that has been performed
- Any co-morbidities
- How the procedure went
- The drugs the patient has received
- Post-operative plan:
  - Are there any immediate concerns
  - Fluid requirements
  - Feeding plan
  - Current vital signs and how often they require re-checking
  - Wound status
  - Bandage requirements
  - Drain requirements
  - Medication requirements
  - Preserved concerns
  - Current pain score

Preparation of Suitable Recovery Accommodation

When preparing accommodation for the post-surgical case, several factors must be considered [15]:

- Location: where is it in relation to the recovery box, and what procedure has been performed? If the horse has had orthopaedic surgery, they will not want a stable at the other side of the practice as walking long distances may cause discomfort. Similarly, if the horse has had an abdominal procedure, they will want a stable in the ICU [8].
- Bedding requirements: does the horse have any specific bedding requirements post-operatively? If dealing with a foal, they may require a straw bed; if the horse is a fracture repair with a cast, the horse may require rubber matting with minimal bedding to enable the horse to ambulate to the box successfully [9].
- Stable fixtures: does the horse have any requirements that need changing in the stable? For example, are they required to be tied up, which would require a hung water bucket and, once awake, access to forage? Does the horse need a dark stable after eye surgery [2]?
- Warmth: post-operatively, horses may struggle to thermoregulate while the anaesthetic agents wear off; this will be more relevant to foals than adult horses but should be factored in for all recovering horses. Heaters, rugs and bandages can be utilised to ensure the patient's temperature is not adversely affected. The patient's temperature should be monitored to ensure that it does not become pyrexic [2].

Observations at Handover

As the horse is being moved from the standing surgery room or the recovery box, they must be monitored for comfort and any signs that they may have sustained a neuropathy or myopathy during the surgery and recovery phase [8].

Once the patient has recovered and returned to the stable, the current pain levels should be assessed. Pain scoring is useful, but accurate patient observation should also be carried out once they have been stabled for a couple of hours and metabolised the rest of the anaesthetic drugs. If dealing with foals or unhandled horses, it may not be possible to use a rug, so heat lamps and, in some cases closing the top door of the stable may help to keep the warmth in. The patient post-surgery or anaesthetic should be evaluated frequently to monitor for complications post-op. This may involve checking patients' vital signs, performing pain scoring and regularly checking the patient by looking over the door of the stable [15].

Treatment Instructions

Depending on the surgeon, how the horse recovered and the post-operative plan, the horse may require a bandage change, fluid therapy or drug treatments following recovery. The RVN needs to read through the post-operative treatment plan and communicate with the theatre team to understand requirements clearly. All equipment required and any treatment rooms needed should be sourced before getting the horse out of recovery [3].

Record Keeping

Finally, hospitalisation charts, nursing care plans and all other records must be kept up to date throughout any patient's stay. This information will provide a complete history of the animal's treatments, nursing interventions and responses so that its progress can be assessed as objectively as possible. Written records must be legible and use only terminology that all staff members understand. Communication is essential for any patient hospitalised as a surgical patient. RVNs ensure that the surgeon and other team members are updated with patient condition changes [8].

12.8 Surgical Nursing and Patient Care for Specific Procedures

The following section will discuss some common equine surgeries and the management of patient within the perioperative period. All surgical patients need to be treated holistically (as a whole) by RVNs, not just for the condition that is present. When dealing with a surgical patient, it can be easy to forget about the individual requirements of the patient and concentrate on the condition or disease process which is present. As an RVN, it is vital to remember that the patient needs holistic care to heal both physically and mentally. The needs of the patient, specified by the vet, need to be met, but the RVN should also think about the enrichment needs of the patient; these should include the following:

- Grooming: if the patient enjoys this, it should form part of the horse's daily routine while in practice. It will help improve the health of the skin and coat, which can help reduce the health problems associated with the build-up of surface grease and debris. It also allows the RVN to assess and examine the horse all over for abnormalities. Grooming also improves mental well-being, as horses in the wild will naturally groom one another. This serves to release endorphins, which improve the horse's mental state.
- Physiotherapy: some horses may require physiotherapy as part of their treatment plan; however, this can also be given as part of the holistic nursing care provided by the RVN under the direction of a vet. When horses are on box rest, it can support their mental well-being and maintain good circulation, prevent muscle tightness and minimise muscle wastage. For more information, see Chapter 17.
- Bandages: stable bandages can be used to support the horse's limbs while they are on box rest. Using bandages can minimise the filling of the limbs associated with restricted movement from box rest. It may also help to support the contralateral limb in painful orthopaedic conditions as the horse may place more weight through the sound limb, and this can lead to complications.
- Environmental enrichment: it is essential that the horse is in a stimulating environment to prevent boredom and reduce the chances of stereotypies developing. Enrichment should be provided in the form of treat balls, hanging licks, horse-safe mirrors and a radio. These can all help to reduce the horse's stress and anxiety.

Spinal Surgery – Dorsal Spinal Process Resection

Dorsal spinal processes (DSPs) impinging on the neighbouring vertebrae are not adequately spaced apart as in the normal spine. This overlapping is commonly referred to as 'kissing spines' and can cause varying pain levels in affected horses. The thoracic and lumbar DSPs are frequently cited as the cause of poor performance and back pain in horses [12]. Radiographs and a thorough clinical examination are used to confirm a diagnosis.

Management

Conservative management may include anti-inflammatory injections around the kissing spine, steroid injections in the spaces between the vertebrae, shock wave therapy and physiotherapy sessions. However, in severe cases, surgery is recommended. The surgeon removes a section of the affected DSP. This can now be carried out in the standing horse with regional nerve blocks. In some cases, the surgeon may opt for a GA; however, this is rarely required as the procedure is well tolerated and there is greater anatomical visualisation in the standing horse. Another surgical procedure is the interspinous ligament desmotomy (ISLD), where the interspinous ligaments are incised to relieve pressure on the ligaments; the surgery can be done with or without the ISLD.

Surgery

Depending on the type of patient, it may be preferred to admit the patient the day before surgery to ensure they can settle in the environment and not have to be sedated immediately. After the horse has settled in the stable, either the day of surgery or the afternoon before surgery the following day, the horse will require radiographs taken of the DSPs. If the practice has up-to-date previous radiographs and the patient has had markers clipped into the hair (when a horse with impinging DSPs is radiographed and a surgical approach is deemed necessary, the radiographer may clip marks into the hair to identify the surgical site/sites clearly), it may not be necessary to radiograph the area for assessment purposes before surgery; however, there will need to be a radiograph taken with metallic markers (often staples) attached to the skin to precisely define the DSP sites to be resected [12]. This process works as follows:

- Stand the horse square either in or outside of stocks – sedation is often required for radiographs of the DSPs; also, if the horse is going straight to surgery, the premedication drugs can be administered at this point.
- The area over the affected DSPs will require clipping in preparation for the staples to be placed prior to the radiograph being taken; this can either be the full surgical clip or just a smaller area over where the staples are to be placed. The staples may be placed directly over the DSPs of interest or to one side of the DSPs, which will be surgeon dependant. This does not have to be a complete surgical preparation; it is just so the skin staples can be placed effectively.
- If doing an up-to-date assessment radiograph, place either barium markers or radiographic markers on the skin in the assumed area of the impingement.
- Take the radiograph – the surgeon can then assess if the markers are in the correct place. Once in the correct position (further radiographs may be required), the staples can be placed (the location of these markers will be the

surgeon dependant; some prefer directly over the DSPs, while some prefer off to the side).

- Once the staples are in place, a final radiograph can be taken to ensure the surgeon is happy with the placement; this radiograph may be required throughout the surgery, so it will either need printing or placing on a screen in the surgery room.
- If going straight to surgery, the whole surgical area can be clipped and prepped according to practice protocol. If the surgery is taking place in the same room as the radiographs, then it is essential to move the horse outside after the clipping and prepping so the room can be cleaned and disinfected, ready for surgery.
- Once the horse is back in the surgery room, local anaesthesia is injected as directed by the surgeon (generally between the first and second surgical preps).
- Complete the final surgical scrub – the horse is now ready for surgery.

The surgery comprises of a longitudinal incision made between the most cranial and caudal of the affected DSPs [12]. Then, the supraspinous ligament is divided sharply and longitudinally and will be elevated from its attachments to the DSPs and retracted abaxially using Gelpi retractors. The dorsal part of the DSP of one or more vertebrae is resected using an oscillating saw, osteotome, Gigli wire or bone-cutting shears. When an oscillation saw is used, Hohmann retractors or self-retraining retractors are necessary to hold the soft tissues away from the exposed DSP. When a Gigli wire with a custom-made wire guide is used, less exposure and dissection are required, which is why some surgeons prefer this technique. Several methods have been described for this procedure, including resection of the entire DSP and subtotal (cranial wedge) ostectomy, a more recent approach [12].

Post-operative Care

Pain Management
These patients can be uncomfortable in the initial postoperative period; however, the standing technique tends to be less painful than the GA approach. Because of this, adequate analgesia is required, which relies on accurate pain scoring assessment performed several times a day (see Chapter 14 for more information).

Dressing
The closure method will determine if a dressing is placed. An increased number of surgeons are using Dermabond Prineo (see Chapter 11 for information), which does not require a dressing as it is a mesh that uses a skin glue to seal, creating a microbial barrier [41]. If this is not used, surgeons may opt for a stent placed over the incision for the

first 24–48, and others may use either a self-adhesive dressing such as Primapore™ or a Melolin™ held in place with something such as Polstaplast™. This area can be challenging to dress, and equine hair can be difficult for the dressing to adhere to, making a dressing hard to maintain.

Stable Requirements
If the surgery is performed during the winter months, the patient may require a heat lamp for the first 24–48 hours to prevent the need for a rug to be placed over the surgical site; however, if this is not possible, the use of clean, freshly laundered rug is favourable while the skin incision is healing.

Discharge
When the horse is comfortable, and the incision is clean and dry, the horse can be discharged from the practice; horses are often given in-hand walking and stretching exercises to assist with the initial recovery period and encourage normal movement.

Laparoscopic Ovariectomy

Equine ovariectomy is a commonly performed elective surgical procedure. Various surgical approaches are used for unilateral or bilateral ovariectomy. The surgical approaches described include vaginal (colpotomy), flank under GA (diagonal, oblique or paramedian) and ventral midline (caudal paramedian) and numerous laparoscopic techniques. The decision as to which approach to use for a particular case depends on the following factors [42]:

- Specific indications for ovariectomy
- Size of the affected ovary
- Surgeon's preference
- Financial constraints imposed by the client
- The temperament of the mare
- Equipment available
- Client expectations

Understanding the benefits and disadvantages of all approaches can aid the vet in selecting the appropriate surgical technique for each patient.

Management
There are many reasons that an ovariectomy might be performed; the most common include [43]:

- Ovarian mass, commonly unilateral
- Tumour
- Ovarian cyst
- Ovarian hematoma
- Ovarian abscess

Tumours of the equine ovary may arise from three tissues of origin [43]:

- Epithelial cell: adenoma, adenocarcinoma, cystadenoma, carcinoma. These tumours are rare but metastasize frequently.
- Germ cell: dysgerminoma (highly malignant), teratoma (incidental).
- Sex cord-stromal tumour: granulosa cell tumour.

An ovariectomy will only be performed after a complete clinical workup, including ovary scans. The patient may have tried hormone treatment first, depending on the cause of the problem.

Surgery

Although there are many reported approaches for this surgery, it is beyond the scope of this book section to discuss all of these approaches; therefore, the most common approach will be discussed, which is a laparoscopic surgery made through the flank of the mare; this has enhanced visualisation compared to others [12].

Patients requiring an ovariectomy must be hospitalised for a prolonged period of starvation before the procedure can occur. Like with many surgical protocols, each practice will have individual policies regarding the length of time; however, generally, it varies between 24 and 72 hours, depending on the source of information [12, 42]. There are also differences in opinions when discussing the starvation protocol; some protocols will involve the removal of forage for a more extended period of time and the removal of concentrates for a shorter period of time. The rationale of the starvation period is to help decrease the amount of ingesta and gas within the GIT, making it easier to exteriorise the ovary and suture the abdominal wall incision [42]. Generally, before the surgery, the vet will perform an abdominal palpation per rectum (with or without ultrasonographic evaluation) to help detect abnormalities associated with the reproductive tract. The results of this evaluation can help dictate the necessary surgical approach based on the palpable size of the ovary to be removed. In addition, identifying pathology, such as adhesions or abscessations associated with the reproductive tract, may provide valuable information regarding the optimal surgical approach [42].

Equipment required for laparoscopic ovariectomy includes:

- Video endoscope camera
- Monitor
- Image capture device
- Light source and cable
- Insufflator and tubing (not always used)

- 0° or 30° 30-cm or 57-cm rigid endoscope
- At least three 10-mm-diameter 15–20-cm-long cannulas with trocars
- Laparoscopic forceps
- Laparoscopic scissors
- Injection needle
- Ligation instrumentation: This can be achieved with either:
  - Ligating loop sutures: in laparoscopic procedures, simple and effective ligating loop sutures facilitate the ligation of pedicles (small stalk-like structures connecting an organ or other part of the body). The ligature consists of a long ligature in a narrow plastic tube at one end and scored at the other, where it is attached. The suture is formed in a ligature loop with a knot. Once the ligature is in place, the scored end is snapped and pulled upward to tighten the loop and secure the knot.
  - Stapling devices: see Chapter 11 for more information on stapling devices.
  - Vessel-sealing device: this technique differs from the conventional coagulating methods that achieve vessel sealing by tissue carbonisation. The heat generated from the bipolar energy determines the fusion of collagen and elastin in the vessel's walls by creating a permanently sealed zone. The system detects the thickness of the tissue to be coagulated and automatically defines the amount of energy required and the delivery time. An acoustic signal informs the surgeon when the vessel obliteration is complete, and its division is possible (typically done with a blade that cuts through the tissue within the instrument itself). This sealing system minimises the thermal effect on the tissues surrounding the sealing line [44].

Once the patient has been starved appropriately, they can be prepared for surgery. Although many surgical techniques exist for removing an ovary, this book section will focus on the flank approach. The individual preference of the surgeon and the diagnosis of the problem will determine whether the patient requires one or both flanks prepared for surgery; an IV catheter will also be necessary during the preparation period; patients should be clipped and prepared as described earlier in this chapter. The patient can then be taken to a clean standing surgery room with a set of stocks and once sedated in the stocks, the following can take place:

- Tail bandage placed – It can also be helpful to tape the horse's tail in a neutral position to the back of the stocks (this can be achieved by using thin electrical tape in a figure of eight around the two uprights at the back of the stocks). This will ensure that if the horse swishes their tail, it does not interfere with the surgical incisions.

- After the tail bandage is in place but before the tail is taped to the stocks, the mare may require bladder catheterisation. This can either be secured in place and left in, or the bladder emptied and the catheter removed.
- The arthroscopy tower is placed in an appropriate place in the room for the surgeon to use it.
- The surgeon injects the site with local anaesthetic, and then the final skin prep can take place.

Post-operative Care

Pain Management

Post-operatively, it is important to monitor these patients carefully for signs of pain; in the initial post-operative period, they may show signs of colic, especially if the surgeon has used an insufflator during surgery as this distends the abdomen and can sometimes lead to discomfort following the procedure. There may also be an increased risk of pyrexia in the initial post-operative period; due to an inflammatory response to the surgery. Pain scoring at least twice a day should be part of the patient's post-operative routine. Clinical parameters should be assessed multiple times throughout the day according to practice policy.

Dressing

The surgeon may place a stent over the incisions for the first 24–48 hours, or they may use a self-adhesive dressing such as Primapore™ or Melolin™ with Polstaplast™. Regardless of the covering method used, the area will require regular checking because the location of the surgery can make it challenging to keep a dressing in place.

Stable Requirements

The patient may require a stable in an ICU for the initial post-operative period. This allows the patient to be closely monitored for signs of pyrexia and allows for careful monitoring during food reintroduction; due to the patient having been starved for an extended period, it is important to reintroduce food slowly and monitor for signs of colic carefully. The foodstuffs selected for this will depend on the individual practice but may consist of small, sloppy, fibre mashes and reduced forage, the amount of which will increase over a set time period. The patient will be expected to be eating normal quantities of normal food before they are discharged from the practice. This will help to reduce the need for re-admission. If surgery is performed in the winter months, it may be beneficial, to place the patient in a stable with a heater, as the surgeon may not want rugs over the surgical incisions; however, if this is not possible, the patient's rugs should be freshly washed to minimise contamination.

Discharge

Patients will need to remain hospitalised until they are eating full rations and there is no sign of initial infection or complications. Generally, horses can be discharged around 3–5 days post-operatively, depending on how they recover and the individual practice policy being followed. The skin incision, providing there are no complications, will take around two weeks to heal and the skin closures will need to be removed at approximately 10–14 days post-operatively. Patients will generally be allowed hand grazing during this period. Surgeons will develop a plan to return to ridden work based on the surgery that was performed and any complications that have arisen.

Enucleation

Horses have large, bulbous eyes located on the sides of their heads and this makes them prone to injury. An enucleation is one of the most common ophthalmic surgeries seen in equine practice; this is where the palpebral margins, nictitans, conjunctiva and globe are all surgically excised [12]. Indications for removal include: blind painful globes, severe corneal or intraocular infection, intraocular neoplasia and traumatised globes not amenable to surgical repair [12]. There are several approaches to enucleation of the equine patient, depending on the condition and surgeon's preference. Owners may also request a prosthesis be used to improve the cosmetic appearance; however, this can increase the chances of post-operative complications as the horse then has an implant [12].

Management

Eye enucleation is used as a last resort when medical treatment has failed, or there has been an untreatable trauma to the eye. In general, horses respond well to the eye being removed; this is especially true if they have been medically treated for an extended period and the eye has been sore; enucleation may be a relief. The patient can be prepared for surgery once the surgeon has done a full workup. If they have not been an inpatient in the lead-up to this decision, this surgery can often be performed as a day patient or at the yard if there is no way of transporting the horse. It is always better to do the procedure in the clean environment of a practice; however, it is possible to carry it out at the horses' yard in some straightforward cases.

Surgery

An IV catheter should be placed to enable appropriate standing sedation protocols to be implemented. This, in turn, will help to facilitate a safer surgical procedure. Appropriate sedation is essential in all standing procedures; however, this is extremely important in surgeries around the head, as this can cause distress to the patient.

Once the horse has been sedated appropriately, the areas around the eye can be clipped and surgically prepared (if the horse has had a subpalpebral lavage (SPL) system, this should be removed before preparation of the skin), and PI solution should be used around the eye at the appropriate dilution rate. The vet will place an anaesthetic block before the surgery; depending on how the enucleation is to be performed, the eyelids may need to be sutured together with 2–0 to 3–0 non-absorbable sutures in a continuous pattern [12]. The equipment used for an enucleation is dependent on the vet performing the surgery but will consist of the following types of instruments:

- Scalpel blade
- Metzenbaum scissors
- Mayo scissors
- Curved artery forceps – type will depend on the surgeon

The eye will be removed as a whole structure; in some cases, the owner will request the placement of an implant (polymethylmethacrylate sphere 34–40 mm in diameter). These have been associated with an increased risk of post-operative infections, and they are contraindicated in cases with infection present or neoplasia left in the remaining tissue [12]. The eye may need to be submitted for histology; this should be discussed with the surgeon before the disposal of any tissue takes place.

Post-operative Care

The patient may require a pressure dressing over the eye after surgery to minimise post-operative swelling and haemorrhage; some surgeons may use a stent in the initial post-operative period. Care should be taken to ensure the patient does not rub the incision on the fixtures in the stable; if the horse shows any signs of this, they should have a protective eye mask placed over the eye to prevent the closures from being dislodged and trauma to the incision. It is important to remember that when dealing with a patient with an enucleation, they should approach from the side that still has the remaining eye, as the horse may be startled if they cannot see the handler.

Pain Management

Pain scoring should be carried out regularly. However, the majority of horses do exceptionally well after an enucleation surgery. Many were so painful with the disease process in the eye that necessitated the surgery that they were considerably less painful immediately after surgery, despite the surgery itself. Most cases will respond well to phenylbutazone twice administered twice daily.

Stable Requirements

The patient must remain stabled until the sutures are removed 10–14 days post-surgery. The stable must be free from protruding objects so the patient does not rub or knock the incision. The stable may require a grid to prevent the patient from rubbing against the side of the stable. Forage should be fed from the floor, so it does not contaminate or irritate the incision.

Discharge

This procedure may be done as a day patient and therefore discharged the same day; if there is a complication during surgery, such as haemorrhage or globe rupture, it may be necessary to keep the patient in for longer for monitoring and potentially, antibiotics may be required. Upon discharge, the owner should be made aware of how to handle the patient to avoid startling them. Owners should be made aware of complications such as SSIs and taught how to identify the symptoms of these. The sutures will need to be removed 10–14 days post-operatively.

Castration

Management

A castration is a standard procedure in equine practice; many other terms may be used, including orchidectomy, orchiectomy, emasculation, gelding and cutting [12]. The procedure sterilises male horses unsuitable for contributing to the gene pool and eliminates masculine behaviour. By removing the primary source of androgens, castration usually renders the horse more docile, even-tempered and manageable [12]. A castration can take place at any age, providing that the testicles are accessible, but due to the ability to keep a stallion and owners being able to deal with behaviours associated with a stallion, most are castrated between 1 and 2 years old. This is sometimes delayed to allow the horse to develop masculine features, such as a crest and musculature, or if the owner is waiting to see if they prove themselves in their chosen discipline. Castration can be performed either with the patient standing or under GA. The surgical methods used may vary according to whether the horse remains standing or is recumbent due to a GA.

Surgery

A general physical examination of the horse should precede castration, including a full TPR and checking of the scrotum; this will typically be done by the surgeon so that they can inspect for inguinal herniation and the presence of both testes. The discovery of inguinal herniation or cryptorchidism (where one or both testes fail to descend from the abdomen into the scrotum) may affect the choice of anaesthesia and the surgical approach. Preoperative sedation of a fractious horse usually permits safe palpation of the scrotal and inguinal areas. It occasionally facilitates palpation of an inguinal testis by causing the cremaster muscles to relax.

Standing Castration

Castration performed with the horse standing can be difficult and dangerous for the surgeon if candidates have an unsuitable character for the procedure. Standing castration of horses with poorly developed testes and ponies can also be complicated. Donkeys and mules can be dangerous to castrate while standing because of their athletic agility and unpredictable reaction to manipulations. Stallions that elicit a hostile or evasive response to genital palpation are best castrated while they are anesthetised. Docile stallions with well-developed testes whose genitalia can be palpated without being sedated are usually the safest candidates for standing castration [12]. All other horses are best anaesthetised for the procedure to maintain the safety of the surgeon and the horse.

Preparation of the patient for a standing castration involves the placement of a short-term IV catheter to enable the safe administration of sedation. There is debate over the safe use of acepromazine in entire male horses and a connection to priapism or penile paralysis; because of this, it should be used with caution or avoided depending on the individual practice policy. Once the horse is sedated, the area can be prepared; colts or stallions undergoing castrations should have a correctly fitted tail bandage to prevent contamination of the surgical field; the requirement for clipping of the surgical site will depend on how much hair the patient has; clipping can be dangerous to achieve in the standing patient, so unless it is essential, it may not be performed. The site will need to be surgically prepared using the methods described above. There will need to be sufficient local anaesthetic available for the vet, around 15–30 ml per spermatic cord; this can either be lidocaine or mepivacaine, typically injected through a 20–22 g needle [12]. However, the vet may also choose to anaesthetise the parenchyma of each testis using an 18-gauge, 1½ in. needle. Using this method, the anaesthetic solution diffuses proximally into each spermatic cord [12].

Careful restraint is essential during this procedure as there is an increased risk to human health due to the location of the surgical site. Adequate sedation should be used throughout. The handler and the vet should wear appropriate personal protective equipment (PPE) and be positioned on the same side of the horse. The vet should be positioned at the horse's shoulder as close to the horse's body as possible. A standing castration can be preferable over a GA, provided the horse is selected appropriately, and local anaesthesia is used to desensitise the area thoroughly.

Recumbent Castration

Castrations are performed in the recumbent horse for many reasons, and the reason for the GA will depend on how it is completed. They can be the preferred method of castration by vets using field anaesthesia, the most critical factor being that a safe flat area is found, and that the horse can be monitored and recovered safely. A combination of injectable anaesthetic agents can be used in conjunction with sedatives to maintain anaesthesia or inhaled agents in a clinical environment (for more information on anaesthesia, please refer to Chapter 10). Once the horse is anesthetised, the site can be prepared; it is easier in the recumbent horse to clip the area if necessary; however, the extent of this will depend on the anaesthetic agents used as some are short-acting, so the procedure needs to run quickly to minimise the need for unnecessary top-ups of anaesthetic agents.

Emasculators

The improved Whites, the Reimer and the Serra emasculators are the most commonly used types. The improved Whites use a similar action to the Serra with a double-crush of the cord and blood vessels followed by a sharp cut, reducing post-op bleeding and infection; this prevents primary and secondary haemorrhage because of the multiple crushing of the spermatic cord and artery. The Reimer emasculator crushes the cord, and a blade operated by a separate handle severs the cord distal to the crushed segment. Because the cord is severed with a separate handle, there is no danger of cutting the cord before it is satisfactorily crushed. The extra handle on the Reimer emasculator makes the instrument somewhat unwieldy for standing castration. The jaws of the Serra emasculator are curved so that the cord is evenly crushed, and the grooves on the crushing blades are oriented parallel to the cord, decreasing the chance of accidentally transecting the cord with the crushing portion of the jaws. Figure 12.29 shows the different emasculators available in veterinary practice.

Although emasculators are not absolutely necessary to successfully castrate a horse, it is often the easiest and quickest way to achieve the result with minimal haemorrhage. Using emasculators reduces the risk of postoperative bleeding and therefore most practices include them as part of the castration kit.

During a castration, the vet will perform the surgery and the RVN may act as a surgical assistant. Within this role, the RVN may be asked to use the emasculators; therefore,

(a)   (b)   (c)

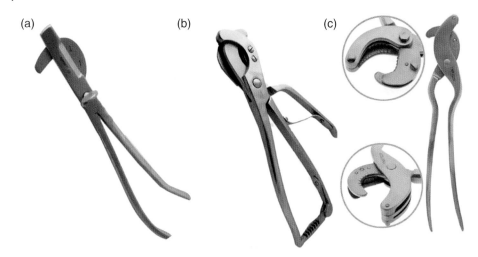

Figure 12.29 Different types of emasculators used in equine practice: (a) the improved Whites, (b) the Reimer, (c) the Serra. *Source:* YNR Instruments Ltd. and Rosina Lillywhite.

it is vital that RVNs understand how to apply emasculators correctly during a castration [12]:

- The emasculator should be applied at a right angle to the spermatic cord, loosely closed to avoid incorporating scrotal skin and slid farther proximally.
- The jaws of the emasculator should then be inspected to ensure that they do not contain any scrotal skin.
- The emasculator should be applied so that the crushing component is proximal to the cutting blade.
- When correctly applied, the wing-nut of the emasculator is oriented distal towards the testis. The emasculator is then said to be applied 'nut to nut'.
- The tension of the cord should be relieved, and the handles of the emasculator should be compressed completely to crush and (depending on the type of emasculator used) sever the cord.
- The time period that should elapse before removing the emasculator varies and will be decided by the vet. Two to three minutes is usually sufficient to achieve haemostasis.

It is also important that RVNs understand how to dismantle, clean and sterilise emasculators correctly. For more information, please see Chapter 11.

Type of Closure

The surgical method used for the castration will often determine how it is closed. Castrations can be closed using open, closed and half-closed techniques. With the open technique of castration, the parietal (or common vaginal) tunic is retained [12]. With the closed and the half-closed techniques, the portion of the parietal tunic surrounding the testis and the distal portion of the spermatic cord is removed. Regardless of the method, the scrotal skin is most commonly left unsutured to heal by second intention [12]. When the skin is left unsutured, the castration is sometimes

called an open castration, confusing the terminology. When the scrotal or inguinal skin is sutured, the castration is sometimes called a closed castration [12]. To avoid confusion, the terms open and closed should be used to describe whether the parietal tunic of each testis was removed and should not be used to describe whether the scrotal or inguinal wound was sutured [12]. Whether a castrate is performed under standing sedation or GA depends on various factors. GA may be recommended for the following considerations:

- Age: horses over the age of 3 due to larger testicle size and increased size of blood vessels.
- Breed: Arabians, some draught breeds, donkeys and mules have a higher risk of eviscerations and haemorrhage following surgery.
- Height: some small breeds may require a GA for logistical reasons.
- Temperament: some horses may be too dangerous to do a standing castrate on.

Post-operative Care

Regardless of whether the horse is kept in the practice or discharged into the owner's care, the immediate postoperative care plan will remain the same. The horse's activity should be restricted for the first 24 hours following castration to prevent haemorrhage from the severed testicular and scrotal vessels. Antimicrobial treatment may be unnecessary if the surgery takes place in clean surroundings. However, a survey of practitioners undertaken to determine the type and frequency of complications after castration, found that horses may be less likely to develop an infection at the castration site if they receive perioperative antimicrobial treatment [12]. It is up to the case vet to prescribe antimicrobials if they believe they are necessary.

Protocols for antimicrobial administration for castrations vary between practices. The individual practice policy and the BEVA ProtectMe guidelines should be taken into consideration for each case (see Chapter 6 for more information). Cold hosing can be used on the site to keep the incision clean and draining; however, the same survey found that horses receiving hydrotherapy after castration may be more prone to develop excessive swelling and infection of the scrotum so this should be done with caution [12].

Pain Management

Post-castration, the patient should not be excessively painful; pain should be manageable with a few days of phenylbutazone orally. Pain levels should be monitored closely using pain scoring, and any increase in pain, swelling or discharge may indicate infection.

Discharge

Due to this being a surgical procedure that can be done in the field, the patient may be discharged back to the client's care after recovering from the sedation or GA. Clients should be made aware that the horse should remain stabled for 24 hours and monitored closely for excessive bleeding. Clients should also be advised to monitor the horse for eventration. This is a potentially fatal complication where a portion of the intestine prolapses through the inguinal canal and out of the scrotal incision. This situation requires immediate intervention. A towel or sheet, ideally dampened with water, should be slung between the hindlimbs of the horse to support the herniated intestines [2]. This will relieve pain caused by the tension on the mesentery caused by the weight of the herniated intestines. Human health and safety should be considered during this process; one person will be required to restrain the horse, and two people will be required to sling the herniated intestines. The horse will require immediate transportation to an equine hospital. Treatment will involve a GA and surgery to clean and replace the herniated intestines [2].

If no complications occur following the initial 24 hours of box rest, the horse can have in-hand walking or long reining to prevent excessive scrotal oedema formation. A large grass field can be ideal for a calm horse to recuperate in; however, it is essential to remember that this does not mean that the horse will be moving around sufficiently to reduce oedema formation; therefore, controlled walking should still occur.

Owners should also be aware that protecting the wound against flies is usually unnecessary, if the horse's tail hairs are long enough to reach the scrotal area; however, applying fly repellent may help as long as it does not come into contact with the surgical site [12]. The horse should be isolated from mares for at least two days after castration.

Ejaculates are highly unlikely to contain sufficient spermatozoa to cause pregnancy after two days following the surgery. The scrotal wound should be nearly healed by three weeks post-op [12].

Laryngoplasty (Tieback Surgery)

Management

A laryngoplasty, or 'tie-back' as it is commonly known, is typically performed alongside a ventriculectomy or 'Hobday' procedure as a treatment for recurrent laryngeal neuropathy (RLN), a condition causing paralysis of the nerve supplying the muscles of the larynx. This is one of the most common causes of increased respiratory noise during exercise, often referred to as 'whistling' or 'roaring' [45]. It almost exclusively occurs in large horses, primarily Thoroughbreds and Warmbloods, and typically only affects the left side. Horses with RLN may present with a history of poor performance and an inspiratory noise, the classic 'roarer', especially during exercise. As in all species, the larynx opens during breathing and closes during eating to prevent water and food from entering the lungs [46]. An opened larynx looks like a diamond-shaped structure; RLN generally affects the muscles of the left side of the larynx, resulting in the inability of the left side to open appropriately. As a result, the amount of air able to travel through the larynx to the lungs is reduced, resulting in exercise intolerance or reduced performance. The roaring or whistling noise comes from turbulent airflow across the vocal cords caused by the narrowed opening to the larynx [46]. Diagnosis is vital for these horses and is based on a clear history, followed by exercise tests, an endoscope-ridden evaluation or a treadmill. Horses can be graded 1–4, with grades 1 and 2 considered within normal limits and grade 4 being abnormal; grade 3 is in a slightly grey area; they may benefit from surgery, but that will depend on the level of competition they are expected to work at as to whether it is worth it.

Surgery

The tieback procedure can be either done under GA but is now more commonly carried out with the patient standing, as this reduces the risks associated with GA, and allows the vet an easier assessment of the degree of arytenoid abduction [12]. The surgery requires an incision over the larynx (laryngotomy) to enable the vet to place suture material between the cricoid and arytenoid cartilage and retract and anchor it in an open position to allow for airflow. The Hobday procedure involves the removal of the horse's vocal cord (typically on the left-hand side) and removing the mucous membrane lining the laryngeal ventricle leading to adhesions between the arytenoid and thyroid cartilages and reduced filling of the ventricles [45]; this is often achieved with the use of a surgical laser. If the tieback is carried out under GA, the Hobday may be carried out standing the following day. It is beyond the scope of this textbook to discuss the Hobday procedure in depth. For further information, please see the further reading section.

Regardless of whether the procedure is carried out under GA or standing, the preparation of the site will remain the same. It may be beneficial to have the IV catheter placed in the opposite jugular vein so that it does not interfere with the surgical site; if this is not possible, a long extension can assist with the use during the surgery. The incision is made over the affected side of the larynx; this means that the cranial part of the neck, including the area between the caudal ½ of the rami of the mandible, requires clipping and surgical prepping. If the surgery is performed under GA, the horse must be placed in lateral recumbency with the affected side up (typically right lateral). The patient's head and neck will need to be extended moderately; this may require tape over the head and neck to maintain the position during surgery [12]. The vet will also require the horse to be scoped during the procedure to ensure that the suture is holding the larynx is under enough tension. This procedure requires strong suture material, which should be ordered and obtained in advance in an appropriate quantity. As well as the specialist suture required for this, the vet may also need titanium washers and/or corkscrew anchors to support the suture and to help prevent the suture from pulling through the surrounding tissues [12].

Post-operative Care

The RVN should be aware, especially after a GA procedure, that laryngeal swelling is possible. Therefore, a tracheostomy kit should be available outside of the recovery stall. This should be left outside the stable for the initial recovery period (around 48 hours) for both GA and standing procedures. For more information on tracheostomies, please see Chapter 14.

Post-operatively, the patient will need to stay at the practice for the first few days to be monitored for signs of infection and any breathing problems associated with the surgery. Feed and water are routinely placed at ground level to reduce laryngeal and upper tracheal contamination. This method of feeding should be encouraged long-term. The patient may prefer soaked hay and soft feeds during the initial recovery as this will promote appetite, as swallowing may initially be sore [12].

Some self-limiting epistaxis may occur post-operatively; the RVN should monitor this and report if it is excessive or becomes non-self-limiting. The laryngotomy wound needs to be cleaned at least twice daily with 1% PI solution or another cleansing agent if left to heal by secondary intention (this is a common method of closure for this

procedure) – the amount of discharge may be quite large due to inflammatory discharge from laryngeal surgery. After cleaning the surrounding tissues, an ointment such as white paraffin or petroleum jelly can be applied to prevent scalding of the surrounding tissues from the discharge. Routine antimicrobials are often unnecessary; however, this will be a practice-led decision.

Pain Management

The patient should receive NSAIDs for 2–3 days postoperatively help to decrease laryngeal oedema and ensure the horse is not in pain following the procedure. The patient's pain levels should be monitored using pain scoring and regular checking of vital signs – any increase in pain may indicate the development of an SSI. There are a few potential complications that should be monitored closely during the recovery stages; these include [45]:

- Infection of laryngotomy surgical site (cellulitis or abscess) may occur in the first 5–7 days:
  - Some vets feel this is more likely if the wound is sutured, particularly as the respiratory tract mucosa cannot be aseptically prepared, and contamination of the wound is inevitable
  - Other vets believe that full closure reduces risk
  - Currently, there is insufficient evidence to suggest either method is without risk of post-operative wound complications
  - Subcutaneous emphysema may occur if there is partial closure.
- Discharge from laryngotomy may attract flies or cause skin scalding:
  - The wound can be sutured to try to assist in healing
  - The surgical wound should be cleaned twice daily.
  - Petroleum jelly can be applied onto the surrounding skin to reduce skin scalding
- Laryngeal oedema and respiratory obstruction:
  - Rarely occurs, especially if peri-operative NSAIDs are used, and there is minimal surgical trauma
  - In severe cases, a tracheotomy tube should be placed, preferably through a laryngotomy incision
  - Severe cases can be treated by spraying the affected area with dimethyl sulfoxide (DMSO)/corticosteroid saline solution via the laryngotomy or nasal catheter once or twice daily.

Discharge

Generally, patients are ready for discharge between 3 and 5 days post-operatively and should remain on box rest for 30 days [12]. A laryngotomy wound should heal in 10–21 days, depending on whether it is sutured or not.

If non-absorbable sutures were placed, these should be removed at 10–14 days post-operatively. Hand-walking is allowed for exercise from the second post-operative week, and the swelling in the laryngoplasty incision area subsides [12]. During the fifth and sixth post-operative weeks (30–45 days after surgery), the horse can be exercised lightly or turned out in a small paddock or round pen. After this, training can resume. The owner should be advised that the horse may develop a chronic cough associated with eating [12].

12.9 Oncological Treatments

Oncology is the study of cancer and its related diseases, with neoplasia meaning 'new growth' and describes the uncontrolled rapid growth of cells. In some cases, this proliferation is of a specific type of cell, such as an epithelial or muscle cell, while in some cases, there can be rapid growth of stem cells that can show no difference.

A tumour is an accumulation of neoplastic cells, and the rate of growth of these cells highly depends on the type of cell involved [43]:

- Benign tumours: Usually well distinguished and grow only on their site of origin. The growth rate and the extent to which they spread to the surrounding tissues can vary.

- Malignment tumours can spread to other areas of the body by invading the blood or lymphatic systems, so organs that filter blood and lymph are most commonly affected, e.g. lungs, liver, spleen and local lymph nodes.

Sarcoids

Sarcoids are fibroblastic skin tumours and are the most common tumour in horses, with some horses having a genetic predisposition to sarcoids. Although the cause is often unknown, there is an association with the bovine papillomavirus. Sarcoids may appear anywhere on the horse but are common on the head (around the eyes), ventral abdomen, udder, sheath, inner thigh and distal limbs [44].

Types of sarcoid include:

- Verrucose: flat, slowly progressive tumours [45]
- Nodular: subcutaneous, slowly progressive tumours [45]
- Fibroblastic: aggressive tumours that may ulcerate (treatment of these may be difficult) [45]
- Occult: superficial, usually causing hair loss [45]
- Malevolent: locally invasive [45]
- Mixed: have the appearance of several sarcoid types [45].

Table 12.9 contains information regarding other commonly occurring equine tumours and their identifiable features.

Table 12.9 Common equine tumours.

Type of tumour	Details	Treatment
Squamous cell carcinoma	Can occur anywhere on the skin but is commonly found on the third eyelid and penis of horses with unpigmented skin	Surgical resection
Granulosa cell tumours	Most commonly seen in the ovaries of older mares	Surgical removal, ideally done laparoscopically
Melanomas	A form of skin cancer, affecting the melanocytes in the skin. These tumours are usually solid black lumps that are locally invasive and slow growing Found commonly on grey horses around the tail and rectum area	Surgical removal, depending on location
Keratoma	Benign tumour of the laminae causing an overgrowth of horn-producing cells of the coronary band. Usually found towards the toe of the foot	Surgical resection, common for reoccurrence
Lymphoma	- *Multicentric lymphoma* – has multiple enlarged lymph nodes. Most common type of lymphoma - *Intestinal lymphoma* – causes intestinal wall thickening - *Cutaneous lymphoma* – tumours under the skin - *Mediastinal lymphoma* – tumours in the thoracic lymph nodes causing respiratory signs and pleural effusions	Treatment ranges from surgical drainage to minimal treatment options depending on where on/in the body

Source: Nicola Rose.

Oncological Treatment

Many treatment options are available for equine tumours; some are more successful than others [47].

Surgical Excision is commonly used for the treatment of tumours and includes

- Sharp surgical excision where the tumour is resected with a blade either standing or under general anaesthetic [48].
- Light amplification by stimulated emission of radiation (LASER) surgical excision is a therapeutic modality that generates an intense beam of light that can be used to cut, seal, or vaporise tissue [48].

Table 12.10 shows the advantages and disadvantages of the surgical excision of equine tumours.

Health and safety implications for surgical excision include the patient's sedation risk and if a GA is involved, the additional risks associated with this. Correct PPE would be essential when using the LASER, including protective goggles and all staff being trained in usage. Signs for all doorways would be needed when using the LASER, and the doors should be fitted with locks [49].

Cryosurgery

Cryosurgery or cryotherapy destroys tissue by application of extreme cold, and for successful treatment, a freeze–thaw cycle is used. The extreme cold destroys tumour tissue by forming intracellular ice, leading to cell membrane rupture. It is most commonly used for sarcoid treatment, and a margin of normal tissue surrounding the lesion should also be treated to reduce the risk of reoccurrence [50]. The tissue is expected to slough around 2–4 weeks after treatment, and depigmentation of the issue is expected. A disadvantage of cryotherapy is that repeated treatments may be required, and complications include severe contraction of the edges of the lesion resulting in a scar. Liquid nitrogen is used as the refrigerant and is contained in a flask-like container with a probe or spray nozzle [47]. Cryotherapy is often used after surgical excision or debulking of tumours where liquid nitrogen is applied to the lesion/s in question. Goggles and

protective gloves should always be worn when handling liquid nitrogen [47].

Topical Treatments

There are many topical treatments for tumours, and they are most commonly used for treating sarcoids. Topical treatments would often be the first line of treatment for many lesions, especially those not around the eye. The advantages of topical treatments are that they are simple, convenient and relatively low-cost compared to many other treatment options. However, their use can be problematic, mainly because the material spreads to the skin around the lesion [51]. Adequate PPE should always be worn when applying these treatments.

Topical treatments used for equine tumours include:

- **Blood root ointment**: this is a herbaceous extract with cytotoxic and immune-modulatory effects on sarcoids, meaning it causes abnormal cells to stop growing and shrink. However, the full mechanism of action of this ointment is poorly understood. Treatment usually consists of daily or twice daily applications of the cream for 7–10 days. Owners can apply the cream, and it is non-toxic. Again, this treatment can help treat relatively small sarcoids but does not work in all cases [52].
- **AW4 LUDES Sarcoid Cream**: formally known as 'Liverpool cream', it is a chemotherapy cream applied to the surface of the sarcoid. It contains the chemotherapy drug 5-fluorouracil, various heavy metals, cytotoxic chemicals and natural plant oils. The cytotoxic nature of the cream makes it dangerous to use and as such, the product should never be left with the client to apply themselves. A typical treatment course involves four treatments over one week [53].
- **Imiquimod (Aldara cream)**: this is an immune response modifier with potent antiviral and antitumour activity used to treat skin cancer and genital warts in humans. A layer of cream is applied over the sarcoid initially three times weekly. It may take 2–4 months of treatment to see a decrease in tumour size, and it is only likely

Table 12.10 Advantages and disadvantages of sharp excision in the treatment of equine tumours.

	Advantages	Disadvantages
Sharp surgical excision	• Traditional method • Can completely remove tumour • Can be used with other treatments	• Without additional therapies has a minimal success rate • Cannot be certain all tumour cells are removed
Laser surgical excision	• Minimised risk of spreading tumour cells during removal • Reduction in haemorrhage during surgery • Reduction in inflammation, promotes fast and efficient wound healing	• Cannot close skin edges • Open wound • Requires specialised equipment and training • Can result in excessive thermal damage

Source: Nicola Rose.

to work on very small/thin tumours (such as occult and verrucose sarcoids). The advantages of this treatment are that owners can apply the cream themselves (wearing gloves) and that it can be used over sensitive areas, for example, joints. However, horses often become sore when this treatment is used and may come to resent the application of the cream [48, 49].

Intertumoral Chemotherapy

- Bacillus Calmette Guerin (BCG) vaccine is also used to prevent tuberculosis; this acts as an immune stimulant that can be injected into the tumour. It is beneficial for treating sarcoids in the eyelids. There is a risk of severe allergic reactions using this drug. At the time of writing, BCG is unavailable due to worldwide supply problems [45].
- Electrochemotherapy (ECT) involves injecting a chemotherapeutic drug (usually cisplatin) into the sarcoid, followed by applying high-voltage electric pulses (electroporation). This increases the drug concentration in the cells of the sarcoid by around 70 times, thereby increasing its effectiveness. Due to the electric shock, the procedure must be performed under a brief GA (usually around 15 minutes). In some cases, it is advised to combine ECT and laser surgery [44].
- Chemotherapy drugs, such as cisplatin and Mitomycin C, can be injected into the tumour. These drugs interfere with deoxyribonucleic (DNA) copying in tumour cells. Repeated injections over several weeks are usually required. The drugs cause inflammation, and the sarcoids often become swollen and sore before they regress [41].

Radiotherapy

Radiotherapy is often considered the 'Gold Standard' treatment for tumours as it is efficient. There are several different ways of performing radiotherapy. Unfortunately, this is a very specialised form of therapy only available at a small number of equine veterinary hospitals in the United Kingdom. Radiotherapy carries significant health and safety risks to people handling horses being treated this way, and it is costly, therefore currently it is rarely used [44].

References

1 Cooper, B., Mullineaux, E., and Turner, L. (2021). *BSAVA Textbook of Veterinary Nursing*, 6e, 429–490. Gloucester: British Small Animal Veterinary Association.

2 Coumbe, K. (2012). *Equine Veterinary Nursing*, 2e, 149. 385–431. Oxford: Blackwell Science Ltd.

3 DeNotta, S., Mallicote, M., Miller, S., and Reeder, D. (2023). *AAEVT's Equine Manual for Veterinary Technicians*, 2e, 305–323. Hoboken: John Wiley and Sons Inc.

4 Ryan, J. and Johnson, J. (2020). The equine nurse's approach to arthroscopic surgery: part 1 – equipment & instrumentation. *Veterinary Nursing Journal* 35 (9): 262–267.

5 Lane, C. (2016). The veterinary nurse's role in nursing an equine surgical colic patient. *Veterinary Nursing Journal* [Internet] Sep [cited 2023 Apr 25] 31 (9): 276–279. Available from https://doi.org/10.1080/17415349.2016.1206457.

6 Horse passports – passports and microchips – services and facilities – practice – RVC equine – Royal Veterinary College, RVC [Internet]. [cited 2023 Apr 25]. Available from: www.rvc.ac.uk/equine-vet/practice/services-and-facilities/passports-and-microchips.

7 Equines and microchips [Internet]. Professionals. [cited 2023 Apr 25]. Available from: www.rcveterinary surgeon.org.uk/setting-standards/advice-and-guidance/code-of-professional-conduct-for-veterinary-surgeons/supporting-guidance/equines-and-microchips.

8 Cooper, B., Mullineaux, E., and Turner, L. (ed.) (2018). *BSAVA Textbook of Veterinary Nursing*, 5e, 738–774. Gloucester: British Small Animal Veterinary Association.

9 Corley, K. and Stephen, J. (2008). *The Equine Hospital Manual*, 1e. Oxford: Blackwell Publishing Ltd.

10 Do you have informed consent? [Internet]. Professionals. [cited 2023 Apr 25]. Available from: www.rcveterinary surgeon.org.uk/faqs/do-you-have-informed-consent.

11 Dugdale, A.H.A., Beaumont, G., Bradbrook, C., and Gurney, M. (2020). *Veterinary Anaesthesia Principles to Practice*, 1e. Oxford: John Wiley and Sons Inc.

12 Auer, J., Stick, J., Kummerle, J., and Prange, T. (2019). *Equine Surgery*, 5e, 143–198. Missouri: Elsevier.

13 Morgan, S. (2016). A nursing approach to the equine standing surgical patient. *Veterinary Nursing Journal* [Internet] Oct 2 [cited 2023 Apr 25] 31 (10): 308–311. Available from: https://doi.org/10.1080/17415349.2016.1215854.

14 Protect me toolkit | BEVA [Internet]. [cited 2023 Feb 27]. Available from: www.beva.org.uk/Protect-Me.

15 Doherty, T., Valverde, A., and Reed, R.A. (2022). *Manual of Equine Anesthesia and Analgesia*, 2e, 720. Oxford: Wiley-Blackwell.

16 Hyperlipaemia in donkeys [Internet]. The Donkey Sanctuary. [cited 2023 Feb 26]. Available from: www.thedonkeysanctuary.org.uk/what-we-do/knowledge-and-advice/for-owners/hyperlipaemia-in-donkeys.

17 Evans, L., Crane, M., and Preston, E. (2021). *The Clinical Companion of the Donkey*. Devon: The Donkey Sanctuary.

18 Brunsting, J.Y., Pille, F.J., Oosterlinck, M. et al. (2018). Incidence and risk factors of surgical site infection and

septic arthritis after elective arthroscopy in horses. *Veterinary Nursing Journal [Internet]* 47 (1): 52–59. Available from: https://doi.org/10.1111/veterinary surgeonu.12699.

19 Burgess, B.A. (2019). Prevention and surveillance of surgical infections: a review. *Veterinary Surgery* 48 (3): 284–290.

20 Surgical safety checklists from concept to implementation [Internet]. The Veterinary Nurse. [cited 2023 Apr 25]. Available from: https://www.theveterinarynurse.com/review/article/surgical-safety-checklists-from-concept-to-implementation.

21 Oxtoby, C., Ferguson, E., White, K., and Mossop, L. (2015). We need to talk about error: causes and types of error in veterinary practice. *Veterinary Record* 177 (17): 426–450. https://doi.org/10.1136/vr.103331.

22 Vetled | Veterinary human factors training and consultancy [Internet]. [cited 2023 Mar 24]. Available from: www.vetled.co.uk.

23 Tool and resources [Internet]. [cited 2023 Apr 25]. Available from: https://www.who.int/teams/integrated-health-services/patient-safety/research/safe-surgery/tool-and-resources.

24 Anesthesia: epidural technique in horses | Vetlexicon Equis from Vetlexicon | Definitive Veterinary Intelligence [Internet]. [cited 2023 Apr 25]. Available from: https://www.vetlexicon.com/treat/equis/technique/anesthesia-epidural.

25 Surgical site infections: prevention and treatment [Internet]. National Institute for Health and Care Excellence; 2019. Available from: www.nice.org.uk/guidance/ng125.

26 Murthy, M.B. and Krishnamurthy, B. (2009). Severe irritant contact dermatitis induced by povidone iodine solution. *Indian Journal of Pharmacology [Internet]*. Aug [cited 2023 Apr 25] 41 (4): 199–200. Available from: https://www.ncbi.nlm.nih.gov/pmc/articles/PMC2875742.

27 Phillips, H. (2018). Surgical skin preparation – best practice protocol for veterinary nurses [Internet]. Australian College of Veterinary Nursing [cited 2023 Mar 21]. Available from: https://vetnurse.com.au/2018/03/07/surgical-skin-preparation.

28 Price, K., Evans, D., and Jayasekara, R. (2017). *Is the Use of Chlorhexidine Contributing to Increased Resistance to Chlorhexidine and/or Antibiotics?* National Health and Medical Research Council.

29 Grzybowski, A., Kanclerz, P., and Myers, W. (2017). The use of povidone-iodine in ophthalmology. *Current Opinion in Ophthalmology* (29): 1.

30 Preventing surgical site infections: equine surgical site preparation [Internet]. The Veterinary Nurse. [cited 2023 Apr 26]. Available from: https://www.theveterinarynurse.com/review/article/preventing-surgical-site-infections-equine-surgical-site-preparation.

31 Surgical skin preparation – are we just going around in circles? [Internet]. The Veterinary Nurse. [cited 2023 Apr 25]. Available from: https://www.theveterinarynurse.com/review/article/surgical-skin-preparation-are-we-just-going-around-in-circles.

32 Knottenbelt, D.C. (1997). Equine wound management: are there significant differences in healing at different sites on the body? *Veterinary Dermatology [Internet]*. [cited 2023 Apr 26] 8 (4): 273–290. Available from: https://doi.org/10.1111/j.1365-3164.1997.tb00273.x.

33 Nixon, A.J. (2020). *Equine Fracture Repair*, 2e, 807–813. Hoboken: John Wiley and Sons Inc.

34 Manso-Diaz, G., Lopez-Sanroman, J., and Weller, R. (2018). *A Practical Guide to Equine Radiography*, 1e, 1–17. Sheffield: 5M Publishing Ltd.

35 Roberts, T.T., Prummer, C.M., Papaliodis, D.N. et al. (2013). History of the orthopedic screw. *Orthopedics [Internet]* Jan [cited 2023 Mar 23] 36 (1): 12–14. Available from: https://doi.org/10.3928/01477447-20121217-02.

36 Lag screw technique [Internet]. Site name. [cited 2023 Apr 26]. Available from: https://surgeryreference.aofoundation.org/orthopedic-trauma/adult-trauma/proximal-tibia/basic-technique/lag-screw-technique.

37 Basic principles of plating [Internet]. Site name. [cited 2023 Apr 26]. Available from: https://surgeryreference.aofoundation.org/orthopedic-trauma/adult-trauma/basic-technique/basic-principles-of-plating.

38 Tooth root abscess [Internet]. [cited 2023 Jan 25]. Available from: https://www.roodandriddle.com/news/education-articles/tooth-root-abscess.

39 von Arx, T. (2011). Apical surgery: a review of current techniques and outcome. *The Saudi Dental Journal [Internet]* Jan [cited 2023 Jan 25] 23 (1): 9–15. Available from: https://www.ncbi.nlm.nih.gov/pmc/articles/PMC3770245.

40 Equine, M.R. (2017). Equine diastemata: abnormal accumulation of food between teeth [Internet]. Mid-Rivers Equine Centre [cited 2023 Jan 25]. Available from: https://www.midriversequine.com/equine-diastemata-abnormal-accumulation-of-food-between-the-teeth.

41 DERMABOND® PRINEO® skin closure system | Ethicon [Internet]. J&J MedTech. [cited 2023 Apr 30]. Available from: https://www.jnjmedtech.com/en-US/product/dermabond-prineo-skin-closure-system.

42 Loesch, D.A. and Rodgerson, D.H. (2003). Surgical approaches to ovariectomy in mares. *Comendium* 25 (11): 862–871.

43 Untangling surgical snags [Internet]. DVM 360. 2008 [cited 2023 May 1]. Available from: https://www.dvm360.com/view/untangling-surgical-snags.

44 Santini, M. (n.d.). An electrothermal bipolar tissue sealing system (Ligasure) in Lung Surgery. [cited 2023 May 1]; Available from: https://www.ctsnet.org/article/electrothermal-bipolar-tissue-sealing-system-ligasure-lung-surgery.

45 Larynx: laryngoplasty technique in horses | Vetlexicon Equis from Vetlexicon | Definitive Veterinary Intelligence [Internet]. [cited 2023 May 9]. Available from: https://www.vetlexicon.com/treat/equis/technique/larynx-laryngoplasty.

46 Laryngeal hemiplegia in horses – respiratory system [Internet]. MSD Veterinary Manual. [cited 2023 May 9]. Available from: https://www.msdvetmanual.com/respiratory-system/respiratory-diseases-of-horses/laryngeal-hemiplegia-in-horses.

47 Knottenbelt, D.C., Patterson-Kane, J.C., and Snalune, K.L. (2015). *Clinical Equine Oncology*. Edinburgh: Elsevier Ltd.

48 Treating tumours in horses [Internet]. Veterinary Practice. 2019 [cited 2023 Apr 27]. Available from: https://www.veterinary-practice.com/article/treating-tumours-in-horses.

49 Equine cancer and sarcoids – Equine Hospital – University of Liverpool [Internet]. [cited 2023 Mar 15]. Available from: www.liverpool.ac.uk/equine/common-conditions/sarcoids.

50 Types of sarcoids in horses [Internet]. [cited 2023 Apr 27]. Available from: https://equinesarcoid.co.uk/types.

51 Tumors of the skin in horses – horse owners [Internet]. MSD Veterinary Manual. [cited 2023 Apr 27]. Available from: https://www.msdvetmanual.com/horse-owners/skin-disorders-of-horses/tumors-of-the-skin-in-horses.

52 Keller, L. (2014). Bloodroot ointment effective treatment option for sarcoids [Internet]. *The Horse* [cited 2023 Apr 27]. Available from: https://thehorse.com/149702/bloodroot-ointment-effective-treatment-option-for-sarcoids.

53 Taylor, S. and Haldorson, G. (2013). A review of equine sarcoid. *Equine Veterinary Education* 25 (4): 210–216.

Further Reading

Ducharme, N.G. and Rossignol, F. (2019). Larynx. In: *Equine Surgery*, 5e (ed. J. Auer, J. Stick, J. Kummerle, and T. Prange), 734–769. Missouri: Elsevier.

13

Medical Nursing and Patient Care

Victoria Gregory and Lyndsey Bett

Glasgow Equine Hospital and Practice, University of Glasgow, Weipers Centre, Glasgow, United Kingdom

Glossary

Acute Severe and sudden
Adiposity Body fat
Asymptomatic Lack of symptoms/clinical signs
Bradycardia Heart rate lower than the normal rate
Bradypnoea Respiratory rate lower than normal rate
Chondroid Firm, dry balls of pus
Chronic Long-term
Degenerative Progressive deterioration.
Diuretic A medication to promote water loss through urine
Dysphagia Difficulty swallowing
Dyspnoea Difficulty breathing
Dysuria Difficulty urinating
Effusion Accumulation of fluid
Empyema Pocket of pus within a body cavity
Encephalitis Inflammation of the brain
Halitosis Bad smelling breath
Hemiplegia One sided paralysis
Hypovolaemia Decreased circulating volume of blood
Idiopathic Cause unknown
Ileus Reduction in intestinal motility
Jaundice Yellowing of the skin and mucous membranes
Mucolytics Medication to help break up mucous
Polydipsia Increased thirst
Progressive disease Gets worse over time, resulting in a general decline in health or function
Purulent Discharge/fluid containing pus
Pyrexia Temperature higher than the normal range.
Quidding Dropping semi-chewed food
Tachycardia Heart rate higher than the normal rate
Tachypnoea Respiratory rate higher than normal rate
Tenesmus Straining to defecate

Introduction

The focus of this chapter is the nursing of medical disorders; however, some cross-over with surgical conditions may occur where more than one form of treatment is an option. Covering every equine medical disorder in detail is beyond the scope of this chapter. Readers are directed to the reference list and further reading section as sources of extra information. Please refer to the glossary for useful information relating to this chapter.

13.1 Commonly Encountered Medical Disorders

Circulatory Disorders

Congenital Heart Disease

A congenital condition is one that a horse is born with. The more common conditions are as follows:

- Ventricular septal defects (VSD), where there is a hole in the septum that separates the two lower chambers of the heart.
- Atrial septal defects (ASD), where there is a hole in the septum that divides the two upper chambers
- Patent ductus arteriosus (PDA) where there is a hole, that links the pulmonary artery and aorta.

These conditions are usually first detected on auscultation of the heart, as an incidental finding, when the veterinary surgeon (vet) is carrying out a routine check and hears a heart murmur. The use of an electrocardiogram (ECG) and echocardiography with Doppler will help to diagnose the severity of these conditions. With VSD and ASD, the larger the defect, the poorer the prognosis, which can lead to

Textbook of Equine Veterinary Nursing, First Edition. Edited by Rosina Lillywhite and Marie Rippingale.
© 2025 John Wiley & Sons Ltd. Published 2025 by John Wiley & Sons Ltd.
Companion website: www.wiley.com/go/equineveterinarynursing

death, but small defects may not affect the horse's life. With PDA, if the ductus arteriosus does not close at all it hinders a horse's growth. It is rare that PDA is the only congenital problem with the foal's heart, ruling out surgical repair, unlike cats and dogs, meaning that euthanasia is required.

Acquired Heart Disease

Acquired diseases are conditions affecting the heart that are not present at birth.

Endocarditis

This is a bacterial infection that causes inflammation of the heart valves or endocardium (the inner most tissue that lines the heart). The bacterial cause may be unknown or be linked to a likely source of bacteria, such as a wound, surgery or an intravenous (IV) catheter.

Clinical Signs
- Heart murmur
- Poor performance
- Inappetence
- Reluctance to move/lameness
- Pyrexia
- Depression

Diagnostics
- A heart murmur may be present on auscultation
- Echocardiogram and Doppler
- Haematology sample to culture for bacteria
- Electrocardiography (ECG)

Treatment
Broad-spectrum antibiotics should be administered until blood culture results are received. The prognosis is usually poor.

Nursing Care
Supportive care, such as encouraging the patient to eat and to interact, will help. Administering medications and helping with diagnostic procedures. There may be some nursing care required linked to the bacterial source if known, such as wound care or bandaging.

Endocardiosis

This disease is a degenerative condition that is seen in older horses. The heart valves, commonly the aortic valve, become thickened and fail to close properly allowing for regurgitation.

Clinical Signs
- Often asymptomatic
- Poor performance

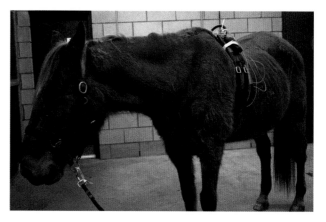

Figure 13.1 Horse wearing an exercise ECG. *Source:* Victoria Gregory.

Diagnostics
- Auscultation for a murmur
- ECG at rest and exercise if safe to do so (Figure 13.1)
- Echocardiogram and Doppler

Treatment
If no other cardiac problems are present, the horse should be able to continue at the level of work it is doing. For human safety, if the horse is ridden or exercised regularly, an exercise ECG should be carried out to check that the heart can cope when asked to work harder and to confirm that the horse is unlikely to collapse during exercise. Regular checks should be carried out to check the progression of the condition and safety for continued exercise.

Pericardial Effusion

The pericardial sac surrounds the heart and provides protection and lubrication. A build-up of fluid in the pericardial sac will reduce the amount of blood able to enter the right ventricle. If the build-up of fluid is acute, it can cause a condition called cardiac tamponade, where the heart is compressed.

Clinical Signs
- Depressed
- Muffled heart sounds
- Painful/reluctant to move
- Inappetence

Diagnostics
- Echocardiography
- Pericardiocentesis

Treatment

This will depend on the amount and aetiology of the effusion. A single-use catheter can be used for pericardiocentesis which involves draining a small amount of fluid from the pericardial sac and then removing the catheter immediately. Larger quantities of fluid, or fluid-looking fibrinous on echocardiography, may need a long stay, wide bore tube placed. This tube can be used for drainage, lavage and administering antibiotics if necessary. The tube must be clamped shut when not in use to ensure that air cannot enter the pericardial sac. Echocardiography can be used to monitor the progress of treatment.

Arrythmias

These are disturbances that can be bradycardic or tachycardic with a regularly irregular rhythm or irregularly irregular rhythm. There is a wide range of disturbances seen in the horse. The following are the most common.

Atrial Fibrillation

This occurs when the atria contracts randomly causing an irregular and sometimes extreme tachycardia. This arrhythmia is described as irregularly irregular as there is no set, predictable pattern associated with it. It may be a primary condition or a clinical finding in a more serious heart condition. Atrial fibrillation may disappear 24–48 hours after exercise or may continue until treatment is started. The longer the condition is left untreated, the harder it is to convert the heart back to a normal sinus rhythm.

Clinical Signs

- Poor performance/not being able to work for as long as usual
- Incidental finding on auscultation
- Respiratory distress

Diagnostics

- ECG
- Echocardiography to check for underlying heart conditions

Treatment

- Administration of quinidine sulphate via a nasogastric tube while the horse is connected to an ECG
- Transvenous electrical cardioversion (TVEC) – usually if quinidine sulphate treatment has failed

Nursing Care

Quinidine sulphate can cause toxicity in the horse, causing clinical signs such as colic, diarrhoea, ataxia, sweating, tachycardia and these can lead to death, so emergency drugs should be kept close by for immediate administration. The vet will need assistance administering the quinidine sulphate

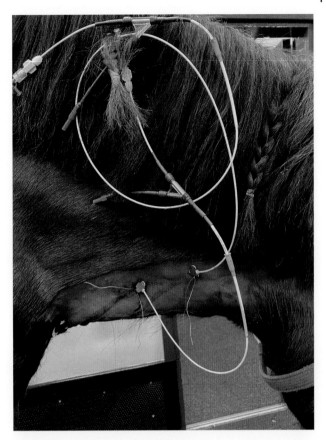

Figure 13.2 Catheter placement for TVEC. *Source:* Dr Claire Dixon.

several times over the day, monitoring the ECG continuously, monitoring the patient closely and continuously for toxicity as described above, and if necessary, administering anti-toxic medications. An IV catheter should always be placed before treatment begins, for rapid venous access [1]. Treatment should stop when the heart has converted to a normal rhythm or toxicity is suspected. The patient will need to wear the ECG monitor for 24–48 hours after the conversion to check that the heart has remained in normal sinus rhythm and should continue to be monitored for quinidine sulphate toxicity after the final dose is administered.

For TVEC, the horse will require a general anaesthetic (GA). A routine jugular catheter will be placed for medication administration as well as electrodes fed through the right jugular to the right atrium and left pulmonary artery (Figure 13.2). Once anaesthetised, the horse will receive shocks at certain points in the ECG trace to encourage the heart to convert back to a normal sinus rhythm. Figure 13.3 shows a horse in lateral recumbency, on low-level cushions, ready to be shocked.

Second Degree Atrioventricular Block

This is a condition often seen in very fit horses at rest. The heart rate will be regularly irregular, missing a beat in a

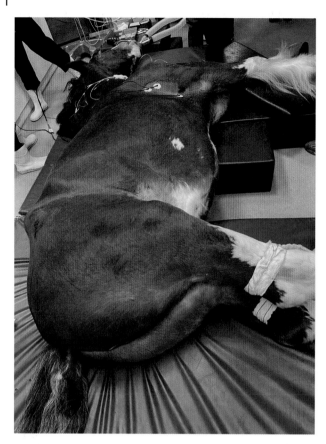

Figure 13.3 Patient positioned for TVEC. *Source:* Dr Claire Dixon.

regular rhythm. This is considered a normal variation. The heart rhythm will return to normal with exercise, stress or excitement.

Clinical Signs

- Asymptomatic

Diagnostics

- Auscultation
- ECG

Treatment

- None required

Atrial Premature Contractions

A regular sinus rhythm is heard with the interruption of a premature beat after exercise. If only heard after exercise, this condition is insignificant, but if the premature beat is heard at rest, combined with poor performance or shows signs of other cardiac disease the condition may be of significance.

Clinical Signs

- Incidental finding on auscultation
- Poor performance

Diagnostics

- Auscultation
- ECG
- Echocardiography to check for underlying heart conditions

Treatment

- None unless there is an underlying condition or affecting performance

Ventricular Arrythmias

These are less common in horses than atrial arrythmias and are commonly linked to other conditions such as colic, toxaemia, electrolyte imbalances and hypovolemia. If it is possible that the arrhythmia is secondary to a non-cardiac condition, this should be resolved first. Otherwise, ECG and echocardiography should be performed to reach a diagnosis.

Lymphatic System Disorders

Lymphangitis

This is inflammation of the lymphatic system, commonly seen in hindlimbs and usually associated with a wound. Bacteria can enter the leg via the smallest of abrasions, causing the lymphatic system to become infected. Once a horse has had lymphangitis, it is at higher risk of developing it again, as there is quite often permanent damage to vessels in that area. The horse can also be left with reoccurring or permanent lameness of the affected limb.

Clinical Signs

- Depression
- Pyrexia
- Swollen limb with pitting oedema (excess fluid build-up that stays indented when pressed)
- Painful to palpate
- Lameness
- Serum oozing through the skin

Diagnostics

- Visualising a wound/bacteria entry point
- Swabbing the wound or oozing skin for culture

Treatment

- Antibiotics
- Non-steroidal anti-inflammatory drugs (NSAIDs)
- Washing the affected limb daily with chlorhexidine

- Cold hosing
- Bandaging
- Exercise

Nursing Care

A registered veterinary nurse (RVN) can administer the medications as directed by the vet and carry out the cold hosing, washing and bandaging of the limb. The limb should be dried before bandaging. The RVN can educate the owner about ongoing care at home and preventative measures to help reduce reoccurrence.

Lymphoma

This is a malignant form of cancer that affects the lymphoid tissue. Lymphoma is the most common cancer found in the horse. The clinical signs will depend on the site where the lymphoma is present. Horses with cutaneous lymphoma, where no evidence of any other lymphoma can be found, will just have the subcutaneous lesion. The lesion should be surgically removed. For multicentric lymphoma, which involves the lymph nodes, gastrointestinal and mediastinal lymphoma the clinical signs are similar.

Clinical Signs

- Weight loss
- Lethargy
- Inappetence
- Oedema
- Enlarged lymph nodes
- Diarrhoea
- Recurrent colic
- Respiratory distress

Diagnostics

- Haematology samples looking for anaemia, neutrophilia (an increase in neutrophils) and increases in fibrinogen and gamma globulin. Hypoalbuminemia (low albumin levels) are often seen.
- Ultrasound
- Radiography
- Biopsy samples of affected tissues

Treatment

Long term prognosis is very poor. Chemotherapy and corticosteroids can prolong life but will be costly to the owner.

Respiratory Disorders

Nasal, Laryngeal and Soft Palate Disorders
Progressive Ethmoid Haematoma

These are benign tumours, made mostly of blood vessels, found in the ethmoid turbinate. Their cause is unknown, and they can reoccur.

Clinical Signs

- Blood-tinged unilateral nasal discharge
- Epistaxis (nosebleed)
- Head shaking
- Noisy breathing at rest
- Facial swelling can occur

Diagnostics

- Endoscopy
- Radiography
- Computed tomography (CT) scan

Treatment

- Inject the haematoma with formalin
- Laser excision
- Cryosurgery
- Surgical resection

Nursing Care

During surgery, there is a risk of blood loss. The patient may need a blood transfusion and intensive care nursing.

Dorsal Displacement of the Soft Palate

During exercise, the soft palate displaces dorsally, above the epiglottis, obstructing the airway. The cause is unknown but can be associated with an underlying respiratory disease, poor fitness (the condition may disappear with improved fitness) or structural abnormalities.

Clinical Signs

- Mouth breathing during exercise
- Upper respiratory noise during exhalation
- Struggling with and possibly stopping during fast exercise

Diagnostics

- Endoscopy at rest and during exercise

Treatment

- Correcting any underlying reason for the displacement
- Improving fitness if unfit
- Surgery using a sharp incision or laser

Nursing Care

If surgery is carried out, the horse will need to be monitored closely during the initial post-operative period for dysphagia

Epiglottal Entrapment

This is when the epiglottis is trapped underneath the sub-epiglottic and aryepiglottic mucosa rather than sitting on top of it. This is usually seen at rest, but some horses only do it during exercise.

Clinical Signs

- Respiratory noise on inspiration and expiration

Diagnostics

- Endoscopy

Treatment

- Standing surgery to cut the mucosa that traps the epiglottis, using a guarded hook knife and endoscopy to visualise the area.

Guttural Pouch Mycosis

Guttural pouch (GP) mycosis is a fungal infection in one or both GPs caused by the *Aspergillus* species. Fungal plaques are formed, which can erode the wall of the internal carotid, external carotid and maxillary arteries. This may result in the horse bleeding to death. Damage to the cranial nerves may also be seen.

Clinical Signs

- Epistaxis at rest
- Dysphagia, caused by damage to the cranial nerves
- Horner's syndrome – this is a condition caused by damage to the sympathetic nervous system displaying clinical signs of a constricted pupil, drooping of the upper eyelid, sunken eyeball and local facial sweating on one side

Diagnostics

- Endoscopy

Treatment

- Surgery to place a balloon catheter, in the affected artery, to stem the flow of blood prior to the damaged wall. This will be removed 10–14 days after placement due to the risk of surgical site infection [2].
- Antifungal topical treatment onto the fungal plaque, either by an indwelling catheter or via an insemination catheter inserted through a fenestration of the mesia septum made using a laser.

Nursing Care

Pre-surgery, intra-operatively and post-surgery the horse is at a high risk of a fatal bleed. A blood donor should be on standby, and a blood collection kit should be ready. Some vets will choose to collect the blood in anticipation of needing it in an emergency. Guttural pouch mycosis surgery is classed as a medium-level emergency [2]. Ideally the horse should be stabilised before the anaesthetic if it has suffered a major bleed but once on site if a bleed starts, surgery should begin to prevent the horse from bleeding to death. Consent for surgery should be sought on arrival at the hospital, and equipment left close to hand should the horse start to bleed.

Guttural Pouch Empyema

The build-up of pus in the GP is usually secondary to an upper respiratory tract infection. Horses presenting with GP empyema should be isolated until culture and sensitivity results are back in case it is *Streptococcus equi*. For the culture and sensitivity testing, a sample of the fluid from the GP can be obtained, using a trach wash tube that will fit down the endoscope. Please refer to Chapter 6 for information on isolation protocols.

Clinical Signs

- Purulent nasal discharge
- Swollen lymph nodes
- Dysphagia
- Pyrexia

Diagnostics

- Endoscopy
- Radiography

Treatment

- Systemic antibiotics
- Daily GP lavage
- Removal of any chondroids with an endoscopic snare or surgery if very large

Airway Diseases
Exercise-induced Pulmonary Haemorrhage

Exercise-induced pulmonary haemorrhage occurs in most breeds undertaking intense exercise. It is not understood why these horses have bleeding from the pulmonary capillaries after exercise. Some horses may have inflammation of the airway, upper respiratory tract obstruction or cardiovascular conditions, but others will have no underlying conditions.

Clinical Signs

- Epistaxis after exercise
- Poor performance
- Sudden death during exercise

Diagnostics

- Endoscopy within 90 minutes of exercise
- Bronchoalveolar or tracheal lavage sample for cytology, within 90 minutes of exercise, usually blood contaminated
- Radiographs of the caudal lung lobe

Treatment
- Rest
- Anti-inflammatory medications
- A diuretic is sometimes administered before intense exercise to reduce the risk of bleeding but is not usually allowed if competing

Equine Asthma

Equine asthma is a relatively new term for a well-known condition describing a spectrum of inflammatory respiratory disorders known collectively as inflammatory airway disease (IAD). Mild to moderate equine asthma was previously known as IAD. Severe equine asthma describes what was previously known as recurrent airway obstruction (RAO).

Severe equine asthma develops due to an allergy to dust particles, fungal and mould spores or pollen is the common cause of flare-ups in this disease. The bronchioles become inflamed, fluid can build-up, which is thicker than normal, and this can cause blockages in the bronchioles. This can then lead to bronchospasms. The disease is a chronic, life-long condition, but the initial pathology can be reversed and kept under control with the correct management and treatment. If left untreated, the damage to the lungs is permanent.

Clinical Signs
- Coughing
- Tachypnoea
- Dyspnoea
- Nasal discharge

Diagnostics
- Management history
- Crackling and wheezing on lung auscultation
- Bronchoalveolar or tracheal lavage sample to look for increased neutrophils
- Rebreathing test

Treatment
- Immediate management change to dust free environment
- Bronchodilators
- Corticosteroids
- Mucolytics
- Dependent on the severity the medications may be given intravenously, by mouth or nebulised

Nursing Care
The owner will need a lot of guidance on how to make the horses' lifestyle as dust-free as possible. Advice should be given on dust-free beddings, feeds, stable location (away from straw/hay use and storage), exercise, equine inhaler use, signs of laminitis if on steroids and signs of deterioration. Some practices will have their own advice sheets for this condition. An RVN could visit the yard to offer individual advice.

Equine Influenza

Equine influenza is a highly contagious upper respiratory tract virus that is airborne and passed on by fomites. The epithelium of the respiratory tract becomes swollen, sore and inflamed. Clinical signs appear one to five days after encountering the virus; therefore, any suspected cases should be isolated immediately, and movement of horses in and out of the yard should be halted until a negative result is received. Vaccination against equine influenza helps to prevent the spread of the disease, and vaccinated horses are less likely to suffer severe clinical signs.

Clinical Signs
- Coughing
- Nasal discharge that becomes purulent after a few days
- Pyrexia
- Lethargy
- Loss of appetite
- Ocular discharge
- Limb swelling
- Enlarged submandibular lymph nodes

Diagnosis
- History of being in contact with an infected horse
- Clinical signs
- Nasopharyngeal swab for virology and polymerase chain reaction (PCR) testing should be collected and submitted within the first week of showing signs as negative results can be seen later in the disease process
- Haematology sample to look at white blood cell counts which may decrease at the onset of the disease but then increase after two weeks
- Paired haematology serum sample taken 10–14 days apart to look for an increase in antibody titres

Treatment
- The horse should be isolated immediately, and strict biosecurity measures should be implemented to decrease the risk of infected other horses. Please refer to Chapter 6 for information on isolation protocols
- NSAIDs may be needed to help with the pyrexia and respiratory inflammation
- Preventative broad-spectrum antibiotics may be given
- Box rest for three to six weeks

Nursing Care

Prevention of the virus is better than cure, so promotion of the vaccination and clinical signs to owners is important. Good stable ventilation is also an important factor. Infected horses should be monitored for signs of secondary conditions such as pneumonia, pleuropneumonia and myocarditis. The horse will need to be isolated and box-rested for a long time, so the owner should be advised on how best to stop the horse from becoming depressed. Depending on the yard setup and the number of horses present, the number of entries into the horses' stable may need to be limited to decrease the risk of spreading the virus. If this is the case when with the horse, interaction is important to prevent boredom and depression. The horse should be groomed regularly. If possible, leave a radio on to provide company and put treat balls or other boredom-relieving items in with the horse to pass the time. A small holed haynet may help to slow the horse's eating speed, making forage last longer.

Equine Viral Arteritis (EVA)

EVA is caused by the equine arteritis virus. It is a contagious disease that is notifiable in the United Kingdom; it should be reported to the Animal and Plant Health Agency (APHA). It can be spread by inhalation, venereal transmission, fomites, contact with aborted foetuses and in utero. It is spread mainly by stallions when mating. Stallions can be permanent spreaders in their semen but show no clinical signs. Stallions and mares should be tested before mating; it is recommended that all stallions are vaccinated and mares if mating with a confirmed spreader stallion. All vaccinated horses will appear positive to the virus after administration, so it is important that a negative blood result is recorded before vaccination can take place. These results should be kept in the passport for future reference.

Clinical Signs

- Pyrexia
- Swelling of scrotum, sheath, mammary glands, limbs and eyes
- Lethargy
- Loss of appetite
- Coughing
- Abortion in mares
- Pneumonia in foals
- Short-term subfertility in stallions

Diagnosis

- History of recent mating or contact with an infected case
- Haematology serum sample for antibody detection
- Ethylenediamine tetraacetic acid (EDTA) haematology sample or semen sample for virus detection

- For abortion or neonatal death, a clinical history of the mare, haematology samples from the mare, placenta samples and the foetus or carcase should be sent to the laboratory

Treatment

- The horse should be isolated for three to four weeks, and strict biosecurity measures put in place. Please refer to Chapter 6 for information on isolation protocols
- Treatment is dependent on symptoms and severity of the condition
- Movement of breeding stock and mating should be halted, and possible vaccination of all breeding stock may need to be implemented

Sinusitis

Sinusitis can be a primary condition, caused by bacteria or a secondary condition caused by an upper respiratory tract infection or a cheek tooth. It most commonly affects the maxillary and frontal sinuses.

Clinical Signs

- Purulent, smelly, unilateral nasal discharge
- Possible facial swelling
- Quidding and halitosis if related to the teeth
- Pain/dull

Diagnostics

- Endoscopy
- Sinoscopy
- Dental exam
- Radiographs
- CT scan
- Sample of fluid for culture and sensitivity

Treatment

- Antibiotics
- Sinus trephine/flap
- Sinus lavage daily
- Any required dental work

Equine Herpes Virus

Please see Chapter 6 for information about this condition.

Urinary

Acute Renal Injury (ARI)

ARI is a sudden decline in kidney function due to a reduction in blood flow to the kidney. This is usually reversible and a secondary condition to hypovolaemia, gastrointestinal disease, endotoxemia or a side effect to medication.

Clinical Signs
- Dull/depressed
- Inappetence
- Increase or decrease in urination
- Polydipsia
- Mild abdominal pain
- Laminitis
- Incidental finding on haematology results

Many of the clinical signs can be mistaken for/confused with other conditions such as colic.

Diagnostics
- Haematology sample, an increase in creatinine, urea or potassium can indicate kidney disease
- Urinalysis, basic tests like visualisation, urine specific gravity and dipsticks can be done in house
- Ultrasound of the kidneys and bladder

Treatment
- Intravenous fluid therapy (IVFT) – care should be taken not to overload the patient with fluids
- Correct any electrolyte imbalances
- Stop any nephrotoxic medications
- Treat the primary condition
- Diuretics

Chronic Renal Failure (CRF)
This is a progressive and fatal disease; the clinical signs do not usually present until the condition is irreversible. It is usually seen in older horses, it can be a caused by ARI, an immune-mediated disease or bacterial infection.

Clinical Signs
- Lethargy
- An increase or decrease in urination
- Polydipsia
- Inappetence
- Weight loss
- Oedema
- Oral ulcers and tartar build-up
- Passing pale urine, lacking in crystals

Diagnostics
- Haematology sample, an increase in calcium, potassium, urea and creatinine and a decrease in sodium and chloride are likely to be seen

- Urinalysis
- Rectal examination to palpate the kidneys for abnormalities
- Ultrasound of the kidneys and bladder

Treatment
Once diagnosed, the horse may be stabilised with treatment, but the condition will still progress. Any nephrotoxic medications should be stopped, and corticosteroids may be used to help reduce intrarenal inflammation. Palliative care should be started, encouraging the horse to eat, and offering plenty of water. If the horse is hospitalised, IVFT can be started.

Nephrosis
Nephrosis is damage to the renal tubules caused by reduced blood flow through the kidneys or nephrotoxins. This condition may lead on to CRF.

Clinical Signs
Presenting signs are the same as for ARI and CRF.

Diagnostics
- Urinalysis
- Haematology sample

Treatment
- IVFT
- Stop any nephrotoxic medications
- Correct any electrolyte imbalances

Lower Urinary Tract Disease
Cystitis
Inflammation of the bladder is usually secondary to urolithiasis, catheter placement or cystoscopy.

Clinical Signs
- Urinating more frequently but with a short stream of urine
- Dysuria
- Blood in urine
- Urine scalding on legs

Diagnostics
- Urine sample for culture and sensitivity
- Cystoscopy (Figure 13.4)
- Ultrasound scan

Treatment
- Antibiotics
- Daily bladder lavage

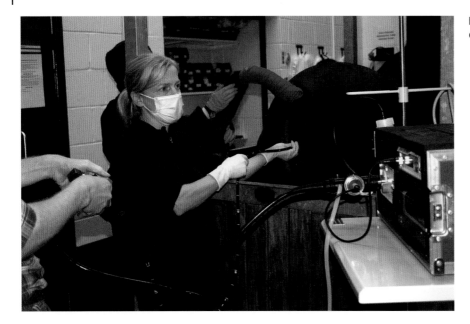

Figure 13.4 A horse undergoing cystoscopy. *Source:* Victoria Gregory.

Urolithiasis

The stones can be found in the bladder or blocking the urethra. Urethral stones are more common in male horses as their urethra is longer. The stones can be made from calcium carbonate, which will break up easily, or have phosphate in as well, making them harder to break.

Clinical Signs

- Stancing regularly but struggling to urinate
- Blood in urine
- Dribbling urine
- Urine/blood-stained legs
- Male horses may not retract their penis for prolonged periods of time

Diagnostics

- Palpation of the bladder
- Urinary catheterisation to check for a urethral blockage and to empty the bladder
- Cystoscopy
- Ultrasound

Treatment

If the stones are small or breakable, they can be removed during cystoscopy using forceps passed through the biopsy channel in the scope, otherwise surgery will be required.

Endocrine Disorders

Pituitary Pars Intermedia Dysfunction (PPID)

PPID is commonly seen in older horses, but it can affect horses as young as 10 years of age. The nerves in the hypothalamus degenerate, progressively, causing insufficient amounts of dopamine to be produced. If the pars intermedia, in the pituitary gland, does not receive enough dopamine, it cannot control the level of hormones it produces. This results in a high level of multiple hormones being produced, including adrenocorticotropic hormone (ACTH).

Clinical Signs

- Hirsutism (long, curly coat)
- Lethargy
- Patchy sweating
- Laminitis
- Polydipsia
- Weight loss
- Recurrent foot abscesses
- Infertility in mares

Diagnostics

- Clinical signs
- Haematology sample to test ACTH levels
- If ACTH results inconclusive a thyrotropin releasing hormone (TRH) stimulation test may be required

Treatment

A dopamine agonist such as pergolide, can be given to balance out hormone levels. To check the horse is receiving the correct dosage, follow-up haematology samples should be taken to check the ACTH level. The horse should stay on these drugs for the rest of their life, and dosage levels should be checked every year. The ACTH result will differ seasonally; the summer solstice relates to the increase of pituitary activity, and the autumn equinox coincides with the decrease in activity [3]. If the horse has laminitis, this will need to be treated and managed long term. Management changes may be required, such as clipping year-round if the horse has hirsutism, nutritional changes to help put weight on but not induce laminitis, and the horse's immune system may be weakened by PPID, making it more important to keep up to date with vaccinations, dental checks and faecal worm egg counts. As the disease progresses, blindness and seizures may occur.

Nursing Care

Most of these patients will be treated at home, but an RVN can be involved in owner education about the condition, collect repeat haematology samples and assist with long-term care and support for the patient and owner.

Equine Metabolic Syndrome (EMS)

EMS is where a combination of insulin dysregulation, obesity and a predisposition to laminitis are evident. It is not known why there is a link between insulin dysregulation and laminitis in EMS. This condition is seen in younger and middle-aged horses and often seen in native pony breeds, but it can affect any breed. Obesity is not always seen.

Clinical Signs

- Regional adiposity – on the crest, shoulders and rump
- Laminitis
- Obesity
- Difficulty losing weight
- Infertility in mares

Diagnostics

- Clinical signs
- Oral sugar test for insulin responses post feeding
- Insulin tolerance test for tissue insulin sensitivity
- Haematology sample for resting insulin concentrations and to rule out PPID

Treatment

- Controlled diet to help with weight loss and reduce the risk of laminitis – The horse will ideally be managed on a forage-only diet, but if still obese, the forage amount should be weighed out, feeding 1.5% of ideal body weight [4]. Any grazing should be considered when calculating feed amounts. Feed companies can analyse forage to ascertain the percentage of non-structural carbohydrates (NSC) present, or owners can soak the hay to reduce the NSC percentage [5].
- Exercise regime to help with weight loss and insulin sensitivity; if there are no orthopaedic concerns – An

exercise programme should be made up to suit the horse that the owner agrees with, can stick to and has the facilities for. The programme should build up to the horse being exercised 5 times a week, for 30 minutes, with an increase in intensity as fitness improves. In humans, regular exercise improves insulin sensitivity in obese insulin-resistant people [4]. Horses with laminitis should not be exercised until the condition has been stabilised.

- Gliflozins are becoming more commonly used in the treatment of EMS. These are SGLT2 inhibitors which block renal glucose reabsorption. This can help to correct hyperglycaemia and reduce high insulin levels to normal or near normal levels. It is suggested to take baseline blood samples to check kidney function and triglycerides and monitor closely before starting gliflozins. This is because these drugs can cause hypertriglyceridemia. It is also important to monitor liver enzymes, kidney function and triglycerides four weeks after first starting the treatment, or if significant weight loss is observed.
- Metformin hydrochloride, is less commonly used now, as in horses, the oral bioavailability is poor and it does not have systemic effects on insulin sensitivity. It was used for its effect on the enterocytes (cells of the intestinal lining) and resulting decrease in enteric glucose absorption [6].
- Levothyroxine has also been used in the past to improve insulin sensitivity [4] and to accelerate weight loss through increasing the metabolic rate [6], alongside an exercise programme.

Nursing Care

A lot of these patients will be cared for at home. An RVN can assist with owner education, foot radiographs where laminitis is suspected, diet and exercise advice, weight clinics and body condition scoring at the yard, and long-term care and support for the owner and patient.

Hypoparathyroidism

This is when the parathyroid glands do not secrete enough parathyroid hormones. Parathyroid hormone regulates and maintains the balance of calcium and phosphorous within the horse; without it, the calcium levels decrease and phosphorous levels increase. It is not known why horses get hypoparathyroidism as a primary condition. Some horses can suffer short term, while others will have the condition for life. Prognosis depends on the response to the initial treatment, but if the horse responds well, the condition can be managed long-term.

Clinical Signs

- Muscle fasciculations
- Tachycardia
- Tachypnoea

- Synchronous diaphragmatic flutter
- Ileus
- Ataxia
- Hyperexcitability
- Seizures
- Cardia arrythmias

Diagnostics

- Haematology sample to check electrolytes
- Assay to check parathyroid hormone levels

Treatment

- IVFT
- Correct electrolyte imbalances
- Vitamin D to help absorb calcium
- Monitoring of ionised calcium levels to decide if long term calcium and vitamin D supplements are required

Neurological Disorders

Seizures

Seizures in adult horses may be caused by several different conditions including, but not exclusive to:

- Trauma
- Tumours
- Encephalitis
- Toxicity
- Metabolic disorders
- Idiopathic

Seizures in adult horses can be very dangerous so human safety and horse welfare must always be a priority when treating these patients.

Clinical Signs

These vary depending on the type of seizure. Partial or focal seizures affect one part of the body such as facial twitching, limb jerking or self-harming. Generalised seizures affect the whole body, and the horse may collapse, become incontinent and salivate excessively. If generalised seizures occur in quick succession, this is called status epilepticus.

Diagnostics

This may depend on any significant known history, such as clinical signs leading up to the seizure, head trauma or known toxicity ingestion. Only if safe to do so, diagnostics may include a CT scan, radiographs, a haematology sample to check complete blood count, electrolytes, specific toxicity, a neurological examination or acquisition of cerebrospinal fluid for analysis.

Treatment

Human safety is paramount when a horse is having a seizure; ideally, a horse should not be approached unless emergency medication needs to be administered. Personal protective equipment (PPE) should be worn in this case, such as a hard hat and steel-toe cap boots. A visual check on entry and exit points should also be carried out before entering the stable, and any plans or concerns should be voiced so that the whole team knows what the plan is and what might go wrong. To control a seizure, diazepam, phenobarbital and pentobarbital may be administered. If a primary condition is diagnosed, this condition should be treated appropriately. For horses who seizure regularly, oral anticonvulsant medications can be prescribed, but this can be costly to the owner.

Cervical Vertebral Stenotic Myelopathy (CVSM)

CVSM, also known as Wobblers syndrome, cervical vertebral malformation and cervical vertebral stenosis, is a developmental condition that causes compression of the spinal cord by the cervical vertebrae. This can be caused by static lesions, which are vertebrae of an abnormal formation and shape, or dynamic lesions, where the vertebrae move abnormally in relation to the other vertebrae. With static lesions, ataxia may be constant but with dynamic lesions ataxia may only be seen when the horse flexes its neck. Clinical signs usually appear between the ages of six months and three years in horses that have a faster growth rate.

Clinical Signs

- Ataxia
- Spasticity
- Stumbling and toe dragging
- Stiff neck
- Standing with a base wide stance
- Overreaching in severe cases

Diagnostics

- History of onset of clinical signs
- Neurological exam
- Radiographs of the cervical vertebrae
- Myelogram
- CT if available
- Ruling out other neurological disorders

Treatment

- Dietary changes to decrease growth rate
- Box rest
- Anti-inflammatory and steroid injections
- Surgery to stabilise the cervical vertebrae

Tetanus

Tetanus is a bacterial infection caused by toxins that are produced by *Clostridium tetani* found in soil. It enters the body via a wound, commonly a puncture wound in the sole of the foot. The toxin travels to the spinal cord where it binds irreversibly to motor neurons and causes spasticity. Tetanus progresses rapidly once signs appear. Horses should be vaccinated against tetanus, and this will help their chance of survival should they contract tetanus.

Clinical Signs

- Stiff and slow gait
- Generalised muscle stiffness and spasms
- Protruding third eyelid
- Strained facial expression due to muscle spasms
- Difficulty chewing and swallowing
- Sweating
- Hyperaesthesia to touch, light and sound
- Unable to open the mouth - lockjaw
- Rigid tail carriage
- Recumbency
- Respiratory failure

Diagnosis

Horses are diagnosed from the clinical signs and their history. If no obvious wound is found, the horse's feet should be checked carefully for hidden puncture wounds. Diagnosis can be confused with colic and laminitis when no wound is found.

Treatment

If diagnosed early the horse can survive but once recumbent the prognosis is very poor.

- Antibiotics – to help to treat bacteria at the wound site
- Muscle relaxants and sedation to help to treat hyperaesthesia
- Tetanus antitoxin – given to neutralise any unbound toxin
- IVFT

Nursing Care

Horses should be stabled in a quiet and dark area away from other horses to avoid stimulation. Feed and water should be offered at chest height so that the horse does not need to stretch for them. Offering food and water at intensive care checks is recommended in case the horse is unwilling to move to the bucket. When entering the stable and handling the horse, the RVN should be quiet and calm but make the horse aware of their presence. If recumbent, the horse will need a very deep bed to try to prevent sores and decubitus ulcers. Pillows or blankets can be placed on the bed to try to prevent trauma to the head and eyes. Food and water should be offered unless dysphagic. Assisted feeding via a nasogastric tube may be required. The patient may need to be managed in a sling. The reader is directed to the Further Reading section for more information.

Spinal Disorders

This usually occurs because of trauma such as rearing over backwards, pulling backwards when tied up, colliding at speed with an object or another horse in the paddock, or falling when jumping. This can cause a fracture of the vertebrae, inflammation around the spinal cord from swelling, haemorrhage, oedema or conditions that develop later, such as arthritis and instability.

Clinical Signs

The type of neurological signs displayed by the horse may indicate which part of the spine is damaged. A cervical fracture or damage to the spinal cord in that area may cause ataxia, weakness or paralysis in all four limbs. Thoracic and lumbar injuries may display as ataxia, weakness or paralysis of the hindlimbs and sacral damage can show signs such as incontinence, hindlimb ataxia, weakness, paralysis and loss of tail tone. There may also be an obvious lesion where the horse is injured.

Diagnosis

- History of a traumatic event, or evidence in the stable or field
- Clinical signs
- Neurological examination
- Radiographs and myelography to identify spinal cord compression
- CT
- Cerebrospinal fluid aspiration to look for an increase in total protein and change in colour

Treatment

- Corticosteroids
- NSAIDs
- Dimethyl sulfoxide (DMSO)
- Physiotherapy

Nursing Care

Minor traumas may not require much nursing care, but if working around ataxic/weak horses, handlers should always work in pairs and be aware that the horse may fall over or collapse. More severe, recumbent cases will require around-the-clock care with regular feed and water offered, assistance to stand with a sling if appropriate and facilities allow, trying to prop the horse in sternal recumbency and changing from left to right lateral recumbency if able.

A urinary catheter may be placed to relieve pressure from the bladder and keep the patient dry. Faeces should be removed regularly for hygiene reasons. The head should be protected with a trauma hat or an adapted, and padded headcollar, to prevent further damage. The eyes should be protected from scratches from the bedding. Human safety must always come first when working with neurological and recumbent horses.

Equine Dysautonomia (Grass Sickness)

Equine grass sickness is a disease of unknown cause that affects the nervous system. Previous suggested causes include poisonous plants, bacterial toxins, insects, fungi and viruses. It is currently believed that toxins produced by the bacterium *Clostridium botulinum* type C may be involved. The most severely affected part of the nervous system is the enteric nerves, which control peristalsis within the gastrointestinal system. It does affect other parts of the autonomic nervous system too; it stimulates salivation controlled by parasympathetic nerves, and within the sympathetic nervous system, it increases the heart rate, inhibits gastrointestinal secretion and promotes adrenaline and noradrenaline release. There are three categories of grass sickness cases: acute, subacute and chronic. About 45–55% of chronic cases will survive, but 100% of acute and subacute cases will be fatal [7]. Although the cause is unknown, some paddocks are known to be linked with several cases of grass sickness. Stabled horses, with no access to pasture, have also been known to have grass sickness. Any horse can be affected by grass sickness, but the most vulnerable categories are horses within the age range of 2–7 years, native Scottish breeds and horses that are overweight. If a paddock has been linked to grass sickness previously, care should be taken if using it for horses in these vulnerable groups.

Clinical Signs

Many grass sickness cases can present like a colic, especially the acute and subacute cases. There are also a wide range of clinical signs, this list will work from most severe to mild signs

- Violent colic signs
- Ileus
- Reflux
- Hypersalivation
- Tachycardia
- Muscle fasciculations
- Sweating or patchy sweating
- Ptosis (drooping of the upper eyelid)
- Dysphagia
- Weight loss

- Tucked up abdomen
- Depressed and lethargic
- Elephant on a box stance
- Rhinitis sicca (abnormally dry mucous membranes in the nose)
- Playing with food and water
- Inappetence
- Decreased faecal output
- Passing dry, mucous covered faeces

Diagnosis

A definite diagnosis can only be made by examining nerve cells from an ileal biopsy or cranial cervical ganglia. The ileal biopsy can be taken standing or under a GA; a GA will be chosen if there is a need to rule out a type of surgical colic. The cranial cervical ganglia can only be accessed at post-mortem. Many other tests and information can be used and put together to rule out other conditions and assume grass sickness, but insurance companies may insist on a biopsy to confirm the diagnosis. Other suggestive diagnostic indicators include:

- Clinical signs, history and paddock history
- Phenylephrine eye test
- Corrugated colon on rectal palpation
- Ileus on ultrasound scan
- Nasogastric tubing to check for reflux
- Dysphagia – a barium swallow test can be carried out
- Endoscopy of the distal oesophagus to check for linear ulceration and reduced motility
- Haematology samples, abdominocentesis and urinalysis can also be used to rule other conditions out

Treatment

Acute and subacute cases should be euthanised as soon as a diagnosis has been made. This may require waiting a couple of days for biopsy results or may be decided using the horses' presenting signs. If awaiting a biopsy result or owner decision to euthanise, the horse should be made comfortable and treated for the clinical signs it is showing, but the welfare of the horse must come first. Treatment for chronic cases will vary massively as each case is very different but can include:

- IV catheter placement and care
- IVFT
- Follow-up haematology sampling
- Nasogastric tubing to administer enteral fluids
- Analgesia if required
- Possibly administering Omeprazole, many of these cases will have gastric ulcers and gastroscopy should be performed if the facilities are available

- Specialist feeding regime
- Water intake monitoring
- Post-operative care if an ileal biopsy was taken
- Lots of grooming, interaction and care

Nursing Care

The RVN plays a key part in the initial work-up, running laboratory tests, setting up equipment and assisting the vet. The most important part of recovery for a chronic case of grass sickness is the nursing care. This may be required within a hospital setting, or for very mild cases and low-budget cases; it may be the owner caring for the horse at home. Some cases require nursing care for more than a year. The owner must be aware of this, willing to care for the horse and willing to learn how to care for the horse, often taught by the RVN. Grass sickness patients can require very intensive, around-the-clock care for long periods of time; nursing care plans and care bundles are a great aid in the recovery of this type of patient, see Section 13.4 for more information. The level of nursing care required will be dictated by the patient and may change frequently but can include and is not limited to:

- Regular intensive care checks
- IV catheter care and monitoring IVFT
- Post-operative care
- Total or partial parenteral nutrition
- Administering medications
- Nasogastric tubing with enteral fluids or food
- Tempting and encouraging to eat if able to swallow – accurate records of how much eaten should be kept
- Monitoring water intake – accurate record kept
- Weighing regularly and keeping a record, this can be used as a tool to monitor recovery or deterioration
- Monitoring for signs of deterioration or secondary conditions such as colic, diarrhoea, choke and aspiration pneumonia
- Grooming
- Hand walking/grazing/turnout
- Cleaning nasal passages if suffering from rhinitis sicca
- Relieving anxiety that may occur due to the increase in adrenaline and noradrenaline release
- Recumbent patient care
- Non-stop tender loving care (TLC)
- Long-term patients may require routine dentals, vaccinations, farriery and faecal worm egg counts/worming
- There is also likely to be lots of owner interaction and care as these cases tend to improve and deteriorate regularly, making it very stressful and upsetting for the owner. The RVN is in a unique position to help the owner navigate these difficult times.

Gastrointestinal Disorders

Colic

Colic is a generalised term used to describe abdominal pain in horses. It can occur due to many different reasons. See Table 13.1 for different types and causes of colic.

Clinical Signs

These may vary from very mild and only noticeable because the owner knows the horse so well, to extremely dangerous. Clinical signs of colic can include, but are not limited to the following:

- Inappetence
- Dull demeanour
- Lethargic
- Pawing at the ground/messed up bedding
- Rolling
- Flank watching
- Stretching, straining to pass faeces and frequently stancing to urinate
- Yawning and teeth grinding
- Sweating
- Dog sitting
- Circling and attempting to lie down but not
- Groaning
- Kicking up at abdomen
- Violently dropping and banging into walls, trauma to face and hips
- Tachycardia
- Tachypnoea
- Increased or decreased borborygmi (gut sounds)
- Pyrexia
- Decreased faecal output
- Bounding digital pulses/heat of hooves

Diagnosis

- Clinical signs and date/time of onset
- In depth history to include current diet, management and exercise levels, any recent changes in diet, management, exercise levels or weather, recent injuries/trauma or medications, last dental check, de-worming protocol, recent travel and when the horse was last seen normal
- Physical examination
- Haematology sample for complete blood count, packed cell volume, total protein, lactate and biochemistry. Further tests may be requested dependent on clinical signs
- Rectal examination
- Ultrasound scan of abdomen
- Abdominocentesis to check for increased white blood cells, total protein and lactate
- Nasogastric tubing to check for reflux

Table 13.1 Different types and causes of colic.

Cause of colic	Description of colic	Treatment options
Diaphragmatic hernia	When the intestines go through the diaphragm into the thoracic cavity	Some cases can be managed medically suffering low grade bouts of reoccurring colic, but most require surgical intervention
Gastric impaction	Food material impacted in the stomach	Medical treatment is the only option due to the location of the equine stomach
Gastric ulcers	Squamous and glandular ulcers found in the stomach	Medical treatment
Parasitic burden	Impactions or damage to the wall linings of the intestines	Medical or surgical dependent on the extent of the burden
Spasmodic colic	Spasms within the intestines	Medical
Strangulating lipoma	The stalk of the lipoma wraps around a piece of intestines, cutting off the blood supply to it	Surgery to remove the lipoma and possibly resect affected intestines
Ileal impaction	Food material blocks the ileum causing gas and fluid to build up in front of the blockage	Surgery to massage the material into the large intestines
Ileocaecal intussusception	This invagination of the ileum can be caused by small masses, foreign bodies or a parasitic burden	Surgery with resection likely
Epiploic foramen entrapment	Small intestines get stuck in the epiploic foramen	Surgery to release the small intestines
Enteritis	Inflammation of the small intestines	Medical but surgery may be required to rule out other types of colic
Tympanic colic	Gas builds up in the large intestines	Medical treatment with enteral fluids and gentle exercise. If still painful surgery may be required
Caecal impaction	Impaction of the caecum	Medical with IVFT and enteral fluids. These are at high risk of rupturing their caecum so surgery should be carried out if the patient is extremely painful or the impaction is very large
Caecal intussusception	The apex of the caecum invaginates due to motility problems. This can include just the caecum or continue to the right ventral colon	Surgery
Pelvic flexure impaction	Impaction at the pelvic flexure where the diameter of the intestines decreases suddenly	Attempt to clear medically with enteral fluids first but surgery if no improvement or pain uncontrollable
Left dorsal displacement of the large colon/ nephrosplenic entrapment	The large colon gets trapped over the nephrosplenic ligament, sitting between the spleen and the body wall	Medical attempts using phenylephrine to shrink the spleen and then gentle lunging exercise to encourage the large colon back into its' normal position. Surgery if not able to correct medically, to replace the large colon to its' correct position
Right dorsal displacement of the large colon	Large colon sits between the caecum and body wall	Some respond to medical management, but most require surgical intervention to replace the large colon to its' correct position
Large colon impaction	Impaction of food in the large colon	Medical with IVFT and enteral fluids. This may take several days so close monitoring is required. Increased pain levels, heart rate and peritoneal fluid changes indicate the requirement of surgery
Large colon volvulus	The large colon twists on itself, cutting of the blood supply. The severity depends on the degree of the twist	Surgery to untwist the large colon
Sand impaction	The horse ingests sand, and it accumulates in the large intestines, it can also be abrasive to the intestines	Medical treatment in mild cases but surgery is often needed to remove the sand
Peritonitis	Infection in the peritoneal cavity	Medical or surgical depending on the severity of infection

Source: Victoria Gregory.

- ± gastroscopy if a gastric impaction is suspected. If gastric ulcers are suspected, the horse's stomach will need to be empty before gastroscopy can be performed
- ± radiography of abdomen if a sand impaction is suspected
- ± faecal worn egg count if a parasitic burden is suspected

Treatment

Depending on the cause of colic the treatment may be medical or surgical. Surgical patients will require medical support after their surgery. The cause of the colic will also determine what treatments are required.

- Intensive care checks. See Figure 13.5 for an example of what an intensive care check may include, to monitor patient improvement or deterioration
- IV catheter placement and care
- IVFT
- Follow up haematology sampling, sometimes multiple times a day
- Nasogastric tubing to administer enteral fluids or remove reflux
- Feet icing to reduce the risk of endotoxin related laminitis
- Analgesia
- Antibiotics dependent on cause of colic
- Specialist feeding regime
- Water intake monitoring
- ± exercise dependent on cause of colic
- ± abdominal bandage change and surgical site care

Nursing Care

RVNs play a vital role in the work-up and care for colic patients. During the work-up and under direction of the vet, the RVN can run laboratory samples, prepare sites for ultrasound and abdominocentesis, and pass the nasogastric tube to check for reflux. If surgery is indicated, a circulating RVN will be required in theatre and possibly one more RVN will be required to assist with the surgery. For medical care, the RVN can place the IV catheter and be responsible for monitoring it, carrying out intensive care checks, setting up and monitoring the IVFT rate requested by the vet and change the fluid bags when required, administer medications as directed by the vet, ice the feet, change the abdominal bandage and reflux or administer enteral fluids. This list is not exhaustive and will differ dependent on the diagnosis. For information relating to the stabilisation of colic patients prior to surgery, see Chapter 10. For information regarding the care of patients following colic surgery, see Chapter 14.

Colitis X

Colitis is inflammation of the colon. Colitis X is a term used to describe an acute, toxic form of colitis with no known cause. Colitis X may be used until a cause of the colitis is known. Colitis X has a guarded prognosis with a high fatality rate. All colitis cases should be treated in isolation until infectious and zoonotic disease test results are confirmed to be negative.

Clinical Signs

- Diarrhoea
- Abdominal pain/colic signs
- Pyrexia
- Tachycardia
- Tachypnoea
- Dull\lethargic
- Cold extremities
- Bounding digital pulses/heat in hooves
- Increased borborygmi (gut sounds)
- Inappetence
- Skin tenting
- Congested/dry mucous membranes
- Capillary refill time >2 seconds

Diagnosis

- Clinical signs
- In depth history, same as for colic
- Full colic work-up to rule out colic
- Ultrasound scan of abdomen to look for inflammation in the colon wall
- Haematology sample for complete blood count, packed cell volume, total protein, lactate and biochemistry. Further tests may be requested dependent on clinical signs
- Faecal samples to test for *Salmonella, Clostridium difficile, Clostridium perfringens*, parasites, Coronavirus and *Lawsonia intracellularis* for yearlings. For *Salmonella*, three faecal samples will be required, taken at 12-hour intervals.

Treatment

- Place IV catheter
- IVFT to correct hydration status
- Correction of any electrolyte imbalances seen on blood results
- Plasma transfusion if blood results show a low protein level
- NSAIDs
- Ice feet – start even if endotoxic signs are not yet seen due to the high risk of toxic laminitis developing
- ± an antibiotic drug effective in the gastrointestinal lumen such as metronidazole
- Nasogastric tubing with toxin binding agents

Intensive Care Record Sheet

Date : _____

Problem List : _____

_____

Student: _____   Weight: _____

Monitoring	8	9	10	11	12	13	14	15	16	17	18	19	20	21	22	23	00	1	2	3	4	5	6	7
Attitude																								
Temp																								
Heart Rate																								
Resp' Rate																								
CRT																								
MM																								
GI Motility																								
Digital Pulses																								
Faeces																								
Urine																								
Appetite																								
Water intake																								
Flush & Check Catheter																								
Reflux																								
Incision																								
PCV																								
Total Protein																								
Pain score																								
Fluid Therapy																								
Type																								
Additives																								
mls/kg/day																								
Litres/hour																								
Drips/sec																								
Est litres received in last 4 hours																								
New bags added																								
Estimated total fluids hanging at end of check																								
Total Fluids In																								
Total Fluids Out																								
CRI Rate																								
Comments																								

STAT IV Giving Set: 10 drops = 1ml   Maintenance = 50ml/kg/day

Figure 13.5 Example of an intensive care record sheet. *Source:* Sammie Feighery & Dr Alexandra. G. Raftery.

Information Box 13.1   Procedure for Transfaunation (Faecal Microbiota Transfer)

Transfaunation Equipment

- Freshly passed faeces from a healthy horse, not on medication, with a good worming history
- Body temperature isotonic solution 1 L/100 kg – this helps to keep the bacteria alive (an isotonic solution can be made by adding 4.5 g table salt and 4.5 g potassium to 1 L of warm water)
- Nasogastric tube and lubricant
- Nose twitch if necessary
- Funnel and jug or stomach pump
- Tubigrip or theatre cap to filter solid particle from faeces
- Examination gloves

Procedure

- Wearing gloves, collect fresh faeces
- Place faeces into a tubigrip made bag or theatre cap

- Wash and squeeze bag of faeces in the isotonic solution to mix the bacteria with the solution, while keeping solid particles separate, to make a transfaunation solution.
- Wring the bag out and dispose
- Pass nasogastric tube and check for reflux
- If no reflux is found, administer the transfaunation solution via the nasogastric tube. It is advisable to keep approximately 500 mL to 1 L of isotonic solution clean to flush the tube with, to ensure that all the transfaunation solution is passed into the horse's stomach, before removing the tube.

Note: Some vets may administer a course of omeprazole to transfaunation patients to reduce the stomach acidity. It is thought that this can make a more suitable environment for the new bacteria to survive in.

Source: Victoria Gregory.

- Transfaunation from a healthy, dewormed horse. This involves taking fresh faeces from a healthy horse's stable to transfer good bacteria into the stomach of a sick horse via a nasogastric tube (Information Box 13.1).
- Anti-diarrheal medications
- Follow up haematology sampling, sometimes multiple times a day
- Intensive care checks to highlight signs of improvement or deterioration

Nursing Care

The RVN plays a vital role in the work-up and inpatient care of these cases. Please see the colic section for more information on this. The tail can be protected from getting covered in faeces by plaiting it up and covering it with a rectal sleeve. The hindlimbs will need to be cleaned daily, and a barrier cream will be applied to prevent skin scalding. The faecal output should be monitored closely, and antidiarrheal medications should be stopped when the diarrhoea stops. Strict isolation measures should be adhered to until an infectious or zoonotic disease has been ruled out. Please refer to Chapter 6 for information on isolation protocols.

Choke

Choke is an obstruction of the oesophagus usually caused by feed material. This can be caused by eating dry feed too quickly, poor chewing due to dental problems or narrowing of the oesophagus from a previous trauma. Horses can choke on grass, so horses that are turned out permanently are also at risk.

Clinical Signs

- Drooling saliva
- Food material and froth seen coming from the nostrils
- Coughing
- Retching
- Abnormal neck extension

Diagnosis

- History – the owner may have witnessed the choke episode start at feed time or seen the horse as normal before feeding
- Clinical examination
- Endoscopy

Treatment

- Heavy sedation
- Administer an antispasmodic
- Attempt to displace the obstruction using a nasogastric tube and warm water to break down the impacted material. The horses' head should be kept low to decrease the risk of aspiration pneumonia
- An endoscope can be used to visualise the obstruction and possibly decrease its size, or dislodge the obstruction, using endoscopic forceps

- If unable to clear the obstruction the procedure may need to be carried out under GA with a cuffed nasotracheal tube
- ± Antibiotics to decrease the risk of aspiration pneumonia occurring

If the choke episode has been going on for a long time, the horse may be dehydrated and require IVFT. In severe cases, there may be damage to the oesophagus, which can be seen once the choke has cleared. All choke cases should be starved for 12 hours after the incident. If possible, the endoscope should be repeated the following day to check for damage to the oesophagus, which may lead to further choke or aspiration pneumonia. If damage is suspected, the oesophagus can be imaged using ultrasound and radiographs taken, after the administration of barium, to see if there are any strictures or damage to the oesophagus. In cases of choke that are unable to be resolved medically, there is an option to perform a surgery called an oesophagostomy. This involves making an incision into the oesophagus and removing the food material. The patient will then need a feeding tube placed until the oesophagus has healed and the horse can eat again. This surgery can cause strictures, increasing the risk of choking in the future. This surgery also carries a high risk of infection due to the opening of a dirty body cavity.

Nursing Care

Once refeeding starts, the horse should be monitored closely for any signs of choking or nasal discharge. The horse should be fed sloppy fibre nut mashes to start, which are very easy to swallow, and then grass can be introduced before hay. If the horse requires IVFT or treatment due to oesophageal damage or aspiration pneumonia, a higher level of nursing care within the hospital will be required.

Diarrhoea

Diarrhoea can be a primary or secondary condition. It may be caused by stress, diet change, parasites, colic, antibiotics, NSAIDs, sand ingestion, anaphylaxis and bacterial infection along with many other reasons. In most cases diarrhoea will self-resolve before a diagnosis is made and a diagnosis may never be found. More severe cases can be fatal.

Clinical Signs

- Diarrhoea
- Dull demeanour
- Pyrexia

Diagnosis

- History – acute or chronic, on any medications prior to diarrhoea starting.

- Check white blood cell levels for indications of infection. Cases with low white blood cell counts and diarrhoea should be isolated immediately in case they have an infectious disease that may also be zoonotic.
- Haematology sample for complete blood count, packed cell volume, total protein, lactate and biochemistry. Further tests may be requested dependent on clinical signs.
- Faecal samples to test for *Salmonella*, *Clostridium difficile*, *Clostridium perfringens*, parasites, Coronavirus and *Lawsonia intracellularis* for yearlings. For *Salmonella*, three faecal samples will be required, taken at 12-hour intervals.
- Full colic work-up, which may be adapted dependent on history.
- Chronic cases may require rectal biopsies to test for inflammatory bowel disease or oral glucose absorption tests for small intestinal causes.

Treatment

This will depend on the cause of the diarrhoea. If the horse was already receiving antibiotics or NSAIDs, these should be stopped. If the onset is acute and the cause unknown, the horse should be treated as having Colitis X. If chronic or acute, anti-diarrheal medications and transfaunation can commence while awaiting test results. IVFT may be required and the administration of plasma or synthetic colloids if hypoproteinaemia develops. Other treatments will depend on the findings during the work-up.

Nursing Care

The horse should have their backend cleaned at least twice daily and barrier cream should be applied to the hind limbs. If willing and allowed to eat, soaked hay and soaked fibre nuts should be offered. If the horse is dehydrated, it may need to have IVFT and therefore careful IV catheter management will be required. Faecal output should be monitored closely, and anti-diarrheal medications stopped when the diarrhoea resolves.

Salmonellosis

Salmonellosis is an infectious and zoonotic disease caused by the bacteria *Salmonella*; strict isolation protocols must be always followed; please refer to Chapter 6 for information on isolation protocols. The bacteria can be spread by water, feed, wildlife on the yard, equine carriers that do not show any symptoms, humans and surfaces contaminated by infected faeces. Stressed horses with compromised immunity are at a higher risk of being infected; this is a major factor in nosocomial cases. Severe cases of salmonellosis can be fatal, but so can the secondary conditions caused during the acute phase of the disease.

Clinical Signs

- Diarrhoea – this can be haemorrhagic
- Pyrexia
- Abdominal pain/colic signs
- Dull/lethargic
- Inappetence
- Tachycardia
- Tachypnoea
- Cold extremities
- Bounding digital pulses/heat in hooves
- Increased borborygmi (gut sounds)
- Skin tenting
- Congested/dry mucous membranes
- Capillary refill time >2 seconds

Diagnosis

- Clinical signs
- In depth history, same as for colic
- Full colic work-up to rule out colic
- Haematology sample for complete blood count, packed cell volume, total protein, lactate and biochemistry. Further tests may be requested dependent on clinical signs
- Faecal samples to test for *Salmonella*, three faecal samples taken at 12-hour intervals will be required

Treatment

- Place IV catheter
- IVFT to correct hydration status
- Correction of any electrolyte imbalances seen on blood results
- Plasma transfusion if blood results show hypoproteinaemia
- NSAIDs
- Ice feet – start even if endotoxic signs are not yet seen due to the high risk of toxic laminitis developing
- ± an antibiotic drug effective in the gastrointestinal lumen such as metronidazole
- Naso-gastric tubing with toxin binding agents
- Transfaunation from a healthy, dewormed horse
- Anti-diarrheal medications
- Follow up haematology sampling, sometimes multiple times a day
- Intensive care checks to highlight signs of improvement or deterioration

Nursing Care

Please see the 'nursing care' section for Colic and Colitis X for more information on this. Strict isolation protocols must be adhered to when nursing zoonotic cases; contact must only be made with the patient when necessary. Any human showing signs of salmonellosis while nursing an infectious case should contact their doctor immediately and self-isolate.

Reproductive Tract Disorders

Endocrine Abnormalities

The ovaries can become enlarged due to the presence of tumours such as Granulosa cell tumours and cystadenoma. Both are slow-growing, benign and usually unilateral. With cystadenoma, the ovary is not usually hormonally active, but the other ovary is normal. With granulosa cell tumours the ovary is usually hormonally active, and the mare may show behavioural abnormalities, including aggression. The other ovary is normally small and inactive but can be normal. In both cases, the ovary with the tumour should be removed. Ovaries naturally become enlarged during pregnancy, so pregnancy must be ruled out if an enlarged ovary is found. Abnormally small ovaries and infertility can be caused by chromosomal abnormalities, old age, PPID and EMS. The ovary size can be palpated on rectal examination.

In male horses, testicles can be retained in the abdomen and not descend into the scrotum; this is called a cryptorchid. It is normal for the testicles to have descended by one year of age, but it may take a bit longer. One or two testicles can be retained. If retained, the testicle does not usually develop properly, and growth is hampered. Retained testicles still produce hormones and can produce fertile semen. If a male horse, who is thought to be gelded, is showing stallion-like behaviour, they may have an abdominal testicle. A haematology sample should be taken by the vet to test the oestrone sulphate or testosterone levels in the blood; the age of the horse will decide which test is used. Abdominal testicles can be removed understanding sedation using a laparoscope, to find and identify the testicular tissue for removal or under general anaesthesia.

Normal anatomy and function of the ovaries and testes can be found in Chapter 4. More information on the surgery involved for retained testicles can be found in Chapter 12.

Disease of Testes, Penis and Prepuce

In some stallions, the spermatic cord can be rotated without causing any pain. This can be an incidental finding on palpation that might cause a decrease in sperm production. If the stallion has a testicular torsion the spermatic cord is usually twisted more than 180 degrees, affecting the blood flow to the testicles and clinical signs can be seen. These signs may be an enlarged and painful scrotum, and signs of colic. Unilateral castration of the affected testicle is usually required.

Masses on the penis and prepuce are quite common in horses. Clinical signs can include visual masses, foul-smelling smegma, difficulty urinating, urine spraying in an unusual direction during urination or dribbling urine, and not retracting the penis. The most common tumour is squamous cell carcinoma, but it can also be warts, sarcoids, melanomas, papillomas, lipomas and fibromas. Depending on the size, position and cause of the mass will decide the treatment. A biopsy can be taken and submitted for histology before treatment or the whole mass may be submitted after removal. Some masses can be removed from the area, but others may require the horse to have a partial or full phallectomy. Inflammation of the prepuce and scrotum can be caused by trauma, especially in breeding stallions and infections.

Prolapse, or paraphimosis, of the penis can be caused by trauma, neurological disease, exhaustion and the use of phenothiazine derivatives such as acepromazine. When the penis does not retract, venous blood flow is affected causing oedema and if left untreated ulcers, infections and necrosis can occur. The penis, and sheath, should be cleaned, cold-hosed, moisturised, massaged and placed into a sling to support the weight of the penis and encourage blood flow. A sling can be made from human tights or a combination of bandage materials. Care should be taken to ensure that the sling does not cause further problems, such as sores between the hind legs or on the horse's back. The horse may require medications such as anti-inflammatories, diuretics or antibiotics depending on the cause and severity.

Abnormal Vulval Conformation

The vulva sits directly below the anus and should be vertical. Most of the vulva should be lower than the level of the pelvic bone. If the anus is sunken, the vulva tilting off vertical or the vulval lips are flaccid, this increases the risk of faeces, air and bacteria entering the vagina and uterus. This can lead to infections and infertility. During pregnancy, if the vulval conformation is poor, this again can lead to infection and abortion. A Caslick vulvoplasty surgery, during pregnancy, can help to reduce the risk of this happening in high-risk mares. A severe loss of body weight, old age, overbreeding and the overuse of Caslick vulvoplasty can all contribute to a poorer conformation of a mare's vulva.

Recto-vaginal Fistula

A recto-vaginal fistula (RVF) can be a congenital anomaly seen in foals but is usually caused during foaling. During foaling, a hole is created in the dorsal vaginal wall, which communicates with the rectum, caused by a foal's hoof.

Clinical signs include faecal matter being seen when urinating, vaginal bleeding and incontinence. A diagnosis can be made on visualisation of the fistula. If the fistula is quite far into the vagina, an endoscope may be needed to assess the tear. The mare should be started on NSAIDs and antibiotics. Surgery will be required but this may be delayed for several weeks dependent on the amount of trauma caused to the mare's vagina. The surgery is likely to be more successful once the swelling has decreased. The mare should be fed a laxative diet pre- and post-operatively to decrease the risk of further tearing.

Musculoskeletal Disorders

Exertional Rhabdomyolysis

Exertional rhabdomyolysis, commonly known as tying-up, is a condition affecting the muscles of the horse after being exercised beyond its' fitness level. It can be seen during the event or immediately after. The muscles cramp commonly the hind quarters, causing a lot of pain, stiffness and muscle breakdown in the horse. These horses are usually dehydrated as well.

Clinical Signs

- Reluctance or stiffness when moving
- Sweating
- Tachycardia
- Tachypnoea
- Firm and painful gluteal, semitendinosus and semimembranosus muscles
- Myoglobinuria (red/brown coloured urine)
- Colic signs
- Recumbency

Diagnosis

- History
- Clinical signs
- Haematology samples for complete blood count and biochemistry to check hydration status, creatine kinase (CK) and aspartate transaminase (AST) levels (an increase indicates muscle damage), and kidney function
- Urine sample

Treatment

- Correction of hydration and electrolyte imbalances
- NSAIDs if no renal damage
- Keep the horse calm and minimise movement
- Keep the horse warm

Nursing Care

The severity of the episode will correlate with how much nursing care is required. The more severe cases will require lots of intensive care nursing, haematology samples to assess hydration and muscle recovery, and checks. If they are recumbent, they will need to be kept comfortable, clean and dry, warm, propped into sternal and offered water and food regularly. Care should be taken to protect the head and eyes when recumbent.

Equine Polysaccharide Storage Myopathy

Equine polysaccharide storage myopathy presents the same as exertional rhabdomyolysis, but the horse has not usually undertaken much exercise, and the condition returns regularly and is progressive. It can be diagnosed on muscle biopsies, which show abnormal levels of glycogen being stored in the muscles and genetic testing. The condition can be managed with an altered diet that is low in digestible carbohydrates and higher in fat, along with a daily exercise routine with suitable warm-up and warm-down exercises. Rest days, stress and a disruption to routine will all increase the risk of muscle cramping.

Azoturia

Azoturia is like exertional rhabdomyolysis but is usually linked to nutrition and rest. Horses at high risk are those that are fed the same high-energy diet on their rest days. The clinical signs, diagnosis and treatment are the same as exertional rhabdomyolysis.

Atypical Myopathy

Atypical myopathy is a fatal disease caused by the ingestion of sycamore seeds, leaves or seedlings. It is a seasonal condition seen when the seeds fall during autumn and winter and germinate in the spring. The horses are poisoned by the hypoglycin A toxin, which slows and stops energy production in the muscles. Horses should be removed from pasture with access to sycamore during spring and autumn to prevent atypical myopathy.

Clinical Signs

- Dull with a low hanging head
- Muscle tremors
- Sore and weak muscles
- Myoglobinuria (red/brown coloured urine)
- Colic signs
- Good appetite
- Sweating
- Breathing difficulties
- ± tachycardia
- ± pyrexia
- ± recumbency
- Sudden death

Diagnosis

- History and known access to sycamore
- Clinical signs
- Haematology samples for Hypoglycin A levels, complete blood count and biochemistry

Treatment

- Correction of hydration and electrolyte imbalances
- IVFT
- Administration of analgesia, antioxidants, anti-inflammatories and multivitamins

Nursing Care

These patients will require lots of nursing care. They will require intensive care checks, with regular medication administration, IV catheter care, IVFT administration, pain monitoring, urine and faecal output monitoring and repeat haematology samples. If recumbent, the horse will need a very deep bed to try to prevent decubitus ulcers. Pillows or blankets can be placed on the bed to try to prevent trauma to the head and eyes. Food and water should be offered at checks, in case the horse is unwilling, or unable, to move to the bucket. If a horse survives the first few days of treatment, this improves the prognosis.

Laminitis

Laminitis is inflammation of the laminae tissue in the hooves, which attaches the pedal bone to the hoof. This inflammation can be caused by several different factors, such as systemic toxicity, metabolic disturbances, steroid administration and excessive weight bearing due to an injury on a contralateral limb. Once the inflammation has occurred the laminae becomes weak allowing for rotation and sinking of the pedal bone. This condition is extremely painful and becomes terminal if the pedal bone sinks through the bottom of the foot. It can affect one or multiple feet.

Clinical Signs

- Reluctance to move
- Stilted gait and painful to turn corners
- Recumbency
- Standing with the weight on the hindlimbs (sawhorse stance)
- Bounding digital pulses
- Hot hooves
- Tachycardia
- Tachypnoea
- Pain on hoof testers

Diagnosis

- History of laminitis episodes, recent management changes or trauma, or conditions linked to laminitis such as PPID and EMS
- Clinical signs
- Radiographs of the feet
- Obesity
- Haematology samples to check for underlying endocrine disorders

Treatment

- Treatment of the primary cause if known
- Cryotherapy in the form of icing the feed should be in carried out in the developmental phase only. The vet will decide if this is appropriate on a case by case basis.
- Remedial farriery or support for the foot
- Administration of NSAIDs and vasodilators to manage the pain and increase the blood supply to the foot
- Bed on sand, if possible, otherwise a deep bed of shavings to the door
- Box rest
- Feed soaked hay, and a low sugar and low starch feed if needed, calculate feed doses and incorporate weight loss if necessary

Nursing Care

Pain management will be a big part of the recovery for horses with laminitis, along with treatment of any primary condition. They will need intensive care checks with regular pain scoring, faecal output monitoring as they will be at risk of impaction colic, repeat radiographs to see the progression of the disease, and assessment of their pain regularly throughout the day. Due to long periods of time spent on box rest, environmental enrichment will be required. Transportation is a painful and stressful event for a laminitic patient; discharge from the hospital may take longer than planned, as the horse will need to be fit to travel. Horses who suffer from an episode of laminitis will always be at risk of having another. RVNs can help to educate owners on preventative measures and long-term management changes.

Navicular Disease

Navicular disease is a progressive condition causing degeneration of the navicular bone. It usually affects both front feet. The cause is not known, but it is known that it can be hereditary. It is thought to be linked to conformation, foot balance and damage to the soft structures surrounding the navicular bone. Navicular syndrome is a generalised term for lameness, diagnosed by nerve block and radiographs, in the heel area of the foot. Now that magnetic resonance imaging (MRI) is available, the damage to the different soft and bony structures can be individually identified and diagnosed.

Clinical Signs

- Lameness
- Landing toe first when walking

Diagnosis

- Palmar digital nerve block or navicular bursa block
- Radiographs
- MRI

Treatment

- Rest
- NSAIDs
- Corrective farriery
- Joint medication with corticosteroids
- Palmar digital neurectomy

The condition can be managed, and slowed down, but not cured. The horse may be able to return to a lower level of work, but consistent, hard work usually worsens the condition.

Tendon Sheath and Joint Infection

In adult horses, joint or tendon sheath infections are caused by bacteria entering via a wound or injection site. The wound can be a puncture wound, from a thorn, so it is important to clip the area and look for any evidence of a bacterial entry point if there is no obvious wound. Foals can have systemic sepsis, where bacteria is circulating in the blood, which causes multiple joint sepsis with no wounds. See Chapter 15 for more information.

Clinical Signs

- Acute lameness
- Wound near a joint/tendon sheath
- Swelling

Diagnosis

- Clinical signs
- History of a wound or injection at the site
- Palpation with a sterile, gloved finger or probe to see where the wound tract leads
- Aspiration of synovial fluid to assess appearance, white blood cell count elevation indicating infection, total protein elevation indicating infection and making a smear to look at under the microscope for which white blood cells

are present. A sensitivity sample is useful to help decide which antibiotics to use

- Radiographs to look for bone damage or foreign material
- Ultrasound to look for soft tissue damage or foreign material

Treatment

Ideally, an arthroscopic examination of the joint, under GA, to flush bacteria and debris out within 24 hours of the wound happening, to increase the chances of recovery. Under GA, the surgeon can also assess any damage in the surrounding area. A standing flush, under heavy sedation, is an option if funds or facilities are limited, but this will decrease the chance of recovery. Repeated surgeries may be needed to eradicate the infection, and still may not cure the horse, resulting in euthanasia. A septic structure left untreated will result in euthanasia due to the amount of damage the infection can do, and the amount of pain that the horse will be in.

Nursing care

The surgeon will require assistance in the workup of the horse, to help with radiographs, lab tests, clipping and prepping the site and obtaining the relevant samples. A circulating RVN will be required during surgery, GA or standing and RVNs can change the bandage in the days following surgery and help if repeated samples or imaging is required.

Disorders of the Sense Organs

Ocular Conditions

Eyelid Abnormalities

Foals can be born with a condition called entropion, where the eyelids roll inwards causing the hairs to rub the cornea. This can be easily resolved by placing sutures at the lid margin to unroll the eyelid. Tumours are common in horses' eyelids, these may be sarcoids, squamous cell carcinomas, melanomas or mast cell tumours. Tumours in the eyelid are not usually noticed until they are quite large. Diagnosis can be made by taking a biopsy of the lump, or diagnosis and treatment may be combined with the tumour being surgically removed and sent away for histopathology. Other treatments may include cryotherapy and chemotherapy. Whichever method is chosen, extreme care must be taken to avoid damaging the eye.

Conjunctivitis

Inflammation of the conjunctiva is common in horses. The cause can be primary or secondary, and the condition can be unilateral or bilateral. Primary causes include foreign bodies, trauma, flies during the summer months and allergens. Secondary causes can be corneal ulcers, uveitis, blocked nasolacrimal ducts and systemic viral and bacterial infections.

Clinical Signs

- Red/pink conjunctiva
- Swollen eyelid
- Excessive discharge from the eye
- Mild discomfort characterised by not fully opening the eye.

Diagnosis

- History and clinical signs, bilateral conjunctivitis is more likely to be linked to a systemic condition
- Ophthalmic examination to rule out more serious conditions

Treatment

This will vary dependent on the cause of the conjunctivitis but may include antibiotic and anti-inflammatory eye drops.

Corneal Ulceration

A corneal ulcer is an inflammatory condition that causes disruption to the epithelial layer of the eye. The ulcer is usually caused by a trauma but can be due to a secondary infection. Horses with corneal ulcers should be seen as an emergency case. Corneal ulcers can lead to enucleation. Secondary uveitis is common, so this should be investigated and treated if diagnosed.

Clinical Signs

- Ocular pain
- Conjunctivitis
- Blepharospasm (abnormal contraction of the eyelids)
- Corneal oedema
- Excessive tearing
- Light sensitivity

Diagnosis

- Clinical signs
- Thorough ocular examination including fluorescein dye, that will stain damaged corneal epithelium green (Information Box 13.2).

Treatment

Corneal ulcers in well-behaved or less painful horses can be treated topically with antibiotics, serum, EDTA and systemically with NSAIDs. Difficult or painful horses and

---

Information Box 13.2 Ocular examination requirements

Environment

For a thorough and effective ocular examination to take place, an area of daylight should be available for the visual inspection of the face and eyes. A darkened area will also be required for ophthalmic examination of the eyes.

Ocular examination equipment

- Pen torch – to test dazzle reflex, pupillary light reflexes and assess pupil size
- Ophthalmoscope – to assess the retina and optic disc
- Slit lamp – to assess the cornea, iris and lens
- Tonometer – to assess intraocular pressure

- Ultrasound scanner – usually performed with the eyelid closed and a probe placed on the upper eyelid, but the probe can be placed directly onto the eye for better images. Used to assess the cornea, aqueous humour, lens, iris, ciliary body, vitreous humour, retina and retro-bulbar space
- Fluorescein stain and saline to rinse the stain out of the eye – to check for corneal ulcers

For in-depth examinations, sedation, topical eye local anaesthetic and nerve blocks are likely to be needed. A soft 6f dog catheter may be used to check for blockage of the nasolacrimal ducts.

Source: Victoria Gregory.

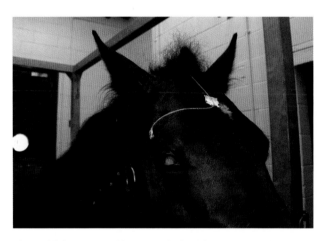

Figure 13.6 Horse with a subpalpebral lavage system in place and fluorescein dye in the eye. *Source:* Victoria Gregory.

more severe ulcers may require a subpalpebral lavage system to be placed to administer medications easily and frequently to the cornea (see Figure 13.6). Treats may still be required to make the administration of medication into a positive experience for the horse. Regular examinations of the eye should be carried out to monitor for any improvement or deterioration of the ulcer, every two to three days. The ulcer may need debriding, or a keratotomy may be beneficial to help with healing. In severe cases, surgery to perform a conjunctival graft or enucleation may be required.

Nursing Care

Ocular conditions are extremely painful, so the patient should be pain-scored regularly. RVNs may be required to teach owners how to apply topical eye medications, or use the subpalpebral lavage system. Eye masks can help

to protect the eye from further damage, but can also cause sores from rubbing on the face and head. The case vet will decide if the use of a mask is appropriate on a case-by-case basis. The stable should be adapted to ensure that the horse cannot cause more trauma to the eye by rubbing it. Due to the pain and administration of opioid medications such as atropine, horses with eye conditions are at a higher risk of developing impaction colic, so their diet should be made up of laxative feeds, and their faecal output monitored.

Keratitis

Keratitis is inflammation of the cornea. In the United Kingdom, there are different types including immune mediated, chronic deep and infectious keratitis that can be viral, bacterial or fungal. Keratitis is likely to only affect one eye but sometimes both eyes, so it is important to examine both eyes regularly.

Clinical Signs

- Ocular pain
- Conjunctivitis
- Blepharospasm
- Corneal oedema
- Excessive tearing
- Light sensitivity

Diagnosis

- Clinical signs
- Thorough ocular examination including culture from the eye before any topical solutions are applied. The culture result can help to distinguish between keratitis and corneal ulcers

Treatment

This will depend on the type and cause of the keratitis. Some types of keratitis can be progressive, so management of the condition is needed. Slow-releasing medication implants can be placed into the eye for long-term treatment.

Nursing Care

This will be the same as for corneal ulceration, please see above.

Cataracts

This is a cloudy area in the lens of an eye, or its capsule, that causes a decrease in vision and can progress to blindness. Cataracts can be unilateral or bilateral and, in some cases, inherited. Some foals are born with, it but acquired causes include inflammation, trauma, toxicity, diet and metabolic conditions. Uveitis can be found in some horses with cataracts.

Clinical Signs

- Cloudiness or opacity of the eye
- Owner concerns of blindness/impaired vision
- Incidental finding on vetting

Diagnosis

- Clinical signs
- Test the horse's vision unsedated by getting them to step over poles and place objects for them to avoid
- Thorough ocular examination to diagnose and assess how much vision has been lost.

Treatment

Mild cataracts will not require treatment. Surgery can be performed for severe and congenital cases. Any underlying trauma or uveitis will require treatment.

Uveitis

Uveitis in horses is a common cause of blindness. The inflammation of the iris, ciliary body and choroid, all part of the uvea, hampers the blood supply to the whole eye. Uveitis can be a secondary condition that is less severe and resolves once the primary condition is treated, but it can also be a primary condition. The cause of primary uveitis is not known, it can be hereditary in some breeds and it can reoccur, known as equine recurrent uveitis (ERU).

Clinical Signs

- Ocular pain
- Excessive tear production
- Blepharospasm
- Corneal oedema
- Conjunctivitis
- Constricted pupil
- Injected blood vessels around the eye
- Light sensitivity

Diagnosis

- Clinical signs
- History of previous uveitis
- Thorough ocular examination

ERU can cause damage to other parts of the eye, including cataracts, retinal degeneration, glaucoma and adhesions.

Treatment

Treatment will depend on the cause and type of uveitis diagnosed, but may include topical and systemic anti-inflammatories, NSAIDs and corticosteroids. Atropine may be used to dilate the pupil. A subpalpebral lavage system may be used to administer medications to the eye carefully and frequently. As mentioned previously, the stable should be made safe so that the horse cannot cause any more trauma to the eye, and the faecal output should be monitored.

Aural conditions

Otitis Externa

Otitis externa is inflammation of the external ear canal, it is not commonly seen in horses. It may be caused by a foreign body, ticks or an allergy.

Clinical Signs

- Head shaking
- Head tilt
- Ear droop
- Rubbing/scratching ear
- Discharge from the ear
- Swelling
- Painful to palpate

Diagnosis

- Clinical signs
- Visual inspection of the ear
- Otoscopy to rule out internal ear problem
- Hearing check – loud clapping out of sight to see their reaction
- Culture of discharge

Treatment

This will depend on the cause and the culture results. All cases should start with topical cleaning of the ear, after the initial examination has been carried out.

Nursing Care

The horse may need daily ear cleaning and medications, this can be done by an RVN, or the RVN can teach the owner if the horse is being treated at home.

Hepatic Disease

Hepatitis

Inflammation of the liver in horses is difficult to diagnose early on as the clinical signs do not start to show until the liver is severely damaged, unable to regenerate and starting to fail. Hepatitis can be caused by toxins, bacteria, viruses, parasites, gastrointestinal disease and serum sickness. Liver disease in horses is often fatal.

Clinical Signs

As previously mentioned, clinical signs do not start to appear until the horse is close to liver failure. These signs include:

- Inappetence
- Jaundice
- Colic signs
- Lethargy
- Ventral oedema
- Diarrhoea
- Weight loss
- Photosensitisation (sensitivity to ultraviolet rays from sunlight) (see Chapter 14 for further information)
- Hepatic encephalopathy (brain dysfunction caused by liver insufficiency)

Diagnosis

- Clinical signs
- Ultrasonography of the liver
- Liver biopsy
- Haematology sample to run biochemistry tests. An increase in glutamate dehydrogenase, aspartate aminotransferase and gamma glutamyl transferase are all indicators of liver disease (see Chapter 8 for further information).

Treatment

Treatment will depend on the cause and the severity of the disease. If there is a known cause, for example, ragwort poisoning, this should be addressed, and field companions may need to be tested also. IVFT, vitamins and antioxidants may be administered. For horses with hepatic encephalopathy, a low dose of sedation may be required to keep them calm and humans safe while treating them. The horse's diet should be adjusted to a low protein and high carbohydrate diet.

Nursing Care

In severe cases these patients will require intensive nursing care and follow up haematology samples to monitor the liver function.

Fluke

Liver fluke is a parasite commonly found in grazing sheep and cattle but can also be found in horses. Immature fluke migrate, causing damage to the liver tissue and the adult fluke can cause damage in the bile ducts. Horses that graze with sheep or cattle are at a higher risk of having liver fluke, so they should be tested regularly as the clinical signs will not present until significant damage to the liver has occurred. There is no routine treatment for liver fluke in horses, so the vet will prescribe medication using the cascade (see Chapter 9 for further information). If liver damage is present, the treatment will be the same as for hepatitis.

Ragwort

Ragwort poisoning is a fatal condition in horses. As with other liver conditions, the damage is not noticed until it is severe. Horses usually ingest the ragwort while out grazing in their paddock or in hay that is fed to them. If the ragwort is in the hay, the owner may not be aware of its presence. The clinical signs will be the same as for hepatitis, and so will the diagnosis. On the liver biopsy, ragwort poisoning can be tested for to give a definitive diagnosis. All horses grazing on the pasture or eating the hay should be stopped from ingesting the suspected food source immediately and have haematology samples taken to test for liver damage. Treatment will be similar to hepatitis cases.

Diseases of the Skin and Coat

Dermatophilus Congolensis

This is a gram-positive bacterium that causes mud fever and rain scald in horses. These conditions are more commonly seen during the winter when the paddocks and tracks are extremely muddy, and the horses' legs, back and rump are exposed to prolonged periods of rain. The bacteria require an entry point, usually caused by moisture, including excessive washing, rough bedding or exercise surface such as stubble fields, fly bites or small cuts and grazes. Feathers can protect from the condition, but can also make the condition worse as the legs will stay moist for longer once wet.

Clinical Signs

- Itchy legs
- Scabs and crusts found on the area affected
- Swelling
- Cracking of the skin
- Pain

Diagnosis

- Clinical signs
- Biopsy for histopathology
- Cytologic examination of the crust

Treatment

- The scabs will need to be removed, this may require sedation or sweat wraps overnight to soften the scabs
- Clipping the affected area
- Bathing the affected area daily, for a week, with dilute chlorhexidine, rinsing and drying thoroughly afterwards
- Applying zinc or antibiotic cream once the leg is dry
- Keeping the horse in a clean and dry environment until healed
- Systemic antibiotics may be required in severe cases

Nursing Care

An RVN can carry out the above treatment if the horse is hospitalised or the owner is unable to carry out the treatment themselves. Preventative care is best so owners should be educated on how to avoid further infection.

Dermatophytosis

Dermatophytosis, otherwise known as 'ringworm' is a contagious fungal infection, caused by *Tricophyton sp.* and *Microsporum sp.*, that enters the skin where it is broken. This is commonly in sweaty areas where tack and rugs have been. Dermatophytosis is zoonotic, so gloves should be used when handling these patients; it can be transmitted directly and indirectly on fomites and will live in wood for many years. In veterinary hospitals, clipper blades can be a common fomite. Immunosuppressed and young horses can be at higher risk of contracting the disease; immunity can occur as the horse gets older.

Clinical Signs

- Ring like raised lesions (can be any shape)
- Hair loss
- Dry and scaly skin

Diagnosis

- Clinical signs
- Skin scarping/hair pluck for microscopy, culture and quantitative polymerase chain reaction (qPCR) testing

Treatment

Dermatophytosis should self-resolve within a few months, but treatment can decrease the severity of the condition.

- Clip the area
- Remove scabs using dilute chlorohexidine
- Bathe in anti-fungal shampoo three times over a one-week period
- Apply anti-fungal topical treatment as directed by the vet

Nursing Care

These patients need to be isolated from others and humans need to take measures to protect themselves. Items used with the patient such as grooming, feeding, mucking out, rug and tack equipment will all need to be disinfected to avoid further spread of the disease. More information on biosecurity can be found in Chapter 6.

Sarcoids

Sarcoids are the most common skin tumours in horses. There are six different types: occult, verrucose, nodular, fibroblastic, mixed and malevolent and they all differ in appearance. The cause of sarcoids is unknown, but it is thought to be a genetic predisposition linked to papillomavirus and insect transmission. Sarcoids commonly start to appear when the horse is between three and six years of age but can develop later. The most common sites for sarcoids to be located are around the eyes and mouth, chest, axilla, ventral abdomen, udder, sheath and inner thigh.

Clinical Signs

- New growths appearing

Diagnosis

- Appearance – biopsy is not advised as cutting into a sarcoid can cause it to grow
- Histology

Treatment

There are many different treatment options with varied success rates. Some sarcoids, such as occult and verrucous, may be best left alone as they can become more aggressive if aggravated. The location of the sarcoid, and its size, will also determine the treatment type. Some treatments may include:

- Surgical removal
- Laser surgery
- Cryotherapy
- Localised chemotherapy
- Electrochemotherapy
- Immunotherapy
- Radiation therapy
- Ligation
- Topical treatment

Nursing Care

Discharge from around the surgery site may need to be cleaned daily following surgery, and a barrier cream applied to the surrounding area to protect it from scalding.

Appropriate PPE measures should be put into place if using chemotherapy, radiation therapy and other toxic medications.

Melanomas

These are tumours that can be benign or malignant and can metastasise. They are most often seen in the skin of grey horses, presenting as firm, nodular lumps that are black. They can occur internally and on any colour horse. Common sites for these to be found are the lips, eyes, ears, guttural pouches, neck, perianal region and the ventral tail. In the perianal region, the tumour can grow larger than a tennis ball. Melanomas are usually only treated if they are causing the horse to have other problems. Large melanomas in the perianal region may cause discomfort when passing faeces and block the rectum. Tumours in the guttural pouches can cause difficulty breathing or impinge on nerves. Treatment can include surgical excision or debulking, laser surgery, chemotherapy, cryotherapy and melanoma vaccination. The vaccination is still in a trial phase and is expensive. There is no cure for melanomas, but they can be managed long-term. Horses should have their melanomas checked regularly to monitor the growth rate and to check for signs of secondary problems. Horses with large perianal melanomas will need to be fed a laxative diet to decrease the risk of rectal impactions.

Infectious Diseases Viral and Bacterial

Streptococcus equi (Strangles)

Streptococcus equi is a gram-positive bacterium that affects horses. It is a respiratory infection that damages the epithelium lining, causes abscesses in lymph nodes and can be systemic, causing abscesses in the abdomen and thorax. The disease is highly contagious, and horses showing clinical signs should be isolated immediately. The infection usually lasts for three to four weeks but some horses can be carriers, and the infection can be present, without clinical signs, for many years. In some cases, the bacteria may spread to produce metastatic abscesses in other lymph nodes and organs. The two main sites affected are the thorax and the abdomen. This leads to a chronic syndrome known as 'bastard strangles' and this may last for several months. Bastard strangles is difficult to diagnose and treat and therefore carries a guarded prognosis.

Streptococcus equi is not airborne but passed by nasal secretions (snorting, coughing, nose-to-nose contact) and by fomites. Horses can be vaccinated against *Streptococcus equi* with two primary intramuscular injections followed by annual boosters.

Clinical Signs

- Purulent nasal discharge
- Pyrexia
- Dull demeanour
- Inappetence
- Lymph node abscesses
- Pus or chondroids in guttural pouches
- Incidental finding on endoscopy

Diagnosis

Diagnosis can be difficult with results returning negative even though the horse has clinical signs. Any horse with clinical signs should be isolated immediately, and no horses in the yard should be moved until the yard is free from infection. A guttural pouch wash, acquired using an endoscope, should be submitted for culture, cytology and PCR testing (Information Box 13.3). A blood sample for serology can be submitted; this may not detect the disease in the first two-week period but will show a rise in antibody response if a paired sample is taken two weeks later. This is useful for diagnosing carriers of the disease. If the horse has an open draining abscess a swab can be taken from this and submitted for culture and PCR. The traditional nasopharyngeal swab is very unreliable; a guttural pouch wash is now preferred.

Information Box 13.3   Procedure and equipment for a guttural pouch wash

Guttural pouch wash equipment

- Endoscope
- Endoscopic flushing catheter
- ± guttural pouch wire
- 30 mL of sterile saline per guttural pouch
- Universal container × 1 or 2 – some vets will submit a sample for each guttural pouch, but others may put both samples into one pot, this may be case dependent
- ± sedation and nose twitch

Procedure

- Pass endoscope
- Enter guttural pouch, you may be able to use the endoscopic flushing catheter to open the flap to guide the endoscope in but if not, you will need the guttural pouch wire
- Flush 30 mL saline into the guttural pouch
- Place end of endoscopic flushing catheter into pool of fluid and draw back on syringe
- Place acquired fluid into universal container
- Repeat for second guttural pouch

Source: Victoria Gregory.

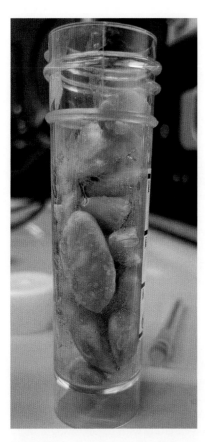

Figure 13.7 Chondroids removed from a guttural pouch using an endoscopic snare. *Source:* Victoria Gregory.

Treatment

Many horses will be treated at the yard with NSAIDs and possibly penicillin, but this is vet dependent. Horses with abscesses should have them hot packed, to encourage maturation and bursting, and if they do not burst by themselves, they will need to be drained or lanced. If a horse starts to show signs of respiratory distress, they may need to be hospitalised and have a temporary tracheostomy tube placed. If the horse has pus-filled guttural pouches, they should be lavaged daily and penicillin mixed with gelatin can be applied topically. Indwelling guttural pouch catheters may be placed for easy daily topical application of medications. Chondroids should be removed by endoscopic snare or basket (Figure 13.7). If they are too large, surgery may be required.

Nursing Care

Strict isolation measures should be adhered to until the horse is proven to be negative for *Streptococcus equi*. Please refer to Chapter 6 for information on isolation protocols. Horses should be monitored for respiratory distress and signs of deterioration. Endoscopy may be required on a daily or less frequent basis to lavage the guttural pouches. Endoscopes and equipment should be cleaned and sterilised appropriately to prevent the infection of other horses. Local owners should be educated on strangles, especially on preventative measures when introducing new horses to the yard.

See Chapter 6 for further information on infectious diseases.

13.2 Pathophysiological States and Common Pathologies Affecting Patients

Sensory Impairment

Blindness

Blindness can be an acute onset caused by trauma to the eye, brain, optic nerve and disease of the central nervous system. A slower onset of blindness may be caused by primary ocular conditions such as equine recurrent uveitis, cataracts, glaucoma or neoplasia. Blindness can also be seen at birth with some congenital conditions. Owners may notice their horse becoming blind when it starts to bump into things or when its behaviour changes. It is not always obvious looking at the eye that the horse is blind. Horses can cope very well with blindness in one or both eyes but should be retired from exercise if blind in both eyes. Enucleation is only necessary if the eye is causing pain to the horse.

Deafness

Equine deafness is rare but can be linked to a congenital condition, head trauma, ear infection and inflammation, old age or ototoxicity caused by gentamicin. A lack of response to loud noises can indicate that a horse is deaf and being startled by things that would not normally have caused a problem, is another sign. Owners may notice these as behaviour changes. A simple clapping or banging, out of sight of the horse, can help with diagnosis of deafness.

Senility

Equine senility can be hard to diagnose because the signs horses display can be signs of pain, blindness, deafness, colic and many other conditions. It is most often linked to old age but can be linked to conditions affecting the brain, such as trauma or encephalitis. Owners report aimless wandering, seeming confused by their normal routine, behavioural changes such as overreacting or underreacting compared to usual, standing facing the corner of the stable, lethargy and not interacting with field companions. There has not been much veterinary research carried out into equine senility, making it harder to diagnose.

Depression

Depression in horses is most often a clinical sign of pain but can be a stand-alone condition. The horse will often look dull with its head hanging low. A change of yard, routine or field/stable mate can all be triggers for equine depression along with stress. The pain is most likely to be chronic, low-grade pain, as opposed to acute, severe, painful colic, laminitis or a fracture that is usually shown more dramatically. Depression can be linked to conditions such as hepatic disease, cardiac disease, colitis, lymphangitis, ocular conditions, dental disease, viruses and atypical myopathy. Pyrexia can also cause horses to look depressed.

Distress

This may also be caused by pain or maybe a behaviour shown as a reaction to a change of yard, routine or field/stable mate. This may be a severe pain linked to colic, or other conditions where the horse cannot cope with the pain when it is stood still. It can also be a sign of a neurological condition. Signs of distress include box walking, yawning, appearing agitated and restlessness.

Reduced Mobility

Lethargy

Lots of conditions may cause lethargy. Clinical signs include looking dull, tired, yawning and lying down or sleeping more often. Again, like depression, these can be linked to conditions such as hepatic disease, cardiac disease, colitis, lymphatic disease, ocular conditions, dental disease, viruses, endocrine disorders and atypical myopathy. Lethargy is commonly associated with pyrexia.

Ataxia

This can be caused by trauma to the brain or spinal cord and conditions such as hypoparathyroidism, cervical vertebral stenotic myelopathy, equine herpes virus-1 (EHV-1) and weakness. The horse appears wobbly with poor coordination and balance.

Paresis

Weakness of the muscles is most often linked to neurological conditions such as diseases or trauma but can be due to malnourishment. It can look like ataxia, with the horse appearing wobbly and uncoordinated.

Paralysis

A single limb paralysis can be caused by trauma to the nerve, from a kick or from poor positioning during a GA. Hemiplegia, paralysis of one side of the body, can be due to nerve damage, a brain tumour or stroke. Fractures and spinal cord damage in the thoracic and lumbar region can cause hindlimb paralysis, while similar damage in the sacral region can also include loss of tail tone and incontinence. Fractures and spinal cord damage in the cervical region can cause paralysis of all four limbs. EHV-1 can cause complete paralysis.

Impaired Nutrition

Anorexia

Equine anorexia, or inappetence, can be due to pain from any part of the horse but abdominal, dental and sinus pain are usually investigated, if no obvious causes of pain are seen externally on the horse. Purulent discharge from the teeth, sinuses and guttural pouches may put a horse off eating, as well as areas of swelling in or near the mouth and throat regions. Some medications, such as metronidazole, can cause anorexia even if they are not being administered orally, as they cause a feeling of nausea. Oral medications being added to feed may cause a horse not to eat that feed, but they are not truly anorexic as they will eat hay and grass or feeds without medications.

Obesity

Excessive body fat accumulation in horses can be caused by EMS, as a side effect of medications such as steroids, or because of poor management. If the risk of obesity is known, due to a medical condition, a reason to stop exercise or medication that is required, it is important that the horse's diet is managed carefully with regular weight monitoring. Obesity can lead to laminitis, which can be fatal, as well as causing damage to organs and joints.

Cachexia

Cachexia is weakness and wasting of the muscles that is caused by an underlying illness rather than nutritional factors on its own. It can be caused by chronic illnesses such as equine dysautonomia (grass sickness), cancer and equine motor neuron disease.

Metabolic Disturbance

Weight Loss

Weight loss can be seen in patients known to be suffering from inappetence, and it can be seen with clinical signs of conditions such as chronic renal failure, PPID, hepatitis and horses with a high worm burden. Horses suffering from weight loss might have dental problems that are causing the weight loss, so their teeth should be examined.

Dehydration

Dehydration can be a primary problem linked to a lack of access to water, in the winter when it freezes, or in the summer when natural water sources dry up, which then leads to problems such as impaction colic. Dehydration can also be secondary in medical conditions where there is an excess loss of fluids and electrolytes due to diarrhoea or sweating, such as colitis-X, salmonellosis, high worm burden, hepatitis, lymphoma and severe pyrexia. Signs of dehydration may include dullness, lethargy, skin tenting, tacky mucous membranes and a high packed cell volume.

Polydipsia

A consistent increase in water intake can be linked to PPID and CRF, but it can also psychogenic due to boredom in the stabled horse. With automatic water drinkers, the water intake cannot be monitored. If a horse is suspected to have polydipsia or a condition linked to it, the water drinker should be sealed off and water offered in buckets instead so that the horse's water intake can be measured. An increase in urine output is usually a sign of polydipsia.

Respiratory Embarrassment

Short, shallow and rapid breathing, at rest, can be a sign pyrexia and pain or linked to an airway trauma or obstruction, diaphragmatic hernia, pleuropneumonia and more commonly severe equine asthma. Horses with dorsal displacement of the soft palate or recurrent laryngeal neuropathy may show respiratory embarrassment post-exercise but not at rest.

13.3 Abnormal Diagnostic Test Results

Laboratory tests are essential in many medical conditions to help to confirm a diagnosis. More information on how to obtain, run and package laboratory samples can be found in Chapter 8.

Adult Clinical Pathology Values

It is important to know the normal range, but it is also helpful to understand what an abnormal result might be indicative of. Results will vary between breed, age and condition, so it is important to think about the horse as an individual. Different machines may use different units of measurement, so it is important to use a reference range that matches up with the laboratory machine in each individual practice. Table 13.2 provides a guide to adult clinical pathology values. This Table is to be used as a guide only, reference ranges vary; it is therefore a good idea for each practice to have a reference range guide that all the vets agree on and use.

Cerebrospinal Fluid

Cerebrospinal fluid (CSF) can be collected from the lumbosacral space, in standing horses, or under a GA from the atlanto-occipital space. Aspiration of CSF is undertaken in horses with neurological signs to help differentiate between trauma and disease. Normal CSF should appear colourless, clear and have low viscosity. The total protein should be between 1 and 12 g/L; an increase will be indicative of inflammation and infection and cause the fluid to become turbid. There are no red blood cells in CSF, but the sample usually contains some due to the way the sample is collected. A red blood cell count higher than 0.6×10^9/L indicates trauma. An increased white cell count indicates infection with the normal range being 0–7/µL. Creatinine kinase, lactate, sodium, potassium and chloride levels can also change during trauma, or disease, and help with diagnosis.

Peritoneal Fluid

Peritoneal fluid analysis is useful when assessing horses showing colic signs as it can help to diagnose peritonitis and to differentiate between a medical colic and a surgical colic (Table 13.3). With peritonitis, the white cell count will be increased and the fluid will be yellow to turbid. In severe cases, the fluid may be too thick to flow through a needle or teat cannula. A culture and sensitivity test is useful for the correct treatment of cases with peritonitis. In medical and surgical cases, the white cell count may be increased due to inflammation. The colour change in surgical cases can reflect blood from the intestines, or even a rupture meaning that gut content is in the peritoneal cavity. Total protein will increase if infection or inflammation is present. An increased lactate is indicative of a strangulating lesion that requires surgery [8].

Synovial Fluid

Synovial fluid is often analysed when there is a suspected communication between a wound and a joint, sheath or bursa. Sepsis can also occur after synovial structure medication or synovial aspiration, so history taking is important as there will be no wound to see. The white blood cell count, total protein, appearance and possibly culture and sensitivity (if the sample is suggestive of infection) will be analysed routinely for these samples. An increase in total protein, from the normal <20 g/L, can relate to inflammation and sepsis. The normal white cell count is $<5 \times 10^9$/L and the neutrophil percentage is <10. Both parameters increase with inflammation and infection, and all three parameters tend to be higher with infection than inflammation. Synovial fluid should be clear, pale yellow and tacky or stringy in viscosity. With trauma and aspiration, the fluid may become serosanguineous or blood-contaminated and may appear turbid if the infection is present.

Table 13.2 Adult clinical pathology values.

Test and unit of measurement	Normal range	Decreased result indicative of examples	Increased result indicative of examples
Total erythrocytes $\times10^{12}$/L	6.2–10.2	Anaemia, haemolysis, chronic disease	Pulmonary disease
Mean cell volume fl	37–55	Iron deficiency, chronic disease	Anaemia, haemorrhage
Mean cell haemoglobin pg	13–19	Anaemia	Intravascular haemolysis
Mean cell haemoglobin concentration %	31–36	Anaemia	Intravascular haemolysis
Haemoglobin g/dl	11–19	Anaemia	Chronic disease, severe equine asthma
Packed cell volume %	32–53	Blood loss, anaemia, decreased erythrocyte production	Dehydration, stress, excitement, endotoxic shock
Total leukocytes $\times10^9$/L	5.5–10	Acute severe infection	Infection, parasites, inflammation, stress
Neutrophils $\times10^9$/L	2.7–7	Excessive demand, endotoxemia, bone marrow suppression	Inflammation, bacterial infection, stress, corticosteroid use
Lymphocytes $\times10^9$/L	1.5–4	Viral infection, stress, corticosteroid use	Viral infection
Monocytes $\times10^9$/L	0–0.5	N/A	Chronic inflammation, tissue damage
Eosinophils $\times10^9$/L	0–0.6	N/A	Disease of intestines, skin, lungs, allergy, hypersensitivity disease
Platelets $\times10^9$/L	100–350	Equine infectious anaemia, lack of production, disseminated intravascular coagulation	Inflammation
Total protein g/L	53–75	Protein losing conditions, excessive fluid therapy, gastrointestinal insults, peritonitis, NSAID toxicity	Dehydration, increased globulin
Serum amyloid A mg/L	0–20	N/A	Inflammation
Creatinine kinase iu/L	110–270	N/A	Rhabdomyolysis, mild increases linked to transportation, exercise, general anaesthesia
Albumin g/L	23–39	Colitis, liver disease, inflammatory disease, malnutrition, parasites, NSAID toxicity	Severe dehydration
Aspartate aminotransferase iu/L	120–340	N/A	Liver disease, liver failure, myopathy, rhabdomyolysis, liver fluke
Urea mmol/L	2.5–8	Liver failure, low-protein diet, anabolic steroid use	Azotaemia, ruptured bladder, renal failure, heart failure
Creatinine μmol/L	85–170	N/A	Azotaemia, ruptured bladder, renal failure, heart failure
Glucose mmol/L	4.3–6	Starvation, malabsorption, septicaemia, liver failure	PPID, EMS, Xylazine administration
Total bilirubin μmol/L	9–39	N/A	Anorexia, haemolysis, liver related obstructions
Sodium mmol/L	134–142	Diarrhoea, reflux, renal disease, peritonitis, ruptured bladder	Dehydration, salt poisoning
Triglycerides mmol/L	0.2–1.2	N/A	PPID, EMS, lipaemia
Calcium mmol	2.9–3.5	Renal failure, lack of food, decreased total calcium concentration, gastrointestinal insults	Chronic renal disease, excessive supplementation, hyperparathyroidism, plant toxicosis, neoplasms

Table 13.2 (Continued)

Test and unit of measurement	Normal range	Decreased result indicative of examples	Increased result indicative of examples
Potassium mmol/L	3–5	Post major surgery, anorexia, gastrointestinal losses, alkalaemia	Urine leaking into the peritoneal cavity (uroperitoneum), oliguria, insulin deficiency
Magnesium mmol/L	0.6–1	Intestinal disease, renal failure	Renal failure, magnesium sulphate overdose
Gamma glutamyl transferase iu/L	1–40	N/A	Liver disease, liver failure, myopathy, rhabdomyolysis, liver fluke
Adrenocorticotropic hormone (ACTH) pg/ml	November–July <30 July–November <50	N/A	PPID

Source: Victoria Gregory.

Table 13.3 Properties of peritoneal fluid.

Feature	Normal range	Medical colic	Surgical colic
Colour	Clear, pale yellow	Slightly turbid, yellow	Clear or turbid, yellow, red, brown
Total protein (g/L)	<25	6.2–20.6	14.6–82.3
White cell count ($\times 10^9$/L)	<5–10	1.1–9.4	1.4–11
Lactate mmol/L	<1	<4	>4

Source: Victoria Gregory.

Pleural Fluid

If pleuritis or pleuropneumonia are suspected, thoracocentesis should be carried out. The pleural fluid aspirated should be reddish yellow in colour, only being able to collect approximately 2–8 mL, with a white cell count of $<5 \times 10^9$/L and a total protein of <25 g/L. With pleuropneumonia there will be excess fluid, which is turbid and may contain fibrinous tissue. Culture and sensitivity should be run on this sample so that a treatment plan can be made. Increased white cell count and total protein are indicative of infection and inflammation.

Urine

Colour and Consistency

Urine can vary greatly between individual horses in its colour and consistency, from pale yellow to brown and clear to turbid. A change in colour can be linked to hydration status or illness. Renal failure can cause pale urine that is lacking in crystals. Dark red/brown urine can be seen in horses with rhabdomyolysis and myopathy due to an increase in myoglobin produced by damaged muscle cells, and blood can be seen in horses with cystitis, urolithiasis and urinary tract trauma. Excess protein and crystals can cause cloudiness in the urine.

Microscopic Analysis

In addition to looking at the urine, to check its colour and consistency, it will also be evaluated under the microscope for casts, cylindrical structures produced by the kidneys suggesting renal tubular disease, white blood cells, red blood cells, epithelial cells and bacteria. An increase in epithelial cells can indicate inflammation or neoplasia; white blood cells and bacteria can increase due to infection and inflammation. An increase in red blood cells will suggest haemorrhage but can be a result of trauma from catheterisation, so this will need to be considered. It can also indicate neoplasia.

Urine Specific Gravity

This is measured on a refractometer and should be between 1.020 and 1.050. Dipsticks can also measure the specific gravity but not as accurately. A low urine specific gravity may indicate renal problems and chronic liver disease. An increased result is indicative of severe dehydration.

Chemicals

These can be tested quickly using a dipstick to check the urine pH, protein levels and the abnormal presence of glucose, bilirubin, ketones, haemoglobin and myoglobin. If these are present, a sample should be submitted for further analysis. A decrease in the normal pH range of 7.0–9.0 can suggest the horse is hypokalemic or has renal tubular acidosis. An increase in proteins can be due to a lower urinary tract infection or renal failure. The presence of glucose can be due to stress or PPID. The presence of bilirubin and ketones are rarely seen in horses. Haemoglobin may be present following trauma or if the horse is suffering from a haemolytic condition. As mentioned previously, horses with myopathies may have myoglobin in their urine.

Faeces

Colour and Consistency

On first appearance, faeces may be very firm or extremely watery indicating an abnormality with the horse, such as impaction or diarrhoea. Endoparasites may be visible in the faeces on rare occasions. If the faecal balls have a covering of mucous, this suggests that the faeces have passed through the gastrointestinal tract (GIT) very slowly due to gastrointestinal disease. This can be a result of a mild case of impaction colic or a more severe condition such as equine dysautonomia that has caused the decrease in gastrointestinal motility. Occult (old/dark) blood suggests an insult towards the beginning of the GIT, whereas frank (fresh) blood could be due to a rectal tear. If a sand impaction is suspected, faeces can be mixed with water in a clear bag or rectal sleeve and hung up for a few hours to settle out. Sand is heavy, so it will fall to the bottom of the mixture. An abdominal radiograph can also confirm the presence, and amount, of sand in the patient.

Microscopic Analysis

This will be used when carrying out faecal worm egg counts. The most common McMaster method will show up strongyle eggs. The accepted range for eggs is <200 eggs per gram. If more are present, the horse will require treatment for parasite burden. See Chapter 8 for more information.

Disease Detection

If a horse has diarrhoea, three faecal samples taken at 12-hour intervals should be submitted for testing. *Salmonella* culture, clostridia toxins and equine coronavirus are all recommended tests for horses with diarrhoea. If submitting samples, these horses should be treated as infectious until the negative results are received.

Respiratory Samples

Tracheal wash samples can help diagnose respiratory inflammation, if there are more than 5% leucocytes present, and help in the diagnosis of the bacteria present, if there is no contamination. The presence of epithelial cells or plant material indicates contamination on entry to the trachea, and so the bacteriology results are of no use. If a patient is suspected to have pneumonia a transtracheal wash should be performed in a sterile fashion. This test decreases the risk of sample contamination from the upper airway. This sample can be submitted for culture and sensitivity to help diagnose the bacteria present and to guide the vet on the correct antibiotic to use. Bronchoalveolar lavage (BAL) samples are used mostly for cytology, as it is impossible to pass the tube without contamination from the upper airway. The sample should have some white foam in, as a result of coming into contact with the surfactant. An increase in leucocytes, in both samples, will indicate inflammation, this may be caused by recurrent airway obstruction, inflammatory airway disease or an infectious lung disease. Exercise-induced pulmonary haemorrhage can be diagnosed from a tracheal wash or BAL, within 90 minutes of exercise, using cytology. When investigating respiratory conditions, both a tracheal wash sample and BAL sample should be collected, in the hope that a good cytology sample and a good bacteriology sample have been obtained.

Skin and Hair

Hair plucks can be used to identify ringworm and rain scald in horses; they can be looked at microscopically and used for bacterial and fungal culture. A dermatophyte (ringworm) qPCR test is also available in the United Kingdom. Skin brushings will be examined using a microscope to look for mites and lice. Skin scrapes can also be used for the identification of ectoparasites, ringworms or rain scalds. If there are fresh scabs on the skin, an impression smear can be made so that the laboratory can test for mud fever and rain scald. *Oxyuris equi* (pinworm) eggs can be collected from the perineum using Sellotape and then identified under the microscope. If there is an open, discharging area, a swab can be used to collect a sample from the site and be submitted for bacterial culture. Fine needle aspirates can be collected from lesions; this can be submitted for cytology to help differentiate between haematomas, seromas, melanomas and sarcoids. The appearance or lack of fluid may also help in the diagnosis when using fine needle aspiration.

Biopsies

Biopsies can be taken and submitted for histopathology from various sites on the horse. The results can diagnose a condition, rule out a condition and help the vet to confirm if they have successfully removed the whole of a sarcoid or tumour. Usually, a few biopsies within the affected site or diagnostic area are sampled, to ensure the laboratory have enough good-quality samples to test and to identify different changes in the tissue from the areas. Some examples of biopsies and relating conditions are skin biopsies to help diagnose tumours, mud fever or rain scald. Ileal biopsies are used to diagnose equine dysautonomia (grass sickness), liver biopsy is used to diagnose ragwort poisoning or hepatitis and rectal biopsy is used to look for intestinal diseases in cases of weight loss. Endometrial biopsies may be taken routinely or when mares are barren to look for signs of inflammation and degenerative tissue. Lymphoma can be diagnosed from lymph node biopsies. Muscle biopsies can be taken when diagnosing exertional rhabdomyolysis, equine motor neuron disease or focal muscle atrophy. If pulmonary or kidney pathology is identified on ultrasound, biopsies from these areas can be taken to help diagnose the type of neoplasia or kidney disease, but they can cause fatal side effects, so these risks need to be considered carefully and discussed fully with the owner.

13.4 Care Plans and Care Bundles

A nursing care plan is a document made following a nursing assessment, identifying actual and potential problems, the nursing care to be implemented and evaluating the process. Care bundles are pre-defined, evidence-based tasks to be carried out for specific conditions, rather than an individual patient and should be used alongside care plans. Nursing care plans and bundles have been slow to be introduced in equine practice, compared to human and small animal nursing. Although many are using standardised medication charts, patient check charts and catheter management checklists rather than a formal personalised care plan. This may be due to the reluctance of RVNs and vets to add in extra work, especially as some equine practices would need to use paper care plans rather than electronic due to lack of resources and finances.

There is also a lack of awareness of what RVNs can do within the remit of the Veterinary Surgeons Act 1966 (see Chapter 3). This can lead to a reluctance to delegate Schedule 3 tasks and fully involve RVNs in the nursing care of the patients. The latter has been acknowledged by the Royal College of Veterinary Surgeons (RCVS), in 2018, stating 'there is some confusion amongst vets and RVNs about the legal framework contained in Schedule 3 of the Veterinary Surgeons Act 1966' [9]. The RCVS is trying hard to educate vets, RVNs and student veterinary nurses (SVNs) about what they can legally do to help improve the nurse's role and lighten the vets' caseload with the patient's welfare at the centre of everyone's role. Finances can also play a part in the number of staff employed by an equine practice,

meaning that RVNs are required to carry out a much larger range of tasks than human or small animal nurses, such as placing orders, managing the equipment care and servicing, updating the billing and invoicing clients, which can divert RVNs away from nursing patients. With this being said, RVNs still have the legal obligation to adhere to the RCVS Code of Professional Conduct for Veterinary Nurses, which states that veterinary nurses must ensure that clinical governance forms part of their professional activities [10]. Under the clinical governance section, continuity of care for patients by having effective systems of case handovers between clinical staff [11] is listed, and this can easily be carried out using nursing care plans.

Application of Nursing Care Plans to Equine Patients

The Medical Model

When starting a care plan, a decision must be made as to which type of nursing care it is going to be centred around. This can be a medical model of nursing where a condition is treated or a task carried out by the RVN, focussing on treating the disease rather than the whole patient [12]. A nursing-focussed model is more about nursing the patient as an individual rather than a task or condition. For this, the client will need to be consulted to find out the patient's individual care needs and what is deemed normal for them [13]. The medical model will have most input from a vet, and is a simplistic model, as they will medically assess the patient and then tell the RVN which tasks they would like carried out and/or which treatment they would like started; the patient will then get better and go home. This model is not ideal for the level of care that patients require and are expected to receive when they are ill, but it is used subconsciously for many recheck patients. With day cases, especially rechecks, the vet will often assess the patient, inform the team of any further procedures that are required, such as radiographs, joint medications, dental checks or cryotherapy. The procedure or treatment is then carried out, and the patient is sent home. There is no formal care plan indicating the medical model has been carried out; it was a horse that was visited briefly, with a condition diagnosed and treated, and some members of the team that assisted with the procedure may not even know the horse's name, just that it was the 'dark bay', in one of the day patient boxes and was lame. Current equine veterinary nursing care is moving away from using the medical model and is advancing towards a more modern, patient-focussed approach.

The Nursing Process

Prior to the use of care plans, the nursing process was introduced in 1967 by Yura and Walsh. This plays a huge part in

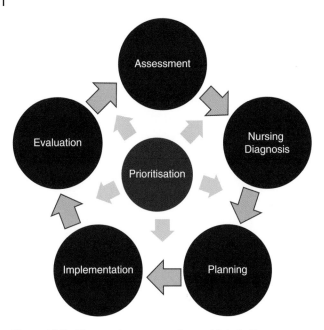

Figure 13.8 The nursing process. *Source:* Victoria Gregory.

the nursing-focussed model of nursing, deciding which nursing care is required for each individual patient, with these decisions being made by nurses and other team members. There are now a few different versions of the systematic framework being used, with a veterinary nursing process including prioritisation all the way through the framework [12], as shown in Figure 13.8. Prioritisation is added in for the nursing process framework as the animal cannot communicate with us, so we need to prioritise what we can see; for example, in an emergency situation is the patient breathing? Are there any visible injuries that could be life threatening? In a non-emergency situation, the patient is likely to be unsure of their new surroundings and may be nervous or excitable.

The stages of the nursing process are:

- Assessment
- Nursing diagnosis
- Planning
- Implementation
- Evaluation

Assessment

Assessment will clearly establish the individual needs of the patient [13]. Taking the time to speak to the owner before assessing the patient gives the opportunity to learn about the patient's behaviour; this may make examining the patient a lot easier for the RVN and the patient. This could also prevent injuries. For example, if the owner knows that

the horse kicks when getting its temperature taken, they can warn members of staff in advance. Assessment is a team effort; if the owner is present, they can be asked about the clinical signs they have been noticing as well as the horse's normal routine, behaviour, feeding plan, medical history and many other appropriate questions. The RVN will need to observe the patient, carry out a clinical examination to highlight any actual nursing problems; these are problems that are already present, such as the patient being recumbent, and discuss with colleagues their findings as someone may have noticed an extra problem. Potential nursing problems, which are problems that can occur as a secondary problem caused by the actual nursing problem, should also be discussed as a team at this point. The potential problems for a recumbent horse might be myopathy, decubitus ulcers and corneal ulcers, to name just a few.

Nursing Diagnosis

Some models now add in nursing decision or nursing diagnosis; this is a specific label for each identified problem related to nursing care [12]. This is different to a medical diagnosis which can only be carried out by a vet.

Planning

This nursing-focussed model includes the nursing diagnosis as part of the planning process, where nursing interventions that are required will be discussed, along with interventions to alleviate actual problems and preventative interventions for potential problems. Goals will be set in relation to solving actual problems during the planning phase.

Implementation

Once the plan, with identified problems, goals and preventative care has been made it can then be implemented by the nursing team. This can be one of the most difficult stages. The key is getting the whole team involved and asking them to contribute to the process. A care plan template can be discussed at a team meeting. This will give all team members a chance to have their say. This in turn contributes to a feeling of ownership within the team and greater levels of concordance with using the care plan. The care plan must be clear and easy to follow so that team members who were not present during the assessment and planning stages can still use it easily.

Evaluation

The evaluation is a vital part of the nursing process. Evaluation involves reflecting upon the nursing process and the outcomes achieved by it [13]. The RVN should ask the question 'have the goals been met?' The RVN can then decide if the nursing interventions are effective or if they need to be revaluated and changed. If the goals were not met it is important to consider if this was a result of a patient issue or a staffing issue. This should then be addressed appropriately. These are all things to consider if the goals have not been met and the nursing process cycle needs to start again. Often, in practice, this process is carried out without any formal documents being produced. This information should be recorded as it is evidence that effective nursing care has been applied. This in turn will contribute to an accumulation of an evidence base for veterinary nursing care.

Models of Nursing Care

There are three main nursing care models used within the veterinary profession:

- The Roper, Logan and Tierney Activities of Living Model (Human)
- Orem's Model of Self-care (Human)
- The Orpet and Jeffery Ability Model (Veterinary)

These can be modified and blended to suit a practice or individual patient's needs.

Roper, Logan and Tierney

The Roper, Logan and Tierney activities of living model is based around 12 activities of living (AL):

1) Maintaining a safe environment
2) Communicating
3) Breathing
4) Eating and drinking
5) Eliminating
6) Personal cleansing and dressing (grooming)
7) Controlling body temperature
8) Mobilising
9) Working and playing
10) Expressing sexuality
11) Sleeping
12) Dying

With this model the consideration must be made as to how the following relate to the 12 AL and care of the patient:

- Age – This will have an impact on many nursing considerations such as what is deemed normal for the age of the patient, their level of independence and mobility, their mental state and what is a suitable environment for them.
- Dependence/independence – This can be affected by the patient's age but also the condition that they require nursing care for. The patient is scored on a dependence/independence scale for each AL and this helps to guide the RVN as to where nursing interventions may be required.

- Factors influencing AL – Psychological, sociocultural, environmental, politico-economic and biological are all factors that Roper, Logan and Tierney identified as having an influence on AL [12]. These may be positive or negative influences.
- Individuality – Although all healthy horses are likely to be able to carry out the 12 AL, they may not all carry them out in the same way, as all patients are individuals.

Taking these points into consideration, a care plan can then be put together using the 12 AL and a nursing assessment, defining any actual and potential problems, nursing goals and interventions, and an evaluation of these 12 AL. Please see Figure 13.9.

Orem's Model of Self-care

Orem's model of self-care looks at eight universal self-care requisites that must be performed in order to achieve self-care. The Orem model then takes into consideration factors that may limit this self-care, how the patient can improve the limitation, and then what nursing interventions are required to help the patient recover, please see Figure 13.10.

The eight universal self-care requisites are:

1) Sufficient intake of air
2) Sufficient intake of water
3) Sufficient intake of food
4) Satisfactory eliminative functions
5) Activity balanced with rest
6) Balance between solitude and social interaction
7) Prevention of hazards to life, human functions and human well being
8) Promotion of human functioning and development within social groups in accordance with human potential, the desire for normalcy (Normalcy)

The concept of balancing self-care requisites with self-care abilities is fundamental to Orem. If these two concepts are balanced, such as in healthy patients, there is no need for any nursing interventions. Orem also identified developmental self-care requisites, which are found in special circumstances associated with development.

The developmental self-care requisites are:

- Intrauterine life and birth
- Neonatal life
- Infancy
- The developmental stages of childhood (foal), adolescence (filly/colt) and adulthood
- The developmental stages of adulthood
- Pregnancy [13]

Orem argued that at each of these stages, the self-care requisites must be considered. An example of a

Patient Details: Mr Biggles – a 7 year old, gelding, Thoroughbred recovering from an emergency laparotomy with a small intestinal resection

Position on Life span: Neonate...X...Geriatric

Activity of living	Nursing assessment	D - dependent I - independent	Patient problem Actual/potential	Nursing goals	Nursing Interventions	Evaluation
Maintaining safe environment	Mr Biggles is unable to do this himself. He needs to be provided with a warm, quiet stable with a rubber floor and deep bed	D.X.........................I	Actual – has some skin sores from rolling pre-surgery Potential – If violently colicking may get more sore or cause dehiscence of surgical incision	Decrease the risk of further sores and damage to the surgical site	Keep bed clean and deep. Keep the surgery incision covered with an abdominal bandage, change and assess daily or more frequently if soiled/slipped. Administer analgesia as directed	A safe environment was maintained. No more sores found and abdominal bandage still in place
Communicating	Able to, calling out when hears other horses. Expressed pain by rolling prior to surgery	D.........................X.I	Potential – becoming too stressed/excitable when hearing other horses, starts to box walk causing movement and potential disruption to the surgical site	Keep levels of stress/excitement at an acceptable level	Always keep another horse in his barn for company, leave the radio on, consider other methods of environmental enrichment, liaise with vet if excessively box walking and administer analgesia and sedation as directed	Mr Biggles has been calm all night, just calling out when he hears the barn door open. No evidence of rolling seen on him or in his bed
Breathing	Able to but reflux seen from both nostrils on arrival to the hospital. Increased breathing rate prior to surgery	D.....................X....I	Actual – Spontaneous reflux observed. Potential – Aspiration pneumonia post spontaneous reflux	Prevent further spontaneous reflux	Reflux every 4 hours via naso-gastric tube, monitor for coughing and nasal discharge and auscultate lungs at checks	No coughing heard. Still getting reflux via the naso-gastric tube but no nasal discharge and lungs normal on auscultation
Eating and Drinking	Able to but not allowed to eat or drink until reflux has stopped	D.X.........................I	Actual – trying to eat shavings, access to food is limited. Potential – dehydration and weight loss	Maintain correct intravenous fluid therapy (IVFT) rate	Keep muzzled to stop him eating shavings, provide IVFT, monitor hydration levels	IVFT running well overnight, packed cell volume and total protein normal, muzzle kept in place
Eliminating	Urinating well, not passed faeces since surgery	D.....X.....................I	Actual – not passing faeces Potential – impaction colic/ileus	Increase intestinal motility to allow normal feeding to commence	Administer prokinetics as directed. Record any faeces on faecal chart	One very small pile of faeces passed overnight but still refluxing. Drops penis to urinate and able to retract
Personal cleansing (grooming)	Skin sores need to be cleaned. Grooming is required.	D.........X.................I	Potential – skin sores and surgical site becoming infected	Decrease the risk of infection. Give TLC by grooming in an attempt to improve demeanour.	Clean sores twice daily and groom once daily. Keep surgical site covered.	The abdominal bandage stayed in place. Sores were cleaned with saline, healing well. Mr Biggles enjoys being groomed.
Controlling body temperature	Able to and within normal limits	D........................X...I	Potential – pyrexia or hypothermia	Maintain normal temperature	Monitor temperature at checks. Shut window and put rug on if cold	Mr Biggles had a normal temperature overnight. It was mild so window left open

Figure 13.9 An example of Roper, Logan and Tierney activities of living model. *Source:* Victoria Gregory.

Mobilising	Able to but restricted to box rest	D...X.....................I	Potential – oedema around surgery site, sheath, and limbs.	Decrease risk of oedema forming	Hand walk during the day	Moving comfortably around the stable. No oedema seen
Working and playing	Has the ability to but not allowed due to the surgery	D...X.....................I	Potential – excitable behaviour in stable due to boredom, becoming excitable when hand walked putting extra pressure on the surgery site	To limit exercise while the surgical site in healing	Hand walk in a bridle. Stop if Mr Biggles is becoming too strong or rearing/bucking and inform the vet	He has been calm in the stable overnight
Expressing sexuality	Gelded	N/A	N/A	N/A	N/A	N/A
Sleeping	Able to but startles easily in his new environment	D.....................X....I	Potential – slower healing due to sleep deprivation	Let Mr Biggles sleep more	Keep barn as quiet as possible with the radio playing relaxing music	Mr Biggles was awake at all checks but could be seen sleeping on CCTV
Dying	At a higher risk than normal	D...................X.......I	Potential – deterioration of condition may lead to euthanasia.	Maintain low levels of reflux in the stomach. Monitor for changes in demeanour and pain	Continue to reflux every 4 hours and perform intensive care checks. Monitor on CCTV and administer analgesia as directed	Mr Biggles was stable overnight with no signs of pain and a consistent heart rate and respiration rate

Figure 13.9   (Continued)

developmental self-care requisite would be temperature regulation in a neonatal foal [13]. This would require extra consideration, as adult horses can generally thermoregulate easily, whereas neonatal foals cannot.

Orem recognised that if a person became ill or injured, the following additional healthcare demands are placed upon them:

- Seeking and securing appropriate medical assistance
- Being aware of and attending to the effects and results of pathologic conditions and states
- Effectively carrying out medically prescribed diagnostic, therapeutic and rehabilitative measures
- Being aware of and attending to or regulating the discomforting or deleterious effects of prescribed medical measures
- Modifying the self-concept in accepting oneself as being in a particular state of health and in need of specific forms of health care
- Learning to live with the effects of pathological conditions and states and the effects of medical diagnostic and treatment measures in a lifestyle that promotes continued personal development [13, 14].

These additional healthcare demands may unbalance the stability of the patient's universal self-care requisites and self-care abilities, and it is at this point where a nursing intervention is required to readdress the balance. An example of this would be a horse with a fractured jaw. This patient would struggle to eat and drink without help. Nursing interventions would need to be implemented in order for the patient to maintain a sufficient intake of food and water [13].

When nursing horses, the RVN may need to teach, guide and direct the owner on how to care for the horse and cope with the condition rather than expecting the patient to do it for themselves.

The Orpet and Jeffery Ability Model

The Orpet and Jeffery Ability model was specifically made for veterinary nursing, taking on the holistic/nursing-focussed approach to nursing rather than the medical model. It looks at 10 abilities of living, the age of the animal and owner factors such as their culture, financial situation and willingness to comply with the suggested treatment plan.

The 10 abilities of living are:

1) Eat
2) Drink
3) Urinate
4) Defecate
5) Breathe normally
6) Maintain body temperature
7) Groom and clean itself
8) Mobilise adequately
9) Sleep and rest adequately
10) Express normal behaviour

Patient Details: Mr Biggles – a 7-year-old, gelding, thoroughbred recovering from an emergency laparotomy with a small intestinal resection

Universal self-care requisites	Self-care abilities	Self-care limitations	Patient actions	Nursing actions
Maintain intake of air	Mr Biggles is able to breath normally but did have spontaneous reflux on arrival	Unable to clean nostrils as wearing muzzle and naso-gastric tube in situ	Breathe	Ensure naso-gastric tube stays in place and does not hinder airway. Remove muzzle periodically to check for nasal discharge and clean if present
Maintain intake of water	Can swallow water but not allowed water due to reflux and ileus	Unable to empty stomach due to ileus	N/A until ileus resolves	Administer intravenous fluid therapy (IVFT), monitor for dehydration, administer prokinetics as directed, continue to reflux via naso-gastric tube every 4 hours
Maintain intake of food	Can swallow food but not allowed food due to reflux and ileus	Unable to empty stomach due to ileus, trying to eat shavings	N/A until ileus resolves	Administer intravenous fluid therapy (IVFT), monitor for dehydration, administer prokinetics as directed, ensure muzzle is in place when unattended, continue to reflux via naso-gastric tube every 4 hours
Manage elimination	Mr Biggles can urinate normally, not passed faeces since surgery	Unable to digest food so gastrointestinal tract empty	Continue to urinate, defecate when ready	Keep bed clean, monitor for defecation or tenesmus. Administer prokinetics as directed
Balance activity and rest	Is able to rest and sleep, will lay down to sleep, able to walk out in hand	Startles easily so wakes up often. On box rest due to surgical incision	Try to relax in new environment to improve sleep. Continue to move around stable and walk out when asked	Keep barn quiet and play relaxing music, Hand walk in a bridle if Mr Biggles is being sensible
Balance solitude and integration	Able to communicate, calling out to other horses	Unable to mix with other horses due to being on box rest after surgery	Continue to communicate	Groom Mr Biggles daily as unable to be groomed by other horses, organise owners to visit
Prevent hazards to life, wellbeing, and functioning	Mr Biggles canfeel pain, move, see and hear normally	He is unable to maintain a clean and safe environment for himself. He currently has no access to food or water	Comply with the administration of medication and walking to aid in his well-being and recovery from ileus	Monitor for signs of improvement or deterioration, provide a deep, clean bed and maintain a safe environment. Continue to reflux Mr Biggles and administer medications as directed
Normalcy	Able to communicate vocally with horses and interact with humans	Unable to mix with other horses due to surgery site and ileus, on box rest	Continue to communicate with other horses and interact with humans in the stable	Provide a calming environment, groom daily, allow owners to visit and promote interaction

Figure 13.10 An example of Orem's self-care model. *Source:* Victoria Gregory.

With this model of nursing care, the assessment phase takes the form of a questionnaire with the owner. The owners are asked about the normal routine for their animal against the 10 abilities of living. The RVN should ask open questions that are likely to give more information than a simple yes or no answer. With the owner's help, the RVN can then identify what the patient is currently not able to do and which clinical signs they have been showing, if any. From the assessment questionnaire, actual and potential problems can be identified, and a plan of nursing care interventions can be put together.

It is important to find out what finances are available for the treatment, what facilities the owner has at home to continue patient care, and what the horse will be required to do following treatment. Owners who have horses simply for pleasure may be happy to care for their horse long term, and if they cannot be ridden again, they can continue with treatment in the hope that the horse can retire. Other owners may require their horses to compete at a high level. In this case, if the horse is not expected to make a full recovery, the owner may consider the horse to be worthless, and euthanasia may be their preferred treatment choice. Some horse's temperament may be the deciding factor; if the owner knows that the horse will not tolerate long-term box rest, it may be safer and better for the horse to choose euthanasia. Once the history and expectations from the owner have been ascertained, a care plan can be made taking these into consideration. The plan will include the horse's normal routine, actual and potential problems and long-term goals, as shown in Figure 13.11.

Using Care Plans in Practice

Criticisms of nursing care plans include the constant need to update the plan, particularly when care is more complex, and time being a limited resource. Another criticism of nursing care plans is the repetition that they generate when the same instructions must be written out for several different patients all suffering from similar conditions [15]. It is also not always easy to adapt a model of nursing care designed for humans to horses, although some of the features of a human-based care plan may be useful and so these can be retained, and new care plans put together. As mentioned previously, these models can be adapted and blended dependent on each individual patient. A patient who has undergone an elective surgical procedure may not require a care plan as in-depth as one for an emergency colic patient with post-operative complications. So, the care plans can be adapted to suit the individual needs of the patients and save time where possible. If care plans are not used properly, by staff on each shift, this reduces the overall benefit of using them. A simpler model, adapted to the individual patient, may encourage their use by all team members, which in turn will benefit the patient's recovery.

Application of Care Bundles to Equine Patients

Care bundles are pre-defined, evidence-based tasks to be carried out for specific conditions, rather than an individual patient. They have been used in human healthcare for many years but are now being introduced into veterinary medicine. Human healthcare started with checklists, and many veterinary practices now have checklists in place for catheter management and surgical procedures under general anaesthesia (Figure 13.12). Care bundles go a step further, looking at recognised symptoms or side effects for a condition or procedure and how to prevent or delay them from occurring. Care bundles should be used alongside care plans, not instead of, to record that certain tasks have been carried out that are proven to help to decrease the risk of morbidity and mortality in that condition. The care plan

will provide the patient-specific care, to ensure that the patient is getting treated as a whole patient and not as a condition, but the care bundle will ensure that condition-specific tasks are also completed.

Care bundles are not specifically nursing-based; they can incorporate tasks to be carried out by vets and grooms as well as RVNs. They may be bundles that are started as soon as a condition is recognised or in preparation for a procedure, such as foal sepsis or IV catheter placement preparation, and finish once the initial treatment/procedure is completed, or they may be used long-term to prevent and recognise complications with IV catheters, limb casts, recumbent patients or patients in a sling. An example of a human care bundle is the ventilator care bundle, which includes specific positioning of the head, regular assessment for extubation, oral care and daily sedation breaks [15]. An example of a catheter site preparation bundle could include hand hygiene, assessing the vein to check its suitability for catheterisation, clipping the area, and following a standardised skin preparation technique. This could go on to include details of the catheter placement and continued aftercare until the removal of the catheter (Figure 13.13). Figure 13.14 shows an example of a care bundle for a recumbent horse.

Implementing veterinary care bundles in practice can elevate the standard of patient care, create a standardised approach and improve patient outcomes [16]. When creating a care bundle, the whole team need to agree on the requirements for the care bundle and the protocols to be put into the care bundle. It is important that everyone understands why they are carrying out each task. This will help ensure that the tasks are carried out correctly and at the required times, and not purposely ignored. Like a care plan, this process will only work if everyone caring for that patient uses the bundle. Once a need and the tasks have been identified, they then need to be researched to find the evidence to support their use. This can then be made into a practice-specific care bundle to suit the patients and environment at each individual practice. Once implemented, it is important that these bundles are monitored and reviewed. Are they being carried out/followed correctly, and if not, why not? Are the reasons for implementing the care bundle being resolved? It may be that the bundle needs adapting as it does not suit the environment it is being used in, or over time, it may become outdated and need updating. It is a good idea to set a review date prior to using the care bundles; the timeframe will depend on the frequency of the bundle use and the caseload of the practice. An IV catheter bundle is likely to be used more frequently than a recumbent horse care bundle, so it should be reviewed sooner. If problems arise before the pre-set review date, the review can be brought forward.

Patient Details: Mr Biggles   **Case number:** 123456
Age: 7 years old   **Weight:** 502kg
Sex: Gelding   **Breed:** Thoroughbred
Condition: Emergency laparotomy with a small intestinal resection, now has ileus
Current medications: IVFT – see ICU sheet for additives and rate
                         Lidocaine IV infusion
                         Metoclopramide IV infusion
                         Penicillin IM Q12hr
                         Gentamicin IV Q24hr
                         Flunixin Meglumine IV Q12hr
                         Metronidazole IV Q8hr

T	37.7	**Warnings:** (allergies, kicks, bites, needle shy etc…)
P	44	
R	12	
MM	P&M	
CRT	< 2 sec	

Notes: Owner aware of post-op ileus, Mr Biggles has exceeded his insurance fee – owner has asked for daily bill updates, owner is in France, she has consented to euthanasia should Mr Biggles re-colic on his current analgesia and we are unable to contact her – form in file. Second surgery is not an option.

Life stage:
Neonate……………………………………………X………………………………………………………………………Geriatric

Activity assessed	Usual routine	Actual problem	Potential problem	Long term goal
Eat	Concentrates twice daily, soaked hay ad-lib	Ileus and refluxing	Gastric rupture, spontaneous reflux	Resolve ileus and return to normal food intake
Drink	From bucket in stable and automatic drinker in field	Ileus and refluxing	Gastric rupture, spontaneous reflux	Resolve ileus and return to normal water intake
Urinate	In stable and field	No problem	Urinating on abdominal dressing	Maintain normal urination
Defecate	In one corner of stable and field	Not passed faeces since surgery, no food due to ileus so intestines are empty	Impaction once feeding restarts	Return to normal once food is reintroduced
Breathe	Normal	None	Aspiration pneumonia due to spontaneous reflux on arrival	Maintain normal functions
Maintain body temperature	Able to	None	Pyrexia or hypothermia	Able to maintain body temperature with rugs
Groom & clean itself	Owner grooms when brings in from field	No owner to groom. Surgery site to be dressed and sores cleaned	Infection of surgical incision and skin sores	Groom daily
Mobilise adequately	In field during the day, hacks out 4 times a week, competes in summer	On box rest due to surgical incision	Oedema forming around surgical site, sheath, and legs	Return to ridden work once surgical incision has healed
Sleep & rest adequately	Lays down in stable at night, rarely lays down in field	New environment, startles quite easily	Slower healing due to sleep deprivation	Normal sleep routine

Figure 13.11   An example of the Orpet and Jeffery ability model. *Source:* Victoria Gregory.

Express normal behaviour	Normally relaxed and calm, plays with field companions. Gets stressed in new and lonely environments	Unable to socialise/be turned-out due to surgical incision. Box walking when hears other horses moving in and out of the barn	Wound breakdown due to extra pressure on incision if excitable in stable	Return to normal environment so that normal behaviour can resume

CARE PLAN					

Patient Name: Mr Biggles				**Date: 02/09/2022**	
Date	**Problem**	**Short term Goal**	**Nursing intervention**	**Reassess/ evaluation**	**Review time/date**
02/09/22	Ileus and refluxing, unable to eat	Improve gut motility with medication and hand walking so that feed can be introduced	Provide intravenous fluid therapy (IVFT) and reflux until able to eat and digest food normally	Still refluxing approx. 4l every 2 hours	02/00/22 8pm
02/09/22	Ileus and refluxing, unable to drink	Improve gut motility with medication and hand walking so that feed can be introduced	IVFT and reflux until ileus resolves. Monitor hydration levels	As above	02/09/22 8pm
02/09/22	Not passing faeces due to ileus and not being allowed to eat	Increase faecal output once feeding resumes	Monitor for faeces and tenesmus	Some faeces passed in the morning	02/09/22 8pm
02/09/22	No companion or owner to groom, wearing abdominal bandage and has skin sores	Maintain coat condition, keep abdominal bandage dry and help skin sore heal	Groom at least once daily, clean skin sores twice daily and change abdominal bandage if wet	Able to groom twice today, coat looks good, abdominal bandage dry, skin sore healing nicely	02/09/22 8pm
02/09/22	On box rest so reduced mobility	Facilitate mobility	Hand walk in bridle 3 times a day	Well behaved while walking	02/09/22 8pm
02/09/22	Not seen sleeping since being hospitalised	Provide a suitable environment for resting	Keep barn quiet and try to avoid walking other patients past Mr Biggles	Appears less anxious today, seen in the same spot for longer periods so hopefully resting	02/09/22 8pm
02/09/22	Box walking	Reduce amount and frequency of box walking	Play calming music and make sure there is always another horse in sight. Inform vet if box walking excessively	Mr Biggles hasn't box walked much today	02/09/22 8pm

Figure 13.11 (Continued)

SURGERY REQUEST						
Horse Name		**Owner Name**		**Patient Number**		
Surgery Date		**Induction Time**		**Surgeon**		
Procedure		**Theatre**	General Ortho Standing	**Horse Position**	DR	LLR
					S	RLR
IV Catheter?	Y / N	**Pre-Clip Sx Site?**	Y / N	**Shoes Off?**	Y	N
Weight	kg			**Other Pre-op Drugs / Procedures** *(specify drug/procedure, route, time etc)*		
Antibiotics *(drug/s, dose, route)*		**Given by:**				
		@ time:				
Analgesia *(drug/s, dose, route)*		**Given by:**				
		@ time:				
Equipment Required	Arthroscopy	Laser	Tourniquet	IVRP	Radiography	Other:
	Laparoscopy	Suction	Hoof knives	Bandaging	Ultrasound	
	V-Pet kit	Cautery	Bone cement	Casting	Endoscopy	

BEFORE INDUCTION				
NURSE / TECH	Mouth rinsed?			**Introductions**
Initials:_____.	All equipment ready and serviceable?			
ANAESTHETIST	All equipment ready and serviceable?			
	All drugs ready and available?			
Initials:_____.	Specific risks pertaining to this patient?			
	Rope recovery? *(discuss with surgeon)*			
SURGEON	Confirm name of patient, procedure and location/s			
	Have the GA risks and potential surgical complications been discussed with the owner?			
Initials:_____.	Anticipated duration and potential complications anticipated with this procedure?			

DURING SURGERY				
INSTRUMENT COUNT	ON		OFF	
SHARPS COUNT *(needles, blades, sutures)*	ON		OFF	
SWAB COUNT (small)	ON		OFF	
SWAB COUNT (large)	ON		OFF	

AFTER SURGERY		
NURSE	Equipment/procedure problems to rectify	
ANAESTHETIST	Equipment problems to rectify	
	Specific post-op concerns	
SURGEON	Specific post-op concerns	
	Post-op plan	

Figure 13.12 Surgical checklist example. *Source:* Victoria Gregory.

Catheter placement and management bundle

Patient name and case number...
Date and time of catheter placement...
Catheter placed by...................................Type of catheter used.................................
Reason for placement...Vein used...................................
Date and time removed...........................Reason for removal....................................

Preparation	Yes - Initials	No – why?
Hands clean and Sterillium used?		
Was vein assessed?		
Area clipped, including extn set sutures?		
Initial scrub with chlorhexidine?		
Local anaesthetic used?		
Chloraprep used?		

Catheter placement	Yes - initials	No – why?
Where procedure took place		
Patient compliance		
Sterile gloves worn?		
Catheter placed aseptically?		
Catheter flushed with heparinised saline?		
Catheter wrap applied?		
Any complications?		

Date	Catheter check task	ü or x and initial					
		12am	4am	8am	12pm	4pm	8pm
	Sterillium hands & wear gloves						
	Catheter wrap clean & in place						
	Extension set firmly attached						
	Catheter patent when flushing						
	Vein visually normal and filling						
	Swelling around catheter site						
	Heat around catheter site						
	Pain or discharge around catheter site						
Date	Catheter check task	ü or x and initial					
		12am	4am	8am	12pm	4pm	8pm
	Sterillium hands & wear gloves						
	Catheter wrap clean & in place						
	Extension set firmly attached						
	Catheter patent when flushing						
	Vein visually normal and filling						
	Swelling around catheter site						
	Heat around catheter site						
	Pain or discharge around catheter site						

Figure 13.13 Catheter site preparation bundle example. *Source:* Victoria Gregory.

Applying an Evidence Base to Care Planning and Delivery

In practice, RVNs are more likely to introduce care plans, checklists and care bundles, but it is important that the whole team agree on the implementation and use. The RCVS state in the code for professional conduct for veterinary surgeons that 'Veterinary surgeons must ensure that clinical governance forms part of their professional activities' [17]. This applies to RVNs also. Clinical governance is defined as a continuing process of reflection, analysis and improvement in professional practice for the benefit of the animal, patient and client owner [11]. As part of this, many practices hold regular morbidity and mortality meetings to discuss potentially avoidable complications or errors that have occurred recently. This is in an attempt to prevent mistakes and accidents happening in the future and to improve patient outcome and human safety. These meetings can be a useful tool for highlighting the need for a care bundle or checklist in relation to a certain situation and for discussing which tasks or protocols are required to help

Recumbent patient care bundle

Patient name and case number...VS in

charge......................Reason for

recumbency...Weight.......................

.....Manual turning or hoist assisted...........................Frequency of turning – every.......................hours

Number of staff required for safe turning.......................

Date	Task	ü or X and initial											
		12am	2am	4am	6am	8am	10am	12pm	2pm	4pm	6pm	8pm	10pm
	Is everyone wearing correct PPE?												
	Talk through turning plan and then turn patient – mark **L** or **R** lateral in box												
	Check IV catheter & fluid lines												
	Apply lubricant to eyes & check head padding												
	Offer water – Allowed water? **Y/N**												
	Offer food – Allowed food? **Y/N**												
	Groom & check for decubitus ulcers												
	Check for urine scalding – clean and apply talcum powder												
	Ensure enough bedding – remove and record faeces												
Date	Task	ü or X and initial											
		12am	2am	4am	6am	8am	10am	12pm	2pm	4pm	6pm	8pm	10pm
	Is everyone wearing correct PPE?												
	Talk through turning plan and then turn patient – mark **L** or **R** lateral in box												
	Check IV catheter & fluid lines												
	Apply lubricant to eyes & check head padding												
	Offer water – Allowed water? **Y/N**												
	Offer food – Allowed food? **Y/N**												
	Groom & check for decubitus ulcers												
	Check for urine scalding – clean and apply talcum powder												
	Ensure enough bedding – remove and record faeces												

Figure 13.14 Example of a recumbent horse care bundle. *Source:* Victoria Gregory.

overcome the problem. However, evidence still needs to be sought to identify why and how these tasks or protocols will improve patient outcomes or reduce risk.

For example, the practice may have identified an increase in IV catheter complications and after a team discussion, it has been suggested that the catheter site is prepared using a new technique and all patients have catheter wraps applied. Following this, research should be carried out to find evidence that supports these new protocols. When training in practice, SVNs are often taught by colleagues and often do not question why things are done a certain way, or if they do the answer may be 'because that is how it's always been done'. If the technique is effective and has no associated complications, then there may be no need to change it, but change can be good and there is no harm in reviewing commonly used techniques and protocols. Creating and adding care plans and bundles can significantly improve patient care if the protocols are researched carefully and implemented by a team who are working harmoniously and synergistically.

The questions 'why am I doing this?' or 'how can I improve this?' should continuously be asked throughout training as an SVN and during a career as an RVN. Seeing practice at other establishments and attending conferences should be encouraged as it will facilitate exposure to other ways of doing things. New findings should be presented to colleagues, with the support of an evidence base as this will make the new ideas more authentic and this is more likely to attract interest and support. The evidence should always be indicative of the change being proposed having a positive outcome, and this does not mean ignoring evidence that disproves the idea. An unbiased approach is required, putting the patient outcome as the priority. There is nothing wrong with suggesting an idea, researching it and then presenting evidence as to why it might not benefit patient welfare and should no longer be implemented.

When conducting research, it is important to know where to look for accurate, reliable and appropriate sources. It has been suggested that there is a significant lack of available published evidence for veterinary medicine and that it can be difficult to access without incurring a fee [18]. Peer-reviewed journals are the best source of evidence; these articles have been scrutinised by a panel of experts. Examples of peer-reviewed journals in the veterinary sector are:

- Veterinary Nursing Journal
- The Veterinary Nurse
- Equine Veterinary Education
- Practice Nurse
- Equine Veterinary Journal
- The Veterinary Record
- UK VET
- Veterinary Evidence
- In Practice

Other sources of information can be the internet, case reports and conferences.

Once gathered, it is important to review the evidence and critically analyse it. The following questions should be considered:

- Was the study carried out in a controlled manner and environment?
- What evidence do the researchers or authors use to back up the claims being made?
- Have inconsistencies or errors been identified during the study?

Research should always be critically analysed before being put into practice. For example, a good, peer-reviewed paper about IV catheter complications may have been identified, but upon closer inspection it may be 20 years old, and the findings may have been disproven by several other more recent papers. The horses used in the study may have been healthy routine surgical cases, but your current complications may be associated with catheters in recumbent foals. Some skin preparation techniques may have been developed following laboratory-based trials, and no research may exist for equine patients specifically. Due to the lack of evidence relating to equine patients, often equine practices need to rely on research from other species and humans. When looking for accuracy and reliability in a source, the author's credentials and the references that they have cited should be checked. For websites, appearances can be important, professional, reliable sites are unlikely to contain spelling mistakes. The website's other pages and links should be checked, and if an 'About Us' page is available, this should be checked also. The domain should be checked to see if the organisation is an education establishment, government site, non-profit organisation or commercial business.

Clinical governance is a continuing process of reflection, analysis and improvement. The result of future morbidity and mortality rounds may suggest that improvement needs to be made on a previously well-researched evidence-based protocol. Changes and improvements should be embraced and implemented effectively. Veterinary medicine is evolving all the time, and nursing care needs to change and progress in order to improve patient welfare and recovery.

13.5 Chronic Wound Care

Classification of Chronic Wounds

This section will focus on chronic wounds. The healing of surgical wounds is covered in Chapter 12. Chronic wounds are wounds that have not proceeded through the stages of healing in an orderly and timely manner to produce

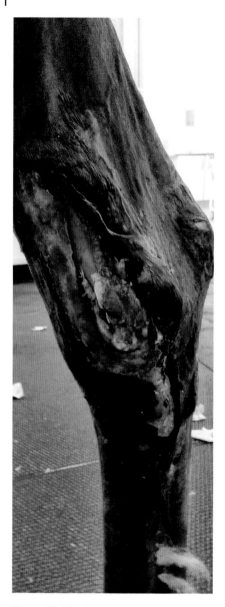

Figure 13.15 A chronic wound. *Source:* Rosina Lillywhite.

anatomic and functional integrity after three months [19]. See Chapter 12 for the stages of wound healing. Figure 13.15 shows a chronic wound.

Factors that Delay Healing

A delay in healing usually occurs due to an undiagnosed disease or because the management of the patient is poor [20]. Some veterinary treatments may affect the rate of wound healing, and this will have to be considered. Treatment plans should be constantly evaluated and adapted if necessary.

Poor Perfusion and Oxygenation

Poor perfusion is a decrease in blood flow to a specific organ or system, in this instance the skin. From the first initial stages of wound healing, it is essential that there is adequate blood flow to the injured area. If the blood flow is reduced, then the wound or site of infection will have a decreased immune response [21]. This immune response relies on the delivery of the essential leukocytes, antibodies, oxygen and nutrients. If these components are not delivered, the wound will have a higher chance of becoming infected or re-infected. In a chronic wound, the decreased perfusion may be related to necrosis of the surrounding tissue or traumatised tissue that has become ischemic. In both circumstances, this tissue must be removed to allow improved perfusion to the surrounding area.

Poor Nutrition

Each individual horse must be looked at as a whole. If the horse is malnourished and lacking certain nutrients, this will have an impact on wound healing; suboptimal nutrition can alter immune function, collagen synthesis and wound tensile strength. The majority of patients are fed a normal diet/ration, which contains all the necessary vitamins and minerals the horse requires for wound healing. However, in underweight or malnourished patients this would need to be addressed. The main macronutrients and micronutrients required for optimum wound healing are proteins, carbohydrates, fats, vitamins A, B complex, C, E and K and minerals such as copper, iron and zinc [22]. These nutrients are generally found in most commercial feeds.

Infection

Infection of a wound is one of the main reasons a wound becomes chronic, and this will result in delayed healing. If the wound does not have a healthy environment, it will not be able to heal. It is important at this point to understand the difference between colonisation and infection.

- *Colonisation*: Virtually all wounds are colonised; in other words, bacteria are present and replicating, but there is no host reaction. This does not necessarily mean that this wound will get infected. In a young patient with an otherwise clean wound, intact immune system and no other pathology, bacteria may colonise the wound without harm. The likelihood of an infection developing depends not only on the ability of the bacterium to cause an infection, but also on whether that host is capable of preventing it.
- *Infection*: Wounds are an ideal environment for bacteria to flourish and, if able to overcome the host's response cause an infection. Infection causes a delay in wound healing as its effects disrupt the migration of fibroblasts and the phagocytic activity of macrophages. In addition, wound edges can be forced apart by accumulating exudate [22]. Clinical signs such as swelling, heat, discharge, pain on palpation and erythema are an indication that infection has

occurred. If the wound has a dressing on it, the discharge may have a distinguished odour to it. Depending the severity of the infection, the discharge may be purulent.

Biofilms

In chronic wounds, biofilms may also contribute to delayed healing. A biofilm is formed when a group of bacteria collaborate by grouping together and generating a polysaccharide matrix that forms an envelope around them. This matrix shields them from passing macrophages and neutrophils, variations in wound temperature, pH, humidity and antibiotics. Stimulated by the presence of bacteria, neutrophils will release a stream of enzymes. These enzymes, unable to penetrate the biofilm, act instead on the wound bed. This leads to chronic low-grade inflammation and degradation of tissue. Biofilms occur more frequently in chronic wounds (60%) than in acute wounds (6%) [22].

Sequestrum Formation

Formation of a sequestrum can contribute to delayed wound healing, especially in the distal limb. A sequestrum forms when a small piece of bone becomes detached, usually as a result of trauma. This small piece of bone can become necrotic, as its blood supply is damaged or disrupted. This can act like a foreign body and lead to an infection. A sequestrum may take a few weeks to develop, therefore the wound may appear to start healing but then show signs of delayed healing. A radiograph of the area will assist in the diagnosis. Initial treatment includes systemic antibiotics and anti-inflammatories. If this initial treatment does not resolve the problem, the sequestrum should be surgically removed, and the wound bed debrided and cleaned. Once the sequestrum has been removed, normal wound healing will be restored.

Antibiotic Resistance

Antibiotic resistance is another factor that must be considered when presented with a chronic non-healing wound. This problem may occur if an ineffective type of antibiotic has been prescribed initially and/or an ineffective dose or the incorrect route of administration has been used. Ideally, every infected wound would be swabbed, and a culture and sensitivity test carried out. An effective course of antibiotics can then be prescribed. For more information regarding antibiotic resistance, see Chapter 6.

Foreign Bodies

Foreign bodies contribute to delayed wound healing. Common foreign bodies seen in equine practice are as follows:

- Metal objects such as nails or wire
- Wood, such as splinters or bits of fencing
- Thorns
- Surgical implants
- Sutures

Diagnostic imaging techniques such as radiography and/or ultrasonography may be required to identify the location of the foreign body. If foreign bodies are left unidentified, they can lead to inflammation and infection. The foreign body must be removed and any inflammation or infection treated for optimal wound healing to occur.

Client Interference

Client interference can be a problem when dealing with non-healing wounds. Clients often act with the best interests of their animal in mind, and do not realise that they might be interfering with or delaying the healing process. Examples of client interference are:

- Cleaning the wound with an inappropriate skin antiseptic.
- Using creams and sprays might delay healing.
- Applying a bandage without the correct technique.
- Not being compliant with discharge instructions. For example, turning the horse out into the field when they should be on box rest.
- Delay contacting the vet in the first instance and trying to treat the wound themselves.

Holding client evenings at the practice and providing information packs to clients would be a useful way to provide education and encourage client concordance with treatment plans. Having a named contact for the owner to liaise with at the practice can also be useful in the management of patients with chronic wounds. This could be a vet or an RVN.

Patient Interference

Patient interference is also a factor that will affect wound healing. If the horse is on box rest, movement should be minimised as this can disrupt the healing process. Box walking should be addressed. Different forms of environmental enrichment should be considered to reduce stress and boredom. The patient may also interfere with the bandage. This repeated trauma can contribute to delayed wound healing and bandage complications. Unpalatable topical solutions can be applied to the outer layer of the bandage to discourage patient interference. A wooden neck cradle or a bib could be used to prevent the horse from reaching the bandage. However, if the patient is continually interfering with the bandage, the cause of this should be investigated. It could be a sign of a complication or discomfort caused by the wound, the dressing or the bandage itself.

Systemic Disease

The main disease that can cause delayed wound healing is PPID (see Section 13.1 for further information). This disease is usually associated with older horses and ponies. If an older horse or pony presents with a chronic wound, it may also be showing other signs of PPID, which include hirsutism, fat deposits around the tail head and crest of the neck, polyuria/polydipsia, recurrent hoof abscesses, laminitis, conjunctivitis, sinusitis and secondary skin infections. PPID is characterised by high serum concentrations of endogenous cortisol that might suppress inflammation to such an extent that healing could be impaired [22]. If suspected, PPID should be diagnosed and treated appropriately.

Poor Wound Management

When a wound first occurs, all the correct procedures and protocols should be put in place to give the patient the best possible chance of healing. These include:

- Correct restraint
- Correct clipping
- Cleaning and lavaging of the wound
- Debridement – surgical or medical as required
- Suturing
- Bandaging

This will all contribute to the main goal of a functional, cosmetic repair. However, when dealing with a chronic wound, it is likely that complications will need to be identified and addressed.

Poor Suturing Technique or Equipment

Sutures are used to close a wound and create an optimal environment for wound healing. Normally, the choice of suture material and the suturing technique will be determined by the vet in charge of the case. An inappropriate choice of suture material or suturing technique can have a negative effect on wound healing. The suture must also be placed at the correct tension; if it is too loose, the wound edges will not properly align, which will disrupt primary intention healing and reduce the strength of the wound. If the sutures are too tight, this may decrease the blood supply to the region and lead to tissue necrosis and wound breakdown. The vet must choose the correct size and type of suture material for each individual wound to try and minimise the chance of inflammation and infection [23].

Historically, the 'golden period' in which to close an accidental wound by primary intention, with little risk of infection, was estimated at 6–8 hours [24]. The concept of a golden period is now largely outdated [24]. The outcome of the wound is now thought to depend on the following:

- The adequacy of the host's immune response
- The virulence of the contaminating bacteria

- Local environmental factors, such as the presence of devitalised or foreign material

This highlights the importance of cleaning and debriding the wound before suturing. A clean work environment is also important to reduce potential contamination. Good personal hygiene is essential when assessing any wound; washing hands, wearing sterile gloves when suturing and using sterile instruments are other factors that must be considered as these can all have an impact on the healing process.

Other Factors that Delay Healing

It is beyond the scope of this chapter section to cover all the factors that delay healing in full detail. Some further factors that delay healing are as follows:

- *Movement*: wounds on areas of high movement, such as joints, are a concern. Movement can reopen wounds and cause dressings to slip and become detrimental to wound healing.
- *Necrotic tissue*: devitalised tendon, muscle or bone disrupts healing. Careful debridement prior to closure can assist healing.
- *Genetic factors*: ponies heal faster than horses [25]. Ponies are believed to have a more effective acute inflammatory response, which can lead to reduced infection rates. Horses are thought to be more prone to exuberant granulation tissue formation, which also slows the healing process [25].
- *Cell transformation*: such as sarcoid formation. This should be considered in chronic non-healing wounds.
- *Drug therapy*: medications such as corticosteroids and chemotherapy drugs can contribute to delayed healing.

Management for Chronic Wounds

Correct Preparation
Clipping

When treating a chronic wound, correct preparation is key. The horse should be safely restrained by a competent handler wearing appropriate PPE. The area around the wound will need to be clipped. Clippers should be clean, and the blades should be sharp and lubricated. Sterile wound hydrogel can be applied to the wound during this process to prevent stray hairs from contaminating the wound [26]. This hydrogel must be removed afterwards so the wound can be thoroughly lavaged.

Lavage

Wound healing is significantly impeded by the presence of microorganisms, necrotic tissue and foreign material. Wound lavage involves the use of fluid to remove loosely attached cellular debris and surface pathogens from the

Table 13.4 Lavage fluids used in equine practice.

Lavage fluid	Details	Comments
Isotonic saline	Is a widely available, non-toxic solution that does not damage tissues. Can be expensive to use in the quantities required to lavage large wounds	Evidence suggests that lavage with isotonic saline is ineffective in reducing bioburden. The use of this fluid in necrotic or heavily infected wounds is therefore questionable
Tap water	Studies have shown that tap water is acceptable for cleansing acute and chronic wounds. Tap water should only be used where a constant supply of portable drinking water is available. Tap water is cheap and readily available	Evidence suggests that lavage with tap water is ineffective in reducing bioburden. The use of this fluid in necrotic or heavily infected wounds is therefore questionable
Povidone iodine (PI)	PI has an antimicrobial effect but can be toxic to tissues. It can be inactivated by blood, serum and other organic matter [27]. PI should be applied in a 0.1–0.2% concentration when used to lavage wounds. This dilution increases the availability of free iodine and minimises the cytotoxic effects [27]	Antiseptics should be used with caution, as their action can compromise healing in some cases. Antiseptics, therefore, should only be used in high-risk wounds such as heavily contaminated or infected wounds
Chlorhexidine gluconate (CG)	CG has an antimicrobial effect but can be toxic to tissues. Advantages include a prolonged residual effect due to its ability to bind to proteins in the stratum corneum [27]. It displays a better activity in the presence of organic matter when compared to povidone iodine. CG should be applied in a 0.05% concentration when used to lavage wounds. CG should be used with caution in periocular wounds and wounds communicating with synovial structures and it is toxic to corneal cells, synovial cells and chondrocytes [27]	Antiseptics should be used with caution, as their action can compromise healing in some cases. Antiseptics, therefore, should only be used in high-risk wounds such as heavily contaminated or infected wounds

Source: Marie Rippingale.

wound [27]. Before use, the lavage fluid should be warmed to body temperature before being applied to the wound [27]. Using solutions at a lower temperature may cause a reduction in wound temperature for up to 40 minutes, and it may take up to three hours for cellular division to recommence [27]. The ideal pressure to deliver the lavage fluid at is no greater than 15 pounds per square inch (psi). If a higher pressure is used, this can cause microorganisms to be driven deeper into the wound. A pressure of 15 psi can be achieved using a 60 mL syringe with a 19 gauge needle attached [27]. There are many solutions used for wound lavage. It is beyond the scope of this chapter to discuss every lavage fluid used in equine practice; however, the most commonly used lavage fluids are summarised in Table 13.4.

The importance of good hygiene in wound care should not be overlooked. Gloves should be worn when examining wounds and changed between patients to reduce the risk of spreading any infection present [22]. If the wound is close to a synovial structure, this should be investigated thoroughly to rule out the risk of infection.

Wound Debridement

Debridement of a chronic wound is essential if the wound is to heal and involves the removal of any necrotic, infected tissue or foreign bodies. This aids in the reduction of the bacterial load, which helps to promote reepithelisation of the wound bed [28]. The type of debridement will depend on the size and the location of the wound and the amount of contamination present. There are various methods of debridement, which include surgical, autolytic, enzymatic, mechanical, hydrosurgical and biosurgical.

Surgical Debridement

The optimal debridement of choice for a chronic wound would be the surgical method. Sharpe debridement is usually carried out using a sharp scalpel blade, scissors or a curette and will rapidly remove any devitalised tissue. When using this method, it is important not to remove any healthy, viable tissue as this may make the wound larger, which in turn will contribute to an increased healing time. Surgical debridement is often combined with pressurised irrigation. Hydrosurgery is a newer technique that combines sharp debridement and irrigation with a Versajet machine (Smith and Nephew) that produces a high-pressure stream of sterile saline to optimise surgical debridement. This technique facilitates the removal of necrotic tissue but preserves viable tissue. Hydrosurgery can be carried out under a GA or standing sedation [29].

Autolytic Debridement

This is the most conservative and least painful method, as this process occurs naturally when the wound is healing. It uses the wound's own enzymes, which have been realised to soften the devitalised tissue. When a wound is chronic, the autolytic process becomes overwhelmed by high levels of endotoxins released from damaged tissue [30]. This natural debridement can be aided by applying hydrogels and dressings to the wound to create a moist environment. A moist environment allows better migration of neutrophils and macrophages than a dry wound environment. Neutrophils and macrophages phagocytise bacteria and debris while releasing enzymes to promote debridement [31].

Enzymatic Debridement

This is the least commonly used method of debridement in equine wounds, as it has limitations regarding large, heavily contaminated wounds. Enzymatic debridement selectively breaks down necrotic tissue or biofilms. Enzymatic formulations include collagenase, papain/urea and streptokinase/streptodornase. It may be used when surgical debridement is not possible or carries a risk, such as wounds that are close to nerves or large blood vessels [25].

Mechanical Debridement

Mechanical debridement uses an external force to help to separate or break down necrotic tissue. This is a nonselective method and can be painful for the patient [30]. Wet to dry dressings are an example of mechanical debridement. With this method, a gauze swab, which has been soaked in sterile saline is placed directly onto the wound. A secondary, non-adherent dressing is placed on top to prevent exudate from soaking through the bandage. This dressing is allowed to dry and then removed taking the devitalised tissue away. This method should be used with caution as it can also remove some of the healthy tissue and cells at the same time. Contraindications include epithelialising wounds and granulating wounds [30].

Biosurgical Debridement

Biosurgical debridement is also known as maggot or larval debridement therapy larval. The larvae of the common green bottle fly *Lucilia sericata* are grown and harvested in vitro. These larvae can be ordered from commercial companies and posted out for next-day delivery to the practice. The action of the larva on the wound is as follows:

- Rapid and selective debridement
- Potent antibacterial action
- The ability to destroy and digest bacteria
- Have an inhibitory effect on the formation of biofilms.

Maggot therapy can stimulate wound healing through increased wound oxygenation and increased wound pH. The action of maggots against methicillin-resistant *Staphylococcus aureus* (MRSA), multidrug-resistant *Pseudomonas aeruginosa* and *Escherichia coli* are of particular interest in chronic wounds [32]. The maggots can be applied directly or indirectly onto the wound. When the maggots are applied directly to a wound a nylon mesh is fixed to the dressing to prevent the maggots from escaping. The wound must be cleaned, and blood or heavy exudate must be removed to prevent the maggots from drowning. When the indirect method is used, the maggots are supplied in a closed polyester net filled with absorbent foam known as a biobag. In a study of 64 human patients, it was concluded that the free-range maggots provided better results than the maggots in a biobag [33].

Antibiotic Therapy

Systemic antibiotic therapy must be considered carefully when treating a chronic wound. Previous antimicrobial resistance should be considered. The wound should be swabbed, and a culture and sensitivity test carried out, to establish which bacteria are present in the wound. The correct course of antibiotics can then be prescribed by the vet with confidence. In heavily infected wounds, regional or local delivery of antibiotics can be useful to target a specific area. Intravenous regional perfusion (IVRP) can be carried out in distal limbs [34]. A tourniquet is required to isolate the infected area, and a sterile butterfly catheter is placed in the selected vein. The antibiotic of choice is then carefully injected into the vein ensuring the vein does not blow or rupture, as this can cause phlebitis and localised tissue necrosis. Once the antibiotic has been administered the needle is removed and a sterile dressing placed over the vein with a light-pressure bandage. The horse must then remain standing for 20–30 minutes without moving.

Creating an Optimal Wound Environment

Moist Wound Healing

Moist wound healing is the practice of keeping a wound in an optimally moist environment to help promote faster healing. It has been shown to promote epithelisation and reduce scarring compared to a dry environment. The benefits of moist wound healing are as follows:

- A moist environment inhibits the formation of a scab. This can aid healing time, as a scab can serve as a barrier to cellular migration, which in turn slows the rate of epithelisation.
- Autolytic debridement is facilitated in a moist environment as it increases the efficiency of the enzymes to break down the necrotic tissue.

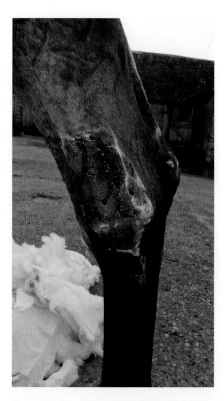

Figure 13.16 The chronic wound from Figure 13.15 beginning to heal following debridement and the application of moist wound healing. *Source:* Rosina Lillywhite.

- The chances of infection are decreased as moist wound healing creates a hypoxic environment which promotes angiogenesis, decreases the pH and helps to create an inhospitable environment for bacteria to grow.
- It promotes the production of collagen by the fibroblasts, reduce pain and scarring.

Hydrogels, manuka honey and certain dressings can be used to aid in moist wound healing. Each wound should be assessed and addressed differently to help create an optimum wound-healing environment for each individual patient (Figure 13.16).

Temperature

The temperature of the wound environment influences wound healing. A reduction in temperature as little as two degrees can affect the healing process as cells and enzymes function optimally at normal body temperature. If the surrounding tissue temperature drops it causes vasoconstriction leading to a decrease in neutrophil, fibroblast and epithelial activity. Once the wound has been assessed and properly debrided, the application of a suitable dressing and bandage can not only help to protect the wound, stabilise and decrease movement, but also helps to maintain the temperature.

Primary Layer Dressings

The primary layer is material that is placed in contact with the wound and usually takes the form of a wound dressing. There are many dressings available on the market, and the best practice is to select one that will provide the most optimal healing conditions for the specific wound being dealt with.

The functions of a primary layer dressing include [20]:

- Debridement of necrotic tissue
- Absorption of fluid from the wound. If fluid is left to collect on the wound surface, it can lead to maceration or tissues or form a reservoir for infection
- Stimulation of granulation tissue
- Promotion of epithelialisation
- Assisting with contraction of the wound

Wound dressings fall into different categories depending on their individual characteristics. Some dressings may fit into more than one category. The main categories are [20]:

- Adherent or non-adherent
- Absorbent or non-absorbent
- Passive – having no action on the wound
- Interactive – responding to the wound environment
- Bioactive – having a biological effect on the wound
- Occlusive, semi-occlusive or non-occlusive – refers to permeability to gas or vapour

It is beyond the scope of this chapter to discuss every wound dressing on the market. The main types of wound dressings used in equine practice are summarised in Table 13.5.

Once an appropriate dressing has been selected for a wound, a bandage will usually be applied. Information on bandaging techniques can be found in Chapter 17.

Topical Wound Treatments

There are several topical wound treatments used in equine practice. Some examples are summarised as follows:

- *Aloe vera*: Has been suggested to possess several potentially beneficial functions, including soothing effect, inhibition of bacterial and fungal growth, anti-inflammatory effects and increased blood flow to name a few [27]. There are no studies evaluating the effects of aloe vera on equine wound healing. However, acemannan (one of the components found in aloe vera) has been shown to demonstrate positive wound-healing effects in dogs [27].
- *Silver sulfadiazine cream*: It is used as a topical broad-spectrum antibiotic treatment. Silver sulfadiazine has been shown to reduce the antimicrobial load in wounds. However, silver sulfadiazine is thought to have very little effect on the rate or quality of wound healing in horses [37]. Further research is required to determine if silver is currently used appropriately in veterinary practice [37].

Table 13.5 Different wound dressings used in equine practice.

Wound dressing type	Specific properties	Commonly uses
Hydrogels (Interactive, occlusive)	Hydrogels provide and maintain a moist wound environment. They donate fluid to the wound and can be used as a filler for a desiccated cavity where they can restore a physiologically sound moist wound healing environment [35]	Used when clipping around the wound to prevent hair contamination. Used in combination with foam dressings in any type of wound where a moist, warm healing environment is required
Manuka honey (Bioactive, interactive, occlusive)	Manuka honey is formulated into medical grade honey, which has prolonged antimicrobial effects. It has debriding, anti-inflammatory and antioxidant properties. Normal honey is not recommended as wound exudate dilutes it quickly, and the dilution reduces the antibacterial effects [35]. Manuka honey has a very low pH, which can cause low to high levels of pain. This would highlight the need for pain scoring and stringent monitoring in patients where this product is used. If signs of discomfort are observed, the dressing should be removed and the area washed	Necrotic or infected wounds
Perforated polyurethane membrane dressings (Passive, non-adherent, non-occlusive)	These dressings do not interact with the wound but provide a protective layer and prevent the secondary layers from sticking to the wound [20]	Typically used over surgical wounds, skin grafts or granulation tissue [20]
Wet to dry dressings (Passive, adherent, non-occlusive)	Can be used to help debridement. A gauze swab which has been soaked in sterile saline is placed directly onto the wound. A secondary, non-adherent dressing is placed on top to prevent exudate from soaking through the bandage. This dressing is allowed to dry and then removed taking the devitalised tissue away. This method should be used with caution as it can also remove some of the healthy tissue and cells at the same time. It can also cause pain on removal	Heavily contaminated or infected wounds
Foam (Passive, absorbent and usually semi-occlusive)	Foam dressings absorb excessive exudate whilst providing a protective layer. Aids moist wound healing, granulation and epithelisation	Wounds producing a large amount of exudate. Granulating wounds
Hydrofibre and hydrocolloid (Bioactive, interactive, adhesive and absorbent, occlusive)	**Hydrofibre dressings:** These are soft, woven pads of sodium carboxymethylcellulose **Hydrocolloid dressings:** These dressings are like hydrofibre dressings, but are a suspension of gelatin, pectin and sodium carboxymethylcellulose which are held in an adhesive polymer matrix [35] Both dressings provide a moist environment for the wound without causing maceration and are designed to soften necrotic tissue. They are said to promote angiogenesis and fibrinolysis, therefore they are useful in the proliferation stage of wound healing. Exudate is absorbed and formed into a gel creating a moist wound environment. Should be used with a secondary foam dressing to keep them in place and prevent loss of fluid [35]	Wounds that require debridement. Wounds that are in the proliferation stage of healing. Should not be used on infected wounds [20]
Alginates (Bioactive and interactive, non-occlusive to semi-occlusive)	Alginates are made from acids obtained from seaweed and are fine, fibrous dressings. Alginates can absorb up to 20 times, or more of their own weight in wound exudate [36]. Exudate is absorbed and formed into a gel creating a moist wound environment. Caution should be used when applying these dressings to wounds on the distal limb of the horse, where excessive granulation tissue can be a problem [35]	Wounds producing a large amount of exudate. Wounds in the inflammatory phase or early proliferative phase of healing [36]
Silver dressings (Interactive, occlusive or semi-occlusive depending on dressing type)	Silver has an antimicrobial effect against many types of bacteria and is used to manage infection in wounds. Various types of silver dressings are available	Infected wounds

Source: Marie Rippingale.

Removal of Dressings

Once a dressing has been applied to a patient, the patient must be closely monitored for signs of complications. Poorly managed dressings can cause a delay in healing [20]. Generally, wounds that are in the inflammatory phase of healing require a dressing change every 24–48 hours. Wounds that are in the proliferation phase of healing require a dressing change every 72–96 hours. However, dressing changes should be carried out according to the individual requirements of the wound and the patient being treated. Reasons to change a dressing are as follows:

- Persistent interference from the patient, e.g. chewing and mutilation
- Foul odour coming from the dressing
- Contamination of the dressing with water or urine
- Exudate or 'strike-through' visible on the outside of the bandage
- Movement of the dressing from the original position [20]

13.6 Effective Home and Follow-up Care for Horses with Long-term Illness

The Importance of Client Concordance in Home Management

It is vital that the owner fully understands what they are taking on when the decision is made to care for a horse at home with a long-term illness. When talking about client concordance in the veterinary sector, it means an agreement between the owner and the veterinary team on how best to treat the patient, with both parties getting equal input and fully understanding the treatment or care to be given. Owner concordance leads to increased levels of care for the patient, as the client has had the opportunity to contribute to the suggested treatment plan and will therefore be more committed to the process.

The welfare of the horse, and owner, should always be a priority. The vet in charge of the case should not suggest home care if they feel that the horse is not well enough to cope at home, or if the horse requires more care and facilities than the owner can provide. It is paramount that the owner fully understands the extent of the horse's condition. Will the horse fully recover? If not, what quality of life can they have? Is there an increased risk of death during the home recovery period? Will the horse ever recover? A conversation discussing all these questions as well as what level of care and facilities the horse will require at home should be held with the owner well in advance of the horse going home. This conversation should be held in a distraction-free environment, away from the horse.

The owner will have lots of questions and concerns, and this conversation may need to be held several times to ensure the owner is prepared to care for the horse at home. If the horse has a progressive or terminal illness, the owner should be educated on the signs of progression or deterioration of the condition and when to phone the vet for assistance.

Long-term illness that the horse may be suffering from can include:

- Laminitis
- PPID
- EMS
- Arthritis
- Severe equine asthma
- Melanomas
- Old age
- Dental disease
- Eye conditions

The owner should be encouraged to attend the practice, if the horse is hospitalised, to help and to learn how to care for their horse. Depending on the horse's condition, the owner may need to carry out daily checks on the horse to include an assessment of temperature, pulse rate, respiration rate and other checks specific to the illness. It may be easier for the owner to implement environment changes if they can see examples within the clinic setting, or if a vet or RVN can visit the home setting, or view a video of the yard, to offer advice on simple changes that may result in significant improvements in the horse's condition. The owner can help with their horse's medications within the practice to learn how to administer the medications correctly and safely. Storage and disposal of the medications should also be discussed. Tips on how to get the perfect consistency for oral medications should be shared. Advice should be given on how to clean and care for equipment such as inhalers, nebulisers, eye masks and reusable bandages, just to name a few. If the owner needs to change the horse's bandage or dressing, they can practice this under guidance, in preparation for going home. Some owners like to video the procedures so that they have a reference to look back on. If the owner can visit the practice, it also helps to build up a bond with the team caring for their horse so that they feel more comfortable phoning for advice once they are at home. It should be made clear who the owner's first point of contact is if they need help with their horse. For care questions, it might be an RVN but for concerns relating to a deterioration, it should be the case vet. This can be confusing for the owner, so recording these details in the discharge instructions, along with relevant phone numbers, may be useful.

The owner should be given plenty of time to obtain any equipment and implement any changes before the horse is

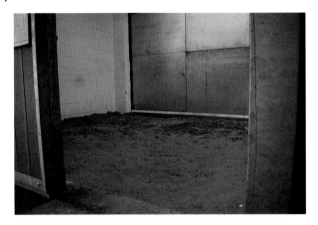

Figure 13.17 A sand box can be used for laminitic patients. *Source:* Victoria Gregory.

discharged. They may require help from suppliers for specialist feed or bedding that has been recommended. Sand is recommended as a bedding material for laminitic cases (Figure 13.17), because it will conform to the solar surface of the hoof and distribute the weight over the solar surface, frog and hoof wall [38]. An environmental change such as this may take a bit longer to organise, as will moving stables at the livery yard, so that the horse is furthest from the hay storage if it is suffering from a condition caused by dust. These changes can also be very costly to the owner. Some conditions may require a large financial outlay at the beginning but then the cost to keep the horse is neutral, whereas other conditions may require years of veterinary or nursing consults, and medication costs, which could increase as the illness progresses. Initial costs and future financial commitments should be discussed when the illness is diagnosed along with the option of euthanasia. The client should be advised to check with their insurer about the costs associated with euthanasia and disposal. Clients should also be aware that insurers may exclude a condition when the policy renews.

Maintaining and Improving Client Concordance with Home Care Plans

When the horse is discharged, the owner should be given a date for a follow-up appointment, either at home or at the hospital or practice. This will help to reassure owners that they will receive continued care and support. The frequency of follow-up appointments will depend on the long-term illness, and which stage the illness is at. This should be discussed during the early stages of the home care planning, and the owner should understand that the frequency of appointments will depend on any improvement or deterioration of the horse's health. Most practices will have client advice sheets for long-term illness conditions

that can be adapted to suit each patient and owner. This information will detail the level of care the owner is expected to give daily at home and what goals, if any, have been agreed upon with the owner. This might be for the horse to lose a certain number of kilograms or be doing a certain amount of exercise by the next consultation. If the horse requires intensive nursing care or regular record keeping, blank templates can be provided for the owner to document clinical findings such as respiratory rate and effort, heart rate, weight measurements and increased lameness. These sheets can also include abnormal parameter guidelines for the individual patient, indicating when a vet should be contacted. It would be helpful if these advice sheets include the names and numbers of the support team and who to contact outside of working hours.

The Ability Model care plan may be suitable for the owner and veterinary team to use with home care cases. An RVN can run through the assessment questions with the owner and explain the use and need for the home care plan. The home care plan can also be based on the care plan used with the patient while they were in the hospital. The RVN can routinely check the patient, onsite or at home, to update the home care plan with the owner. Some updates can be carried out over the phone, and new home care plans can be sent electronically for the owner to use. More information regarding care plans can be found in Section 13.4.

Nurse clinics are growing in popularity and can be carried out at the practice, or out on yards. The use of RVNs on an ambulatory basis is also increasing. This is ideal to give extra support to owners who are caring for horses at home. RVNs can assist with the following:

- Regular weighing and body condition scoring
- Taking haematology samples
- Checking owner-kept records
- Geriatric care
- Administration of medication
- Pain scoring
- General health checks
- Dressing changes
- Radiographs
- Sedating for allied professionals under the direction of the case vet[1]
- Clipping
- Transporting
- Environment enrichment

---

1 Sedation may only be carried out by an RVN if the patient in question is under the care of the vet directing the treatment and the dose is agreed by the vet beforehand. Incremental dosing must be prescribed by the directing vet.

Figure 13.18 An example of a SMARTER goal plan. *Source:* Victoria Gregory.

SMARTER goals example

Specific: To decrease Leo's weight over the next three months to decrease the risk of his laminitis reoccurring.

Measurement: This will be measured in kgs using the university weigh scales on a weekly basis. He should lose approximately 100kg in three months. The grooms will be responsible for Leo's weekly weight examination and fill in his weight chart.

Achievable: This can be achieved by reducing Leo's hay ration to 1.5% of his body weight daily. He will receive 10kg (dry weight) of hay that has been soaked for 24 hours. When other horses are fed, he can have a small handful of chaff to stop him kicking at the door. Leo can be lunged 3 times a week for 5 minutes, monitoring for any signs of lameness, and be turned out regularly in the indoor school. If no lameness is seen, lunging can increase by 5 minutes per week until a maximum of 30 minutes per session is reached. If Leo is unable to exercise, the diet should be monitored to assess weight loss. If no weight loss is seen, rations may need to be decreased further to have an effect.

Relevant: This is relevant for Leo as he is obese and has evidence of laminitic changes on radiographs.

Time-bound: In three months Leo should weigh approximately 600kg

Exciting: Leo will start to feel healthier, fitter and find exercising easier once he has lost some weight. His cheeky behaviour should start to reappear.

Rewarding: Once Leo has reached his goal weight, he can start turned out in the paddock for one hour per day. His weight should still be monitored weekly, and his exercise plan should be continued.

RVNs can help with worming regimes by performing faecal worm egg counts, offer nutritional advice and continue educating the owner on the care of their horse as the horse's condition progresses. Nurse clinics are a good way of keeping regular contact with the owner and the horse, at little extra cost to either party, outside of their regular consultations, showing how much the team care for the horse and want to support the owner. This can also relieve time pressure as the RVN can assist the owner with nursing tasks, which then allows the vet to perform more vet-related tasks.

As the horse continues to be cared for at home, there may be many different reasons for goals being changed and adapted. A specific, measurable, achievable, realistic and time-bound (SMART) goal tool may be useful to set goals and monitor if the long-term goal is being achieved. A SMART goal can be used in many different aspects of life to set personal and business goals but can also be patient based. An E and R can be added on to the end for 'exciting' and 'rewarding' [39]. The goal must be specific such as lose X amount of weight to decrease the risk of laminitis, you must be able to measure the result, in this case it can be measured as weight loss in kilograms. An achievable goal should be set that the owner will be able to manage, this can be helped by supplying the amount of feed the horse should be receiving per day and an exercise plan that the owner can fit into their busy day. Weight loss goals can be broken down into weeks or months, depending on how often the horse can be weighed, rather than one large, potentially overwhelming, goal. The goal is relevant because obesity is linked to an increased risk of laminitis [40]. A time limit can be put on the goal such as lose X number of kilograms by the recheck date in two weeks' time. This can be exciting for the owner because losing weight may mean that the horse can be ridden again, this may be rewarding enough for the owner or maybe they have their own SMARTER goal of attending a competition and winning a prize as their reward. An example of a SMARTER goal is shown in Figure 13.18 for a horse who is obese (Figure 13.19).

As the seasons change, it will become harder to keep weight on some horses and weight off others; in the winter months, it may become difficult to exercise the horses or turn them out; the horse's diet will need to be adapted to accommodate these things. The goal may be reached quicker than expected meaning that other plans and future goal timelines can be brought forward. For personal reasons, the owner may no longer be able to spend as much time working towards goals that have been set previously or may just feel overwhelmed by the task when they get home. The owner should be reassured that any small changes in the right direction will help, and they should be supported to break the goal down into smaller, simpler steps that will benefit the horse. If

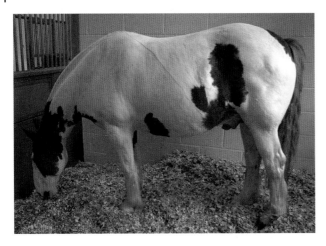

Figure 13.19 An obese horse. *Source:* Victoria Gregory.

the owner is liaising with a consistent, patient and understanding team, they are more likely to be honest if they are struggling to accommodate the changes at home that are required to achieve the goals.

Palliative Care for Equine Patients

Owners who are providing palliative care at home for their horses will need a lot of veterinary support but also emotional and mental health support. If a good rapport has been built between the owner and the veterinary care team, it is easier to identify if the owner has the appropriate support for themselves whilst caring for their horse and following the horse's death. When visiting or holding nurse clinics for terminally ill patients, a big part of the job will be supporting the owner and preparing them for the death of their horse. There are lots of pet bereavement specialists, as well as mental health charities, that the practice can signpost the client to. Owners should be introduced to quality-of-life (QOL) assessments early on in their horse's illness, so they become familiar with assessing their horse and knowing what normal behaviour is for that individual horse. Lots of equine charities have QOL assessment materials available online. Livery yard peers, riding instructors and people on the internet will all have different opinions about whether a horse is suffering or not. Regular and correct use of an owner aimed QOL assessment, taught by a member of the veterinary team, may help to reassure the owner that they can identify if their horse is suffering or not and help to remove emotions from any difficult decisions. QOL assessments can be used to recognise the improvement as well as any deterioration in a condition. Owner-aimed QOL assessments tend to be based on open questions rather than a numerical scoring system that the vet may use. It is thought that a numerical scoring system is unlikely to help clients make decisions and may make clinicians seem cold and uncaring [41].

As a horse gets older or a health condition deteriorates, the horse's needs will change. A horse that lives out all year-round may need a field shelter or no longer be able to cope with being out during the winter months, or a horse that is usually stabled may need to be turned out more to help with a respiratory condition. Horses may find it harder to stand up, after rolling or laying down, so a deeper bed and rubber mats should be provided to help prevent injury when trying to stand. If stabled for long periods, or permanently, a dust-free environment furthest from the hay store is ideal, with good ventilation. Horses are herd animals, so it can be beneficial if the full-time stabled horses can be in view of each other to help to reduce stress and improve QOL. Owners may need help with accommodation changes, such as advice on how to settle anxious horses and make their environment safer for them. Some horses may not cope with the changes and so compromises will need to be made. Accommodation changes will most likely mean nutritional changes as well, and possibly an increased risk of impaction colic. Advice on these management changes for geriatric horses or horses with long-term illness can be discussed in nurse clinics or on information sheets provided by the practice.

If the horse is no longer able to socialise, they may start to show signs of boredom, dullness and depression. Boredom-relieving items may help to improve the horse's demeanour such as treat balls, fine-holed haynets so that forage lasts longer, hanging vegetables in the stable, horse-safe mirrors or getting another animal as a companion in the stable or field. If food is used, this must be accounted for in the horse's daily rations. Regular grooming and human interaction may help the horse's demeanour as they are social animals and like to mutually groom when access to a companion allows. While grooming, the owner may also notice any new melanomas, oedema, swelling or signs of deterioration in the horse's condition. As the horse ages and/or the condition progresses its nutritional requirements will change, this can be for several different reasons, and it may be that the horse is struggling to maintain their weight due to difficulty chewing long strands of fibre, as a side effect of medication or carrying too much weight due to decreased exercise or the progression of the illness.

Regular assessment of the patient with body condition scoring and weigh tapes or attending weight clinics can help the owner to manage their horse's nutritional requirements. It is difficult for the owner to be objective about the horses' weight if they see them daily. Regular monitoring and recording of any observations may make it easier to identify any changes in the horse's weight. It is likely the horse will require increased monitoring and record keeping as it ages or any health problems progress. Again, these are processes that can be taught and discussed at nurse clinics or visits and can help the owner to recognise when, or if, the horse needs to be hospitalised or euthanised, along with the

QOL assessments. If the horse is hospitalised, palliative care may consist of intensive nursing care, pain scoring resulting in added pain relief, IVFT, enteral tube feeding, surgical intervention to prolong life and increase comfort levels, dressing or bandage changes and eventually euthanasia.

References

1 Durando, M. and Corley, K. (2008). Monitoring and treating the cardiovascular system. In: *The Equine Hospital Manual* (ed. K. Corley and J. Stephen), 440–441. Chichester: Blackwell Publishing.

2 Freeman, D.E. (2019). Surgical site infection after occlusion of the internal carotid artery with a thrombectomy catheter: Can this be prevented? *Equine Veterinary Education* 31 (1): 45–48. Available from: https://doi.org/10.1111/eve.12774. (accessed 13 August 2022).

3 Durham, A.E. (2014). Further observations of seasonality of pars intermedia secretory function in 30,000 horses and ponies [Internet]. https://sites.tufts.edu/equineendogroup/files/2013/10/Equine-Geriatric-Workshop-II-DRH-2014.pdf (accessed 13 August 2022).

4 Frank, N., Geor, R.J., Bailey, S.R. et al. (2010). Equine metabolic syndrome. *Journal of Veterinary Internal Medicine* 24 (3): 467–475. Available from: https://doi.org/10.1111/j.1939-1676.2010.0503.x. (accessed 13 August 2022).

5 Morgan, R., Keen, J., and McGowan, C. (2015). Equine metabolic syndrome. *Veterinary Record* 177 (7): 173–179. Available from: https://doi.org/10.1136/vr.103226. (accessed 13 August 2022).

6 Durham, A.E., Frank, N., McGowan, C.M. et al. (2019). ECIEM consensus statement on equine metabolic syndrome. *Journal of Veterinary Internal Medicine* 33 (2): 335–349. Available from: https://doi.org/10.1111/jvim.15423. (accessed 13 August 2022).

7 Pirie, R.S. and McGorum, B.C. (2018). Managing the chronic grass sickness case. *UK-VET Equine* 2 (3) Available from: https://doi.org/10.12968/ukve.2018.2.3.76: (accessed 02 January 2023).

8 Henderson, I.S.F. (2013). Diagnostic and prognostic use of L-lactate measurement in equine practice. *Equine Veterinary Education* 25 (9): 468–475. Available from: https://doi.org/10.1111/eve.12033. (accessed 13 August 2022).

9 RCVS (2018). Navigating schedule 3 delegation in practice: some case studies [Online]. Available from: https://www.rcvs.org.uk/news-and-views/features/case-studies-for-navigating-schedule-3-delegation-in-practice/ (accessed 30 August 2022).

10 RCVS (2022). Code of professional conduct for veterinary nurses [Online]. Available from: https://www.rcvs.org.uk/setting-standards/advice-and-guidance/code-of-professional-conduct-for-veterinary-nurses/#animals (accessed 30 August 2022).

11 RCVS (2020). 6. Clinical governance [Online]. Available from: https://www.rcvs.org.uk/setting-standards/advice-and-guidance/code-of-professional-conduct-for-veterinary-nurses/supporting-guidance/clinical-governance/ (accessed 30 August 2022).

12 Ballantyne, H. (2018). *Veterinary Nursing Care Plans Theory and Practice*. Boca Raton: CRC Press.

13 Jeffery, A. and Ford-Fennah, S. (2020). The nursing process, nursing models and care plans. In: *BSAVA Textbook of Veterinary Nursing*, 6e (ed. B. Cooper, E. Mullineaux, and L. Turner), 291–309. Gloucester, British Small Animal Veterinary Association.

14 Gonzalo, A. (2021). Dorothea Orem: self-care deficit theory [Online]. Available from: https://nurseslabs.com/dorothea-orems-self-care-theory/ (accessed 30 September 2022).

15 Ballantyne, H. (2016). Beyond the nursing care plan: an introduction to care bundles. *Veterinary Nursing Journal* 31: 43–46. Available from: https://members.bvna.org.uk/blog/view/Beyond_the_nursing_care_plan_an_introduction_to_care_bundles_by_Helen_Ballantyne_wSX. (accessed 30 September 2022).

16 Waxman, C. (2022). The evidence for checklists and patient care bundles in veterinary nursing. *Today's Veterinary Nurse* Spring. Available from: https://todaysveterinarynurse.com/emergency-medicine-critical-care/the-evidence-for-checklists-and-patient-care-bundles-in-veterinary-nursing/ (accessed 30 September 2022).

17 RCVS (2022). Code of professional conduct for veterinary surgeons [Online]. Available from: https://www.rcvs.org.uk/setting-standards/advice-and-guidance/code-of-professional-conduct-for-veterinary-surgeons/ (accessed 10 October 2022).

18 Barry, L. (2021). Evidence based veterinary medicine: a practice-based example. *Veterinary Nursing Journal* 36: 217–220. Available from: https://members.bvna.org.uk/blog/view/Evidence_based_veterinary_medicine_a_practice_based_example_by_Lydia_M_Barry_fkH. (accessed 30 September 2022).

19 Dubhashi, S.P. and Nunan, R. (2015). A comparative study of honey and phenytoin dressings for chronic wounds. *Indian Journal of Surgery* 77 (Suppl. 3): 1209–1213.

20 Anderson, D. and Smith, J. (2020). Small animal surgical nursing. In: *BSAVA Textbook of Veterinary Nursing*, 6e (ed. B. Cooper, E. Mullineaux, and L. Turner), 792–793, 800–801. Gloucester: British Small Animal Veterinary Association.

21 Orsini, J.A., Elce, Y.A. and Kraus, B. (2016). Management of severely infected wounds. In: *Equine Wound*

Management, 3e (ed. Theoret, C. and Schumacher, J.), 452. Wiley: Oxford.

22 Dart, A.J., Sole-Guitart, A., Stashak, T.S. et al. (2016). Selected factors that negatively impact healing. In: *Equine Wound Management*, 3e (ed. C. Theoret and J. Schumacher), 30–46. Oxford: Wiley.

23 Dart, A.J., Sole-Guitart, A., Stashak, T.S. et al. (2016). Management practices that influence wound infection and healing. In: *Equine Wound Management*, 3e (ed. C. Theoret and J. Schumacher), 68. Oxford: Wiley.

24 Zehtabchi, S., Tan, A., Yadav, K. et al. (2012). The impact of wound age on the infection rates of simple lacerations repaired in the emergency department. *Injury* 43: 1793.

25 Wilmink, J.M., van Weeren, P.R., Stolk, P.W. et al. (1999). Differences in second-intention wound healing between horses and ponies: histological aspects. *Equine Veterinary Journal* 31: 61–67.

26 Pritchard, P. (2015). The nurse's role in the management of equine limb wounds. *The Veterinary Nurse* 6: 90–98.

27 Jacobsen, S. (2016). Topical wound treatments and wound-care products. In: *Equine Wound Management*, 3e (ed. C. Theoret and J. Schumacher), 76. Oxford: Wiley.

28 Biagio, M., Nahirniak, P., and Morrison, C.A (2022). Wound Debridement [Online]. Available at: https://www.ncbi.nlm.nih.gov/books/NBK507882/ (accessed 22 January 2023).

29 Skarlina, E.M., Wilmink, J.M., Fall, N. et al. (2015). Effectiveness of conventional hydrosurgical debridement methods in reducing *Staphylococcus aureus* inoculation of equine muscle in vitro. *Equine Veterinary Journal* 47 (2): 218–222.

30 Broadus, C. (2013). Debridement options: beams made easy [Online]. Available at: https://woundcareadvisor.com/debridement-options-beams-made-easy_vol2-no/ (accessed 22 January 2023).

31 Hendrickson, D.A. (2004). *Wound Care Management for the Equine Practitioner*, 46. Wyoming: Teton NewMedia.

32 Lepage, O.M., Doumbia, A., Perron-Lepage, M.F. et al. (2012). The use of maggot debridement therapy in 41 equids. *Equine Veterinary Journal* 44 (S43): 120–125.

33 Steenvoorde, P., Jacobi, C.E., and Oskam, J. (2005). Maggot debridement Therapy: free-range or contained? An in-vivo study. *Advances in Skin and Wound Care* 18: 430.

34 Biasutt, S.A., Cox, E., Jeffcott, L.B. et al. (2021). A review of regional limb perfusion for distal limb infections in the horse. *Equine Veterinary Education* 33 (5): 263–277.

35 Packer, M. and Devaney, J. (2011). Dressings used in equine traumatic wound care. *The Veterinary Nurse* 1: 162–171.

36 Jacobsen, S. (2016). Update on wound dressings: indications and best use. In: *Equine Wound Management*, 3e (ed. C. Theoret and J. Schumacher), 114. Oxford: Wiley.

37 Freeman, S.L., Ashton, N.M., Elce, Y.A. et al. (2021). BEVA primary care clinical guidelines: wound management in the horse. *Equine Veterinary Journal* 53: 18–29.

38 Mitchell, C.F., Fugler, L.A., and Eades, S.C. (2014). The management of equine acute laminitis. *Veterinary Medicine (Auckl)* 6: 39–47. Available from: https://doi.org/10.2147/VMRR.S39967. (accessed 12 September 2022).

39 Zeltman, P. (2019). Do you want to get stuff done? Make your goals smarter [Internet]. [cited 2022 Aug 24]. Available from: https://www.veterinarypracticenews.com/do-you-want-to-get-stuff-done-make-your-goals-smarter/ (accessed 12 September 2022).

40 Rendle, D. (2020). Obesity and laminits: looking beyond lockdown. *UK-Vet Equine* 4 (5): 144–146. Available from: https://doi.org/10.12968/ukve.2020.4.5.144. (accessed 12 September 2022).

41 Parker, R.A. and Yeates, J.W. (2012). Assessment of quality of life in equine patients. *Equine Veterinary Journal* 44 (2): 244–249. Available from: https://doi.org/10.1111/j.2042-3306.2011.00411 (accessed 12 September 2022).

Further Reading

Blood, D.C. and Studdert, V.P. (1999). *Saunders Comprehensive Veterinary Dictionary*, 2e. London: Elsevier Saunders.

Corley, K. and Stephen, J. (ed.) (2008). *The Equine Hospital Manual*. Chichester: Blackwell Publishing.

Mair, T.S., Love, S., Schumacher, J. et al. (ed.) (2013). *Equine Medicine, Surgery and Reproduction*, 2e. London: Saunders Elsevier.

Reed, S., Bayly, W., and Sellon, D. (2016). *Equine Internal Medicine*, 4e. St Louis: Elsevier Saunders.

Reeder, D., Miller, S., Wilfong, D.A. et al. (2009). *AAEVT's Equine Manual for Veterinary Technicians*. Iowa: Wiley-Blackwell.

Ryan, J. and Johnson, J.P. (2022). Long-term nursing care of the equine patient in a sling. *Veterinary Nursing Journal* 34 (4): 34–39.

Theoret, C. and Schumacher, J. (ed.) (2016). *Equine Wound Management*, 3e. Oxford: Wiley.

White, N. and Edwards, B. (1999). *Handbook of Equine Colic*. Oxford: Butterworth Heinemann.

14

Emergency and Critical Care Nursing

Bonny Millar[1], Phillippa Pritchard[2], Marie Rippingale[3], and Rosina Lillywhite[4]

[1] *Equicomms, CVS House, Norfolk, UK*
[2] *Liphook Equine Hospital, Liphook, Hampshire, UK*
[3] *Bottle Green Training Ltd, Derby, UK*
[4] *VetPartners Nursing School, Petersfield, UK*

14.1 First Aid

First aid is the provision of initial care for an illness or injury. Within The Veterinary Surgeons Act (VSA) (1966), a dispensation is given for first aid to be carried out without veterinary supervision by an unqualified person in an emergency situation to save a life or relieve pain or suffering [1]. The key aims of first aid are as follows [1]:

- Preserve life
- Prevent suffering
- Stabilise the patient's condition and prevent further harm
- Promote recovery

First aid differs from emergency veterinary treatment.

- First aid: This can be carried out by a layperson; however, if a more qualified staff member is available, then this person should take the lead on first aid. Delegation to lay people, regardless of expertise, is at the discretion of the veterinary surgeon (vet) [2]. The provision of first aid may include techniques such as cold hosing, application of pressure to a bleeding wound, applying a basic bandage and moving the patient to a safe area.
- Emergency veterinary treatment: May only be carried out by a vet, registered veterinary nurse (RVN) or student veterinary nurse (SVN). At the time of writing this text, RVNs and SVNs may only carry out emergency veterinary treatment under the direction of their veterinary surgeon employer. SVNs must be appropriately supervised as stated in Schedule 3 of the VSA (see Chapter 3). Emergency veterinary treatment may include techniques such as placing an intravenous (IV) catheter

and administering pain relief, antibiotics, sedation and IV fluids (prescribed by the treating vet).

The Royal College of Veterinary Surgeons (RCVS) Code of Conduct for Veterinary Surgeons; states that all vets in practice must take steps to provide 24-hour emergency first aid and pain relief to animals according to their skills and the specific situation [3]. 'In practice' means offering clinical services directly to the public or to other vets. Taking steps can include the provision of emergency cover with vets cooperating with each other to provide 24-hour care, either by sharing any on-call duties with local practices or a dedicated out-of-hours emergency service clinic. Terms of arrangements should be made in writing between the veterinary practices prior to services being carried out. According to the Animal Welfare Act, a person becomes responsible for an animal by virtue of ownership or when they have been said to have assumed responsibility for its day-to-day care. This includes those who assume responsibility for the animal on a temporary basis, for example, keepers and carers such as owner's friends, neighbours and relatives and staff at boarding premises and animal sanctuaries [3]. When the owner, keeper or carer is concerned that the animal is suffering or requires attention and contacts a vet, they then place the onus of decision-making on to the vet [3].

The provision of first aid and pain relief is to allow initial assessment of an emergency patient to prevent undue suffering and facilitate euthanasia if appropriate [3]. The RCVS Code of Conduct for Veterinary Nurses states that RVNs and SVNs must make animal health and welfare their first consideration when attending to animals; they must keep within their area of competence and refer cases if required. The nursing care provided should be appropriate and adequate. RVNs in practice must take steps to provide emergency first aid and pain relief according to their skills and specific situations [4]. Providing pain relief by administering medication can only be carried out under the direction of a vet. The RCVS Code of Conduct for Veterinary Surgeons states that vets and RVNs should ensure that support staff for whom they are responsible conform to the following [3]:

- Are competent, courteous and properly trained
- Do not suggest a diagnosis or clinical opinion
- Are advised to pass on any request for urgent attention to a vet
- Are trained to recognise those occasions when it is necessary for a client to speak directly to a vet

Advice for Owners on Administering First Aid

- Advice for owners regarding first aid should be given with caution. It is not always possible to assess the client's ability from a telephone call. In a first aid emergency situation, it is important to advise the owner not to put themselves at risk. Human safety is a paramount consideration, and this should be made clear to the owner as a priority [5].

Some examples of relevant advice to give to clients are as follows:

- If a foreign body is present, it is acceptable to ask for the object not to be removed prior to the arrival of the vet, for example, a solar penetration [5]. Advice can be given on bandaging to allow the patient to stand without causing more damage to the area, such as taping something that is bigger than the object to the hoof, so that the object remains in place for the vet to see the direction of entry [6].
- If the patient is haemorrhaging, the owner should be asked to describe the nature of the bleeding, as it is important to find out if an artery has been damaged. If excessive bleeding is present, regardless of whether it is arterial or venous, the owner can be asked to apply pressure by applying a basic bandage or by holding a clean towel or jumper on the area [5]. If the bleeding seeps through the padding layer, further layers should be applied if this can be done safely.
- If a horse has colic and is rolling violently, the owner should be advised to put the horse in a safe area, for example, a stable with deep bedding, a small paddock or sand school and observe it until the vet arrives. The owner should be advised not to put themselves at risk under any circumstances.

First Aid Techniques

Haemorrhage and Wounds

Haemorrhage can be either internal or external; external, for obvious reasons, is much easier to identify as the blood is visible, while internal haemorrhages, such as those caused by a kick to the abdomen or a clotting problem, are more difficult for the vet to diagnose. If the haemorrhage is severe, it can lead to hypovolaemic shock. Cardiovascular function can be assessed by monitoring the heart rate, respiratory rate, colour of mucous membranes, capillary refill time (CRT) and checking for cold extremities. The nature of the bleeding should be investigated:

- Arterial bleeding – is bright red in colour and spurts from the wound; this can result in rapid blood loss and in extreme circumstances, death. Arterial blood spurts in time with the rhythm of the heart rate.
- Venous and capillary bleeding – is darker red in colour and oozes rather than spurts from the wound.

It is sometimes difficult to accurately measure the amount of blood loss, so the patients' parameters should be carefully monitored. Packed cell volume (PCV) can be measured following a large bleed. However, the results should be interpreted cautiously as the PCV may remain the same for several hours due to splenic contraction in response to the blood loss. In these circumstances, it may take up to 24 hours following the injury to observe a significant drop in the PCV [7].

Techniques used to control haemorrhage can include:

- Applying pressure with a clean/gloved hand for five minutes.
- Pressure bandage – Application of an absorbent bandage (towel/cotton wool, gamgee) or similar secured with cohesive bandage [5].
- Pressure points – Requires knowledge of anatomy and requires firm pressure that may not be possible in the equine patient due to temperament or muscle mass. The brachial artery, femoral artery or coccygeal artery can be used.
- Tourniquets – These can be makeshift in the form of a belt if an Esmarch bandage is unavailable and should be positioned proximal to the wound. Tourniquets should be applied with extreme caution due to the risk of causing ischemia and necrosis if used incorrectly.
- Using artery forceps (if available) to occlude the bleeding vessel if this can be done safely.

Musculoskeletal Injuries

The severity of a wound is difficult to judge from external appearance; small puncture wounds can easily penetrate

Table 14.1 Classification of wounds [5].

Classification	Description	Notes and potential causes
Incised	Clean cut caused by a sharp object	Most commonly seen in surgical wounds, may cause profuse bleeding
Lacerated	Tearing of tissue and uneven edges	Barbed wire or electric fencing, bleeding less profuse. Higher risk of contamination
Abrasion (graze)	Superficial wound, full skin thickness not penetrated	Embedded dirt and foreign bodies may be present. Can be caused by falling or sliding on concrete or gravel
Contusion (bruise)	Blunt force that ruptures capillaries below the skin surface	Stones in feet or kick wounds. May be associated with deeper injuries, e.g. fractures
Puncture	Small external wounds often associated with significant deeper damage	Standing on a nail or stake wound from running into a fence. Blackthorn penetration

Source: Phillippa Pritchard.

underlying synovial structures on the limbs, causing sepsis. See Table 14.1 for the classification of wounds. First aid treatment can include covering the wound with a dressing to prevent further contamination and control of haemorrhage, as mentioned above. If possible, sterile wound hydrogel can be applied to the wound and the surrounding area can be clipped. This will allow the vet to easily visualise the area of interest. The sterile wound hydrogel will prevent further contamination of the wound from the clipping process. If the wound is highly contaminated with minimal haemorrhage, then flushing the wound with a low-pressure hosepipe is acceptable first aid for most wounds [5].

Fractures

Adequate support or coaptation is essential in equine fracture first aid. If a fracture is inappropriately supported before treatment can be instigated, it can result in displacement of the fracture, which will lead to euthanasia in most cases. A Robert Jones bandage (RJB) is the mainstay for fracture support. If a wound is present, this should have an appropriate dressing applied, which should be held in place with orthopaedic padding. The RJB then consists of multiple layers of padding, such as cotton wool or gamgee, held in place and tightened by a densely knitted conforming bandage, that allows for support and compression of the fracture. Each layer is applied more tightly than the previous one, increasing the compression across the fracture. The outer layer of a RJB is made up of a layer of self-cohesive or self-adhesive bandage according to practice protocol. The finished RJB for a normal-size horse requires 10–15 rolls of cotton wool or gamgee. Its diameter should be at least three times the diameter of the limb and should make the limb cylindrical in appearance.

Fractures can be classed as open (those involving a wound) or closed (those not including a wound). Simple fractures involve one fracture line, and comminuted fractures involve more than one fracture line and an element of distance between the fracture lines [8]. For more information regarding fractures and RJBs, see Chapter 12.

Splints can improve comfort and the outcome of a fracture; they are commonly used in conjunction with the RJB for radius or tibial fracture stabilisation. For these, there should be a lateral splint applied that extends to one joint proximal to the suspected fracture. The splint should be padded to ensure that there is contact with the scapula/rump, respectively, to prevent the abduction of the limb [9]. Splints can be made from a variety of materials that may be available in the field; a rail from a post and rail fence or a plastic drainpipe of an adequate size are both reasonable materials that can be used. Commercial splints such as the Kimzey leg saver splint and the Monkey splint are easy to apply and support lower limb fractures for transport to a practice for treatment. For more information regarding splinting, please see Chapter 12.

Cast Horse

A horse described as 'cast' is recumbent, stuck with their legs up against the wall of the stable/fence line and unable to right themselves. This is commonly seen when horses are housed in stables that are too small or in horses that roll too close to the wall. Human safety is paramount in the case of a cast horse. At least three people will be required to free the horse safely. All personnel should wear personal protective equipment (PPE) in the form of steel toe-capped boots, hard hats and gloves. It is important to ensure that all personnel can get out of the stable at any time. One person should place a hand on the horse's head and neck to prevent them from struggling; this depends a bit on the position of the horse and whether it is safe to do so. One person should attempt to loop (not tie) long ropes or lunge lines around the patient's lower limbs, ideally just above the fetlock. One rope should be used for the hindlimbs, and one should be used for the forelimbs. Once the ropes are in place, all personnel should position themselves close to the exit point. The person restraining the head and neck should move away to a safe distance, and then the two other people should pull at the same time to move the horse over onto its other side.

The horse should be allowed to stand before the ropes are removed, and the patient checked over for any visible signs of injury. The horse should also be checked for signs of colic, as this may explain why the horse was rolling in the first place. The provision of banks in the stable is often enough to discourage most horses from rolling close to the wall.

Severe Abdominal Pain

Described as colic, a horse suffering from abdominal pain can show several symptoms depending on the severity of the pain. Some equine patients such as native ponies and donkeys may show pain less readily. They are therefore often described as stoic. These patients can be in severe pain but only show mild signs outwardly. In contrast, some horses show signs of pain more readily, even if the pain is mild or moderate, for example, Thoroughbreds. The main first aid treatment for a horse showing signs of abdominal pain is to ensure they are in a safe and secure area; feed should be withheld until the patient has been assessed by a vet. A stable is a suitable place to house the patient during this time, so long as there are minimal stable fixtures and pieces of equipment present as these can present as a source of injury. A reasonable amount of bedding should be provided to protect the patient from sores due to rolling or lying down during this period. Hand walking may help, but only if it is safe to do so; if the horse remains unsettled and tries to roll while walking, it is safer for the horse and the handler if they return to the stable [10].

Identification and Treatment of Burns

Table 14.2 displays the most common types of burns seen in veterinary practice. Burns in horses are relatively uncommon and mostly occur during hot weather (radiation) or following a stable fire (thermal). The other burns described in Table 14.2 are less commonly seen.

Sunburn is commonly seen in horses with pink skin, especially around the muzzle or occasionally seen on limbs. First aid treatment would involve removing the horse from the source of the problem, so moving the horse to a stable. If a horse is 'prone' to sunburn, factor 50 sun cream should be applied if the horse is turned out during the day, and

Table 14.2 Types of burns and potential causes [11].

Type of burn	Cause
Ice burn (Frostbite)	An ice burn occurs when ice or other extremely cold objects come into contact with and damage the skin tissue. The water in the skin cells freezes, forming sharp ice crystals that can damage the skin cell structure. Blood vessels constrict, reducing blood flow and the amount of oxygen delivered to the area. Blood clots can form, further restricting the flow of oxygen. Bleeding may occur if the cold temperature affects blood-clotting proteins
Thermal burns	Thermal burns occur due to heat sources which raise the temperature of the skin and tissues. This causes tissue cell death or charring. Hot metal, scalding liquids, steam and flames can cause thermal burns when they come into contact with the skin
Radiation burns	Radiation burns occur due to prolonged exposure to ultraviolet rays of the sun or to other sources of radiation such as X-rays
Chemical burns	Chemical burns occur due to strong acids, alkalis, detergents or solvents coming into contact with the skin or eyes
Electrical burns	Electrical burns occur due to an electrical current, either alternating current (AC) or direct current (DC)

Source: Phillippa Pritchard and Rosina Lillywhite.

UV-blocking rugs could be used [12]. Alternatively, only turning the horse out at night may be an effective solution.

Sunburn should not be confused with photosensitisation, which occurs when the UV rays of the sun react with photoproducts in the skin of certain horses. Primary photosensitisation can occur following ingestion of certain plants such as St John's wort, clover and perennial ryegrass. The administration of medication such as phenothiazines, thiazides and sulfonamides may also make a horse more prone to developing primary photosensitisation. Secondary photosensitisation may occur due to underlying conditions such as liver disease, which will require further investigation and treatment [13]. See Chapter 13 for more information.

First aid for other burns involves removing the source of the problem and cooling the area with cool or lukewarm water for at least 20 minutes, being careful not to overcool the patient [14]. Cooling should be carried out immediately following the injury. The damaged skin should then be covered with a non-adherent dressing or cling film and wound hydrogel. Creams should not be applied to burns in the first instance, and blisters should not be popped [15]. Foam dressings that are impregnated with honey or silver can be used to reduce the microbial population on the burn site and will be less likely to stick to the skin underneath it [16]. Analgesia is essential in most cases, and IV fluids may be required if the damage is extensive, but this will be assessed on arrival of the vet. Cooling is the most important first aid treatment for burns [5].

The seriousness of a burn depends on the depth and size of the area affected [11]:

1) **First-degree (superficial) burns:** First-degree burns affect only the epidermis. The burn site is red, painful, dry and there are no blisters present. An example would be mild sunburn. Long-term tissue damage is rare.
2) **Second-degree (partial thickness) burns:** Second-degree burns involve the epidermis and part of the dermis layer of skin. The burn site appears red, blistered and may be swollen and painful.
3) **Third-degree (full thickness) burns:** Third-degree burns destroy the epidermis and dermis. There may also be damage to the underlying bones, muscles and tendons. When bones, muscles and/or tendons are also burned, this may be referred to as a fourth-degree burn. The burn site appears white or charred. There is no feeling in the area as the nerve endings have been destroyed.

Thermal burns can be seen in foals that have had heat pads placed under them to keep them warm during surgery or if they are recumbent. Care should be taken to ensure that heat pads are not too hot and are not in direct contact with the skin. As well as thermal injuries, there is a possibility of tissue damage from friction burns, chemical burns or freeze damage (from ice therapy). Generally, the worse the burn, the larger the area it affects, and the greater the likelihood of shock, dehydration and infection.

Burns covering up to 50% or more of the body are usually fatal, although the depth of the burn also influences mortality. Wound infection is challenging to prevent because of the difficulty of maintaining a sterile wound environment. Long-term care is required to prevent continued trauma because burn wounds are often pruritic, and self-mutilation is common. Burns can cause disfigurement, which can affect athletic function. Therefore, the athletic use of the horse should be considered when deciding on an appropriate treatment programme.

Smoke inhalation can be seen alongside burns, especially if a horse has been in a stable fire. The patient should be removed from the smoke cloud during the initial assessment. Smoke inhalation can cause severe respiratory distress, and admission into an equine practice or hospital for intensive support and oxygen therapy may be required. It can take 24–36 hours to know the full extent of the damage for both smoke inhalation and burns, so close monitoring is required [14].

Poisons

Poisonous Plants

Table 14.3 displays some of the commonly encountered plants that are poisonous to horses. First aid treatment of poisoning cases includes removing the patient from the areas with the plants in, for example, moving them to a stable or field shelter. Monitoring these patients and identifying the plant involved is essential so the vet can initiate treatment on arrival. Treatment may include analgesia, nasogastric tubing to empty the stomach and administration of activated charcoal to absorb any remaining toxins. IV fluids may also be required, and the patient may need to be admitted to a practice for further treatment and monitoring.

Prevention is always better than cure. Owners should be advised to carry out the following [17, 19, 21, 22, 24, 25]:

- Supplementary feeding of horses with forage during times of minimal grazing as this will reduce the chance of horses eating inappropriate plants.
- Fence off poisonous trees and plants to reduce intake.
- Ensure fencing is in good working order to prevent horses from accessing poisonous plants.
- Move horses to separate grazing during abundant times, for example, autumn for acorns and sycamore seeds and spring for sycamore saplings.
- Check fields and paddocks daily for poisonous plants and seeds and remove them immediately.

Ragwort is restricted under the legislation 'The Weeds Act (1959) and The Control of Ragwort Act (2003); it is not an offence for ragwort to grow; however, landowners must control the plant in high-risk areas within 50 m of grazing land or arable farms [17]. It is advisable to wear PPE in the form of gloves and a face mask when removing these plants from the pasture, and the plant should be disposed of carefully to prevent the spread of seeds. Incineration is commonly used to dispose of ragwort, but checks should be made with the local authority to ensure that the burning of garden waste is allowed [17].

Herbicides

These substances are used to control plants: most are synthetic and selective, with low toxicity to mammals. However, some may contain arsenic, which is less selective and more toxic to mammals. Vegetation treated with herbicides at the proper dilution rates poses a low risk to horses, especially when the product has dried. Runoff of these agents into water sources may be a source of poisoning or if used in excessive quantities, withdrawal periods (animals on grazing) should be adhered to prevent toxicity. Whether acute or chronic, the symptoms will rarely lead

Table 14.3 Poisonous plants [17–23].

Plant	Poisonous parts	Symptoms	Toxin involved	Body system involved
Ragwort	All parts, even if wilted or dried	• Depression • Lethargy • Jaundice (yellowing of mucous membranes) • Photosensitisation • Diarrhoea • Abdominal pain • Weight loss More severe symptoms can include neurological signs: • Head pressing • Loss of coordination, circling • Seizures • Aggression	Pyrrolizidine Alkaloids (PAs), ingestion of these cause toxic by-products to be produced in the liver that disrupt DNA function in liver cells	The liver, can regenerate until 70% becomes damaged. The damaged cells then lose the capacity to regenerate, and no treatment can reverse the damage caused [17]
Yew	All parts. Yew is an evergreen tree or shrub that has needle-shaped leaves and often has red berries	Symptoms of poisoning are similar across species and include: • Ataxia • Pupil dilation • Abdominal pain • Muscle weakness • Convulsions At first, it may cause tachycardia but can proceed to bradycardia, bradypnoea and/or death [18]. Treatments can include gastric lavage; however, death can occur rapidly [19]	Toxic alkaloids known as taxine A and B	Cardiovascular – Taxine B is a calcium channel antagonist which interferes with heart muscle contraction [19]
Leylandii (Leyland cypress)	All parts are potentially poisonous [20]	• Diarrhoea • Ulcerated mucous membranes	Unknown, limited literature on effects or causative agents [21]	Affects the gastrointestinal system. It also irritates the mucous membranes
Sycamore	Leaves, seeds and saplings especially, but all parts are poisonous	Often fatal muscle disorder that causes symptoms such as: • Muscle weakness • Muscle tremors • Myoglobinuria (dark brown/red coloured urine) • Colic • Recumbency. Some horses are affected by lower quantities of the toxin than others	Commonly referred to as atypical myopathy, caused by the toxin Hypoglycin A	Muscular (including the muscles used for breathing and heart muscle) – is fatal in three-quarters of the cases seen [22]
Oak	Acorns – seeds of the oak tree. Some horses may actively seek out acorns, and anecdotally they appear to become 'addicted'; each individual has a different tolerance of the tannins. Leaves of the oak tree are also poisonous	Symptoms include: • Lethargy • Depression • Colic • Haemorrhagic diarrhoea • Dehydration • Inappetence	Tannic acid and other tannins	Affects the gastrointestinal system. Tannins are astringents and so draw water out of body tissues. Haemorrhagic diarrhoea is caused by the destructive effect tannins have on the intestinal lining [23]. Tannins can also cause liver and kidney damage

Source: Phillippa Pritchard.

to a diagnosis; gastrointestinal signs are common, as well as death; if poisoning with a herbicide is suspected, then identification of the product that has been ingested would aid in the treatment [23].

Rodenticides

Rodenticides may be poisonous to horses if accidentally ingested. As with herbicides, identifying the toxic element involved is essential in order to provide appropriate treatment. Rodenticides are often coloured, but the assumption of the ingredient by the colour should be avoided as this may change during digestion. Rodenticides may contain anticoagulants, bromethalin (neurotoxin) and cholecalciferol (which disrupts calcium and phosphorus homeostasis), among other ingredients [26]. First aid would involve preventing further access to the rodenticide, calling the vet and monitoring the patient until the vet arrives.

Pheasant Feed

Pheasant feed can cause grain overload, resulting in acute laminitis, colitis and in some cases, sudden death. First aid involves the immediate removal of the patient from the feed source. Other treatments may include:

- Cryotherapy: The application of ice to horses' feet remains controversial. During the prodromal stage (the period before clinical signs develop), cryotherapy is thought to be beneficial as the resulting vasoconstriction may reduce the delivery of vasoactive and inflammatory substances to laminar capillaries, which in turn, reduces the activity of tissue-degrading enzymes [27]. In contrast, icing following the clinical manifestation of the disease may reduce oedema formation but potentially aggravate ongoing ischaemic vascular events. To minimise tissue temperature in the horses' feet effectively, ice boots should incorporate the entire distal limb up to the carpus/tarsus [27]. The cryotherapy must be in place for at least 72 hours following the ingestion of the feed to be effective [28]. The decision on whether cryotherapy is appropriate or not will be made by the treating vet.
- Grain substances should be removed from the horse's diet.
- The horse should be stabled with a deep of shavings.
- The vet may lavage the stomach and administer activated charcoal.
- Analgesia should be administered as required according to the vet's instructions.
- Prior to the administration of antibiotics, anti-endotoxic medication may be considered. Polymyxin-B and endotoxin-specific antibodies may be used [27].
- Ongoing IV fluids may be required along with intensive monitoring.

Immediate treatment supportive care is similar for all poisoning cases and includes removal of the toxic substance, monitoring and identifying the substance to allow the vet to instigate specific treatment.

The Veterinary Poisons Information Service

Veterinary Poisons Information Service is a member-only 24-hour service that provides veterinary professionals with advice on poisoning cases. There is also an animal poison line for owners to enquire about possible cases of poisoning as well; they have an extensive database of previous cases to be able to provide appropriate advice and/or treatment options [29]. Contact details for the Veterinary Poisons Information Service can be found in the 'Useful Links' section at the end of this Chapter.

14.2 Work-up of the Emergent Patient

Triage

Triage comes from the French word 'trier', which means to pick, choose or sort. In a veterinary sense, triage is defined as the process of rapidly classifying patients according to their clinical priority, allowing identification of those patients that might need urgent, lifesaving help and ensuring that this occurs immediately and before patients with less severe problems. [30]. In equine veterinary nursing, triage is crucial in efficiently managing horses' diverse range of conditions and emergencies. For triage to occur successfully, information must be gathered from the patient's history and initial clinical examination in a referral situation; this information may be gathered by the client care advisor (CCA) or RVN over the telephone prior to arrival. On arrival, an initial assessment can occur where the RVN quickly assesses the horse, noting vital signs, behaviour, and obvious signs of distress or injury. They gather information from owners or handlers regarding the horse's history and the circumstances leading to the current situation.

Triage is normally associated with a colour scheme taken from human disaster response teams to quickly identify the agency of a patient's medical needs. Using this system, triage can be broken into colour-coded brackets, as shown in Table 14.4.

This table can help identify different triage categories, which helps prioritise cases from immediate to non-urgent. This is a guide, and all practices will follow their own procedures. Generally, all patients in practice will be seen on arrival; however, if this is not possible, triage based on the type of case is the best way to proceed.

Table 14.4 Emergency triage categories for equine practice.

Colour	Urgency	Target waiting time	Examples of cases
Red	Immediate	0 mins	Acute colic, full collapse, respiratory collapse, heat stress, active haemorrhage, collapsed foal, atypical myopathy, dull or unusually quiet donkey.
Orange	Very urgent	15 mins	Eye trauma, diarrhoea, fracture, severe wound, mild colic, septic joint or tendon sheath
Yellow	Urgent	30–60 mins	Chronic illness, minor wounds, choke, foot abscess
Green	Standard	120 mins	Acute mild lameness, cough, acute skin conditions, sarcoids, a nosebleed that has stopped
Blue	Non-urgent	240 mins	Mild lameness, poor performance, routine surgical procedures, chronic medical investigation

Source: Rosina Lillywhite.

Often, the first opportunity for the RVN or CCA to ascertain whether an emergency is life-threatening or not is through the initial telephone call made to the practice by the client. It is important to remember that the client may be distressed during this interaction. A calm, reassuring approach should be adopted during this exchange. Practice protocols for handling emergency telephone calls should be followed if available. If the emergency is identified as severe and life-threatening, two options are available.

- A vet can be sent out to the patient's location.
- The patient can be brought into the practice.

It is important to consider what is most appropriate for the patient and the client. The client may not have access to transport, the patient may not be used to being loaded or the patient may not be in a safe condition to transport. On the other hand, it may be quicker for the client to transport the patient to the practice, and if the patient is in an appropriate condition to travel, this may be the best option. More information on transporting critically ill horses can be found in Chapter 5.

Emergencies for which an examination by a vet should be advised without delay would include, but are not limited to, the following [30]:

- Colic
- Non-weight bearing lameness
- Fracture
- Severe bleeding
- Respiratory distress
- Collapse or unconsciousness
- Sudden onset of severe neurological abnormalities
- Severe diarrhoea
- Extreme pain

- Ocular injury
- Acute laminitis
- Significant wounds
- Puncture wounds
- Dystocia
- Sick foal
- Dull, unusually quiet or sick donkey

In other situations, the RVN may need to question the client further to determine if the patient needs to be seen immediately or if an appointment can be made in the immediate future. Examples of this include, but are not limited to, the following [30]:

- Minor wounds
- Mild diarrhoea
- Mild lameness

It is advisable to take the name of the client and the patient and a contact telephone number at the start of the call. If first aid advice is required, this should be given according to existing practice protocols. The client's safety should be considered during these calls. The administration of first aid measures should not be encouraged if there is a chance that this may result in injury to the client or the patient.

General rules for handling emergency telephone calls include the following [30]:

- When answering the phone call, the operator should state their name and the name of the practice.
- The operator should remain calm and polite at all times.
- It should be ascertained as quickly as possible whether this is a life-threatening emergency.
- The timing and nature of the injury should be ascertained along with the details of any treatment given and the response of the animal to this.

- Details regarding the condition of the animal should be gathered, such as vital signs, degree of ataxia or ability to stand, any haemorrhage, discharge and estimation of pain levels.
- Give the client clear instructions and directions if they have decided to transport their horse to the practice.
- Ensure there is easy access at the practice to contact details for several transport companies and a horse ambulance service. The client may require these if they do not have their own transport.
- Advice regarding the safe transportation of the patient should be given.
- Obtain an estimated arrival time if the patient is coming to the practice.
- Obtain the client's contact details, including a mobile phone number and repeat this information back to the client to ensure it is correct.
- Obtain detailed directions and a postcode for the yard if a vet is to attend. A code for What3words will also help the vet to find the yard.
- A financial quote should be given to the client for consideration.

When an emergency telephone call is taken, the RVN or CCA should inform the rest of the team if the patient is coming into the practice. This will allow for preparations to be made for the patient's arrival.

A capsule history should also be obtained from the owners of emergency patients. This history focuses on the essential information that could alter the early management of the patient [30]. This history can be taken during the initial phone call or when the patient arrives at the practice. Important questions to ask regarding a capsule history are as follows [30]:

- What is the age and sex of the animal?
- If the animal is male, is he castrated?
- Is the animal on any medication? If so, when was the last dose given?
- Has the animal been diagnosed with any long-term medical problems?
- What is the animal's vaccination status?
- Does the animal have any known allergies?
- Has the animal had any access to known toxins?
- When was the last time the animal ate or drank?
- When was the last time the animal passed faeces and urinated? Was it normal?
- How long has the animal been showing signs of the current problem?
- Has this problem got better, worse or stayed the same since it was first noticed?
- Have there been changes to the way the animal is usually managed recently?

Preparing for the Admission of an Emergency Case

Careful preparation is the key to treating emergencies successfully [30]; as many things as possible should be prepared in advance. Paperwork, such as consent forms, should be completed as much as possible before the patient arrives. Additional members of staff should be organised as required. A designated area should be prepared before the patient's arrival; this could be an examination room, radiography room, isolation unit, intensive care stable or foal unit, depending on the emergency being admitted. For all emergency cases, this area should be easily accessible from the car park or at least have access for a horsebox or trailer. This will prevent a debilitated patient from unnecessarily walking a long distance.

Examination Area

An examination area could include a radiography room, an examination room, a standing surgery suite or a set of stocks. Regardless of the areas selected, the working space should be cleared of unnecessary clutter, and the following should be prepared:

- Relevant equipment as required, such as a stethoscope, thermometer, ophthalmoscope, needles, syringes, blood tubes, clippers and a nasogastric tube.
- Relevant diagnostic aids such as an ultrasound scanner, radiography equipment and/or an endoscope.
- Depending on the patient's condition, the crash box should be placed in close proximity (see Chapter 10 for further details).
- Medication such as sedation and analgesics.
- Consumables such as IV catheters, IV fluids, swabs, dressings and bandage materials.
- Equipment to facilitate the administration of oxygen.

The Operating Theatre

If required, the operating theatre should be prepared as follows:

- The surgical table should be positioned ready for the patient.
- The anaesthetic machine and circuit should be set up and leak tested.
- Appropriate endotracheal tubes should be selected, and leak tested.
- The surgical kit should be prepared.
- Gloves and gowns should be laid out ready.
- Swabs and a suitable skin antiseptic should be set up ready for the surgical scrub.
- Appropriate lighting and heating should be set up ready.

Further information relating to preparing the operating theatre for use can be found in Chapter 11.

Immediate Care Upon Arrival, Stabilisation and Resuscitation

Any patient with a potentially life-threatening condition should be taken to an appropriate area of the practice upon arrival, where a primary survey will be carried out [30]. The primary survey starts with an assessment as to whether cardiopulmonary cerebral resuscitation (CPCR) is required. This requirement is rare in equine emergencies, but a primary assessment should only take 30 seconds to carry out and may help to identify specific areas of concern. The mnemonic DRABC should be followed:

- D: Danger – before doing anything else, the first aider must assess the danger of the situation and check that it is safe to proceed
- R: Response – the first aider must test if the patient is responsive or not. If the patient is classified as unresponsive, the first aider should proceed through the ABC steps outlined below.
- A: Airway – does the patient have a patent airway?
- B: Breathing – is the patient making useful breathing efforts?
- C: Circulation – does the patient have evidence of spontaneous circulation (heartbeat and pulses)?

If CPCR is required, this should be instigated immediately, and a vet should be alerted to attend. The process of CPCR and the different roles required are covered in Chapter 10. If it has been established that CPCR is not required, a major body system assessment should be carried out. Within this assessment, the three main body systems are [30]:

- Cardiovascular
- Respiratory
- Neurological

To assess the cardiovascular and respiratory systems, clinical parameters should be assessed and quantified as described in Chapter 17. Neurological function can be evaluated by observing the patient's gait and mentation [30]. Once the primary survey has been completed and treatment for any major body system abnormalities has been initiated, a secondary survey should be carried out. This involves a head-to-tail systematic examination of the patient. Areas that should be examined are as follows [30]:

- Nose
- Mouth
- Eyes
- Ears
- Limbs
- Hooves
- Thorax
- Abdomen
- External genitalia
- Tail

When dealing with any acute emergency, the RVN will play a significant role within the veterinary team. The RVN should be familiar with the equipment and medications that are likely to be required and have these ready and easily accessible. A proactive approach is required, and the RVN must think ahead to facilitate the developing situation [1]. This approach may include preparing an intensive care stable for the patient following the initial assessment. In this case, factors such as heating, comfort and the provision of appropriate food and fluid should be considered. Drug doses for medication prescribed by the case vet should be carefully worked out, prepared and administered as required. The RVN may be required to place an IV catheter and start the patient on IV fluids as directed by the vet. Oxygen may need to be administered, which should be set up quickly and efficiently, always considering patient and human safety. The RVN may also be required to assist in theatre in several roles, such as:

- Scrubbing in to assist with the surgical procedure
- Acting as a circulating nurse
- Monitoring the anaesthetic under the direction of a vet or assisting a vet with this process

As well as carrying out clinical procedures on the patient, the RVN may have a role in the organisation of the general area. This role may include managing people and equipment, keeping track of sharps and ensuring the health and safety of the patient and all staff members. The RVN may also take on the role of record-keeping during emergency procedures. This will include noting clinical parameters, pain scoring, medication administered, timings for procedures, and if required, filling in the anaesthetic record. Accurate record-keeping is essential for the case vet to use as a reference and for the practice to use in the case of litigation [1].

14.3 Accommodation for Critically Ill Patients

Critical Care Unit Design

Equine-specific critical care units are becoming an essential part of equine hospitals. Critical care stables are now designed and built with specific characteristics to suit the needs of the patient and their condition. This overview of the principles informing design is intended to highlight some of the key decisions made about the planning, layout, equipment, staffing and operation of accommodation for critically ill patients.

Environmental Considerations

- **Space:** Patients housed in a critical care or foal unit will require a high level of monitoring. Therefore, one of the biggest challenges is providing sufficient space for not only the patient but for a variety of equipment and the number of personnel moving through it. The British Horse Society (BHS) has set out stable size recommendations (see Chapter 5) to ensure the comfort and safety of the occupant is not compromised while they are on box rest. These recommendations may not be spacious enough for the hospitalised patient who, due to their clinical condition, requires prolonged box rest or is recumbent much of the time. In an ideal world, it is best to provide stables of differing sizes to accommodate the various sizes of the patients to be treated and to meet the needs of the individual [31].

- **Purpose:** The area being built should be designed to meet the needs of the practice for years to come. If a high number of sick foals are to be treated, it may be advisable to build a specialised foal unit [31]. This would include building a number of large stables with removable barriers in them. This would allow the mare and foal to interact and would also increase the safety of the staff treating the foal. For both foal and adult critical care stables, it would be prudent to consider facilities for heating, fluid administration, oxygen administration, electrical supply points and easy observation [31].

- **Location:** Critical care stables may be physically separate from other buildings, in a quiet corner of a busy hospital or they may adjoin a nursing station. It is often useful to locate critical care boxes near the anaesthetic recovery boxes as sick post-operative patients may need supportive therapy following surgery [31].

- **Safety:** Safety of the patient, equipment and people must always be considered. Within the design of specialist stabling, the predictable threats to safety must be reduced in the design. Floor surfaces must be non-slip throughout to the benefit of patients and staff, and the stable design and services must follow local building regulations when constructed.

- **Sustainability:** Durability and ensuring a long life that is fit for purpose will be part of a sustainability plan. Stables constructed in a rush may not be robust enough or suitable for multiple years or decades of use. Adapting and converting existing structures is commendable, but these structures

may not hold up to the high level of cleaning and disinfecting that is required in critical care accommodation.

Building Materials and Facilities
Floors and Walls

Floors in stables and ancillary treatment areas must be hard-wearing, non-slip, non-porous, easy to clean and durable. They should be seamless so fluid, and debris cannot underrun the floor covering; such spaces form natural reservoirs that can harbour pathogenic organisms. Concrete blocks are an ideal building material for stable walls due to their strength and long-lasting resilience to wear. Ideally, these walls need to be covered in impervious coatings that will not encourage bacterial adherence or fluids to saturate the surface. Insulating the cavities of stable walls and subfloors is recommended to prevent internal condensation from forming on surfaces. This also helps to maintain a constant temperature without heat loss in winter or heat retention in the summer months. This adds a considerable cost to the construction of the stables, but creates a better environment for the patient, care team and the equipment that occupies it.

Drains

Drains are essential for the removal of the large amounts of water used during the disinfection process once the patient has been discharged. Drains can be situated in the stable (usually centrally located) or along the edge of the door (channel drain). They need to be planned for and built into the floor, or else they will be very costly to retrofit. The camber (slope) of the stable floors should be designed to prevent the pooling of liquid in the stable, with all runoff directed to the door leading outside and away from the neighbouring stables. Unfortunately, drains create the perfect environment for bacterial colonisation, which can be problematic to eliminate unless drain covers and waste collection reservoirs are easily dismantled and disinfected. If they are installed, they must be cleaned and disinfected daily, especially if they regularly become clogged up with bedding and faeces. Secure drain covers must be fitted to ensure the safety of both the patient and staff members.

Bedding

Bedding for critically ill patients must provide a cushioning, non-slip, warm surface that absorbs waste and does not impede recovery (see Chapter 5 for general information on bedding).

Certain bedding types recommended for specific conditions are as follows:

- Pregnant broodmares, who are hospitalised for assisted parturition, should be kept on a deep bed of good quality, dust-extracted straw. This is the bedding of choice for most stud farms as it is perceived to be warmer and cleaner for the new-born foal. Shavings are more likely to be ingested or inhaled by a foal that spends considerable time in recumbency.

- Horses with open wounds that cannot be bandaged should be kept on shredded paper or cardboard bedding. This material is less likely to adhere to wounds and is more easily removed by lavage.
- Colic patients are routinely starved and box rested and will attempt to eat bedding when they are feeling better in the recovery phase. To discourage this, dust-free shavings are the bedding of choice to prevent intestinal impaction complications.
- Horses in limb casts can find it difficult to ambulate freely around the stable. Straw bedding can impede their movement as it can wrap around the cast [31]. With shavings, they are less hindered and can move more easily. Rubber matting and a thin layer of shavings are recommended for these cases.
- Horses with laminitis will require soft, supportive bedding such as shavings. As these horses also like to lie down frequently, rubber matting should be used with a deep bed on top [30]. The bedding should be continued all the way up to the door, and food and water situated close together.

Ventilation

Ideally, critical care accommodation will be well-ventilated and will prevent cross-contamination by having a separate air space from any other stable blocks in the practice. While it is preferable to provide filtered air changes through ventilation systems designed for veterinary operating and exam rooms, this is rarely practical.

The two main types of ventilation are as follows:

Passive Ventilation

Heat radiating from the horse rises when surrounded by cool air drawn in from lower surroundings. It pushes the lighter warm air upwards to the ceiling. This is known as the stack effect. Air vents at peak level in the roof allow the removal of warm and stale air enabling the circulation of fresh air below. In individual stables, the top doors can be kept open as this aids the circulation of fresh air, with vents at the gutter line under the roof overhang functioning to remove odours and stale air (see Figure 14.1).

Active Ventilation

Also known as mechanical ventilation, this includes air conditioning and hot air extractors. These units are mechanically powered and actively draw fresh air into the stable and then help to expel warm air from roof spaces. They work with and accelerate natural air flows, improving circulation faster than

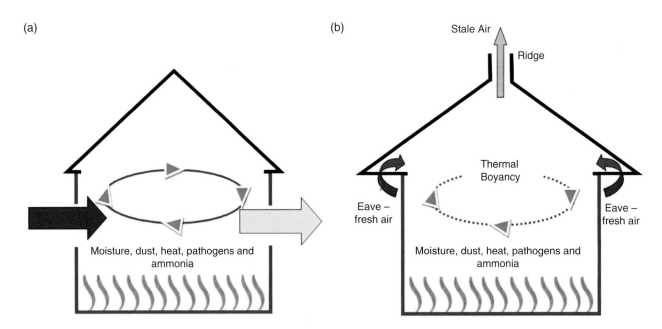

Figure 14.1 The stack effect. Figure (a) shows a stable with inadequate ventilation; this system relies on windows or air bricks to draw fresh air through the front and allow the stale air, once circulated, to escape out of the back. Figure (b), on the other hand, shows how the warm air is less dense and more buoyant than the colder air and can rise to the roof of the stable, where it can escape through the vents within the ridge of the stable. The vents within the eves of the stable allow fresh air to enter the stable. Stables should also have windows to maximise the ventilation available to the horse. *Source:* Rosina Lillywhite.

can naturally occur. To work efficiently, the stables and supporting rooms must be sealed from the outside environment.

Heating

If they are connected, there are often noticeable room temperature fluctuations between critical care stabling and the rest of the practice. If this can be minimised and attempts can be made to eliminate drafts, temperature variations between stables and treatment rooms will be easier to manage. A combination of constant ambient background heat and instant, concentrated heat sources (heat lamps) provides a selection of options according to the patient's changing needs. Any heating supply that is within the stable must have an integrated circuit breaker as a safety measure to limit damage caused by an overcurrent or short circuit.

Heating facilities are commonly required for the following patients:

- Post-operative colic patients
- Mares following a caesarean
- Sick foals
- Critical care patients, for example, atypical myopathy
- Chronically debilitated, underweight patients, e.g. dysautonomia (chronic grass sickness)

Lighting and Electrical Outlets

An important aspect of good critical care is the provision of adequate lighting so every area of the patient can be clearly examined. Installing several protected, waterproof and adjustable ceiling lights will help the veterinary care team examine the patient effectively. Adjustable lights allow for dimming when equipment like ultrasound machines are used in the stable. Night lights also assist the veterinary care team in making observations of inpatients at night, creating a calm atmosphere, especially around mares and foals, without disturbing them.

Mare and foal stables require many electrical outlets for the variety of infusion pumps and monitoring equipment that is needed to support a critically ill foal. These will need to be kept well out of reach of the mare and foal and encased in waterproof protective covers to prevent interference.

Features of lighting suitable in stables and adjoining passageways are as follows:

- Bright, dimmable lights without shadows
- Natural lighting with artificial options
- Skylights in covered passageways
- Lights that are waterproof to IP65 (Ingress Protection) rating for outdoor lighting. An IP65 rating means that the product is dust-tight with protection against low-pressure water jets from any direction.

- Waterproof light switches and sockets positioned outside stables, out of reach of the patient.

Health and safety should be considered at all times. Exposed electrical cables or surface-mounted trunking in or near the stable should be avoided as this can be chewed by the horse. Dangling electrical extension leads, or cables should be avoided as these could present as trip hazards and lead to injury.

Biosecurity

More now than ever, after witnessing a worldwide pandemic, hospital design and function should incorporate biosecurity measures that focus on preventing nosocomial (hospital-acquired) infections.

This may include:

- Training of all personnel involved on the basic biological principles of infectious disease and prevention.
- Dedicated care teams that solely treat critical care patients and do not treat patients in other areas of the hospital.
- A thorough pre-admission discussion with the client and referring vets to assess whether it is safe for them to be admitted to the practice.
- Adherence to admission biosecurity protocols for all-day cases and inpatients (for example, vaccination status).
- A stable layout that prevents the spread of disease and keeps immunosuppressed patients safe from additional infectious agents.

Facilitating Movement

Critically ill patients are often debilitated, weak, maybe recumbent and might need to be moved to different areas of the practice for diagnostic or surgical procedures. Having wide corridors and stable doorways for using large animal rescue slides, foal stretchers and trolleys makes the movement around the practice easier for the care team and provides space for equipment such as oxygen cylinders, electrocardiogram (ECG) equipment and emergency kits that may accompany the patient. Viewing windows with impact-limiting Perspex and grills enables the caregiver a good opportunity to monitor and assess the patient without disturbing them.

Fixtures and Fittings

Stainless-steel fluid bag hangers are essential in critical care stables and must be securely fixed to the centre of the stable ceiling. A rope is fixed to the hanger via a swivelling ball bearing, goes through a pulley system, travels along the ceiling, through the wall and is fixed outside the stable, away from possible interference by the occupant. If

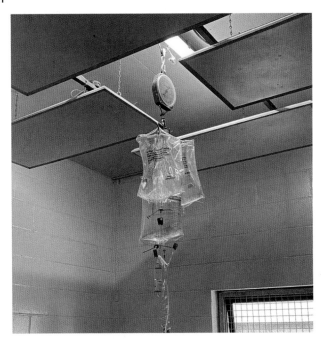

Figure 14.2 IV fluid hanger. *Source:* Marie Rippingale.

installed correctly, this will support several 5-l fluid bags and permit the raising and lowering of the whole system for bag changes (Figure 14.2).

Closed-circuit television (CCTV) surveillance allows viewing from other areas of the practice and enables video capture if unusual clinical behaviour is observed. Regularly recording all monitored patient observations is essential, and these should be documented on critical care forms or on the practice's software systems.

Patient Care Records

Documentation of patient care is essential for the following reasons:

- Provides a basis for care planning and treatment.
- Enables communication between the vet and nursing teams.
- Patient care records can act as legal documents.
- It can be used for billing and is essential for quality audits.

It is important to have protocols in place to preserve clients' rights by handling and storing their personal data safely following General Data Protection Regulations (GDPR) [32]. Practically, this means ensuring that patient records are not in an area that the general public can access. See Chapter 2 for more information regarding GDPR.

14.4 Nursing Requirements of the Critically Ill Horse

Breathing and Cardiovascular Function

Treatment and care of cardiovascular disease should be specific to the disease. Medical therapy can manage some conditions, with the aim to limit damage to cardiac muscle, control the fluid accumulation in the lungs, improve circulation and regulate the heart rate and rhythm. For the clinically unstable, giving intranasal oxygen can improve oxygenation and support cardiac function. Heart rate, pulse rate and respiratory rate should be monitored regularly (see Chapter 17). All patients suffering from cardiovascular disease should be encouraged to maintain a comfortable position that optimises breathing and oxygen delivery to tissues. This can be assisted by keeping weakened and recumbent patients, no matter what size, maintained in sternal recumbency. Maintaining a recumbent patient in sternal recumbency will also reduce the chances of hypostatic pneumonia developing [33]. Physiotherapy techniques can be used to promote circulation to the affected areas [33] (see Chapter 17). The goal is for the treatment to return heart and respiratory rates to normal and even if there is no cure, for the horse to have a good quality of life. These patients require intensive nursing and regular monitoring.

Parenteral Nutrition

For a short period of time, the sick patient can have its caloric needs met by IV crystalloid infusions with dextrose and by utilising its internal stores. If it remains anorexic or consumes nothing orally (nil by mouth) for a sustained period of time, it will need the addition of lipids, amino acids and electrolytes to provide nutritional support. There are several gastrointestinal conditions where the critically ill patients may require partial parenteral nutrition (PPN) or total parental nutrition (TPN) to prevent loss of body condition and a detrimental state of catabolism. These methods are designed to enable IV feeding to sustain life, bypassing the usual process of ingestion and digestion.

The two options are as follows:

- PPN: formulas meet some but not all of a patient's daily nutritional requirements.
- TPN: formulas provide all the required nutritional needs, in a constant 24 hours/ day IV infusion.

Some clinical teams are reluctant to implement TPN because of the knowledge and equipment required, the environmental setting needed for compounding, the high cost and the complications the patient can experience. The TPN solution must be mixed in an area of the practice away from stables and bedding, preferably in a lab setting with an exhaust hood. The area and countertop must be clutter-free, dust-free and clean. If required, a refrigerator dedicated to TPN storage should be situated nearby. Mixing of the TPN solution should take place under sterile conditions with the operator wearing a mask, sterile gloves and a sterile gown, with an assistant to open the fluid containers, mixing bags and supplements. Once the bags are filled, air trapped in them is expelled; they are labelled with the date and time of mixing and stored in the fridge. Solutions should be discarded if not used within 24 hours of being stored [34]. It is best to formulate the mixture just before it is due to be infused.

TPN should be protected from light during administration to prevent photodegradation of its components. Several components of TPN, such as certain vitamins such as vitamin A, riboflavin, certain amino acids, and lipid emulsions, are sensitive to light. Exposure to light, especially ultraviolet (UV) light, can lead to chemical degradation or alteration of these components, rendering them less effective or even harmful. For example, exposure to light can lead to the breakdown of lipid emulsions, causing the formation of peroxides and other harmful compounds that may contribute to oxidative stress when infused into the patient.

Additionally, photodegradation of certain components may result in the formation of toxic by-products or loss of potency, which can compromise the safety and efficacy of TPN therapy. For instance, degradation of vitamins in TPN solutions may lead to decreased nutritional value and potentially contribute to deficiencies in patients who rely on TPN for their nutritional needs.

Therefore, protecting TPN from light by using light-resistant infusion tubing, bags, or covers during administration is essential to maintain the stability and integrity of its components.

TPN should always be administered through a non-thrombogenic IV catheter in a large vein, this is usually the jugular vein [34]. Large volume or rapid administration of TPN is not possible due to the osmolarity of the solution and high glucose concentrations. Therefore, crystalloid fluid therapy is usually administered concurrently to maintain fluid balance [34]. Due to the potential for bacterial growth in TPN solutions, a dedicated IV catheter or catheter port that is used only for the TPN solution should be identified and maintained [34]. Administration sets should be changed daily. The components of TPN contain lipids and dextrose, the perfect media for the proliferation of bacteria. Therefore, a scrupulous aseptic technique must continue once the bag is connected to the patient. If the giving set is disconnected and inadvertently contaminated for any reason, it must be replaced. Figure 14.3 shows TPN mixed and ready to be infused. For more information on mixing

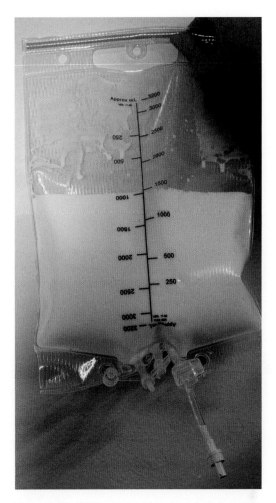

Figure 14.3 TPN mixed and ready to be infused. *Source:* Rosina Lillywhite.

and administration of TPN, please see the further reading list at the end of this chapter.

Mobility and Physiotherapy

Patients with limited mobility, accompanied by generalised weakness may require physiotherapy to prevent contractures or laxities while convalescing. Deep beds help to provide support and padding while recumbent, but the addition of soft mats to pad hips and shoulders to prevent decubital ulcers (pressure sores) may help. Basic physiotherapy techniques are covered in Chapter 17.

Modern versions of support slings are now used more frequently, having been redesigned to support the whole body in a balanced manner, without exerting pressure on the thorax and skeletal protuberances. It takes skill and experience to manage the horse in a sling, and their use is not without risks. It is important to understand the mechanics of how they function and to know how to dismantle them in an emergency to release the horse. Nursing care includes:

- Preventing friction rubs and pressure sores
- Monitoring orthopaedic comfort
- Providing mental stimulation
- Performing passive physiotherapy in preparation for removal from the sling
- Keeping the stable scrupulously clean

See the further reading section for more information regarding managing equine patients in slings.

Hygiene

Maintaining good patient and stable hygiene is important in critically ill horses as there are many ways where exposure to environmental factors could cause delays and complications in healing. Equipment used for cleaning stables and grooming should not be used on other patients, and staff working with critically ill patients should not handle the transient population of horses that enter the practice. Implementing reverse barrier nursing techniques will help prevent opportunistic infections that could devastate the immunosuppressed patient. See Chapter 6 for further information on biosecurity and infection control techniques.

Skincare

Maceration occurs when the skin has softened and broken down due to continual exposure to moisture. This could be associated with highly exudative dressed wounds and discharge from open wounds and drains. With critically ill patients that are recumbent for much of the time this is a concern, as these patients will often lie in their own urine, faeces and sweat without the ability to move away from these secretions. Such patients will require regular grooming and sponge baths of the areas affected. After the area has been thoroughly dried off, absorbent pads should be placed under the macerated areas to help prevent the formation of decubital ulcers [33]. Frequent turning and mucking out of recumbent horses will help to limit the exposure to waste materials that could cause macerated skin. Recumbent horses should be turned once every four hours as a minimum and encouraged to stay in sternal recumbency as much as possible [33]. Grooming is a good time to examine the skin and coat closely for any new lesions. If new lesions occur, they should be treated quickly by drying the affected area and applying an emollient cream [33]. Manes and tails can be plaited to prevent matting.

Maintaining Body Temperature

A healthy horse can thermoregulate, meaning they are able to maintain a constant body temperature in the presence of fluctuating environmental conditions. In a horse suffering from shock, systemic infection or other diseases, this ability may be impaired, leaving them unable to maintain a normal body temperature. To assist in keeping them warm, stable rugs and bandages are applied and stables are fitted with heat lamps. If the patient becomes pyrexic this may be counterintuitive, as they will not be able to cool themselves under thick rugs. A light-moisture wicking cooler that moves moisture away from the body will help them to cool their body temperature without getting chilled.

To actively lower a high temperature, a continuous application of water by sponge or spray will rapidly cool a horse as it removes heat by conduction, transferring the heat from the horse to the water. Eventually, the water coming off the horse is closer in temperature to the horse. The water should not be scraped off as evaporation is much slower compared to conduction. The water must remain on the body surface to make conductive heat removal effective. See the further reading section for more information on efficient cooling techniques for horses.

Compared to humans, healthy horses have a wider thermoneutral zone and do not feel cold until environmental temperatures drop below 5 °C, or even lower if sheltered from wind and rain. The horse's winter coat has insulating properties in sustained cold weather as long as it stays dry. The hairs will stand on end, trapping warmth from the body against the skin. Most practices will have stables equipped with heat lamps and take measures to prevent drafts from travelling through stable blocks. If a horse is not shivering, then warming methods are rarely needed. If the rectal temperature is subnormal, then drying the horse prior to rugging is recommended. The usual peripheral measures (rugging and bandages) are ineffective in restoring the body temperature to normal in these cases unless the patient has its core rewarmed. The administration of warmed IV fluids and warm water enemas can help to achieve this.

Stables must be equipped with enough bedding to prevent drafts and provide a layer of protection to the horse when it lies down. The use of rubber mats can enhance this but should not be used without a thick layer of bedding on top. The choice of bedding used depends on the condition being treated and the preference of the clinical team.

14.5 Critical Care Techniques for Respiratory Disorders

Oxygen Administration

For some disorders, it may be necessary to administer oxygen to the patient. Face masks are not routinely used in equine practice as they are difficult to keep in place and rarely seal well enough for the patient to receive sufficient oxygen. Intranasal oxygen insufflation, through a flexible oxygen tube fixed to the side of the headcollar with tape is an easily tolerable and recommended method for administering oxygen to equine patients. A flow rate of 15 L/min is recommended for adult horses [1].

Tracheostomy

Occasionally, an obstruction in the horse's upper respiratory tract can lead to restricted air intake and respiratory distress. A tracheostomy is performed to open the airway, bypassing the pharynx to enable unobstructed breathing. The surgical procedure creates an opening in the trachea, enabling a tube to be fitted between the tracheal rings. Depending on the condition, it can be a temporary or permanent solution to the condition.

Different types of tracheostomy tubes are available for use in horses. Ideally, they should be made of a material that is easy to clean, non-irritating and well tolerated by the horse. Short-term cuffed and uncuffed silicone J-type tubes are easy to fit in an emergency and can be secured with umbilical tape around the neck. Metal self-retaining tubes have two interlocking flanges that fix it in the tracheal lumen without the need for tape ties.

Performing an emergency tracheostomy is an act of veterinary surgery and should be carried out by a vet, but the RVN can play an important role in preparing the equipment and the patient. In some circumstances, this is a life-saving procedure. Therefore, it is essential that the surgery takes place as quickly and efficiently as possible. It is a good idea to have an emergency tracheostomy kit prepared beforehand. Contents of this kit should be as follows [1]:

- Tracheostomy tube (ideally two different sizes)
- Clippers
- Surgical scrub, spirit and swabs
- Sedation
- Local anaesthetic
- Scalpel blade and handle
- Suture material and needles

The case vet will decide if sedation is appropriate for the individual case being treated. The patient should be restrained effectively. The RVN should clip and aseptically prepare the ventral aspect of the neck. The site for tube placement is the junction of the upper and middle thirds of the neck [1].

The tracheostomy procedure will then be performed by the vet as follows [1]:

- A line of local anaesthetic is infiltrated subcutaneously at the site of tube placement.
- A vertical incision of approximately 5–7 cm is made through the skin and extended to the surface of the trachea.
- A horizontal incision (no greater than one-third of their circumference) is made between two trachea rings.

- The tracheostomy tube is then inserted between the rings of the trachea and directed distally.
- The tube is secured in place. The method of this will depend on the type of tube being used.

Management of an indwelling tracheostomy tube requires a sustained commitment to maintaining the new open airway, preventing infection and obstructions. With a tube in place, secretions are increased and threaten to block the tube as the body responds to having a foreign object in place. The tube must be removed, cleaned and disinfected twice daily. While the tube is removed, the wound can be cleaned with any secretions removed by suction if needed. In the initial period following placement, a dressing may be placed between the skin and the tube to prevent ulceration while the wound starts to heal. These patients are prone to lower respiratory tract infections because their breathing bypasses the normal filtration of particles and contaminants through their sinuses.

A dust-free, stable management regime is important with these horses. Initially, they will need to be box rested for monitoring of the tube, the initial adjustment to having the tube fitted. Dust-free bedding, ideally a type that cannot be inhaled through the tube, is preferred, with all hay soaked and offered from the ground. Concentrates should not be offered from a feed manger or bucket as the horse may be able to dislodge the tube on the sides. Feeding off the floor in wide rubber tubs is preferable. These patients benefit from being stabled near busy corridors where people can frequently walk by and observe them, checking that the tube has not been dislodged.

Thoracic Drains

The insertion of large bore chest drains enables the removal of thick pleural fluid, fibrin and cellular debris that otherwise could not be withdrawn through needles. If effusion persists, they can be sutured into place and used for continued pleural lavage and drainage.

The materials used for the placement of a chest drain include:

- Ultrasound scanner
- Local anaesthetic
- Fenestrated chest tubes with a blunt trocar ranging in size (16–32 French)
- Scalpel blade
- Haemostat
- Nylon suture
- Heimlich valve or non-lubricated condom

The horse is sedated and manually restrained as requested by the vet. The location for the tube insertion should be at the most ventral aspect of the pocket of fluid, avoiding the heart and confirmed by ultrasonography.

The site is clipped, and aseptic skin preparation is carried out. The area will be rescrubbed after being blocked with a local anaesthetic. The vet will make a stab incision through the skin, and the chest drain with the blunt trocar is carefully advanced through the intercostal muscle. When the tube enters the pleural cavity, the resistance suddenly ends. The tube is advanced, so all the fenestrations are in the pleural cavity and the trocar is removed, with the free flow of fluid confirming the correct placement. A haemostat is used to clamp off the tube to prevent air ingress, while the tube is sutured in place. Purse-string and Chinese finger trap sutures are placed to secure the tube in place. A Heimlich valve or a non-lubricated condom with the end cut off, is fitted on the distal end of the tube to prevent ingress of air; frequent cleaning below the drainage site is required as well as the application of a barrier cream. If a rug is worn, a large kennel liner can be attached to its underside to absorb any discharge without wicking through to the rug. Stable bandages can be applied to the distal limbs of the patient to prevent scalding from the draining fluid as the horse ambulates around the stable. This can also help to minimise fluid build-up and swelling in the distal limbs, which can be uncomfortable and limit mobility.

14.6   Management of the Patient with Critical Thoracic Trauma

Thoracic trauma is uncommon but can result in serious life-threatening injuries including:

- Pneumothorax
- Haemothorax
- Pleuritis
- Diaphragmatic hernias
- Lacerations to the lungs, heart and major blood vessels

The most important objective is to rapidly assess the patient, determine their immediate needs and administer treatment that will stabilise their condition. This may mean providing oxygen, resuscitation fluids and treating shock. The horse will need to be kept in a quiet environment to limit further haemorrhage and be closely monitored on an hourly basis until its condition stabilises. Surgical or invasive treatments should be performed only after its condition improves, and the signs of shock are diminishing.

Chest wounds can penetrate into the pleural cavity and can create a life-threatening pneumothorax. Horses with pneumothorax can become distressed and develop tachypnoea and laboured breathing [1]. With a thoracic wound, if pneumothorax is suspected, a sterile, airtight bandage should be fitted to prevent further aspiration of air [1]. In an emergency, plastic kitchen wrap can be used ideally with a sterile bandage [1]. This will help to stabilise the patient until definitive treatment can be administered.

14.7   Intensive Nursing Requirements for Horses

Equine intensive care nursing has undergone significant advancement and increased specialisation in recent decades. Trauma is often accompanied by emergency conditions that require an informed and rapid nursing response.

Haemorrhage

Haemorrhage is often the result of trauma, with external bleeding from the body being visually apparent. Acute and significant blood loss is associated with pale mucous membranes, marked tachycardia, colic and weakness that can lead to rapid deterioration and collapse. PCV can be measured to try to investigate blood loss. However, the results should be interpreted cautiously as it may take up to 24 hours following the injury to observe a significant drop in the PCV [7]. The treatment aims to prevent haemorrhagic shock and stem or limit further blood loss. In many cases, no further treatment is required once the blood loss has been controlled.

Resuscitative IV fluid therapy to treat the resulting hypovolaemia may be necessary, with careful monitoring of haematology parameters. Shock doses of up to four times the blood loss can be administered, which improves oxygenation even with a decreased packed cell volume. There are different approaches to fluid therapy, with some clinicians limiting the volumes to maintain a lower blood pressure in an attempt to slow haemorrhage. This could lead to poor tissue perfusion and oxygenation and subsequent cardiovascular collapse. Others will risk further haemorrhage by administering larger volumes of crystalloid and colloid fluids to maintain a normal blood pressure and prevent hypovolaemic shock.

As discussed earlier in this chapter, with external bleeding, direct pressure with sterile dressings and/or bandaging is the recommended method to slow blood loss from distal limbs. If the blood continues to seep through the bandage, to prevent dislodging newly formed clots, it is best to place another pressure bandage over the one in place. Tourniquets can be placed to help to stem heavy bleeding and should be positioned proximal to the wound. Tourniquets should be applied with extreme caution due to the risk of causing ischemia and necrosis if used incorrectly.

What is less evident is trauma-induced internal bleeding. It can occur within the guttural pouches, lungs, thorax, abdomen, retroperitoneal region, intestinal lumen, musculature and pelvis due to arterial ruptures. Internal bleeding is more difficult for the vet to diagnose and requires the use of ultrasonography, haematological and biochemistry analysis, cytological evaluations and exploratory laparotomy if the patient stabilises. As discussed earlier, if the thoracic cavity has been penetrated, plastic kitchen wrap can be used to prevent ingress of air into the thorax as a first aid measure.

Treatment options are limited due to the inaccessibility of the traumatised area, but keeping the horse box rested in a quiet environment helps to limit further bleeding. If the patient is hypoxic as a result of the blood loss, intranasal oxygen should be administered. Oxygen lines can be fixed to the horse's mane and run up through the fluid hanger in the stable, then to the outside of the stable. The oxygen canisters should be safely stored out of reach of the horse. A blood transfusion may be required if blood loss has been severe. See Section 14.9 for further information.

Wounds

Detailed wound healing and management content can be found in Chapters 12 and 13.

Traumatic wounds are dealt with in a similar manner as haemorrhages. Wounds often result in bleeding and should receive first aid pressure bandages in the first instance. With the cessation of bleeding, the wound can be flushed, debrided and assessed to identify the structures involved.

After the initial assessment, primary wound closure with sutures or staples may be attempted. A delayed primary closure may be indicated in the presence of contamination, contused or swollen soft tissues. When suturing traumatic wounds, correct skin preparation is vital. All wound edges need to be anatomically apposed, using the least number of sutures necessary to limit the chance of infection being tracked below the skin. Choosing the right suture material and technique affects the success of the closure, with synthetic monofilaments being less reactive and adding strength.

Older wounds that have a compromised blood supply make primary closure difficult, and these often need to heal by second intention. With second-intention healing, the wound defect relies on epithelisation and contraction to close, which will significantly add to the healing time. This may also include wounds to the body that have significant skin deficits. These wounds will still require covering with innovative ways to secure dressings and bandages to prevent contamination.

Effective nursing care contributes positively to wound healing as it aims to:

- Prevent contamination and provide optimal conditions for wound healing through effective dressing selection and bandaging.
- Prevent self-mutilation of the wound through effective bandaging and instigating nursing interventions if required.
- Promote favourable conditions for good wound healing for example, dry, clean environmental conditions, rubber flooring, suitable bedding and an appropriate feeding regime.
- Help the patient cope with prolonged box rest by providing mental stimulation and environmental enrichment.

Luxations

A joint luxation is a complete dislocation or complete separation between the bones that normally articulate to form a joint (Figure 14.4). A joint subluxation is a term that refers to a partial dislocation of the joint where there is still some contact between the articular ends of the bones.

With a joint luxation, the severity can range from complete instability of the joint with complete inability to bear weight on the limb to limited misalignment of the joint and a weight-bearing capacity. Once a veterinary diagnosis has been confirmed and reduction of the luxation is performed, external coaptation for stabilisation of the

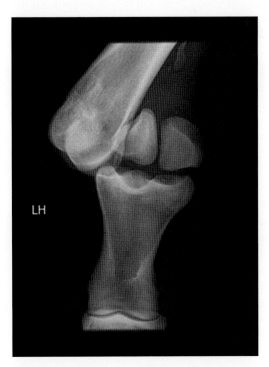

Figure 14.4 Radiograph showing a joint luxation.
Source: Rosina Lilllywhite with permission from Liphook Equine Hospital.

dislocated joint is compulsory. If an open dislocation exists, the prognosis is guarded and may require numerous cast changes to enable access to the wound for treatment.

Depending on the severity, the horse may return to work, but osteoarthritis is a common complication even with effective immobilisation, box rest and convalescence. If reduction of the luxation cannot be sustained in the correct anatomical position, the joint becomes non-mobile and arthritic, causing significant and chronic pain.

Foreign Bodies

Foreign bodies are objects or materials found in the body that do not originate there. They can be microorganisms like bacteria and viruses or objects that enter a body part through trauma via ingestion or inhalation. Horses are frequently treated for the removal of foreign bodies that they step on or are impaled by. They range in size from blackthorns to large stakes, and all must be managed in a way that limits further injury during investigation and removal. Those that penetrate sterile body cavities such as synovial structures, the peritoneum, intestines or the pleural cavity are of the greatest concern. Items that frequently penetrate the hoof, such as nails or wire barbs, are commonly contaminated with soil, faeces and rust. These serve as a transfer mechanism for bacteria, which can lead to severe infection.

Obtaining a detailed history will help to determine if the injury needs to be treated as an emergency that often necessitates referral. Owners should be made aware that keeping the item in situ is recommended until a vet can see the horse; a bandage should be applied around the wound using a padded ring of bandage padding, so the pressure is focused on the surrounding area and not on the foreign body itself, as this would cause further damage and deeper penetration. If a foreign body is removed before the horse is admitted to the hospital, the client should be advised to bring the object with them. The vet can examine the item to determine if any fragments remain in the wound.

Recovery can be prolonged depending on the severity of the wound and what structures are involved. The patient may be box rested to restrict mobility and encourage wound healing with limited complications. Medicinal therapy administered would be prescribed by the case vet according to the individual injury. This may include antibiotics and non-steroidal anti-inflammatory drugs (NSAIDs), with regular monitoring of inflammatory markers and haematology values to gauge the success of treatment. The bandage will need to be changed according to the injury and the requirements of the wound. The bandage should be monitored carefully for any damage or strike-through of exudate. The horse's overall comfort will need to be assessed, and regular pain soring should be carried out. As the horse is on box rest, offering plenty of forage and fibre-based feedstuffs will help to maintain intestinal motility and help to prevent impactions. Gastrointestinal function will need to be monitored closely. Environmental enrichment should be provided, and the horse could be groomed regularly to encourage interaction, if appropriate for that individual case.

Thoracotomy

Surgery on the thoracic cavity is rarely performed due to the low incidence of disorders affecting the thorax, the poor prognosis of many conditions and the cost of the procedure and its recovery period.

Thoracotomies in patients with pleuropneumonia or abscesses in the thorax can respond favourably to this invasive surgery if medical management has had limited effect. It is achieved in the standing horse with sedation and the administration of intranasal oxygen and IV fluids. This procedure allows the removal of fibrin, purulent material and abscess debris from the pleural cavity. Sometimes, this procedure is facilitated by a rib resection to enable better access to the affected areas. Thoracotomies can also be carried out to remove neoplastic masses and partial lung resections. Scrupulous management of chest drains is vital, with measures taken to prevent air ingress and avoid infection at the insertion site. The insertion site will need to be monitored for any localised reactions, pain and swelling.

In neonates, rib fractures can be repaired by internal fixation using plates, cortical screws and cerclage wire. These foals usually incur thoracic trauma at birth or during rough handling, resulting in rib fractures or dislocations at the costochondral junction. Complications associated with rib fractures are haemothorax, pneumothorax, myocardial lacerations and contusions, with rapid death if the rib fragments perforate the heart. Internal fixation limits the damage if there are mobile fragments present but must be followed by intrathoracic suction to alleviate pneumothorax. Post-operative nursing care includes:

- Oxygen administration
- Ambulatory support
- Administration of analgesia and antibiotics as prescribed by the vet
- Regular blood gas monitoring
- Surgical wound management
- Cautious handling

These foals should be allowed to rest in a position that they feel most comfortable in and quickly learn to lie down unaided.

Laparotomy

Laparotomy in the horse is the most common surgical procedure associated with colic and gastrointestinal disease. A general anaesthetic (GA) with the horse in dorsal recumbency is required to allow full access to the abdominal organs, with a ventral midline incision. While all the intestinal organs are palpable, only about ¾ can be exteriorised for resections or repairs. Following recovery, the horse should be placed in a critical care box with heat lamps and the provision to administer IV fluids. The stable should have a deep, clean bed of shavings and be well ventilated. Any medication required will be prescribed by the case vet depending on each individual case. Post-operative colic patients require extensive, intensive care treatment and nursing care, which may include:

- Regular critical care checks (according to practice policy) to monitor pain and progress. All body systems are assessed, and clinical parameters are taken. See Chapter 17 for further information.
- IV catheter site checks as these patients are more prone to developing thrombophlebitis. See Chapter 17 for further information.
- Gastric decompression to relieve excess gas and fluid, such as enteral reflux.
- IV crystalloid fluids may be required as many postoperative colic patients require limited oral fluid intake. The amount and type of fluid should be prescribed by the vet, and the amount required worked out carefully. The patient should be monitored closely. Daily serum electrolyte tests may indicate the need for supplementation.
- Prokinetics drugs such as lidocaine to stimulate gut movement and prevent ileus.
- Analgesia, may include NSAIDs such as phenylbutazone or flunixin meglumine and/or opioids such as morphine, to reduce pain and inflammation [35].
- Antibiotics help to prevent and treat any infection. These should be prescribed by the case vet after careful consideration of the British Equine Veterinary Association (BEVA) ProtectMe guidelines and the individual practice policy for reducing antimicrobial resistance.
- Polymyxin-B to help to treat endotoxaemia [35].
- Repeated haematology and biochemistry analysis, including frequent lactate measurements.
- Surgical wound and abdominal support management. Depending on the wound closure method used, this may include changing a belly band.
- Environment enrichment to include grooming and walks if appropriate
- Periodic mouthwashes with fresh water if the patient is being starved for any length of time [35].

- Reintroduction to eating in the form of offering grass around 48 hours post-op, but only if the clinical parameters are improving.

Colic patients are usually discharged from the practice 5–14 days following surgery. Each patient should be treated as an individual when it comes to a home care plan, but generally, the horse will require a period of box rest for around two months before being allowed small paddock turnout. Full turnout and ridden exercise may be introduced approximately four months following surgery depending on progress [35].

Caesarean Section

Dystocia in the mare is a true emergency and can be life-threatening to the mare and foal. A rapid veterinary assessment with obstetrical manipulation should be carried out, moving quickly onto a controlled vaginal delivery or a caesarean section under GA if a conscious delivery is not possible. Mares have an explosive second stage of labour, and if the foal is not delivered within 90 minutes of chorioallantoic membrane rupture, its chance of survival is minimal. For this reason, some hospitals will perform a caesarean section immediately upon the mare's arrival, forgoing the time it would take to attempt a controlled vaginal delivery.

The post-surgical care is similar to that of a colic patient and includes monitoring and administering IV fluid therapy and medications. There may be the added challenge of having a neonate in the stable; thus, attention must be directed towards ensuring the foal does not become entangled in fluid administration lines. Abdominal dressings and support bandages help limit the formation of oedema and discourage the foal from nudging the surgical site when searching for the udder. The placenta must be removed soon after recovery, preferably within three to five hours and examined thoroughly to prevent complications from retained foetal membranes. The consequences of this are potentially life-threatening and may lead to endotoxaemia, endometritis, peritonitis and laminitis. As a precaution, the mare may have her feet iced or placed in cold boots to assist in preventing laminitis. An abdominal drain can be placed cranial to the incision during surgery to use for large volume peritoneal flush postoperatively. Analgesia and antibiotics will be administered according to the treating vet's instructions. Regular pain scoring and critical care checks are required.

Obstetrical treatments will include uterine flushing with a sterile isotonic solution twice daily until the syphoned-out fluid runs clear. Extra care must be taken to limit the flush volumes as it could strain the uterine incision, risking leakage into the peritoneum. The foal should be monitored carefully, and treatment provided as required. For more information on foals, please see Chapter 15.

Hypocalcaemia

Hypocalcaemia or low blood calcium is a relatively uncommon condition but can lead to synchronous diaphragmatic flutter if left untreated. This is because the function of the phrenic nerve as it passes over the right atrium, is compromised from the electrolyte imbalance. It is stimulated and contracts the diaphragm at the same time as atrial depolarisation. These contractions cause the horse to have what looks like 'hiccups'; this unique clinical sign is often referred to as 'the thumps'. The abnormal stimulation of the phrenic nerve results in a synchronised heart and respiration rate.

Causes can include:

- Endurance exercise, particularly in hot weather
- Lactation from two weeks prior to foaling up to a few days post-weaning
- Dehydration
- Transportation
- Intestinal disease
- Trauma
- Endocrinology disorders
- Renal failure
- Endotoxemia and sepsis

Hypocalcaemia is diagnosed by low serum calcium (4–6 mg/100 ml:1–1.5 mmol/L) concentrations [36]. Low serum magnesium may be found in transit cases. Treatment is with calcium borogluconate IV (given to effect) added to isotonic IV fluids [36]. The heart should be auscultated during therapy. If left untreated, the horse can develop seizures, but with urgent electrolyte rebalance, the condition is easily corrected.

Shock

Shock is defined as inadequate tissue oxygenation resulting in decreased perfusion to vital organs. The consequences of untreated shock are severe as a lack of oxygen supply to the tissues will have significant effects on all organs, in particular the brain, heart and kidneys [5]. If the state of shock is prolonged, it may lead to organ failure and death [5]. Please see Table 14.5 for the different classifications of shock.

Table 14.5 Different classifications of shock [37].

Classification of shock	Cause	Associated conditions
Hypovolaemic shock	Caused by tissue hypoperfusion resulting from blood loss, leading to decreased circulating blood volume	Haemorrhage: Middle uterine artery bleed, laceration of a large artery associated with a fracture or wound Fluid loss: Diarrhoea associated with colitis, gastric reflux associated with enteritis, sweating in response to exercise, fluid leakage associated with extensive burns Third space loss: Pleural or peritoneal effusions, fluid trapped in the large colon secondary to a large colon volvulus
Cardiogenic shock	Caused by a failure of an effective cardiac pump. Is rare in equine patients	Cardiomyopathy. Arrhythmias such as third-degree atrioventricular (AV) block and ventricular tachycardia. Valvular dysfunction such as chordae tendineae rupture
Distributive shock	Caused by an insufficient circulating volume due to vasodilation and decreased systemic vascular resistance	Conditions such as endotoxaemia, sepsis and anaphylaxis lead to the release of cytokines and inflammatory mediators that can result in distributive shock. Endotoxaemia can occur secondary to a variety of diseases including colitis, pleuropneumonia and retained foetal membranes
Obstructive shock	This is rare in equine patients but is often attributed to an obstruction of blood flow. It can occur in response to a massive pulmonary thromboembolism	Diseases that restrict the ability of the heart to expand such as pericardial effusion and restrictive pericarditis. Diseases that compress large vessels such as tension pneumothorax or large colon volvulus
Metabolic shock	Is not related to altered blood flow but is instead a problem with blood oxygenation, tissue uptake of oxygen, cell utilisation of oxygen or cell demand for oxygen	Anaemia or respiratory diseases resulting in poor oxygen exchange. Carbon monoxide toxicity, cyanide toxicity and sepsis

Source: Marie Rippingale and Bonny Millar.

Stages of Shock

The stages of shock are defined by how well the body is able to adapt to the conditions that result in shock, by trying to meet the energy demands of the cells [37]. This response is focused on meeting the demands of the most vital body organs, such as the brain and the heart.

Compensatory Mechanisms

The first reaction of the body when faced with conditions which cause shock is to initiate certain compensatory mechanisms. It is important to remember that these compensatory mechanisms are not without consequences. For example, decreasing perfusion to less vital organs, such as the gastrointestinal tract, will eventually become exhausted [37]. These compensatory mechanisms include multiple physiologic responses that are triggered when the body detects a decreased oxygen delivery, circulating volume and mean arterial blood pressure, including [37]:

- Fluid moves from the interstitial space into the vascular space causing an increase in blood volume.
- Decreased mean arterial blood pressure triggers the release of catecholamines, which causes arterial and venous constriction, increased myocardial contractility and an increased heart rate. It also results in increased antidiuretic hormone (ADH) secretion, which stimulates an increase in water reabsorption in the kidney to increase blood volume.
- Decreased arterial pressure in the kidney results in activation of the renin–angiotensin–aldosterone pathway, which results in systemic vasoconstriction to increase blood pressure and increased sodium and therefore, water resorption to increase blood volume.
- Catecholamine and adrenocorticotrophic hormone (ACTH) release leads to increased circulating cortisol, which stimulates glucogenesis and protein catabolism to meet increased cellular energy demands.

Stage I: Compensated (Hyperdynamic) Shock

Compensatory mechanisms discussed above are able to maintain blood flow to the brain and heart. Clinical signs include tachycardia, tachypnoea, congested mucous membranes, decreased CRT and bounding peripheral pulses [37].

Stage II: Early Decompensated Shock

Compensatory mechanisms are unable to meet the energy demands of tissues, which results in anaerobic metabolism, lactic acidosis and organ dysfunction. Clinical signs include [37]:

- Progressive tachycardia and tachypnoea
- Prolonged CRT

- A toxic line on mucous membranes
- Cold extremities
- Decreased urine production
- Altered mentation

Stage III: Late Decompensated (Irreversible) Shock

As anaerobic metabolism continues, sympathetic arterial and venous constriction is overwhelmed, resulting in blood pooling in venules, fluid leaking into interstitium and activation of inflammatory cells. This eventually leads to organ failure and death. Clinical signs include [37]:

- Marked hypotension
- Bradycardia
- Circulatory collapse
- Pale/grey mucous membranes
- Organ failure

Even with aggressive treatment, this stage is often fatal [37].

Treatment

The treatment of shock is mainly directed at improving oxygen delivery to tissues and correcting the underlying disease. IV fluid resuscitation is the mainstay of therapy for shock. A variety of fluid types can be used, and a combination of fluid types is often required for the best result. The case vet will prescribe the appropriate fluids to be administered to the patient:

Isotonic Crystalloids [37]
- Can be administered at a 'shock dose' of 60–90 ml/kg.
- Initially, a bolus of ¼ of this dose can be given, and then the status of the patient reassessed.
- Rapid administration of IV fluids can be difficult in horses. Due to redistribution to the extravascular space, only 25% of the volume administered remains in the intravascular space after one hour.

Hypertonic Saline [37]
- Can be administered as an IV bolus to rapidly increase intravascular volume at a dose rate of 2–4 ml/kg.
- Hypertonic saline achieves this by drawing fluid out of the interstitium, though this fluid eventually redistributes resulting in a short-term volume expansion of less than one hour.
- In order to maintain the volume expansion and rehydrate the interstitium, large volumes of isotonic crystalloids (10 l for every 1 l hypertonic saline) must be given concurrently.

Colloids [37]

- These are fluids that have a high oncotic pressure due to high-molecular-weight molecules. These molecules remain within the intravascular space and help to expand the circulating volume.
- Dose rates of 10–20 ml/kg can be used.
- Synthetic or natural colloids can be used. Please see Section 14.8 for further information.

Administration of fluids is not without risk in patients with shock; frequent, stringent monitoring is required to identify any adverse reactions or deterioration in the patient's condition. Regular blood pressure measurements will determine if fluid replacement is effective; if not, then cardiac support drugs such as pressors or inotropes may be required. Treatment with pressors or inotropes will require intensive monitoring and care [37]. Intranasal humidified oxygen therapy, administered in one or both nostrils depending on the level of hypoxia, can assist in raising oxygen saturation and can be monitored with arterial blood gases.

Broad-spectrum antibiotics, anti-inflammatory medications and endotoxin inhibitors may be prescribed by the case vet depending on the individual case. Critical care monitoring, pain scoring and frequent haematology and lactate analysis will be required to determine how the disease is progressing. The patient may require assistance with thermoregulation in the form of rugs, bandages and heat lamps. Mental stimulation and environmental enrichment should also be provided to improve demeanour and assist with recovery. Success in therapy depends on early and aggressive veterinary interventions and presents a challenging situation for the nursing team as complications that can arise from shock are complicated to manage.

14.8 Fluid Therapy

Indications for Fluid Therapy

Fluid administration for maintenance or replacement purposes is one of the foundations of equine critical care and must be readily available for use in any equine practice. Its main purpose is to restore circulating volume and improve cardiac output, which will in turn, improve tissue perfusion and correct imbalances in electrolyte and acid–base abnormalities.

Fluid therapy is beneficial for:

- Maintaining adequate levels of hydration when disease or circumstances prevent the patient from drinking and sustaining hydration themselves.
- Restoring deficits that have caused dehydration.
- Replacing continuing fluid losses when a disease process continues.
- Overhydrating for treatment of a condition that requires increased fluid retention, for example, softening a large intestinal impaction.

Clinical signs of dehydration may include the following:

- The horse may appear quiet and dull
- Mucous membranes may be congested (dark red) and tacky to touch
- Increased CRT (over two seconds)
- Tachycardia
- Poor skin turgor
- Decreased urine output
- Slower jugular refill time

Haematological analysis may suggest a high PCV and an increased total plasma protein. Horses with dehydration can have biochemistry abnormalities associated with dehydration like an increased urea, creatinine and lactate. The percentage of dehydration relates to the amount (%) of body weight lost. Clinical signs relating to dehydration can be seen as follows [37]:

- Less than 5% dehydration: Clinical signs may not be apparent.
- 5–7% dehydration: Clinical signs may include tacky or dry mucous membranes, a prolonged CRT and mild depression.
- 8–10% dehydration: Clinical signs will present as above with the addition of prolonged skin tenting, weak peripheral pulses, cool extremities, moderate tachycardia and depressed mentation.
- 10–12% dehydration: Clinical signs will present as above with the addition of cold extremities, obtunded mentation, severely prolonged skin tenting and severe tachycardia.
- 12% dehydration and over: Clinical signs will present as above and the patient may be moribund or comatose, recumbent and have severe tachycardia or bradycardia.

Dehydration ranging over 10–12% is fatal if not addressed rapidly and aggressively.

Types of Fluids

A decision on what type of fluid to administer needs to be determined based on biochemistry analysis and the disease state. The standard baseline electrolyte solutions used in equine practice are 0.9% sodium chloride (saline) and balanced electrolyte solutions.

There are two categories of IV fluids routinely used in equine practice:

- Crystalloids
- Colloids

Crystalloids

Crystalloids contain water, sodium or glucose, plus other electrolytes and a buffer to maintain a stable pH. The fluid may be hypotonic, isotonic or hypertonic in relation to plasma. Crystalloids move easily between intravascular (25%) and interstitial spaces (75%) within an hour following administration. This results in a 250 ml increase of plasma volume for every 1 l of fluid infused. This benefits the patient when it is dehydrated and hypovolaemic, but care must be taken not to exceed the recommended amount as this could lead to tissue oedema [37].

Movement of fluid into the intravascular space will result in decreased total plasma protein through dilution, which may be beneficial or detrimental depending on the clinical condition and desired outcome. This should be considered when formulating a fluid plan.

Isotonic Polyionic Fluids (Lactated Ringers, Hartmann's, 0.9% Sodium Chloride)

These are the most commonly used crystalloid solutions in equine practice and have a similar osmotic pressure to blood. These fluids largely move into extracellular fluid (2/3) and plasma (1/3), which aids in restoring plasma volumes. Only 25% of the infused volume will remain in the intravascular space one hour after infusion [37]. Therefore, almost three times the volume replacement is needed to return the hydration level to a normal balance. The electrolyte composition of these fluids is similar to plasma; however, it has a lower potassium composition making it not uncommon for the patient to require potassium chloride additives. Isotonic saline (0.9%) is hypernatraemic and hyperchloraemic when compared to plasma and lacks other electrolytes. It is not used as a maintenance or resuscitation fluid but may be indicated for the treatment of hyponatraemia and hypochloraemia.

Hypotonic Solutions (5% Dextrose)

In the bag, the osmolarity of 5% glucose solution is close to being isotonic [38]. However, once administered to the patient, the glucose is rapidly taken up by the cells and metabolised. Therefore, giving 5% glucose solutions is equivalent to giving free water, which has a lower osmotic pressure compared to blood and will distribute evenly to all fluid compartments [38]. It is limited in its ability to reverse cardiovascular collapse. It cannot be given in large volumes as it lacks electrolytes and can cause hyperglycaemia. The consequence of this leads to excess diuresis, which results in more fluid loss. It is, however, useful in patients with high circulating sodium and chloride levels.

Hypertonic Solutions (7.2% Sodium Chloride)

These are used in small volumes and as a temporary fix in emergency situations. Due to having greater osmotic pressure compared to blood, they encourage the transfer of fluid from the cells into circulation. This results in fast plasma volume expansion, but this effect is temporary and can lead to dehydration. Following the administration of hypertonic saline, isotonic fluids need to be given at a rate of 10 l to every 1 l of hypertonic saline to counteract dehydration [37]. Hypertonic fluids can be administered to patients requiring emergency surgery as a rapid treatment for haemoconcentration and hypovolaemia and will support cardiovascular function during GA.

Colloids

Colloids are solutions that contain large molecules of starch and protein compared to crystalloids, which contain large volumes of water and salts. The advantage is that they expand the plasma volume by a greater amount and stay in circulation for 8–10 hours. This enables rapid volume replacement, improving vascular perfusion with less risk of tissue oedema. They are commonly used in the treatment of hypovolaemia. Types of colloids available in the United Kingdom are as follows:

Plasma

This is the noncellular portion of whole blood collected from a compatible donor. It has had the cells removed by centrifugation. Albumin is the main component of plasma and is responsible for preventing fluid from leaking out of intravascular circulation. It is rarely used for rehydration due to the vast volume required but is beneficial in replacing immunoglobulins, clotting factors, platelets and anticoagulants. Hyperimmune plasma is commercially available in one-litre bags but can be expensive. Plasma can be separated in practice, but it takes specialist materials to ensure the cells are separated from the plasma.

Whole Blood

This is indicated for treating hypovolaemia in patients with severe and rapid haemorrhage or acute haemolysis. If time permits, using a crossmatched and blood-typed donor is preferred. If the recipient risks dying before receiving the blood, an alternative donor could be a healthy gelding of the same breed. Usually, crossmatching is not carried out for the first transfusion, but the donor's serum can be mixed with the recipient's red blood cells and vice versa to look for signs of clumping, indicating agglutination. As universal donors do not exist, crossmatches should precede additional transfusions [39]. Horses receiving plasma or whole blood infusions must be closely monitored throughout the process as they can exhibit signs of hypersensitivity leading to anaphylaxis at any time during the transfusion. This can include tachycardia, tachypnoea, agitation, pruritis, pyrexia and urticaria. If adverse signs become apparent, the transfusion must be stopped and supportive anti-inflammatory therapy might be necessary. See Section 14.9 for more information.

Gelofusine

This is a synthetic plasma substitute containing gelatine and sodium chloride. It is indicated for the treatment of hypovolaemia, shock and the prevention of hypotension when the condition cannot be treated with crystalloids alone. It will pull fluid into circulation and expand the blood volume as well as increase the oncotic pressure. Because of their desired effect, only small volumes of colloids are needed in comparison to crystalloids. Gelofusine is expensive; therefore, it is used sparingly in equine practice and not licensed for use in horses. However, it can be used under the prescribing cascade, which allows vets to prescribe specialised products that would not be available for critically ill patients otherwise (see Chapter 9 for further information). There is a small risk of adverse reactions (anaphylaxis) with administering gelofusine, and patients require close monitoring by an experienced nursing team.

Infusion Pumps and Syringe Drivers

Fluid infusion pumps used in human medicine have long been utilised in equine practice (Figure 14.5). They are calibrated medical devices that draw IV solutions from a standard fluid bag through a giving set, past pumps that use a peristaltic action to deliver the fluid to the patient. They are set to a predetermined infusion rate and have mechanisms in place to prevent air ingress, as well as alarms to signal when there are disturbances to the fluid flow. They can be safely used in foals and horses of all sizes because their veins are large enough to cope with the pressures that the pump delivers on them without risk of vessel damage and extravasation. Some infusion pumps can save the total volumes infused over a specified time on their software, making it easier for the veterinary team to calculate gains against losses. The maximum rate is 999 ml/hour, which is not sufficient for maintenance infusions in the adult horse but is very useful for foals, smaller infusions and administering TPN.

Syringe drivers are also medical devices that can be used in equine practice. Smaller volumes of solutions and

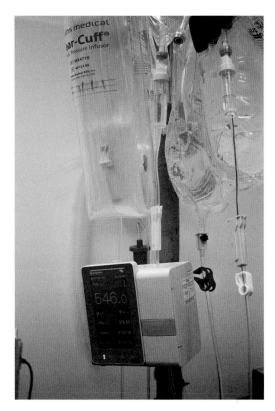

Figure 14.5 An infusion pump in use. *Source:* Rosina Lillywhite.

medications are mixed in syringes and secured to the driver. An actuator is programmed to push the syringe plunger at a set rate, delivering controlled and constant volumes to the patient.

Enteral Fluids

In some cases, enteral fluids will be required. Enteral fluids may be administered via a nasogastric tube.

The main advantages of giving enteral fluids by nasogastric tube are as follows:

- Less expensive than IV fluids
- Does not require sterile supplies
- Absorption via the gastrointestinal tract is a natural process and physiologically normal, making fluid imbalances unlikely.

Horses can comfortably receive a bolus of 6–8 l, although it is not uncommon for the stomach to accommodate about 20 l or more when gastric reflux is present. Due to the small size of the equine stomach, care should be taken not to overload the patient with fluids, as discomfort and rupture can occur. Hypovolaemia amplifies absorption in the gastrointestinal tract, and the fluids administered will enter the circulation within an hour. Administering fluids by this method is contraindicated in the presence of ileus, intestinal obstructions or marked bowel inflammation. An oral fluid delivery system can be constructed that utilises gravity-fed administration into a soft (silicone) nasogastric tube that is fixed in place. It delivers a continuous 'trickle' rate of fluids into the stomach. This is only advised with patients who are standing and not showing signs of colic. Careful monitoring is required with the use of oral fluid delivery systems, as the position of the tube within the stomach can alter, and this can change the rate of fluid administration.

Administering tap water via a high enema is effective in rehydrating horses that are unable to drink. Because the permeability of the rectal mucosa is good and this method is easily tolerated, rectal fluid therapy could benefit patients who cannot tolerate nasogastric fluid administration. Sterile fluids are not required, and the risk of fluid overload is low with this method.

Indications for enteral fluids:

- Increase fluid absorption of gastrointestinal ingesta, for example, to soften large intestine impactions.
- Correct electrolyte imbalances
- Maintain a zero-balance state
- Treat dehydration in the presence of ongoing losses
- Trigger the gastrocolic reflex, which in turn stimulates intestinal motility.

For more information regarding nasogastric tubing, see Chapter 17.

Fluid Balance

Because water is the body's most essential nutrient, clinicians must attempt to keep patients in a zero-fluid balance. This means maintaining a state where the amount of fluid excreted from the body is exactly equal to that which is introduced, resulting in an equilibrium. In veterinary practice, daily fluid balance is measured by calculating the difference between all intakes, such as IV fluids, enteral and/or parental nutrition, and all outputs, for example, waste excreted and losses, not including insensible losses. Insensible fluid losses are the volumes of body fluids lost in daily physiological functions that cannot easily be measured, mainly from respiration, perspiration and the water in faeces. When fluid balance is disrupted, it can lead to an altered balanced state. Negative fluid balance results in clinical dehydration as there is insufficient water content in the interstitial space. This results in less water intake than the output from faeces, urine, sweat and respiration.

Fluid overload or positive fluid balance is not perceived to be a great concern in the adult horse but should be closely monitored in neonates during fluid therapy. The most common cause is overhydration with IV fluids, which results in the presence of excess water in the interstitial and intracellular spaces. This can be a desirable effect in the presence of large intestinal impactions. Systemic overhydration from large-volume fluid therapy forces water into the ingesta, promoting colonic secretion, which enables it to soften and exit the body. Urinary output will be increased at this time, with a diluted concentration, but should normalise once the fluid rate is returned to normal.

Other causes include an increase in total body sodium concentrations with an associated rise in extracellular water, which occurs in some disease states. These may include congestive heart failure, kidney failure, oliguria and liver failure.

Hypoperfusion

Fluid therapy is most effective in treating hypoperfusion or shock, where there is inadequate, blood circulation, and therefore oxygen to tissues and organs. The early, compensatory signs of shock include tachycardia, a weakened pulse, pale mucous membranes with decreased CRT, and cool extremities such as cold ears and legs. This is when the body is still capable of compensating for fluid loss. As it progresses into decompensated shock, the signs include low blood pressure, tachypnoea, shivering and hypothermia, agitation and altered mentation. This is when the body can no longer compensate for the decrease in oxygen delivery to tissues.

Hyperperfusion

Increased tension and perfusion of blood to tissue and organs. It is also associated with clots that form in the major vessels, resulting in congestion of blood to the organs affected by the embolism. Embolisms are rare in the horse, so if hypertension does exist, further investigation of its cause is needed.

Fluid Calculations

Calculating fluid requirements is estimated and depends on the clinical signs, the laboratory data and the expected characteristic of the disease condition. It considers the maintenance, deficits and projected losses over a 24-hour period, while the horse is regularly monitored. Neonates have different daily maintenance requirements because they have greater body fluid content in proportion to the adult. Their extracellular fluid space (ECF) is also greater when compared to an adult. This, along with a higher metabolism, rapid growth and fluid losses, results in larger fluid requirements per kilogram.

Daily maintenance requirements of adult horses and foals are as follows [37]:

- Adults: 40–60 ml/kg/24 hours
- Foals: 80–100 ml/kg/24 hours

The percentage (%) of dehydration must be determined through haematology testing. Once the % dehydration has been determined, the litres of deficit can be calculated using the following equation:

Body weight (kg) × % dehydration = litres of deficit

Add the deficit and maintenance together to get the amount to be needed for 24 hours.

Example 1 A 400 kg horse with diarrhoea is 6% dehydrated. The vet has requested that the horse receives maintenance crystalloid fluids for 24 hours at a rate of 50 ml/kg/24 hours in addition to replacing the fluid deficit. Calculations required for this patient include:

- The total daily maintenance
- Fluid deficit
- Total of maintenance and fluid deficit added together

Maintenance requirement over 24 hours:

400 kg × 50 ml = 20 l

Deficit or losses due to the diarrhoea:

400 kg × 0.06% = 24 l

Maintenance and deficit volumes:

20 + 24 = 44 l

The horse needs 44 l of fluid over 24 hours if the disease state continues. The deficit should be replaced quickly but carefully, usually within a few hours. Some clinicians will replace half the deficit, given as a shock dose, then reassess the patient to determine how it has responded to treatment and will readjust the subsequent volumes accordingly.

The drip factor, which is printed on the giving set packaging, states the number of drops in one millilitre (mL) of solution delivered by gravity. The rate is determined by counting the number of drops that fall in the drip chamber per minute. This is not always a useful way to monitor fluid therapy in adult patients, as it can be almost impossible to count the drops accurately due to the speed and volume of fluid being administered. However, it can be a useful to work out how many drops per minute are required when administering fluids to foals. Giving sets with a drip factor of 20 drops/ml are most commonly used for foals (see Example 2).

Example 2 The vet has requested that a 60 kg foal receive maintenance crystalloid fluids for 24 hours at a rate of 100 ml/kg/24 hours. Calculations required for this patient include:

- The total daily maintenance
- ml per hour
- ml per minute
- The fluid administration rate in drops per minute

The drip factor is 20 drops per minute.

Daily Maintenance

The daily maintenance fluid requirement for this foal is 100 ml/kg/24 hours

Therefore, the daily fluid requirement for this foal is 100 (ml/kg) × 60 kg (bodyweight) = 6000 ml or 6 l to be administered over 24 hours.

ml per hour = amount of fluid ÷ 24

6000 ml ÷ 24 hours = 250 ml/hour

ml per minute = ml/hour ÷ 60

250 ÷ 60 = 4.2 ml/min

Drops per min = ml/min × 20

4.2 mls/min × 20 = 83.3 drops per min.

This can be rounded down to 83 drops per minute.

For more information on fluid therapy in foals, see Chapter 15.

Gravity Fed Infusions

The majority of fluid delivery devices used in equine practice are gravity-fed systems that are hung from the ceiling of the stable. In its simplest form, 5 l sterile fluid bags are hung from the centre of a stable with a fluid administration set attached, with a flexible and expandable line attached to the catheter extension set. If the pulley system is securely fixed to the ceiling joists, it can support 4–5 bags of 5 l fluids and an infusion pump if required. Before installation, it is important to check that the parts and ropes have been weight-tested by the manufacturer.

While giving IV solutions using gravity-fed systems is commonplace, the following complications should be considered:

Disconnection of the fluid line:

- This can cause a break in sterility, contaminating the giving and catheter extension sets.
- If the fluid line is disconnected, the horse is not getting the fluid replacement it needs, which can compromise welfare and recovery.

- This can increase the risk of an air embolism occurring or bleeding from an open catheter/extension set if one-way valves are not present.

Trauma to the fluid line:

- Foals accompanying mares can chew fluid lines within their reach.
- The patient can rub the catheter against a wall, damaging the catheter and the giving set.
- If the patient is showing signs of colic, it can become entangled in the fluid line and disconnect or break it.
- If the patient is box walking, they can twist the fluid line so tightly that it occludes the lumen and prevents fluid flow.

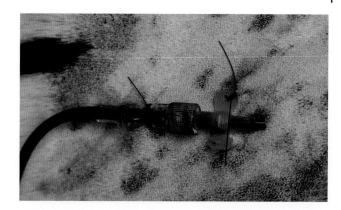

Figure 14.6 A kinked catheter. *Source:* Rosina Lillywhite.

Intravenous Catheter Complications Associated with Intravenous Fluid Therapy

Patency

The continuous flow of fluids through a fluid line prevents blood from pooling in the administration set and clots forming in the catheter. When fluid lines are to be disconnected for any length of time, the catheter must be flushed with normal or heparinised saline. The catheter must be checked for patency and flushed four times a day if it is not used for continuous infusions. Even with frequent flushing, catheters can still form clots or kinks, affecting patency.

Blood clots in the catheter hub can sometimes be removed by aspiration with a syringe. The catheter should be flushed with heparinised saline following this. There is a risk that smaller clot fragments can be pushed into the narrower tip of the catheter and cause complete occlusion or enter the bloodstream. There may still be some patency with partial occlusion, but the desired drip rate may be intermittently disrupted. Ideally, when a clot is suspected, the catheter should be removed and replaced in a different vein to ensure optimal patency.

Intravenous Catheter Damage

Kinks in catheters are common and can affect fluid rates and limit the ability to give medications (Figure 14.6). The skin at the insertion site has a fair amount of elasticity and can move away from where the catheter has entered the vein. This causes kinks near the hub where it is fixed in the skin with sutures, while the subcutaneous space has more mobility. Improperly sutured catheters can cause a reduction in the infusion rate, risking lower volumes being administered. This issue commonly occurs in the jugular vein when the patient changes their neck position. The hub must be re-sutured to help straighten the catheter and improve the patency. If this is unsuccessful, the catheter

will need to be replaced with care taken to suture it properly to maximise its effectiveness.

Venous Spasm

A venous spasm can also be defined as vasoconstriction and is characterised by a narrowing of the blood vessel. The smooth muscle lining of the vessel walls contract in response to injury, and the response of the nervous system to pain. The vasoconstriction is caused by a substance called thromboxane A_2, which is activated by platelets, damaged epithelial cells and vascular smooth muscle caused by needle sticks [40]. This can make catheterisng the vein difficult, especially after repeated attempts.

Extravasation

Extravasation is defined as the leaking of blood, lymph, fluids or drugs, from a blood vessel into the surrounding space. There is a slight risk when catheters are situated in smaller peripheral veins, namely that the pressure exerted on the vessel by a fluid pump can cause extravasation of fluid. The vein is damaged, or fluid leaks from the insertion site. A fluid pump will not recognise that it is delivering fluids into the subcutaneous space; therefore, no alarm will sound and it will continue pumping until an increased pressure forces an alarm. Extravasation can also occur when there have been repeated needle sticks in the vein or when the catheter tip abrades the vessel wall. Some drugs can irritate the blood vessels, causing erosion and leaking if they are not administered as recommended.

Signs of extravasation:

- Oedema at or below the catheter insertion site
- Erythema around the catheter insertion site
- Pain or tenderness when the area is palpated
- A reduction in patency of the catheter
- Infusion flow is intermittent or ceases completely

- Cool skin temperature below the insertion site where subcutaneous fluids have been collected

For more information relating to IV catheter placement and care, please see Chapter 17.

14.9 Blood Products

Fresh or frozen equine plasma and freshly collected whole blood are commonly used in equine critical care as life-saving therapies.

Types of Blood Products

Plasma

Plasma is predominantly used to treat:

- Hypoproteinaemia and shock to support a stable oncotic pressure.
- Coagulopathy as it provides clotting factors.
- Endotoxaemia and sepsis as it contains anti-endotoxic antibodies for immune support.
- Neonates that are at risk of failure of passive transfer, delivering immunoglobulins that were lacking at birth. Hyperimmune plasma is collected from donor herds that are hyperimmunised to provide antibodies at high concentrations. See Chapter 15 for more information.
- Thrombocytopaenia in horses who are not anaemic. Fresh plasma is transfused when active platelets are needed, but not the red cells.

Plasma is administered through a blood-giving set, with a filter integrated within the drip chamber.

Whole Blood

Whole blood is an exact replacement intended to replenish deficits in the recipient's oxygen-carrying capability in the presence of haemorrhage, anaemia and shock. Fresh whole blood may also be used for its clotting factors and platelets.

In neonates, washed erythrocytes are administered when the foal is diagnosed with neonatal isoerythrolysis. Before the foal receives the mare's blood, the plasma is removed and the cells are washed repeatedly. This removes the antibodies contained within the mare's plasma that adversely react to the foal's erythrocytes.

A whole blood transfusion is required if the patient has a packed cell volume of 12% or less and is continuing to decrease in the presence of continued haemorrhage or anaemia and is clinically unstable. Other reasons to transfuse are haemoglobin levels below 6 g/dl and blood loss that exceeds 25% of the patient's total blood volume [39]. If these levels fall further, weakness and dyspnoea at rest are evident, with the added risk of heart failure as oxygen delivery to tissues is impaired.

Blood Donors

If the recipient has not had a prior transfusion, one can be safely performed in an emergency, without crossmatching. The ideal donor is as follows:

- A young, healthy gelding, preferably of the same breed
- Good temperament
- Over 500 kg
- Fully vaccinated
- Known medical history
- Not have travelled outside the country
- Not previously had a blood transfusion.

Broodmares are not good blood donors as they may have developed alloantibodies, through exposure to foreign red blood cell antigens, through breeding and foaling. If the patient requires a subsequent transfusion, cross-matching is recommended to confirm compatibility. Further transfusions increase the possibility of adverse anaphylactic reactions; therefore, they must be approached with caution and with a full understanding of the patient's clinical status.

Blood Typing and Crossmatching

Horses are known to have eight blood groups with seven internationally recognised – A, C, D, K, P, Q and U. Each group matches a specific surface antigen known as a factor. At present, over 30 different factors are recognised. When the seven different groups match in multiple combinations with a factor, this results in over 400,000 blood type possibilities with no true universal donors. The blood types are named using both group and factor identification. The first letter is in upper case to represent the group, followed by a lower-case letter to state the factor, for example, Qa or Aa [39]. Rapid blood typing tests are not available for general practice use yet, so blood must be sent to a specialist testing lab.

Many larger referral hospitals will do their crossmatching and use this to identify the presence of antibodies that might be incompatible with the recipient. The procedure cannot be carried out quickly, as accessing donor horses that do not reside on the premises is time-consuming, and samples must be collected each time a crossmatch is performed. Time is needed for the incubation of crossmatch reactions to trigger haemolysis (destruction of red blood cells) if there is limited or no compatibility.

Crossmatching is effectively a test transfusion carried out in the lab to see how the recipient's blood will react with the potential donor's blood. It is a method of detecting any significant antibodies in either the recipient's or donor's blood without causing harm to the recipient. There are two types of cross matches:

- **Major crossmatch:** Involves mixing the donor's erythrocytes (red blood cells) with the recipient's serum and observing haemolysis or agglutination (clumping of red blood cells) in the presence of antibodies.
- **Minor crossmatch:** Involves mixing the donor's plasma with the recipient's erythrocytes to determine if there are antibodies present that might cause agglutination or haemolysis of the recipient's red cells.

The following is an example of the basic method for performing a major crossmatch:

1) After removing the serum, prepare a saline cell suspension of the donor's red blood cells.
2) Prepare a sample of the recipient's serum by removing the erythrocytes.
3) On a glass slide, mix one drop of donor red cells, one drop of the recipient serum and one drop of saline.
4) Gently rock the slide, encouraging the samples to mix and observe microscopically for agglutination and visually for haemolysis.
5) The donor and recipient are compatible if the sample mixes without agglutination occurring.

Donor blood that is compatible should not show agglutination in either the major or minor crossmatch. Blood showing clear incompatibility during cross-matching should not be transfused, as the donor cells will undergo lysis in the presence of the recipient's plasma antibodies.

Incompatibility with a minor crossmatch means the transfusion can still proceed, but with caution. This is because the donor's serum antibodies will be diluted and cause less of a reaction when added to the recipient's own plasma. However, if the donor's serum is likely to add significant volume to the recipient's plasma capacity, the donor serum should be removed as it increases the likelihood of an adverse reaction. The packed red cells are then washed in the lab, under sterile conditions and reconstituted with isotonic saline.

Transport of Whole Blood and Plasma

Whole blood and washed red cells that have been cooled must be transported in temperatures between 2 and 10 °C. If this temperature is not maintained, its oxygen-carrying capabilities may be reduced once it is transfused. The presence of the anticoagulants prevents clotting during storage and transit until the time of transfusion. Blood or plasma that has been unintentionally exposed to warm temperatures risks bacterial proliferation. Every effort should be made to keep frozen plasma in the same frozen condition

so it can be transferred to a storage freezer without large temperature fluctuations on arrival.

Packing boxes and materials must be designed for this purpose and equipped to collect all the leaked fluid, without escaping the box, in the event of damage to the container. The shipping boxes have insulated inserts with tight-fitting lids to maintain the temperature. Dead space in the box should be minimised; cold packs or ice should not be allowed to come into direct contact with the blood bags. All transport containers must be appropriately labelled, stating what the contents are and with any warnings or instructions added. All packaging must comply with the requirements of the postal service used. The transit time for all blood products should not exceed 24 hours.

Equipment, Collection and Administration for Blood Transfusions

When going out on a visit to collect blood from a donor, a pre-prepared catheter kit is useful to take to ensure no supplies have been left behind. The donor's jugular vein will need to be clipped and aseptically cleaned. Using an accepted IV catheter placement technique (see Chapter 17), a 10–12-gauge, 3-inch. catheter is placed with the catheter tip directed cranially (retrograde placement) (Figure 14.7). This enables faster blood collection using

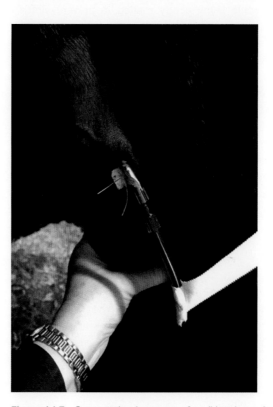

Figure 14.7 Retrograde placement of an IV catheter for blood collection. *Source:* Bonny Millar.

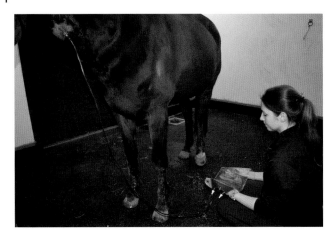

Figure 14.8 The blood bag should be held below the catheter to enable rapid collection of blood. *Source:* Rosina Lillywhite.

gravity flow. The whole blood is collected in commercially available collection bags that are pre-loaded with the correct proportion of citrate–phosphate–dextrose–adenine (CPDA-1) anticoagulant. This anticoagulant, is preferred for extending the shelf life and preserving the cell morphology of the stored blood. The bag's integrated collection line is attached to the catheter, and the jugular vein is occluded. The bag is held below the catheter to enable rapid collection of blood while being gently rotated to prevent clotting and ensure an even mix of blood and anticoagulant (Figure 14.8). Vigorous movement of the blood should be avoided as this will cause lysis (disintegration) of the erythrocytes. The bag can be weighed to confirm the correct proportion of blood to anticoagulant has been collected.

Whole blood can be administered immediately if it is not to be stored. When correctly stored and refrigerated at 4 °C, whole blood can have a shelf life of 30–35 days, and fresh frozen plasma, up to three years. Stored whole blood and plasma need to be warmed to body temperature prior to administration. Whole blood is given through a blood-giving set, with a filter integrated within the drip chamber.

Calculating Transfusion Volumes and Rate

In the horse, 8–10% of its body weight is blood. This equates to approximately 45 l in a 500 kg horse. A healthy donor can safely give 20–25% of blood if they receive IV isotonic fluids post-infusion. There are a number of ways to calculate the estimated blood volumes needed by the recipient. The following formulae are accurate and consider the donor's PCV, the recipient's need and body weight [39]:

Litres of whole blood

$$= \frac{\text{desired PCV} - (\text{Recipient's PCV} \times 0.08 \times \text{body weight in kg})}{\text{PCV of donor}}$$

Another method to estimate the amount of blood the recipient needs, assuming the donor's PCV is 40%: Give 2.2 ml of whole blood/kg body weight, to increase the recipient's PCV by 1%.

Preparation and Administration of Fresh and Frozen Plasma

To make plasma, whole blood collected from the donor is run through a cell separator in a technique called plasmapheresis. The blood enters a sterile canister and begins centrifuging. While the canister is spinning, the blood cells are returned to the donor with replacement fluids, and the plasma is extracted and collected into sterile bags with anticoagulants. During filling, the bags are weighed to ensure they all fill with equal volumes. Plasma samples are removed for bacteriology cultures and for use in future cross matches. At this point, the plasma can be administered to the patient, or if it needs to be stored for future use, the bags should then be labelled and placed in a freezer.

Frozen plasma should be thawed just prior to administration. The best method for defrosting the plasma is thawing it in a temperature-controlled water bath. If the water is too hot, above 40 °C, the plasma proteins can denature and the fibrinogen can separate causing a precipitate to form. Nothing should be added to the plasma bag, and it must be administered through a filtered blood-giving set. Plasma that has been thawed can be stored at 4 °C for up to 20 days if it has not been warmed. See Chapter 15 for more information regarding plasma transfusions in foals.

Patient Monitoring During a Transfusion

A baseline clinical examination of the recipient is performed prior to the transfusion and documented so comparisons can be made with subsequent checks. The transfusion is ideally carried out on a patient who is not sedated and can be monitored closely throughout the procedure. The transfusion begins at a rate of one drop per second, ensuring the drip is clearly distinguishable in the drip chamber of the blood-giving set. Temperature, pulse and respiration (TPR) readings are taken every five minutes in the early stages of the transfusion and then every 15 minutes if there are no changes to the TPR parameters after 30 minutes. These readings should be recorded along with the batch number for the plasma in case of a transfusion reaction. The drip rate can be increased as required if the vital signs remain consistent.

Adverse reactions are not uncommon during a blood or plasma transfusion and typically occur within the first 10–15 minutes of the start of the transfusion, although some delayed reactions can arise at the end of the procedure or even days later. Immune-mediated haemolytic reactions are the most common and quite concerning, often of a febrile nature. Their incidence also increases significantly if the recipient receives subsequent transfusions or when the administration of all blood products is not slow or carefully monitored.

Nonimmune-mediated transfusion reactions are less common, and are generally associated with problems during blood collection, handling, administration and storage, in conditions where contamination was possible. It is essential that all stages of blood collection, preparation and administration are conducted in aseptic conditions.

Clinical signs may include the following:

- Mild pyrexia
- Tachycardia
- Tachypnoea
- Dyspnoea
- Fasciculations
- Urticaria (Figure 14.9).
- Severe anaphylaxis

Beginning with a baseline rectal temperature with continued measurements, primarily in the early stages of the transfusion, aids in recognising the early signs of adverse reactions. If diarrhoea becomes apparent during the transfusion, this can be a clear sign of impending anaphylaxis. Therefore, the infusion should stop, and systemic support should be offered immediately.

Allergic reactions of any severity are treated by immediate discontinuation of the transfusion with the administration of an antihistamine or corticosteroids if indicated. Some clinicians use dexamethasone, but its immunosuppression properties may be a concern in some critically ill patients. In severe allergic reactions, resulting in anaphylaxis, the administration of epinephrine may be lifesaving.

Transfusion Overload

While extremely uncommon in adult horses, transfusion overload can be a concern in neonates or miniature ponies. It can lead to signs of a positive fluid balance, respiratory distress, hypertension, pulmonary oedema and associated circulatory complications. Monitoring the central venous pressure (CVP) is useful as it assesses cardiac function, intravascular volume and vascular tone. Adhering to the recommended transfusion rates and volumes while being aware of the patient's circulatory limitations will help to prevent fluid overload.

Young neonates receiving multiple whole blood transfusions, in quick succession, are at a higher risk of iron overload and hypervolaemia. Due to their small size, they are taking on a larger volume in comparison to adult horses. The amount of iron transfused can exceed the normal iron concentration in the foal's circulatory system. It can lead to a compromised liver that fails to metabolise the excess iron, resulting in hepatopathy. Depending on the severity, treatment may include keeping the patient in sternal recumbency and administering diuretics and oxygen therapy to support cardiac function.

Donkey Factor

All donkey red blood cells have an antigen specific to their species, known as 'donkey factor'. This is not present in horses; therefore, they are naturally donkey factor negative, making it unsafe to transfuse donkey blood into a horse, but donkeys can be safely transfused with horse blood [38]. When horses are exposed to donkey factor antigens, their antibodies cause haemolysis and agglutination. This can result in an increased risk of neonatal isoerythrolysis in mule foals. That risk far exceeds what is recognised in horses, so it is important to cross-match mule neonates to any multiparous mare, before it is allowed to nurse. Donkeys can tolerate horse plasma transfusions as long as the usual precautions are taken. For more information about donkeys, see Chapter 16.

14.10 Pain Assessment in Equine Patients

Monitoring Patients for Pain and Stress

Pain is defined as an unpleasant sensory and emotional experience associated with actual or potential tissue damage or described in terms of such damage [41]. The inability to communicate in no way negates the possibility that an

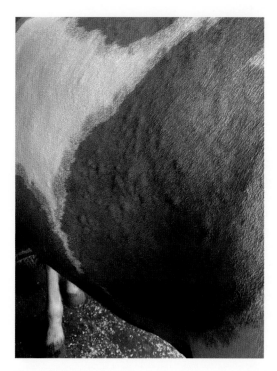

Figure 14.9 Horse with urticaria. *Source:* Marie Rippingale.

individual is experiencing pain and needs appropriate pain-relieving treatment [41]. Acute pain can be beneficial as it can help to protect against injury and enable healing. Chronic pain, however, can be detrimental to health, physiologically, immunologically and psychologically, and it can result in suffering and distress [41]. Chronic pain such as this is referred to as maladaptive pain. Prey species such as equids tend to hide pain. It is not in their best interests to express pain, as predators are more likely to target sick or injured animals [41]. This can make pain recognition difficult for vets and RVNs in practice.

There are different types of pain [42]:

- 'Physiological' pain acts to protect the body by warning of contact with tissue-damaging stimuli. This type of pain is produced by stimulation of nociceptors innervated by high threshold (Group III) and unmyelinated C (Group IV) fibres.
- 'Clinical' (nociceptive) pain, by contrast, is produced by peripheral tissue injury or damage to the nervous system.

Clinical pain can be categorised as inflammatory or neuropathic pain. Inflammatory pain is further categorised as either visceral (thoracic and abdominal viscera) or somatic (skin, joints, muscles or periosteum) in origin [42].

- Visceral pain is poorly localised and described as cramping or gnawing. It may be referred to cutaneous sites far from the site of injury.
- Somatic pain is more easily localised and is described as aching, stabbing or throbbing. It is generally acute. Somatic pain includes cutaneous or incisional pain after operation and is frequently referred to as superficial (skin) or deep (joints, muscle and periosteum).
- Neuropathic pain occurs as a direct result of damage to peripheral nerves or the spinal cord and is described as burning, stabbing, intermittent and is often unresponsive to treatment.

Both inflammatory and neuropathic pain can produce the following [42]:

- Allodynia: Pain caused by a stimulus that does not normally cause pain.
- Hyperalgesia (primary and secondary): This is a heightened sensitivity to pain.
- Central nervous system (CNS) and peripheral sensitisation to external stimuli.

Idiopathic pain is pain that has no specific or determinable cause. Idiopathic pain is often excessive and can be accentuated by activation of the sympathetic nervous system (SNS) due to emotional stress or excitement. For more information about pain pathways, please see Chapter 10.

Horses show signs of pain and stress in a variety of ways. These can range from dullness and inappetence to violent rolling and non-weight-bearing lameness. Knowing as much as possible about what is normal for each individual patient is important. This will help to inform observations and nursing interventions to ensure that the patient receives effective, individualised care. During the admission process, it is important to talk to the owner about the horse as an individual. It is often useful to fill in a patient assessment form (see Chapter 13 for further details) to record what is normal for that patient when they are at home. Having a baseline knowledge of what is normal for each horse will facilitate the identification of abnormalities. For example, if a patient is usually bright and friendly but has been dull and uninterested since admission, this would require assessment and intervention.

The overall condition and demeanour of the patient should be assessed, and the findings recorded. This assessment could include:

Coat, Eyes, Nose, Ears and Skin

- The coat should be shiny without evidence of parasitic activity or flaky skin; a dull staring coat can be a sign of poor nutrition or poor health.
- In the healthy horse, the eyes should be bright and clear; they should be fully open with no signs of cloudiness or discolouration of the globe. There should be no evidence of discharge around the eyes, although a small amount of crustiness may appear at times, which is normal; if it becomes thick, sticky and yellowish or green this is abnormal [43].
- The nostrils should be clean and free from excessive amounts of mucous; a trickle of clear liquid is normal.
- Ears should be mobile and move with the noise in the environment; a dull or painful animal will often have less mobile ears, or ears that sit out to the sides [43].

Weight and Body Condition Score

- To get the most accurate weight for a patient, a mobile weighbridge can be used; if this is not available or if a simple monitoring tool is required, then a weigh tape can be useful to monitor a reduction in girth width, for example.
- Body condition scoring is a simple and easy tool that can be used to monitor the distribution of fat across the body. The patient is scored on specific parts of the body and is given an overall numerical score. The assessment can then be periodically repeated and the new score compared with the old one (see Chapter 5 for further information).

Table 14.6 The most common stereotypies seen in equids [45].

Stereotypies	Description	Comments
Box walking/fence walking	Obsessive walking of the stable or fence line in a field	May accentuate lameness and become more manic during times of stress. Can be caused by frustration or the desire to escape
Crib biting/windsucking	Holding and/or sucking on an object	May be related to feeding practices for example, reduced forage
Weaving	Frequent and on occasions rapid movement from side to side in the doorway or within the stable itself	May be caused by frustration and /or a desire to escape. Can accentuate lameness or existing problems in the forelimbs
Head nodding	Frequent and on occasions rapid movement of the head up and down	May be related to frustration. No particular medical consequence although true head shaking should be investigated and treatment options considered
Wood chewing	Chewing of wooden furniture within stable, stable doors or fencing/trees surrounding fields	May be caused by inadequate quantity of forage in the diet. Can cause damage to the incisors and or mucous membranes. Expensive for owners to replace damaged areas

Source: Phillippa Pritchard.

Water Intake and Appetite

- It is important to gain information from the owner as to how much the horse eats and drinks and what foods constitute their diet.
- The owner will be able to give information regarding appetite, which may be important. For example, that horse may always eat all concentrates feed but may not always eat all forage given; therefore, if the patient stops finishing the concentrated feed, then this may be a sign of pain or stress.
- It is often useful to ask the owner to bring concentrate feeds and forage from home if the horse has an unpredictable appetite.
- It is important that the patient maintains a healthy intake of food and water while they are at the practice. Intake should be monitored carefully.

Behaviour and Body Language

- The behaviour and body language shown by a patient in the practice should be compared with what the owner reported as normal for the horse at home.
- Research has been carried out into behaviours that are common among horses that are showing signs of pain. This research lead to the development of the horse grimace scale (HGS) [44]. See the section on pain scoring for further information.
- Other changes in behaviour may be seen in response to pain, including aggression, compulsive behaviours and agitation.
- It has been noted that 20–30% of domesticated horses practice some form of stereotypic behaviour; this is classed as repetitive unvarying behaviours that have no apparent function.
- These behaviours can include box-walking, crib-biting/windsucking and weaving. Most stereotypic behaviours are noted in horses that are confined with a lack of forage within their diet causing the horse to seek out a coping mechanism.
- The most common stereotypies seen in equine patients are displayed in Table 14.6.

Clinical Parameters

- Clinical parameters should be assessed as discussed in Chapter 17. Each horse will have different resting parameters, so it is important to know what is normal for each individual.
- Pain can cause an elevation in clinical parameters such as heart rate and respiratory rate. However, these parameters on their own are non-specific for the presence and severity of pain since they may be influenced by other factors. Therefore, they should be taken into account along with other observations.

Levels of Consciousness

- Consciousness levels are not as deliberately assessed in equine patients as much as in other species. Despite this, it is important to assess the mental state of the horse regularly.
- Mentation is a description of the patient's mental activity and can be described as follows:
- Normal: Bright, alert and responsive (BAR).

- Obtunded: Reduced response to the environment, which can be:
- Mild – may be mistaken for lethargy. This may only be noticed by the owner with a mild decrease in auditory stimulus.
- Moderate – still responsive to voices such as their name and noises, but stronger stimuli may be required, and the animal's response may not be considered normal by the owner.
- Severe – Usually causes the patient to be non-ambulatory but still responsive to loud noises and hand clapping.
- Comatose – Unconscious, patient is unable to be aroused despite stimulus.

Pain Scoring for Equine Patients

Pain scoring systems are used to assess patients as individuals and ensure that pain management is as effective as possible. Using a pain scoring system ensures a reflective approach, and this helps to improve standards, identify problem areas and optimise patient care [46]. There are several different types of pain scoring systems.

Simple Descriptive Scale
In a simple descriptive scale (SDS), after pain assessment, the observer rates the pain as follows [46]:

- No pain
- Mild pain
- Moderate pain
- Severe pain

Descriptors can be used to assist the observer in categorising the pain observed. This system is rudimentary but is simple to use in veterinary practice.

Simple Numerical Rating Scale
Another system is the numerical rating scale (NRS), with behavioural descriptors attached to each number. The observer assesses the degree of pain being experienced by a patient and then assigns a number appropriate to the degree of pain. This can also be used to grade lameness, according to a 0–5 or 0–10-point scale. This system is simple to use and has proven to be accurate when used across multiple observers.

Visual Analogue Scale
The visual analogue scale (VAS) is a scoring system in which a mark is placed on a 10 cm line, the extreme left representing no pain, the extreme right the worst pain imaginable. An advantage of this system is that the result can be quantified numerically by measuring the distance of the mark along the line from the 0 mm end. However, VAS has been found to be less reliable when more than one assessor is used. It is therefore more commonly used for research studies carried out by a single assessor rather than in clinical practice [46].

The simple scales can be effective but are highly dependent on observer training for their consistent application, and often underestimate severe pain.

Multidimensional or Composite Pain Scales
Specific pain scoring systems have used the inclusion of multiple pain-associated parameters. These take the form of multidimensional or composite pain scales (CPS) and include the measurements of selected 'items' that may include interactive, behavioural and physiologic parameters. CPSs are multi-factorial scales where the measured 'items' are scored according to a simple descriptive scale, and these scores are then combined to generate a CPS score. Published studies describing various CPS systems in the horse have demonstrated excellent inter-observer reliability [47]. There are a number of CPS published for horses, donkeys and more recently, foals. However, they can be time-consuming to carry out and require trained personnel to perform them.

Facial Expression of Pain
Recently, the value of recognising facial expressions as an indicator of pain has been acknowledged. The work started in the field of rodent pain and has now expanded to horses, donkeys and foals. The HGS was developed by Dalla Costa et al. after the observation of horses following castration. The study identified six facial action units (FAUs) as follows [44]:

- Orbital tightening
- Ears held stiffly backwards
- Tension above the eye area
- Prominent strained chewing muscles
- Mouth strained and pronounced chin
- Strained nostrils and flattening of the profile

When assessing each FAU, a score from 0 to 2 is assigned to each: 0 for not present, 1 for moderately present and 2 for obviously present. The pain score is then added up to an overall score out of 12. Grimace scales are considered to give several advantages over other routinely used methods of assessing pain in animals [44]:

- Grimace scales are less time-consuming to carry out.
- Observers can easily and rapidly be trained to use them.
- Grimace scales may utilise the human tendency to focus on the face when scoring pain.

- Grimace scales can be used to effectively assess a range of painful conditions, from mild to severe pain.
- The safety of the observer can be increased when assessing pain in horses, as grimace scales do not require the observer to approach the subject and palpate the painful area for the assessment.

Work carried out on facial expressions of pain in horses led to descriptors for 'the equine pain face' [47] (Figure 14.10). Facial pain scales are also now available for donkeys and foals. It is important that these scales are applied where possible, as there are variations in the

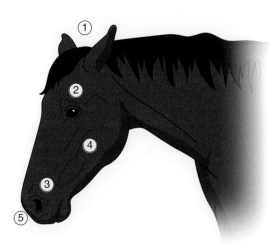

The Equine Pain Face	
Number	Signs to Look for in the Horse
1	Ears – The distance between the ears increases at the base. Both ears are lower and turn outwards; this may look asymmetric
2	Eyes – Contracted muscles around the eye give the upper eyelid an angular appearance. The sclera of the eye may be more prominent in the medial canthus. With intense pain, the stare may become intense and withdrawn.
3	Nostrils – The medial aspect of the nostrils dilates towards the medial plane. This leads to the nostrils looking more square in appearance.
4	Facial Muscles – These become tenser throughout the side of the face.
5	Muzzle – There is increased tension in the chin and lips, resulting in the muzzle edges becoming more shaped.

Figure 14.10 The equine pain face [47]. *Source:* Rosina Lillywhite.

way that horses, donkeys and foals display pain (see Chapter 16 and the further reading section for more information).

It is now common for CPS systems to have a facial assessment component either embedded in them or developed to be used alongside them. The combination of these two pain scoring systems allows the assessment of both physiological parameters and behavioural components, and the hope is that this produces a more reliable outcome for the observers and the patients.

The Role of the RVN in Pain Scoring

RVNs are in a unique position to carry out pain scoring effectively. RVNs tend to spend increased amounts of time with patients, whether that be making a clinical assessment, grooming or generally observing them in the practice environment. RVNs could be an important asset when it comes to objective pain scoring due to their close relationship with the patients. Furthermore, this also highlights the importance of talking to owners about the individual patients, what they like and dislike, to get an idea of personality and behaviour. Again, RVNs are in a good position to gain this information during the admit procedure. This also shows the owner that their horse will receive individualised care and treatment while at the practice, which would hopefully lead to an increased sense of comfort, and trust.

Using Pain Scoring in Practice

There are many different methods available in practice to pain score equine patients; however, implementing pain scoring can be difficult. The initial introduction of new ideas can be met with scepticism and resistance. One way to address this is to introduce the idea at a meeting and allow the whole team to have their say. Different pain scoring methods could be presented at the meeting, but it should be up to the veterinary team present to select an accurate method that will work moving forward in the individual practice in question. If every team member should be given the opportunity to put ideas forward, as then they will feel more invested in the process, which will ultimately increase overall concordance. This in turn will contribute positively to the welfare of the equine patients at the practice.

References

1 Smith, M. and Haylock, S. (2012). Basic first aid. In: *Equine Veterinary Nursing* (ed. K. Coumbe) 134, 137, 149–150. London: Wiley-Blackwell.

2 RCVS. (2017). 19. Treatment of animals by unqualified persons – professionals [Internet]. http://Rcvs.org.uk. Available from: www.rcvs.org.uk/setting-standards/advice-and-guidance/code-of-professional-conduct-for-veterinary-surgeons/supporting-guidance/treatment-of-animals-by-unqualified-persons.

3 24-Hour emergency first aid and pain relief [Internet]. Professionals. 2023 [cited 2023 Jan 9]. Available from: www.rcvs.org.uk/setting-standards/advice-and-guidance/code-of-professional-conduct-for-veterinary-surgeons/supporting-guidance/24-hour-emergency-first-aid-and-pain-relief/#:~:text=3.1%20The%20RCVS%20Code%20of%20Professional%20Conduct%20states,What%20does%20it%20mean%20to%20be%20%E2%80%98in%20practice%E2%80%99%3F.

4 Code of professional conduct for veterinary nurses [Internet]. Professionals. [cited 2023 Jan 9]. Available from: www.rcvs.org.uk/setting-standards/advice-and-guidance/code-of-professional-conduct-for-veterinary-nurses/.

5 Boag, A. and Nichols, K. (2011). Small animal first aid and emergencies. In: *The BSAVA Textbook of Veterinary Nursing*, 5e (ed. B. Cooper, E. Mullineaux, and L. Turner), 590–631. Gloucester England, Gloucester: British Small Animal Veterinary Association.

6 Basic first aid for your horse and preparing for emergencies [Internet]. extension.umn.edu. Available from: https://extension.umn.edu/horse-health/basic-horse-first-aid-and-preparing-emergencies.

7 Fielding, C. and Magdesian, K. (2011). Review of packed cell volume and total protein for use in equine practice. *AAEP Proceedings* [Internet] [cited 2023 Jan 14]; 57:318–321. Available from: https://aaep.org/sites/default/files/issues/proceedings-11proceedings-318.PDF.

8 Deidre, M.C. Fractures in horses [Internet]. Vcahospitals. [cited 2009]. Available from: https://vcahospitals.com/know-your-pet/fractures-in-horses.

9 Emergency management of equine fractures [Internet]. Veterinary Practice. [cited 2023 Feb 6]. Available from: https://www.veterinary-practice.com/article/emergency-management-of-equine-fractures.

10 Horse colic prevention and management [Internet]. Blue cross. [cited 2023 Feb 18]. Available from: www.bluecross.org.uk/advice/horse/health-and-injuries/horse-colic-prevention-and-management.

11 Burns and wounds [Internet]. [cited 2023 May 10]. Available from: https://www.hopkinsmedicine.org/health/conditions-and-diseases/burns.

12 Highlander plus sun shade fly combo rug | Shires equestrian [Internet]. http://shiresequestrian.com. [cited 2023 Feb 18]. Available from: https://shiresequestrian.com/highlander-plus-sun-shade-fly-combo-rug-9313.

13 Photosensitization in horses – horse owners [Internet]. MSD Veterinary Manual. [cited 2023 Feb 18]. Available from: https://www.msdvetmanual.com/horse-owners/skin-disorders-of-horses/photosensitization-in-horses.

14 Jenkins, G. How to manage thermal burn wounds. Improve Veterinary Practice [Internet]. 2018 Jul 28 [cited 2023 Jan 15]. Available from: https://www.veterinary-practice.com/article/how-to-manage-thermal-burn-wounds.

15 NHS Choices (2020). *Recovery – Burns and Scalds* [Internet]. NHS Available from: https://www.nhs.uk/conditions/burns-and-scalds/recovery/.

16 Wound care after burn injury | MSKTC [Internet]. http://msktc.org. Available from: https://msktc.org/burn/factsheets/wound-care-after-burn-injury.

17 Ragwort | The British Horse Society [Internet]. www.bhs.org.uk. Available from: www.bhs.org.uk/horse-care-and-welfare/health-care-management/pasture-management/ragwort/.

18 PubChem. Taxine [Internet]. http://pubchem.ncbi.nlm.nih.gov. [cited 2023 Feb 18]. Available from: https://pubchem.ncbi.nlm.nih.gov/compound/Taxine#section=Information-Sources

19 Poisonous plants | The British Horse Society [Internet]. www.bhs.org.uk. Available from: www.bhs.org.uk/horse-care-and-welfare/health-care-management/pasture-management/poisonous-plants/.

20 Atypical myopathy fact file – fact files – information and advice – RVC Equine – Royal Veterinary College, RVC [Internet]. www.rvc.ac.uk. [cited 2023 Feb 18]. Available from: www.rvc.ac.uk/equine-vet/information-and-advice/fact-files/atypical-myopathy#panel-key-points.

21 Acorn poisoning | The British Horse Society [Internet]. www.bhs.org.uk. Available from: www.bhs.org.uk/horse-care-and-welfare/health-care-management/horse-health/equine-diseases/acorn-poisoning/.

22 Identifying ragwort | The British Horse Society [Internet]. www.bhs.org.uk. [cited 2023 Feb 18]. Available from: www.bhs.org.uk/horse-care-and-welfare/health-care-management/ pasture-management/ragwort/identifying-ragwort/.

23 Herbicide poisoning in animals – toxicology [Internet]. Veterinary Manual. Available from: https://www.msdvetmanual.com/toxicology/herbicide-poisoning/herbicide-poisoning-in-animals.

24 Common horse, pony & donkey poisons | RSPCA [Internet]. www.rspca.org.uk. [cited 2023 Feb 18]. Available from: www.rspca.org.uk/adviceandwelfare/pets/horses/health/poisoning/common.

25 Bates, N. (2021). A brief overview of acute poisoning in sheep. *Livestock* 26 (6): 292–299.

26 Overview of rodenticide poisoning in animals – toxicology [Internet]. MSD Veterinary Manual. [cited 2023 Feb 18]. Available from: https://www.msdvetmanual.com/toxicology/rodenticide-poisoning/overview-of-rodenticide-poisoning-in-animals?query=rodenticide%20poisoning.

27 Schramme, C.A. and Labens, R. (2013). Orthopaedics 2: Diseases of the foot and distal limbs. In: *Equine Medicine, Surgery and Reproduction*, 2e (ed. T.S. Mair, S. Love, J. Schumacher, et al.), 333. London: Saunders Elsevier.

28 Eps, A.W. and Pollitt, C.C. (2009). Equine laminitis model: cryotherapy reduces the severity of lesions evaluated seven days after induction with oligofructose. *Equine Veterinary Journal* 41 (8): 741–746.

29 Webmaster, V. *Common Poisons. Veterinary Poisons Information Service [Internet]*. Veterinary Poisons Information Service Available from: https://www.vpisglobal.com/common-poisons/.

30 Boag, A. and Marshall, R. (2020). Small animal first aid and emergencies. In: *BSAVA Textbook of Veterinary Nursing*, 6e (ed. B. Cooper, E. Mullineaux, and L. Turner), 599–601. British Small Animal Veterinary Association: Gloucester.

31 Greet, T. (2008). Hospital design and organisation. In: *The Equine Hospital Manual* (eds. K. Corley and J. Stephen), 292–293. West Sussex: Wiley-Blackwell.

32 GOV.UK. (2023). Data protection. Available at: https://www.gov.uk/data-protection (accessed 1 April 2023).

33 Snalune, K. and Paton, A. (2012). General nursing. In: *Equine Veterinary Nursing*, 2e (ed. K. Coumbe), 173. Oxford: Wiley-Blackwell.

34 Stratton-Phelps, M. (2008). Nutritional management of the hospitalised horse. In: *The Equine Hospital Manual* (eds. K. Corley and J. Stephen), 292–293. West Sussex: Wiley-Blackwell.

35 Boys Smith, S. and Millar, B.M. (2012). General surgical nursing. In: *Equine Veterinary Nursing Manual* (ed. K. Coumbe), 388–392. Oxford: Blackwell Science Ltd.

36 Nout, Y.S. and Jeffcoyy, L.B. (2013). Neurology. In: *Equine Medicine, Surgery and Reproduction*, 2e (ed. T.S. Mair, S. Love, J. Schumacher, et al.), 230–231. London: Saunders Elsevier.

37 Hart, K.A. and Epstein, K.L. (2013). Common problems and techniques in equine critical care. In: *Equine Medicine, Surgery and Reproduction*, 2e (ed. T.S. Mair, S. Love, J. Schumacher, et al.) 561–562, 564–568. London: Saunders Elsevier.

38 Boag, A. and Hughes, D. (2018). Fluid therapy. In: *BSAVA Manual of Canine and Feline Emergency and Critical Care*, 3e (ed. L.G. King and A. Boag), 36. Gloucester: BSAVA.

39 Divers, T.J., Radcliffe, R.M., Cook, V.L. et al. (2022). Calculating and selecting fluid therapy and blood product replacements for horses with acute haemorrhage. *Journal of Veterinary Emergency and Critical Care (San Antonio)* 32 (S1): 97–107. Available at: 10.1111/vec.13127 (accessed 1 October 2023).

40 Rucker, D. and Dhamoon, A.S. (2022). Physiology, thromboxane A2 [Online]. Available at: https://www.ncbi.nlm.nih.gov/books/NBK539817/#article-30114.s2 (accessed 1 October 2023).

41 Dugdale, A.H.A., Beaumont, G., Bradbrook, C., and Gurney, M. (ed.) (2020). Chapter 3: Pain. In: *Veterinary Anaesthesia Principles to Practice*, 19–20. Oxford, Blackwell Publishing.

42 Muir, W.W. (2005). Anaesthesia and pain management in horses. *Equine Veterinary Education* 15 (S7): 20–25.

43 Lenz, T. (2019). Signs of a healthy horse | AAEP [internet]. http://Aaep.org. Available from: https://aaep.org/horsehealth/signs-healthy-horse.

44 Dalla Costa, E., Minero, M., Lebelt, D. et al. (2014). Development of the Horse Grimace Scale (HGS) as a pain assessment tool in horses undergoing routine castration. *PLoS One* 9 (3).

45 Nicol, C. (2010). Understanding equine stereotypies. *Equine Veterinary Journal* 31 (S28): 20–25.

46 Murrell, J.C. and Ford-Fennah, V. (2020). Anaesthesia and analgesia. In: *BSAVA Textbook of Veterinary Nursing*, 5e (ed. B. Cooper, E. Mullineaux, and L. Turner), 680. BSAVA: Gloucester.

47 Gleerup, K.B. and Lindegaard, C. (2015). Recognition and quantification of pain in horses: a tutorial review. *Equine Veterinary Education* 28 (1): 47–57.

Further Reading

Jamieson, C.A., Baillie, S.L., and Johnson, J.P. (2022). Blood transfusion in equids – a practical approach and review. *Animals (Basel)* 12 (17): 2162. https://doi.org/10.3390/ani12172162. PMID: 36077883; PMCID: PMC9454663.

Lanci, A., Benedetti, B., Freccero, F., Castagnetti, C., Mariella, J., van Loon, J.P.A.M., and Padalino, B. (2022). Development of a composite pain scale in foals: a pilot study [Online]. Available at: https://www.mdpi.com/2076-2615/12/4/439 (accessed 15 May 2023).

Ryan, J. and Johnson, J.P. (2022). Long-term nursing care of the equine patient in a sling. *Veterinary Nursing Journal* 34 (4): 34–39.

Takahashi, Y. et al. (2020). A comparison of five cooling methods in hot and humid environments in thoroughbred horses. *Journal of Veterinary Science* 91: 103–130. Available at: https://www.sciencedirect.com/science/article/abs/pii/S0737080620302215 (accessed 30 January 2023).

Van Dierendonck, C., Burden, F.A., Rickards, K., and van Loon, J.P.A.M. (2020). Monitoring acute pain in donkeys with the equine Utrecht University Scale for Donkeys Composite Pain Assessment (EQUUS-DONKEY-COMPASS) and the Equine Utrecht University Scale for Donkey Facial Assessment of Pain (EQUUS-DONEKEY-FAP) [Online]. Available at: https://www.researchgate.net/publication/339452639_Monitoring_Acute_Pain_in_Donkeys_with_the_Equine_Utrecht_University_Scale_for_Donkeys_Composite_Pain_Assessment_EQUUS-

DONKEY-COMPASS_and_the_Equine_Utrecht_ University_Scale_for_Donkey_Facial_Assessmen (accessed 15 May 2023).

http://VetFolio.com (2023). Treating Thoracic Injuries [Online]. Available at: https://www.vetfolio.com/learn/ article/treating-thoracic-injuries (accessed 29 Jan 2023).

Useful Links

Veterinary Poisons Information Service
  Website: https://www.vpisglobal.com
  Phone (vets): 0207 305 5055
  Phone (owners): 01202 509 000

15

Equine Reproduction, Parturition and Neonatal Nursing Care

Sarah Baillie

Equine Veterinary Medical Center, Doha, Qatar

15.1 Equine Reproduction and Breeding

Principles of Genetic Inheritance and Define Terms

Genetic inheritance is the passing of genetic information from parent to offspring. This is the way in which traits such as coat colour, height and behavioural characteristics are repeated from generation to generation.

Some definitions of important terms used when describing genetics include:

- **Gene:** A gene is a segment of deoxyribonucleic acid (DNA) and is the unit which transfers traits. This is the physical unit which is passed from parent to offspring. Each gene contains the data for a specific characteristic. Genes are arranged within chromosomes, and the point on a chromosome where the gene is located is known as the gene locus. Chromosomes are found in the nucleus of the cells of the body, and different species have different numbers of chromosomes. Horses have 32 pairs of chromosomes, which are numbered from 1 to 31, with the final pair identified as X and Y.
- **Allele:** Alleles are versions of the same genes, and a foal will inherit one allele from the mare and one from the stallion.
- **Homozygous:** When a foal inherits the same gene from both parents, it is known as homozygous. If a foal inherits the identical mutated gene for a certain genetic condition, then that foal is at high risk of developing that condition.
- **Heterozygous:** Conversely, when a foal inherits different versions of a gene from each parent, they are known as heterozygous.
- **Genotype:** An individual's genotype is the specific collection of genes they have or their genetic makeup.

- **Phenotype:** The way in which an individual's genotype is expressed physically is their phenotype.
- **Dominant:** When a foal receives two different versions of a gene from its parents, the gene which is expressed is known as the dominant gene. It is also possible for two alleles to be different, and both to be expressed and this is known as co-dominant.
- **Recessive:** In contrast to dominant genes, the allele which is not expressed is known as recessive. This means that the trait for which that gene is coded will not be present in that animal.
- **Mutation:** Changes or disruptions in a DNA sequence are known as mutations. Mutations usually occur due to a mistake in copying of DNA during the cell division process. Mutations can also be caused by exposure to radiation or certain chemicals or viruses. Mutations that occur within the egg or sperm can be passed on to the offspring, and these are known as germ-line mutations. Mutations which occur elsewhere in the body are not passed on, and these are known as somatic mutations.
- **Sex-linked gene:** When a gene that controls a characteristic is located on a sex chromosome (x or y chromosome), it is known as sex-linked. Sex-linked genes are more frequently present on an x chromosome as x chromosomes are much longer and therefore contain more genes. As females have two x chromosomes, they have the chance of a gene on the other x chromosome being dominant. This means that males more often express sex-linked traits than females, for example, haemophilia.
- **Lethal gene:** When a gene that is essential for growth and development is mutated in a way that results in the death of the animal, this is known as a lethal gene. Dominant lethal alleles need only be present in one copy to be fatal, whereas identical recessive lethal alleles from each parent must be passed to the offspring to be fatal.

Textbook of Equine Veterinary Nursing, First Edition. Edited by Rosina Lillywhite and Marie Rippingale.
© 2025 John Wiley & Sons Ltd. Published 2025 by John Wiley & Sons Ltd.
Companion website: www.wiley.com/go/equineveterinarynursing

To understand genetic inheritance, Mendel's first and second laws are used. Mendel's first law, the law of equal segregation, relates to the chances of specific alleles being passed to a parent's offspring. The copy of the allele for each gene from each parent is chosen at random, meaning that the chance of an allele being passed to the offspring is 0.5, because one is passed from each parent and each parent has two potential alleles to pass on.

Mendel's second law, the law of independent assortment, states that the segregation of each gene pair happens independently from other pairs. Genes dictating different characteristics are inherited independently of each other, and this means that whether a foal is chestnut is unrelated to how tall the foal will grow.

To identify how alleles move through generations, a monohybrid cross is used. A monohybrid cross is the study of the inheritance of a single characteristic. The monohybrid cross shows the alleles for one characteristic and the dominant relationship between those alleles. It is commonly demonstrated in a genetic diagram where the dominant allele is represented by a capital letter and the recessive allele by a lowercase letter. Figure 15.1 demonstrates a monohybrid cross for brown coat colour. B represents the dominant allele for a brown coat colour, and b demonstrates the recessive allele for a chestnut coat colour.

Equine Breeding Cycles

From 12 months of age colts can begin to produce spermatozoa and puberty occurs between 18 months and 2 years of age. However, full sexual maturity does not occur until 3–5 years of age in most stallions with some stallions remaining fertile into their 20s. Stallions produce new

	MARE b	MARE B
STALLION **b**	FOAL b/b (Chestnut)	FOAL b/B (Brown)
STALLION **B**	FOAL b/B (Brown)	FOAL B/B (Brown)

Figure 15.1 Monohybrid cross for brown coat colour. *Source:* Sarah Baillie.

spermatozoa daily, and it takes approximately 57 days for the sperm to fully mature [1].

Although it is possible for a stallion to breed all year-round, there are several seasonal changes in their reproductive physiology. Production of sperm is affected by daylight hours and reduces during winter months by up to 50%; however, exposure to artificial light has been shown to increase spermatozoa production [2]. Although the sperm output decreases in winter, the quality and motility are unaffected. During the breeding season, a stallion's testicles are larger and have a greater volume than outside of the breeding season. In some but not all stallions, libido is reduced during the non-breeding season.

Mares are fertile and can be bred from 4 years of age, reaching peak fertility around 6 years of age. Fertility declines from 15 years onwards, and most mares become completely infertile from 20 years of age. Mares are seasonally polyoestrous; they have an oestrous cycle, which consists of ovulation followed by an interovulatory phase, and this cycle is affected by day length. The phase during which the mare ovulates is called oestrus and during this phase the mare is receptive to the stallion. Oestrus typically lasts 3–6 days, but can last longer at the start of the breeding season, due to lower levels of luteinising hormone (LH). The period between the end of one oestrus cycle and the start of the next oestrus cycle is called dioestrus and is also sometimes known as the luteal phase; this phase lasts 15 days typically but varies based on the length of oestrus to maintain a 21-day cycle. During the short daylight hours of winter, the mare's ovaries do not function, and this period is called anoestrus. The transition from anoestrus into the breeding season is called the vernal transition, or alternatively, it may be referred to as a spring transition. Spring transition is triggered when daylight hours increase and subsequently exposure to light increases. This stimulates the hypothalamus to produce gonadotrophic-releasing hormone (GnRH), which in turn stimulates the pituitary gland to release follicle-stimulating hormone (FSH), triggering follicle growth in the ovary. The transition back to anoestrus is called the autumnal transition. The hormones involved in the oestrus cycle of the mare can be seen in Figure 15.2.

Ovulation marks the beginning of dioestrus, and the mare stops being receptive to the stallion. Following ovulation, a corpus haemorrhagicum and then a corpus luteum (CL) forms in the ovary, and this secretes progesterone. The high levels of progesterone decrease LH, and ovarian function is reduced so that the mare cannot reproduce during this time. During dioestrus, a group of follicles within the ovary start to develop and, towards the end of dioestrus, one follicle becomes larger than the rest. This is known as the dominant follicle and can usually be identified

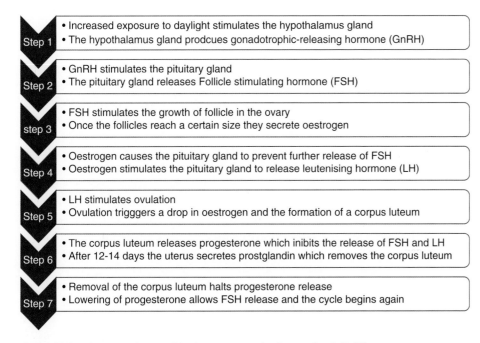

Step 1
- Increased exposure to daylight stimulates the hypothalamus gland
- The hypothalamus gland prodcues gonadotrophic-releasing hormone (GnRH)

Step 2
- GnRH stimulates the pituitary gland
- The pituitary gland releases Follicle stimulating hormone (FSH)

step 3
- FSH stimulates the growth of follicle in the ovary
- Once the follicles reach a certain size they secrete oestrogen

Step 4
- Oestrogen causes the pituitary gland to prevent further release of FSH
- Oestrogen stimulates the pituitary gland to release leutenising hormone (LH)

Step 5
- LH stimulates ovulation
- Ovulation trigggers a drop in oestrogen and the formation of a corpus luteum

Step 6
- The corpus luteum releases progesterone which inibits the release of FSH and LH
- After 12-14 days the uterus secretes prostglandin which removes the corpus luteum

Step 7
- Removal of the corpus luteum halts progesterone release
- Lowering of progesterone allows FSH release and the cycle begins again

Figure 15.2 Hormones involved in the oestrus cycle. *Source:* Sarah Baillie.

ultrasonographically approximately a week before ovulation. During dioestrus, the uterus is firm, without oedema and the cervix is tightly closed.

At the start of oestrus, the CL regresses, progesterone levels drop, the uterus becomes soft and oedematous, and the dominant follicle increases in size. Growth of the follicles produces oestrogen, which induces the behavioural characteristics of oestrus and makes the mare receptive to the stallion. These behavioural changes are the key indicators of oestrus, and identifying them can be assisted by the use of a teaser stallion. The mare is introduced to the teaser stallion, usually with a fence or wall between them, to see how the mare responds to his presence. If the mare shows signs of aggression to the stallion, like pinning her ears back or kicking, she is not in oestrus. Conversely, If the mare is receptive to him by lifting her tail and urinating, she is in oestrus. The follicles increase in size, and the largest follicle tends to be the one to ovulate. Immediately before ovulation, the dominant follicle enlarges to peak size and softens. Within the ovary is an ovulation fossa, and when ovulation occurs, the oocyte leaves the ovary via this fossa. The follicle rapidly decreases in size due to the expulsion of fluid, and the cycle begins again.

Anoestrus is the period of the year during which mares do not reproduce. In the United Kingdom and most of the northern hemisphere, this occurs over the winter months and is an evolutionary adaptation to ensure foals are not born in adverse, cold conditions. In countries with less distinct seasons or year-round warm weather, mares can reproduce at any time of year.

While the breeding cycle of horses remains fairly consistent, it can be intentionally manipulated to create potentially better breeding outcomes, and it can be unintentionally affected by other factors. As previously discussed, the breeding cycle of both mares and stallions is affected by exposure to daylight and consequently seasonal changes in day length. In some countries, including the United Kingdom, Thoroughbred racehorses and other disciplines compete in age groups with a universal birthday (for example, 1st January for UK Thoroughbreds). This means that it is beneficial for foals to be produced as early in the year as possible, so they are more developed than their later-born competitors. The relatively short period of long daylight hours within a year means there is a restricted window in which mares can be bred, and if a mare takes multiple attempts to conceive, this time limit may become a problem. For these reasons, systems have been developed to extend the breeding season by exposing horses to artificial light during shorter days, usually to bring forward the start of the breeding season. It appears that daylight is the seasonal factor that most affects the equine breeding cycle rather than ambient temperature. Although an increase in body temperature prior to ovulation has been identified in one study [3], increased ambient temperature does not appear to advance the onset of the breeding season [4]. It is still commonly believed that ambient temperature affects the breeding cycle and without further research, it seems reasonable to assume that both daylight and temperature play a role, as they have been shown to in other species [5].

The breeding cycle may also be affected by food availability and feeding patterns. Minor changes in body condition score do not appear to affect the breeding cycle [4]; however, the ability to access food frequently and trickle feed as horses naturally do in the wild is important. Mares that have constant access to roughage are significantly more reproductively efficient than mares that are fed the same amount of roughage but in restricted time blocks [6]. Access to quality feed in sufficient amounts is especially significant in older mares, past their peak breeding age.

It is possible to manipulate the breeding cycle of the mare with medication to increase the chances of successful breeding. Manipulation of a mare's cycle can assist in timing ovulation around the availability of the selected stallion, make breeding techniques such as embryo transfer possible, allow more frequent attempts at conception and control the behavioural aspects of oestrous.

Some commonly used hormonal preparations include:

- **Prostaglandin:** This is used to synchronise oestrus in line with stallion or semen availability. It is also used to shorten the interovulatory period (also known as 'short-cycling') to decrease time to repeat insemination or from foal heat.
- **Gonadotropin-releasing hormone:** This is used to speed up or induce ovulation.
- **Human chorionic gonadotropin:** This is also used to speed up or induce ovulation.
- **Altrenogest:** This is a synthetic progesterone that halts oestrus effectively keeping the mare in dioestrus until the medication is discontinued.

There are several methods available for breeding horses, including natural covering, artificial insemination and embryo transfer.

Natural covering involves introducing the stallion to the mare when she is in oestrus and receptive. This can be done with both horse's leads in hand or by turning them out in a paddock. Some mares can be initially aggressive towards the stallion before allowing him to mount her even during oestrus, and may require further restraint such as twitching or hobbling. It may be an appropriate precaution for the mare to wear covering boots; felt boots which cover the hoof and protect the stallion from injury should she kick him. Natural covering has the benefit of being the least time and resource-consuming breeding method; however, it restricts stallion selection to a smaller number available within travelling distance. For Thoroughbreds, where the offspring is intended to be raced, natural covering is the only method permitted by Weatherbys.

Artificial insemination (AI) involves introducing fresh, chilled or frozen semen into the uterine body as close to ovulation as possible. The mare's cycle is closely monitored by frequent ultrasound examinations, to ensure insemination occurs close to ovulation, to increase the chance of successful conception. Fresh semen must be used as soon as it is collected. This is only really used when the mare and stallion are at the same stud, but the mare cannot be covered due to her behaviour, risk of injury or presence of a young foal. The decision to use chilled or frozen semen largely depends on the choice of stallion and what is available. When using chilled semen, insemination must take place within 24–48 hours; this restricts selection to stallions within Europe for mares in the United Kingdom. Insemination with frozen semen has the advantage of increasing the number of stallions to choose from. The semen can be transported from anywhere in the world and stored indefinitely. Therefore, it can be ready and available at any time. Frozen semen needs to be inseminated within 12 hours of ovulation, so monitoring for ovulation is frequent. The data on pregnancy success rates is mixed, with some papers [7, 8] reporting lower success rates with frozen semen and some studies [9, 10] finding similar success rates between the two semen types. Factors such as experience with the type of semen for insemination, transportation conditions of the semen, stallion selection and mare reproductive health and anatomy may affect the success rates, and it is not as simple as one semen type is better than another.

Embryo transfer (ET) is the process of removing an embryo from the biological dam and placing it in the uterus of a recipient mare, to carry the pregnancy and birth the foal. This method can be utilised for mares that are not reproductively fit and able to carry a pregnancy to full term, and give birth or mares with other pre-existing conditions that preclude this, such as laminitis. The main use of embryo transfer is to produce foals from valuable competition mares while allowing the mare to continue competing. One further benefit is that it allows more than one foal to be bred from one donor mare in a season.

The advantages and disadvantages of natural covering, AI and ET are laid out in Table 15.1.

While it is possible to surgically transfer an embryo laparoscopically via a flank incision, a non-surgical technique is much more widely used. Successful transfer requires careful planning and chemical manipulation of the donor and recipient mares' cycles to ensure they are both in oestrus at the same time. Recipient mares are selected based on reproductive and general health, age, size and proven record of carrying foals to term, producing sufficient milk and demonstrating strong maternal instinct. It is beneficial to have several recipient mares available to ensure the synchronisation of cycles. Stallion selection is also important,

Table 15.1 The advantages and disadvantages of natural covering, AI and ET.

	Advantages	Disadvantages
Natural covering	Lowest cost	Limited stallion selection
	No restrictions on breed registration	Risk of injury to the mare and stallion
		Risk of injury to handlers
Artificial insemination	Greater stallion selection including stallions who had semen stored before death	More expensive than natural covering
	Allows assessment of semen quality	Specialist equipment and training required
	Decreased risk of spread of venereal disease	Storing semen by any method may reduce its viability
		Requires frequent transrectal ultrasonography so the mare needs to be amenable to that (or frequently sedated)
Embryo transfer	Allows mares to stay in competition/work	Expensive and time consuming
	Possible to produce more than one foal a year from a mare	Requires specialist equipment and further training
	Allows mares which are unable to carry a pregnancy to term to reproduce	

Source: Sarah Baillie.

and semen should be from a stallion with a proven record of high fertility and retaining semen quality when it is chilled or frozen. Most donor mares are artificially inseminated rather than naturally covered and fresh or chilled semen is preferable over frozen in this instance.

Once the donor mare has been successfully inseminated, approximately 1 week from ovulation the embryo is flushed from the donor mare's uterus via a filter that catches the embryo (Figure 15.3). The embryo is then transferred to a dish, where it is evaluated and washed. The embryo is then transferred into an empty, sterile semen straw and inserted into the uterus of the recipient mare using an insemination gun. In the recipient's uterus, the embryo is able to develop, as normal, to full term and be delivered and raised by the recipient mare. Recipient mare selection is very important, and using a mare which is significantly different in size can adversely affect foal development; however, once this is accounted for, foals born by ET will grow and progress in the same way a foal born to its biological dam would [11].

With all breeding methods, there are several signs and methods of pregnancy diagnosis in the horse. Behaviourally, the mare should not show further signs of oestrus and not become receptive to the stallion again; however, some mares do. The embryo will travel to the uterus around 6 days after fertilisation and will move between horns, which helps in maternal recognition of pregnancy. Around day 16, the embryo will settle in one place, and this is when pregnancy diagnosis starts to be possible. The most commonly used and accurate method of pregnancy diagnosis in the early stages is a transrectal ultrasound examination of the reproductive tract, and this allows confirmation of

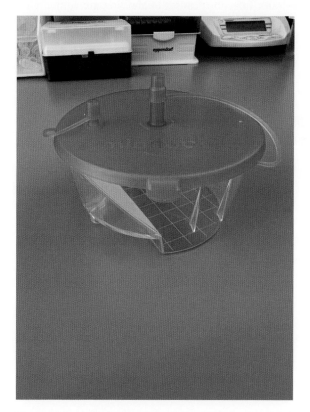

Figure 15.3 An embryo collection filter. *Source:* Sarah Baillie.

pregnancy from 16 days or sometimes even as early as 10 days. Transrectal ultrasound examination is also beneficial for early detection and reduction of twin pregnancies and assessment of foetal viability. Pregnancy may also be diagnosed by transrectal palpation of the reproductive tract and visual inspection of the vagina and cervix. Pregnancy diagnosis via blood test is possible, and the type of test depends on the stage of pregnancy. Equine chorionic gonadotropin (eCG), which is produced by the placenta from 45 to 90 days gestation can be detected in maternal blood. After 90 days of gestation, oestrone sulphate is produced by the foetus itself, and this can be tested from a maternal blood sample.

Despite the effort and cost invested in getting a mare pregnant, sometimes the pregnancy does not reach full term and terminates before the foetus is able to survive outside the uterus. Causes of abortion in horses can be split broadly into infectious and non-infectious. Bacterial infection is the most common cause of abortion in the mare and occurs when the placenta comes into contact with bacteria. Usually, this is an ascending infection. A fungal infection via the same route is also possible, but it is much less common. Another infectious cause of abortion is equine herpes virus 1 (EHV-1), which is a virus most commonly transmitted via direct or very close contact with an infected horse. Other rarer infectious causes of abortion are equine viral arteritis (EVA) and equine infectious anaemia (EIA).

The most common non-infectious cause of abortion is twinning, and abortion usually occurs in late gestation due to placental insufficiency to support two pregnancies. It is very rare for twins to be delivered at full term, and even rarer for them to survive, with the chances of both twins being born alive at 1:10,000. Another non-infectious cause is umbilical cord strangulation, which causes a disruption or complete cessation of the supply of blood, oxygen and nutrients to the foal. Uterine torsion is another cause of late-term abortion. The exact cause of uterine torsion is unknown, but it can sometimes be corrected by rolling the mare with pressure on her abdomen. Most commonly, surgical correction is required and this can be achieved via flank incision understanding sedation or midline laparotomy under general anaesthesia. Uterine torsion, which is not corrected, can restrict blood and oxygen flow to the foetus, resulting in abortion.

Essentials of Ante and Post-partum Care

Gestation length in horses is variable but usually lasts between 335 and 342 days and a foal born before 320 days of gestation is considered premature. The equine foetus develops almost completely over the first 107 days as follows:

- *Day 15*: The primitive beginnings of the optical and nervous system form. Limbs begin to form. Cartilaginous tissue is present.
- *Day 19*: The spinal cord begins to form.

- *Day 25*: The tail starts to develop.
- *Day 25*: Hooves begin to form.
- *Day 28*: The heart is divided into two chambers.
- *Day 34*: The lungs and trachea start to take shape. The limbs are fully formed.
- *Day 35*: Vascularisation of the dermis begins. The forebrain, hindbrain and midbrain are distinguishable.
- *Day 36*: The diaphragm is identifiable.
- *Day 38*: The oesophagus and tongue develop. The heart is fully formed.
- *Day 40*: The nasal cavity, sinuses, nasopharynx, trachea and other structures of the upper respiratory tract develop.
- *Day 48*: Bones begin to ossify.
- *Day 80*: Mammary glands begin to form.
- *Day 97*: Hair is present on the skin.
- *Day 107*: Limbs have prominent joints and hooves.

After this initial rapid development, the foetus is an almost fully formed miniature version of a foal and the rest of gestation is focussed on growth.

Around 16 days from conception the embryo fixes in place in the uterus and develops an extraembryonic membrane surrounding it and this is the chorioallantois. By day 20, the allantois begins to develop over the chorioallantois and quickly grows to encase the embryo and chorioallantois. The allantois then becomes the primary provider of blood supply. From day 40, these membranes begin to attach to the endometrium and the placenta continues to develop to full maturity over the next 100–110 days.

Progesterone is a steroid which is essential in the maintenance of pregnancy, and progesterone levels increase in the first half of gestation before dropping around mid-gestation. Progesterone drops again immediately prior to parturition, and this induces uterine contractions. The other significant steroid hormone in pregnancy is oestradiol, which rises in the second half of gestation and increases the contractility of the uterus ready for parturition. The CL formed at ovulation is responsible for maintaining pregnancy initially; however, this is taken over by the endometrial cups from day 40. The endometrial cups are a collection of cells formed on the placenta, and they produce large amounts of eCG, which in turn, stimulates the ovaries of the mare to form additional CLs, releasing more progesterone to further support the pregnancy in the first trimester.

It is advised that pregnant mares are kept on the fat side of good condition, with a body condition score of 6–7/10; however, obesity can have a negative impact on the foal, as well as pose a health risk to the mare. Over the first eight months of pregnancy, the mare's nutritional requirements are the same as that of a non-pregnant mare, and energy requirements gradually increase over the final three months as the foal grows to full-term size. Mares in late gestation require an increased amount of dietary protein and adequate provision of calcium and phosphorus for foetal development. Lactating mares have higher energy requirements than during pregnancy as they produce milk at 2–3% of their body weight. Dietary protein requirements are also higher during lactation than pregnancy, but calcium and phosphorus requirements are the same as during late gestation.

It is recommended that the pregnant mare should be moved to the foaling location no later than 4 weeks before her due date. This is important not only to ensure the mare is relaxed and settled into her environment before foaling, but also to expose her to the pathogens endemic to that location, so that antibodies are formed and ready to be passed on to the foal. The mare should also be checked for the presence of a Caslick's. A Caslick's procedure involves suturing closed the vulval lips to prevent contamination of the reproductive tract. Once the sutures are removed or have dissolved, the vulva remains sealed and this should be cut well in advance of foaling to prevent injury. During the final 4 weeks of pregnancy, the mare should be checked daily for signs of impending foaling.

These signs include:

- Increased udder size
- Relaxing of the pelvic ligaments and vulva
- Vulval discharge
- Secretions or 'waxing' of the teats

If the mare produces and drips or streams milk before the foal is born, it is important to make provisions for supplementary feeding of colostrum as soon as the foal is born. Prematurely streaming of milk means the limited amount of colostrum produced at the beginning of milk production is likely to run out before the foal is born.

Normal parturition involves three distinct stages. Stage one can last between 30 minutes and 4 hours and is the preparatory stage for the expulsion of the foal. During stage one, the mare will become restless, and this can be mistaken for colic. The mare will repeatedly lay down and stand back up, sweat up, lift and swish her tail and flank watch. During this stage, the mare should be prepared by wrapping her tail and washing her vulva and udder. The handler should be prepared that the mare may be unpredictable during this time and take care when preparing the mare not to become trapped or injured as she lays down or stands up.

Stage two begins with the rupture of the chorioallantois and the expulsion of a large volume of allantoic fluid. This stage is fast-moving and should take no more than 30 minutes. The mare will usually stay lying down throughout most of stage two and will push as her uterus contracts to expel the foal. Immediately after the rupture of the chorioallantois, one of the foal's front feet will appear followed by the other and this slight difference in position of the two forelimbs allows the shoulders to pass through the mare's pelvis more easily. The forefeet are closely followed by the nose. The front legs, head and neck are delivered first, then the torso and hindlimbs. It is advisable to stay close by to observe but not intervene unless necessary. The mare will usually rest for a while, often with the foal's hind feet still in the vagina. The umbilical cord should be left to break naturally as the mare stands. Cutting the cord should be avoided as this may result in haemorrhage.

Stage three of parturition involves the expulsion of the foetal membranes, and this should occur between 30 minutes and 3 hours after foaling. The placenta should be tied up above the hocks to prevent the mare stepping on it. Failure of this process is known as retained foetal membranes and can be due to uterine inertia and hormonal dysregulation. Retained foetal membranes are a potential source of uterine infection and, if left untreated, can lead to septicaemia, metritis, endotoxaemia, laminitis and death. Treatment may include uterine lavage and oxytocin administration to induce uterine contractions. When caring for patients with retained foetal membranes it is important to monitor closely for signs of infection or septicaemia such as increased temperature and dark red mucous membranes. Digital pulses should also be checked regularly and comfort levels assessed, in order to identify the signs of laminitis.

The two most common complications during foaling are premature placental separation (also known as 'red bag' delivery) and dystocia. Premature placental separation is observed as a failure of the chorioallantois to rupture and the appearance of the red velvety chorioallantois rather than the bluish-white membranes of the amnion. This is a life-threatening emergency for the foal as oxygen delivery has been compromised. The chorioallantois must be cut immediately, using blunt-ended scissors, to allow safe delivery of the foal.

Dystocia is difficulty foaling and can be due to incorrect positioning of the foal, malformation of the foal, oversize of the foal or delivery of twins. Dystocia is a time-sensitive and life-threatening emergency for both the mare and the foal. Once the cause of dystocia has been established, the most appropriate intervention can be selected. In some cases of foetal malpositioning, it may be possible to manipulate the foal into the correct position with the mare standing. Alternatively, the mare may be anaesthetised to allow controlled vaginal delivery. The mare is positioned in dorsal recumbency with the hind end elevated by hoisting the hindlimbs upwards (also known as the Trendelenburg position). The foal can then be pushed back into the birth canal and manipulated into the correct position. Ropes or chains can be attached to the foal's limbs and head to pull the foal out. If the foal cannot be delivered vaginally, then caesarean section is indicated. This requires general anaesthesia and a midline laparotomy to incise the uterus and remove the foal via the abdomen. Caesarean section requires a large, experienced team and a well-equipped operating theatre. Alternatively, if the foal is dead or not viable, then fetotomy may be performed. This involves using embryotomy wire on handles to dissect and remove the dead foetus in sections.

Once the placenta is passed, it should be checked thoroughly to ensure it is intact and healthy. The placenta should be handled with gloves and immediately disposed of after inspection, as anatomical clinical waste. If any part of the placenta is retained in the mare, endometritis can develop. This is an inflammation of the uterus, which can become septic, and lead to the development of septicaemia and laminitis if left untreated. The mare should be monitored closely postpartum for complications. Regular physical examination can help identify early signs of issues. The udder should be checked for milk. One sign of inadequate milk production, and need for medication such as domperidone, is a foal that constantly butts at the udder, repeatedly attempts to nurse and does not lie down to rest after nursing. A serious potential complication postpartum is uterine artery rupture, which can cause fatal haemorrhage. Signs of uterine artery rupture include pale mucous membranes and abdominal pain. The condition is diagnosed based on rectal palpation of the uterus and abdominal ultrasound examination. Uterine tear or rupture is also a possible postpartum complication and presents as general colic signs. If left untreated; this can lead to peritonitis. Uterine prolapse is a rare complication post-foaling and is easily identified by the appearance of the uterus protruding from the vulva. Mares are at increased risk of many gastrointestinal lesions post-foaling, and close monitoring for signs of colic is advisable.

15.2 Normal Foal Physiology and Development

Key Differences Between the Major Body Systems of Neonates, Foals and Adult Horses

There are many key differences between neonates, foals and adults, and it is important not to think of foals as identical, smaller versions of adult horses. A comparison of

Table 15.2 A comparison of clinical parameters for neonates, foals, weanlings and adults.

	Neonate	Foal	Weanling	Adult
Heart rate (beats per minute)	60–120	60–80	40–60	32–40
Respiratory rate (breaths per minute)	30–60	20–40	8–20	8–16
Temperature (°C)	37.7–38.8	37.5–38.7	37.5–38.6	37.5–38.6

Source: Sarah Baillie.

clinical parameters for neonates, foals, weanlings, and adult horses can be found in Table 15.2.

Differences can be identified within the body systems as follows.

Cardiovascular System

In a foetus, oxygenated blood enters the circulation from the placenta via the umbilical vein and through the ductus venosus, which bypasses the liver. The blood then travels via the caudal vena cava into the right atrium of the heart and through the foramen ovale to the left atrium. Some blood also passes through the right ventricle to the pulmonary artery via the ductus arteriosus. This allows the blood to bypass the not-yet-functional lungs. Over the first few weeks of life, the neonate transitions to the normal circulation mechanism of an adult, blood flow through the foramen ovale gradually reduces and the ductus arteriosus closes. It is common to hear cardiac murmurs in neonates during the first week of life, and these are caused by the sound of blood flowing through the foramen ovale and ductus arteriosus before they close. Transient dysrhythmias in the first 30 minutes of life are common and unconcerning unless they persist. The heart rate reduces in the foal as it grows and ages but, in some horses, does not reduce to that of a mature adult heart rate until two years or older.

The neonate's immature sympathetic nervous system means they have lower vasomotor tone, decreased peripheral vascular resistance and lower stroke volume than older foals and adults. This combination of poorly developed mechanisms means the neonate is highly susceptible to hypotension and poor perfusion. Foals have a higher blood-brain barrier permeability, which decreases as they age meaning that lower dosages of some medications may indicated in neonates to prevent overdose or unwanted side effects.

Respiratory System

The foetal lungs are collapsed and fluid filled. During the birth process, the majority of the fluid is expelled from the lungs, and the foal takes its first breath, which fills the lungs with air. The remainder of the fluid forms respiratory surfactant. Initially, the neonate's respiratory rate is high, up to 80 bpm for the first hour, as it adapts to extra-uterine life, but it decreases by around half over the first few days of life. As the foal ages and grows in size, the respiratory rate continues to decrease much like the heart rate. Unlike older foals and adults, neonates do not respond to hypoxia by increasing their respiratory rate, and this can further compound hypoxia. Respiratory function is further challenged in the neonate by a more compliant chest wall compared to older foals and adults. Neonates have a higher demand for oxygen than older foals and adults, requiring 12 ml/kg/hour compared to 5–8 ml/kg/hour for an adult.

Renal System

The urine production of a neonate is 148 ml/kg/day [12] compared to 15 ml/kg/day for an adult horse [13] and is very dilute due to their primarily fluid diet. The neonatal renal system adapts from excretion via the placenta in utero, to producing and excreting urine in the first few hours of life. It matures to the full renal function seen in older foals and adults over the first few weeks of life. Colt foals tend to pass the first urine sooner than fillies, but both should have passed urine by 12 hours after birth. The urachus is a tubular structure which removes waste from the foetal bladder via the umbilical cord in utero, and after birth, the urachus closes as urine is excreted via the urethra. Patent urachus is the failure of the urachus to close, and some urine continues to be excreted from the urachus. This is common in neonates who have received fluid therapy, particularly those who have received aggressive fluid resuscitation and is almost always self-limiting.

Reproductive System

The female reproductive system is developed completely by birth, and a filly foal has all of the reproductive organs of an adult mare. The only difference is that until the female horse transitions through puberty, the hormonal controls of the reproductive system are not functional. In the colt foal, the reproductive organs are present at birth; however, the testes are located in the foetal abdomen and begin to move into the scrotum within the final month of gestation. Over the first two weeks of life, the testes should fully descend into the scrotum, and the path from the abdomen closes.

Gastrointestinal (GI) System

During the first 24 hours of life, intestinal permeability allows the foal to absorb immunoglobulins from ingested colostrum and after the first day the gut wall closes off this permeability. The neonate's tendency for poor perfusion means mucosal blood supply is also poor, and this increases the risk of gastric ulceration despite the neonate's higher gastric pH than older foals and adults. Gastric pH decreases over the first 30 days of life and remains consistent from then onwards. The GI tract at birth is sterile and as the neonate ingests milk and explores its environment, microorganisms are introduced into the GI system establishing a GI microflora. Healthy foals should have a natural instinct to eat the mare's faeces, and this helps them to ingest bacteria which colonise in the gut much like the transfaunation procedure utilised in the treatment of diarrhoea (see Chapter 13 for further information). Following the passing of the meconium, the faeces of a neonate are very soft and unformed as their entire intake is milk. When the foal is a few weeks old, it may begin to eat some hay and pick at the mare's feed. This change in diet can cause transient diarrhoea, which is known as 'foal heat' diarrhoea, as it coincides with the onset of the mare's first oestrus post foaling. As the foal ages and eats more roughage, the faeces become similar to that of an adult horse.

Other Differences

Neonates and foals have a higher normal body temperature range than adults. Around 6 months of age the foals' body temperature decreases to the same range as an adult horse. Foals' soft, fine hair coat, fragile skin and low levels of body fat mean they are more prone to decubitus ulcers (pressure sores) than adults. Foals under 6 weeks old are much more vulnerable to hypothermia than older foals and adults. This is due to a combination of low body weight to surface area ratio, low levels of subcutaneous fat, poorly matured 'thermostat' in the medulla, poorly developed shivering mechanisms and limited metabolic reserves. Corneal sensitivity is lower in foals and neonates than that of adult horses. This means foals may not always demonstrate signs of pain, such as ptosis and protective closing of the eyelids, when a corneal ulcer is present. Foals have higher proportional body water than adults, and as such, require higher doses of water-soluble drugs. Foals also have lower body fat levels than adults, which means fat-soluble drugs are redistributed less causing higher plasma concentrations, which increases sensitivity to both the intended effect and side effects of the medication.

Development of Immunity in Equine Neonates

Foals are born almost entirely agammaglobulinaemic meaning insignificant amounts of immunoglobulins are present in neonatal serum before ingesting colostrum. Passive immunity is essential for the newborn foal, as it has virtually no active immunity at this stage. Transfer of passive immunity from the mare occurs via ingestion of colostrum. The mare produces colostrum for the first 12–24 hours after parturition before milk production takes over. This coincides with the foal's ability to absorb immunoglobulins and other sources of passive immunity via the temporary permeability of the gut. Colostrum contains immunoglobulins immunoglobulin G (IgG) and, in smaller quantities, immunoglobulin A (IgA) and immunoglobulin E (IgE). There are seven types of IgG, all of which have slightly differing functions for immunity. Peak immunoglobulin concentrations are reached at 8–12 weeks of age for most immunoglobulins; however, some IgG types do not reach adult levels until after one year of age [14]. Colostrum also contains inflammatory cytokines, which have a poorly understood but significantly positive effect on the development of immunity in equine neonates.

While exposure to environmental antigens is important in the development of immunity in the equine neonate, consideration must be made for foals born in a hospital environment or admitted within the first few weeks of birth. The neonate's immature immune system leaves it extremely vulnerable to nosocomial infections when housed in a practice where multiple, potentially antibiotic-resistant pathogens are present. Close attention to cleanliness and hygiene is essential, and it is not unjustified to establish a protocol for reverse barrier nursing of all neonatal inpatients. As a minimum, gloves must be worn at all times when handling neonates; equipment must be sterilised between patients (especially feeding equipment such as bottles and teats), and disinfectant foot dips/mats should be used when entering and leaving the stable.

Vaccination of the mare during late gestation is recommended for its benefits of increasing immunity in the foal. Tetanus vaccination 4 weeks before parturition allows placental transfer of immunity to tetanus, to protect the vulnerable neonate after birth. Tetanus antitoxin may also be administered to the foal immediately after birth to increase protection. Tetanus antitoxin is used short-term as a treatment or for a very short period of protection, whereas tetanus vaccination is used to prevent tetanus infection in the long term. Influenza vaccination of the mare at the same time as tetanus vaccination is recommended. Vaccination against EHV is required three times during pregnancy; this initially protects the mare from the virus and subsequently prevents abortion. Another EHV vaccination at nine months of pregnancy allows placental transfer of immunity to the foetus. Some veterinary surgeons recommend vaccination against rotavirus in populations with larger numbers of foals, where exposure to rotavirus is higher.

Common Conditions Affecting the Neonatal Foal

Neonatal Maladjustment Syndrome (NMS)

NMS, also known as Hypoxic Ischaemic Encephalopathy (HIE) or dummy foal syndrome, is one of the most common reasons for hospitalisation of the equine neonate in the first few days of life [15]. The exact pathogenesis of the disease is still not fully understood; however, increasing research is being carried out, and more information is becoming available. The primary pathway of NMS appears to be a compromise to the oxygen supply to the foetus or neonate either through premature placental separation, or a prolonged or abnormal parturition. This causes cerebral hypoxia and consequent ischemia. Recent research has identified the role of a neurosteroid in NMS and has found that increased plasma progestogen concentrations in affected foals have a role in suppressing the central nervous system. This suppression is what creates the depression and dull demeanour associated with NMS [16]. Development of the Madigan foal squeeze technique is based on this premise, and the foal is squeezed with a rope around the thorax for 20 minutes to mimic the process of passing through the birth canal, which starts the neurological process that lead to the reduction in neurosteroid levels (Figure 15.4). A similar syndrome exists in human neonates, which has been more thoroughly researched and disappointingly, the only intervention which has been found to have a consistent positive effect on outcome is therapeutic hypothermia [17]. As seen in foals, intensive nursing care, prevention of infection, symptomatic treatment and time are the key factors in supporting a human baby with NMS.

Madigan foal squeeze step-by-step

- Make a fixed loop at the end of a long rope
- Place the rope around the foal, between the front legs and over the withers ending with the fixed loop on the withers
- Pass the rope around the foal's thorax and half hitch it behind the fixed loop
- Repeat this a second time further back on the thorax
- Pull all of the loops snug and take the remaining rope behind the foal
- Pull on the end of the rope until the foal lies down
- Maintain the same pressure for 20 minutes then remove the rope

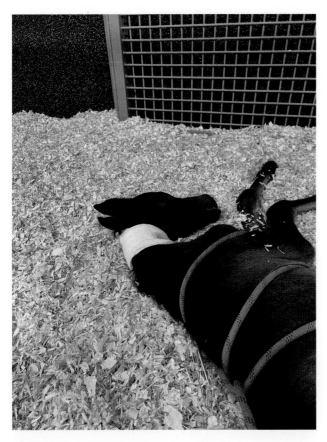

Figure 15.4 Positioning the rope on a foal for the Madigan foal squeeze. *Source:* Sarah Baillie.

Prematurity

Foals born before 320 days of gestation are categorised as premature and can display multiple physical traits of immaturity. If no concurrent conditions exist, then foals may well finish maturing ex-utero and develop normally, although they are usually smaller in size than mature foals of the same age. Foals born at full term, which display these same traits of immaturity are known as dysmature and the same principles apply. In both premature and dysmature foals an important diagnostic test to be carried out is a radiographical examination of the carpi and tarsi. Incomplete ossification of the cuboidal bones is common in these foals, and the degree of incomplete ossification correlates with potential for athletic performance. However, rest and restriction of load bearing through the limbs can help, prognosis for function as an adult is guarded [18].

Meconium Retention

Meconium retention is a common condition of the equine neonate, occurring more frequently in colts than fillies, where the first faeces of the foal, containing waste material from foetal life, are retained in the GI tract. Usually, it is relatively easy to treat, and the first (and often second) attempt at resolving meconium retention is administration of a phosphate enema. Some breeders and veterinary professionals choose to administer a phosphate enema after birth routinely as a preventative measure. Soapy water enemas are also utilised by some practitioners and can be very effective. Failure of phosphate or soapy water enema to resolve meconium impaction requires administration of a retention enema. This procedure consists of passing a foley catheter rectally and administering an acetylcysteine solution, which is left in place for 20–30 minutes with the foal in lateral recumbency and the hind end raised (Figure 15.5). This usually requires sedation of the foal although the author has found it useful to perform retention enema during a foal squeeze procedure, if both are required, as foals tend to become very relaxed during the squeeze. In some cases, meconium impaction cannot be resolved medically and surgery to remove the impaction via midline laparotomy is required.

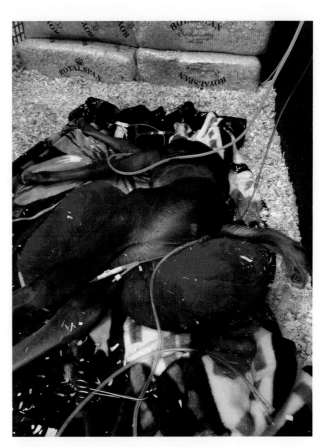

Figure 15.5 A foal receiving an acetyl cysteine retention enema. *Source:* Sarah Baillie.

Septicaemia

Septicaemia, commonly referred to as sepsis, is one of the most common causes of disease in neonatal foals, and if left untreated it will inevitably be fatal. Bacteria, or less commonly viral pathogens, enter the bloodstream and spread throughout the body to the organs and joints. The most common entrance points for pathogens are the umbilicus, GI tract, intravenous catheter sites or wounds. Septicaemic foals may become depressed, hyperthermic, tachycardic, tachypnoeic and progress to recumbency. Septicaemia often results in synovial infections affecting multiple joints (also known as joint ill), and without systemic antimicrobial treatment, aggressive lavage and local antimicrobial administration to the affected joints, a performance and life-limiting lameness is a distinct possibility. Blood culture and culture of synovial fluid of affected joints (if any) are important for pathogen identification. Antimicrobial sensitivity testing should be utilised to ensure correct antimicrobial selection.

In foals, unlike adults, primary septic arthritis is usually due to haematogenous spread from bacteria that have entered the bloodstream. Treatment is the same as described previously for joint illness. Neonates with septic arthritis will typically be very lame, and often require assistance to stand. It is useful to check the mare's udder frequently to assess whether the foal has been getting up to nurse.

Bacterial infection may also cause diarrhoea, which can be debilitating in the neonate. Diarrhoea can cause significant electrolyte and metabolic derangements, which require close monitoring and aggressive treatment with fluid therapy. Neonates with severe diarrhoea may benefit from constant rate infusion of fluids with the addition of tailored electrolyte additives based on serial blood testing.

Pneumonia

Bacterial and viral pneumonia is common in foals, and some frequently observed pathogens include EHV, influenza and Rhodococcus. Endoscopic examination of the upper airways and collection of a tracheal wash sample can be beneficial in identifying the specific pathogen; treatment can then be tailored accordingly. Foals with pneumonia, especially those with Rhodococcus pneumonia, are prone to periods of hyperthermia and may require active cooling measures. Cooling can be achieved by utilising some or all of the following:

- Provision of fans
- Cool water or alcohol baths
- Administration of cooled intravenous fluids.

Nebulised administration of antimicrobials (in combination with systemic administration) or mucolytic agents can be very beneficial for foals with pneumonia.

Atresia Ani

Atresia ani is an uncommon birth defect affecting neonates, which is the absence of a fully formed rectum and anal opening. Foals are unable to pass faeces and develop colic. Surgical correction is the only treatment option and prognosis is guarded especially in cases where there is no anal opening and a large defect.

Umbilical Hernia

An umbilical herniation is a relatively common and manageable congenital condition in foals, and scrotal or inguinal hernias may also be present at birth in colt foals, although they more commonly develop later. It may be possible in neonates to manually reduce a small hernia by frequently digitally manipulating its contents back into the abdomen, and many umbilical hernias resolve spontaneously in time. Some small umbilical hernias may be treated by manipulating all of the intestine from the hernial sac back into the abdomen and applying a tight band (lamb castration ring) to the empty sac to allow the body to close the body wall defect. Larger or persistent hernias may require surgical correction. Occasionally, the intestine contained in a hernia may become constricted with a compromised blood supply. This is a surgical emergency requiring immediate midline laparotomy and possible resection of the compromised gut.

Entropion

Entropion is a fairly common congenital condition seen in neonates where the eyelid (usually the lower lid) turns inwards with the lashes in direct contact with the cornea. Untreated entropion can lead to corneal ulceration. It is common to see entropion exacerbated by dehydration and often simply correcting hydration leads to spontaneous correction of the entropion. In some cases, frequently rolling the eyelid out can resolve entropion; however, it may be necessary to suture the eyelid in the correct position.

Congenital Jaw Malocclusions

Congenital jaw malocclusions, overbite (parrot mouth) or underbite (monkey or sow mouth) can occur in foals and cause issues once they mature enough to start foraging and grazing. Application of tension wire and bite plates can be used to correct these conditions, and treatment is more successful if it is initiated at a younger age.

Wry Nose

A wry nose is a congenital deformity of the nasal bones and septum, which presents as asymmetry of the nose and in some cases can prevent the foal from nursing. Mild cases may not require correction, and it is possible that the foal can grow into a normal adult with the only requirement for additional care being increased necessity of dental check-ups. In severe cases when airflow is compromised, or the foal is unable to obtain adequate nutrition, surgical correction is indicated.

Angular Limb Deformities (ALDs)

ALDs are a relatively common finding in foals and can be corrected with exercise restriction, shoeing or surgical intervention. ALDs are categorised as either valgus, where the limb deviates outwards below the affected joint, or varus with the limb deviating inwards below the joint. ALDs are most commonly seen in the carpus and tarsus, but the fetlocks may also be affected. Congenital flexural limb deformities are also seen in neonates and are either hyperextension of a joint (laxity) or hyperflexion of a joint (contracture). As with ALDs, controlled exercise and shoeing may correct these deformities. Splints may be beneficial in some cases, and oxytetracycline administration may be cautiously used in the treatment of hyperflexion. Surgical treatment is indicated in some cases.

Cleft Palate

The cleft palate is a congenital developmental defect of the soft and sometimes the hard palate, which prevents covering of the trachea when the foal swallows. Usually, the first sign of cleft palate is a visualisation of milk coming from the nostrils and/or a gurgling noise during nursing. Although this condition is relatively rare, if unaddressed it can lead to aspiration pneumonia. Therefore, it is prudent to check all neonates admitted to the hospital by digitally palpating the soft palate orally. Confirmation of cleft palate can be made endoscopically, and surgical correction is an option for these foals.

Congenital Cardiac Abnormalities

Several congenital cardiac abnormalities may be seen in the equine neonate, and these include:

- Ventricular septal defect is an opening in the septum between the ventricles and is the most common congenital heart defect in horses.
- Atrial septal defect is an opening in the septum between the atrium and ventricle.
- Patent ductus arteriosus is the failure of the closing of the foetal vessel, which allows blood circulation to bypass the lungs.
- Truncus arteriosus is the failure of the separation of the foetal vessel into the aorta and pulmonary artery.
- Tricuspid atresia is a partially or fully closed-off tricuspid valve.

Microphthalmia

Microphthalmia is a congenital condition affecting the eye. The eye is small in size with a prominent third eyelid. In mild cases, the eye is only slightly reduced in size, and it is visual; however, in severe cases, the eye is tiny and non-visual. The condition may be unilateral or bilateral, and there is no treatment possible.

Ruptured Bladder

Ruptured bladder in the neonate usually occurs during parturition but can occur after birth as a consequence of trauma or urinary tract obstruction and is most commonly seen in colt foals. A ruptured bladder leads to uroperitoneum and causes abdominal distension, colic and dribbling of urine from the penis or vulva. Surgical repair of the bladder and lavage of the abdomen is the only viable treatment. Uroperitoneum should be treated as a medical emergency, and the foal should be stabilised before surgery is carried out.

Failure of Passive Transfer (FPT)

FPT is a common condition of the equine neonate and occurs when the foal fails to ingest an adequate amount of good-quality colostrum within the first 12 hours of life. Reasons for this may include:

- Physical inability to latch on and nurse
- Lack of drive to nurse
- Inadequate colostrum production by the mare
- Mare 'running milk' before parturition
- Rejection of the foal by the mare.

If any of these issues are noted within the first 12 hours of life, colostrum can be administered via nasogastric tube (NGT) to prevent failure of passive transfer. FPT is diagnosed by testing the level of IgG present in the foal's blood. Specific, quantitative laboratory tests are available; however, the commonly used snap test kits are accessible, simple to use and reliable (Figure 15.6). IgG can only accurately be tested after 12 hours at which point the GI tract of the foal may no longer be permeable and oral administration of colostrum is ineffective. Therefore, the most effective treatment for FPT is the administration of IgG-rich plasma. Several brands of commercially produced plasma products are available and following administration, IgG should be rechecked within 24 hours to confirm whether adequate levels have been reached in case further plasma transfusion is required. Table 15.3 displays IgG readings in relation to the requirement for a plasma transfusion.

Neonatal Isoerythrolysis (NI)

NI is a haemolytic disorder in which the foal inherits a red blood cell (RBC) antigen from the stallion, which the mare

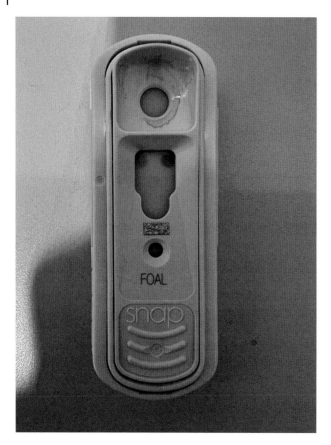

Figure 15.6 A snap test showing failure of passive transfer. *Source:* Sarah Baillie.

Table 15.3 IgG readings and levels of passive transfer.

Level of passive transfer	IgG (g/L)	Plasma transfusion
Failure of passive transfer	<4	Required
Partial failure of passive transfer	4–8	Advised
Successful passive transfer	>8	Not required

Source: Sarah Baillie.

does not have, but has developed antibodies against due to previous exposure either during previous foaling or via blood transfusion. When the foal ingests the antibody-rich colostrum, it inherits the antibodies the mare has produced against the RBC antigen it possesses, and so, the antibodies begin to destroy the RBCs of the foal. Foals appear normal when born; however, following ingestion of colostrum, they become weak and lethargic, stop nursing and present with jaundice and anaemia. In foals with severe clinical signs and/or a packed cell volume below 15%, blood transfusion is indicated. Transfusion may be of donor blood from a cross-matched donor or with washed RBCs from the mare. RBCs are washed using saline in a specifically designed system to remove the mare's defensive antibodies.

Fell Pony Syndrome

This is also known as foal immunodeficiency syndrome, is a fatal genetic disorder caused by a chromosomal mutation specific to the Fell breed. Ongoing research is being carried out to better understand the syndrome; however, there is currently no available treatment, and the condition is usually fatal within 3 days of birth.

Normal Adaptive Behaviour and Reflexes of a Neonatal Foal

The neonatal foal is born with several innate behaviours and reflexes, while others develop later in the foal's life. The first of these reflexes is evident within 2 or 3 minutes of birth when the foal moves into sternal recumbency, and this is known as the righting reflex. This is followed closely by another innate reflex, which is the suckle reflex, an important adaptive behaviour that ensures the foal nurses as soon as possible and ingests adequate colostrum and nutrition. The suckle reflex is usually present well before the foal attempts to stand or gets close to the udder. The foal's next instinct is to attempt to stand, and this may take many attempts over the first 30 minutes of life, but the foal should be standing unassisted by 1 hour from birth. As soon as the foal is able to stand, it should instinctively begin to search for the udder, latch on, and nurse within 2 hours of birth. The foal will instinctively push at the udder to induce milk let-down and quickly learn to do this when it is hungry.

A fully developed pupillary light reflex and partially developed palpebral reflex are present at birth in foals. However, the menace response is a learned behaviour over the first 2 weeks of life, and this should be remembered when assessing vision in neonates. Another reflex that foals are born with is the kick reflex, although they do not always display this instinct fully until they are a few days old. Digital pressure running along the spine from the pelvis to withers should invoke forward movement and bucking or kicking behaviour. Similarly, if the mare nips at the foal's tail base when it is nursing, it is a normal response for the foal to kick. Imprinting occurs shortly after parturition and is the process through which a mare and foal form an attachment. The mare and foal quickly learn to identify each other using scent, and this helps them stay together. The foal is unable to visually identify the mare during the first few weeks of life.

Normal findings and progression of a newborn foal include:

- First urination within 12 hours of birth, with colt foals usually urinating around 6 hours from birth and fillies taking around 11 hours.
- The first faeces (meconium) is usually seen within the first 3 hours following birth
- The meconium should be fully passed within 12 hours of birth, and failure to pass meconium within 24 hours combined with frequent straining is indicative of meconium impaction.
- Immediately after birth, the heart rate may be as low as 40 bpm, increasing to 120 bpm before decreasing to 80–100 over the first week of life.
- Transient cardiac arrhythmias are often identified in the minutes after birth but should resolve over the first 2 hours of life.
- Cardiac murmurs are a common and unconcerning finding during the foal's first week of life.
- The respiratory rate of a neonate ranges from 30 to 60 bpm, reducing to 20–40 bpm after the neonatal period.
- Crackles and other loud lung sounds are a normal finding on chest auscultation immediately after birth as the foal expels and absorbs fluid from the lungs.
- The healthy, ambulating neonate should have clear lung auscultation. However, it is normal to hear transient crackles in the dependent lung of a recumbent foal or a foal which has recently stood up.

In the assessment of neonates, an APGAR scoring system may be utilised (Table 15.4). APGAR is an acronym made up of the first letter of each parameter assessed, and those are appearance (of mucous membranes), pulse, grimace (response to tactile stimulation), activity (muscle tone) and respiration. Each parameter is assigned a score, and the combined total is used to quantify the effects of perinatal asphyxia. A normal, healthy neonate should have an APGAR score of 10.

15.3 Foal Nutrition and Feeding

Lactation in the Mare

It is important to remember that once the mare has successfully carried to term and birthed a live foal, she still has an essential role in keeping that foal alive by providing nutrition in the form of milk. Lactation is a process that demands a lot of energy. The amount of milk produced by a lactating mare is up to 3% of her body weight, and the mare's calorific requirement is 1.5–1.7 times that of a barren mare. Consideration must be made for the provision of an adequate amount of dietary protein to allow the mare to produce high-quality milk. Mare's milk is high in protein and in order to replace this lost protein, she requires an intake of almost double that of a barren mare. Lactating mares also have an increased demand for calcium and phosphorus, which are passed from milk to the foal to ensure its optimal development.

The alveoli of the udder are lined with lactation cells called lactocytes, which initiate and control the synthesisation and secretion of milk. Nutritional components of milk are supplied from the mare's blood via the mammary vessels and cross into the alveoli. The equine mammary gland is composed of two mammae, each with a corresponding teat. The mammae are separated by a septum, and each mammae consists of two lobes. Lactation is controlled by three hormones: prolactin, oestrogens and progestogens. Prolactin is the primary hormone in milk production and let-down as well as being responsible for ductal

Table 15.4 APGAR scoring system for newborn foals.

	Score 2	Score 1	Score 0
Appearance: mucous membranes	Pink	Pale pink	Grey or blue
Pulse: Heart rate and rhythm	>60 bpm, regular	<60 bpm, irregular	Absent
Grimace: Nasal stimulation	Sneeze	Grimace	No response
Ear stimulation	Head shake	Ear flick	No response
Activity: Muscle tone	Able to maintain sternal recumbency	Able to flex limbs	Limp
Respiratory function	Regular	Irregular	Absent

Score 0–2: Implement resuscitation protocol.
Score 3–5: Utilise vigorous tactile stimulation, ensure airway patent, provide supplemental oxygen.
Score 6–7: Utilise vigorous tactile stimulation and ensure airway patent.
Score 8–10: No intervention, monitor.
Source: Sarah Baillie.

development in the mammary gland. Oestrogens and pro-gestogens are also responsible for milk production and let-down; however, neither hormone has any effect without the presence of prolactin. Progestogens only have an effect in the presence of both prolactin and oestrogens.

The main constituents of mare's milk are:

- Fats, although mare's milk contains considerably less fat than cow's milk or human's milk.
- Proteins, mainly whey and casein.
- Lactose is the sugar component of mare's milk.
- Vitamins and minerals.
- Water forms the bulk (almost 90%) of milk and is the neonate's sole source of hydration.

Colostrum contains the same constituents as milk but just in different quantities. Colostrum has a much lower water content and higher protein content. The protein content of colostrum is significantly different as rather than consisting of whey and casein; the proteins are the immunoglobulins required for immunity. Protein content of colostrum is 13% compared to 3% in milk.

Agalactia is the name for failure to produce milk or colostrum when it is required, for example, immediately after giving birth, whereas inadequate milk production is known as dysgalactia. The underlying cause should be established and addressed, and some common causes include:

- Inadequate nutrition
- Systemic disease of the mare
- Lack of bonding with the foal
- Mastitis.

Once the cause has been addressed, both conditions may be treated by provision of extra food and administration of lactogenic medication such as domperidone.

Mastitis is inflammation and infection of the mammary gland. This is uncommon in the mare prior to weaning as the constant suckling of the foal keeps milk flowing and prevents ascending infection. Mares with mastitis may present with:

- A hot swollen udder, often with dry and cracked skin which is very painful to touch.
- Fever
- Dullness
- Inappetence
- Apparent hindlimb lameness or reluctance to walk due to pain when moving the hindlimbs.

Lactation tetany (also known as hypocalcaemic tetany or eclampsia) is a condition caused by increased calcium loss in milk, which is not adequately replaced in the diet. Signs of lactation tetany include:

- Anxiety and excitability
- Muscle rigidity and tremors
- Prolapse of the third eyelid
- Inability to chew and hypersalivation
- Synchronous diaphragmatic flutter (also known as thumps) is a rhythmic spasming of the diaphragm in time with the heartbeat caused by electrolyte imbalance
- Cardiac arrhythmias.

Untreated, the condition can progress to recumbency, seizures and death. See Chapter 14 for further details.

Milking technique for the mare is quite different to milking a cow. The teat should be gently grasped at the proximal join with the udder, between the thumb and first two fingers of one hand, and a squeezing action combined with gently pushing up into the udder will release the milk. It is important to be patient and gentle. Milk let-down is often not spontaneous, and it is helpful to manipulate the udder briefly first to mimic the way a foal would induce milk let-down. Hygiene is important and hands should be washed, and gloves worn when handling the udder. The udder should also be wiped clean before milking. A negative experience of milking for the mare can be very detrimental as she may begin to associate the experience with discomfort and become aggressive or stressed when her udder is touched. To milk mares with very small or inverted teats a milking pump may be useful, and if a pump is not available, one can be created by cutting the end from a 50ml syringe and reinserting the plunger in the cut-off end (Figure 15.7). Pumps, whether commercial or homemade, should be used with caution to prevent injury to the udder.

Foal Weaning

Weaning is the process of physically separating a mare and foal and consequent cessation of the provision of nutrition via nursing. It is common practice for foals to be weaned at around 6 months of age; however, it is possible to wean foals earlier than this. The process can safely take place once the foal consumes an adequate intake of roughage and feed. In the wild, foals have been noted to naturally wean at 9–10 months of age, [19] and this fits with the timing of GI tract changes, which means foals are no longer able to utilise lactose from milk in the same way younger foals can. If the foal is small for its age or somehow developmentally stunted it may be beneficial to delay weaning whereas, if the mare is in poor condition or systemically diseased, early weaning may benefit her by reducing her energy demands from lactation. If weaning is required before the foal is able to acquire adequate nutrition from non-milk sources, then the provision of donor milk or milk replacer may be required. To prepare the foal for weaning,

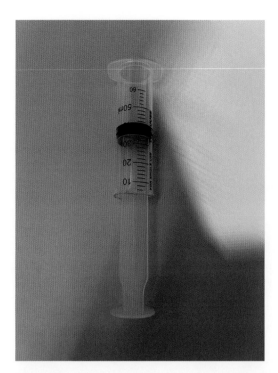

Figure 15.7 A homemade syringe milking 'pump'. *Source:* Sarah Baillie.

it may be useful to increase the amount of food they eat by introducing creep feed. This can be initiated from as young as one month of age and allows accurate assessment of when the foal is eating adequate amounts to be safely weaned. Weaning may be carried out abruptly by simply removing the mare or foal to another area where they cannot see or hear each other; however, this approach causes significant stress to both the mare and the foal. Gradual weaning involves removing the mare or foal for increasing lengths of time until permanently separating them. Although still stressful, it seems to cause less distress to the mare and foal. Traditionally, in the stud environment, foals are weaned at the same time and housed together for company, which appears to alleviate some of the stress of weaning. Moving the foal to live with another, unrelated adult horse has also been found to alleviate weaning stress [20]. It is important to monitor the foal throughout the weaning transition and beyond to ensure physiological and behavioural development is progressing correctly.

One area that is particularly important to monitor is growth, and this can be achieved via several methods. Visual assessment and photographic records can give a useful indication of how the foal is progressing. In some facilities, it may be possible to weigh the foal regularly, on an electronic weighbridge, which gives a very accurate representation of growth over time. Perhaps the most practical method of monitoring growth could be a combination of visual assessment, body condition scoring and measurement with a weigh tape. As foals grow, are exposed to novel environments, and gradually shift from an entirely milk-based diet to eating roughage and grazing, their intestinal flora develops, and this helps to prevent GI upset during the changes over weaning. The foal's method of digestion changes in time with its diet and by 2 months of age the foal has begun to develop function in the caecum and large colon, which eventually will lead to hindgut fermentation as a way of breaking down food for energy. This process is complete by 6 months of age and so often coincides with weaning age.

Conditions Affecting Suckling Foals

Severe Combined Immunodeficiency Disease (SCID)
This is a genetic, congenital condition affecting Arabian foals and Arabian crosses. Although the condition is congenital, affected foals do not show symptoms until around 2 months of age. Affected foals do not develop active immunity and so, once passive immunity is no longer functional the foal has no defence against disease-causing pathogens. Most foals with SCID succumb to respiratory infection and die of pneumonia. The condition is fatal, and no treatment is available; however, genetic testing is available for potential breeding pairs.

Equine Gastric Ulceration Syndrome (EGUS)
Gastric ulceration is common in foals after the neonatal period with a prevalence of more than 22% increasing to 98% 2 weeks after weaning perhaps due to the combination of stress, dietary change and management differences [21]. Conversely, to adult horses, foals have a higher incidence of glandular and duodenal ulceration than squamous ulcers. Reducing stress as much as possible, especially during weaning and dietary changes can help with prevention of EGUS, as well as making management changes very gradually. Treatment with omeprazole is indicated in older foals, and the addition of sucralfate may be beneficial in cases of glandular ulceration.

Parasitism – Strongyloides Westeri
This is an infection in the mare can lead to migration of the parasites through the milk to the foal, and although this rarely causes disease in foals, it has been reported that threadworm infection can lead to diarrhoea and weight loss. Parascaris equorum infection is a threat to grazing foals as the commonly found and increasingly resistant parasite is ingested by the foal, and infestation can cause serious intestinal impaction as well as migrating larvae causing respiratory disease. The immunologically naïve foal is

vulnerable to all parasites commonly affecting adult horses. Parasite control in foals is described in Section 15.4.

Tyzzer's Disease

This is a clostridial, bacterial infection most commonly seen in foals around one month of age. Lactating mares fed on a high protein diet ingest the bacteria and excrete it in their faeces, which the foal then ingests. The disease causes necrotic liver lesions and is rapidly fatal in young foals. Older foals with more developed immune systems and increased exposure may also be affected with less severe symptoms. Successful treatment is difficult, but aggressive supportive care, including fluid therapy is required and antimicrobial administration is also indicated. Reducing stress for foals and reducing the amount of protein in mares diets may help in prevention.

Orphan Foals

In this context, the term orphan refers to any foal without access to the mare which carried it. Foals may be orphaned due to any of the following:

- Loss of the mare either in the parturition process
- Loss of the mare due to complications post-partum
- Loss of the mare through elective terminal caesarean section
- Rejection by the mare
- Inability of the mare to produce milk

The first and arguably most important consideration for an orphan foal is meeting nutritional requirements followed by consideration of socialisation and normal behavioural development. The ideal solution for an orphan foal is to be fostered onto another lactating mare and allowed to develop as it would have with its mother. Grafting foals onto foster mares is a laborious but rewarding process. Correct mare selection is critical and is dictated primarily by her character and maternal instinct. The foster mare must be good natured, with a very strong maternal instinct and consistent milk production. Various methods of grafting a foal onto a foster mare have been described and it is something of an art, so personal preference for technique can be developed. Some techniques the author has found useful are rubbing the mare's faeces on the foal so when the mare sniffs it; she smells a familiar scent, generous positive reinforcement with food and treats for the mare and skipping a feed of the foal to ensure it is hungry and driven to latch on and nurse. If the orphan foal has never nursed before, it is useful to teach the foal to drink from a bottle so that the bottle can be used to guide the foal to the mare's udder (Figure 15.8). Historically, it was believed that dead foal of the foster mare should be skinned,

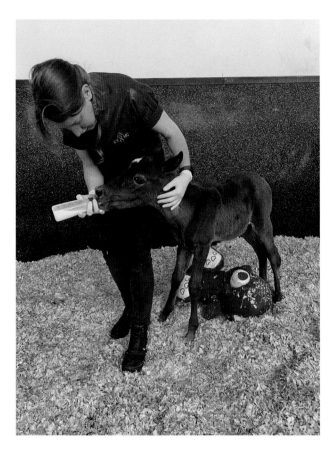

Figure 15.8 A foal learning to drink from a bottle before being fostered. *Source:* Sarah Baillie.

and the skin placed on the foster foal to give it the dead foal's scent. Thankfully, this practice is now becoming less and less popular.

If fostering is not an option, then the foal will need to be hand reared. Hand rearing is an around-the-clock job, and clients must be made aware of the task they are taking on in raising an orphan foal. During the neonatal period, the foal must be fed every 2 hours with the frequency of feeding reducing very gradually as the foal ages. The ideal feed for an orphan foal is milk from a donor mare; however, this is rarely possible. Instead, milk replacers are commonly used, and several commercial brands are available, which are ideal because they contain the necessary macro and micronutrients required by the foal. Care should be taken to only add the required amount of water for reconstitution, as adding excess water can cause diarrhoea, as can provision of overly concentrated milk replacer. In the absence of milk replacer, goat's milk may be used as it is similar in fat and glucose content to mare's milk. Cow's milk may also be used. However, cow's milk is much higher in fat and lower in glucose than mare's milk, so semi-skimmed milk should be used with the addition of 20 g/L of dextrose.

The temptation to bottle-feed an orphan foal should be avoided. Bottle feeding is more labour intensive than bucket feeding, increases risk of aspiration of milk and consequent pneumonia, and increases the association of humans with milk for the foal, which has negative behavioural consequences. The foal should first be taught to drink from a bowl, and this is usually a very simple process especially if the foal has never nursed before (Figure 15.9). If the foal has nursed previously and is having difficulty adapting to the bowl, it can be helpful to guide them to the milk with a bottle teat and place it in the milk so the foal 'finds' the milk. Warming the milk replacer can also help encourage foals to drink from the bowl. As soon as the foal is used to drinking from a bowl, it should be moved to bucket feeding to reduce human interaction. A bucket is hung at chest height and at feeding time the milk is poured into the bucket and the foal is left to find and drink the milk by itself. Milk pellets can be offered in addition to milk replacer, and these can be mixed with water to create a 'soup' to introduce them to the foal. After this, the water content of the soup is gradually reduced until the foal is eating the pellets dry. Hay can be offered to the foal from a few weeks of age and turnout in a paddock allows the foal to learn to graze. During the transition from milk only to a milk and a roughage diet, the foal's faeces will noticeably change from the soft, pale brown milk faeces to something similar in consistency to an adult horse's faeces. Changes in faecal consistency may also be seen if switching from one brand of milk replacer to another or exchanging milk for milk replacer. If these changes need to be made, it is a good idea to switch gradually by mixing the two products, starting by adding a small amount of the new product to the old, and gradually adjusting the ratio until the mix only

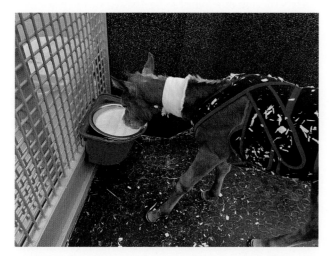

Figure 15.9 An orphan foal drinking milk from a bucket. *Source:* Sarah Baillie.

contains a small amount of the old product. This allows the foal's GI tract time to adapt and prevents the onset of diarrhoea. The orphan foal should be weighed and measured regularly to ensure it is growing at the correct rate. Young foals should gain approximately 1 kg bodyweight per day.

The importance of reducing the association between humans and milk and keeping human interaction to a minimum cannot be stressed enough. Serious behavioural issues develop commonly in hand-reared foals due to the lack of appropriate socialisation as a foal. An ideal solution to this problem is to house the foal with a calm and tolerant barren mare, or a good-natured pony or donkey, who will teach the foal how to interact with other equids. Socialisation with other foals can also be very helpful. In the absence of other equids for socialisation, housing the foal with other species can be beneficial, and goats or sheep can make good companions for orphan foals.

As with any foal, good hygiene is important and the orphan should be kept in a clean and safe environment. Attention should be paid to washing of feeding utensils between use and, particularly when the foal is a neonate, utensils should be thoroughly cleaned and soaked in bottle sterilising fluid. Foals are small, agile and inquisitive and as such, likely to escape their housing if given the opportunity. The accommodation should be checked carefully for any protrusions that may cause injury.

15.4 Routine Veterinary Care of Normal Foals

Requirements for Handling and Foot Care

Early and appropriate handling of foals is essential in ensuring normal behavioural development and a safe and handleable horse as it ages. Handling the foal should begin from the first days of life although care should be taken not to disrupt bonding between the mare and the foal. Mares can react unpredictably to people handling their foal. Therefore, an extra handler for the mare should be present while others focus on the foal. Handlers should always wear appropriate personal protective equipment (PPE) such as a hard hat, gloves and steel toe-capped boots. The foal should be handled frequently, and become used to being caught, gently restrained and examined. Care should be taken in catching a young foal to ensure it causes as little stress as possible. It may be useful to have two handlers to catch a particularly exuberant, healthy foal. If the mare is amenable, she can be useful in this process. The mare can be positioned with her hind quarters against a wall, close to a corner, and the foal corralled into the space between the mare and wall to be caught. Foals are naturally inquisitive, and this can be useful when it comes to catching them. If the handler squats down in the stall and remains still, a bold, inquisitive foal will come to investigate, and may be more easily caught this way. Knowing the foal's personality is very useful when it comes to catching and restraint. Some foals require a 'less is more' approach and become distressed and boisterous when restrained with more force. For examination of the joints and umbilicus or monitoring vital signs, an arm around the chest and one around the rump, or a gentle hold on the tail base will be sufficient. For collecting blood samples or administering intravenous injections, the foal should be restrained by looping one arm under the chin and grasping the opposite ear and with the other hand, firmly grasping the tail base (Figure 15.10).

Some procedures such as intravenous catheter placement may require the foal to be restrained in lateral recumbency. Young foals are generally very amenable to being laid down. Smaller foals may simply be lifted and laid in position, whereas larger foals may be 'folded' by placing a hand across the bridge of the nose, grasping the tail base and pushing the head away from the handler towards the foal's torso. Once laid down, pressure on the shoulder should keep the foal there, but it may also be necessary to hold the foal's legs in place to prevent kicking of the handlers.

Once the foal is comfortable with being caught and restrained, routinely palpating the limbs, lifting the feet and cleaning the feet out is advisable. The earlier the foal becomes accustomed to this handling, the easier the transition to footcare will be. At around 2 months of age, the foal should have its first trim by a farrier. It's likely that

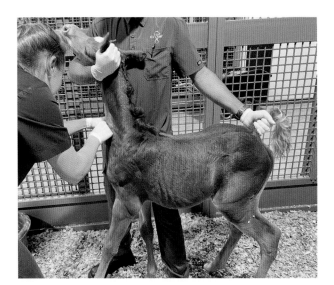

Figure 15.10 A foal being restrained for blood sample collection. *Source:* Sarah Baillie.

the hoof will not need much work; however, starting and maintaining regular visits from the farrier from this point will help the foal to get used to routine foot care. It is important to make this process as positive an experience as possible for the foal to prevent behavioural issues later on. A patient farrier who is experienced in handling foals is essential. Foals' hooves grow more rapidly than older horses, and normal hoof growth is around 1.5 cm per month. For this reason and for regular monitoring of correct limb growth, it is recommended that the farrier attends every month.

Congenital limb deformities can be divided into two categories: angular limb deformities (ALDs) and flexural limb deformities (FLDs). ALDs are a deviation of the limb from below a joint, and FLDs are hyperextension or hyperflexion of a joint.

- *Carpal or tarsal valgus*: The limb deviates outwards from the knee or hock and may be corrected with a glue-on extension on the medial side and trimming the lateral side of the hoof.
- *Fetlock valgus*: The limb deviates outward from the fetlock and is treated in the same manner as carpal and tarsal valgus.
- *Carpal or tarsal varus*: The limb deviates towards the midline from below the joint, and this may be corrected by fixing an extension to the lateral hoof wall and trimming of the medial side.
- *Fetlock varus*: The limb deviates inwards from the fetlock and is treated in the same manner as carpal and tarsal varus.
- *'Windswept' foals*: This is a combination of varus in one joint and valgus in the opposite joint, and it is treated as above for the specific deviation on each limb.

Hyperflexion of a joint can be assisted by the placement of a toe extension to prevent knuckling over when walking and to put pressure through the toe to push the joint toward extension. Toe extensions appear to be most useful in fetlock hyperflexion. Periodic application of a splint can be very useful in treating hyperflexion; however, these should never be left in place for more than 8 hours, and great care should be taken in applying appropriate padding to prevent pressure sores. Hyperextension of a joint may be improved by the application of a heel extension to manipulate the joint into a more normal position. Controlled exercise is also very beneficial in these cases.

Parasite Control Protocols for Foals

Foals are vulnerable to all of the parasites that commonly affect adult horses and are more susceptible to their effects as the body has not been able to develop any resistance to them. The two main endoparasites of concern are thread-worms and ascarids. Threadworms are the endoparasites which first affect foals because they pass in the milk from the mare via vertical transmission. Threadworms rarely cause disease in foals; however, there are some reports of diarrhoea and colic and much more rarely, haemorrhage from damage to vessels as the worms migrate through the liver and lungs. Ascarid infection is a much more common and concerning event for young foals. Ascarids are very large in relation to the size of the foal's GI tract, and an ascarid impaction is a serious and potentially life-threatening problem. The migrating larvae of ascarids can also cause respiratory disease in foals. Tapeworms are rarely noted to be a problem in foals.

Ectoparasites may also affect foals, and it is important to ensure the mare and other horses on the premises are free from ectoparasites to protect the foals. Ticks are not host-specific and any tick will attach to a foal. Ticks seek areas of thin skin to attach to, and so foals make a particularly good host for them. The tick can cause local inflammation and more worryingly anaemia, which foals are more vulnerable to due to their relative size. Ticks also spread Lyme disease and, outside of the UK, other serious diseases such as tick paralysis. Foals may also be affected by lice, the same species which affect adult horses (*Damalinia equi* and *Haematopinus asini*) but the foals fine coat and thin skin mean the effects of self-mutilation can be more severe. While it is theoretically possible for foals to be affected by demodectic mange, it has not been widely reported.

Control of threadworms is centred around the treatment of the mare to prevent galactic transfer to the foal, so the first worming treatment of the foal itself is aimed at reducing ascarid burden. First anthelmintic treatment in foals is recommended at around 6 weeks of age although this varies from 2 weeks to 12 weeks between practitioners. Treatment with fenbendazole, which is licensed from 2 weeks of age, is recommended as the first dose. 6 months later a faecal worm egg count (FWEC) may be carried out to determine if further treatment is required. In autumn, it is recommended to administer a dose of moxidectin (licensed in foals over 4 months of age) to reduce the risk of larval cyathostomiasis.

Grazing management is of increasing importance as anthelmintic resistance grows. Arguably the most important aspect of this is regular removal of faeces, and this should be carried out at least twice a week, to ensure larval parasites excreted in the faeces do not spread throughout the pasture. Other useful grazing management strategies are:

- Eliminating rough patches of long grass when horses tend to defecate in a small, concentrated area
- Keeping muck heaps well away from grazing areas

- Co-grazing horses with small ruminants such as sheep or goats.

Rotational grazing is useful but cannot be relied upon as a sole method of parasite control unless paddocks are to be left empty for a year or more, as endoparasites can survive in the pasture for extended periods. Strongyles, for example, have been found to survive for up to 9 months on grazing land in cold conditions [22]. For more information regarding endoparasites and ectoparasites, see Chapter 5.

Vaccination Protocols for Foals

Tetanus vaccination is essential for all horses and foals to prevent the fatal condition. The first tetanus vaccine should be administered after five months of age, and it is often combined with weaning. A second tetanus vaccine is required 4–6 weeks later, followed by a booster one year later. After this initial booster, doses are administered every two years.

Vaccination against influenza is highly recommended, and the initial dose is usually administered at the same time as the first tetanus vaccine at six months of age. A second dose is administered between 21 and 92 days later and can be given at the same time as the second tetanus vaccine dose. A third dose is administered a further 150–215 days later followed by yearly booster doses.

Equine herpes virus (EHV) 1 and 4 are the only herpes viruses currently vaccinated against. As with tetanus and influenza vaccination, the initial vaccine dose is also required after five months of age with a second dose 4–6 weeks later. A booster is then required within six months of the second vaccination, and boosters every six months thereafter are required to maintain vaccination coverage.

Current advice from the horse racing levy board (HBLB) is that only breeding stallions require vaccination against equine viral arteritis (EVA) [23]. In some cases, vaccination of breeding mares is also recommended due to the primarily venereal spread of the disease.

Protocols and Requirements for Breed Registration

It is a legal requirement for all horses in the United Kingdom to have a passport and to obtain one the horse must be registered either in the general stud book, Weatherbys non-Thoroughbred register or with a specific breed society. In order to apply for a passport, the foal must be microchipped by a vet, and this is a legal requirement that must be carried out before the foal reaches 6 months of age. The following list is a summary of the main passport-issuing agencies and their requirements for registration.

- *Weatherbys*: Weatherbys maintain the general stud book, a record of all racing Thoroughbreds in the United Kingdom. They also maintain a non-Thoroughbred register and issue passports. All Thoroughbred brood mares and stallions must be registered with Weatherbys in order to register the foal if it is intended for racing. Weatherbys require notification within 30 days of birth or the foal will not be eligible to race when older. Once this notification has been made the foal can be registered. To register a Thoroughbred with Weatherbys a vet must record the markings of the foal and collect a DNA sample to be submitted with the application. The foal must also be microchipped at the time of DNA sample collection, and this must be carried out before the foal reaches 4 weeks of age.
- *Anglo European Studbook (AES)*: The AES maintain two studbooks for foals intended to compete in show jumping, dressage or eventing. To register a foal on the main studbook, the owner must be able to prove three generations of the foal's lineage on both the mare and stallion's side. If this is not possible, the foal may be registered on the auxiliary studbook. AES requires a record of the foal's markings completed by a vet at the time of microchip implantation, and a covering certificate from the stallion's owner or agent.
- *Breeders Elite Studbook*: The Breeders Elite studbook is a register of sport horses bred in the United Kingdom. A main and auxiliary studbook are maintained and registration on the main studbook requires proof of three generations of the foal's lineage on both the mare and stallion's side much like AES. Registration with Breeders Elite requires a record of the foal's markings completed by a vet at the time of microchip implantation, before weaning and a covering certificate from the stallion owner or agent.
- *Sport Horse breeding of Great Britain (SHB(GB))*: SHB(GB) allow registration of any foal which is expected to exceed 14.2hh as an adult. As with the previous two societies, there is a main studbook requiring proof of lineage and an auxiliary studbook.

There are many breed-specific societies with which foals can be registered, including:

- The Welsh Pony and Cob Society
- Arab Horse Society
- British Connemara Pony Society
- Dales Pony Society
- Dartmoor Pony Society
- Exmoor Pony Society
- Fell Pony Society
- Highland Pony Society
- New Forest Pony Breeding and Cattle Society.

15.5 Nursing Requirements of Sick Foals

Accommodation Requirements for Nursing Foals

There is some debate about the most appropriate bedding for young foals. Some prefer a deep straw bed, while others feel shavings on a rubber-matted floor are better. Paper or cardboard bedding may be appropriate especially if any personnel are prone to dust allergies. Whichever substrate is used, it is important that the stable is mucked out regularly to maintain good levels of hygiene for the immunologically vulnerable nursing foal. A deep bed is important, and foals should never be allowed to lay on a hard, uncovered floor as their fine coat and thin skin make them prone to pressure sores and rubs. Any break in the skin is a potential entry point for infectious pathogens. Foals with flexural limb deformities may struggle to move around in a very deep bed as they cannot lift their limbs high enough to clear the bedding. This is especially the case when the foal is wearing a cast to correct limb deformities, as the limb is fixed in place and unable to bend at the joints. For these patients, a shallower bed is required; however, they are still just as prone to skin damage, and maybe even more so, as they spend long periods lying down. For this reason, the best bedding combination for these foals is a reasonably shallow covering of shavings or paper on a rubber mat-covered floor, which is very regularly skipped out to ensure the foal does not lay in faeces.

When nursing foals with diarrhoea, the stable will have to be cleaned out many times a day, as these foals produce copious amounts of diarrhoea, and will most likely have an indwelling intravenous catheter as a potential route for infection. Efforts should also be made to regularly clean diarrhoea from the walls and fixtures of the stable, with particular attention to door handles and other commonly touched areas to prevent the spread of contaminants. Diarrhoea is commonly caused by infectious agents, which are spread in the diarrheic faeces, and some of these pathogens are zoonotic meaning personnel are at risk as well as other patients. Consideration must be made as to how to dispose of contaminated bedding. In a neonatal intensive care unit (NICU) or practice where multiple vulnerable foals are housed, each stable should be mucked out individually, the contaminated bedding disposed of before moving to the next stall, and utensils replaced or cleaned between stables. Contaminated bedding for foals with diarrhoea must be disposed of as infectious clinical waste until there is confirmation of negative culture results for all potential infectious causes.

Access to patient accommodation is an important and often overlooked consideration. It is important to be able to observe and monitor the foal as much as is required for the condition. To maintain the mare and foal bond, keeping interference to a minimum is useful and being able to monitor from a distance is key. In-stable closed-circuit television (CCTV) cameras are immensely useful for this task, and some systems allow remote movement of the camera and zoom functions, which can even facilitate observation of respiratory rate and pattern. Accommodation for nursing foals should be physically separated from other patients, and inpatients should not be able to make direct contact. Therefore, stables with solid walls are ideal rather than connecting walls with bars, for example, which allow horses to touch noses. The accommodation should also facilitate separation of the foal from the mare (Figure 15.11). This is important for foals which are not ambulatory and could be stepped on and injured by the mare, foals with an aggressive mare which cause a danger to the foal and/or handlers, foals which require constant rate infusion of medication or fluids or supplemental oxygen, and foals which are not permitted to nurse from the mare for example before surgery, if identified as at risk of neonatal isoerythrolysis or in some cases of diarrhoea.

A veterinary hospital is a high-risk place for an immunologically immature foal, and this risk becomes greater when the foal is systemically ill. The high number of potential pathogens and constantly changing population are a considerable threat to the neonate. Simply separating the foal physically from other patients is not enough, and they also must be protected from indirect spread of disease by considering PPE and equipment such as mucking out tools, feed and water buckets, and grooming kit should ideally be used only for the specific patient. If a lack of available equipment prevents this, then all items should be cleaned and disinfected between patients. Monitoring equipment should also ideally be utilised for one foal only, but if this is not possible, then equipment should be very thoroughly cleaned and disinfected between patients. This is especially important as most monitoring equipment comes into direct contact with the patient. Consumables or pieces of equipment which can be disconnected should be changed between patients. For example, if using an indirect blood pressure monitor, each foal should have its own cuff, which is not used for any other foal. The monitor itself can then be cleaned and then wiped down with disinfectant between uses, and the foal's specific cuff attached. Perhaps the biggest risk to the foal is unintentional transfer of pathogens via personnel.

The use of PPE can greatly reduce this and in a NICU setting it is not unreasonable to utilise full PPE such as gowns or overalls, double gloves, shoe covers and potentially even hair covers and masks. As a minimum, gloves must be worn at all times when handling foals and changed between patients and when contaminated. A disinfectant foot dip should be positioned at the stable door and stepped in before entering the stable. Staff may be used to stepping in the foot dip on the way out of the stable of a patient with an infectious disease, and it should be made clear that the measures are in place to protect the foal from the outside world, and everyone should enter the stall as clean as possible. It is important that the disinfectant used is one which is effective against the pathogens commonly found in veterinary hospitals. Foot dips must be emptied and replenished regularly to ensure that they remain effective.

Figure 15.11 A foal separated from the mare within the same stable. *Source:* Sarah Baillie.

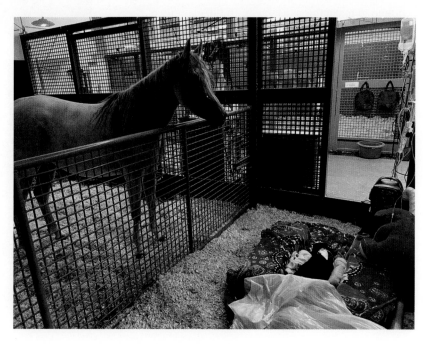

Practices should put in place specified, written, distributed and displayed protocols for the management of foals, and these must be followed and enforced. Risk assessments must be carried out, communicated and acted upon in relation to both common conditions or reasons for admission of foals, as well as handling scenarios for both foals and their mares. This also applies to the use of equipment and cleaning products. Care should be taken to follow the manufacturer's instructions for the use of equipment and cleaning products to ensure safe use and prevent injury to operators or patients or damage to equipment. Correct dilution rates are important in the use of disinfectants to ensure they have the required action and to protect the foal from disease.

When considering the accommodation requirements of a nursing foal, it is vital not to overlook the requirements of the mare. The goal should be to allow the mare and foal to live in as similar a way as possible to that in which they would live at home, if the foal were healthy. If the foal is ambulatory, it should spend as much time as possible with the mare in order to learn, nurse in a natural pattern and develop behaviourally. Foals that are not able to stand or ambulate normally require individual assessment and support, which will be discussed in detail in the next section of this chapter. Separating the mare and foal causes stress to both of them and should only be done if absolutely necessary. If the foal is not allowed to nurse, use of a muzzle should be considered before separation. Some mares are naturally very protective of their foal, and the increased handling required during hospitalisation and treatment may exacerbate this.

Careful assessment of the mare's character and behaviour will dictate how this is managed, and a sound understanding of body language, behaviour and maternal instinct is required to make this assessment. In the majority of cases, the mare will remain somewhat calm if allowed to stay very close to the foal while it is handled, and care is taken not to stand between the mare and foal blocking her access to it. If the mare bites but does not carry out any other acts of aggression, then it may be useful to place a muzzle on her and allow her to remain close by. If the mare is dangerously aggressive, then steps must be taken to protect handlers and the foal from injury, and this usually involves temporary removal of the mare or foal. This can, however, exacerbate the situation by reinforcing her belief that humans wish to remove her foal from her, and it may be more appropriate to utilise restraint methods to keep the mare with the foal while protecting personnel and equipment. It is a difficult balance, and the correct course of action will depend on the characteristics of the mare, the experience level of the handlers, and the requirements of the procedure being carried out. The priority though should always be safety of personnel with the mental and physical well-being of the mare and foal a close second.

Nursing Requirements of Recumbent Foals

Nursing a recumbent foal is a labour of love. It is incredibly time- and energy-consuming but equally, if not more, rewarding. The first consideration to make is the reason for recumbency. The condition which prevents the foal from being able to stand and ambulate dictates the requirements for nursing care.

Reasons for recumbency include:

- Neonatal maladjustment syndrome (NMS)
- Sepsis
- Prematurity/dysmaturity
- Traumatic injury
- Limb deformities

This section will describe nursing care of recumbent neonates affected by NMS unless otherwise stated.

Correct positioning is crucial for recumbent neonates for several reasons. Firstly, the foal must remain in a sternal position to be able to maintain adequate respiratory function (Figure 15.12). Positioning in lateral recumbency drops the foal's partial pressure of oxygen (PaO_2) (a marker of oxygenation) by 14 mmHg [24]. Foals with NMS have

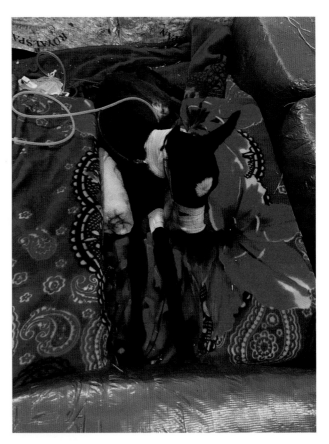

Figure 15.12 A foal in a sternal support. *Source:* Sarah Baillie.

already faced a hypoxic insult, and almost all continue to face challenges maintaining oxygenation levels throughout recumbency, so maintaining a position which assists with effective ventilation is very important. The best way to keep a foal in sternal recumbency is by situating it in a sternal support. The sternal support is a simple device consisting of two cushions joined together to prevent them from being pushed apart. These can be sourced from commercial manufacturers of veterinary positioning aids or manufactured to specific requirements by a marine upholsterer. Blankets, vetbeds or duvets can be utilised to pad the sternal support before the foal is placed in it. If the foal is slightly smaller than the sternal support is designed for, a rolled-up towel or small pillow placed at each shoulder can hold the foal in position. Care should be taken when positioning the foal so that no undue pressure is placed on the foal's chest by pushing the shoulder supports too far back. The foal has a very compliant chest wall and requires room to expand the chest fully for effective respiratory function. Foals with displaced rib fractures should not be placed in a sternal support due to the risk of pushing the fractured rib into a lung or the heart. Because friction of the fractured rib against the surface of the lung negatively affects lung health, the lung is less efficient at gaseous exchange. For this reason, foals with unilateral rib fractures should spend more time laid with the affected lung positioned down to allow the healthy lung to fully expand and allow the foal to oxygenate well.

The other consideration for positioning is that the fine, soft coat (which is often more pronounced in premature or NMS foals) gives little protection to the fragile skin of a neonate and this, in combination with their low level of subcutaneous fat, makes them highly susceptible to decubitus ulcers. The combination of an extended period in one position, hair dampness caused by urine contamination and application of liquids to the coat (for example, a contact medium for ultrasound examination), and friction when moving means recumbent neonates almost inevitably will develop some decubitus ulcers in time despite the best efforts. When this happens, covering the lesion with a hydrocolloid dressing prevents contamination, keeps the ulcer from drying out and provides a layer of cushioning protection to prevent progression. Prevention of decubitus ulcers requires keeping the foal clean and dry by controlling its environment. This means preventing the foal from urinating onto itself, which is only practically achievable by urinary bladder catheterisation. If an ultrasound examination is required, the foal should be moved out of its bed to another area, and following the procedure, any contact gel or other liquid should be thoroughly dried from the foal's coat. Baby powder can be applied to soak up any residue. Some clinicians use alcohol on the patient's coat to help with probe contact; it is not advisable to do this with sick

neonates as they are unable to regulate their body temperature sufficiently, which can lead to hypothermia. Baby oil is an appropriate alternative as it does not affect the foal's temperature, and it creates a protective layer over the skin and hair. The bedding on which the foal is positioned must be changed regularly and should be changed every time it is soiled to ensure the foal stays clean and dry. The foal should be turned every two hours to ensure pressure is distributed between both sides and that each lung is dependent for equal amounts of time (except in cases of displaced rib fractures as described above).

As previously mentioned, neonates are poorly developed to thermoregulate effectively, and this is further exacerbated by the lack of movement in a recumbent foal and difficulty maintaining adequate perfusion to produce sometimes profound hypothermia. Addressing the underlying cause of hypothermia is essential, and usually, poor perfusion is the issue which requires cardiovascular support with fluids and medication. While addressing the cause, it is important to prevent further heat loss, and this can be done in several ways. Firstly, the ambient temperature of the foal's accommodation should be warm enough to prevent further loss, and this can be controlled by ensuring doors and windows are kept closed and utilising heat lamps. Ideally, ambient temperature should be maintained slightly above 24°C for sick foals due to their increased metabolic demands and poor thermoregulatory controls. Caution should be employed with the use of heat lamps and they should be both properly secured so they do not fall onto the foal, and set up at a suitable distance to prevent accidental burning. Blankets, duvets and rugs may all be useful in keeping a recumbent foal warm and because perfusion is so often an issue in these foals, wrapping the legs to warm the extremities can be very helpful. A forced air-warming device such as a Bair Hugger can be very useful for these foals if one is available (Figure 15.13).

Gentle movement is important for recumbent foals for stimulation as well as maintaining muscle mass and limb function. If the foal is conscious and able to move its limbs, it can be helpful to manipulate the limbs regularly. Pushing the limbs into a flexed position and applying gentle pressure on the bottom of the hoof for the foal to push back against is a useful physiotherapy technique. The importance of regular standing should not be underestimated even in foals which are unable to support their own weight. Every two hours, when repositioning the foal, it should be lifted to a standing position with its feet on the ground. This helps to wake the foal up, improve cognitive function, decrease lung collapse, strengthen muscles and improve GI function. If the foal can support its own weight or even walk a few steps, it should be encouraged to do so. These foals should be gently encouraged to do as much as they

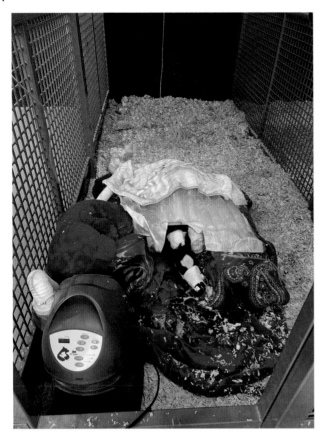

Figure 15.13 A foal under a Bair Hugger forced air warming blanket. *Source:* Sarah Baillie.

are capable of to ensure that they make progress towards becoming fully ambulatory.

Recumbent foals are obviously not able to ambulate and nurse independently, and all recumbent foals require some form of nutritional support. For a foal which is recumbent due to limb deformities but has normal cognitive function, this is as simple as physically holding the foal up at the udder and allowing it to nurse. Typically, foals born with severe limb deformities tend to be quite large, so this can be physically demanding on the handlers. Positioning the foal and resting the foal's torso on a bale of shavings can help to take some of the strain. For recumbent foals with neurological dysfunction, this is not so simple. Some foals may be able to support their own weight for short periods or even take a few steps. These foals should be taken to the mare, and if they cannot nurse yet, they should be fed beside the udder. This process helps the foal to associate the feeling of fullness with being at the udder and is a helpful step towards the ultimate goal of a foal, which can stand and nurse for itself. Foals which are unable to stand for the duration of feeding should be positioned securely in sternal recumbency for feeding to prevent milk reflux and aspiration pneumonia. If the foal is conscious and able to drink from a bowl, this is an ideal feeding method. However, it is rare that a foal with NMS, which is recumbent, is able to bowl feed. In this case, feeding via NGT is indicated.

Placement of an indwelling NGT is preferable to the frequent passing of a tube. Severely affected NMS foals may be unable to tolerate enteral feeding due to compromised GI function and in this situation the use of total parenteral nutrition (TPN) may be indicated. Care should be taken when administering TPN to maintain impeccable hygiene both in the handling of the TPN, the associated giving set and in maintenance of the intravenous catheter. The combination of lipids, glucose and amino acids and a warm environment makes an ideal breeding ground for bacteria. Dual lumen intravenous catheters are useful in TPN administration so that one lumen can be dedicated to TPN. TPN fluid lines must be changed every 24–48 hours, and once open, TPN should not be used after 48 hours. Fluid therapy is tailored to the needs of the patient based on hydration status, blood pressure, perfusion, and electrolyte and acid/base status. It is not uncommon for the recumbent NMS patient to have multiple constant rate infusions (CRIs) set up concurrently (Figure 15.14).

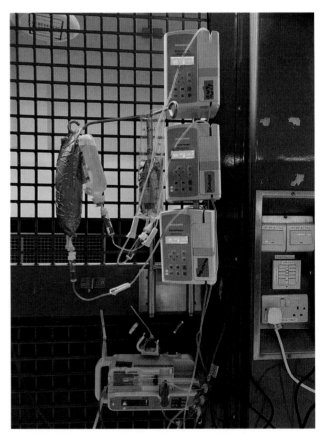

Figure 15.14 Multiple CRIs ensuring accurate administration of fluids and medications to a sick foal. *Source:* Sarah Baillie.

The umbilicus is a common site of entry for disease-causing pathogens, and foals which have undergone aggressive fluid therapy resuscitation are at increased risk of a patent urachus. This means that the umbilicus of these patients is constantly exposed to urinary contamination as well as laying with the umbilicus in contact with the bedding. Therefore, umbilical care is very important. The umbilicus should be dipped in 0.5% chlorhexidine or 2% iodine every six hours and kept as clean as possible. Iodine tincture is sometimes recommended as an umbilical dip as it is believed to dry out the stump, and aluminium spray is also used on some studs for the same reason. Whichever product is used, it is important to ensure that it does not cause further contamination. Therefore, dips should be changed daily, and spray caps kept clean and debris free. The author prefers to make and label a pot of umbilical dip for each patient and apply it using a clean syringe to maintain cleanliness and good hygiene. Daily ultrasound examination of the umbilicus is advisable for early identification of sepsis.

The neonatal cornea is less sensitive than that of an adult and the menace response has not yet developed, so when a foal is recumbent and often unable to control movements of its head, it is both susceptible to cornea ulceration and does not display signs of pain obviously. For this reason, a daily eye examination is required, and the eye should have a fluorescein stain applied to check for the presence of a developing corneal ulcer. Adequate padding around the head of the recumbent foal, as well as frequent application of eye lubricants can reduce the risk of corneal ulcer formation. Foals showing seizure activity may benefit from a padded head protector to prevent eye trauma.

Urinary bladder catheterisation is highly recommended in the recumbent NMS foal, and the benefits outweigh the risk of ascending infection, which can be minimised with scrupulous hygiene. Catheterisation keeps the foal clean and the bedding far less contaminated, especially in colt foals. It allows accurate measurement of urinary output and hydration status, both of which can change rapidly in neonates with serious consequences. Changes in diet, like the switch from mare's milk to milk replacer, can induce transient diarrhoea or have the opposite costive effect. The often-compromised GI function of foals with NMS may mean an absence of faecal output for long periods. Foals nutritionally supported entirely with TPN may not pass faeces at all, and that is not surprising as their GI tract is empty and functioning poorly. Foals without GI compromise, which are enterally fed and do not pass faeces for more than 24 hours, should receive an enema as described earlier in Section 15.2 relating to meconium impaction.

The recumbent equine neonate is an ideal candidate for utilising nursing care plans. Their care is complex and involves multiple body systems with numerous potential problems to consider. The care plan will require frequent evaluation and reassessment of nursing care interventions as these foals improve and deteriorate rapidly with new problems developing all the time. For this reason, accurate record-keeping is essential. These foals require almost constant monitoring and accurate, detailed records can help identify subtle but significant changes in patterns that may otherwise have been missed. Each foal with NMS differs slightly, and records of baseline normal for that foal are much more useful than published parameters.

15.6 Nursing Support of Foals Undergoing Investigations and Supportive Therapies

To collect venous blood from a foal the external jugular vein is the most accessible venepuncture point. Blood can be collected with a needle and syringe or a vacutainer system, although the vacutainer system is rarely practical in young foals due to their small size and difficulty accessing venepuncture sites. The low level of body fat and superficial position of the foal's jugular vein mean visualisation is often easier than in adult horses, and the behaviour and energy levels of the foal are usually the biggest challenge to the procedure. If collection from the jugular vein is not possible, then the cephalic or saphenous veins can be utilised. If a jugular catheter is in place, it is advisable to avoid the opposite jugular vein for repeated blood sampling in order to preserve its patency in case of compromise to the catheterised vein. Common limb venepuncture sites in the foal are the cephalic vein on the inner forearm and the saphenous vein on the inside of the proximal hindleg. It is possible to collect blood from the lateral thoracic vein and other veins of the foal, although this is rarely required in practice. If a small amount of blood is required, then the facial sinus is a useful site for blood collection. To obtain a drop of blood for serial glucose testing, an ear or gum prick with a very small needle can be performed in order to preserve the veins for larger blood samples. To collect an arterial sample for blood gas analysis, the dorsal metatarsal artery below the hock on the outer hindlimb is often utilised. This is a useful site for arterial blood collection, as the artery runs separately from any veins at that point, so accidental venous blood collection is avoided. In very mobile foals, the hindlimb may be difficult to restrain for sample collection, and other sites may be more appropriate such as the brachial artery of the forelimb, an ear or tail artery.

Some foals may require diagnostic imaging, such as radiography or ultrasound. If the procedure is short and the patient tolerant, little support other than adequate restraint is required. Unlike adult horses, young foals tend to lie down when sedated and require relatively lower doses due to their immature central nervous system and more permeable blood–brain barrier. Benzodiazepines such as diazepam or midazolam are commonly used for the sedation of neonates, as these agents cause less suppression of the cardiovascular system than other sedatives, and provide adequate sedation for most procedures. In older foals, alpha2 agonists such as xylazine are routinely used, as benzodiazepines provide less effective sedation in older foals. Butorphanol is also commonly administered in conjunction with xylazine to provide pain relief for some procedures. For procedures which require the foal to be sedated and restrained, especially in lateral recumbency, it may be prudent to administer supplemental oxygen, especially if the procedure is predicted to take a long time.

Many hospitalised foals require the administration of intravenous fluid therapy. Maintenance requirements for foals where there are no excessive losses are estimated at 80–120 ml/kg/day. Hypovolaemia and electrolyte derangements are indications for fluid therapy, and the signs of these should be understood by the equine registered veterinary nurse (RVN). Hypovolaemia is usually demonstrated as tachypnoea, tachycardia, weak peripheral pulses and cold extremities. Mucous membrane appearance and skin tent are very unreliable measures in foals and should not be relied upon for assessment of hydration. Blood tests are the most useful way to assess hydration and electrolyte levels in combination. Crude tests such as urine specific gravity are also cheap, simple and effective ways to assess hydration. Blood parameters, including packed cell volume, total protein and lactate, can be used to assess hydration, and all three of these parameters increase in dehydrated foals. Serum electrolyte levels can also be measured from a blood sample and show the type and severity of electrolyte derangements.

Hypokalaemia is a common electrolyte derangement, especially in foals which have not been nursing well. Hypokalaemia occurs rapidly in the inappetent foal and can require aggressive supplementation to reverse it. Intravenous administration of potassium chloride must be undertaken with caution though as it is a relatively small amount given rapidly, it can cause a fatal overdose. Oral administration of potassium in the form of lo salt can also help to restore potassium levels in the foal. Signs of hypokalaemia are weakness and reduced GI function, which are usually already present in the sick foal, so regular blood testing is useful for early identification. Hypocalcaemia is another common electrolyte derangement in the foal, and signs include tachycardia and abnormal cardiac rhythms, tachypnoea, ataxia, muscle fasciculations and seizures. This can be addressed by supplementation of intravenous fluids with calcium. Hyponatraemia is a less common

electrolyte derangement in foals, which can be responsible for seizure activity. Administration of sodium-rich fluids can correct this derangement. Respiratory alkalosis and respiratory acidosis are both fairly common acid–base imbalances in sick neonates, and metabolic acidosis and alkalosis may also be seen. Sick foals with diarrhoea sometimes present with a metabolic acid–base deficit due to electrolyte losses through diarrhoea.

As previously discussed in this chapter, the transfer of passive immunity from mare to foal via immunoglobulins in the colostrum is essential to the foal's survival. Failure of passive transfer leaves the neonatal foal vulnerable to infection, as active immunity has not developed yet, leaving the body unable to fight off pathogens. Therefore, it is important to check the foal's IgG level 12–24 hours following birth and, if low IgG levels are detected, the administration of immunoglobulin-rich plasma is indicated. If a foal is known to not have access to good quality colostrum, then donor colostrum should be administered via a NGT in the first 12 hours of life. If failure of passive transfer is not identified and treated, it is extremely likely that the foal will develop an infection within a few weeks. This could be a respiratory infection or most likely septicaemia, which can spread to multiple joints. Treatment of septicaemia and joint infection is expensive and time-consuming, and it can be very difficult to get the infection under control. This has long-term implications for the foal's health and may well lead to permanent damage to the joints, negatively affecting future athletic ability.

The hospitalised foal may require nutritional support in the form of supplemental feeding. If milk from the mare is not available, it may be necessary to feed the foal with a milk replacer. Commercial milk replacer powders and pellets are widely available and nutritionally balanced. The manufacturer's recommendations for preparation should be followed to ensure the preparation is not over or under diluted. There is an exception to this rule though in introducing a previously very GI-compromised foal to milk replacer. It may be beneficial to first introduce a half-strength milk replacer, i.e. use half the amount of powder to the normal amount of water. Some practitioners recommend the preparation of a milk replacer with boiling water and then allowing it to cool slightly above room temperature before feeding. Using boiling water should destroy at least some bacteria that may be present in the powder. Both prepared milk replacer and collected mares' milk should be stored in the fridge and either discarded after 24 hours or frozen for longer storage. As discussed in the earlier section on feeding orphan foals, bowl feeding is the best technique for supplemental feeding (Figure 15.15). It allows the foal to drink without the presence of a human and, if the bucket is positioned at an appropriate height, has a

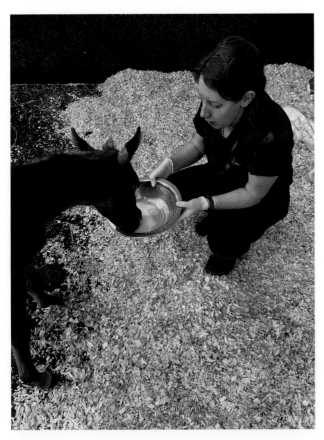

Figure 15.15 A foal drinking milk from a bowl. *Source:* Sarah Baillie.

low risk of aspiration. Bottle feeding is not recommended unless transitioning a foal from bucket feeding to nursing from an udder. The technique for bottle feeding is important due to the risk of the foal aspirating milk and developing pneumonia. The foal should have free movement of its head, and the bottle should be tilted so the milk sits in the teat but does not pour from it; this way, the foal sucks the milk from the teat and controls the flow. In foals with NMS, it is important not to attempt bottle feeding until the foal has a very strong suckle reflex and demonstrates independent udder searching behaviours.

Sometimes, feeding via a NGT is indicated and placement of an indwelling tube is required. The NGT selected should have the smallest bore size possible to help prevent damage to the oesophageal mucosa. The tube can either be sutured in place or secured to a sutured nasal oxygen cannula if one is present. Securing it to the oxygen cannula has the benefit of being able to move the NGT to check for reflux; however, it comes with a much higher risk of the NGT accidentally being pulled out. The author's preference is to bend and tape the NGT around a tongue depressor at the nostril to prevent kinking of the tube, and to suture the tube securely to the non-cartilaginous part of the nostril. Very narrow

NGTs with a guidewire are excellent for indwelling use and are relatively easy to place with practice. Due to the narrow bore of the tube, it cannot be externally visualised or palpated in the oesophagus, and confirmation of correct placement should be carried out by endoscopy or radiography. Before each feed, gentle negative pressure should be applied to the tube using a syringe to check for the presence of reflux. Milk should be allowed to flow into the tube by gravity only and should never be forced through the tube. A small amount of warm water run through the tube after feeding will prevent blockage of the tube with milk.

As neonates have a higher demand for oxygen than adults, supplemental oxygen is more frequently required. A nasal oxygen cannula can be placed in the nasal cavity to facilitate this. A small human NGT known as a Ryles tube or a small foley catheter may be used as an oxygen cannula. The distance should be measured from the nostril to the medial canthus of the eye, and this is the length of tubing which should be inserted, via the ventral meatus, into the nose. The tube can be taped around a tongue depressor to prevent kinking and sutured to the non-cartilaginous portion of the nostril. Oxygen, either from a portable tank or a wall-mounted unit, can then be connected via long tubing to the oxygen cannula. Oxygen administered to foals should always be run through a humidifier to ensure it does not dry out and damage the fragile mucous membranes. A flow rate of 5–10 l per hour is usually sufficient for a neonate depending on respiratory function. Ideally, supplemental oxygen should be titrated to effect assessed by serial arterial blood gas analysis.

Urinary bladder catheterisation comes with a risk of ascending infection, and placement of a catheter should be carried out using an aseptic technique. The foal should be restrained in lateral recumbency, and the vulva or penis and prepuce should be thoroughly cleansed with chlorhexidine and rinsed with sterile saline; sterile lubricant should be applied to the foley catheter, and the person carrying out the procedure should don sterile gloves. In fillies, one finger is inserted into the vagina to palpate the pelvic bones and urethral opening. It is not often possible to feel the opening itself, but the finger can be used to guide the foley catheter towards where the urethral opening should be, and the catheter is gently advanced. If the catheter slides in smoothly, then it is most likely in the correct place; if resistance is felt, then it should be withdrawn to the pelvic bones and attempted again. Successful placement is confirmed when urine is seen in the catheter, and gentle aspiration with a catheter-tipped syringe may be required to start the flow. In colts, a non-sterile assistant is required to grasp and extrude the penis and the lubricated catheter is passed into the urethral opening and advanced into the bladder. Once the foal is catheterised, the cuff should be inflated, and the catheter may be sutured in place. A urine collection bag is useful in a non-ambulatory foal to collect and measure urine and maintain hygiene. If the foal is too mobile for a collection bag, then the end of the catheter should be covered with a condom with the end cut off, which protects the catheter from contaminants but allows urine to flow freely out. It is important to regularly check the catheter for patency and blockages may be resolved by flushing with warm sterile saline. Failure to recognise and remove blockages could result in bladder rupture if the foal is unable to urinate around the catheter.

During admission of a sick foal or when changes in their condition occurs, several diagnostic procedures may be required. In order to carry out these procedures safely the foal must be correctly restrained. To restrain a foal in a standing position for procedures which are well tolerated such as physical examination, radiography or ultrasound the foal can be held with one arm across the chest and the other around the rump or gently grasping the tail. Alternatively, two people can hold the foal. One person can hold the chest, and one person can hold the hips or tail. For less well-tolerated procedures such as blood sample collection, the handler should loop one arm under the throat and grasp the opposite ear to have control of the head, and lift and drop the chin to facilitate vein visualisation; the other hand is used to firmly grasp the tail base. Procedures such as intravenous catheterisation for fluid therapy, insertion of a nasal oxygen cannula or urinary bladder catheterisation are usually less stressful for the foal if carried out while restrained in lateral recumbency. This also makes it easier to maintain adequate sterility for procedures than starting a procedure standing and the foal then lying down once it becomes tired. The number of available handlers dictates how this is achieved. If only one handler is available, then they should sit with one leg straight under the foal's neck, hold the head and place the other leg gently over the foal's chest, placing the foot behind the foal's elbow and taking care not to put any pressure on the chest wall. If more handlers are available, then one person should sit straddling the hind limbs, and put gentle pressure on the foal's hip with their hand if required. The second person should straddle the front legs and put gentle pressure on the foal's shoulder with their hand. This gives control of the legs, prevents personnel and equipment from being kicked and protects the foal from injury.

It may often be necessary to administer plasma or other blood products to sick foals, and these should be given with caution. A transfusion reaction can occur as a result of administering these products, and the risk is increased if the foal has received a dose of these products previously. The heart rate, respiratory rate and temperature should be measured before administration and throughout the procedure. A marked increase in any of the parameters warrants cessation of administration as they indicate onset of a transfusion reaction. Other signs include urticaria, muscle tremors and convulsions. Parameters should be diligently recorded along with the batch number of the plasma product (Table 15.5). This means if a reaction were to occur, an accurate record of the procedure exists along with batch information to pass on to the plasma manufacturer in case

Table 15.5 Plasma transfusion guide.

Equipment required	What to monitor and record	Administration process	Signs of reaction	What to do in event of reaction
Warm water and thermometer for defrosting	The batch number of the plasma	Defrost the plasma in a warm water bath no warmer than 38°C	Increase in heart rate	Stop the transfusion
Equipment for IV catheter placement if the foal does not already have one in place	Heart rate before and every 5 minutes during transfusion	Place a short-term IV catheter if the foal does not already have one in place	Increase in respiratory rate	Inform the responsible veterinary surgeon
A filtered blood giving set	Respiratory rate before and every 5 minutes during transfusion	Separate the foal from the mare or have someone restrain the mare safely	Increase in temperature	If reaction is mild the transfusion may be restarted very slowly and/or with a different bag of plasma
Flush for the IV catheter	Temperature before and every 5 minutes during transfusion	Insert the filtered giving set into the bag of plasma and attach to the foal's catheter	Urticaria	If the reaction is severe the foal may require administration of adrenaline, corticosteroid and/or IV fluids
Someone to restrain the foal and someone to restrain the mare if necessary	Rate of plasma administration	Administer the plasma over 20–30 minutes starting at a slow drip and increasing if no signs of reaction noted	Muscle tremors or convulsions	Record all parameters, timings and medications administered

Source: Sarah Baillie.

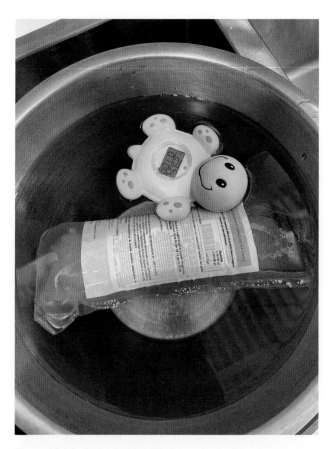

Figure 15.16 Plasma defrosting monitored with a baby bath thermometer. *Source:* Sarah Baillie.

Table 15.6 Normal clinical parameters for foals.

	Immediately post partum	1 day old	1 week old and over
Heart rate	40–80 bpm	100–140 bpm	80–100 bpm
Respiratory rate	60–80 bpm	20–40 bpm	20–40 bpm
Temperature	37.7–38.8c	37.7–38.8c	37.7–38.8c

Source: Sarah Baillie.

of a batch fault. Recording the batch number is also useful in case further plasma administration is required, as using the same batch reduces the risk of a reaction. Blood products must always be administered via a filtered giving set. A baby bath thermometer is useful for defrosting frozen plasma as the thermometer floats in the water and beeps and flashes if the temperature is too high (Figure 15.16). When administering any medication, it is important to follow the manufacturer's instructions, understand the drug's potential side effects and ensure you are aware of the correct administration for that medication. Before administering any medication, it is a good idea double check the dose and route of administration.

15.7 Monitoring Techniques for Sick Foals

Normal clinical parameters for foals are displayed in Table 15.6.

Other parameters measured are capillary refill time, which should be less than 2 seconds; mucous membrane colour which should be pale pink, blood pressure, which should maintain a mean arterial pressure (MAP) above 60 mmHg; and oxygen saturation, which should be 99–100%.

Foals can display pain and distress in slightly different ways to adults, although they are similar in many ways. Generally, pain is expressed through tachycardia, tachypnoea and reluctance to nurse. A foal which is lame may be more reluctant to stand and nurse and could require encouragement to do so. Often, cessation of nursing is the first or only sign a foal shows in response to pain, and this may go unnoticed for some time. Regularly checking the mare's udder can inform whether the foal is nursing well, and a foal which is frequently seen at the udder but has a milk-stained face, is a sign that it is not nursing but rather standing at the udder out of habit as the mare drips milk onto it. Foals experiencing abdominal pain, especially due to EGUS, will frequently roll onto their back and lay in dorsal recumbency, rather than exhibiting the typical behaviours of an adult horse with colic.

Faecal output should be monitored and recorded, and a normal nursing foal should pass faeces several times a day. The faeces produced by a foal, which is drinking milk only, are soft and pale brown and as the foal's diet starts to include more roughage, the faeces become darker and more formed. An absence of faeces is a sign of poor GI function, ileus or impaction and should be investigated. A foal's intake of milk and/or other feed and water sources should also be monitored and recorded. These should correlate with the faecal output. The foal's weight should be measured daily to ensure it is growing at an appropriate rate. The foal should gain approximately 1kg bodyweight per day.

Urine output is an important parameter to monitor in sick foals. A sudden decrease in output is often the first sign of hypovolaemia or cardiovascular dysfunction. If a urinary catheter is in place with a collection bag attached, the urine output should be recorded and used in conjunction with recording of amounts of fluids administered intravenously, and enteral milk feeding. The fluid should be balanced with the urine (and reflux if collected) amount to ensure there are no ongoing fluid losses. Urine appearance should also be noted, and urine specific gravity (USG) can be used to assess hydration. Normal foal urine should appear pale yellow and clear, with a USG of 1.001–1.025. Young foals consuming only milk and nursing frequently usually have a USG below 1.015. It is useful to remember that some medications alter urine colour; for example, rifampicin colours urine red, and it may be mistaken for blood or myoglobin in the urine.

The foal's demeanour, level of consciousness and neurological state should also be monitored and recorded. The RVN should assess whether the foal is bright and interacting with people and the mare and performing normal behaviours such as udder seeking. If the foal is dull, inappetent and reluctant to interact this should be noted and communicated to the rest of the team if it is a new development. If the foal appears to be unconscious or is very dull or moribund then the response to tactile and pain stimulus should be checked. Some signs of NMS are very subtle at first, and a good understanding of normal behaviour will help identify small changes. Signs of NMS include:

- Reluctance to nurse
- Lack of affinity for the mare
- Disorientation
- Reluctance to stand or walk
- Reduction in urine output
- Reduction in faecal output
- Collapse
- Seizures

There are different types of seizure activity in foals. There may be small, subtle, focal seizures, which are expressed with licking and chewing, or abnormal jaw movements while the foal remains standing or laying in a normal position. Another common seizure activity is paddling of the legs while laying down. Star gazing, extending the head and neck out and up, is often a precursor to greater seizure activity. Grand mal seizures are dramatic and violent and can easily result in injury to the foal. Some foals will have a single seizure and never display any seizure activity again. Others may continue to have repeated episodes and require control with medication such as diazepam or midazolam, phenobarbital or levetiracetam. It is important to be vigilant for seizure activity, especially in high-risk foals such as NMS foals, foals with hypoxia, foals with electrolyte derangements, and Arabian foals. If there are any concerns about a foal developing seizure activity or if a foal has already displayed seizure activity, it is useful to ensure the area they are housed in is free from protrusions and hazards and pad the walls if possible. A barrier of shavings bales can be an accessible option for protection.

References

1 Johnson, L. and Thompson, D.L. (1986). Seasonal variation in the total volume of Leydig cells in stallions is explained by variation in cell number rather than cell size. *Biology of Reproduction* 35 (4): 971–979.

2 Deichsel, K., Schrammel, N., Aurich, J., and Aurich, C. (2016). Effects of a long-day light programme on the motility and membrane integrity of cooled-stored and cyropreserved semen in Shetland pony stallions [Online]. Available at: https://reader.elsevier.com/reader/sd/pii/S0378432016300483?token=B846E4F776EE22C587A50418C4934B90EB0D0612DE7329A1C323F2ACBC7F7A6305CE2E8679C13D461E41CACB1F76058D&originRegion=eu-west-1&originCreation=20220217091223 (accessed 17 February 2022).

3 Bowman, M.C., Vogelsang, M.M., Gibbs, P.G. et al. (2007). Utilizing body temperature to evaluate ovulation in mares. *The Professional Animal Scientists* 23 (3): 267–271.

4 Dini, P., Ducheyne, K., Lemahieu, I. et al. (2019). Effect of environmental factors and changes in the body condition score on the onset of the breeding season in mares. *Reproduction in Domestic Animals* 54 (7): 987–995.

5 Verhagen, I., Tomotani, B.M., Gienapp, P., and Visser, M.E. (2020). Temperature has a causal and plastic effect on timing of breeding in a small songbird [Online]. Available at: https://journals-biologists-com.ezproxy.lib.gla.ac.uk/jeb/article/223/8/jeb218784/223853/Temperature-has-a-causal-and-plastic-effect-on (accessed 23 February 2022).

6 Benhajali, H., Ezzaouia, M., Lunel, C. et al. (2013). Temporal feeding pattern may influence reproduction efficiency, the example of breeding mares. *PLoS One* 8 (9): e73858.

7 Samper, J.C. (2001). Management and fertility of mares bred with frozen semen. *Animal Reproduction Science* 68 (3–4): 219–228.

8 Katila, T. (2003). Effects of hormone treatments, season, age and type of mares on ovulation, twinning and pregnancy rates of mares inseminated with fresh and frozen semen. *Pferdeheilkunde* 19: 619–624.

9 Lewis, N., Morganti, M., Collingwood, F. et al. (2015). Utilization of one-dose postovulation breeding with frozen-thawed semen at a commercial artificial insemination center: pregnancy rates and postbreeding uterine fluid accumulation in comparison to insemination with chilled or fresh semen. *Journal of Equine Veterinary Science* 35 (11): 882–887.e1.

10 Crowe, C.M., Ravenhill, P.J., Hepburn, R.J., and Shepherd, C.H. (2008). A retrospective study of artificial insemination of 251 mares using chilled and fixed time frozen-thawed semen. *Equine Veterinary Journal* 40 (6): 572–576.

11 Peugnet, P., Mendoza, L., Wimel, L. et al. (2016). Longitudinal study of growth and osteoarticular status in foals born to between-breed embryo transfers. *Journal of Equine Veterinary Science* 37: 24–38.

12 Brewer, B.D., Clement, S.F., Lotz, W.S., and Gronwall, R. (1991). Renal clearance, urinary excretion of endogenous substances, and urinary diagnostic indices in healthy neonatal foals. *Journal of Veterinary Internal Medicine* 5 (1): 28–33.

13 Rumbaugh, G.E., Carlson, G.P., and Harrold, D. (1982). Urinary production in the healthy horse and in horses deprived of feed and water. *American Journal of Veterinary Research* 43 (4): 735–737.

14 Perkins, G.A. and Wagner, B. (2015). The development of equine immunity: current knowledge on immunology in the young horse. *Equine Veterinary Journal* 47 (3): 267–274.

15 Bernard, W.V., Reimer, J.M., Cudd, T., and Hewlett, L. (1995). Historical factors, clinicopathologic findings, clinical features, and outcome of equine neonates presenting with or developing signs of central nervous system disease. *American Association of Equine Practitioners USA* [Online]. Available from: https://scholar.google.com/scholar_lookup?title=Historical+factors%2C+clinicopathologic+findings%2C+clinical+features%2C+and+outcome+of+equine+neonates+presenting+with+or+developing+signs+of+central+nervous+system+disease&author=Bernard%2C+W.V.+%28Rood+and+Riddle+Equine+Hospital%2C+Lexington%2C+KY.%29&publication_year=1995 (accessed 25 February 2022).

16 Madigan, J.E., Haggett, E.F., Pickles, K.J. et al. (2012). Allopregnanolone infusion induced neurobehavioural alterations in a neonatal foal: is this a clue to the pathogenesis of neonatal maladjustment syndrome? *Equine Veterinary Journal* 44 (s41): 109–112.

17 Sakr, M. and Balasundaram, P. (2022). Neonatal therapeutic hypothermia. In: *StatPearls*. [Online]. Available from: http://www.ncbi.nlm.nih.gov/books/NBK567714/ (accessed 25 February).

18 Coleman, M.C. and Whitfield-Cargile, C. (2017). Orthopedic conditions of the premature and dysmature foal. *The Veterinary Clinics of North America. Equine Practice* 33 (2): 289–297.

19 Henry, S., Sigurjónsdóttir, H., Klapper, A. et al. (2020). Domestic foal weaning: need for re-thinking breeding practices? *Animals* 10 (2): 361.

20 Henry, S., Zanella, A.J., Sankey, C. et al. (2012). Adults may be used to alleviate weaning stress in domestic foals (Equus caballus). *Physiology & Behavior* 106 (4): 428–438.

21 Elfenbein, J.R. and Sanchez, L.C. (2012). Prevalence of gastric and duodenal ulceration in 691 nonsurviving foals (1995–2006). *Equine Veterinary Journal* 44 (s41): 76–79.

22 Nielsen, M.K., Kaplan, R.M., Thamsborg, S.M. et al. (2007). Climatic influences on development and survival of free-living stages of equine strongyles: implications for worm control strategies and managing anthelmintic resistance. *Veterinary Journal* 174 (1): 23–32.

23 Horserace Betting Levy Board. (2022). Code of practice: prevention [Online]. Available from: https://codes.hblb.org.uk/index.php/page/53 (accessed 25 February 2022).

24 Stewart, J.H., Rose, R.J., and Barko, A.M. (1984). Respiratory studies in foals from birth to seven days old. *Equine Veterinary Journal* 16 (4): 323–328.

Further Reading

Rendle, D., Austin, C., Bowen, M., Cameron, I., Furtado, T., Hodgkinson, J., McGorum, B., and Matthews, J. (2019). Equine de-worming: a consensus on current best practice roundtable [Online]. Available at: https://horsetrust.org.uk/wp-content/uploads/2019/12/UK-VET_EQUINE_2019_Equine_Worming_Roundtable-Equisal-Web.pdf (accessed 26 January 2023).

16

Donkeys

Dominique Doyle[1], Chloe Skewes[1], and Marie Rippingale[2]

[1] The Donkey Sanctuary, Sidmouth, Devon, UK
[2] Bottle Green Training Ltd, Derby, UK

The contents of this Chapter have been approved by The Donkey Sanctuary

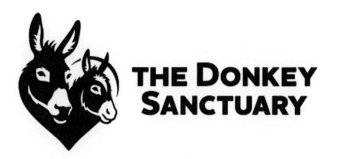

Introduction

Donkeys have been serving mankind for 5000 years [1]. The phrase 'beasts of burden' describes their utility as pack animals and in many parts of the world, they play a significant economic and social role. In the United Kingdom, most donkeys are kept, unlike the horse, as pets. Their increased popularity means that they are seen more frequently for treatment in equine practice. There are several anatomical and physiological differences between donkeys and horses. **Donkeys are not just small horses with big ears!** Therefore, donkey-specific protocols should be put in place and adhered to in equine veterinary practice. By following donkey-specific protocols, Registered veterinary nurses (RVNs) can ensure that donkeys receive individualised, species-specific nursing care and therefore have an optimum chance of recovery.

16.1 Behaviour

General Behaviour

Donkeys are highly intelligent and capable of learning; however, this is often overlooked, and donkeys are commonly referred to as stoical or stubborn [2]. These labels must be understood to make the handling and monitoring of donkeys safer and more efficient in practice. Stoicism is predator-avoidance behaviour typically exhibited by prey species. Illness and injury make prey species such as the donkey vulnerable to predators and the ability to hide weaknesses made them less likely to be targeted [2]. Stoic behaviour can make reading the signs of discomfort and pain in donkeys difficult in practice. A sick or injured donkey may show no obvious clinical signs until their condition is severe. **A dull or unusually quiet donkey is a veterinary emergency and requires immediate attention [2]**. It is therefore imperative that RVNs understand general donkey behaviour when it comes to monitoring and assessing comfort levels. See Section 16.6 for information about pain scoring.

So called 'stubborn behaviour' is associated with donkeys, and this is often a misunderstanding in relation to their stoical nature. Donkeys showing caution will often be misinterpreted as being stubborn [3]. Fear will often produce a defensive reaction from a donkey, and they will often try to escape. This behaviour should be recognised as fear and not misinterpreted as the donkey being stubborn or uncooperative [2]. Fear can produce 'flight', 'fight' and/or 'freeze' responses, and these can result in defensive behaviour.

Flight responses may include the following:

- Tail tucking and clamping
- Increased muscle tension, especially in the muzzle
- Turning the head away from the handler
- Stepping sideways slowly to avoid being caught

Fight responses can pose a health and safety risk to donkeys and people. These may include [2]:

- Head tossing
- Stamping, pawing and striking out
- Leaning or pushing into the handler. This can be dangerous when the handler is standing against a solid object.
- Biting
- Kicking. Unlike horses, donkeys can be very effective at kicking forwards with their hindlegs.

A freeze response can include:

- The donkey refusing to move and 'planting' themselves in one place.
- This behavioural response has led to donkeys being incorrectly associated with stubborn behaviour. It is important to remember that a frozen donkey is in fact scared and not being stubborn.
- See Table 16.1 for further information.

RVNs working with donkeys in practice should be able to recognise the signs of fear as this will facilitate intervention at an early stage. This will help to reduce stress to the donkey and the risk of injury to handlers.

Bonding and Bereavement

Donkeys form strong bonds for life with their companions. For this reason, donkeys should always be admitted to the practice with their companion(s). Separating donkey companions can lead to stress, anorexia, hyperlipaemia and death. If a donkey has a closely bonded companion(s), the companion(s) should be kept close by during any examinations and treatment [2]. Due to their tendency to form strong bonds, it is beneficial for the RVN to spend time with a sick donkey and their companion(s) (Figure 16.1). Tender loving care (TLC) in the form of grooming, petting and hand feeding can contribute enormously towards reducing stress and promoting recovery [4].

RVNs, in practice, should know how to manage a situation in which donkey companions are separated by death. If one of the donkeys dies or is euthanised, it is essential that the surviving companion(s) are allowed to remain with the body of their companion until they have lost interest [5]. The bereaved companion(s) should be closely monitored for several weeks afterwards, as bereavement stress can manifest itself up to three weeks after the death. If it is appropriate for all the animals involved, another quiet donkey could be introduced to the pair at home over a fence prior to euthanasia. This will mean that the survivor is left with a companion within its visual field [2]. After the euthanasia, a structured introduction can then be made between this pair. This process should be managed carefully. RVNs and veterinary surgeons (vets) can make a big difference in the quality of life of the remaining companion and the owner by offering advice and support during this process. If a surviving donkey is alone following bereavement, the RVN and vet should assess the requirement for a new companion. Individual donkeys may react differently to bereavement and may not need a new companion immediately [2].

16.2 Handling and Restraint

RVNs working in equine practice may be required to assist with the handling and restraint of donkeys either in the hospital or during out-on-yard visits. Regardless of the reason for handling or restraint, all involved should make sure that this is a positive experience for the donkey. This will help to reduce stress and the risk of injury to both the donkey and the handlers. It is always a good idea to consult the owner in these situations. It can be beneficial to have the owner present, as the donkey will already have a trusting relationship with them. Where this is not possible, the owner should be consulted as to which handling and restraint techniques might work best. If the donkey has a bonded companion, they should be present and remain in eyesight of their friend for the duration of the procedure [2]. When handling donkeys, appropriate personal protective equipment (PPE) should be worn, such as a hard hat, gloves and steel toe-capped boots. Table 16.1 presents different handling and restraining techniques for situations that may be encountered in equine practice.

Any handling or restraint should be made to be a positive experience for the donkey. Therefore, following the application of any restraint, the handler should spend some time with the donkey to provide some reassurance [2]. Food can be given as a reward as well as wither scratches if appropriate [2].

The need to use a twitch should be considered very carefully. A nose twitch applied to the top lip of the donkey may be effective, although each individual will react differently to this. Twitches should only ever be applied under veterinary supervision where there is no other option [2]. Twitches should not be used for procedures such as farriery, dental or routine veterinary treatments. They should never be left in place for more than five minutes. **Ear twitching in donkeys is not recommended.** It is painful and can result in defensive behaviour [2].

Behaviour modification can be approached with techniques such as shaping plans. The best way to help a donkey

Table 16.1 Handling and restraint techniques for donkeys.

Situation	Environmental considerations	Handling considerations	Physical restraint	Comments
Fearful donkey: A fearful donkey may employ flight behaviour and try to escape from the handlers. This behaviour is seen as barging, pulling away and dragging handlers. It is important to remember that this is a fear response and should be dealt with calmly and with the least physical restraint possible	• Quiet, calm environment • Remove anything that could cause injury • Have companion present • Have owner present if appropriate	• Ensure the donkey is wearing a correctly fitted headcollar • Stroke or fuss the donkey to provide reassurance [2] • Offer fibre feed in a bucket or a salt lick • Block the donkey's view of the clinician/procedure with hand or body position [2] • Do not put fingers or thumbs inside the headcollar during restraint as they could become injured if the donkey struggles [2]	• Stand on the left side of the donkey facing their head • Place your left arm over the top of the donkey's nose and hold their head into your body • Put your right arm over the donkey's head and place your hand against the edge of the cheekbone • Hold the head into your body • Lean your hip or leg into the donkey's brisket • Place your feet a comfortable width apart and remain stable if the donkey pushes forward [2] (Figure 16.2)	• Sedation may be required if the donkey poses a health and safety threat [2]
'Frozen' donkey: Donkeys may 'freeze' and become unwilling to move when they are fearful of new situations. It is important to allow the donkey time to assess the situation. Patient, sensitive handling is required [2]	• Remove unfamiliar objects • Turn lights on in dark areas • Open doors and gates as widely as possible • Spread straw or shavings on unfamiliar surfaces [2] • Have companion present • Have owner present if appropriate	• Walk the patient's companion in front of their friend and encourage them to follow • Use food incentives such as ginger biscuits • Back the donkey through doorways or into the stocks • Use a broad webbing strap around the donkey's hindquarters to encourage forward momentum • Blindfolds can be used but only if appropriate as this can cause panic [2]	• Always remain calm • Only apply small amounts of pressure where appropriate • Increasing levels of restraint and force will only heighten the donkey's fear and escalate their behaviour [2]	• Sedation may be required if the donkey poses a health and safety threat [2]

Source: Marie Rippingale.

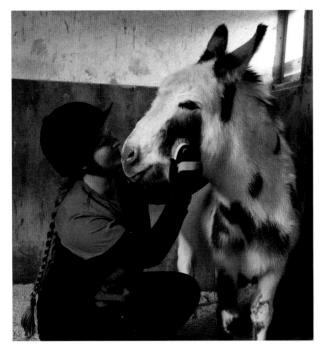

Figure 16.1 Grooming and spending time with donkeys can contribute significantly to their recovery. *Source:* Dr Francis Boyer.

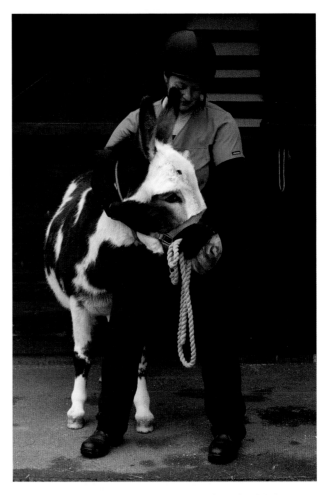

Figure 16.2 Physical restraint technique for a fearful donkey. *Source:* Dr Francis Boyer.

learn is to use the process of shaping behaviour [6]. Shaping is a process where the desired behaviour is broken down into small steps or learning blocks for the donkey to process. The small steps are then added together through training to build the final desired behaviour [6]. For example, behaviour shaping could be implemented to achieve a calm, safe farrier visit [6]. The steps involved in behaviour shaping can be written down to create a shaping plan that is easy to follow. If the plan is written down, it makes it less likely that steps will be missed out or misinterpreted and this will make the process more positive and efficient for the donkey and handlers involved. Further resources and information can be found by accessing The Donkey Academy. This is virtual learning environment provided by The Donkey Sanctuary. Please see the useful links section at the end of this chapter.

16.3 Nutrition

The domestic donkey is descended from African wild asses that evolved to live in semi-arid environments with only poor quality, sparse vegetation. To increase their potential food sources, donkeys have evolved as browsers as well as grazers with woody shrubs and trees being potential food sources when grasses and other low vegetation are not abundant [7]. Donkeys are highly efficient at digesting poor

nutritional quality fibre and possess a superior digestive efficiency compared to horses when digesting forages such as straw [8]. The donkey's natural adaptations to survive on poor quality feed when compared to ponies means that when donkeys are treated as mini horses or kept in the same way as their horse companions, they may become obese and subsequently develop serious health problems. This is a serious consideration for RVNs when caring for donkeys in practice.

Donkeys require a diet high in fibre and low in calories and will eat the equivalent of 1.3–1.8% of their body weight in dry matter each day. This equates to a standard-sized donkey of 180 kg in weight being fed 2.5–3.5 kg of good-quality barley straw over 24 hours [9]. This is dependent on the season, with the lower value being required in the summer. This value is also calculated assuming that the donkey has no dental issues. Donkeys with poor teeth may require further alterations to their diet. Straw should form the majority of the diet for most donkeys as it is high

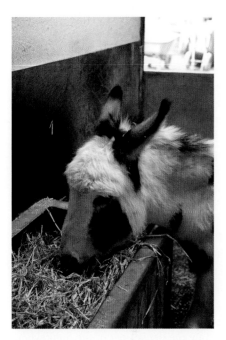

Figure 16.3 Good quality barley straw is ideal to feed to donkeys with good teeth. *Source:* Dr Francis Boyer.

in fibre and low in sugar. Good quality barley straw is ideal for feeding donkeys with good teeth (Figure 16.3). Oat straw is better suited to old or underweight donkeys with good teeth as this has a slightly higher nutritional value than barley straw [10].

A RVN working in equine practice should source the appropriate feed for donkeys if they are admitted. If the donkeys eat straw at home, it is important to keep their diet the same to avoid gastrointestinal upset. If straw cannot be sourced, the owners should be asked to bring in forage from home to avoid an abrupt dietary change. A feed balancer should also be fed to provide extra vitamins and minerals. The RVN could also give the donkeys access to an equine mineral lick.

Following a full veterinary examination, diagnosis and, based on a treatment plan, an inappetent, poorly donkey should be tempted with anything it will eat. These patients should be hand fed with bread, carrots, apples and/or ginger biscuits. Donkeys with poor teeth may struggle to chew these. In this case, carrots and apples can be grated and added to the feed. If this is not practical, mashed tinned carrots or small amounts of apple sauce could be used [9]. It is important to avoid feeding cereal-based coarse mixes to donkeys as they do not require the high sugar and starch levels provided by such feeds. Problems such as gastric ulceration, laminitis and obesity could occur as a result of overfeeding [9]. An anorexic, very sick donkey must be managed according to the condition being treated and in consultation with the case vet.

Water

A clean supply of water should always be available to donkeys. Water intake will vary but is on average about 4–9% of body weight per day during rest. Donkeys prefer clean water, so in the hospital, the RVN should ensure that water is changed at least daily. If it is very cold, tepid water can be offered to encourage water intake. If tepid water is offered, the temperature should be checked beforehand to make sure it is safe for drinking. Fruit juice and mint can be added to drinking water to encourage consumption. Clean, fresh water should always be offered separately.

16.4 Differences in Anatomy and Physiology

There are several anatomical and physiological differences between donkeys and horses. These differences should change how donkeys are viewed from a treatment and nursing care perspective.

Physiological Parameters

The physiological parameters of the donkey are different when compared to those of the horse. Table 16.2 shows the normal parameters for horses and donkeys.

Hooves

A major difference between the horse/pony and the donkey is their hooves. Donkeys have upright pasterns, with their hoof wall being between 5% and 10% steeper. Additionally, their hoof wall is a constant thickness from heel to toe. The appearance of the donkey's sole is likened to a U-shape, with a narrow, more developed heel contributing to an overall cylindrical shape as opposed to the conical shape hoof of a horse or pony. While the donkey has a more developed heel with a slight flare, it is paired with a broader frog that does not extend as far proximally in their hoof compared to horses and ponies. This means that the frog does not give the same support to the donkey's pedal bone.

Table 16.2 Normal parameters for donkeys and horses [2].

Parameter	Donkey	Horse
Temperature	36.5–37.8 °C	37–38.5 °C
Pulse rate	36–52 beats per minute	24–40 beats per minute
Respiration rate	12–38 breaths per minute	8–16 breaths per minute

Source: Chloe Skewes and The Donkey Sanctuary.

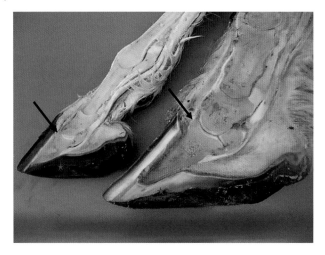

Figure 16.4 This image displays a cross section of a normal donkey hoof (left) and normal horse hoof (right). The black arrows indicate the level at which P3 begins, note the donkey's pedal bone is roughly 1 cm below the coronary band whereas the horse's is level. The red stars indicate how far forward the horses frog extends towards the toe providing support to the horse's pedal bone compared to the donkey. *Source:* The Donkey Sanctuary.

Therefore, the use of frog supports for a laminitic donkey is not appropriate [2].

These differences in hoof anatomy, combined with an underdeveloped pectoral muscle and a donkey's overall smaller size and stature, give them a noticeably narrower gait when stationary and mobile compared to the horse or pony. The internal anatomy of their hooves is different in that their pedal bone begins just 1 cm below the coronary band (Figure 16.4). When handling donkeys for procedures like foot radiographs, it is important to be aware that they have a lower centre of gravity when compared with horses. When picking up their feet to place or position them for radiographs, they need to be held lower and closer to the ground for them to be comfortable and balanced. This also applies when picking out their hooves [2].

The donkey's hoof has a higher moisture content compared to horses or ponies; this difference serves them well when living in a dry, rocky environment. However, in the humid, wet conditions experienced in the United Kingdom, this characteristic means their hooves are more pliable, permeable and at a higher risk of hoof pathologies. For instance, white line disease and abscess formation are common in donkeys [2].

Coat

The donkey's coat does not possess the waterproofing abilities of horses as they do not produce the same quantities of natural grease. In a study that compared the coat properties of horse, donkeys and mules, it was discovered that donkeys had significantly lower hair weight and hair length than horses, both in the winter and in the spring [11]. There were also large seasonal changes in hair weight and length for both horses and mules, but not for donkeys [11]. These differences make donkeys less able to tolerate wet and cold weather. Donkeys should be provided with suitable shelter all year around. Secondary to providing shelter, additional support can be provided in cold weather conditions with appropriate rugging [9]. When nursing donkeys, it is vital to be aware of their susceptibility to cold. General anaesthesia, standing sedation and recovery can put them at greater risk of hypothermia in comparison to horses or ponies.

Donkeys should be checked over carefully for the presence of ectoparasites and sarcoids, the signs of which can be hidden be long, dense coats [2]. Donkeys can be affected by the same ectoparasites as horses and ponies, and these are diagnosed and treated similarly. It is important to be aware that topical application of treatments for ectoparasites may be affected by the dense coat of the donkey and this may limit effective distribution of the treatment [2]. For more information regarding ectoparasites, see Chapter 5. For more information regarding sarcoids, see Chapter 12.

Injection Sites

When blood sampling or placing intravenous (IV) catheters in donkeys using their jugular vein, it is important to note their prominent cutaneous coli muscle, which lies along the middle third of the jugular groove. This makes the upper and lower third the best sites for injection. Additionally, a steeper angle of introduction is required for accurate access to the jugular vein in comparison to horses or ponies. Due to donkeys having thicker skin, it is recommended to use local anaesthetic and a cut down for IV catheterisation (Figure 16.5). When choosing a site for intramuscular (IM) injection, the pectoral muscle is not appropriate because it is underdeveloped compared to horses or ponies alternative, more appropriate injection sites should be used [2] (Figure 16.6).

Nasolacrimal Duct

The anatomical positioning of the nasolacrimal duct in donkeys is different to its location in a horse or pony. The donkey's duct is found on the upper aspect of their nares whereas in the horse this opening of the duct is found on the lower aspect of the nostrils. The reason for this could be that the dorsolateral position of the duct opening in the donkey could reduce its likelihood of becoming blocked from sand or dust in the desert environment the donkey originates from [2].

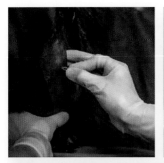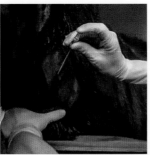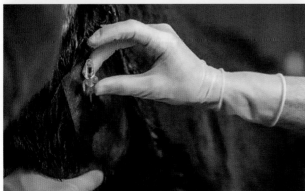

Figure 16.5 This series of images demonstrate intravenous catheter placement in the donkey. The first image shows a sterile cut down of the skin following a local anaesthetic bleb. Note the steeper angle of introduction when introducing the catheter in the second image. *Source:* The Donkey Sanctuary.

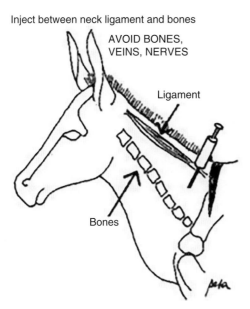

Inject between neck ligament and bones

AVOID BONES, VEINS, NERVES

Ligament

Bones

Figure 16.6 This image shows one of the appropriate intramuscular injection sites in the donkey. *Source:* The Donkey Sanctuary.

Number of Vertebrae

The number of vertebrae differs slightly between donkeys and horses. Table 16.3 provides a comparison between the donkey and the horse. The donkey has one fewer lumbar vertebra and four fewer coccygeal vertebrae when compared to the horse or pony [12]. It is useful to note that the site for epidural injections is more caudal compared to horses due to the ease of access in this location.

Table 16.3 Normal number of vertebrae for horses and donkeys.

Vertebrae type	Donkey	Horse
Cervical	7	7
Thoracic	18	18
Lumbar	5	6
Sacral	5	5
Coccygeal/Caudal	15–17	15–21

Source: Chloe Skewes.

Differences in Medications and Drug Metabolism

Very few drugs are licensed specifically for donkeys. Drug dosages used in horses are often transferable under the cascade for use in the donkey. As there are physiological differences between donkeys and other equids, there are also differences in pharmacokinetics, meaning that drug doses and frequency of administration may need adapting for the donkey. Although it is not a definitive rule, donkeys' drug metabolism is generally faster than in horses or ponies. This is because donkeys have adapted by evolving to live in arid and sparse environments with a reduced water supply. They can recycle water more efficiently to cope better with dehydration compared to horses.

Donkeys can maintain their blood plasma volume when up to 20% dehydrated [13]. This affects drug distribution and contributes to both the clearance rate and the half-life of medications being shorter in the donkey. Recommendations are to reduce the dosing interval of medications instead of increasing the dose itself. An accurate weight is essential, and the best practice is to weigh the donkey using an electronic weighbridge. Alternatively, the dedicated donkey weigh tape and nomogram, which accounts both a donkey's height and heart girth measurements can be used to estimate weight. An accurate weight is important to ensure effective dosing is achieved and to reduce the risk of toxicity [2].

There is variation in metabolism within the species, donkeys of different sizes can metabolise some medications at different rates [2]. For example, miniature donkeys metabolise phenylbutazone faster, and they require more

Table 16.4 Drugs and dosages used in donkeys with key donkey specific information.

Name of drug	Dose	Route	Comments for use in the donkey
Carprofen	0.7—1.3 mg/kg q24hrs	IV PO (orally)	Give IV as a single dose. Metabolised more slowly in donkeys
Etorphine			MUST NEVER BE USED IN THE DONKEY
Ketamine	2.2—2.8 mg/kg bwt	IV	Cleared more rapidly in donkeys, especially miniature donkeys. More frequent top-ups required for total IV anaesthesia
Meloxicam	0.6 mg/kg	IV	Not advised for use in donkeys – very short half-life
Phenylbutazone	2.2 mg/kg—4.4 mg/kg q12hr in standard. q8hr in miniatures	IV, PO	More rapid clearance than in horses. Administer twice daily to donkeys and three times daily to miniature donkeys
Flunixin	1.1 mg/kg q12hrs	IV, PO	
Fentanyl			Larger dose patch on mg/kg basis required to achieve comparable plasma levels of fentanyl; analgesic levels achieved more rapidly; more frequent patch changes required. Accurate dose rates not confirmed
Tramadol		PO	Poor oral bioavailability (reported as 11.7%). Not recommended for use in donkeys
Gentamicin	66 mg/kg SID (once per day)	IV	Care in mammoth asses: volume of distribution is lower so take care to avoid toxicity: A lower dose should be used in hypovolaemic animals but a shorter dosing interval may be required to keep levels above minimum inhibitory concentration
Oxytetracycline	5-10 mg/kg q12—24hrs	Slow IV	Shorter elimination half-life. Dosing interval should be half that recommended for horses. More data required
Na Penicillin G	20,000 IU/kg IV q4—6hrs	IV	Shorter dosing intervals required in donkeys for beta-lactam antibiotics. More comparative studies required
Trimethoprim sulphamethoxazole	30 mg/kg q12hrs	PO	Volume of distribution and elimination rate of trimethoprim differs to that of sulphonamides, therefore ratio may not be optimal for donkeys. However, commonly used effectively in donkeys
Danofloxacin			Does not achieve effective plasma concentrations in donkeys at 1.25 mg/kg
Marbofloxacin	0.33—2.6 mg/kg q24hrs	Slow IV	Slower elimination in donkeys. 0.33 mg/kg for Enterobacteriaceae sp. 2.6 mg/kg Staphylococcus aureus
Norfloxacin			Not suitable for use in donkeys: IV administration at 10 mg/kg has induced seizures, IM has caused local swelling, and oral administration has low availability
Buprenorphine	5-10 µg/kg q8hrs	IV	
Detomidine	0.01—0.04 mg/kg 0.04—008 mg/kg 0.04 mg/kg	IV IM Oral gel	Donkeys may require larger doses to achieve adequate sedation IM dose 1.5—2× IV dose. Maximal effects in quiet, unstimulating environment after injection
Firocoxib		PO	Good oral bioavailability, shorter half-life than in horses and ponies. More research needed to determine optimum dosing interval
Dexamethasone	0.05—0.2 mg/kg q24hrs	IV, IM or PO	Contraindicated in hyperlipidaemic animals
Guaifenesin	To effect ~50—110 mg/kg needed for induction	IV	Metabolised more rapidly in donkeys than horses and ponies but donkeys show greater sensitivity. For a donkey specific 'triple drip' recipe see Chapter 17: Sedation, Anaesthesia and Analgesics
Heparin sodium	100—200 IU/kg q8—12hrs	IV	May be used in hyperlipaemia. Check clotting factors before initiating treatment
Imidocarb dipropionate	2 mg/kg q24hrs for Babesia caballi 4 mg/kg q3 days for four treatments for B. equi	IM IM	DO NOT USE IMIDOCARB DIHYDROCHLORIDE IN DONKEYS. Take care with imidocarb dipropionate as it can cause muscle necrosis, central nervous signs and death at higher doses

Source: The Donkey Sanctuary.

frequent dosing intervals of three times daily or every eight hours. Standard-size donkeys are dosed every 12 hours with phenylbutazone. There are other anti-inflammatories used in horses that are also given to donkeys; for instance, Flunixin meglumine every 12 hours is used as a first-line peri-operative choice with phenylbutazone for ongoing analgesia. Whereas these anti-inflammatories can be suitable for use in horses every 24 hours, they should be administered to donkeys every 12 hours due to their faster metabolic rate. Phenylbutazone can be started at a loading dose of 4.4 mg/kg but should then be reduced to a maintenance dose of 2.2 mg/kg after the initial loading period. Although Meloxicam is used as an anti-inflammatory in horses, it is not recommended for use in the donkey as they metabolise it too quickly [2].

Donkeys metabolise sedatives more quickly than horses and can require higher doses to achieve adequate levels of sedation. Table 16.4 provides information on drugs and dosages used in donkeys.

16.5 Common Donkey Disorders

It is beyond the scope of this chapter to discuss every disorder that affects donkeys. Therefore, the most common disorders will be discussed in the hope that this will give the reader a good foundation of knowledge to build on. The reader is directed to the further reading section for more information.

Hyperlipaemia

Causes

Hyperlipaemia is a common complication that donkeys, are particularly susceptible to as both a primary and secondary condition. It is a result of a negative energy balance, for instance, when the body's energy reserves are limited. Primary hyperlipaemia is usually caused by internal factors to the donkey such as existing insulin resistance. Secondary hyperlipaemia is usually caused by an extrinsic factor such as a stressor and this means that a donkey who is inappetent, anorexic, starved or not provided with sufficient nutrition for their body to function, for example, during pregnancy or a disease state, is at an increased risk. Other risk factors associated with hyperlipaemia are obesity, a heavy worm burden, rapid weight loss and increased age. Donkeys over 18 months are more commonly affected [14]. Alongside these risk factors, hyperlipaemia is exacerbated by stress, which can result from illness, changes to their routine, including their individual or group management, turnout or dietary change and a change in environment or transportation.

Unlike horses, donkeys are not often familiar with travelling, this can elevate their stress levels, which indefinitely increases the risk of them developing hyperlipaemia or worsening their condition. Therefore, when preparing for the hospitalisation of donkeys, the RVN must focus on making the hospital environment as suitable for them as possible. Stabling areas should be large enough to accommodate one donkey and a companion. If this is not possible, their companion should be stabled next to the patient to allow physical contact. Being aware that donkeys are smaller than horses is important; the ability to lower stable doors or make safe adaptations will reduce their stress levels. Donkeys are often not familiar with horses or ponies; stabling without other equids nearby is more suitable for donkeys and their companions. Being aware of possible stresses for donkeys while hospitalised is vital as they do not always display signs of stress outwardly. Prevention of stress and making changes to reduce stress are proactive ways to nurse donkeys effectively.

It is often difficult for the vet to diagnose the primary cause of hyperlipaemia in many cases, leading to symptomatic treatment in the absence of a definitive diagnosis. The Donkey Sanctuary recommend testing at risk presurgical patients for hyperlipaemia. The survival of donkeys post colic surgery have been observed to be lower when compared to horses due to hyperlipaemia.

Pathophysiology

A negative energy balance triggers the body to overmetabolise triglycerides from fat reserves, a process that donkeys' body systems cannot efficiently switch off (Figure 16.7). When a large amount of fat is circulating

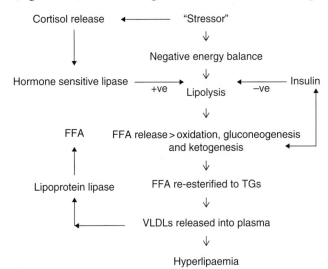

Figure 16.7 Pathway for mobilisation of fats stored in adipose tissue as an energy source. FFA = free fatty acids; VLDL = very low-density lipoprotein; TG = triglyceride. *Source:* The Donkey Sanctuary.

in the blood, it results in fatty infiltration of organs, including the liver, pancreas and kidneys, leading to irreversible damage and multiple organ failure [2]. Early detection and treatment in the initial stages are paramount to reducing the chances of mortality.

Clinical Signs

Hyperlipaemia is often hard to identify. Clinical signs that a donkey is entering a hyperlipidaemic state are often non-specific and can be triggered by other conditions [2]. RVNs should be aware that any hospitalised donkey post-surgery or tooth extraction, for example, or those with untreated dental conditions, colic or choke, may develop hyperlipaemia. Therefore, if donkeys present any of the following clinical signs, they should be considered a clinical emergency and a vet should be informed immediately:

- Dullness
- Inappetence
- Anorexia
- Reduced gut motility
- Halitosis
- Reduced faecal output
- Faeces that are dry or mucous-covered

Diagnosis

Diagnosis requires an urgent biochemistry blood sample prior to results confirming high triglycerides; a visual interpretation of the blood and whether the serum appears milky may be an initial indication to begin supportive treatment and nursing interventions immediately (Figure 16.8).

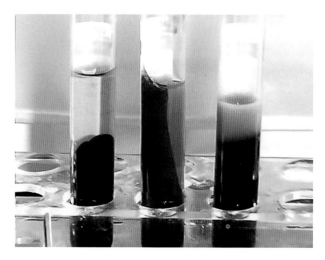

Figure 16.8 Clotted blood samples. From left to right. The first sample shows a normal clear serum. The second is beginning to become cloudy when triglycerides are moderately elevated and the third milky coloured serum indicates severely elevated triglycerides. Source: The Donkey Sanctuary.

Treatment
Pharmacological Intervention

Analgesia management in the form of non-steroidal anti-inflammatories (NSAIDs) is important combined with administering gastro-protectants.

Severe Cases

The severity of the patient's state of hyperlipaemia and the clinical picture determined by the vet will impact how frequently a RVN is required to provide critical care monitoring to the patient. All inappetent patients will require a minimum of two hourly checks with those receiving IV fluids and parental nutrition being more frequent. Monitoring of patients should include taking their temperature, heart rate, including pulse quality and respiratory rate (TPR), mucous membrane colour and capillary refill time check as well as auscultating borborygmi (gut sounds) and checking for digital pulses. Both composite and facial pain-scoring using specific donkey pain scales is hugely important combined with an assessment of the patient's demeanour and interaction with their companion (see Section 16.6). These factors contribute to a holistic nursing approach and assist in monitoring a patient's progression.

Mild Cases

Mild cases of hyperlipaemia may not require hospitalisation; the vet will assess the patient and may decide that support in the form of glucose supplementation is required; dosages can be calculated and administered via dosing syringe or added to a feed by an RVN, given that a vet has authorised the dose. Supplementation following this method will only be possible if the patient has some voluntary appetite. Donkeys that present with some voluntary appetite may require less frequent nursing observations, but it is important to check how much they are eating to assess whether they require additional nutritional support. RVNs need to be aware of and be able to identify when a donkey may be 'sham' eating. This is where donkeys will appear to perform mastication of feed but actually ingest very little [2]. Weighing the forage or feed offered and eaten is an accurate method of monitoring what the patient is ingesting.

Supplementary Feeding and Fluids

Patients who are inappetent may require immediate energy via a nasogastric tube administered 2–3 times per day. The mixture would consist of a fibre-rich product like micronised oat-based breakfast cereal or liquidised pellet feed with additional electrolytes and glucose. At times, an RVN may be required to administer these feeds orally via a dosing syringe, depending on patient compliance. Feeding via nasogastric tube is only appropriate where there is no ileus, otherwise this can lead to bloat and tympany. In some cases, a vet may decide that enteral feeding methods should be combined with IV fluid therapy. In extreme cases, a donkey may be admitted for IV fluids for rehydration alongside parental IV nutrition to restore a positive energy balance [2]. These patients require close monitoring and strict IV catheter care. RVNs should perform a visual inspection of the catheter site, clean the immediate area if contaminated, regularly flush the catheter with heparin saline at a minimum of four hourly intervals, and disinfect the catheter port before administering medications if a self-disinfecting bung is not used. Donkeys, like horses, are at increased risk of jugular vein thrombophlebitis from long-term catheterisation or irritation from injectable medications.

RVNs and patient care assistants (PCAs) can tempt patients to eat from their hands as opposed to large buckets as they will often be refused [2]. Using tempting foods such as the following can encourage donkeys to eat:

- Fresh or dried mint
- Mint cordial
- Bananas and their skins
- Grated ginger
- Carrots
- Apples
- Ginger biscuits.

If a donkey is refusing feed but can be led to a nearby hedgerow with their companion, their natural instinct to browse can stimulate a donkey's appetite (Figure 16.9). Allowing patients this opportunity to browse can be hugely beneficial, and its importance can be overlooked at times [2]. If access to a hedgerow is not possible, cutting a selection of brambles, hazel and other non-toxic shrubs to offer the donkey in the stable can be a suitable substitute. Examples of toxic shrubs, trees and plants that should be avoided are:

- Bracken
- Oak
- Elder
- Laurel
- Ivy
- Hemlock
- Sycamore

A factsheet regarding poisonous plants and trees is accessible on The Donkey Sanctuary website for further reading [15]. Donkeys recovering from hyperlipaemia can also benefit from browsing to help maintain their appetite. Once a patient's appetite has returned, they will require support to maintain this. RVNs should always remain conscientious of subtle changes in the appetite or demeanour of their patients. Hospitalised donkeys must have access to their usual diet as they may favour it over other feed available to them. Additionally, RVNs should record and give a visual description of faecal output in addition to gut sounds. If these are reduced, a vet must be informed, as patients receiving NSAIDs while stabled in a hospital setting are at risk of developing ileus or an impaction [2].

Laminitis

Laminitis is the inflammation of the soft tissue connecting the hoof and pedal bone called the laminae. When these structures get damaged, it causes the pedal bone to move, rotate and or remodel. These changes to the bone are often irreversible, and the pain associated can be extreme, with euthanasia in severe cases being necessary.

Causes

Causes and contributing factors of laminitis are the same as in horses and ponies, although some possibly have increased significance in donkeys. The causes can be allocated into three broad categories [16]:

- *Category one is supporting limb laminitis*: This is seen in donkeys that have acute, uncontrolled painful lameness in one limb that causes them to overload the contralateral limb. Management changes such as transportation or walking on hard ground can cause a bout of acute laminitis on top of a previously undiagnosed case of chronic laminitis.
- *Category two is toxic/inflammatory related laminitis*: This has not been extensively researched in donkeys but is expected to have the same mode of action as in other

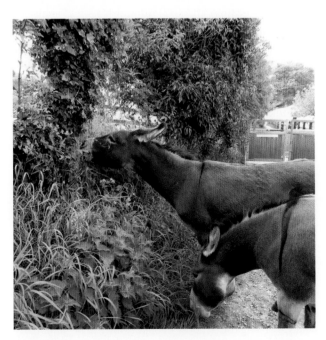

Figure 16.9 Donkey patient and companion browsing freely while supervised. *Source:* The Donkey Sanctuary.

equids. At The Donkey Sanctuary, endotoxin-induced laminitis has been observed in cases of septicaemia, associated with acute typhlocolitis and other septic processes. Inappropriate nutrition leading to obesity can also contribute to the development of laminitis. For example, having access to lush grass or cereals is a risk factor and a common cause of laminitis in donkeys with or without underlying metabolic disease.

- *Category three is endocrinopathic causes of laminitis*: This can occur secondary to other hormonal imbalances or disturbances due to conditions like equine metabolic syndrome (EMS) and pituitary pars intermedia dysfunction (PPID). With these patients, obesity is a serious problem. Reduced energy requirements and chronic food overload result in hyperinsulinaemia.

Clinical Signs

Donkeys are known for their stoical nature, which affects the way they behave with foot pain in comparison to horses, and do not tend to show the classic equine stance as horses do unless severely affected. Donkeys can suffer from acute and chronic laminitis as other equids can. Donkeys that present with acute laminitis display sudden pain affecting both forelimbs and sometimes a positive response to hoof testers. However, if a donkey does not respond to hoof testers, it does not mean they are not affected by laminitis; this could be due to donkeys generally having thicker soles but also due to large hoof testers not always being appropriate for their smaller hooves. Further clinical signs include:

- Increased periods of recumbency
- Shortened gait
- Subtle weight shifting to alleviate pain between each hoof
- Altered weight distribution
- Strong digital pulses
- Heat in the hooves [2].

Digital pulses should be assessed daily in hospitalised donkeys to allow early identification and treatment should laminitis occur.

Donkeys suffering from chronic laminitis do not display a sudden lameness in their forefeet but may display a pain response to hoof testers. Donkeys with chronic laminitis can show an altered gait with a shortened stride, but when these subtle mobility changes occur over time it can be harder to notice. Physically, their external hoof may display structural changes, for example, laminitic rings in the hoof wall, which spread out towards the heel, a flat, dropped sole and often a stretched white line. Chronic laminitis also causes clinical signs that are not visible externally, which require radiographs to be taken. These are changes in the internal structures of the hoof. As mentioned, the pedal bone can move or sink in the hoof in relation to the coronary band, in addition to it possibly rotating or remodelling.

Diagnosis

Diagnosis of acute laminitis by a vet is based on the donkey's presenting clinical signs, which are relevant to laminitis, together with observing their behaviour and pain score. Blood testing and radiography are part of the diagnostic process, which can be helpful in determining if the donkey is suffering from chronic laminitis. Blood testing is advised when laminitis cannot be given a mechanical or inflammatory cause, as this could indicate an underlying contributing disease factor.

Treatment

Management and Husbandry

Treatment for laminitis in a donkey is similar to that of a horse or pony. Initially, box rest on deep, non-edible bedding with footpads provides some initial relief. Supporting both forelimbs with pads is an advisable precautionary measure that could reduce the chances of overload laminitis if both limbs are not already affected [16]. When box resting a donkey, they should have a bonded companion resting with them or nearby to avoid exacerbating their stress [16].

Pharmacological Intervention

Analgesia will be prescribed by a vet to reduce the pain caused by laminitis; multimodal analgesia is preferable, and a combination of NSAIDs, paracetamol and opioids are found to be most effective. Administration of analgesia should be followed by consistent and regular pain scoring, including noticing subtle changes in behaviour. This is extremely important as it means vets and RVNs have a consistent scale in order to effectively detect acute pain and monitor the donkey's individual response. This ensures the donkey is receiving adequate pain relief.

Cryotherapy

Cryotherapy uses cold temperatures to reduce inflammation. It can make a significant difference in the donkeys' prognosis when utilised at the onset of first clinical signs. At The Donkey Sanctuary, RVNs aim to begin cryotherapy within one hour of a vet examining a donkey with suspected acute laminitis. It is important to act promptly within a few hours as after this timeframe cold therapy is unlikely to be effective with a risk of being detrimental to the patient. Determining when to begin cryotherapy in donkeys is challenging. Initial clinical signs can be very subtle, causing the window of opportunity to be potentially shortened. Donkeys should be monitored closely for any of the clinical signs listed previously. Cryotherapy should only be utilised in cases where a vet has confirmed acute laminitis and authorised the treatment to begin. This treatment method is not to be applied to donkeys suffering from chronic laminitis because the aim of cold therapy is to reduce the inflammation of the laminae during an acute episode. It will not improve the physical deterioration of chronic laminitic cases and can be detrimental. The Donkey Sanctuary uses 'ice boots' made from empty 3-l fluid bags filled with ice and tied so that the hoof and pasterns are fully submerged (Figure 16.10). Specialised boots can be sourced; however, they are not always the best fit for smaller donkeys. To be most effective, the therapy should keep the hoof wall surface at a temperature of 7–10 °C for 48 hours; this will require regular ice refills. Donkeys usually tolerate this therapy very well in comparison to other equids, and a reduction in their pain scores can often be seen within 24 hours.

When managing donkeys for laminitis, it is important to ensure they have access to enrichment activities to help keep them occupied while on box rest. At The Donkey Sanctuary, box-rested donkeys are provided with a selection of treats picked from hedgerows. These include any non-toxic plants and shrubs, for instance, brambles, hazel branches and gorse. These can be tied or hung in bunches for the donkey to browse (Figure 16.11).

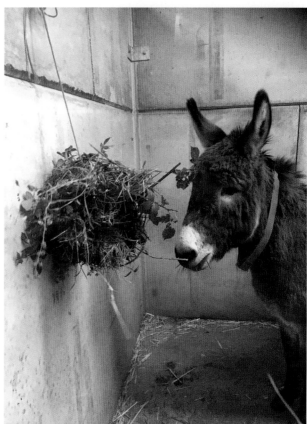

Figure 16.11 Hospitalised donkey and companion enjoying enrichment while on box rest. *Source:* The Donkey Sanctuary.

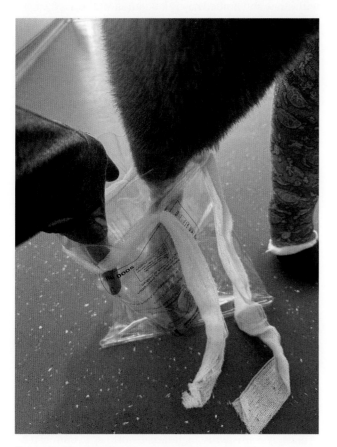

Figure 16.10 Repurposing empty fluid bags to utilise them as ice boots, more suitably sized for donkeys. The hoof is submerged in ice ensuring the donkeys sole is flat in the bottom of the boot not unbalanced on ice as this can cause discomfort. Conforming bandage is used to secure the boot. *Source:* The Donkey Sanctuary.

Remedial Farriery

Radiographs will provide information on the condition of the inner hoof and can guide further treatments. The vet can decide if and what type of remedial farriery is required. For example, in donkeys, rim shoes are found to be beneficial. Farriers apply rim shoes by using polyurethane composites often in the form of fast-drying glue, to build a shoe around the hoof wall in layers, which is then rasped into shape. The purpose of a rim shoe is to reduce the pressure on a thin sole. Although rim shoes are used in donkeys, shoes with frog supports known as heart bars are not suitable for donkeys. This is because heart bars are designed to support a horse or ponies' frog, which in turn supports their pedal bone beneath, whereas a donkey's frog is broader at the heel and does not extend as far forward towards their toe. In the acute stages of laminitis, a thick cotton foot pad covering the entire frog and sole is recommended, as this provides complete solar support and helps to distribute the load evenly throughout the hoof. Alternatively, rim shoes made from acrylic and filled with gel inserts can be applied for longer-term solar support and comfort for laminitic donkeys. Chronic laminitis can cause a donkey's sole to become abnormally thin resulting in increased sensitivity, so the gel inserts work to provide additional protection. Rim shoes are lightweight and better suited to donkeys compared to traditional steel shoes that may be used for horses or ponies.

Dietary Management

These physical treatments for laminitis in donkeys should be combined with essential changes in dietary management. In acute cases, the donkey must be removed from the pasture and provided with a change in diet as specified above. The donkey's appetite, gut motility and faecal output must be monitored closely when nursing these patients because reduced movement from box rest could result in hyperlipaemia or impaction colic [17]. Straw is an appropriate dietary option, but for donkeys with a dental disease requiring a special diet, a short-chopped feeding equivalent with a low non-structural carbohydrates (NSCs) is required. Hay often has a higher NSC, which makes it unsuitable for laminitics whereas haylage can be appropriate if it is high in fibre content and a declared NSC level. Haylage often has a lower sugar content when compared to hay as it is fermented. In the short-term, forage with a NSC level of less than 10% is most suitable [2].

Donkeys must maintain an appetite, so if their usual diet is ab-lib grass, it is not always appropriate for them to be given only straw or stover (an alternative fibrous forage similar to straw usually harvested from maize/corn) immediately, as despite it being an ideal long-term diet, it could cause them to become inappetent. Dietary change, box rest and analgesia can all contribute to an intestinal impaction being detected late, so careful monitoring of faecal output and gut sounds is required. Providing a very small amount of hay could help to ease the transition and assist in maintaining a voluntary appetite. The energy level of hay can be easily reduced by soaking it for 6–8 hours, as this will reduce the sugar content and will help to provide some extra water in the diet also. When nursing any hospitalised donkey, not just those who are laminitics, maintaining hydration and encouraging water intake is important. Warming drinking water can be helpful, and flavouring it with fruit juices or mint can encourage compliance, as well as being a source of enrichment. Clean, fresh water should always be offered separately. If a donkey's appetite is reduced, unmolassed, wet, beet feed can be used for laminitics to help maintain fluid intake in addition to being a palatable feed, which is useful for mixing in oral medications.

Laminitic donkeys require a high-fibre and low-sugar diet, meaning a food source low in NSC is required. Donkeys are more efficient at digesting fibre when compared to horses, which means that they maintain well on a lower nutritional fibre like straw or stover [18]. This diet should be combined with a controlled weight loss programme if the donkey is overweight. Weight loss and changes to diet must be implemented slowly, as excessive dietary restriction or starvation can trigger hyperlipaemia [2]. Making dietary changes for patients suffering from acute or chronic laminitis is an essential part of a treatment and prevention plan.

A maintenance diet for a donkey at risk of laminitis is one that an obese or overweight donkey would require: low NSC, including sugars preferably this would be straw or stover, given that a dental check suggests their oral health is satisfactory. Donkeys in warmer climates should be maintained on straw and limited access to grazing, ideally less than 0.2 acres per donkey and not in excess of 0.5 acres. In colder climates, less than 10 °C, they should be provided with straw and limited hay [2]. Rotating and correctly managing pasture that donkeys graze is important as grass that has been stressed by being overgrazing is at risk of having a higher NSC and sugar content that is similar to lush or frosty grass [2].

In a hospital environment, it is important to make appropriate changes to a sick patient's diet, as those who are recovering or healing may require increased energy.

Pituitary Pars Intermedia Dysfunction (PPID)

PPID, or equine Cushing's disease (ECD), is a hormonal disorder that affects the pituitary gland in the brain, specifically the pars intermedia. The nerve fibres supplying the gland become damaged, which causes the release of excess hormones, mainly adrenocorticotropic hormone (ACTH). The condition progresses with age as the damage to the nerve fibres increases when uncontrolled.

Clinical Signs

Clinical signs of the condition between donkeys and other equids can differ; donkeys rarely present with hirsutism (the classic hairy coat), excessive sweating, drinking and urination, which is typical of horses and ponies [19]. Common symptoms seen in donkeys include:

- An increased susceptibility to endo and ectoparasite burdens. A consistently high faecal worm egg count can be an indication of PPID.
- Change in body shape, weight loss, loss of muscle mass and abnormal fat deposition combined with insulin resistance.

- Lethargy and a poor demeanour may occur. However, these are not often easy symptoms to spot.
- Unexplained or recurrent bouts of laminitis must be recognised as a possible result of PPID, as this condition can cause hyperinsulinaemia, which has a direct association with laminitis in donkeys and ponies [2].
- Immunosuppression can result in complications with wound healing. It is important to be aware of this when nursing or managing donkeys with both surgical and traumatic wounds [20].

Diagnosis

Diagnostic testing for PPID involves a blood sample to check the basal ACTH levels following the same protocol as utilised in horses and ponies. The diagnostic ranges for ACTH differ depending on the time of year; between November and June, the range is 2.7–30.4 pg/ml, and between July and October, it is 9.0–49.1 pg/ml. These are donkey-specific reference ranges that The Donkey Sanctuary has developed for donkeys between the ages of 3 and 20. Readings in excess of these ranges could suggest that a donkey has underlying PPID [2]. Severe stress or pain can alter the results as a result of general anaesthesia, sedation, illness or acute laminitis. Although older equids are susceptible to PPID, there is evidence to suggest younger donkeys are also affected, so monitoring for clinical signs in all ages is advised.

Treatment

Treatment is the same as used in horses and ponies and includes medicating with pergolide. When observing donkeys who are beginning pergolide treatment, it is important to monitor their appetite because the medication is administered orally in tablet form, which can be refused. Disguising the tablet in a sandwich of bread or ginger biscuits, with a small amount of jam or marmite, can make medications more palatable, as can adding the medication directly to a piece of apple or carrot. Another option is to try disguising the medication in a forage ball, which can be made from a small amount of soaked forage balancer moulded into a ball and offered by hand or in a bucket.

Alternatively, dissolving the tablet in a small amount of water or squash in a dosing syringe enables it to be mixed into a small feed or administered as an oral drench, although the latter is not a sustainable long term as daily oral drenching can cause donkeys to become resentful of intervention, handling or eating as they can become suspicious of being medicated and unfamiliar tastes. A reduction or loss of appetite can consequently induce secondary hyperlipaemia more easily in donkeys than in horses [2]. In addition to medicating with pergolide, The Donkey Sanctuary promote regular remedial farriery and clipping if hirsutism is present, although excessive coat growth is less commonly seen in PPID donkeys. Donkeys can have a thicker coat compared to horses, so this clinical sign may not be so obvious. Donkeys do not often present with polydipsia with PPID; however, adlib water should be provided for donkeys as it can be hard to assess if they are drinking excessively due to PPID.

Asinine Metabolic Syndrome (AMS)

Causes

AMS (known as equine metabolic syndrome in horses) is recognised by apidosity, elevated insulin levels, insulin dysregulation and a tendency to develop laminitis. Long-term insulin elevation as a result of AMS can cause chronic changes for the donkey, such as irreversible damage to the hooves due to secondary laminitis. Donkeys are at an increased risk of being insulin resistant compared to horses and ponies, due to their thrifty genotype as an adaptation to an environment where food is scarce. This genotype when combined with lack of exercise and abundant food, make donkeys kept as companion animals more prone to developing AMS.

Clinical Signs

Clinical signs to note in donkeys and ponies are, recurrent or acute laminitis and regional adiposity, which is defined as fatty deposits on the rump and/or crest.

Diagnosis

Baseline insulin blood tests assist the vet in diagnosing the condition. However, entire starvation is not recommended in donkeys. Access to straw overnight is recommended to reduce the risk of hyperlipaemia. If a donkey's basal insulin level is increased, this is indicative of insulin dysregulation. The reference range basal insulin in donkeys is 0–15.1 uIU/ml; these figures have been developed by The Donkey Sanctuary. In some cases, insulin blood can be ambiguous, so a vet may decide to perform a dynamic challenge test, otherwise known as a karo-light test. This follows the standard protocol used for horses. Corn syrup is administered orally, which is followed by a blood sample for serum insulin levels 75 minutes post-administration. If tolerated and appropriate for the individual donkey, a blood sample for basal insulin and blood glucose prior to administering the corn syrup is the best practice [16].

Treatment

A combination of changes in diet and exercise is most effective for a donkey with AMS. They should be managed following the same dietary programme as a potential laminitic or overweight donkey. When altering a donkey's diet to facilitate weight loss, changes must be gradual to ensure that the risk of hyperlipaemia is minimised [2]. In more challenging cases where dietary and exercise modifications are not effective on their own, medication may be required. Gliflozins can be used and these are SGLT2 inhibitors which block renal glucose reabsorption. This can help to correct hyperglycaemia and reduce high insulin levels to normal or near normal levels [21]. In donkeys, it is suggested to take blood samples to check for liver values and monitor closely before starting gliflozins. This is because these drugs can cause hyperlipidaemia, which is raised lipids in the blood, not necessarily hyperlipaemia which is the clinical syndrome. Blood samples are recommended to be taken at 1, 2 and 4-weeks post treatment and a tapered withdrawal is usually recommended.

Levothyroxine can be utilised in donkeys, horses or ponies when other treatment options have been exhausted, although it should always be an adjunctive therapy combined with dietary management. Metformin is no longer recommended for use due to poor bioavailability and limited efficacy.

When managing endocrine disorders in equids, especially donkeys, preventative measures and proactive nursing care are recommended. Maintaining a fit and healthy body condition score or providing appropriate intervention to work towards this is important. Managing obesity in donkeys can reduce their susceptibility to laminitis and its association with both PPID and AMS, in addition to the risk of secondary hyperlipaemia. When nursing donkeys in a hospital setting, it is important to ensure they are receiving correct and appropriate nutrition. For long-term cases, regular body condition scoring and weighing are vital in order to maintain optimum weight and condition.

Common Dental Conditions

It is important to know when caring for donkeys, in comparison to horses, that they can have a good body condition score despite having poor dental health. Loss of weight or condition is not always a reflection of a donkey's oral health. Owners should regularly body condition score their donkeys using the dedicated chart devised by The Donkey Sanctuary (Figure 16.12). This is important as donkeys do not carry weight or fat in the same places as horses, and their coats can also disguise poor condition. Condition scoring can help to manage all aspects of a donkey's health, including their dentition. A donkey's stoical nature means that they often hide pain or discomfort and will continue to eat even when suffering from severe oral pain. Prophylactic dental care is vital to prevent dental conditions or diseases from developing or worsening. Donkeys should not be left

until they are displaying the obvious signs of dental disease, such as excess saliva, quidding, a foul oral smell or nasal discharge. Additionally, the combination of prophylactic dental examinations and proactive nursing interventions are essential in helping to reduce the number of equines affected by the systemic disease. As a result of untreated disorders of the teeth, donkeys with dental complications are at risk of having poor body condition, hyperlipaemia and impaction colic [22].

Donkeys are prone to having overcrowded mouths as a result of having the same number of teeth as their larger equine relatives, but in a much smaller space. Donkeys are at an increased risk of developing dental disorders that go unnoticed because unlike other equines used for ridden work, they are not often required to wear bits. This means that owners of companion donkeys are unlikely to realise that there is an issue or any need for dental care. Subsequently, donkeys do not often receive regular dental checks as it is assumed that if they are eating, there is no necessity for them. The domesticated donkey frequently develops sharp enamel overgrowths, this is due to the difference in the environment in which they evolved and the environment they find themselves in the United Kingdom. An arid landscape with limited grass and harsh vegetation is vastly different from the lush green fields found in the United Kingdom. The Donkey Sanctuary promotes regular dental examinations for donkeys and mules. This is at least once or twice yearly but can be as frequent as every three months, depending on the individual case. Qualified Equine Dental Technicians (EDTs) should complete routine dental checks and rasping, referring cases as necessary to a vet for advanced dental treatments, working alongside them in the ongoing care of each patient.

Advanced dental procedures in donkeys consist of managing conditions such as:

- Displaced teeth
- Diastemata
- Caries
- Fractures of the tooth
- Apical infections
- Retained deciduous teeth
- Abnormalities in the occlusal surface
- Both simple and complex extractions.

Often, radiographs are utilised to assist with the diagnosis. RVNs are required to assist with these procedures both in the home and hospital setting. Nursing roles consist of monitoring patients receiving standing sedation, preparing for nerve blocks, preparing equipment and materials, for instance, the dental endoscope and diastema putties, and assisting with or taking the radiographs.

Donkeys are more likely to develop sharp enamel points or overgrowths, mainly in their cheek teeth. When left unmanaged, these can cause lacerations and ulcers to the cheeks and tongue. In combination with these enamel points, other types of overgrowths, hooks, steps and shear mouth can cause severe oral pain. Periodontal disease (PD) is a pathological process causing inflammation and infection of the structures surrounding the teeth [22]. PD ranges in severity and can be secondary to the occurrence of overgrowths that are causing food entrapment or packing [23]. Quidding can be seen as a clinical sign of dental disease. This occurs when the equid chews the food, and before swallowing, drop partially masticated food falls from the mouth. It is important to visually inspect the ground around the donkey's feeders to ensure that any potential quidding is identified, as it is a clear indication of dental problems, and can lead to impaction colic in some cases.

PD most frequently occurs due to food stasis, which can be caused by diastemata formation. 90% of cheek teeth in donkeys that were diagnosed with PD were directly caused by diastemata [22]. Diastemata are spaces between the teeth. They can be categorised as open or valve. An open

FACTSHEET: Owners

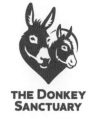

THE DONKEY SANCTUARY

CONDITION SCORING AND WEIGHT ESTIMATION OF THE DONKEY

Keeping a regular record of your donkey's condition scores and estimated weight measurements can be very useful for monitoring their health and management.

For donkeys over 2 years of age their weight can be estimated using The Donkey Sanctuary's weight estimator. For donkeys less than 2 years of age, height cannot be used to help estimate the donkey's weight but the table at the bottom of the following page can be used instead. Please note that the estimator is not accurate for miniature or mammoth donkeys. In order to estimate your donkey's weight you will need to know their height and heart girth measurements (in centimetres).

MEASURING YOUR DONKEY

To measure your donkey's height, stand him/her on a hard level surface and measure from the ground up to the highest point of their withers. Once a donkey is over four years of age this measurement will only be required once and the same measurement can be used in future weight estimations. A height measuring stick is ideal but a broom handle marked at the height of the donkey's withers can be measured to give an accurate reading.

The heart girth measurement can be taken using an ordinary tailor's tape measure. The tape measure should pass around the bottom of the donkey's chest as far forward as possible and as close to the front legs as possible. The tape measure should cross the top of the donkeys back approximately 10 centimetres (a hands width) back from the withers. The front of the cross can be quite a good guide to the position of the withers. The tape should be pulled firmly but carefully around the donkey and the reading taken in centimetres.

The heart girth measurement should always be taken in the same location preferably by the same person to ensure a continuity of the measurements taken. Both height and heart girth measurements can then be marked on the weight estimation chart and the donkey's weight read off the centre scale by drawing a line between the two measurements.

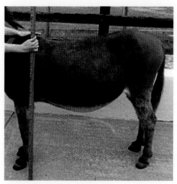

Measuring height (cm)

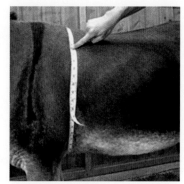

Measuring girth (cm)

Figure 16.12 Donkey weight estimator guidance. *Source:* The Donkey Sanctuary.

DONKEY BODY CONDITION SCORE CHART

Accurate Body condition scoring is a hands-on process for feeling the amount of muscle and fat that are covering the donkey's bones. Using this chart as a guide, feel the coverage over the bones in five specific areas listed below. Fat deposits may be unevenly distributed especially over the neck and hindquarters. Some resistant fat deposits may be retained in the event of weight loss or may calcify (harden). Careful assessment of all areas should be made and combined, to give an overall score. When deciding on the correct course of action following condition scoring, you might have to take into consideration the age of the donkey and any veterinary conditions they have. Aged donkeys can be hard to condition score due to lack of muscle bulk and tone giving thin appearance dorsally with dropped belly ventrally, while overall condition may be reasonable. If in doubt, get advice from your vet.

Condition score	Neck and shoulders	Withers	Ribs and belly	Back and loins	Hindquarters
1. Poor (very thin)	Neck thin, all bones easily felt. Neck meets shoulder abruptly, shoulder bones felt easily, angular.	Dorsal spine and withers prominent and easily felt.	Ribs can be seen from a distance and felt with ease. Belly tucked up.	Backbone prominent, can feel dorsal and transverse processes easily.	Hip bones visible and felt easily (dock and pin bones). Little muscle cover. May be cavity under tail.
2. Moderate (underweight)	Some muscle development overlying bones. Slight step where neck meets shoulders.	Some cover over dorsal withers, spinous processes felt but not prominent.	Ribs not visible but can be felt with ease.	Dorsal and transverse processes felt with light pressure. Poor muscle development either side of midline.	Poor muscle cover on hindquarters, hip bones felt with ease.
3. Ideal	Good muscle development, bones felt under light cover of muscle/fat. Neck flows smoothly into shoulder, which is rounded.	Good cover of muscle/fat over dorsal spinous processes, withers flow smoothly into back.	Ribs just covered by light layer of fat/muscle, ribs can be felt with light pressure. Belly firm with good muscle tone and flattish outline.	Can feel individual spinous or transverse processes with pressure. Muscle development either side of midline is good.	Good muscle cover over hindquarters, hip bones rounded in appearance, can be felt with light pressure.
4. Overweight (fat)	Neck thick, crest hard, shoulder covered in even fat layer.	Withers broad, bones felt with pressure.	Ribs dorsally only felt with firm pressure, ventral ribs may be felt more easily. Belly over developed.	Can only feel dorsal and transverse processes with firm pressure. May have slight crease along midline.	Hindquarters rounded, bones felt only with pressure. Fat deposits evenly placed.
5. Obese (very fat)	Neck thick, crest bulging with fat and may fall to one side. Shoulder rounded and bulging with fat.	Withers broad, bones felt with firm pressure.	Large, often uneven fat deposits covering dorsal and possibly ventral aspect of ribs. Ribs not palpable dorsally. Belly pendulous in depth and width.	Back broad, difficult to feel individual spinous or transverse processes. More prominent crease along mid line fat pads on either side. Crease along midline bulging fat either side.	Cannot feel hip bones, fat may overhang either side of tail head, fat often uneven and bulging.

Figure 16.12 (Continued)

diastema means that the gap is the same width along with its entire depth, whereas a valve diastema means that the gap tapers towards the surface of the tooth; in some cases, the gap is completely closed at the surface. Valve diastemata are more problematic as food or foreign bodies for instance shavings or other bedding, become trapped within the space. If closed, the food cannot exit, leading to gingivitis, mechanical irritation and PD. It is very important to maintain routine dental care of donkeys and other equids as they age due to the likelihood of diastemata formation increasing as a result of anatomical changes [2]. As a result of this, donkeys between the ages of 15 and 20 should receive more frequent prophylactic examinations, at least twice annually. Diastemata can be caused by developmental disorders or secondary due to acquired conditions like displaced teeth.

Dental displacements are variations in the position of teeth from their normal eruption space; these are most commonly identified in the mandibular molars [2]. They are often caused by inadequate space during the eruption stage, which may not be noticed while the donkey is juvenile, and or incorrect orthodontic forces in the oral cavity. For example, when these teeth continue to erupt unequal pressures are applied when the donkey is chewing food. This increases the severity of the displacement, making it more easily identified. Six monthly examinations of a donkey's teeth throughout its juvenile years, between 0 and 5 years of age, is the best practice as this is when the exchange between deciduous and permanent teeth occurs so developmental conditions can be proactively identified and monitored [2]. The timescale of when a donkey's permanent teeth erupt is typically six to eight months later than this process occurs in horses and ponies [22].

Regular dental care should always be provided to donkeys and other equids. Dental overgrowths, in most cases, are managed by qualified EDTs using various rasping techniques; they will also identify other dental conditions like diastemata and displacements. Diastemata can be appropriately managed by vets using short and long-term techniques; the application of putties or the widening of the diastema with a specialised burr. Dental displacements are managed according to their severity and the patient's individual condition; some displacements require strategic extraction of teeth as determined by the vet.

RVNs should be aware of clinical signs associated with dental disease in equids:

- Asymmetry of the head
- Presence of ocular or nasal discharge
- Lesions of the lips or tongue
- Pain or discomfort on the application of cheek pressure, tongue/hyoid pressure and temporomandibular pressure
- Oral malodour

- Food pocketing
- Signs of quidding
- Difficulty eating
- Excessive salivation or drooling
- The presence of long food fibres or undigested cereals in faeces

Dental disease is the second most common problem in donkeys following disorders of the hoof and is known to have the ability to cause severe pain and discomfort. In donkeys specifically, this pain can go unrecognised due to their stoic nature and instinct to eat despite the pain [22]. It is vital that RVNs can proactively identify pain in donkeys utilising the specialised composite pain assessment as an additional tool, alongside other indicators of pain in equines. For instance, an increase in their temperature, pulse and respiratory rates, reaction to nociceptive pressure tests and changes in their demeanour. It is essential to monitor a donkey's appetite when nursing them following any dental procedure. Early intervention with nutritional support is important when their appetite is reduced. Most donkeys should be offered soft feeds to ensure they are eating adequately once they recover from sedation. If nerve blocks have been administered, then an appropriate time should be allowed before offering feed to prevent harm caused to the tongue when eating. RVNs may also be required to perform flushing of non-packed extraction sockets, for instance following incisor extractions.

16.6 Pain Recognition in Donkeys

RVNs can play a vital role in recognising and scoring pain in their patients. It is widely accepted that recognising pain in prey animals, such as donkeys, can be challenging. The stoical nature of this species can make it difficult to identify signs of pain or discomfort. Severe pain can be missed in donkeys due to behaviours such as sham eating. In donkeys, any signs of pain, no matter how subtle, should be taken seriously.

Over a decade ago, the importance of recognising pain in horses and donkeys was reported [24, 25]. Although studies have been carried out assessing pain in donkeys, it was not until recently that a study was performed to develop and validate pain scales specifically for this species. The University of Utrecht has constructed two pain scales that have been validated for use in assessing acute pain in donkeys. 'The Equine Utrecht University scale for donkey composite pain assessment' and 'The Equine Utrecht University scale for donkey facial assessment of pain' can both be downloaded and used within the hospital environment. In practice, RVNs will find these scales particularly useful as part of their daily monitoring of patients. By using these scales, RVNs can have a direct positive impact on donkey patient welfare. Both scales are quick and simple to use with many of the questions based on observation alone.

Signs of pain in donkeys include the following:

- Lack of interest in the external environment
- Lowered head position
- Weight shift more frequently
- Show reduced ear movement and are often held horizontally or facing backwards
- Sham eating
- Spend more time recumbent
- Tooth grinding or moaning
- May startle easily or headshake at rest
- Episodes of tail flicking or pawing at the floor
- Altered posture

These signs can range from being very subtle to more obvious. RVNs should observe patients for 5–10 minutes as this will help to identify more subtle signs and in particular, picking up on sham eating. When using 'The Equine Utrecht University scale for donkey composite pain assessment', the observer should work from left to right. The first 15 questions are purely observational. These questions are answered by gaining information from observing the donkey outside the stable. This reduces that change of the donkey being influenced by the presence of the observer. The next stage involves a physical examination of the patient. Once this has been completed, a score should be added up. If the patient scores **five or above**, then the vet should be contacted regarding analgesia. For 'The Equine Utrecht University scale for donkey facial assessment of pain', a score of **three and above** requires the vet to be contacted regarding analgesia.

During the study to develop these scales, it was found that the donkey composite pain scale was most useful when assessing orthopaedic pain and post-surgical pain. The facial pain scale was most useful when assessing head-related pain and acute colic episodes. However, in the authors' experience, the composite scale is most useful in the hospital environment, assessing various causes of pain, including post-dental extractions. RVNs can be instrumental in developing protocols for using these scales in practice.

16.7 The Role of the RVN in Facilitating Owner Concordance

Owner concordance is extremely important to ensure that donkeys and other equids receive correct and effective care at home. The term concordance refers to an agreement being reached between the client and the vet or RVN regarding a treatment plan. The agreement is expected to incorporate the wishes and beliefs of the client in the decision-making process. The veterinary team should strive to achieve concordance with treatment plans; otherwise, these plans will not be successful and patient welfare could be compromised. RVNs are a vital communication link between vets and owners. Their skills and knowledge are key in helping owners to understand why their donkey's health is paramount, and what they can do to ensure they are providing correct care specific to their donkey's individual needs. The Donkey Sanctuary team are enthusiastic about educating their Guardian homes about all aspects of donkey-specific care and behaviour; this is a huge part of achieving owner concordance with treatment plans. An RVN can support owners with preventative healthcare such as advice on vaccination and worming programmes. Many donkeys do not receive correct preventative healthcare, and this is mainly down to a lack of education on the part of the owner. RVNs can discuss the importance of vaccination and worming programmes with the owner, including the discussion of infection control procedures and management strategies to reduce or prevent the spread of endoparasites (see Chapter 5 for further information). In consultation with the case vet, the RVN and the owner can identify and implement an effective preventative healthcare programme for each donkey, treating them as an individual.

RVNs, in practice, can teach owners regarding donkey-specific behaviour traits such as stoicism and the relevance of this, for example, hiding pain, displaying only subtle signs and often mimicking normal behaviours to disguise themselves within their group of companions. Demonstrating how to conduct a pain score on their donkey can help owners to understand and link specific behaviour changes to the way their donkey may display pain or discomfort, as these signs can differ from other equines. RVNs can demonstrate to owners how to be aware of and notice how their donkey's behaviour may change when receiving treatment using the points within the composite pain scale. This is an important part of the process of developing an owner's understanding of long-term benefits when intervention or medication is provided consistently. RVNs can be extremely beneficial in helping owners to understand underlying conditions even when there are no obvious clinical signs. For instance, in cases of AMS, if the donkey presents as lame with acute or recurrent laminitis, once the inflammation has been controlled and the donkey is sound, owners may be inclined to cease management or dietary changes. However, RVNs can educate owners as to how continued changes make a huge difference in the donkey's long-term health in relation to reducing the deterioration, or progression of endocrine diseases.

Alongside demonstrating and supporting owners with pain scoring, RVNs could also ensure they are aware of the specific donkey body condition score (BCS) chart (Figure 16.12) and how to utilise it on a regular basis. Both when visiting a donkey in the home or when discharging them from the hospital. This is a good time to encourage owners to become familiar with the BCS chart and to ensure they know what score their donkey is currently. Often, owners are unaware that their donkey is overweight until they are visually and physically able to conduct a BCS with an RVN's assistance. Conducting a BCS is relatively quick once those using it are familiar with the key steps, so time should not be a limiting factor. When donkeys are undergoing a management and weight loss programme, it is necessary for a BCS to be performed once a month, and ideally weighed using an electronic weighbridge. However, at times when physically weighing the donkey is unachievable, a donkey-specific weight tape which uses both the donkey's heart girth measurement and height to estimate their weight can be used. RVNs could combine BCS training and the correct use of a donkey-specific weight tape and nomogram devised by The Donkey Sanctuary (Figure 16.13) for owners who are unfamiliar with this method of weight checking.

DONKEY WEIGHT ESTIMATOR

To estimate a donkey's weight using the diagram below mark the height and heart girth measurements on the correct axis. Then draw a line between the two. The donkey's weight is indicated by where the line crosses the weight axis. For example, a donkey 104 cm tall (a) and with a heart girth 122 cm (b) should weigh 181 kg (c).

DONKEY WEIGHT ESTIMATOR

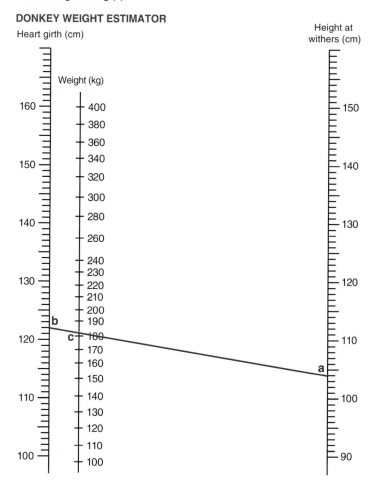

Whilst the weight estimator is an effective tool to estimate weight it's accuracy cannot be guaranteed.

Weight estimation table for donkeys under 2 years

Heart Girth (cm)	75	76	77	78	79	80	81	82	83	84	85	86	87	88	89	90	91	92	93	94	95	96	97	98	99	100
Weight (kg)	46	47	49	51	53	55	57	59	61	63	65	67	69	71	74	76	78	81	83	86	88	91	94	96	99	102

Research and Operational Support I © The Donkey Sanctuary I Published: 2013 I Revised: November 2018 I Phone: 01395 578222

Figure 16.13 Donkey weight estimator guidance. *Source:* The Donkey Sanctuary.

RVNs could conduct follow-up visits to donkeys in the home or on yards to provide advice about donkey-specific dietary and management requirements and assist owners with weight checking and BCS examinations. RVNs could also provide visits for taking follow-up blood samples for ongoing PPID and AMS cases when requested by a vet.

RVNs can also be helpful in supporting owners to assess their donkey's quality of life during ambulatory visits and this can be especially helpful to the owners of geriatric donkeys. If euthanasia is not immediately indicated or accepted by the owner, it is a valuable exercise to monitor changes or progressive decline by examining and recording specified parameters [2]. The RVN can give the owner a monitoring sheet to record the health and welfare of their donkey such as the 'Monitoring your donkey's quality of life' that has been produced by The Donkey Sanctuary and is free to download. The owner should complete the sheet on a daily or weekly basis and discuss the findings with the case vet or RVN. The parameters included in the sheet give a good indication of the health and, importantly, the welfare of the donkey, and will enable the owner to see any progress or decline. If the quality of life of the donkey is considered to be poor and treatment options are limited by severity of disease or financial considerations, then euthanasia is likely to be the best outcome for the donkey's welfare. Euthanasia should not be considered a failure, but the last good thing that can be done for the donkey [2]. It is important that the case vet and RVN support the client through the process of euthanasia. This can involve helping the client to manage the donkey's companion, help find a new companion, and offering details of bereavement services.

16.8 Conclusion

Donkeys are not just small horses with big ears! There are many physiological differences to consider in comparison to horses. An RVN working with donkeys must be able to recognise these differences and cater for them. Donkey specific protocols should be put in place and adhered to. Special areas of consideration such as strong bonding, specific nutrition, different drug metabolism and different clinical parameters should all be taken into account, along with the tendency for donkeys to develop hyperlipaemia. By following protocols specific to donkeys, the RVN can ensure that these patients receive individualised, species-specific nursing care, and therefore have an optimum chance of recovery.

Acknowledgement

The editors would like to thank Dr Alex Thiemann from The Donkey Sanctuary for her assistance and support with writing this chapter.

References

1 Ali, M., Baber, M., Hussain, T. et al. (2014). The contribution of donkeys to human health. *Equine Veterinary Journal* 46: 766–767.

2 Evans, L., Crane, M., and Preston, E. (2021). *The Clinical Companion of the Donkey*, 2e, pp. 11–13, 15, 19–23. Leicestershire: Matador.

3 McLean, A.K., Navas, F.J., and Canisso, I.F. (2019). Donkey and mule behaviour. In: *Diseases of Donkeys and Mules* (ed. T.J. Divers and R.E. Toribio), 576. Pennsylvania: Elsevier.

4 Dabinett, S. (2008). Nursing care. In: *The Professional Handbook of the Donkey*, 4e (ed. E. Svendsen, J. Duncan, and D. Hadrill), 342–351. Wiltshire: Whittet Books Limited.

5 The Donkey Sanctuary (2016). *Donkey Care Handbook*, 5e. Sidmouth: The Donkey Sanctuary.

6 Hart, B. (2022). Shaping behaviour: why small steps are the key to success. https://www.thedonkeysanctuary.org.uk/news/shaping-behaviour-why-small-steps-are-the-key-to-success (accessed 20 April 2024).

7 Lamoot, I., Callebaut, J., Demeulenaere, E. et al. (2005). Foraging behaviour of donkeys grazing in a coastal dune area in temperate climate conditions. *Applied Animal Behaviour Science* 92: 93–112.

8 Wood, S.J., Smith, D.G., and Morris, C.J. (2005). Seasonal variation of digestible energy requirements of mature donkeys in the UK. *Pferdeheilkunde* 21: 39–40.

9 The Donkey Sanctuary (2014). Feeding the elderly donkey. Available at: https://www.thedonkeysanctuary.org.uk/sites/uk/files/2017-08/feeding-the-elderly-donkey.pdf (accessed 18/05/2021).

10 The Donkey Sanctuary (2015). *Donkey Care Handbook*, 4e. UK: The Donkey Sanctuary.

11 Osthaus, B., Proops, L., Long, S. et al. (2018). Hair coat properties of donkeys, mules and horses in a temperate climate. *Equine Veterinary Journal* 50 (3): 339–342.

12 Herman, C. (2009). The anatomical differences between the donkey and the horse. https://www.ivis.org/library/veterinary-care-of-donkeys/anatomical-differences-between-donkey-and-horse (accessed 13 June 2022).

13 Grosenbaugh, D., Reinemeyer, R., and Figueiredo, M. (2011). Pharmacology and therapeutics in donkeys [Online]. Available from: https://aaep.org/sites/default/files/issues/eve-23-10-523-530.pdf (accessed 2 June 2022).

14 The Donkey Sanctuary (2018). Factsheet: hyperlipaemia [Online]. Available at: https://www.thedonkeysanctuary. org.uk/sites/uk/files/2019-02/Hyperlipaemia-for-vets.pdf (accessed 13 June 2022).

15 The Donkey Sanctuary (2017). Poisonous plants and trees [Online]. Available from: https://www. thedonkeysanctuary.org.uk/what-we-do/knowledge-and-advice/for-owners/poisonous-plants-and-trees#main-content (accessed 13 June 2022).

16 Thiemann, A.K., Buil, J., Rickards, K., and Sullivan, R.J. (2021). A review of laminitis in the donkey [Online]. Available at: https://beva.onlinelibrary.wiley.com/doi/ abs/10.1111/eve.13533 (accessed 13 June 2022).

17 Burden, F.A., du Toit, N., Hazell-Smith, E., and Trawford, A.F. (2011). Hyperlipemia in a population of aged donkeys: description, prevalence, and potential risk factors. *Journal of Veterinary Internal Medicine* 25 (6): 1420–1425.

18 Thieman A and Doyle D. (2021). Donkey nursing [Webinar]. CPD Video on Demand. BVNA.

19 The Donkey Sanctuary (2017). Endocrine disorders in donkeys [Online]. Available at: https://www. thedonkeysanctuary.org.uk/what-we-do/knowledge-and-advice/for-owners/endocrine-disorders-in-donkeys (accessed 2 June 2022).

20 Thiemann, A. (2019). EMS and PPID in donkeys [Online]. Available from: https://www.thedonkeysanctuary.org.uk/ research/paper/2688 (accessed 12 June 2022).

21 Kellon, E.M. and Gustafson, K.M. (2022). Use of the SGLT2 inhibitor canagliflozin for control of refractory equine hyperinsulinemia and laminitis. *Open Veterinary Journal* 12 (4): 511–518.

22 The Donkey Sanctuary (2020). *The Clinical Companion of Donkey Dentistry*, 1e. Matador: Kibworth Beauchamp.

23 Dacre, I., Dixon, P.M., and Gosden, L. (2008). Dental problems. In: *The Professional Handbook of the Donkey*, 4e (ed. E. Svendsen, J. Duncan, and D. Hadrill), 62–81. Wiltshire: Whittet Books Limited.

24 Ashley, F.H., Waterman-Pearson, A.E., and Whay, H.R. (2010). Behavioural assessment of pain in horses and donkeys: application to clinical practice and future studies. *Equine Veterinary Journal* 37 (6): 565–575.

25 Robertson, S. (2010). The importance of assessing pain in horses and donkeys. *Equine Veterinary Journal* 38 (1): 5–6.

Further Reading

Evans, L., Crane, M., and Preston, E. (2021). *The Clinical Companion of the Donkey*, 2e. Leicestershire: Matador.

Divers, T.J. and Toribio, R.E. (ed.) (2019). *Diseases of Donkeys and Mules*. Pennsylvania: Elsevier.

Useful Links

The Donkey Academy
https://www.thedonkeysanctuary.org.uk/donkey-care/ donkey-academy

17

Practical Equine Veterinary Nursing

Marie Rippingale[1], Kate Lambert[2], Cassie Woods[3], Tamsyn Amos[4], and Bonny Millar[5]

[1] Bottle Green Training Ltd, Derby, UK
[2] Pool House Equine Hospital, Crown Inn Farm, Lichfield, UK
[3] Lower House Equine Clinic, Plas Cerrig Lane, Shropshire, UK
[4] Priestwood Physiotherapy, Sitterlow Farm, Parwich, Ashbourne, UK
[5] Equicomms, Norfolk, UK

17.1 Clinical Examination

Introduction

Registered veterinary nurses (RVNs) should have a good knowledge of the normal clinical parameters for equine patients. This facilitates the recognition of abnormalities, which can then be recorded, and a treatment plan can then be created accordingly. A common approach includes following a system known as SOAPIER, which stands for:

- **Subjective:** A subjective assessment is based on an opinion or feeling relating to an individual's perspective or preferences. A preliminary assessment of the patient should be completed before handling the horse. This visual assessment should include aspects such as body condition, demeanour, temperament, posture, general coat condition and wounds or swellings [1].
- **Objective:** An objective assessment is unbiased and is based on observable or verifiable facts. This includes assessing the patient's vital parameters monitoring their food and fluid intake. A pain score should also be carried out. See Chapter 14 for more information.
- **Assessment:** Results of the subjective and objective assessments should be documented during this stage. Ideally, these results would be documented on a clinical parameter record sheet or a care plan assessment record.
- **Plan:** Nursing interventions are documented in this section. Ideally, these would be recorded on a nursing care plan. See Chapter 13 for more information.
- **Intervention:** After the nursing care plan or treatment plan has been created, nursing interventions should be put into practice. These interventions should be documented.

- **Evaluation:** The effectiveness of the nursing interventions needs to be evaluated. If goals, not objectives, were achieved or not achieved, this should be noted during this stage.
- **Re-assessment:** The care or treatment plan is reassessed and changed according to the results of the evaluation stage.

When using the SOAPIER system, both subjective and objective findings should be recorded clearly. A nursing care plan can then be formulated in conjunction with the veterinary treatment plan [1].

Clinical Parameters

The clinical parameters that should be assessed in equine patients include temperature, pulse, respiration (TPR), digital pulses, mucous membrane colour, capillary refill time and gut sounds (borborygmi) (Table 17.1). These readings should be taken twice daily; however, they may be required more frequently in critically ill horses.

During a clinical patient examination, a competent handler wearing personal protective equipment (PPE) such as a hard hat, steel toe-capped boots and gloves should restrain the patient. The RVN examining the patient should also wear appropriate PPE. Clinical parameters should be taken in a quiet environment, and the patient should be relaxed to get the most accurate readings. Terms associated with clinical parameter readings can be found in Table 17.2. When conducting a clinical examination on a horse, it is important to order the stages of assessment to yield the most accurate results. For example, taking the temperature last as this may be stressful for the horse and lead to elevations in heart rate and respiratory rate.

Table 17.1 Normal clinical parameters for the horse, donkey and foal.

Equid	Temperature (°C)	Pulse (beats per min)	Respiration (breaths per min)	Mucous membrane colour	Capillary refill time	Gut sounds	Digital pulses
Horse	37–38.5	24–40	8–16	Pale pink	>2 secs	++ | ++ ++ | ++ Noise present in all 4 quadrants	Nothing abnormal detected (NAD)
Donkey	36.5–37.8	36–52	12–38	As above	As above	As above	As above
Foal (1 month of age onwards)	37.7–38.7	60–80	20–40	As above	As above	As above	As above

Source: Marie Rippingale.

Table 17.2 Terms associated with clinical parameter readings in the horse.

Term	Meaning	Associated conditions
Hyperthermia	High temperature	Infection
Hypothermia	Low temperature	Shock, general anaesthesia
Tachycardia	Increased heart rate	Pain, infection, stress
Bradycardia	Decreased heart rate	Shock
Tachypnoea	Increased respiration rate	Pain, infection, stress
Bradypnoea	Decreased respiration rate	Shock
Dyspnoea	Difficulty breathing	Severe equine asthma (formerly known as recurrent airway obstruction or RAO)
Apnoea	Cessation of breathing	General anaesthesia and death
Cheyne-Stokes	Alternating periods of deep, rapid breaths, followed by shallow breathing and apnoea.	Hypoxia and death
Hypoactive gut sounds	Reduced borborygmi	Intestinal impaction or torsion
Hyperactive gut sounds	Increased borborygmi	Spasmodic colic, colitis, or enteritis

Source: Marie Rippingale.

Respiratory Rate

Normal Reading

- Horse: 8–16 breaths per minute

Method

- The respiratory rate can be counted by watching the abdomen move with each breath.
- The number of breaths should be counted over one minute.
- This can be done from outside the stable to avoid disturbing the horse.

- An alternative method is to feel the expiratory breaths at the nostrils. However, some horses may find this stressful, which will elevate the respiratory rate and make it inaccurate [1].
- The lung sounds should also be assessed. The trachea and both sides of the thorax should be auscultated, on inspiration and expiration, listening for abnormal harshness, crackling or wheezing (Figure 17.1).
- The presence of laboured breathing should also be noted.
- The horse has 18 ribs, with the lungs extending, when fully expanded, to the 16th rib. To identify the 16th rib, a straight line should be drawn from the point of the

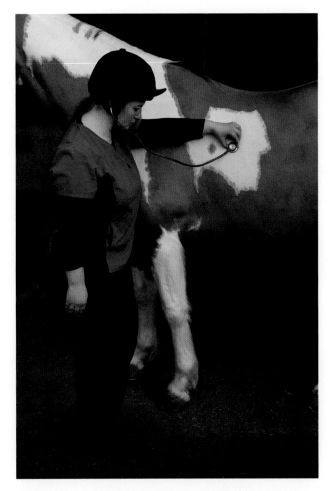

Figure 17.1 The thorax should be auscultated as part of a respiratory examination. *Source:* Dr Francis Boyer.

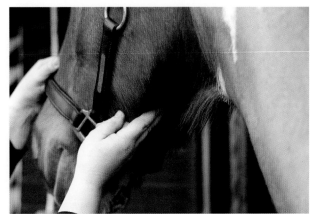

Figure 17.2 The pulse is most commonly taken using the facial artery. *Source:* Dr Francis Boyer.

elbow up to the point of the hip. This will mark the caudal boundaries of the lung field to auscultate.

- The nostrils should be examined for evidence of nasal flaring and discharge, with any distinguishing characteristics noted.
- Both nostrils should be checked to ensure that they have a free airflow.

Pulse Rate

Normal Reading

- Horse: 24–40 beats per minute

Method

- The arterial pulse is the difference between systolic and diastolic blood pressure waves and can be counted by palpation of any superficial artery [1].
- The most common place to take a pulse rate is the submandibular artery, which is palpated on the medial side

of the mandibular ramus, just in front of the muscular section of the ventral cheekbone (Figure 17.2).

- Once the artery is located with the fingertips, the pulse rate should be counted for one minute.
- RVNs should be familiar with other locations for taking the pulse (Figure 17.3) in case the submandibular artery is inaccessible, for example, during surgery.
- Other suitable arteries are:
- Transverse facial
- Lingual
- Carotid
- Saphenous
- Coccygeal
- Metacarpal and metatarsal
- Digital
- A normal pulse should be strong and regular. A horse with compromised cardiovascular function may have a weak and irregular pulse.
- The heart and pulse rates should be synchronised, with the pulse strength and rhythm patterns noted.
- A pulse deficit is apparent when the pulse rate is slower than the heart rate. This is common in patients with atrial fibrillation (see Chapter 13).
- Sinus arrhythmia is a normal finding where the heart rate increases during inhalation.
- The jugular veins should be observed and palpated for distention, thickening or pulsing that may indicate cardiovascular disease or thrombosis (Figure 17.4).

Digital Pulses

Normal Reading

- Horse: Mild or non-palpable pulse

Method

- In healthy horses, digital pulses should be hard to find.

(palpable in a depression
just caudal to the eye)

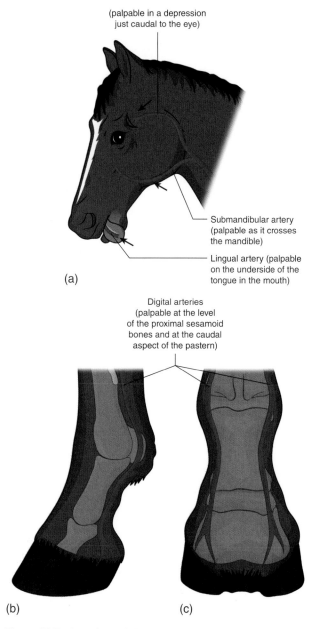

Submandibular artery
(palpable as it crosses
the mandible)

Lingual artery (palpable
on the underside of the
tongue in the mouth)

(a)

Digital arteries
(palpable at the level
of the proximal sesamoid
bones and at the caudal
aspect of the pastern)

(b)   (c)

Figure 17.3 Locations of the arterial pulses. (a) Diagram of the head showing the locations where pulses are palpable. Diagram of lateral (b) and palmar/plantar digital arteries (c). Image reproduced with kind permission from Wiley Publishing © Wiley. [2].

- The digital arteries are located and palpated in the distal limb at the level of the proximal sesamoid bones and the caudal aspect of the pastern (Figure 17.3).
- The fingertips are used to palpate the pulse and assess its strength.
- A strong or 'bounding' pulse can be an indication of inflammation in the distal limb.
- Strong digital pulses are associated with several conditions, such as laminitis and foot abscesses.

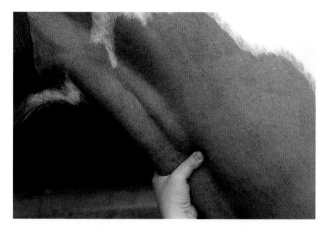

Figure 17.4 Jugular veins should be observed and palpated to check for abnormalities. *Source:* Dr Francis Boyer.

- It is important to monitor digital pulses in patients who are at risk from endotoxemia, as laminitis can occur as a secondary complication

Heart Rate
Normal Reading
- Horse: 24–40 beats per minute

Method
- Auscultation of the heart is a crucial component of a clinical examination.
- The heart rate should be auscultated just behind the elbow in the axillary region (Figure 17.5).
- Moving the forelimb forward can facilitate ideal positioning for the stethoscope.
- A systematic examination involves listening to both sides of the thorax [1].
- The number of beats should be listened to for at least one minute, to allow time for any abnormalities to be detected. Once the heart rate is stabilised, the beats over 15 seconds can be counted and multiplied by four to give the beats per minute.
- There are four heart sounds that can be heard, and these are designated S1, S2, S3 and S4 (Table 17.3).
- The sound designated S4 is the first sound to be heard in the cardiac cycle.
- The normal sequence when all heart sounds are audible is: S4, S1, S2 and S3, although frequently, only two or three sounds are heard [1].
- The normal heart sounds something like b-lup-dup-p, although often it is only S1 and S2 sounds that are identified making a 'lup-dup' sound [1].
- Close attention should be paid to murmur sounds or the presence of an arrhythmia.

• An arrhythmia is described as an abnormal rhythm, and if clinically significant, an electrocardiogram (ECG) may be necessary to determine the cause.

Abdominal Auscultation

Normal Readings

• Continual noise should be heard in all four quadrants. Gut sounds or borborygmi are recorded, as seen in Table 17.1. The cross represents the four quadrants of the abdomen, and the + signs indicate how much noise is heard in each quadrant.
• Hyperactive gut sounds are recorded as three pluses.
• Normal gut sounds are recorded as two pluses.
• Hypoactive gut sounds are recorded as one plus.
• If gut sounds are absent, no pluses are recorded and a treatment plan must be devised and implemented immediately.

Method

• Abdominal assessment and auscultation are critical in the examination of the horse. Most abdominal abnormalities in the horse are associated with the digestive system and involve a change in gastrointestinal motility [2].
• The horse should be observed for abdominal distention and asymmetry on both sides of the abdomen.
• Auscultation of the gastrointestinal tract is performed with a stethoscope across four quadrants:
• Upper left: Left paralumbar to midflank (Figure 17.6).
• Lower left: Left midflank to the ventral abdomen (Figure 17.7).
• Upper right: Right paralumbar to midflank.
• Lower right: Right midflank to ventral abdomen [2].
• The ventral midline area can also be assessed.
• Each quadrant should be auscultated for 1–2 minutes.
• On the left side, large intestinal borborygmi sounds are less pronounced because the spleen sits transversely against the body wall and in front of the intestines.
• Time should be spent auscultating the lower left quadrant as this is the area where the pelvic flexure sits (see Chapter 4 for more information).
• The pelvic flexure is a common site for impactions, and these can occur commonly as a secondary complication in hospitalised horses. Any reduction in borborygmi in this area should be noted and communicated to the case veterinary surgeon (vet).
• On the left side, the small intestines are easier to auscultate and normally sounds like the quiet gurgling of a stream.
• In a normal horse, loud, gassy borborygmi can be heard on the right side as gas moves through the liquid ingesta of the large colon.

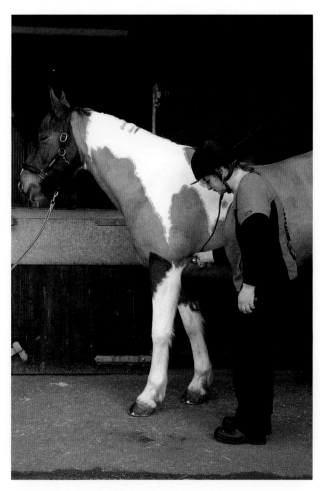

Figure 17.5 The heart rate should be auscultated just behind the elbow in the axillary region. *Source:* Dr Francis Boyer.

Table 17.3 Normal heart sounds in the horse.

Heart sound	Activity in the heart
S1	Relates to the start of systole and the emptying of the heart [1]. This makes a 'lub' sound.
S2	Occurs as the semi-lunar valves in the arteries close at the end of systole [1]. This makes a 'dub' sound.
S3	Sound made by the fast phase of blood flow into the ventricles during diastole (the filling of the heart) [1]. This makes a 'd' sound.
S4	Composed of the noise of the atria contracting just before systole begins and the closing of the mitral and tricuspid valves [1]. This makes a 'b' sound.

Source: Marie Rippingale.

• A murmur is described as any sound in the cardiac cycle that should not be present. An echocardiogram may be required to determine the cause of a murmur, which is of clinical significance.

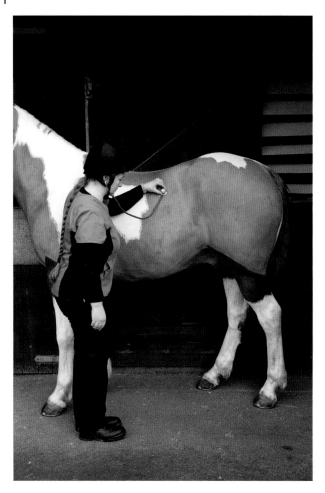

Figure 17.6 Assessment of borborygmi in the upper left quadrant of the abdomen. *Source:* Dr Francis Boyer.

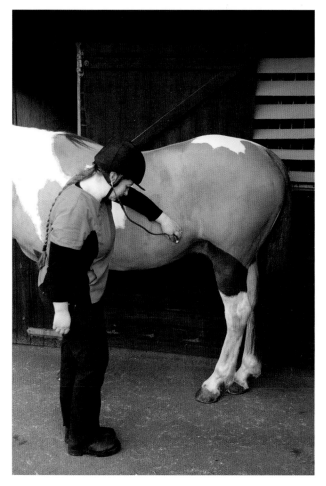

Figure 17.7 Assessment of borborygmi in the lower left quadrant of the abdomen. *Source:* Dr Francis Boyer.

- Caecal emptying sounds, or 'the caecal flush', are unique and heard on the right paralumbar fossa. They sound like water flushing down a drainpipe and occur every 1–2 minutes in the normal horse.
- In colic patients, gas can accumulate dorsally in the paralumbar fossa, and with enough distension, gut sounds can be heard cranially into the ribcage.
- Decreased or complete cessation of gut sounds may suggest serious and detrimental changes to the intestine. This is often described as a 'quiet' abdomen. 'Pinging' high-pitched sounds indicate trapped gas in the caecum or large colon and will often be associated with tympanic colic.
- Hypermobile gassy and fluid gut sounds may indicate an episode of spasmodic colic, impending colitis or enteritis.

Mucous Membrane Colour and Capillary Refill Time
Normal Readings
- Mucous membrane colour: pale pink
- Capillary refill time: fewer than 2 seconds.

Method
- Mucous membranes should always be assessed in good natural light.
- The mucous membranes in the mouth are most commonly assessed and can be visualised by parting the lips of the horse.
- The mucous membranes in the mouth should be uniformly pink and moist.
- Any colour change must be noted, as this can indicate deterioration in the horse's condition. See Table 17.4 for further information.
- To assess the capillary refill time, a finger can be used to press the gum to blanch the tissue (Figure 17.8). The pressure should then be released, and the time taken for the tissue to return to a normal colour observed.
- A delayed return of colour to the mucous membranes over two seconds reflects reduced tissue perfusion and dehydration.

Table 17.4 Mucous membrane colour and associated conditions.

Term	Meaning	Clinical signs	Associated conditions
Cyanotic mucous membranes	Deoxygenated mucous membranes	Blue mucous membranes	Shock, severe equine asthma, heart failure
Blanched mucous membranes	Under perfused mucous membranes	White mucous membranes	Anaemia, hypotension, shock
Congested mucous membranes	Highly perfused mucous membranes	Bright red mucous membranes	Dehydration, endotoxaemia, sepsis
Jaundiced (icteric) mucous membranes	Increased bilirubin in blood stream	Yellow mucous membranes	Liver disease
Petechial haemorrhages	Focal haemorrhages	Red dots on mucous membranes	Disseminated intravascular coagulation

Source: Marie Rippingale.

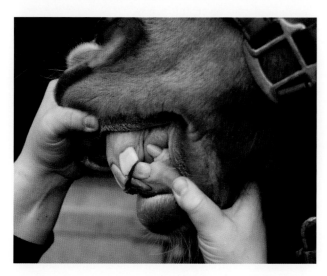

Figure 17.8 To assess the capillary refill time, a finger can be used to press the gum to blanch the tissue. The time taken for the colour to return should then be noted. *Source:* Dr Francis Boyer.

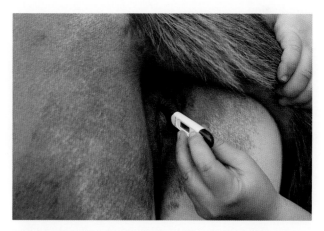

Figure 17.9 The thermometer should be inserted about 2 inches into the rectum and held against the rectal wall. *Source:* Dr Francis Boyer.

Temperature
Normal Reading
- Horse: 37–38.5°C.

Method
- The horses' temperature is typically taken rectally.
- The result may be slightly lower than expected if the horse has just passed faeces.
- Caution should be employed when taking temperatures in horses due to the need to stand behind the patient.
- If the temperament of the patient is not known, a set of stocks can be used to reduce the risk of injury.

- A competent handler wearing PPE should restrain the patient.
- The end of the thermometer should be lubricated. This is especially important in neonates.
- The RVN should stand to one side of the patient to take the temperature.
- The RVN should make the patient aware of their presence by using their voice and running their hand slowly along the horse's back and hindquarters.
- The base of the tail should be gently grasped and elevated.
- The lubricated end of the thermometer should be inserted about 2 inches into the rectum and held against the rectal wall to avoid contact with faecal material, which may cause an inaccurate reading [1] (see Figure 17.9).

- Once the thermometer alarm sounds, the thermometer should be carefully removed, the reading noted and the thermometer should be turned off and disinfected.

Conclusion

RVNs should be confident in carrying out a thorough clinical assessment of a wide range of patients. Results should always be recorded and communicated to the rest of the veterinary team. Changes to treatment or nursing care plans can then be made quickly and effectively, leading to a high standard of patient care and an optimum chance of recovery.

17.2 Administration of Medication

Introduction

The administration of medication is often delegated to RVNs by the treating vet. Therefore, RVNs should have a good knowledge of the effects of these medications, the correct routes for administration and how to recognise and manage complications safely if they occur.

Oral Medication

Oral medications include liquids, suspensions, solutions and syrups. The simplest way to give oral medication is to mix it into feed. Some patients may need extra encouragement to eat medication; if this is the case, succulents such as garlic, carrots and apples may be offered. Adding molasses to the feed may increase palatability also. Feeds containing molasses may not be an option for horses on a diet, with laminitis or metabolic conditions such as pituitary pars intermedia dysfunction (PPID), also known as equine Cushing's disease (ECD) and equine metabolic syndrome (EMS). For these patients, water from sugar beet pulp could be used; this has a low sugar content but will add flavour. Medications should only be added directly before feeding. Leaving medications in feeds for some time can cause the stability of the drug to change, which can affect the efficacy of the drug. Not all oral medications can be given in feeds; detomidine gel is an oromucosal gel that must be administered sublingually to be effective. RVNs should always read the manufacturer's instructions before administering any medication.

How to Administer Drugs Using a Dosing/Catheter Tipped Syringe

Some horses may not eat medication that has been put in their feed, so the medication may need to be administered using a dosing syringe. The technique for this is as follows [3]:

- A competent handler wearing appropriate PPE is essential for adequate restraint
- After checking the mouth is empty, the tip of the syringe should be inserted into the mouth, pointing up towards the back of the tongue
- The medication should then be introduced directly onto the tongue
- The horse's head should be held up, and its mouth should be carefully monitored to ensure the medication is not expelled and wasted

Potential Complications [3]

- Difficulty ensuring complete dose is ingested.
- Aspiration of medication, which may cause aspiration pneumonia; however, this is rare.
- Injury to nervous horses and/or their handler.

Topical Medication

Topical medications include creams, ointments, shampoo and gels.

- When applying to the skin, ensure the area is cleaned prior to application.
- Clipping may be required in some breeds to ensure good skin contact.
- Gloves should be worn.

Advantages

- Delivering a high concentration of medication locally can lead to a lower quantity of medication required overall compared to that required systematically to achieve the same effect.
- Depending on the patient, topical medication can be easier to apply than oral medication.
- Topical medications can be applied by an owner.

Potential Complications

- Too much hair in the area can prevent good contact.
- Horses may rub or lick topical medications off; if this is the case, light bandages, muzzles or a neck cradle may be required to prevent the horse from gaining access to the affected area.

Eye Drops/Ointments

Eye conditions may require medication to be delivered directly onto the corneal surface. It is crucial to ensure the tip of the application bottle or syringe does not come into contact with the corneal surface, as this can cause further trauma, and bacteria can be transferred from the applicator to the eye. Occular medications often require multiple applications throughout the day, so it is essential to make the experience as stress-free and positive for the horse as possible. Otherwise, they can become head-shy and start to resent treatment. Scratches, grooming and treats can be used to help the horse to develop a positive association with the treatment. General tender loving care (TLC) and grooming should be provided for every patient regardless of their condition to encourage interaction and promote psychological wellbeing.

Subpalpebral Lavage (SPL)

If horses strongly resent the application of eye medication or if frequent doses are required, then a subpalpebral lavage (SPL) may be placed. A SPL is an indwelling lavage system placed under the upper or lower eyelid; the lavage system is sutured to the skin, and the tubing is then threaded through the mane, so the injection port is at least midway down the horse's neck. The injection port should be changed daily to minimise contamination [4]. The volume of medication administered can vary from 0.1 to 0.5 ml [4]. Air should be administered following the medication to ensure that it reaches the eye and does not sit in the SPL tubing. The horse should be observed for blinking or for the medication to be seen entering the eye. It is important to determine how much air is needed to follow the medication to ensure it reaches the eye. Both medication and air should be administered slowly through the lavage system so the horse does not become sensitised to it. Five minutes should be left between medications to allow time for the medication to be absorbed [4]. Rewards such as treats, scratches and/or licks should be given to the horse following medication to make this a positive experience for the patient.

Nursing Observations

Horses with eye conditions often need to be kept in a dark stable away from direct sunlight; if this is not possible, then an ultraviolet (UV) fly mask may be required to protect the eye. Haynets should be removed from the stable to prevent the horse from rubbing its eye, and a stable grill may be required to prevent rubbing on the stable door. Sometimes, the headcollar is left on the horse to facilitate catching. In these circumstances, the headcollar should be made of leather and be padded, especially around buckles and metalwork to prevent rubbing and the development of sores on the face. Specially designed eye masks are now commercially available for horses. They have rubber cups that further protect the eye, which can help to prevent rubbing.

Injectable Medication

Patient Restraint

For injections to be given successfully, safely and effectively, patient restraint should be considered. This will prevent excessive movement and help to avoid improper injection [5]. As a minimum, all horses receiving an injection should be restrained using a headcollar and lead rope. The handler should wear PPE such as a hard hat, steel toe-capped boots and gloves. Treats or a lick may be offered to the patient if appropriate to help to make the procedure a positive experience. Extra restraint may be necessary in the form of stocks or sedation for fractious or needle-shy horses. Each case should be evaluated on an individual basis. If sedation is required, this must be prescribed by a vet.

Drawing Up Medication

Medication must be drawn up carefully and aseptically. The following steps should be followed [5]:

- Hands should be clean, and gloves worn. This will contribute towards reducing the spread of nosocomial infections and preventing contamination of the medication and injection site.
  The following should be verified as correct:
  – Patient
  – Medication
  – Route
  – Dosage
  – Timing
  – Expiration date
  – Broach date
  – Storage of the medication prior to injection
- If appropriate, the medication should be gently inverted to make sure it is mixed thoroughly.
- An appropriate needle and syringe should be selected.
- The needle should be attached to the syringe without contaminating the hub of the needle or the tip of the syringe. This will help to maintain asepsis.
- The rubber bung on the medication should be disinfected using a gauze swab soaked in 70% alcohol (not appropriate for vaccines). This will help to reduce contamination.
- The needle cap should be removed carefully. The needle should be inserted aseptically into the rubber bung on the bottle. The needle should not be touched as it is inserted into the bottle, as this could lead to contamination.
- The correct amount of medication should be drawn back into the syringe. The needle and syringe should be carefully removed from the bottle.
- The needle and syringe should be held vertically, and the syringe should be tapped to dislodge any air bubbles. These should then be removed.

- Horses can tolerate 0.25 ml/kg of air before showing clinical signs. Even so, removing excessive air bubbles will help to reduce the risk of an air embolism developing, especially during an intravenous (IV) injection.
- The amount of medication remaining in the syringe should be checked. More medication should be withdrawn if required.
- Recapping needles is a hazard and should be avoided. The needle can be removed using artery forceps or using the lid of a sharps bin.
- A new needle should be applied to the syringe.
- The syringe should be labelled with the drug name, drug concentration, time and date. This will help to mitigate errors.

Intramuscular (IM) Injections
Sites for IM Injections
Note: Images for this section are to be used as a guide only. Each horse should be assessed individually when locating an appropriate injection site.

- The main sites for IM injection in horses can be seen in Figure 17.10.
- *Trapezius muscle*: The landmarks form a triangle 4″ above the dorsal border of the cervical vertebrae, 4″ cranial to the cranial border of the scapula and 4″ below the border of the crest of the neck [5] (Figure 17.11).
- *Pectoral muscle*: Located in the cranial most part of the chest, craniomedial to the thoracic limbs [5] (Figure 17.12).
- *Gluteal muscle*: The injection site can be found in the centre of a triangle formed by the tuber coxae, tuber ischium and tuber sacrale (Figure 17.13).

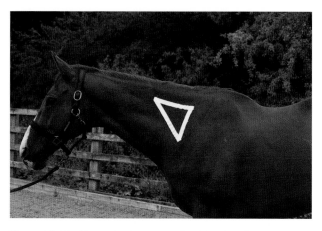

Figure 17.11 Trapezius intramuscular injection site. *Source:* Dr Francis Boyer.

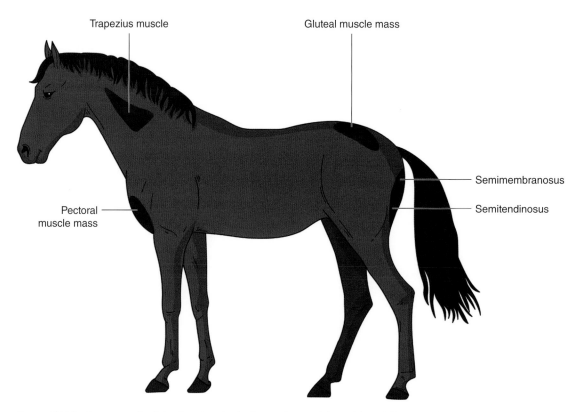

Figure 17.10 Intramuscular injection sites in the horse. *Source:* Adapted from Wiley. © Wiley.

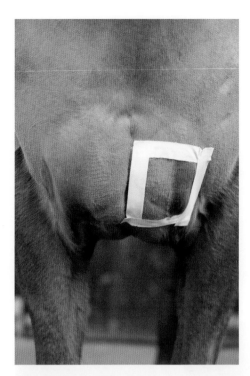

Figure 17.12 Pectoral intramuscular injection site.
Source: Dr Francis Boyer.

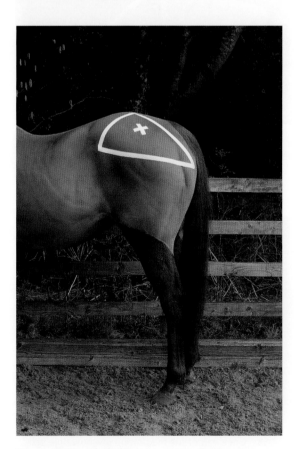

Figure 17.13 Gluteal intramuscular injection site.
Source: Dr Francis Boyer.

Table 17.5 Needle size for different routes of medication administration in adult horses.

Route of administration	Recommended needle size	Comments
Intravenous (IV)	18–20g × 1–1.5 inch needle [4]	Depends on viscosity of medication to be delivered.
	23–25g × 5/8 inch	For packed cell volume (PCV) measurement only.
Intramuscular (IM)	20–18g × 1.5 inch needle [4] Gluteals -18g × 1.5 inch Pectorals - 20g × 1.5 inch Trapezius – 21g × 1.5 inch	Depends on viscosity of medication delivered.
Subcutaneous (SC)	20–22g × 1.5 inch needle [4]	N/A

Source: Kate Lambert.

- An 18–21 g × 1.5-inch hypodermic needle and a syringe should be used in most horses [3]. See Table 17.5 for details of needle sizes.
- A 20 g × 1-inch needle should be used for foals [3].
- Ideally, no more than 5–10 ml should be delivered per injection site [6]. This is not the case for gluteal muscles. Any amount up to 20 ml can be administered into the gluteal muscle. However, if the volume of medication is larger than 20 ml, the medication should be split into more than one location [4].

Method for IM Injections

Restraint of the horse is important to ensure the safe administration of medication.

- The injection site should be swabbed with a suitable skin preparation to remove any superficial contamination (Figure 17.14).
- Tapping the horse with the backside of your hand two to three times will desensitise the area first and make the injection less of a shock to the horse (Figure 17.15). This will make the procedure safer as the horse is less likely to react to the needle.
- For injection into the gluteal muscle, the person administering the injection should stand as far cranially and close to the horse as possible to prevent them from being kicked.
- The needle should be inserted without the syringe attached (Figure 17.16). Once the needle is in, the syringe should be attached and aspirated. This is **ESSENTIAL** to

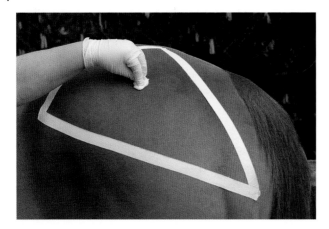

Figure 17.14 The injection site should be swabbed with a suitable skin preparation to remove any superficial contamination. *Source:* Dr Francis Boyer.

ensure no blood vessels have been penetrated (Figure 17.17).

- If no blood is visible, the medication can be injected. If blood is present on aspiration, **DO NOT INJECT**; the needle should be redirected, and the syringe aspirated again.
- If no blood is present on aspiration, it is safe to inject the medication.
- Once half of the medication has been injected, the syringe should be aspirated again to make sure the needle is still in the correct place (Figure 17.18). If no blood is present, the full dose of medication can then be administered.
- Once the medication has been administered, the needle and syringe should be removed.
- The injection site should be swabbed and checked for any bleeding.

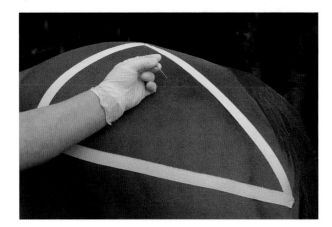

Figure 17.15 Tapping the horse with the backside of your hand two to three times will desensitise the area first and make injection less of a shock to the horse. *Source:* Dr Francis Boyer.

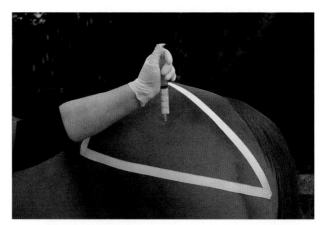

Figure 17.17 Once the needle is in, the syringe should be attached and aspirated to check for venepuncture. *Source:* Dr Francis Boyer.

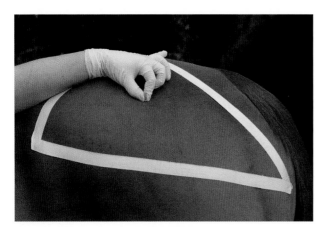

Figure 17.16 The needle should be inserted without the syringe attached. *Source:* Dr Francis Boyer.

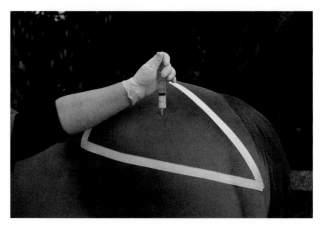

Figure 17.18 Once half of the medication has been injected, the syringe should be aspirated again to make sure the needle is still in the correct place. *Source:* Dr Francis Boyer.

- If the volume of medication is bigger than 20 ml, the medication can be split into more than one location. Alternatively, with a gluteal injection, the needle can be redirected halfway through the injection. Following re-direction, the syringe must be aspirated to check for venepuncture. The muscle group and side used for the injection should be recorded. This is important to facilitate the rotation of muscle groups, to prevent heat or swelling at an injection site.

Potential Complications

- Injury to horse or handler.
- Inadvertent puncture to other structures, especially blood vessels, can cause severe reactions, including seizures which is classically associated with the injection of procaine penicillin [6].
- Inadvertent puncture of vertebrae or nuchal ligament (neck injections).
- Inadvertent puncture of the sciatic nerve (in the hind limb).
- Localised swelling, especially when injecting into the pectoral muscles.
- Pain, stiffness or abscess formation at the injection site [3].
- Abscess formation is an occasional complication. A disadvantage to using neck or gluteal muscles for injection is that should abscessation occur; these are more difficult sites to drain [6].
- Muscle soreness is a common complication. Rotating the sites used can avoid this, especially if the medication is to be administered twice daily [6]. If muscle soreness occurs, no further injections should be administrated at that site, and topical heat packs might provide some relief for this problem [6].
- The horse's behaviour and temperament should be considered. Sometimes, it is not possible or safe to inject horses via the IM route. In these cases, oral or IV medication can be administered instead.
- *Anaphylaxis.* This can occur in the form of a seizure. If this happens, the handler and RVN should consider human safety as a priority. A vet should be alerted immediately.

Nursing Observations

- Reaction after medication, ranging from urticaria (itchy skin lumps/rash) to seizures and/or collapse.
- Sore injection sites following repeated injections: if this is the case, then a change in muscle groups and/or hot packing of the sore area can be implemented.

- The horse's behaviour should be considered. If the horse is becoming more difficult to inject as time goes on, then positive enforcement, clicker training or possibly changing the route of medication may be required.

Handler Observations

While restraining the horse for an injection, the handler should look out for the following signs of a reaction:

- Dilation of the pupils
- Rapid sedation/excitement
- Muscle twitching
- Horse's head quickly lifting into the air followed by excitable behaviour

The handler should inform the vet or RVN of any behavioural changes straight away, to allow the handler and the person giving the medication time to move to a safe place. A vet should always be informed if a change in behaviour occurs.

Intravenous (IV) Injections
Sites for IV Injections

- *Jugular vein*: Most commonly used vein for IV injections. Jugular veins are large and easily accessible. If a complication occurs in one jugular vein, the lateral thoracic should be used as an alternative rather than the other jugular vein. If both jugular veins become compromised, this can disrupt venous drainage to the head, which can have life-threatening consequences.
- *Lateral thoracic*: Commonly used as an alternative to the jugular vein, especially if a complication has occurred. Easy to access and attach IV fluids to in critically ill patients.
- *Cephalic vein*: Rarely used due to location. More commonly used in foals than in adult horses.
- *Saphenous vein*: Rarely used due to location and health and safety implications.

Method

- See Table 17.5 for details of needle sizes.
- Make sure the horse is well restrained by a competent handler wearing PPE.
- IV injections should be given in the cranial third of the neck as the carotid artery is less superficial there.
- The injection site should be swabbed with a suitable skin antiseptic to remove any superficial contamination.
- The vein should be raised (Figure 17.19), and the needle inserted at an angle of 30 degrees to the skin, pointing upwards (Figure 17.20).

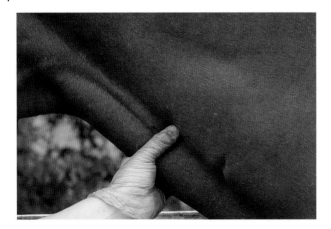

Figure 17.19 The vein should be raised.
Source: Dr Francis Boyer.

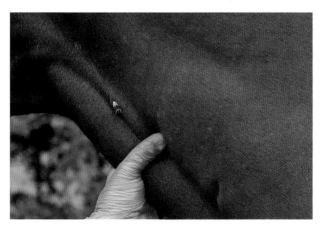

Figure 17.21 Blood should be seen indicating correct needle placement. The blood should be dark in colour and slow-flowing (dripping). *Source:* Dr Francis Boyer.

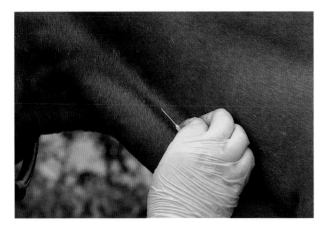

Figure 17.20 The needle was inserted at an angle of 30 degrees to the skin pointing upwards. *Source:* Dr Francis Boyer.

- Blood should be seen, indicating correct needle placement. The blood should be dark in colour and slow flowing (dripping) (Figure 17.21). If bright red, fast-flowing (spurting) blood is seen, this is an indication that the needle is in the carotid artery (Figure 17.22).
- If the needle is thought to be in the carotid artery, **THE MEDICATION SHOULD NOT BE INJECTED**; the needle should be removed, and pressure should be applied. Another injection site should be selected for the medication.
- Once the needle is confirmed to be in the vein, the syringe should be attached and aspirated to ensure the needle is still in the correct place before injecting the medication (Figure 17.23).
- The medication should be given slowly, and the syringe should be intermittently aspirated to ensure that the needle is still in the correct place.

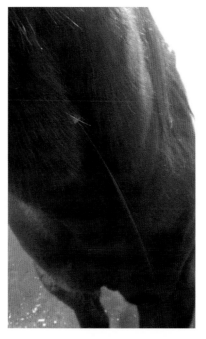

Figure 17.22 If bright red, fast-flowing (spurting) blood is seen, this is an indication that the needle is in the carotid artery. *Source:* Marie Rippingale.

- Pressure can be applied once the needle is removed using a gauze swab or a gloved hand to prevent a haematoma (Figure 17.24).

Potential Complications

- Injury of horse or handler.
- Self-injection. If this happens, medical attention should be sought immediately [7].
- Inadvertent puncture of other structures, for example, the carotid artery. This often happens when a needle is

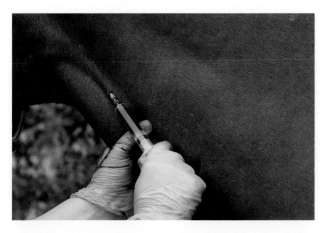

Figure 17.23 Once the needle is confirmed to be in the vein, the syringe should be attached and aspirated to ensure the needle is still in the correct place before injecting the medication. *Source:* Dr Francis Boyer.

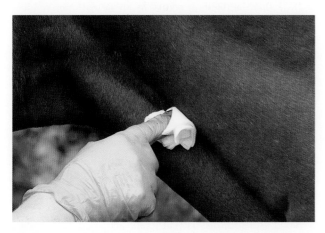

Figure 17.24 Pressure can be applied once the needle is removed using a gauze swab or a gloved hand, to prevent a haematoma. *Source:* Dr Francis Boyer.

inserted too deeply. Bright red blood will spurt out of the needle. **Medication should never be injected into the artery, as this can cause severe reactions such as collapse and seizures.**

- Extravascular injection can cause pain, inflammation, infection and tissue sloughing [7].
- Anaphylaxis can occur in the form of a seizure. If this happens, the handler and RVN should consider human safety as a priority. A vet should be informed immediately.

Nursing Observations

- Swelling of the vein. This could be indicative of a thrombus.
- Pain around the vein could result from a reaction to drugs or be a sign that some medication has been given perivascularly rather than intravenously.

- Change in behaviour, such as increased and sudden levels of sedation, and seizures if the sedation is accidentally administered into the carotid artery.
- Previous signs of catheter placement, scaring or trauma to the vein can make it more difficult to inject at that site.

Phlebotomy (Taking a Blood Sample)

Blood samples are most commonly obtained from the jugular vein in horses. The process follows the procedure for needle placement as described for IV injections above. There are two methods used for obtaining a blood sample: Using a needle and syringe and using a vacutainer system.

Needle and Syringe

- Once the needle has been confirmed as being in the jugular vein, a syringe can be attached and aspirated so that blood flows back into the syringe.
- The vein should be raised during this process.
- If blood stops flowing at any point, the syringe should be disconnected, and the needle should be carefully redirected until blood flow is restored [7].
- Once the blood sample has been obtained, the vein should cease to be raised and the needle should be withdrawn.
- Pressure can be applied once the needle is removed using a gauze swab or a gloved hand, to prevent a haematoma.
- The blood sample should then be quickly decanted into an appropriate vacutainer or sample pot.

Vacutainer System

- Once the needle has been confirmed as being in the jugular vein, the vacutainer should be pushed firmly onto the piercing needle [7] (Figure 17.25).
- Care should be taken not to move the needle within the vein.

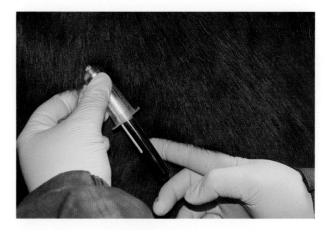

Figure 17.25 A blood sample being taken using the vacutainer system. *Source:* Rosina Lillywhite.

- The vein should be raised until the vacutainer is full.
- If blood stops flowing at any point, the vacutainer should be pulled off the piercing needle, and the sleeve and needle redirected [7].
- The vacutainer should then be pushed back onto the piercing needle [7].
- Once the blood sample has been obtained, the vein should cease to be raised and the needle should be withdrawn.
- Pressure can be applied once the needle is removed using a gauze swab or a gloved hand, to prevent a haematoma.

Subcutaneous (SC) Injections
Method for SC Injections
- SC injections are often given in the neck just in front of the scapula.
- The injection site should be swabbed with a suitable skin antiseptic to remove any superficial contamination.
- A handful of skin should be grasped, and a 21-gauge × 1.5-inch needle should be placed (with a syringe attached) into the base of the handful of skin (Figure 17.26).
- The syringe should be aspirated to ensure a blood vessel has not been accidentally punctured. If no blood is seen, then it is safe to inject the medication.

Complications
- The needle could be placed through the skin and out the other side
- The injection can be difficult and slow in thick-skinned horses.

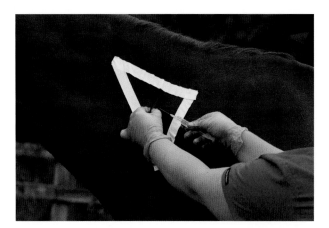

Figure 17.26 Administration of a subcutaneous injection. *Source:* Dr Francis Boyer.

17.3 Intravenous Catheter Placement

Introduction

IV catheters are commonly used in equine practice; however, this can lead to complications such as thrombus and thrombophlebitis. RVNs should be vigilant when placing IV catheters and monitoring catheter sites so that complications can be prevented.

Indications

Indications for placing an IV catheter include:

- *Fluid therapy (crystalloids, blood and or plasma)*: Placing an IV catheter allows the administration of large amounts of fluids over an extended period of time. See Chapter 14 for more information.
- *Drug therapy*: Having access to an IV catheter reduces the need for repeated venepuncture if medication needs to be administered regularly throughout the day. This reduces trauma to the vein and is more pleasant for the patient.
- *Total parenteral nutrition (TPN)*: This requires the provision of a dedicated IV catheter, which must be treated aseptically.
- *Measurement of central venous pressure (CVP)*: Used to assess cardiac function and to monitor fluid therapy. A long saline-filled catheter is advanced through the jugular vein into the right atrium, and the pressure is then measured.
- *Blood transfusions:* IV catheters are used to facilitate blood collection and administration during a transfusion.

Points of IV Access

The jugular vein is most commonly catheterised as they are large and easy to access (Figure 17.27). If IV catheter complications occur in one jugular vein, catheterising the contralateral jugular vein is contraindicated due to concerns over disruption of venous drainage. Swelling of the head and cervical region can then lead to a life-threatening airway obstruction. Other IV catheter sites used in the horse include the lateral thoracic (Figure 17.28) and cephalic veins, but these sites are more prone to catheter complications from patient interference and movement. Saphenous veins can be catheterised, but due to the location, catheter placement and handling may be dangerous [8]. The IV catheter site should be chosen carefully depending on the individual patient and the reason for placing the IV catheter.

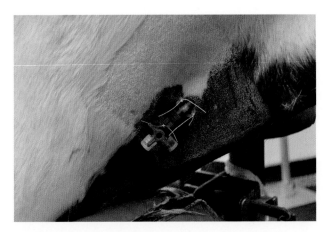

Figure 17.27 A jugular catheter placed in a retrograde orientation. *Source:* Marie Rippingale.

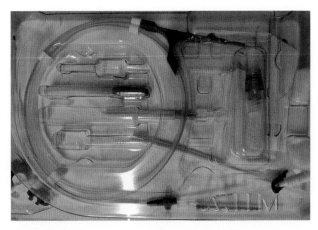

Figure 17.29 An over-the-wire catheter. *Source:* Rosina Lillywhite.

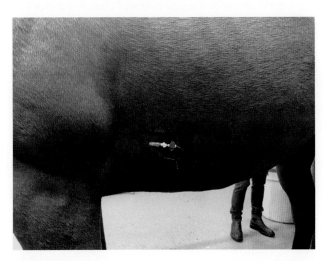

Figure 17.28 A lateral thoracic catheter. *Source:* Elaine Packer.

Catheter Selection

The choice of catheter depends on several factors, including [8]:

- Volume and rate of fluids
- Type of fluid
- Patient's potential to develop a thrombosis
- The expected duration of catheterisation
- Finances

Catheter Material

IV catheters are available in a number of different materials, and these need to be considered before a choice is made. Different materials include:

- *Tetrafluoroethylene (Teflon)*: These are the most thrombogenic catheters and are prone to kinking and cracking

with long-term use. They are usually termed 'short stay' catheters and should only be left in situ for a maximum of 24 hours. Teflon catheters tend to be the cheapest.
- *Polyurethane*: These are less thrombogenic than Teflon catheters as they are softer and more flexible. They are usually termed 'long stay' catheters and can be left in situ for up to 21 days if monitored and handled correctly. Polyurethane catheters are more expensive than Teflon catheters.
- *Silicone*: These are the least thrombogenic of the IV catheter materials. They are long and flexible. Often used for over-the-wire catheters and can be left in place for one to two months if required (Figure 17.29). Over-the-wire catheters are most commonly used for critical care and patients requiring TPN. These catheters tend to be the most expensive.

All IV catheters are thrombogenic to a degree. So, careful selection is important to minimise the risk of complications.

Catheter Size

The size of the catheter should also be considered:

- A 10–12-gauge catheter is recommended for severely hypovolaemic adult horses and donor horses when giving blood for a blood transfusion. The disadvantage of this is that large bore catheters are more thrombogenic.
- A 12–14-gauge catheter is recommended for moderately hypovolaemic adult horses.
- 14–16-gauge catheters should be used for horses requiring frequent medication.
- 16-gauge catheters are sufficient for hypovolaemic weanlings and Shetlands or miniature horses [9].

Direction of Placement

There are two directions for catheter placement in the horse:

- *Retrograde* (Figure 17.27): The catheter is placed 'up the way' or against the direction of blood flow. This technique minimises the risk of air embolism if the catheter or hub gets disconnected. This argument does not apply if the catheter is fitted with a haemostatic valve [8]. Retrograde placement can lead to catheter complications during high-rate IV fluid administration due to increased turbulence of blood flow and irritation of the endothelium.
- *Antegrade* (Figure 17.30): The catheter is placed 'down the way'. Or with the direction of blood flow. This direction increases the risk of air embolism if the catheter of cap becomes disconnected. This direction of placement does however decrease the risk of catheter complications during high-rate IV fluid administration due to decreased turbulence of blood flow and reduced irritation of the endothelium. This allows for more rapid administration of IV fluids [8].

There is no right or wrong direction to place an IV catheter in as long as all of the risks have been considered to inform the final decision.

Placing an IV Catheter

Equipment Required

Placing an IV catheter in an equine patient requires an aseptic technique. To facilitate this, all equipment should be prepared beforehand. Equipment required includes [10]:

- Clippers with a clean size 40 blade attached
- Surgical scrub – usually 4% chlorhexidine
- Sterile swabs
- Surgical spirit spray
- Non-sterile exam gloves for surgical scrub
- Sterile exam gloves to wear during insertion of the catheter
- 2 ml local anaesthetic with a 23G needle
- Over-the-needle IV catheter. Usually 14G for adult horses or 16G for foals
- 10 ml heparinised saline flush
- Suture material
- Injection cap/3-way tap
- Extension set filled with heparinised saline
- Sterile surgical blade (optional)

Technique for Placing an Over-the-needle Catheter

The most commonly used catheters in equine practice are the over-the-needle catheters. The technique for placing these catheters is described below:

- Aseptic preparation of the catheter site is essential as horses are prone to catheter complications, which can prove to be life threatening.
- Correct surgical skin preparation solutions and scrubbing techniques are discussed in detail in Chapter 12. The reader is directed there for further information.
- An area of skin should be clipped over the cranial two-thirds of the jugular vein (Figure 17.31). Catheters should not be placed at the distal one-third as inadvertent carotid puncture is more likely to occur here.
- The clipped area should then be surgically scrubbed with the operator wearing exam gloves.
- A subcutaneous bleb of local anaesthetic solution should be deposited over the vein (Figure 17.32).

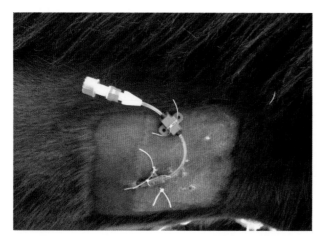

Figure 17.30 A jugular catheter placed in an antegrade orientation. *Source:* Marie Rippingale.

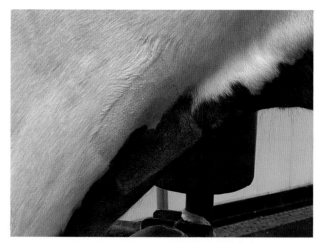

Figure 17.31 An area of skin should be clipped over the cranial two-thirds of the jugular vein. *Source:* Marie Rippingale.

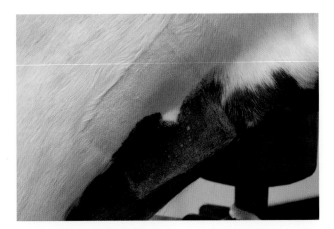

Figure 17.32 Local anaesthetic should be injected subcutaneously to form a bleb over the vein. *Source:* Marie Rippingale.

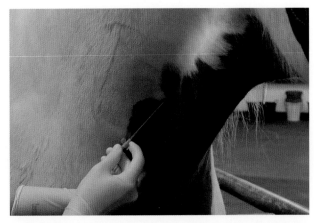

Figure 17.33 The catheter should be advanced through the skin into the vein at a reasonably acute angle (about 45°) until blood wells in the hub. *Source:* Marie Rippingale.

- This area should again be surgically scrubbed with the operator wearing exam gloves.
- Surgical spirit should be sprayed on the area.
- A small stab incision can be made through the skin at the incision site. This is known as a 'cut down'. This reduces skin drag and lowers the risk of inadvertent carotid artery puncture. This is an optional step that tends to be clinician dependent.
- A sterile tray should be set up to contain the IV catheter and injection cap/extension set.
- The person placing the catheter should don sterile surgical gloves.
- The jugular vein should be raised with one hand, and the catheter should be held by the hub with the other hand.
- The bevel of the stylet should face the person placing the catheter.
- The catheter should be advanced through the skin into the vein at a reasonably acute angle (about 45°) until blood wells in the hub (Figure 17.33).
- If inadvertent puncture of the carotid artery occurs, the catheter should be withdrawn, and pressure applied to the area for at least 5 minutes.
- Once venous blood is observed, the angle of advancement is reduced so that the catheter lies almost parallel with the skin (20–30°). The catheter and stylet are advanced together into the vein. The stylet can be withdrawn at any point but should never be re-inserted. The catheter should be advanced until the hub meets the skin.
- The 'clean hand' should advance the catheter, and the hand that raised the vein should hold the stylet (Figure 17.34).
- Once the catheter has been placed, a sterile bung, 3-way tap or extension set can be attached.
- The catheter should then be stitched to the skin (through the local anaesthetic bleb) (Figure 17.35).

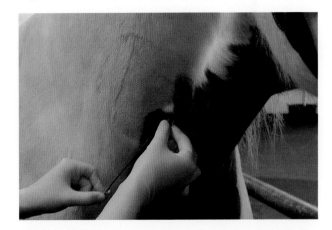

Figure 17.34 The clean hand should advance the catheter, and the hand that raised the vein should hold the stylet. *Source:* Marie Rippingale.

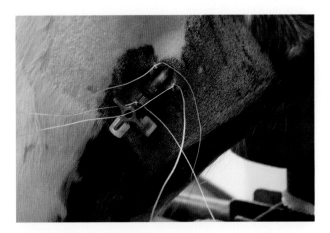

Figure 17.35 The catheter should then be stitched to the skin (through the local anaesthetic bleb). *Source:* Marie Rippingale.

- The loose ends of the suture material should be cut to an acceptable length (Figure 17.27).
- The catheter should then be flushed with the heparinised saline, and the bung, 3-way tap or extension set cleaned.
- The use of an extension set decreases direct handling of IV catheter parts close to the skin and this helps to reduce the chance of complications occurring.

Over-the-wire Catheter Placement Technique

It is beyond the scope of this section to discuss all types of catheter placement in depth. However, the following is a short description of the technique for placing an over-the-wire IV catheter [9]:

- Preparation is the same as for an over-the-needle catheter, including surgical skin preparation and the placement of a local anaesthetic bleb.
- In ponies and donkeys with thick skin, a small stab incision is made through the skin at the site of the catheter.
- The vein is raised, and venous access is gained with a needle from the catheter kit placed through the skin at an angle of 30–40°.
- Once blood is seen, the angle of the needle is changed to 5–10° and advanced to the hub.
- A guidewire is passed through the catheter into the vessel leaving 5–10 cm of wire exposed.
- **It is crucial not to let go of the wire in the standing adult horse as gravity may take the wire into the vein completely. This can cause a fatal wire embolism.**
- The needle is withdrawn out of the skin and off the wire completely.
- A dilator is fed over the wire and pushed through the skin to create a tunnel.
- The dilator is removed, and the catheter is fed over the wire.
- The guidewire is finally removed, and the IV catheter is sutured in place and flushed with heparinised saline.

IV catheters are also placed using the through-the-needle catheter placement technique. The reader is directed to the further reading section for more information.

Risks and Complications

With any IV catheter placement, there are risks and complications that the RVN must be aware of and monitor to ensure high standards of patient care.

- *Venous trauma*: During placement of the IV catheter, the vein can become traumatised making it more prone to developing further complications. Catheter placement should take place carefully to avoid unnecessary trauma

as this may lead to venous spasm, which would make further attempts to catheterise the vein difficult.
- *Catheter tip laceration (Figure 17.36)*: Once an over-the-wire catheter has been placed and the stylet removed, the stylet must never be replaced back into the catheter. This can cause the end of the catheter to shear off and act as a foreign body. If the broken catheter tip dislodges from the rest of the catheter, it can lodge in the heart or the lungs of the patient with potentially fatal consequences.
- *Phlebitis*: This is inflammation of the vessel wall and may appear as erythema (reddening) of the skin at the catheter site. Pain, heat and swelling may also occur with phlebitis [11].
- *Thrombosis*: This is the formation of a blood clot in the vessel. This can occur as a result of catheter placement, excessive catheter movement or extended duration of catheter placement [8]. Thrombus formation is more common in horses who are endotoxaemic or septicaemic, therefore extra care is required with these patients.
- *Thrombophlebitis*: This is defined as a thrombus formation and inflammation or the vein, which has the potential to get infected. Life-threatening septicaemia can

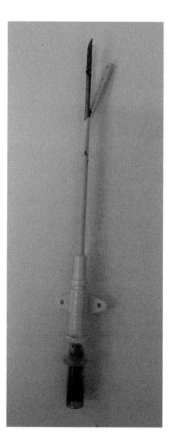

Figure 17.36 Catheter tip laceration. *Source:* Marie Rippingale.

develop if left untreated [8]. Clinical signs include heat, pain and swelling of the catheter site and hardening of the vein. If thrombophlebitis is suspected, the catheter should be removed immediately, and the catheter tip sent away for culture and sensitivity testing.

- *Extravasation*: This occurs when an IV catheter becomes dislodged, allowing fluid to enter the surrounding tissues. This is undesirable as some medication is irritant to perivascular tissue and can cause inflammation and sloughing.
- *Kinking (Figure 17.37)*: The degree of kinking will depend on the movement, softness and construction of the hub of the catheter [8]. Kinking may occur when the catheter has not been stitched in correctly and this may predispose to irritation, thrombosis, blocking of the catheter, extravasation and catheter breakage [8].

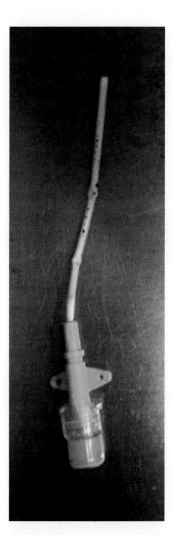

Figure 17.37 A kinked catheter. *Source:* Marie Rippingale.

Care of IV Catheters

Hygiene

IV catheters and the surrounding sites require vigilant monitoring from the RVN. Strict hygiene measures should be followed. Hands should be washed following the World Health Organisation (WHO) handwash method (see Chapter 6), and exam gloves should be worn every time the catheter or the surrounding site is touched. If catheter caps are used, they should be changed daily. Alternatively, self-disinfecting catheter caps impregnated with 70% isopropyl alcohol can be used to improve hygiene and help to reduce contamination of the catheter.

Flushing with Heparinised Saline

The IV catheter should be checked at least three times a day for the presence of heat, pain or swelling. Venous patency should also be checked; the vein should be raised and should fill the full length of the neck [10]. Every time a catheter is used for drug administration, it should be flushed with 10 ml of heparinised saline (10,000 IU heparin in 1 l Ringer's solution or saline to give a final concentration of 10 IU/ml) [8]. This will ensure that the whole volume of the drug has been flushed into the vein. It will also help to prevent blood clot formation and therefore occlusion of the catheter [8]. IV catheters should be flushed with heparinised saline at least four times daily if they are not being used for fluid therapy or regular drug administration. To check for patency, a syringe containing heparinised saline should be attached to the catheter and aspirated. If the catheter is patent, blood will flow back into the syringe. If the catheter is blocked, no blood will be seen and the catheter should be investigated.

Bandaging Catheter Sites

There are conflicting reports on the use of bandages and antimicrobial-impregnated dressings on IV catheter sites in horses. One argument is that it may protect the catheter site from environmental contamination for example, in a patient with colic who is frequently rolling, as the catheter site could get contaminated from the pathogens and dust in the bed. The opposing argument is that neck bandages are difficult to maintain on adult horses can often become displaced. This can cause irritation to the catheter site and cause complications to occur. Neck bandages may be easier to maintain in foals, which is useful, as these patients tend to spend more time lying down in a contaminated environment when compared to adult horses. Careful selection of appropriate patients is key here. If neck bandages and dressings can be successfully maintained in colic patients and foals, they may be useful in reducing contamination of the catheter site and therefore catheter site complications.

Ultrasonographic Monitoring of Catheter Sites

Ultrasound scanning is a useful tool in the early detection of thrombophlebitis in equine patients with IV catheters [12]. In one study, subclinical signs of thrombophlebitis were identified in 27% of horses. This would suggest that regular ultrasound scanning of intravenous catheter sites could identify early signs of thrombophlebitis and facilitate early preventative treatment. High hygiene standards should be observed while carrying out ultrasound scanning of IV catheter sites in horses to ensure no contamination occurs. RVNs could carry out regular ultrasound examinations of IV catheter sites as part of evidence-based nursing practice. It would be more practical for RVNs to carry out the ultrasound scans, and the presence of a vet would not be required, further reducing the cost of the procedure. RVNs could acquire images, but no diagnosis would be made. The images would be interpreted by a vet, who would then make a diagnosis and collaborate with the RVN to produce and an effective treatment plan.

IV Catheter Care Bundle for Horses

Prevention is better than cure in relation to IV catheter complications in horses. The development of evidenced-based IV catheter care bundle for horses could help to reduce the incidence of IV catheter complications and improve overall welfare for equine patients.

As part of the care bundle, high-risk patients could be identified, such as those who are endotoxaemic or septicaemic. These high-risk patients should then have the following nursing interventions implemented:

- Left and right jugular veins could be assessed via ultrasound before the insertion of a catheter.
- Measurements could be taken taken and then compared to ultrasound scans taken once the IV catheter was in situ.
- Placement of a long-stay catheter made from polyurethane or silicone as they are the least thrombogenic.
- Regular assessment and monitoring of IV catheters and catheter sites.
- Regular flushing of IV catheters to maintain patency and reduce the incidence of phlebitis.
- Self-disinfecting catheter hubs applied as standard.
- IV catheter site scans to be carried out once daily to assess for subclinical signs of thrombophlebitis.

More information about care bundles can be found in Chapter 13 and the further reading list.

Conclusion

Strict monitoring of catheter sites is essential in equine patients to try to reduce potential complications. The RVN is in an ideal position to monitor catheter sites and implement preventative strategies. The application of an equine IV catheter care bundle could facilitate evidence-based nursing practice and raise the standards of care for equine patients. Clinical audits could be used alongside the implementation of an IV catheter care bundle to provide an unbiased means of monitoring protocol changes, and this would serve to ensure that patient welfare is not compromised.

17.4 Bandaging Techniques

Introduction

Wounds are frequently seen in equine practice. Therefore, it is important for RVNs to know how to treat wounds and bandage patients correctly. Information relating to wound care and dressings has already been covered in Chapters 12 and 13. This section will focus solely on correct bandaging techniques.

The Role of the Bandage in Equine Practice

Bandages have several roles, such as [13]:

- Control of haemorrhage
- Prevention and reduction of swelling
- Prevention of patient interference
- Reduction in pain
- Immobilisation
- Prevention of wound contamination

Many of these roles are involved in preventing the 12 factors that delay healing (see Chapter 12). This makes a properly applied bandage a powerful tool for the RVN in practice when assisting with optimal wound healing. Unfortunately, a poorly applied bandage can assist in some of the 12 factors that delay healing. Examples include:

- A bandage that has been applied too tightly can exacerbate a poor blood supply and poor oxygenation.
- A bandage that has been applied too loosely can facilitate movement at the site of a wound.
- A bandage that has slipped down can allow the patient/bacteria access to the wound. This can lead to continuing trauma and infection.

It is imperative that bandages are applied correctly and monitored closely. This will help to assist in optimal wound healing reduce the risks of any complications developing. All patients should be treated as individuals when it comes to bandaging. Horses with different temperaments will tolerate different bandaging techniques. The bandage should be adapted to suit the patient without compromising its original function.

Layers of a Bandage

Bandages are made up of three layers: a primary layer, a secondary layer and a tertiary layer.

The Primary Layer

Wound dressings form the first part or primary layer of the bandage. See Chapter 13 for detailed information regarding wound dressings. It is well known that wounds heal best in a warm, moist environment and the application of a wound dressing can assist with this. There are many dressings out on the market now, and the best practice is to select one that will provide the most optimal healing conditions for the specific wound being dealt with. Gloves should be worn before handling dressings to avoid contamination. Dressings should be picked up from the back, and no fingers should touch the front or wound-facing side. The dressing should then be applied straight to the wound the correct way around (wound facing side to the wound).

The Secondary Layer

The secondary layer is essentially used to keep the primary dressing in place, provide protection and absorption of discharge, as well as to help to prevent movement. Materials used for this include soft rolls of orthopaedic padding and gamgee or cotton wool. These padding materials are held in place with stretchy, conforming, mesh bandages such as Knitfirm™. Care should be taken when applying the conforming layer bandage. It should never be applied directly to the skin as it can cause damage. An inch of padding should be visible above and below the bandage once the conforming layer has been applied to protect the skin of the patient. The conforming layer should be held in place with strips of tape, as tucking it into the layers of the bandage can create a pressure point.

Bandage sores are commonly seen in equine practice on the lower limb of the horse. The lower limb of the horse does not contain any muscle; therefore, bandages are often applied over large bony prominences such as the the accessory carpal bone at the back of the carpus and the calcaneus (point of the hock). Bandage sores develop when pressure is applied over the thin skin in these areas. The following are some suggestions for preventing bandage sores:

- Applying extra padding in the secondary layer such as cotton wool can help to prevent bandage sores.
- 'Doughnuts', made from rolled-up orthopaedic padding, can be applied directly over bony prominences to help to pad and protect them.

- Using bandaging materials that are at least 15 cm wide is thought to reduce areas of focalised pressure that can predispose to the formation of bandage sores.
- Each layer of bandage applied should overlap the previous layer by 50% to achieve an even pressure.
- Apply enough pressure, but not too much. This comes with practice, but bandages do not need to be applied tightly; a good, firm and even pressure is what is required.
- A figure-of-eight bandaging technique can be applied over the carpus and tarsus with the aim of reducing pressure over the bony prominences [14].

For most bandages in equine practice, two layers of cotton wool and conforming mesh bandage are applied over one layer of orthopaedic padding. However, the bandage should be applied to suit the wound being treated and the temperament of the patient. For a Robert Jones bandage (RJB), which is used to immobilise fractures, the bandage should end approximately three times the width of the original limb being bandaged [13]. For more information regarding RJBs, please see Chapter 12.

The Tertiary Layer

This protective outer layer is usually achieved by using self-adhesive, conforming bandages such as Vetwrap™ or adhesive bandages such as Tensoplast™. These bandages are applied carefully as they are stretchy, so it is easy to put them on too tight. The aim is to get a neat, even finish with no areas of focalised pressure or creases. If a self-adhesive conforming bandage has been used as a tertiary layer for the majority of the bandage, an adhesive bandage can be applied at the top and bottom of the bandage to help keep it in place and to prevent any bedding from getting down the top and contaminating the wound.

Procedure for Applying a Multi-layered Bandage to a Distal Limb

1) Ensure the patient is adequately restrained by a handler wearing appropriate PPE.
2) All required bandaging materials and equipment should be prepared, unwrapped and placed in a clean tray ready for use (Figure 17.38).
3) Gloves should be worn. The dressing should be picked up from the back. The front of the dressing should not be touched (Figure 17.39).
4) The dressing should be applied with the correct side facing the wound (Figure 17.40). The dressing should be held in place with orthopaedic padding (Figure 17.41). The bandage should be applied working from distal to proximal.
5) A layer of gamgee or cotton wool should be applied (Figure 17.42).

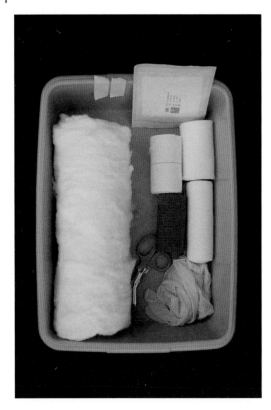

Figure 17.38 All equipment should be prepared and unwrapped beforehand. *Source:* Dr Francis Boyer.

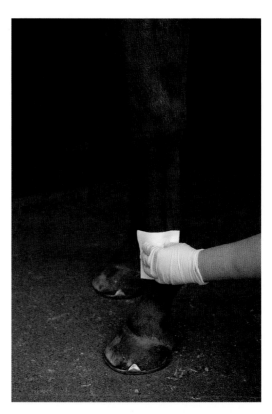

Figure 17.40 The dressing should be applied with the correct side facing the wound. *Source:* Dr Francis Boyer.

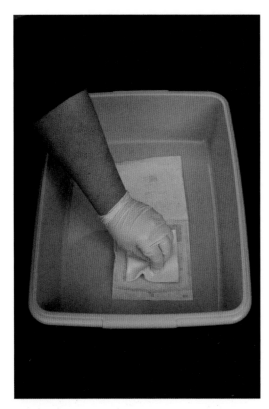

Figure 17.39 Dressings should be picked up from the back, and no fingers should touch the front or wound facing side. *Source:* Dr Francis Boyer.

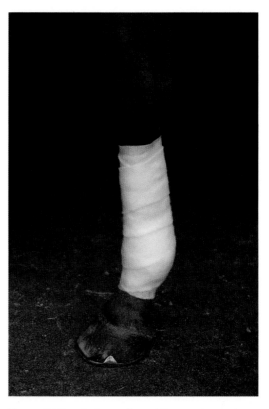

Figure 17.41 Orthopaedic padding can be used as part of the secondary layer to hold the dressing in place. *Source:* Dr Francis Boyer.

6) A stretchy, conforming, mesh bandage should be used to hold the padding in place. This should ideally be fixed with pieces of tape. One inch of padding should be visible at the top and bottom of the bandage (Figure 17.43).

7) Additional layers of cotton wool and conforming bandage can be added at this stage depending on the size of bandage required.

8) A self-adhesive, conforming bandage is applied. Again, one inch of padding material should be visible at the top and bottom of the bandage (Figure 17.44).

9) An adhesive bandage can be used to secure the top and the bottom of the bandage (Figure 17.45).

10) The bandage should be checked to make sure it is neat and of an even pressure.

Pressage Bandage

A pressage bandage is a reusable, elasticated stocking with a zip fastening [14] (Figure 17.46). Pressage bandages are available in several sizes for the tarsus, carpus and fetlock regions. They are used to apply even pressure to wounds and reduce oedema in superficial wounds [14]. A wound dressing and a secondary padding layer are applied first,

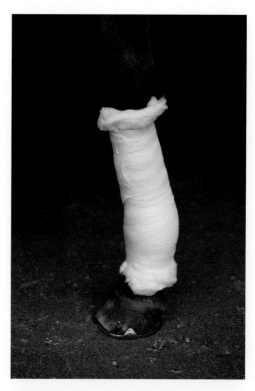

Figure 17.43 Secondary layer padding materials are held in place with a stretchy, conforming, mesh bandage. An inch of padding should be visible above and below the bandage following application. *Source:* Dr Francis Boyer.

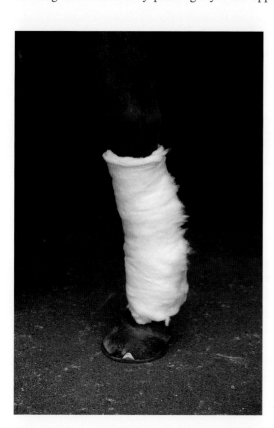

Figure 17.42 Cotton wool can be used as part of the secondary layer to provide padding. *Source:* Dr Francis Boyer.

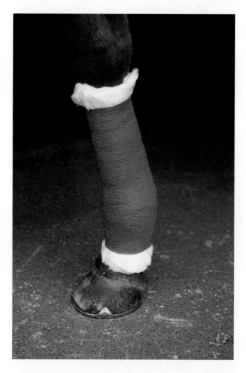

Figure 17.44 Self-adhesive, conforming bandages can be used as part of the tertiary layer. *Source:* Dr Francis Boyer.

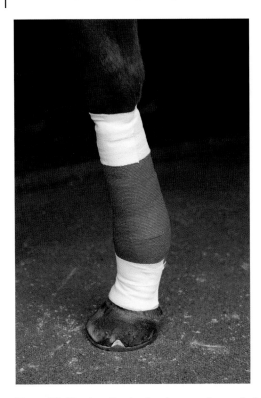

Figure 17.45 An adhesive bandage can be applied at the top and bottom of the bandage to help keep it in place. *Source:* Dr Francis Boyer.

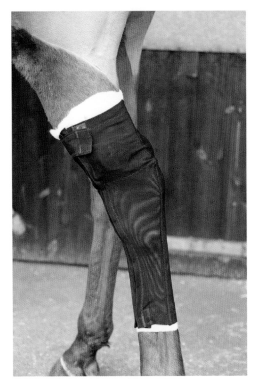

Figure 17.46 A pressage bandage. *Source:* Dr Francis Boyer.

and the pressage bandage is used as a tertiary layer. It is sometimes useful to apply a stable bandage with gamgee below the pressage bandage, and some adhesive bandage above the pressage bandage to help to keep it in place. Pressage bandages are sometimes useful for young horses who resent the pressures produced by a traditional bandage, as this can sometimes result in self-mutilation and destruction of the bandage. Pressage bandages are reusable, so they can help in cases where owner finances are a concern.

Foot Bandages

There are some instances where the foot may need to be bandaged. The most common reason for this would be a foot abscess. To prevent the poultice or dressing from moving upwards over the pastern, the bandage should incorporate both the heel and sole of the foot. Strong tape can be made into a pad and can be used to reinforce the bottom of the bandage. The coronet band and the skin surrounding it should not be covered with tape, as this can cause sweating, irritation and trauma to these areas [14].

Foot bandages should be checked regularly to make sure that they are intact and have not become wet or contaminated. Bags can be used to cover foot bandages to make them waterproof [14]. This is not recommended as a long-term solution, as this can cause the foot to become hot and sweaty, which can cause further complications [14]. Metal hospital plates may be fitted following certain surgeries, such as a pedal bone scrape. This can make the application of hoof bandages easier and reduce the amount of bandaging material required.

Procedure for Applying a Foot Bandage

There are many ways to apply a foot bandage or a poultice. This method can be varied, and different materials used if required.

1) Ensure the patient is adequately restrained by a handler wearing appropriate PPE.
2) All required bandaging materials and equipment should be prepared, unwrapped and placed in a clean tray ready for use (Figure 17.47).
3) The poultice material should be applied as required (Figure 17.48).
4) Padding material in the form of cotton wool should be applied on top of the poultice material (Figure 17.49).
5) The padding material should be held in place by the application of a self-adhesive conforming bandage. This bandage should be applied using a figure of eight technique (Figure 17.50).

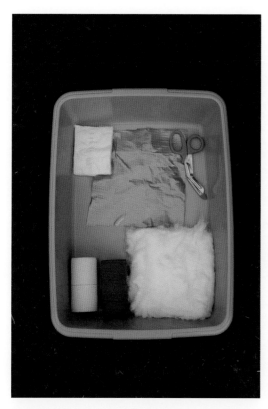

Figure 17.47 All required bandaging materials and equipment should be prepared, unwrapped and placed in a clean tray ready for use. *Source:* Dr Francis Boyer.

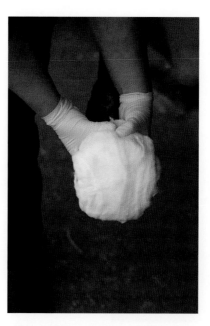

Figure 17.49 Padding material in the form of cotton wool should be applied on top of the poultice material. *Source:* Dr Francis Boyer.

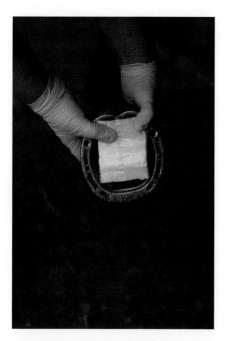

Figure 17.48 The poultice material should be applied as required. *Source:* Dr Francis Boyer.

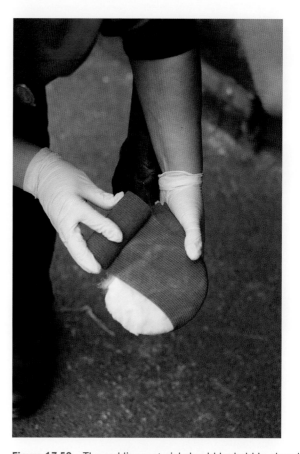

Figure 17.50 The padding material should be held in place by the application of a self-adhesive conforming bandage. This bandage should be applied using a figure-of-eight technique. *Source:* Dr Francis Boyer.

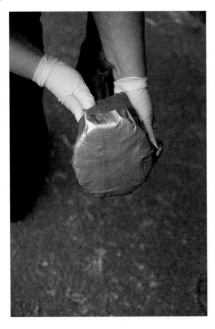

Figure 17.51 Once half of the self-adhesive conforming bandage has been used, the tape pad can be applied and stuck down firmly. *Source:* Dr Francis Boyer.

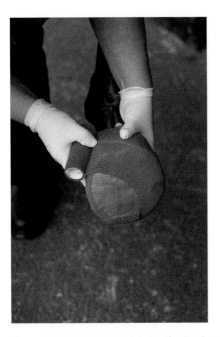

Figure 17.52 The rest of the self-adhesive conforming bandage can be used to cover the tape and secure the bandage. *Source:* Dr Francis Boyer.

6) Once half of the self-adhesive conforming bandage has been used, the tape pad can be applied and stuck down firmly (Figure 17.51).
7) The rest of the self-adhesive conforming bandage can be used to cover the tape and secure the bandage (Figure 17.52).

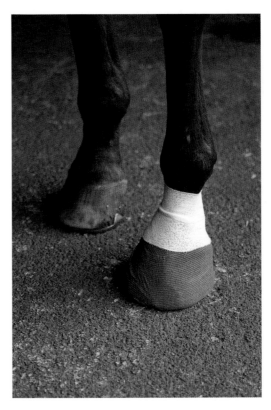

Figure 17.53 Adhesive bandage can be applied to the top of the bandage to stop any dirt or bedding getting in. *Source:* Dr Francis Boyer.

8) Adhesive bandage can be applied to the top of the bandage to stop any dirt or bedding getting in (Figure 17.53).
9) The bandage should be checked to ensure that it is even and not too tight in any area.

Abdominal Bandages

An abdominal support bandage or belly band can be applied following colic surgeries or caesareans to assist in the management of abdominal wounds. Abdominal bandages are particularly useful for heavily pregnant mares, mares with a foal at foot or where wound complications have occurred [15]. Abdominal bandages should be changed at least once daily, and the surgical wound should be assessed for signs of infection or dehiscence. Care should be taken in male horses so that urine does not contaminate the bandage, and therefore the wound [15]. Some clinicians prefer to use stents on an abdominal wound. Stents are sterile absorbent dressings that are sutured in place. This is a useful technique for highly discharging wounds and wounds that require extra pressure [16]. Usually, an absorbable dressing would be used on an abdominal wound. There are various types

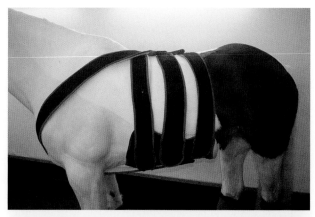

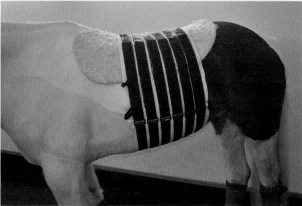

Figures 17.54 and 17.55 Commercially available abdominal bandages. *Source:* Rosina Lillywhite.

of commercially made re-useable abdominal bandages on the market (Figures 17.54 and 17.55). These are washable and easy to apply. However, they are expensive to purchase, so standard bandaging materials may be used instead [16]. Abdominal bandages are usually applied using an adhesive bandage such as Tensoplast™ as this helps to prevent the bandage from slipping (Figure 17.56). Further supports can also be made from soft material and attached around the chest and neck to prevent slipping. The bandage should be applied with an even tension around the abdomen, and extra padding should be applied at the withers to prevent pressure sores [16]. Care must be taken not to apply these bandages too tightly, and they should be monitored carefully to check for rubbing at the stifles or the elbows [16].

Conclusion

A bandage is a powerful tool used by RVNs in veterinary practice to help patients to achieve optimal wound healing. However, it is essential to have a good working knowledge of wound healing and factors that may interfere with this process. A poorly applied bandage can often do more harm than good. Therefore, rules and standards must be adhered to in order to achieve optimal healing for patients.

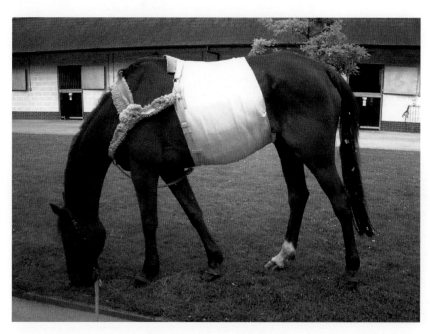

Figure 17.56 An abdominal support bandage applied with an adhesive bandage. *Source:* Reproduced with permission from Coumbe et al. [48] / John Wiley & Sons, Inc.

17.5 Nasogastric Intubation

Introduction

Nasogastric intubation is a procedure that is often used in equine practice, both in the hospital and out on ambulatory visits. It is an important skill to develop and can be useful for a variety of cases. The passing of a nasogastric tube is commonly performed for the following reasons [17]:

- Assessing and removing reflux from the stomach
- Gastric decompression
- Administering water and electrolytes/magnesium sulphate to treat impactions
- Providing fluid for hydration
- Delivering medications directly into the stomach
- Assessing and correcting obstructions in the oesophagus
- Aiding in the passing of a gastroscope
- Feeding dysphagic cases such as chronic grass sickness
- Enteral feeding

Equipment List

The following equipment will be required (Figure 17.57):

- Stomach tube – This can be made from silicon or urethane material. These are available in different sizes
- Lubricant
- Warm water
- Two buckets – one for fluid to be administered, and one to catch reflux
- Pump or funnel
- Sedation
- Twitch (if necessary)
- Electrolytes/Magnesium sulphate or desired additives
- Gloves

Technique

- The horse should be restrained with a headcollar and held by a competent handler wearing PPE.
- A twitch or sedation can be used for further restraint if required.
- The correct size of tube should be selected for the size of the patient.
- The handler should stand on one side of the horse while also holding the twitch if used. The person passing the tube should stand on the opposite side of the horse.
- The tube should be lubricated at the end to help it pass smoothly.
- One hand should be placed on the nostril, with the other hand on the end of the tube allowing some length available to pass.
- The tube should be inserted into the nostril and passed ventrally through the ventral meatus.
- The hand on the nostril can guide the tube ventrally by using a finger on the tube to direct it downwards while the tube is carefully advanced (Figure 17.58).

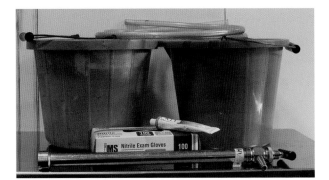

Figure 17.57 Equipment required for nasogastric tubing. *Source:* Rosina Lillywhite.

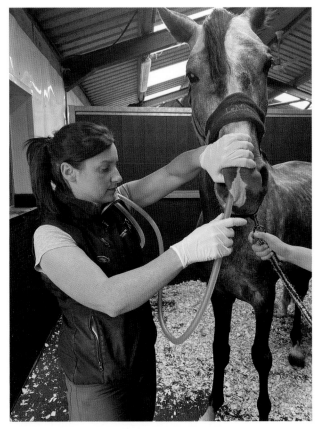

Figure 17.58 The hand on the nostril can guide the tube ventrally by using a finger on the tube to direct it downwards while the tube is carefully advanced. *Source:* Dr Simon Woods.

- Keeping the tube ventral will help to avoid the risk of contact with the ethmoid turbinates, which could cause a haemorrhage. It also facilitates easier passage into the oesophagus.
- The tube should be advanced carefully until the pharynx is reached, where resistance can be felt.
- Flexing the horse's neck downwards can facilitate the correct passage of the tube into the oesophagus. At this point, the tube should be moved swiftly forward to encourage the horse to swallow and allow the tube to enter into the oesophagus.
- The tube will need to be advanced several inches confidently in order to aid the horse in swallowing.
- The action of the horse swallowing can be felt against the tube. Dramatic coughing would indicate that the tube has gone into the trachea, and care should be taken to avoid this. However, the horse will not always cough especially when sedated and therefore checks must be carried out each time.
- The placement of the tube can be observed by looking at the neck on the left side, where the outline of the tube should be visible close to the left jugular groove. The tube may also be palpated here. The tube can then be gently advanced down to the cardia and into the stomach.
- Prior to administering any fluids, the stomach contents should be assessed, firstly to check that the tube is in the stomach, and also to check for reflux.
- This is done by placing a small amount of fluid into the stomach and then draining it back out again into a bucket.
- If there is any doubt as to the location of the tube, it must be removed immediately and replaced as stated above.
- Once the tube is confirmed to be in the stomach, any reflux should be drained out. The amount should then be measured.
- Fluid can then be administered either using a jug and funnel or a pump.

Safety Checks
- The tube should be passed ventrally.
- The tube should be visualised on the left side of the neck at the jugular grove.
- Any air felt on exhalation could indicate that the tube is in the trachea. If this is the case, the tube should be withdrawn immediately.
- Passing down the oesophagus should feel resistant, whereas the trachea will feel smooth.
- Once the tube is in the stomach, the smell of gastric contents can be an indicator that the tube is correctly positioned.

- Stomach sounds can also be heard by placing an ear to the tube.
- Sucking on the tube should create negative pressure when in the oesophagus; however, care should be taken when doing this due to the risk of zoonosis such as salmonella. Using a stomach pump is a safer method.
- Blowing on the tube should be possible and create a bubble of air that can be seen in the oesophagus.
- Coughing from the patient, indicates the tube is in the trachea; if this is the case, the tube should be immediately removed to avoid the risk of fluid entering the airway.

Complications Seen When Passing a Nasogastric Tube
- *Haemorrhage*: The tube should be withdrawn, and the bleed should be assessed to ascertain the extent and severity. If copious, it should be allowed to clot; packing with gauze may be necessary. The other nostril may then be used once this is under control.
- *Pharyngeal/oesophageal trauma*: The tube should be removed, and the proceeded halted. The vet may then wish to carry out a further assessment with the use of a video scope.
- *Stomach rupture*: This may become apparent following the procedure, and therefore, horses should be monitored closely following the passage of a nasogastric tube. The horse may become distressed and show colic symptoms. The vet will carry out a further assessment of the horse.
- *Inadvertent intratracheal placement*: The tube should be removed, and any administration of fluids should cease immediately. This may cause the horse to cough. The vet should be consulted.
- *Aspiration pneumonia*: This may not be evident for a few days; the horse should be monitored closely for any clinical signs such as an increased temperature, lethargy and increased respiratory effort.
- *Colic*: This may present shortly after fluids have been administered; horses may show signs of pain and should be monitored closely immediately following tubing.

Feeding Tubes
Nasogastric tubes can be used as and when required, but for more regular treatments can also be sutured in place. Tubes made out of silicone are preferred as mucosal trauma is less likely to occur; however, polyurethane tubes are also suitable [18]. If the horse is closely supervised in a hospital setting, most nasogastric tubes can be left in place for up to eight days [18]. The fibre content of the enteral diet dictates the size of the nasogastric tube used for infusion [18]. The tube with the smallest internal diameter should be selected to decrease pharyngeal and oesophageal irritation.

Fibre-free diets can be administered through an 18 Fr, 250 cm feeding tube. Diets containing fibre should be administered through a tube with an internal diameter of at least 0.65 cm [18].

Indications

Feeding tubes are more suited to patients who require timely and regular feeding that needs to be maintained over a duration of time. Types of cases include, but are not limited to [19]:

- Horses who are unable to eat
- Oral problems
- Oesophageal problems
- Post oesophageal surgery
- Botulism or tetanus
- Cases of dysphagia
- Horses who will not tolerate the frequent passing of a nasogastric tube

Indications for foals:

- For administering colostrum
- For foals who have not had a passive transfer of immunity
- Orphaned foals
- Foals who do not suckle
- Foals whose dams have low immunoglobulin levels in their colostrum
- For congenital defects such as persistent epiglottic frenulum or congenital oesophageal stenosis
- For neonatal maladjustment syndrome, when foals are not suckling from the dam

In some cases, usually as a last resort, an oesophagostomy tube may be used when feeding cannot bypass the nasal passages, pharynx or proximal oesophagus [20].

Placement of a Feeding Tube

The placement of these tubes can be technically demanding, as the tube is smaller in diameter and less rigid in comparison to a nasogastric tube. Therefore, difficulty may arise in getting to the larynx, passing into the oesophagus and maintaining a fluent passage down into the stomach. Indwelling tubes are usually fitted with a guide wire, and prior to starting the procedure, it should be confirmed that the guidewire is easily removed. Lubricating the wire, can aid a smoother removal [21]. A third person is required for this procedure as the passage of an endoscope for visualisation purposes is key to an easier placement. Sedation may be used, but for foals, sedation may depress the swallow reflex. Polyurethane feeding tubes are specifically designed for the long-term use in foals.

- To begin, the endoscope is passed down one nostril until the larynx is visualised.
- The second person can then begin to pass the tube following guidance from the scope operator.
- Ideally, a monitor will be used so that all parties can view the passage of the tube.
- Once the tube reaches the larynx, the horse can be stimulated to swallow by introducing a small amount of water via the endoscope.
- Following passage down into the stomach, the wire can then be removed.
- Checks should then be carried out to ensure that the tube is in place.
- This includes the removal of a sample of stomach fluid. Once in place, the tube should be marked at the nostril once it is confirmed that placement is correct.
- This makes it easier to assess if any dislodgement has occurred [19].
- To ensure the tube remains clean, the proximal end of the tube is then closed. The tube can then be attached to the headcollar with tape to prevent dislodgment.
- Tubes may also be stitched in place.
- Radiography can be carried out to check the placement of the feeding tube when using a radiopaque polyurethane tube.

Maintenance of Feeding Tubes

The following maintenance should be carried out on a feeding tube prior to feeding and after feeding:

Prior to Feeding
- Check sutures or tape is in place
- Check mark on tube is still at the exit of the nostril
- Remove end cap and wipe the end
- Check that the tube is still correctly positioned by removing a sample of stomach contents
- Flush with water to check for a blockage in the tube.

After Feeding
- Flush the tube with water to remove any build up from the tube
- Wipe the end
- Replace the proximal end cap

Frequency, Amount and Type of Feed

Pelleted feeds can be used with indwelling feeding tubes. The advantages are that they are inexpensive and already nutritionally balanced. An alfalfa pellet-based slurry made from alfalfa pellets is a suitable option. A vitamin and mineral balancer should be added if the pelleted feed being used is not a complete feed. Pelleted diets must be dissolved before administration. This can be achieved by griding the pellets down before water is added or by processing the pellets in a blender after they have been soaked in warm water [18]. The quantity of water required for each pelleted feed will vary; however, the amount of water added should be recorded as part of the horses' daily fluid intake. This amount should be subtracted from the daily fluid requirement of the horse to ensure that overhydration does not occur [18].

Enteral diets can be formulated if no commercial diet is available or if a special formulation is required to meet the nutritional needs of the horse. One enteral diet recipe called the 'Naylor Diet' has been published. This formulation provides 12.2 Mcal DE and requires a daily volume of the following [18]:

- 900 g dextrose
- 900 g casein
- 2000 g dehydrated alfalfa meal
- 21 l of water
- 230 g of a mineral mixture (see further reading for more information).

The nutritional requirements of the patient should be worked out carefully before an enteral diet is formulated. Diets that are formulated should be done so with care. Diets with high concentrations of oil or dextrose should be avoided as they can increase the risk of digestive and metabolic disturbances [18]. When the nutrition is first administered to the patient, the following protocol should be followed to avoid metabolic and gastrointestinal complications that can occur with rapid re-feeding [18]:

- Feed 25–30% of the total volume on days 1–2
- Feed 30–60% of the total volume on days 2–3
- Feed 60–100% of the total volume on days 3–4

Enteral feedings should be divided into at least 2 treatments per day. In a hospital setting, it is preferable to divide feedings into 4–6 treatments per day. No more than 6 l of fluid should be administered per feed in an adult horse weighing over 450 kg [18]. Amounts may need to be reduced for smaller patients.

Complications Seen with Indwelling Feeding Tubes [19, 21]

- Haemorrhage from the initial passing of the tube. The tube should be withdrawn, and the bleed should be assessed to ascertain the extent and severity. If copious, it should be allowed to clot; packing with gauze may be necessary. The other nostril may then be used once this is under control.
- The tube may move out of the oesophagus and into the pharynx, which may cause aspiration pneumonia.
- The tube may become blocked. This can be cleared with water, or a small amount of fizzy drink.
- Aspiration pneumonia may occur as a result of food or substances inhaled into the lungs. Horses with indwelling feeding tubes placed should be monitored intensively to include temperature readings and the assessment of lung sounds. A backflow of food or substance may also indicate this problem. If this is suspected, the feeding tube should be removed.
- Laminitis can be a potential side effect due to a low-fibre, high-carbohydrate diet. The horse should be monitored intensively to include digital pulses and the ration formulated to the horse's size and requirement. Additionally, insulin levels could also be monitored.
- Colic may present shortly after the feed has been administered; horses may show signs of pain and should be monitored closely immediately following tubing.
- Diarrhoea or constipation may occur. The horses' faecal output should be monitored, as well as borborygmi (gut sounds). The quality and quantity of the faeces should be recorded.
- Rhinitis may occur in response to placement of the tube. This may cause the foal or horse to rub at the tube, which may lead to displacement.
- Hyperglycaemia may occur following feeding that has been too aggressive. This is more common in critically ill foals. Regular measurement of glucose can help with monitoring. The patient should also be monitored for increased urination, thirst and lethargy.
- Laryngeal or pharyngeal trauma may occur following tube placement or movement. The tube should be removed, and the proceed halted. The vet may then wish to carry out a further assessment with a video scope.
- Oesophageal ulceration may occur. It is important to ensure that the correct size tube is used and that the tube is inserted gently and secured. Oesophageal ulceration may lead to complications in feeding once the tube is removed, and may stop that patient from wanting to eat. Following removal of the feeding tube, the vet may want to scope the oesophagus.
- Tube damage may occur if the patient tries to remove the tube.

Return to Voluntary Feeding

During the time that the enteral liquid diet is administered, small amounts of fresh feed should be offered to the patient [18]. Suitable feeds can include:

- Fresh grass
- Grass hay

- Oat hay
- Alfalfa leaves
- Succulents such as apples and carrots

Supplemental feeds that contain a high concentration of non-structural carbohydrates should be avoided during the re-feeding period. Once the horse is deemed ready, they can be weaned off the liquid enteral diet over a 2–3-day time period [18].

Cleaning of Tubes

The cleaning of nasogastric tubes and enteral feeding tubes must be carried out as soon as possible after use, to prevent build-up of food material within the tube.

The tube should be rinsed with warm water on the inside and outside. Enzymatic cleaner can then be used to break down any contents within the tube, as per the manufacturer's instructions. Using a tube feeding brush enables a thorough clean of the inside of the tube. The tube should then be rinsed again, submerged and left to soak in an appropriate disinfectant, again according to the manufacturer's instructions. After the required time, the tube should be removed from the solution and rinsed thoroughly before being hung to dry. Care should be taken not to store tubes with any moisture inside, as this can encourage the growth of mould.

17.6   Urinary Catheterisation

Introduction

In equine practice, urinary catheters are more commonly placed for either brief periods for example to collect a urine sample, or to drain urine during surgical procedures in the standing or anaesthetised patient. Indwelling catheters in horses are more prone to irritation and inflammation than other species; this is due to the calcium content of equine urine and the possibility of crystal formation along the catheter [22]. For this reason, catheter placement should be carefully considered, especially when dealing with indwelling catheters. However, the use of catheterisation in equine surgical cases contributes to a smooth anaesthetic as the horse is less likely to be stimulated by the need to urinate.

Minimising Stress and Distress

Prior to placing the urinary catheter, for patient welfare, ease of placement and colleague safety, the patient should be sedated. During standing surgery, this is often carried out during the pre-operative preparation when the patient is settled in a set of stocks. It is recommended during standing procedures that PPE in the form of a hard hat is worn when placing a urinary catheter. During general anaesthesia, this is normally carried out once the horse is anesthetised and on the operating table, during the pre-operative preparation stage prior to the commencement of surgery.

Urinary Catheterisation in Mares

Placing a urinary catheter in a mare follows a different process to placing a urinary catheter in a male horse. The equipment required is as follows:

- Cotton wool
- Warm water
- Rectal glove (ideally sterile)
- 2% chlorhexidine scrub
- Disposable gloves
- 500 ml Sterile saline
- Sterile gloves
- Water based lubricant
- Mare urinary catheter
- Vet wrap or vetcling
- Catheter tip syringe (to use if suction is required)

Preparation

The mare's tail should be wrapped using either a vetwrap or vetcling. The tail can then be tied back to the rear of the stocks using a quick-release tie technique. It is important to remember to remove this as soon as possible afterwards, as it can cause damage to the dock. A general clean of the perineal area should be carried out in a non-sterile manner, any dirt or build-up should be gently removed. Any faecal matter should be removed from the area to reduce the risk of contamination. Sterile gloves should be donned, and a gentle sterile scrub should be carried out using the 2% chlorhexidine solution, working from the centre of the vulva towards the periphery. It is beneficial to have one hand to hold the skin back while using the other hand to clean. Having the cleaning solution and cotton wool on a trolly at waist height reduces the need to move around and helps to maintain sterility. Using the same dirty-clean hand technique throughout ensures there is no contamination from the dirty area to the clean area. Once the area is fully cleaned, it should be rinsed with sterile saline from the top to the bottom, which will help to reduce any irritation from the chlorohexidine scrub solution [23].

The Catheterisation Process
- A sterile rectal glove should be worn on the inducing arm and sterile gloves on both hands.

- The assistant should first open and pass the sterile catheter in an aseptic manner.
- The assistant should then open a sterile packaged lubricant and apply to the inducing hand of the operator and also to the catheter. Lubricating the catheter will help to prevent trauma.
- One hand is placed into the vulva to locate the urethral opening. This is located on the floor of the vagina, a hand's length further cranial to the pelvic brim.
- Once located, digital manipulation can be used to slightly dilate the urethral opening and cause the urethral sphincter to relax. This hand is then kept in position (Figure 17.59).
- The catheter should then be introduced through the vulval opening with the other hand, directing the tip of the catheter underneath the first hand, guiding it between the fingers of the inducing hand to maintain control.
- Once the inducing hand has guided the tip into the urethral opening, the second hand introduces the catheter further along the urethra into the bladder. Once the bladder is reached, urine will flow spontaneously and the stylet can be removed. Flow can also be yielded by aspiration with a syringe.

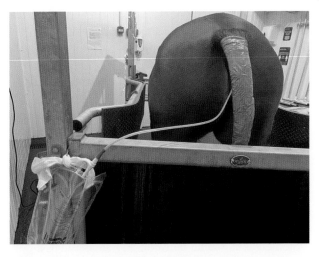

Figure 17.60 Once placed, the catheter should be securely attached to a urine collection bag. *Source:* Dr Simon Woods.

- The catheter should be securely attached to a urine collection bag (Figure 17.60).

It is important to acknowledge the proximity of the anus when inserting catheters into mares during surgery, as this poses an additional risk of bacterial infection, which could lead to a post-operative complication.

Urinary Catheterisation in Male Horses

Placing a urinary catheter in a male horse follows a different process to placing a urinary catheter in a mare. The equipment required is as follows:

- Cotton wool
- Warm water
- 2% chlorohexidine scrub
- Rectal glove (ideally sterile)
- Disposable gloves
- 500 ml Sterile saline
- Sterile gloves
- Water based lubricant
- Stallion urinary catheter
- Vet wrap or vetcling
- A catheter tip syringe (to use if suction is required)

Preparation

The gelding or stallion's tail should be wrapped to help maintain sterility. In order to facilitate placement, sedation (prescribed by a vet) should be administered to allow the penis to be extended. The penis should be gently but firmly held to prevent retraction. Using a mild/dilute chlorohexidine solution and cotton wool, the distal penis, the urethral and urethral fossa should be cleaned gently, ensuring that

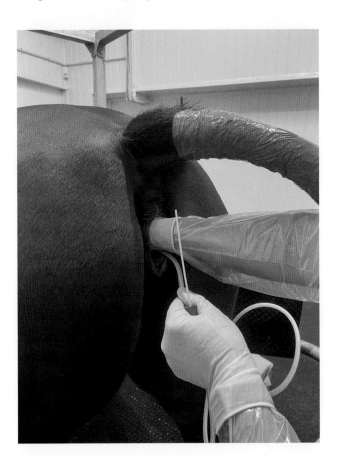

Figure 17.59 Placing a urinary catheter in a mare. *Source:* Dr Simon Woods.

during the cleaning process the penis does not return to the sheath. The use of gauze swabs should be avoided as they can be abrasive to this sensitive area. One hand should be used to hold the penis, which is the 'dirty' hand and the other hand should be used to clean the area of interest, this is known as the 'clean' hand. The diverticulum and fossa should be cleaned carefully as there may be a smegma build-up in these areas. This is a good opportunity to also remove any smegma beans that could cause the horse discomfort in the future. Once the area has been cleaned, the penis can be rinsed with sterile saline.

The Catheterisation Process

- Sterile gloves should be worn, and an assistant will be required to pass equipment.
- Sterile rectal sleeves may be worn underneath the gloves.
- The assistant should first open and pass the sterile catheter in an aseptic manner.
- In order to protect any damage to the urethra and to assist with an easier passage, water-soluble sterile lubrication should be applied to the end of the catheter by the assistant, again in a sterile manner. Single packet lubrication is recommended as this can be used per individual case.
- One hand again should be used as the 'dirty' hand, which is used to hold the penis; it is recommended that this be the non-dominant hand of the operator.
- The catheter can then be introduced into the urethral opening and gently advanced ensuring no resistance is felt. The horse at this stage may attempt to retract the penis, and this should be prevented. It may be easier to have a second person hold the penis.
- The catheter should be advanced further until a flow of urine is achieved. The advancement should be smooth; however, there may be a small amount of resistance.
- The passage should be monitored for any increased resistance, which could suggest there are kinks in the tube. Once entering the bladder, a small loss of resistance may be felt. Once the bladder is reached, urine should spontaneously flow, and the stylet can be removed. Flow can also be yielded by aspiration with a syringe [24].
- The catheter should be securely attached to a urine collection bag (Figure 17.61).

Catheters Types

A flexible catheter is more commonly used in equine practice. This can be in the form of a stallion flexible catheter, a mare flexible catheter or a foley catheter. Metal urinary catheters can be more traumatic and are therefore avoided. In the event that an indwelling urinary catheter is needed, a foley catheter would be the preferred choice.

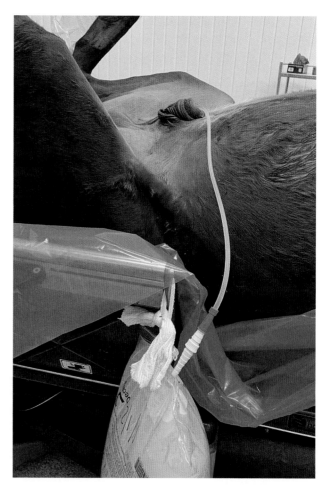

Figure 17.61 The catheter should be securely attached to a urine collection bag. *Source:* Dr Simon Woods.

Methods of Avoiding Patient Interference

Urinary catheterisation is most commonly used during surgical procedures in adult horses. Because of this, interference from the patient is limited, and the catheters are removed prior to the patient leaving the procedure room. Often, repeat catheterisation is chosen in place of indwelling urinary catheters due to potential complications such as urinary tract infections and placement security. However, there are some instances in which indwelling catheters may be required, such as foals in intensive care. More information on this can be found in Chapter 15.

Monitoring and Cleaning Urinary Catheters

When dealing with indwelling catheters, the catheters should be cleaned twice daily, around the point of the exit from the body and the catheter itself. This can be carried out with a dilute chlorhexidine solution and rinsed with sterile water. During surgery, the area should also be monitored closely when using a short-stay urinary catheter. It is important to monitor the urine output and avoid any backflow by changing the collection bag before it gets full. With mares, the catheter may sit very close to the anus, and therefore ensuring this area is clean is crucial to avoid any risk of infection. The amount and appearance of the urine should be reported to the anaesthetist and recorded on the anaesthetic record.

The following steps should be carried out while nursing a patient with an indwelling urinary catheter:

- *Use a closed system*: This consists of a urinary catheter attached to a receptacle for urine collection, such as a sterile fluid collection bag [25]. The use of an anti-reflux valve, which prevents a backflow of urine back to the patient is recommended.
- Ensure good hygiene is maintained throughout.
- Regular emptying of the urine collection bag.
- Monitoring the area for any redness/swelling/irritation.
- Monitoring patient comfort levels.
- Monitoring urination frequency and appearance.

Equine Urine Output and Appearance

Urine output can increase and decrease depending on various conditions. Normal urine output values are as follows:

- Adult horses: 2.0 mL/kg/hour [26]
- Foals: 4.0–8.0 ml/kg/hour [26]

Clinical conditions that may affect urinary output include the following [26]:

- Renal disease
- Water deprivation
- Dehydration
- Polydipsia (excessive drinking) (due to other medical conditions and some side effects of certain medications)

The normal appearance of equine urine is pale to dark yellow in colour. It can be clear or appear cloudy if large quantities of calcium carbonate crystals are present. Red or dark brown urine is abnormal and should be investigated immediately. Equine urine is alkaline with a pH range of 7.0–9.0 [26]. Urine should be assessed immediately after collection or stored in an airtight container due to the presence of pyrocatechin. This is an oxidising agent and will turn urine dark brown or red when exposed to air.

Relevant Conditions

Reasons for the use of urinary catheterisation in practice include:

- Catheterisation during surgery: either standing surgery or during general anaesthesia, to provide patient comfort and as part of multimodal anaesthesia.
- Collection of urine for urine analysis.

- For intensive care foals to monitor urine output and prevent skin scalding.
- For bladder drainage where a micturition is prevented by a physiological condition.
- Lavage of the bladder for cases such as sabulous cystitis.
- For contrast administration for imagining of the urinary tract.

  For medical investigations such as bladder stones, cystitis and urethral blockage.

17.7 Physical Therapy Techniques

Introduction

The aim of physical therapy is to manage pain, optimise healing and maintain or maximise the function of the horse. This should not be limited to orthopaedic or musculoskeletal cases but can be beneficial in rehabilitating a range of conditions, especially if a period of box rest is to be prescribed [27]. Physical therapy should always be carried out with the treating vet's consent and guidance. Where necessary, assistance from a veterinary physiotherapist should be sort. All physical therapy treatments carried out should be well documented to include the type, duration and frequency of each exercise or modality. Good documentation allows for all people involved in the horse's care to continue with the program and easily see where improvements or deteriorations occur, to allow the program to be adjusted accordingly [28].

Health and Safety
Practice protocols for health and safety should be adhered to at all times.
PPE should be worn as required and includes:

- A riding hat.
- Sturdy or steel-toe-capped boots.
- Gloves if holding or leading the horse.

Equipment for restraining the horse dependent on activity:

- Headcollar and leadrope
- Bridle
- Chifney
- Lunge line
- A second person to hold the horse rather than having them tied up

Environment:

- Be aware of external stimuli that may spook or unsettle the horse, i.e. vehicles moving, horses out in the field and doors opening.

- Surfaces should be swept clean and be level and non-slip.
- There should be enough room to complete exercises safely.

Active Exercise

The most common component of physical therapy in rehabilitation is controlled exercise. The diagnosis, whether lameness, injury or illness, will dictate the type, duration and intensity of exercise prescribed [29].

Stable Exercises

Muscle is metabolically a very greedy tissue; if not used, muscle atrophy can occur quite rapidly. This should be a consideration in the following:

- The recumbent patient
- Long-term box rest or a cross-tied patient

- An immobilised area for example, where a RJB has been applied
- A non-weight-bearing limb.

When there has been sufficient healing that the horse is able to move freely around the stable, then simple stable exercises can commence to begin to activate and strengthen muscles prior to introducing more strenuous exercise. These exercises can be done twice daily. Figures 17.62–17.65 demonstrate some simple stable exercises.

Straight Line Walking

Any walking exercise that the patient will be allowed to do is totally dependent on the illness/injury and the stage of healing [30]. Following surgery or an injury, walking is usually started in five-minute sessions, twice a day; this is

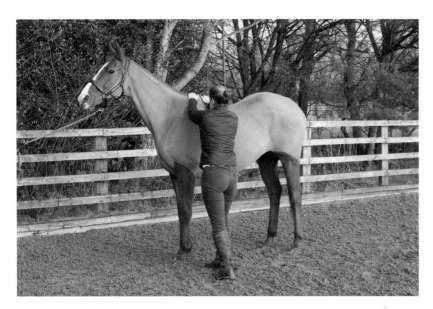

Figure 17.62 Wither rock. Stand close to the horse, hand on top of wither and gently rock side to side: targets thoracic sling musculature. *Source:* Dr Francis Boyer.

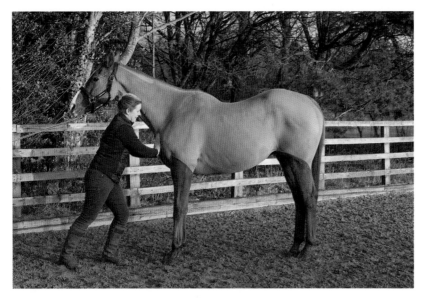

Figure 17.63 Caudal sternum push. Place hand on most cranial aspect of sternum and gentle rock backwards: targets epaxials and hypaxial, and hamstrings. *Source:* Dr Francis Boyer.

Figure 17.64 Lateral tail pull. Hold the tail below the dock and pull (gently) to the side: targets Quadriceps/Obliques. *Source:* Dr Francis Boyer.

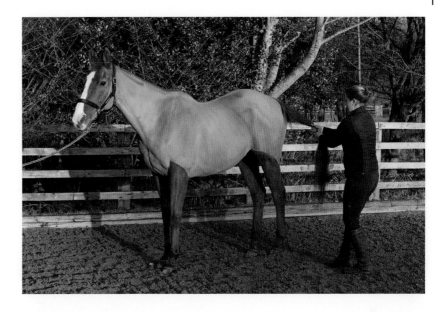

Figure 17.65 Caudal tail pull. Hold tail well below the dock and pull tail straight back (if safe to do so), then gentle release: Targets epaxials. *Source:* Dr Francis Boyer.

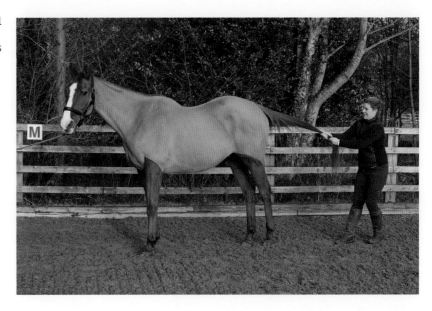

commonly increased by five minutes a week, but this is totally dependent on the individual patient's case.

When walking the horse, it should be encouraged to walk in a forward but relaxed manner. Bearing in mind a horse on box rest is likely to be fresh and excitable when walking out, correct restraint equipment such as a bridle is often necessary to maintain control safely.

Pole Work

Pole work increases the activation of hypaxial and epaxial muscles (Figure 17.66). It also encourages the horse to use an increased range of motion in its lower limb joints [31]. The intensity of pole work will vary depending on each case and the stage of healing.

Management of the Lower Limb
Stable Bandages

Stable bandages are a soft bandage consisting of some form of padding, gamgee for example, and a soft non-stretch or fleece bandage (Figure 17.67). Their purpose is to provide protection, warmth and some degree of support to the lower limb; they can also be used to help manage oedema. Stable

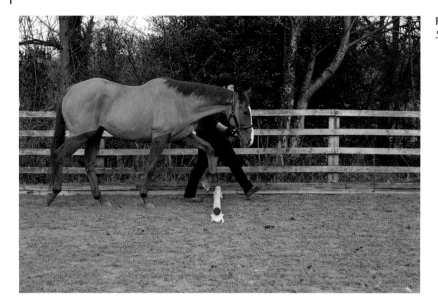

Figure 17.66 Pole work. *Source:* Dr Francis Boyer.

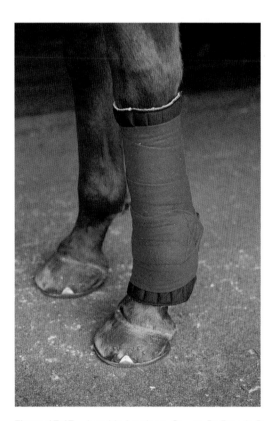

Figure 17.67 A stable bandage. *Source:* Dr Francis Boyer.

bandages are soft, and so should not to be used for immobilisation of the limb.

A hospitalised horse may be recumbent or lying down more than normal due to injury and/or illness, so stable bandages can provide some protection from bruising and abrasions from the floor and their own limbs/hooves. Horses on reduced exercise or box rest are more likely to experience oedema in the lower limb; the compression effect of a stable bandage can prevent or reduce this. They can also be applied to the contralateral limb to provide support. Prior to application, the horse should be safely restrained or held in a clean area with any bedding swept out of the way. The limb should be clean, dry and free of any bedding debris. Stable bandages should cover from the coronet up to the proximal metacarpus/metatarsus; the bandage should not extend any higher as this will limit the movement of these joints. The padding should be held to lie flat and wrinkle-free against the leg while the bandage is applied snuggly with even tension over the top, taking care not to over-tighten the fastening. Once applied, the tension should be checked. A finger should be able to fit comfortably underneath the bandage [32].

Splinting

Splinting can be used as first aid when a fracture or severe soft tissue injury is suspected to prevent any further damage to the area and allow the horse to be transported for further diagnostics and treatment. It is also a treatment in its own right to immobilise a fracture or soft tissue while an injury heals.

There are several commercially available coaptation splints for the lower limb, such as the Monkey splint or Kimzey leg saver splint (Figure 17.68). These are applied over the top of a thick bandage; the hard part of the splint lies over the cranial aspect of the limb, and straps hold it

Figure 17.68 Commercially available splints. (a) Kimzey leg saver splint. (b) Farley compression boot. *Source:* Reproduced with permission from Coumbe et al. [48] / John Wiley & Sons, Inc.

(a)

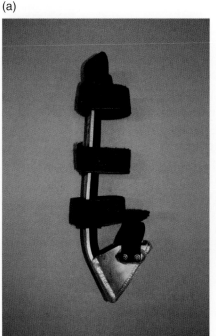

(b)

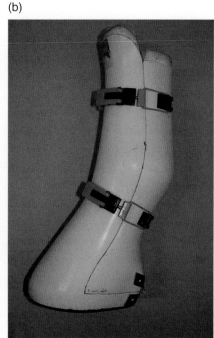

snug. Another prefabricated splint is the Farley compression boot; this splint consists of two moulded plastic halves that can be strapped around the lower limb to immobilise it. A well-applied, thick bandage underneath these splints is vital to provide further support and prevent pressure sores [33].

Ice Boots

There are many types of ice boots on the market; the ones that contain frozen gel or ice are more effective at cooling than those that are just soaked in water (Figure 17.69). Ice boots cool the legs via conduction and also have a compressive effect. They can be used to help manage inflammation, pain and oedema in the lower limb.

If the boots are applied straight from the freezer and are not manufactured with a layer of fabric over the ice pack, it is advisable to use a layer of thin material or a tubigrip underneath to prevent ice burns. A well-fitting ice boot should cover the lower limb from pastern up to the metacarpus/tarsus and be fastened snugly so it does not slip down or move. Cross-tying or tying the horse up will prevent the horse from pulling off the boots themselves or moving around so much that they slip down.

Ice boots should be applied for 15 minutes at a time. For the first 48 hours after injury, they can be applied every few hours and then three or four times a day afterwards. Providing precautions have been taken to avoid ice burns, ice

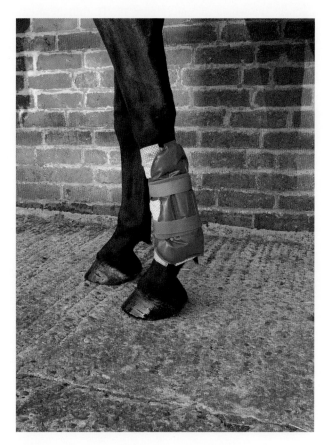

Figure 17.69 An ice boot. *Source:* Tamsyn Amos.

boots are a safe treatment tool. The main contradictions are actively haemorrhaging wounds and burns.

Manual Rehabilitation Techniques

Coupage

Coupage is a form of respiratory physical therapy; it can help to loosen bronchial and pulmonary secretions and stimulate expectoration. It is more successful in foals and miniature breeds due to their smaller size. Coupage is more effective following nebulisation and can be carried out standing or in lateral recumbency with an assistant to help to restrain the patient. If the horse or foal is recumbent, it is important to remember to turn them to alternate the side that coupage is performed on. Coupage is carried out with a cupped hand, to achieve the correct shape curve the fingers and palm into a 'C' shape and close the thumb to the index finger to complete the cup shape (Figure 17.70). Coupage is ineffective with a flat hand as it is the trapped air between the cupped hand and the horse that creates the vibration at a frequency that can modify the mucus to a consistency that is easier to expel.

Coupage is achieved by repeatedly thumping the cupped hand against the horse's side over the ribs, with firm but not painful pressure. The position of the hand should be moved to cover the whole ribcage (Figure 17.71). Initially, treatment should begin with 30-second sessions, building up to five minutes three or four times a day. If the patient's condition allows, following coupage with gentle exercise such as walking can further help with expectoration.

Stretching Exercises

All movement is dependent on the range of motion available at a joint and its limiting factors. This includes the physiological design of the joint (hinge versus ball and socket), capsuloligamentous structures and joint pathologies (such

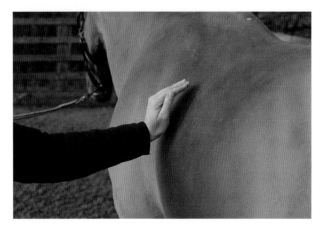

Figure 17.70 Coupage hand position. *Source:* Dr Francis Boyer.

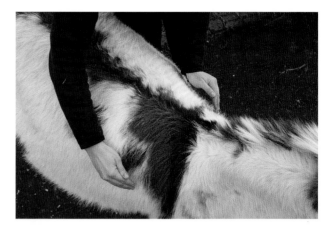

Figure 17.71 Coupage on a donkey. *Source:* Dr Francis Boyer.

as osteophyte formation within a joint). Muscles can also inhibit range of motion due to tension or shortening.

Both passive and dynamic stretching can be used as part of a physical therapy program to increase range of motion. These can be very effective techniques, but it is important that they are only used at the appropriate time depending on the stage of healing. For example, a horse that is cross-tied while a fracture heals should not be doing any stretches that would cause it to move or create torsion through the affected limb. In comparison, a horse that has had an interspinous ligament desmotomy can begin its stretching program within a few days of surgery to activate the muscles that support the spine.

Handler safety should be an important consideration at all times; these techniques require one person to correctly restrain the horse and another to perform the stretch. Care should be taken if the horse has been sedated. Stretching exercises should only be performed once the sedation has fully worn off, as this will decrease the risk of the patient losing their balance. With passive stretching, the handler should also take into consideration their own posture, bending at the knee, not the back and not interlocking their fingers around the limb in case the horse pulls away. During dynamic stretching, the handler should be aware of their position relative to the horse; if the horse needs to adjust its position during the stretch, the handler must have sufficient room to step back out of the way.

Passive stretching is used as a treatment to increase the range of motion at a joint, lengthen soft tissue and relax muscle spasm. In a working horse, a regular stretching regime is used to assist in injury prevention, but it is equally important for the box-rested horse that does not have the opportunity to move around, graze and roll to stretch for itself. Stretching should be carried out on warmed-up muscles. If possible, a 10–15-minute walk is a sufficient warm-up, or if the horse is not able to exercise, or is recumbent, a heat pack can be applied to the area being stretched for 10 minutes. Once in the correct position for the stretch, and the horse is relaxed into it, hold for 30 seconds and repeat each stretch three times [34]. Figures 17.72–17.75 demonstrate a range of passive stretches.

Dynamic stretches are also known as carrot or baited stretches. Unlike passive stretches, they give the horse complete control of the movement, which makes them safer to carry out as there is less risk of the horse over stretching. Dynamic stretches have a twofold effect on the body. To complete the movement, one set of muscles is stretched and another set is activated; this is a particularly useful way of activating core musculature in a horse with back pain or following spinal surgery [35]. Figures 17.76–17.80 demonstrate a range of dynamic stretches. Ballistic stretching, the bouncing or snatching at the end of a stretch has been linked to injury so should be avoided where possible. Stretches should be kept smooth and controlled.

Thermotherapy

Thermotherapy is the application of heat to increase tissue temperature to encourage:

- Increased metabolic activity.
- Reduced muscle spasm.
- Localised vasodilation.
- The provision of analgesia.

Figure 17.72 Forelimb protraction stretch. *Source:* Dr Francis Boyer.

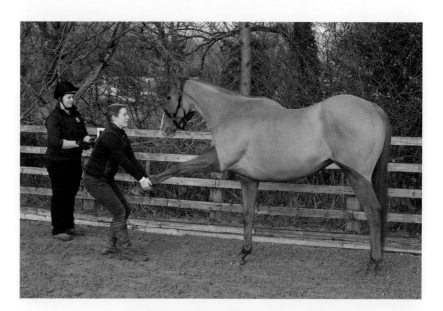

Figure 17.73 Hindlimb protraction stretch. *Source:* Dr Francis Boyer.

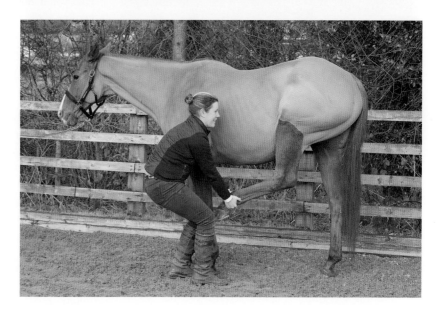

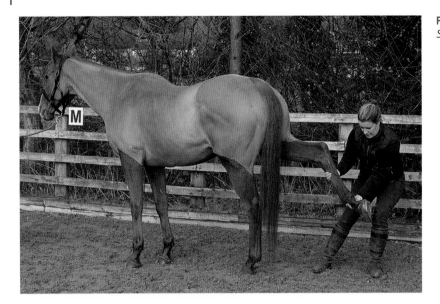

Figure 17.74 Hindlimb retraction stretch. *Source:* Dr Francis Boyer.

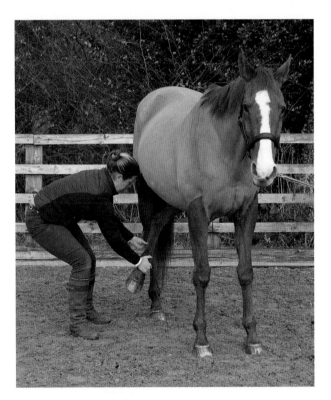

Figure 17.75 Hindlimb adduction stretch. *Source:* Dr Francis Boyer.

A heat pack is the most common method of application; once heated, it should be comfortable to touch but not hot enough to burn [35]. The heat pack should be applied for up to 15 minutes at a time (Figure 17.81).

Cryotherapy

Cryotherapy is the local or general application of a cold temperature. Cryotherapy. causes the following physiological effects that make it an extremely useful treatment technique:

- Analgesic
- Hypometabolic
- Vasoconstrictive
- Reduces muscle spasm.

There are several methods of applying cryotherapy: ice boots, cold water hosing, ice water immersion, ice packs and ice massage. Ice water immersion (Figure 17.82) and cold-water hosing (Figure 17.83) are the most effective at cooling [36]. The choice of method is usually down to the ease and safety of application. Cold water hosing and ice water immersion are easy and safe for the lower limbs and hooves; however, if cryotherapy needs to be applied on the horse's body, or near to a surgical site, an ice pack or ice massage may be easier and potentially pose less of an infection risk (Figure 17.84). If working with a young or nervous horse, or one that needs to remain immobile, an ice pack may be better tolerated than hosing or being made to stand in a bucket of water. An icepack can be used directly from the freezer but it should be wrapped in a layer of thin material to prevent ice burns. It should be held on to the required area for 10–15 minutes.

Massage

Massage is a general term that covers a range of techniques; it is a treatment tool with many applications which are as follows [37–39]:

Figure 17.76 Nose to chest.
Source: Dr Francis Boyer.

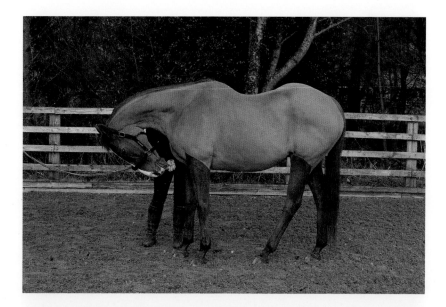

Figure 17.77 Nose between fetlocks.
Source: Dr Francis Boyer.

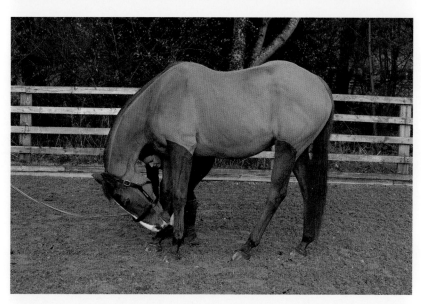

Figure 17.78 Nose to girth.
Source: Dr Francis Boyer.

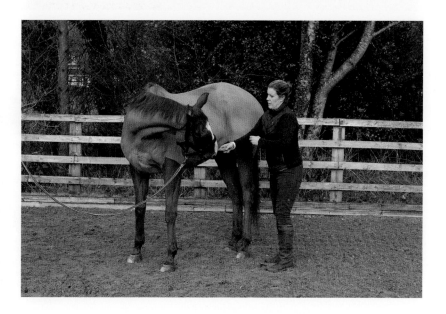

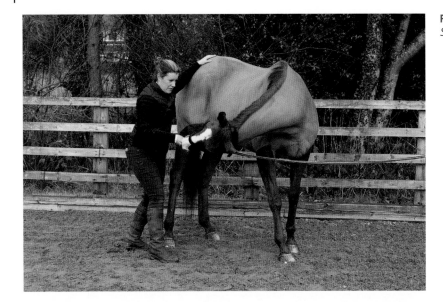

Figure 17.79 Nose to flank.
Source: Dr Francis Boyer.

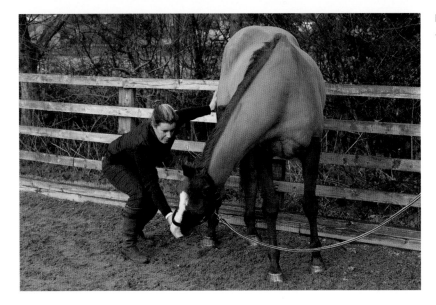

Figure 17.80 Nose to hind fetlocks.
Source: Dr Francis Boyer.

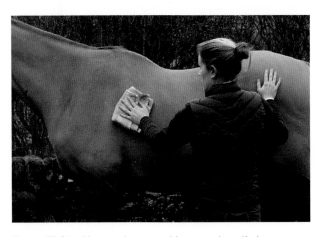

Figure 17.81 Heat pack wrapped in a towel applied over a muscle. *Source:* Dr Francis Boyer.

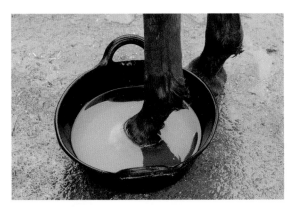

Figure 17.82 Ice water immersion. Select a rubber bucket with no handle and fill it to the required depth with cold water. Lift the horse's limb into the bucket and encourage it to stand. Add ice to the water and swirl it around the leg periodically. Keep in place for 10–15 minutes. *Source:* Dr Francis Boyer.

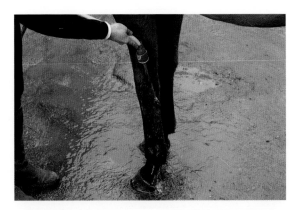

Figure 17.83 Cold hosing. Hold the hose above the area requiring cryotherapy so the water runs down over it. Keep in place for 10–15 minutes. *Source:* Dr Francis Boyer.

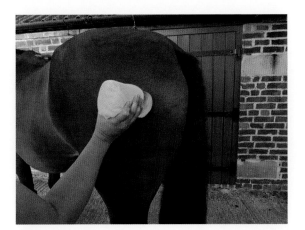

Figure 17.84 Ice massage. Make a large ice cube or ball using a paper cup or plastic bag. Once fully frozen, break the ice cube out and apply with gentle pressure in a circular motion over the area required for up to 15 minutes. *Source:* Tamsyn Amos.

- Assists with the reduction of pain memory/fear.
- Pain relief.
- Reduction of muscle spasm.
- Increased superficial circulation.
- Assists lymphatic drainage.
- Improves the appearance of scar tissue.

The most basic massage techniques are called effleurage and petrissage. Effleurage is long, slow, rhythmical strokes of even pressure used only over muscle. Petrissage encompasses a range of techniques, including kneading, stretching and squeezing. These techniques warm up superficial tissue, increase localised vasodilation, assist with lymphatic drainage and have a local analgesic effect.

Massage is a well-tolerated treatment modality. However, there are contraindications to its use, which are as follows:

- Over fractures
- Over wounds
- Infection
- Malignancy
- Pregnancy
- Acute injuries

Case Examples

The cases displayed in Tables 17.6–17.9 give examples of how to plan a treatment program with a problem list, goals and appropriate techniques. Suitability of each treatment technique and the point in recovery at which it is used will vary between individual cases, so good clinical reasoning and awareness of contradictions are essential. All treatments should be carried out with the treating vet's consent and guidance.

Table 17.6 Physiotherapy treatment program for a recumbent patient.

Recumbent patient	Clinical considerations	Treatment goals	Treatment technique
	Pressure sores/limb injuries	Protect limbs and maintain circulation	- Stable bandages - Passive limb stretches - Massage
	Respiratory complication	Optimise lung function	- Coupage - Regular turning and positioning
	Muscle spasm/soreness	Reduce spasm and discomfort	- Turn and reposition regularly - Massage - Thermotherapy - Cryotherapy
	Muscle atrophy	Maintain/improve muscle mass	When patient is able to stand or in supported standing in sling: - Baited stretches - Stable exercises

Source: Tamsyn Amos.

Table 17.7 Physiotherapy treatment program for a laminitic patient.

Laminitic patient	Clinical considerations	Treatment goals	Treatment technique
	Laminitis risk in systemically sick patient	Decrease risk of laminitis	• Ice water submersion of hooves (only in initial stages – once clinical signs appear icing the hooves can be detrimental)
	Compensatory muscle soreness due to posture (offloading fore limbs)	Relieve soreness and help reduce postural changes	• Heat pack • Massage • Static stable exercises (lateral tail pulls) • Initially no exercises that increase load to forelimbs
	Stiffness and muscle atrophy due to prolonged period of box rest	Maintain and/or improve available range of motion and muscle mass	Once condition is stable enough and horse is comfortable to start loading forelimbs: • Baited stretches • Stable exercises When able progress to: • Passive limb stretching • Straight line walking • Pole work

Source: Tamsyn Amos.

Table 17.8 Physiotherapy treatment program for a patient following a dorsal spinous process osteotomy.

Dorsal spinous process osteotomy	Clinical considerations	Treatment goals	Treatment technique
	Pain around surgical incision	Decrease pain	• Gentle massage to surrounding area – NOT over incision. • Ice massage to surrounding area – NOT over incision
	Muscle spasm/Soreness elsewhere in back	Decrease spasm and discomfort	• Massage • Thermotherapy (heat pack) • Baited stretches
	Muscle atrophy from box rest (possibly from pre surgery if long term problem)	Increase and/or maintain muscle mass and strength	• Straight line walking • Stable exercises (tail pulls, etc.) • Baited stretches Progression when able: • Pole exercises
	General stiffness from box rest (possibly from pre surgery if long term problem)	Improve and/or maintain joint range of motion	• Baited Stretches • Passive limb stretching Progression when able: • Pole exercises

Source: Tamsyn Amos.

Table 17.9 Physiotherapy treatment program for a patient following colic surgery.

Surgical colic	Clinical considerations	Treatment goals	Treatment techniques
	Weakness of abdominal muscles due to incision and inactivity	Maintain and/or improve muscle mass and strength	Once incision has healed sufficiently: • Baited stretches and (abdominal muscles engage to balance the body as the head and neck move). An easier stretch not asking the horse to reach so far requires less muscular effort so initially just head turns and then build up to a full stretch over time • Short amounts of controlled straight-line walking • Active stable exercises

Table 17.9 (Continued)

Surgical colic	Clinical considerations	Treatment goals	Treatment techniques
			When able progress to: • Build up distance straight-line walking • Walking over poles
	General stiffness and muscle atrophy due to prolonged period of box rest	Maintain and/or improve available range of motion and muscle mass	Once incision has healed sufficiently: • Baited stretches • Active stable exercises
			When able progress to: • Passive limb stretching • Straight line walking • Pole work
	Swelling/oedema in the lower limbs	Disperse/prevent swelling	• Stable Bandages • Active stable exercises that encourage weight shift between limbs • Straight line walking • Massage
	Post-surgical muscle discomfort from position during surgery or being lifted to/from surgery	Reduce pain	• Massage • Thermotherapy • Cryotherapy

Source: Tamsyn Amos.

17.8 Euthanasia

Introduction

Euthanasia, defined as a good death, provokes strong emotions that, together with issues of equine welfare and human safety, can make this a stressful procedure [40]. Before the procedure, it is essential that the clinician has obtained informed consent from the clients and insurers. This should be written consent but in emergencies this may have to be verbal. RVNs may be required to discuss consent for euthanasia and euthanasia options with clients. The British Equine Veterinary Association (BEVA) has produced guidelines to assist with the decisions involved with euthanasia of horses. These guidelines include advice on insurance implications and can be a useful source of information to discuss with clients or direct them to [41]. See the further reading section for more information.

Methods of Euthanasia

There are two main methods of euthanasia in the horse.

- Shot by free bullet
- By injection

Shot by Free Bullet

- A headcollar and leadrope will be required to restrain the horse with.

- If unsettled or stressed, the horse may require sedation (prescribed by a vet).
- A safe location for shooting should be considered.
- All humans and other animals should be removed from the area.
- If an assistant is holding the horse, they should stand behind the person operating the gun [41].

Method

In horses, the brain is situated high in the head. The shot should be aimed in the middle of the forehead. Two imaginary lines should be drawn from the middle of each eye to the base of the opposite ear. The horse should be shot approximately 2 cm above the point where the lines cross [42]. The shot should be aimed slightly down into the brainstem and the back of the head [43]. The bullet is discharged into the brain of the horse to cause death.

Advantages [40]

- Death is rapid
- It is inexpensive
- The carcass can be disposed of easily

Disadvantages

- Aesthetically unpleasant
- Can be dangerous
- A gun licence will be required.

Injection of Quinalbarbitone Sodium and Cinchocaine Hydrochloride – Somulose®

Injection of Somulose® causes a rapid loss of consciousness and cessation of respiration followed by a cardiac arrest, which leads to the death of the patient.

Method

- Move the patient to an appropriate area
- Restrain with headcollar and leadrope/halter
- Give food if appropriate
- Administer sedation if required (prescribed by a vet)
- Place a 14-gauge jugular catheter (see Section 17.3).
- Inject calculated volume of Somulose® over about 15 seconds [40, 41].
- Handler to gently keep the horse's head low to prevent it from flipping over backwards.
- Collapse will occur 35–45 seconds after the start of the injection.
- Handler to gently guide the horse into lateral recumbency.
- Death will occur within two minutes of the Somulose® injection being administered.
- Death is to be confirmed by the absence of spontaneous respiration, and cardiac output. The chest should be auscultated to check that heart sounds are absent before death is confirmed.

Advantages

- Euthanasia can be performed anywhere.
- It is considered safer than shooting.
- Owners often find this technique less distressing.
- A gun licence is not required.

Disadvantages

- Catheter or needle placement is required and this could be problematic with horses that are needle shy.
- If the horse's blood pressure is very low, this can prolong the euthanasia process.

The Euthanasia Process

Preparing the Clients for Euthanasia

Discussing options for euthanasia with the client is important, so they know what to expect and so the best option can be selected for the horse.

The following points should be discussed thoroughly with the client:

- The procedure and exactly what it involves.
- The client should be given the option to be present for the procedure. They should be asked if they wish, to be present for the whole procedure or just part of it. Some clients may want to leave once the horse has been sedated.
- The client should be asked if they would like to spend time with the horse following euthanasia (so the carcass collectors are not kept waiting).
- What happens following euthanasia, such as collection and types of disposal.
- What they would like to happen with the horse's belongings, and if they would like any keep sakes.
- Costs should be discussed, including agreeing to settle the bill at an appropriate time.

Environment

The environment in which a horse is euthanised is very important and should be considered. Ensuring a nice quiet environment for both horse and owner can make the procedure much less stressful. In a practice environment, taking the patient to a quiet area will keep the horse relaxed and allow the client some time to spend with their horse before the procedure commences. By letting other members of the team know that euthanasia is taking place, the environment can be kept as calm and quiet as possible. The area chosen for euthanasia in the practice should be clutter-free with plenty of room. An important factor to consider in equine practice is to make sure a vehicle can gain access to collect the carcass after the procedure, so it should be near a well surfaced track to enable the collection process to be successful all year round, in all weather conditions.

Timing is also important; if it is not an emergency, picking a time of the day when there are fewer clients and horses moving around, will create a better atmosphere prior to euthanasia. The appointment list for the day should be checked, and an appropriate time slot should be selected. An entrance and exit route should be carefully prepared for the client so they can leave quickly following the procedure. The client should not have to walk through the whole practice and past other horses when they are upset. A quiet room should be made available in case the client would like to stay onsite for a short while following the procedure. This obviously cannot be achieved in all practices, but it is worth considering what can be done to improve the client experience at such a sad and distressing time.

Staff Involved

The procedure should involve as few staff members as possible. This will help to create a more relaxed atmosphere. The horse should be restrained in a headcollar by a competent handler wearing PPE. Bridles and chifneys should only be used until the horse is sedated, and then they should be removed. Allowing clients to hold their own horses for euthanasia is not recommended for health and safety reasons. Clients should be allowed to watch, and a discussion as to what to expect will help make the experience less traumatic. For home visits, a discussion should be had with the client regarding an appropriate area for the procedure, an appropriate person to hold the horse and options for the collection of the carcass. The vet and the person collecting the carcass can then arrange to meet at the same time to make the whole process as smooth as possible.

Equipment Required

Equipment required for the procedure should be set up in advance. This includes:

Shooting
- Consent form
- Sedation
- Gun and bullets
- Stethoscope

Injection (Figure 17.85)
- Consent form
- Sedation
- Stethoscope
- Catheter
- Suture material/super glue
- Extension set
- Heparinised saline
- Euthanasia solution drawn up in advance such as Somulose® calculated at 10 ml per 100 kg [41]
- A blade and swabs to remove the catheter after the procedure

Extras
- Food for the horse. This may not be appropriate in all cases and should be checked with the case vet first.
- Plaiting bands and scissors for obtaining mane and tail keep sakes.
- Shoe removal kit if shoes are required for keep sakes.
- The horse's belongings gathered together in a bag so the owner does not have to wait around after the procedure.

Other Considerations

Not all horses are mobile enough to make it to the euthanasia area; these horses may be kept in the stable or moved to a recovery box that is closer. If the procedure is being carried out in a stable, the yard should be kept as quiet as possible. Client visits should be avoided during this time. Haynets and water buckets should be removed as this may allow more room, making the environment safer for both staff and the horse. Although this is a sad part of veterinary nursing, making sure the euthanasia is carried out as calmly and smoothly as possible is a skill which both horse and owner will appreciate.

Carcass Disposal Following Euthanasia

Options include:

- *Hunt kennel*: The carcass is collected by the hunt kennels and is then fed to the hounds. This is often the cheapest disposal method. This option is not appropriate if Somulose® has been used for euthanasia.
- *Cremation*: Mass or private. A mass cremation is when the carcass is cremated with other carcasses; often, ashes

Figure 17.85 Equipment to be prepared for euthanasia by injection. *Source:* Rosina Lillywhite.

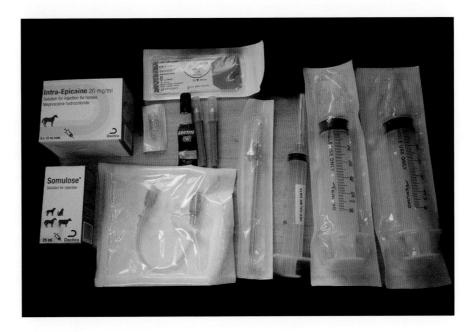

are not returned to the owner. Private cremation is for that individual carcass only; the client often receives the ashes back in a casket of their choice; this method is significantly more expensive.

- *Burial*: This will require appropriate permission [40], usually from environmental health, due to the risk of the carcass contaminating water sources.

If an appointment and time are made for euthanasia, then organising a time that suits both the vet and the carcass disposal company is recommended. Once the client has made their decision regarding disposal, normally, the practice will communicate with the disposal company on behalf of the owner. For private cremation, it is important to get all the correct contact details from the client.

Client Support Following Euthanasia

In practice, following euthanasia, the owner is often left with a member of staff, and this is often an RVN who has the time to sit with the owner, offer them a warm drink and some emotional support. It is also important that owners are offered further support if they need it once they leave the practice. For home visits, extra time should be booked out for the vet if possible, as this will allow them time to offer some support to the owner following euthanasia.

Billing for euthanasia can be a difficult subject to discuss with an owner at such a sensitive time. For planned euthanasia, it is recommended that payment is made prior to the procedure so that no further communication will be required following the procedure, allowing the owner time and space to grieve. This is not always possible in emergency situations; if the client is registered, then they can be billed for the procedure a few weeks later, allowing them time to grieve. If they are not a registered client, then a credit card payment may be required, but this needs to be handled in a sensitive manner.

Sometimes, euthanasia can be unexpected, and the vet will have to break bad news to the client. Support from staff (often RVNs) is needed during this time, as well as discussing the procedure, disposal of the carcass and making sure that the owner understands the procedure. Offering to call family or friends for the client, staying with them and offering them a drink and a quiet room until family members arrive is often appreciated. In unexpected and sudden cases of euthanasia, there may not be time to get written consent from the owner. In these cases, verbal consent should be given on either a recorded phone line or witnessed by another member of staff, and the conversation accurately recorded on the patient's notes. The vet should ask to see the horse's passport so that they can check identification of the horse. The microchip number or passport sketch can be checked to ensure it matches the horse that has been presented before euthanasia is carried out.

Following euthanasia, some practices phone the client to check on them a few days later. Sympathy cards can also be sent to the client; these are often signed by the case vet and any members of staff who were involved with the horse during their treatment programme.

Bereavement Counselling

Bereavement, grief and loss can cause many different symptoms and affect people differently [44]. Owner should be encouraged to talk to friends, family members, health professionals and councillors if required. A few charities offer bereavement counselling free of charge. Owners should be made aware of these services.

The British Horse Society (BHS) offers support to horse owners before the procedure is carried out, and discusses the following:

- The current health of the horse.
- Worries and concerns.
- Euthanasia and disposal options.
- How to organise euthanasia/disposal.
- How the BHS can offer emotional support.

The BHS also offers support on the day of euthanasia and the day after the procedure [45]. The Blue Cross offers a free and confidential Pet Bereavement Support Service by phone, email or webchat [46]. World Horse Welfare also offers support and has made leaflets available for owners, one to give the facts about euthanasia, and the other to help owners make a plan long before they will need it [47]. RVNs can help owners by making them aware of these services and how to access them.

References

1 Snalune, K. and Paton, A. (2012). General nursing. In: *Equine Veterinary Nursing Manual*, 2e (ed. K. Coumbe) pp. 155, 158–159. Oxford: Blackwell Science.

2 Costa, L.R.R. (2018). History and physical examination of the horse. In: *Manual of Clinical Procedures in the Horse* (ed. L.R.R. Costa and M.R. Paradis), 52. Hoboken: John Wiley & Sons.

3 Roberts, C.A., Loines, L., and Tillett, K. (2012). Medicines and their management. In: *Equine Veterinary Nursing*, 2e (ed. K. Coumbe), 196–200. Oxford: Wiley.

4 Barr, B.D., Javsicas, L., and Zimmel, D. (2009). Nursing care. In: *AAEVT's Equine Manual for Veterinary Technicians*, 1e (ed. D. Reeder, S. Milner, D. Wilfong, et al.), 283–284. Iowa: Wiley-Blackwell.

5 Chapman, A. (2018). Injection techniques. In: *Manual of Clinical Procedures in the Horse* (ed. L.R.R. Costa and M.R. Paradis), 72–73. Hoboken: John Wiley & Sons.

6 Stephen, J. (2008). Intramuscular injections. In: *The Equine Hospital Manual*, 1e (ed. K. Corley and J. Stephen), 13–14. Oxford: Blackwell Publishing.

7 Corley, K. (2008). Collection of blood samples and intravenous injection. In: *The Equine Hospital Manual*, 1e (ed. K. Corley and J. Stephen), 10–12. Oxford: Blackwell Publishing.

8 Copas, V.E.N. and Boswell, J.C. (2012). Fluid therapy. In: *Equine Veterinary Nursing Manual*, 2e, pp. 237, 238 (ed. K. Coumbe). Oxford: Blackwell Science.

9 Corley, K. (2008). Jugular catheterisation. In: *The Equine Hospital Manual* (ed. K. Corley and J. Stephen) p. 28, 30. West Sussex: Wiley-Blackwell.

10 Millar, B. (2010). Step-by-step guide to intravenous catheter placement in the horse. *Veterinary Nursing Journal* 25 (2): 23.

11 Taylor, R., Holmes, P., and Jasani, S. (2012). Small animal fluid therapy. In: *BSAVA Textbook of Veterinary Nursing*, 5e (ed. B. Cooper, E. Mullineaux, L. Turner, and T. Greet), 644. Gloucester: BSAVA.

12 Geraghty, T.E., Love, S., Taylor, D.J. et al. (2009a). Assessment of subclinical venous catheter-related diseases in horses and associated risk factors [online]. *Veterinary Record* 164: 227–231. Available from: http://veterinaryrecord.bmj.com/content/164/8/227.full.html (accessed 6 October 2022).

13 Smith, M. and Haylock, S. (2012). Basic first aid. In: *Equine Veterinary Nursing* (ed. K. Coumbe), 138. London: Wiley-Blackwell.

14 Chandler, S. and Middlecote, L. (2012). Principles of general nursing. In: *BSAVA Textbook of Veterinary Nursing*, 5e (ed. B. Cooper, E. Mullineaux, L. Turner, and T. Greet), 418. Gloucester: BSAVA.

15 Boys Smith, S. and Millar, B.M. (2012). General surgical nursing. In: *Equine Veterinary Nursing* (ed. K. Coumbe), 390. London: Wiley-Blackwell.

16 Rossdales (2015). Bandaging techniques for horses [Online]. Available at: https://www.rossdales.com/assets/files/Bandaging-techniques-for-horses.pdf (accessed 5 February 2023).

17 Ethell, M.T., Dart, A.J., Hodgson, D.R., and Rose, R.J. (2000). Alimentary system. In: *Manual of Equine Practice* (ed. D.R. Hodgson and R.J. Rose). West Philadelphia: Saunders.

18 Stratton-Phelps, M. (2008). Nutritional management of the hospitalised horse. In: *The Equine Hospital Manual* (ed. K. Corley and J. Stephen), 278–284. West Sussex: Wiley-Blackwell.

19 Harris, P.A. (2012). Clinical nutrition. In: *Equine Veterinary Nursing*, 2e (ed. K.M. Coumbe) pp. 122, 123. West Sussex: Wiley-Blackwell.

20 Gajanayake, I., Lumbis, R., Greet, G., and Girling, S. (2011). Nutrition and feeding. In: *BSAVA Textbook of Veterinary Nursing*, 5e (ed. L. Turner, B. Cooper, and E. Mullineaux). Gloucester: BSAVA.

21 Dunkel, B. (2008). Passage of a nasogastric tube and indwelling nasogastric tube. In: *The Equine Hospital Manual* (ed. K. Corely and J. Stephen) p. 15. Oxford: Blackwell Publishing Ltd.

22 Hendrickson, D.A. and Rubio-Martinez, L.M. (2021). Complications of urinary surgery. In: *Complications in Equine Surgery* (ed. D.A. Hendrickson and L.M. Rubio-Martinez), 571. Hoboken: John Wiley and Sons Inc.

23 Sponseller, B. and Sponseller, B. (2018). Urinary catheterization of mares. In: *Manual of Clinical Procedures in the Horse* (ed. L.R.R. Costa and M.R. Paradis), 504–509. Hoboken: John Wiley & Sons.

24 Sponseller, B. and Sponseller, B. (2018). Urinary catheterization of adult male horses. In: *Manual of Clinical Procedures in the Horse* (ed. L.R.R. Costa and M.R. Paradis), 499–503. Hoboken: John Wiley & Sons.

25 Bloor, C. (2023). The use and management of closed urinary catheters. *The Veterinary Nurse* [Online]. Available at: www.magonlinelibrary.com (accessed 1 November 2022).

26 Toribio, R.E. (2007). Essentials of equine renal and urinary tract physiology. *Veterinary Clinics Equine Practice* 23 (3): 533–561.

27 McGowan, C., Stubbs, N., and Jull, G. (2007). Equine physiotherapy: a comparative view of the science underlying the profession. *Equine Veterinary Journal* 39: 90.

28 Phillips, A., Stiller, K., and Williams, M. (2006). Medical record documentation: the quality of physiotherapy entries. *The Internet Journal of Allied Health Sciences and Practice* 4 (3): 4.

29 Davidson, E. (2016). Controlled exercise in equine rehabilitation. *Veterinary Clinics of North America: Equine Practice* 21 (1): 159–165.

30 Abrantes, J., Atalaia, T., Clayton, H., and Prazeres, J. (2021). Equine rehabilitation: a scoping review of the literature. *Animals* 11 (6): 1508.

31 Mackechnie-Guire, R., Murray, R., Newton, R. et al. (2022). Effect of ground and raised poles on kinematics of the walk. *Journal of Equine Veterinary Science* 115: 104005.

32 Watson, R. (2016). Bandaging for protection and support. *Equine Health* 2016 (27): 35–37.

33 Wright, I. (2017). Racecourse fracture management. Part 2: Techniques for temporary immobilisation and transport. *Equine Veterinary Education* 29 (8): 440–451.

34 Kaneps, A.J. (2016). Practical rehabilitation and physical therapy for the general equine practitioner. *Veterinary Clinics of North America: Equine Practice* 32 (1): 167–180.

35 Clayton, H., Hauptman, J., Kaiser, L., and Stubbs, N. (2011). Dynamic mobilisation exercises increase cross sectional area of musculus multifidus. *Equine Veterinary Journal* 43 (5): 522–552.

36 Marlin, D. (2019). Evaluation of the cooling efficacy of the different equine leg cooling methods. *Comparative Exercise Physiology* 15 (2): 113–122.

37 Crook, T. and Hill, C. (2010). The relationship between massage to the equine caudal hindlimb muscles and hindlimb protraction. *Equine Veterinary Journal* 38: 683–687.

38 Hemmings, A., McBride, S., and Robinson, K. (2004). A preliminary study on the effect of massage to reduce stress in the horse. *Journal of Equine Veterinary Science* 24 (2): 76–81.

39 Scott, M. and Swenson, L.A. (2009). Evaluating the benefits of equine massage therapy: a review of the evidence and current practices. *Journal of Equine Veterinary Science* 29 (9): 687–697.

40 Murrell, J.C. and Ford-Fennah, V. (2012). Anaesthesia. In: *Equine Veterinary Nursing*, 2e (ed. K. Coumbe), 459. Oxford: Wiley.

41 Walker, A. and Lane, C. (2016). Equine anaesthesia. In: *Aspinall's Complete Textbook of Veterinary Nursing*, 2e (ed. N. Ackerman), 591–592. London: Elsevier.

42 The Humane Slaughter Association (2022). The humane killing of livestock using firearm [Online]. Available at: https://www.hsa.org.uk/humane-killing-of-livestock-using-firearms-positioning/horses1#:~:text=The%20shot%20should%20be%20aimed,they%20cross%20(Figure%209) (accessed 8 October 2022).

43 Knottenbelt, D.C. (2012). Humane destruction. In: *Saunders Equine Formulary* (ed. D.C. Knottenbelt and F. Malalana), 317. Liverpool: Elsevier.

44 NHS (2022). Grief after bereavement or loss [Online]. Available at: https://www.nhs.uk/mental-health/feelings-symptoms-behaviours/feelings-and-symptoms/grief-bereavement-loss/ (accessed 7 August 2022).

45 British Horse Society (2022). Friends at the end [Online]. Available at: https://www.bhs.org.uk/our-work/welfare/our-campaigns/friends-at-the-end (accessed 4 May 2022).

46 The Blue Cross (2022). Pet bereavement and pet loss [Online]. 2022 [cited 2022 May 10]. Available at: https://www.bluecross.org.uk/pet-bereavement-and-pet-loss (accessed 10 May 2022).

47 World Horse Welfare (2022). Equine end of life [Online]. Available at: https://www.worldhorsewelfare.org/advice/management/end-of-life (accessed 4 May 2022).

Further Reading

BEVA (2023). Euthanasia [Online]. Available at: https://www.beva.org.uk/Guidance-and-Resources/Routine-Healthcare/euthanasia#checklist (accessed 12/02/2023).

Costa, L.R.R. and Paradis, M.R. (ed.) (2018). *Manual of Clinical Procedures in the Horse*. Hoboken: John Wiley & Sons.

Rippingale, M.C. and Fisk, N.K. (2013). Factors causing thrombophlebitis in horses: methods of prevention 1. *The Veterinary Nurse* 4 (4).

Rippingale, M.C. and Fisk, N.K. (2013). Factors causing thrombophlebitis in horses: methods of prevention 2. *The Veterinary Nurse* 4 (5).

Corley, K. and Stephen, J. (ed.) (2008). *The Equine Hospital Manual*. West Sussex: Wiley-Blackwell.

18

Exam Technique and Revision Aids
Susan L. Holt

University of Bristol, Bristol, United Kingdom

18.1 Preparing to Study

To ensure you are ready for productive study and can perform to the best of your ability in examinations, there are fundamental concepts for you to consider before you begin. Understanding and improving your general state of well-being, resilience, and developing an understanding of stress, will have a positive impact on your level of engagement and consequently, your achievements.

Maintaining Good Mental Health and Resilience

The World Health Organisation describe mental health as,

> … a state of mental well-being that enables people to cope with the stresses of life, realise their abilities, learn well and work well, and contribute to their community. It is an integral component of health and well-being that underpins our individual and collective abilities to make decisions, build relationships and shape the world we live in.

Resilience is defined by the American Psychological Association as,

> … the process and outcome of successfully adapting to difficult or challenging life experiences, especially through mental, emotional and behavioural flexibility …

These are ever changing states for everyone, but it is important to take the time to identify how you are feeling physically and mentally, especially as you approach the exams.

There may be simple changes you can make to improve your well-being and resilience; it may be that you feel you need to reach out for support to help you manage. Protective factors for developing resilience include the ability to ask for support and connect with others when required, rather than trying to cope alone [1]. Connecting with others is first on a list of five steps to improving mental health and well-being and is embedded throughout the other factors.

The National Health Service (NHS) suggest five key steps you can take to improve your well-being and help you to feel more positive:

1) Connecting with other people
   - Helps you build a sense of belonging and self-worth
   - Gives you an opportunity to share positive experiences
   - Provides emotional support and allows you to support others
2) Being physically active
   - Raises your self-esteem
   - Helps you set goals or challenges and achieve them
   - Causes chemical changes in your brain which can help to positively change your mood
3) Learning new skills
   - Boosts self-confidence and raises self-esteem
   - Helps you to build a sense of purpose
   - Helps you connect with others
4) Giving to others
   - Creates positive feelings and a sense of reward
   - Gives you a feeling of purpose and self-worth
   - Helps you connect with others
   - Can be small acts of kindness that fit with your study commitments
5) Paying attention to the present moment (mindfulness)
   - Can help create a better understanding of yourself
   - Can help you appreciate and enjoy life

Your college or university may have a subscription with a well-being app for your phone, free to you as students, such as FIKA, so do make enquiries. The Headspace app subscription is free for students with a Spotify account (at the time of writing this chapter). There are features on Headspace that are free for all to use and comes highly recommended.

Dealing with Exam Stress

Revision, assignment deadlines and examination periods are inherently times of increased stress for most students. However, do not always assume this to be a negative situation, it is distinct from being in distress. Firstly, stress is an inherent part of daily life, which is impossible to avoid. Stress that we encounter as part of our normal daily routine can be good for developing our personal resilience. Consider that each time we encounter a stressful situation and successfully cope with that situation (this includes when we reach out for help), we develop new strategies and build resilience. Next time a comparable situation arises, you will be better prepared to cope and have an increased level of resilience. Conversely, if we try to avoid stress, we switch developing long-term resilience strategies with short-term comfort. This strategy can create low resilience in the future. It is important to remember that the presence of stress does not automatically have negative consequences. We can choose to view stress as a positive motivator that exists to help us prepare and perform to our peak ability.

Focussing on the Positives

Realising the difference between what is currently known and what we are expected to learn could function as a stressor. This can be a positive motivator for learning success. Eustress is described as a healthy response to stress and perceived stress has been associated with increased levels of achievement in human nursing students [2]. Stress can be beneficial when preparing for exams as it acts to motivate individuals to learn and improves performance in study and assessments [3]. However, prolonged exposure to stress without positive and adaptive strategies can lead to distress and will negatively impact health and well-being, consequently impacting your ability to perform well [4].

When you recognise a stressor such as an exam, firstly, keep things in perspective. Exams are not '*everything*' and results do not define you, or mean that you cannot go on and be successful, should you not achieve the result you were aiming for the first time. See the signal of stress as a positive sign that you are getting ready to adapt and rise to the challenge. Consider next what it is you need to do

in order to achieve. Get organised, and plan to break down your task into small, achievable chunks. Problem-solving is a positive reaction to a stressor. Do not set yourself unachievable goals, be realistic with your plans. Ensure you still make time to unwind and relax too, including getting a good night's sleep, exercising and eating healthily. Continue to look after your health and well-being, following the five-step NHS plan above, avoid stimulants such as caffeine. Reach out for support with friends, family, tutors and other students. Do take time to reflect on all you have achieved to date and use past achievements to silence any doubts of your ability to be successful.

Study Environment

Before you begin your study tasks and revision, it is important to ensure you create a suitable environment to work in. Here are tips to consider when setting up your study space:

1) Create your own space
   This does not need to be a permanent area; consider the best space in your home environment (Figure 18.1), but also stay mobile. Libraries, college or university spaces and outdoor areas can also be valuable resources for productive study while reducing distractions. A tidy, clutter-free space with natural lighting, low noise and an ambient temperature of around 20–22°C [5], will all be beneficial for your productivity.

2) Avoid distractions
   We can all be guilty of procrastination. Try to recognise your key distractors and make a list, how can you avoid each one? Do you need to put your phone in another room, for example? Let friends and family know when you have planned to study so you will not be disturbed. Have drinks and snacks available in your study space, as

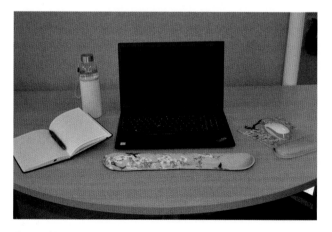

Figure 18.1 Example of a suitable desk space for home study. *Source:* Rosina Lillywhite.

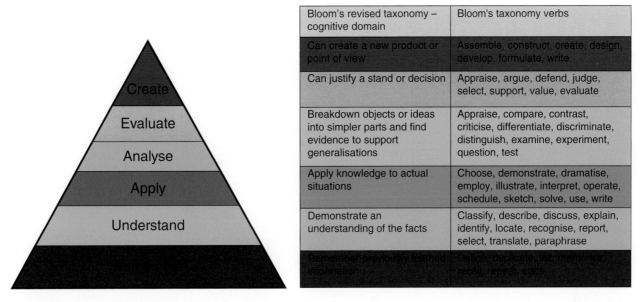

Figure 18.2 Bloom's Revised Taxonomy. *Source:* Rosina Lillywhite [8].

the act of sourcing these may turn into a procrastination exercise.

3) Breaks and rewards

Once you feel you have achieved a goal you have set, reward yourself, e.g. time on your phone, watching a favourite TV show or going out for a walk. This will be individual to you. Think, what will motivate me? Do take regular breaks, we are not machines and you will be more productive if you take a 10–15 minute break every 30–40 minutes. Ensure you change your posture regularly, to avoid musculoskeletal strain [6].

18.2 Revision

We all have the right to an education, and you have chosen to take the opportunity to complete a pathway to become an equine registered veterinary nurse (RVN). This comes with the responsibility to take ownership of your learning and become actively engaged in this process.

Metacognition is described as the ways that students direct and monitor their learning. Self-regulated learning (SRL) is described as students taking responsibility for their learning with an active role [7]. Metacognition, or thinking about your thought processes, will help you decide and plan what is required, what will work best for you and when. SRL is then putting this into action by completing the tasks you have set. There is a strong body of evidence that suggests that students who are able to practice metacognition and SRL will be able to increase their attainment [7].

When considering and planning your learning journey it can be useful to refer to Bloom's Revised Taxonomy (Figure 18.2), in order to build and develop your learning from simple recall of facts (at the bottom of the pyramid) towards the ability to analyse and evaluate ideas and concepts (at the top of the pyramid). This is a higher level of learning that leads to deeper, long-term understanding. For example, recalling the skeletal anatomy of the horse would be a task at the bottom of the pyramid, whereas understanding what factors can increase the risk of laminitis and how this is managed and explained to an owner, would require engagement higher up the pyramid.

Planning and Organisation

Planning is the key to exam success and being prepared and organised will also reduce the level of stress you experience. This starts with timing; work back from your exam period, planning how much you need to achieve in each week, then you can decide when to start your revision. Consider this sooner rather than later during your course.

Evaluate each topic, it can be common to prioritise subject areas that we are more confident with as this is more enjoyable. However, within each topic, assess yourself to ascertain your level of understanding and identify areas that you need to prioritise during your revision.

Once you have established when to start and what you need to prioritise, you need to plan a structure of how to achieve this. A revision timetable can be useful but does not need to be overly complex. In fact, keep it simple if this serves you, a tick list each week may be sufficient. There are free online sites to help you create your revision timetable, e.g. getrevising.co.uk. Just make sure designing your timetable does not become your reason to procrastinate; you

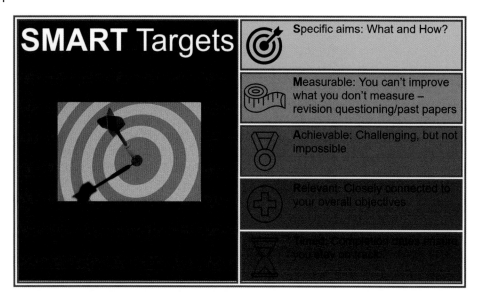

Figure 18.3 SMART targets. *Source:* Susan L. Holt.

must put your plans into action. Remember also to plan rest breaks, fun activities and rewards.

Creating specific, measurable, achievable, relevant and timed (SMART) targets will be best to make your planning appropriate and realistic. An example of a SMART target might be, 'This week, I am going to create a mind map and flash cards to revise the cardiovascular system and then ask my friends to quiz me on Friday' (Figure 18.3).

Learning Techniques

There is no single perfect way to learn, even though we may all have our own preferences. Which method is best will not only depend on our own preferred style but also on the information we are trying to learn, remember and understand. Only ever using one method may limit your ability to retain the required information for the varied topics within veterinary nursing programmes.

When learning factual concepts, including those around anatomical structure and veterinary terminology, time-spaced repetition is key. Examples such as creating flash cards and quizzes to share with peers will create a good set of activities to complete and repeat, with time intervals in between. This will support your recall of these facts for the examination. The positive effects of this learning technique are grounded in scientific evidence [9]. Leaving it all until the night before is not a suitable strategy for this type of learning.

In addition to factual recall, during your training you will also be required to understand a variety of more complex theories and concepts. These may require you to take a different approach to ensure you understand the topic and can evaluate and appraise the content. In this situation, creating patient or client scenarios can be useful, such as creating a patient case to develop an appropriate care plan. There are also two strategies developed by scientists to help you understand complex theories, the Feynman Technique and the ADEPT approach. These strategies can be used together to help support your revision as follows:

1) In your own way, without consulting the literature, write an explanation of the concept, making it as simple as you can, use the following ADEPT activities:
   - **A**nalogy: Demonstrate the concept with a suitable comparison
   - **D**iagram: Draw or illustrate the concept
   - **E**xample: Give a simple, contextualised example
   - **P**lain English: Describe the concept in everyday words
   - **T**echnical definition: Provide more formal, detailed information
2) Which aspects did you have trouble explaining in step number 1? Repeat step 1 for those elements you found challenging.
3) When you feel you have completed steps 1 and 2, try to further simplify your explanations as if teaching to someone new, without losing any of the key information. Review any areas of this you find challenging.

Peer Support

Do not underestimate the benefits of learning alongside your peers. Your fellow students are an excellent source of support and motivation during your studies, having the same goals as you. Try to develop a peer study group and plan meetings in your revision diary. If each person in the study group identifies an area they are struggling with, you can share topics to each explain to your study group. This jigsaw style of learning means you get to discuss multiple topic areas, while you only review one for the group. Writing questions for others in your peer group has a similar effect. Writing appropriate questions and answers requires a good understanding of the topic. If you then share the bank of questions, you will have a fantastic way to measure your revision aims. Your college or university may also have access to an online question writing forum called Peer Wise, which is a repository for multiple choice questions, so do ask your tutors about this too.

Revision Tools

- Flash cards – useful for condensing notes about specific topics, stating terms on one side and definitions on the other, or writing a question on one side with the answer on the other. These cards can be shared with peers and can be helpful for revision supported by family and friends.
- Mind maps – good to help you understand connections between concepts and ideas. These can be colourful and designed by hand or electronically to suit you.
- Quizzes, past papers, essay writing – required to measure the effectiveness of your revision and track your progress.
- Study groups – helps to break up the workload on creating the resources listed above. Peer discussions and support will enhance your learning and revision success.
- Rhymes, stories or mnemonics – can be helpful when learning facts, e.g. '**A D**elicious **PIE**' is a mnemonic that can be used to remember the steps of the nursing process, **A**ssessment, **D**iagnosis, **P**lanning, **I**mplementation and **E**valuation.

18.3 Written Exam Technique

Firstly, there are some obvious factors to consider, but they are important, nonetheless. Get a good night's sleep, eat well and do not start cramming the night before. Ensure you have the equipment you require, check your exam instructions carefully, do you need a calculator for example? Ensure that you are fully aware of the exam timetable and locations. Where do you need to be and when? Ensure you leave yourself plenty of time to arrive early without causing yourself time stress before you even start your examination. Take care not to mingle with students who may be a source of stress to you before the examination. Instead, seek out the company of students who can support

a feeling of calm and confidence. Exams can consist of a variety of question styles, including multiple choice, short answer and long answer questions. Regardless of the question type, before you start take a deep breath, relax and follow these few simple steps:

1) Read the exam instructions carefully, ascertain how many questions you are required to answer and in what sections.
2) Read the whole paper carefully before you start the first question, making a note of the marks available for each. This will help you plan how much time should be spent on each area of the exam.
3) Now you can start, read the question carefully, note the 'command word', e.g. state, list, describe, explain, appraise or evaluate, this reveals the type of answer that is required by the question.
4) Do not linger on a question if you are struggling to recall the information, move on and come back once you have completed the other questions. This will help you relax and build your confidence.
5) Avoid the temptation to leave too early. Check back through your answers, have you answered the questions fully, according to the marks available and the command word? Check any calculations. Have you answered **ALL** the required questions?

18.4 Practical and Oral Assessments

The **Objective Structured Clinical Examination (OSCE)** is the well-known staple assessment that is part of all current Royal College of Veterinary Surgeons (RCVS) accredited veterinary nursing courses and is considered the summative assessment for the RCVS Day One Skills (DOS).

During any course, there may also be oral assessments such as role play tasks or presentations that form your formative or summative assessments. The **professional discussion** is a requirement in Further Education (FE) for **some apprenticeship students** and consists of a 45-minute assessment with a trained assessor under controlled conditions.

Demystifying the OSCE

Firstly, those of you heading towards your OSCE will have completed (or very nearly) your online log of clinical skills and a registered veterinary professional will have already deemed you competent in the range of tasks that the OSCE is testing. Do not get caught up in the 'urban myths' that surround this examination. There are no tricks or special magic elements required to pass, just practice and revision related to the methodologies detailed by your education provider, which will be enhanced by an understanding of evidence-based nursing techniques. Do ensure that you focus on the instructions from your **own** university or college, as OSCE protocols and stations will vary between them. Remember, these are day-one nursing skills that you have been undertaking since enrolling as a student veterinary nurse, you can do them. Examiners involved in the OSCE will be standardised and trained by your institute to ensure the objective nature of the marking within the examination. They will be there to support you while ensuring a standardised approach for each student. The OSCE exists to ensure you are a **safe** and **effective** practitioner via a summative controlled assessment, prior to registration as a veterinary nurse, no more, no less.

While it is appreciated that this examination can trigger a greater level of anxiety due to the nature of being watched by an examiner, students who are prepared for the examination should have few problems performing appropriately, despite any nerves on the day. Consider again your reaction to that initial feeling of nervous stress, discussed at the start of this chapter.

OSCE Format

Each awarding body will have stipulated to you how many OSCE stations you are required to perform and how many you need to pass, in order to pass the exam overall. For example, there may be a total of 10 or 12 stations for you to undertake and you may be required to pass a minimum of 8 to pass the OSCE overall. This will vary between institutes, so get your information from the horse's mouth, not a third party.

Each station will contain exactly what you need to perform the task, plus there may be distraction equipment to ensure that you are able to make informed decisions around the equipment you select. For example, if you are required to select 10 correct surgical instruments, there may be a total of 15 instruments with 5 being 'distractors' to the correct choices. Figures 18.4 and 18.5 display examples of the standard set up for two OSCE stations. You will move between stations with time to read your scenario before performing each task. While you may be afforded additional time for reading, the time allowed to complete each task will be standardised for all students. This is usually 6 minutes per station.

Practice Makes Perfect

Firstly, as soon as the OSCE task methodologies are made available to you, begin to incorporate them into your daily nursing tasks. They are based on evidence-based practice, and you should be constantly striving to perform nursing

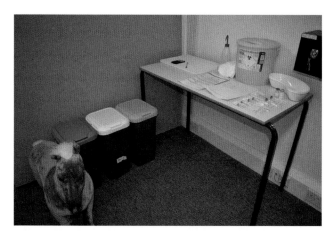

Figure 18.4 Example of a general nursing OSCE station. *Source:* Rosina Lillywhite.

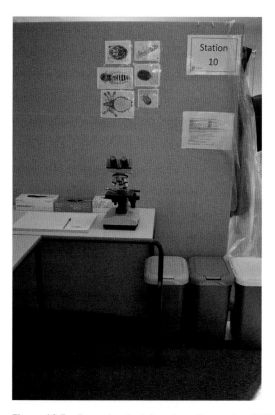

Figure 18.5 Example of a laboratory diagnostics OSCE station. *Source:* Rosina Lillywhite.

techniques for the benefit of your patients, so why wouldn't you use them now? Consider, 'Why do I perform the task this way?' This will develop deeper learning and understanding and stand you in good stead on the examination day.

Ensure you have a critical friend, not a close friend necessarily, but someone who will be happy to give you a critical appraisal of your performance. As you approach the examination, get used to being watched and having feedback around your performance. Did you clearly achieve all aspects of the gowning and closed gloving task for example, or was there an aspect that needs improving or refining? Get used to performing the task in the 6-minute period.

The Day of the OSCE Exams

Hopefully, you will awake after a good night's sleep and have breakfast, which will give you energy for the day. Ensure that you have read all the instructions fully. Again, double-check the time and venue for your examination. If this is planned somewhere new to you, consider travelling to the venue before the exam to remove this additional hurdle and uncertainty from the actual day. Consider carefully what is required in terms of appearance, e.g. appropriate clothing, hair tied up, nails well manicured, jewellery removed, as well as any additional items required such as pens, calculators and identification.

You will receive a briefing before entering the examination, usually read by the senior examiner or administration staff. This will also give you the chance to ask any last-minute queries before the start of the examination.

Once you enter the examination room, you will be instructed on which station you will be starting and which way around the room you will progress. Do take five slow, deep breaths if you are feeling nervous, this will help you to remain calm and focussed. Read carefully through your first scenario twice and you can then start to plan how you will perform the task. Do remember, it is unlikely that you are required to pass every station to pass overall. Therefore, if you have a station that you feel has gone poorly, do not then carry this feeling with you to the next station. More commonly, students who assume they have failed a station have actually performed better than they have perceived, so do not let your negative thoughts cloud your ability to perform in subsequent stations. Do not assume that you have failed any one station, this will not serve you.

After the examination, avoid the temptation to 'dissect' each station with your peers. This only serves to cause you anxiety while awaiting your results. Just know that you have done your best on the day and do something relaxing and fun. Ensure that you do not discuss the stations with students yet to attempt their examination; this is very unlikely to help them, and you may give them misinformation, as aspects of stations will be changed between cohorts of students. This will also be viewed as academic misconduct by your institute and treated accordingly.

Oral Assessments

Like the OSCE, an oral assessment can evoke a greater nervous response than a written examination due to the added element of being directly observed. Remember all that we covered at the start of this chapter to support your coping strategies and embrace your nervous energy.

Review the assessment criteria provided, paying full attention to all the details. Ask for any example questions from your institute to help you understand the requirements and help you plan your revision and preparations. Revision techniques here are the same as previously discussed, but do remember, you also need to practice speaking aloud. This can be to yourself at first, use a mirror if you find this helpful. Standing up when you speak and shifting your weight onto your lead foot can also help you feel more confident. It is also highly advisable to practice aloud in front of peers, friends or family. This will really give you confidence ahead of the assessment. It will also help you form your answers and practice the skill of speaking to an audience. The acronym **LIPS** can help you remember the key stages during the assessment:

- **L**isten – Pay full attention to your assessor and actively listen.
- **I**nterpret – Did you understand the question? You can ask for clarity where needed.
- **P**ause – Take a short pause here to begin to formulate your thoughts into your answer.
- **S**peak – Deliver your answer slowly and concisely, convey your confidence.

Avoid over preparation, as this can make you less adaptable in the assessment, remember to listen actively and answer appropriately. Revise the required topics and run through two or three scenarios related to your assessment. If you are delivering a specific presentation you have prepared, practice your performance and timing aloud until your speech flows with confidence and in the set time frame. Ensure you arrive in plenty of time so you can be as relaxed as possible when you start.

For those students undertaking the **end-point professional discussion** as part of an apprenticeship scheme, the specific information is available here:

ST0343_Vet Nursing_L3_QM_Annotated_AP_C12 (instituteforapprenticeships.org)

18.5 Summary

Do take time to review how you are currently feeling mentally and physically and do not be afraid to ask for help. Well-being and resilience do not come without support from your tutors, peers, family and friends, help is available, so ensure you use it.

Planning in advance will be key to your examination success. Use multiple learning strategies and set yourself SMART targets to achieve and review your revision goals regularly. These are all part of active learning; metacognition and self-regulated learning are proven to improve attainment.

Remember all you have achieved to get to this point; you have a proven record already. Everyone around you wants you to succeed, including your tutors and examiners and they will be happy to offer help and support as required. So, relax and enjoy your learning journey, you have an exciting career ahead of you.

Example Questions

Multiple Choice Questions

1 Schedule 3 of The Veterinary Surgeons Act 1966 states exemptions whereby those other than veterinary surgeons may perform specified tasks relating to animal treatment.

Under what circumstances may a registered veterinary nurse induce anaesthesia under a veterinary surgeon's direction?
   a Administration of medicine incrementally to induce anaesthesia for routine surgery
   b Administration of specific quantities of medicine to induce anaesthesia
   c Incrementally in an emergency under direction of a veterinary surgeon
   d When anaesthetising a patient prior to euthanasia

2 The use of the correct fire extinguisher to control a fire in the initial stages can significantly reduce the risk to people.

Which device would be most suitable to use on live electrical equipment?
   a Carbon dioxide extinguisher
   b Foam extinguisher
   c Water extinguisher
   d Wet chemical extinguisher

3 In the cardiovascular system, blood enters the heart into the right atrium after circulation around the body.

Which blood vessel leads into the right atrium?
   a Brachiocephalic artery
   b Caudal vena cava
   c Aorta
   d Pulmonary artery

4 In the image below, identify the structure labelled with the letter A:

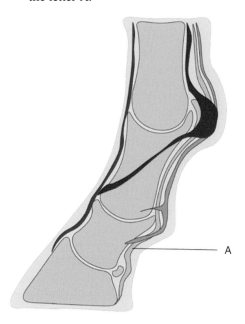

Image *source:* Rosina Lillywhite

   a Superficial digital flexor tendon
   b Suspensory ligament
   c Deep digital flexor tendon
   d Common digital extensor tendon

5 Which two structures are bound to move together by the reciprocal apparatus in the hindlimb of the horse?
   a Coffin joint and the fetlock
   b Fetlock and the tarsus
   c Tarsus and the pastern
   d Tarsus and the stifle

6 What is the normal range for the heart rate of a resting adult horse in beats per minute?
   a 10–15
   b 16–23
   c 24–40
   d 51–56

7 When preparing a mare for a caesarean section, what is the most appropriate position for the mare to be placed into post induction prior to the commencement of surgery?
   a Dorsal recumbency
   b Left lateral recumbency
   c Standing
   d Ventral recumbency

8 When calculating intravenous fluid therapy for the horse, what is the daily maintenance requirement in ml/kg?
   a 5
   b 25
   c 50
   d 500

9 When preparing a urine sample for sediment examination under the microscope, what is the correct revolutions per minute (rpm) setting for the centrifuge to spin the sample for 5 minutes?
   a 1000–1200 rpm
   b 1500–2000 rpm
   c 2500–3000 rpm
   d 3500–4000 rpm

10 How long is the average duration of oestrus in a mare?
   a 3–6 days
   b 7–9 days
   c 10–14 days
   d 15–20 days

11 When preparing the surgical site of a horse undergoing blepharoplasty, what would be the most appropriate disinfectant preparation for the surrounding skin?
   a Chlorhexidine 0.1%
   b Chlorhexidine 5%
   c Povidone-Iodine 1%
   d Povidone-Iodine 0.1%

12 What is the main route of transmission for the equine influenza virus?
   a Contact with urine
   b Indirect transmission
   c Inhalation of aerosols
   d Via fomites

13 When preparing a foal of under 4 weeks of age for general anaesthesia, how long prior to induction is it appropriate to starve without risking hypoglycaemia?
   a 15–30 minutes
   b 35–50 minutes
   c 55–80 minutes
   d 85–100 minutes

14 During equine anaesthesia what is an appropriate mean arterial blood pressure to maintain during the procedure to minimise the risk of post-anaesthetic myopathy?
   a 30–45 mmHg
   b 60–70 mmHg
   c 85–100 mmHg
   d 110–125 mmHg

15 In the stages of wound healing, what stage is described by the following statement?
   'Development of granulation tissue, involving endothelial cells laying down new blood vessels and epithelial cells which migrate over the top of the wound'
   a Inflammatory phase
   b Maturation phase
   c Proliferation phase
   d Remodelling phase

Short Answer Questions (SAQ)

1 Bacteria can grow and reproduce very quickly in the right environmental conditions. It is vital for a veterinary nurse to understand this process and how to reduce this to maintain an appropriate hospital environment. (10 marks)
   a List **THREE** environmental conditions required for bacterial reproduction and growth (3 marks)
   b Briefly describe the reproductive process of bacteria. (4 marks)
   c What stain can be used in the rapid identification of bacteria and what indications will this stain provide to aid identification? (3 marks)

2 An inexperienced owner wants information about breeding from their mare. (10 marks)
   a Describe an overview of the natural annual breeding cycle of the mare in the United Kingdom. (4 marks)
   b Name and describe the three phases of the mare's oestrous cycle. (6 marks)

3 The veterinary nurse plays a vital role in managing theatre equipment and ensuring sterility is achieved and maintained. (10 marks)
   a Briefly describe the process for cleaning a pair of Olsen Hagar needle holders following use in theatre (3 marks)
   b What steps are required next before packaging the instrument for sterilisation? (4 marks)
   c Describe the appropriate autoclave cycle with temperature, pounds per square inch (PSI) and time for this piece of equipment once packed (3 marks)

MCQ Answers

Question number	Answer
1	b
2	a
3	b
4	c
5	d
6	c
7	a
8	c
9	b
10	a
11	c
12	c
13	a
14	b
15	c

SAQ Model Answers

Question 1

a Any THREE of: A supply of nutrients (1), optimum temperature (1), correct pH (1), water (1), correct gaseous environment (1).

b Bacteria reproduce asexually by dividing two daughter cells, a process known as binary fission (1). The time between successive divisions is called the generation time (1); this time can be short from around 20 minutes in some bacteria (1); in appropriate conditions, growth is exponential; one bacterium produces two, then two produce four and so on (1).

c Gram stain (1), whether the bacteria is gram-positive or gram-negative (1), allows the structure of the bacteria to be observed (1).

Question 2

a The mare is seasonally polyoestrous (1) with cyclical ovarian activity occurring during the spring, summer and autumn (1). This seasonality means that foals are born naturally in the spring and early summer (1), with the highest pregnancy rate between May and July (1).

b The follicular phase (oestrus) (1) is when the mare will stand for the stallion with raised tail (1). In the luteal phase (dioestrus) (1), the mare is not receptive to the stallion (1). Anoestrus (1), is a period with no ovarian hormonal activity during the winter months (1).

Question 3

a Soak initially in cold water or chemical cleaning solution (1), using a stiff bristled brush under running water (1) clean paying attention to joints, ratchets and serrations (1).

b The instrument should be dried (1). It should be inspected for sharpness (1) and checked for distortion (1). It should be lubricated (1).

c 134 °C (1) at 30 psi (1) for 3.5 minutes (1).

References

1 Stainton, A., Chisholm, K., Kaiser, N. et al. (2019). Resilience as a multimodal dynamic process. *Early Intervention in Psychiatry [Internet]* 13: 725–732. Available from: https://doi.org/10.1111/eip.12726. (cited 24 October 2021).

2 Rudland, J.R., Golding, C., and Wilkinson, T.J. (2020). The stress paradox: how stress can be good for learning. *Medical Education [Internet]* 54: 40–45. Available from: https://doi.org/10.1111/medu.13830. (cited 30 October 2021).

3 Gibbons, C. (2010). Stress, coping and burn-out in nursing students. *International Journal of Nursing Studies [Internet]* 47: 1299–1309. Available from: https://www.sciencedirect.com/science/article/pii/S0020748910000830 (cited 24 October 2021).

4 Labrague, L.J., McEnroe-Petitte, D.M., Papathanasiou, I.V. et al. (2018). Stress and coping strategies among nursing students: an international study. *Journal of Mental Health [Internet]* 27: 402–408. Available from: https://doi.org/10.1080/09638237.2017.1417552. (cited 24 October 2021).

5 Wargocki, P., Porras-Salazar, J.A., and Contreras-Espinoza, S. (2019). The relationship between classroom temperature and children's performance in school. *Building and Environment [Internet]* 157: 197–204. Available from: https://www.sciencedirect.com/science/article/pii/S0360132319302987 (cited 28 November 2021).

6 National Health Service. (2019). How to sit at your desk correctly [Internet]. NHS. Available from: https://www.nhs.uk/live-well/healthy-body/how-to-sit-correctly/ (cited 10 January 2022).

7 Muijs, D. and Bokhove, C. (2020). *Metacognition and Self-regulation: Evidence Review*. Education Endowment Foundation. ERIC.

8 Armstrong, P. (2010). Bloom's taxonomy [Internet]. Vanderbilt Univ. Teach. Available from: https://cft.vanderbilt.edu/guides-sub-pages/blooms-taxonomy/ (cited 12 December 2021).

9 Versteeg, M., Hendriks, R.A., Thomas, A. et al. (2020). Conceptualising spaced learning in health professions education: a scoping review. *Medical Education [Internet]* 54: 205–216. Available from: https://doi.org/10.1111/medu.14025. (cited 28 November 2021).

Further Reading

Heywood, A. (2017). OSCEs hints, tips and tricks for students and clinical coaches. *Veterinary Nursing Journal* 32 (2): 54–56. https://doi.org/10.1080/17415349.2016.1259843.

Yon, E. (2020). OSCEs: do you know how? *Veterinary Nursing Journal* 35 (9–12): 269–271. https://doi.org/10.1080/17415349.2020.1849235.

Links

https://www.nhs.uk/mental-health/self-help/guides-tools-and-activities/five-steps-to-mental-wellbeing/.

https://www.nhs.uk/mental-health/self-help/guides-tools-and-activities/breathing-exercises-for-stress/.

https://www.nhs.uk/mental-health/self-help/guides-tools-and-activities/tips-to-reduce-stress/.

https://www.studentminds.org.uk/examstress.html.

Revision Timetable Maker/Study Planner (getrevising.co.uk).

ST0343_Vet Nursing_L3_QM_Annotated_AP_C12 (instituteforapprenticeships.org).

19

Career Progression

Sarah Baillie

Equine Veterinary Medical Center, Doha, Qatar

Introduction

Becoming a registered veterinary nurse (RVN) is a significant achievement which requires years of dedication and study. But career development does not stop at gaining the RVN qualification. There are many ways to improve and evolve either within the RVN role or by using the RVN qualification to work in other roles and to achieve further qualifications. Gaining the RVN badge and joining the Royal College of Veterinary Surgeons (RCVS) register for veterinary nurses is just the start of what can be a life-long and exciting career journey.

19.1 Progression Within Clinical Practice

Many RVNs discover a passion for a particular area of practice and wish to focus on this, for example, an RVN may find the precision and attention to detail of surgical nursing appealing. It is common for larger equine practices and university hospitals to split their caseload into distinct departments overseen by specialist veterinary surgeons and RVNs are allocated to a particular service. This allows them to develop skills in that area and gain a deeper understanding of that field of practice. An example may be a practice divided into surgery, internal medicine, lameness, reproduction and diagnostic imaging allowing RVNs to work within their department of interest.

Radiographer or Diagnostic Imaging Technician

One distinct area which some RVNs choose to develop is diagnostic imaging. A practice with a high lameness caseload may have scope for a dedicated radiographer and some hospitals also offer advanced imaging modalities such as magnetic resonance imaging (MRI), computed tomography (CT) and nuclear scintigraphy. Diagnostic imaging RVNs can be utilised for the daily operation and maintenance of the equipment and machines involved in these different imaging modalities. A variety of diagnostic imaging continued professional development (CPD) courses are offered for RVNs with an interest in this area and manufacturers of specialised imaging equipment offer training tailored to their products.

Equine Neonatal Intensive Care Unit (NICU) Nurse

A small number of equine practices have a dedicated NICU due to having a high caseload of sick neonates. These practices tend to be in areas with a dense population of breeding stock, usually Thoroughbreds and are surrounded by studs. The NICU is seasonally busy and often extra RVNs are taken on for the foaling season. Foals in the NICU require very intensive nursing (Figure 19.1). The NICU RVN is able to develop practical skills, such as arterial blood sampling, rapidly due to the frequency of requirements for such procedures. Undertaking a seasonal role like this is a good way to experience life in other countries without committing to emigrating permanently. Sometimes, seasonal RVNs are offered permanent positions at the end of the season, and this is a great way to spend a few months experiencing what it is like at a practice before taking on a permanent role.

Senior Nurse

Experienced RVNs may take on a senior role within a practice which involves greater responsibility without traditional management duties. A senior RVN may be responsible for a specific area or department, mentor junior team members, provide a channel of communication between

Textbook of Equine Veterinary Nursing, First Edition. Edited by Rosina Lillywhite and Marie Rippingale.
© 2025 John Wiley & Sons Ltd. Published 2025 by John Wiley & Sons Ltd.
Companion website: www.wiley.com/go/equineveterinarynursing

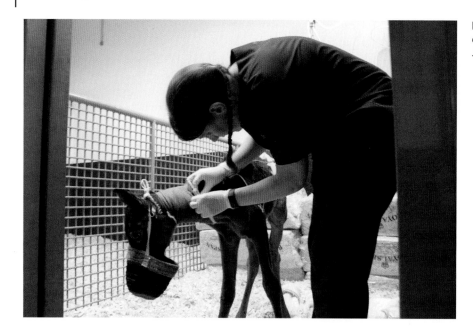

Figure 19.1 A NICU nurse, carrying out an intravenous injection. *Source:* Sarah Baillie.

management and the nursing team, or take on extra areas of responsibility.

Nurse Clinics

Some RVNs find interacting with horse owners rewarding, enjoy client education and as such are drawn to providing nurse clinics. Clients can make an appointment to bring their horse to see an RVN, much like they would for a vet appointment. Procedures such as repeated blood sampling for monitoring chronic conditions, weight checks and nutritional advice or dressing changes can be offered as well as many other services. This role can give RVNs a greater sense of autonomy while still having the security of being based at a practice.

Ambulatory Nursing

In addition to nurse clinics, there is also scope to offer an ambulatory nursing service and this area is rapidly growing in popularity, as its benefits are becoming more widely recognised. Providing nursing care at the patient's home means less stress, no requirement for transportation and convenience for the client. RVNs may be utilised to expand the service provided by the ambulatory team as well as sharing the established workload. Appointments may be offered for tasks such as taking radiographs, collecting blood samples, dressing changes, rehabilitation treatments and medication administration or demonstrations. Ambulatory RVNs could also offer appointments for behavioural issues and help clients and their horses with issues such

as fear of clipping, needle-shy patients or difficulty in administering oral medications.

Dental Technician

An area that some RVNs may wish to develop is dentistry and if this is something that they are passionate about, they may decide to undertake formal training to become a British Association of Equine Dental Technicians (BAEDT) qualified Equine Dental Technician (EDT). This qualification can be utilised in a hospital setting providing routine treatment alongside a more comprehensive dental service, or it could be used to provide an ambulatory dental service. Some veterinary surgeons choose to focus on dentistry as their preferred area of practice and offer a wide range of advanced dentistry procedures. Some RVNs may find they enjoy assisting with this type of work and might choose to undertake further training to develop skills and understanding of the procedures, as well as training on the use and maintenance of the specialist equipment.

Laboratory

Often, the RVN role involves some laboratory work and it is possible to develop this as an area of interest. In equine practice, it is more common for large laboratories to be attached to hospitals rather than stand-alone as is common in small animal practice. Therefore, there may be more practical opportunities for RVNs to develop their interest in laboratory diagnostics. The laboratory technician role encompasses operating haematology and biochemistry machines as well as manual testing such as faecal worm egg counts, logging

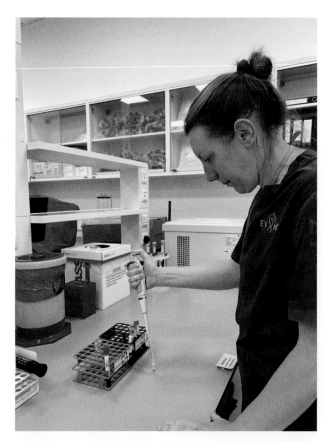

Figure 19.2 An RVN preparing a blood sample for biochemistry testing in a laboratory. *Source:* Sarah Baillie.

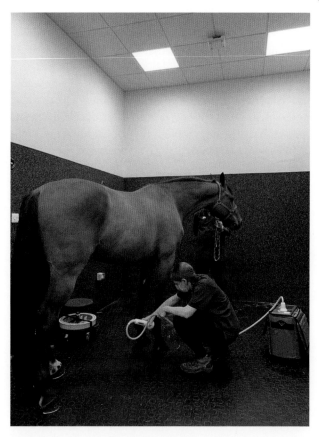

Figure 19.3 An RVN performing shockwave therapy as part of the rehabilitation process for a competition horse recovering from an injury. *Source:* Sarah Baillie.

samples and recording results (Figure 19.2). In undertaking laboratory duties, an RVN may find an interest in a particular area, such as microbiology or polymerase chain reaction (PCR) testing and wish to focus on this and learn more about the technical aspects and how it relates to clinical practice.

Rehabilitation Nurse

Some conditions and treatments require an extensive rehabilitation period and while there is no longer a requirement for hospitalisation, it may not be possible for the care required to be given at home. In this case an RVN may be the ideal person to provide the extra care required. This role may be offered as an ambulatory service at the patient's home, at the veterinary practice, or at another location such as a livery yard with useful facilities for rehabilitation, that are not available at the patient's usual stabling. The role of the rehabilitation nurse may include hand walking, long-reining, bandaging, administering medications or provision of therapies such as magnetic diathermy, K-wave laser or shockwave (Figure 19.3). It is possible that this role could be encompassed within the ambulatory nursing role.

Physiotherapist

Further to the rehabilitation nurse role, it is possible to obtain a physiotherapy qualification which could be complemented by the knowledge and understanding an RVN has. To practice physiotherapy, you must obtain a qualification, and this can be achieved in one of three ways. Either a degree in veterinary physiotherapy, a human physiotherapy degree followed by further veterinary-specific training, or a postgraduate certificate in veterinary physiotherapy, are required to practice as a physiotherapist for horses [1]. The equine physiotherapist's role involves visiting and treating patients in their home environment, at a practice, or at a competition venue.

Pharmacy Roles and Suitably Qualified Person (SQP)

An interest in medication, stock control and dispensary management may lead RVNs to a role in their practice pharmacy or dispensary. An RVN may wish to undertake a further qualification to become an SQP which allows them to prescribe and dispense certain medications from a licensed premises. Registration with the Veterinary Medicines Directorate (VMD) and an approved body, following successful completion of examinations set by that body, is required to become an SQP [2]. Once qualified, an SQP is required to undertake regular CPD which is applicable and relevant to the role. The role of veterinary pharmacist is one which appears to be more prolific in the United States but is also increasingly seen in the United Kingdom. General Pharmaceutical Council (GPC) registered pharmacists receive some training on veterinary medications and are legally allowed to dispense and prescribe some veterinary products [3]. It is possible for an RVN with a veterinary nursing or animal science degree to undertake a veterinary pharmacy postgraduate course from postgraduate certificate to master's degree level. Courses are also offered in veterinary pharmacy management if a master's degree is not accessible, but this is an area you wish to pursue.

Clinical Supervisor (formally known as a clinical coach)

The role of clinical supervisor allows experienced RVNs to teach and mentor student veterinary nurses (SVNs) in a clinical setting. To become a clinical supervisor, an RVN must be employed within an RCVS-accredited training practice and is required to undertake a clinical supervisor training course. Most veterinary nurse training providers offer clinical supervisor training for free or reduced cost if the supervisor's SVN is enrolled with that training provider. Clinical supervisor training courses typically last one day and attendance of a refresher standardisation course is required every year. A clinical supervisor's role involves working closely with the SVN, teaching skills, observing, supporting and assessing progress. The clinical supervisor is required to record in an online central skills log, the SVNs progress and performance in relation to specific clinical skills. The clinical supervisor should arrange regular meetings with their SVN and allocate teaching time, assessment time and regular practice sessions for clinical skills to support the student to obtain their veterinary nursing qualification.

Locum Nurse

While not as commonplace as in small animal practice, opportunities do exist for equine RVNs to work as locums. Locum nursing involves working at more than one practice for short-term periods usually covering for maternity leave, sick leave or staff shortages. Some benefits of locum work can include:

- Freedom to select when and where you wish to work.
- Chances to experience different practices and facilities.

- Often a higher rate of pay than permanent roles.
- An opportunity to work in a practice and assess its suitability before committing to a permanent role.

Some negatives to this type of work could be:

- Lack of stability and regular income.
- Having to learn to work with new equipment, people and protocols frequently.
- A requirement to travel far from home depending on where demand is.

Locum RVNs may choose to be self-employed, work under an umbrella company or make other arrangements with the practices they work for. When working under an umbrella company, many elements are taken care of such as invoicing, tax and insurance. However, the umbrella company will collect a fee for this. When working in a self-employed capacity, it is important to check the most up to date requirements for insurance, tax, national insurance and invoicing. It may also be pertinent to consider income protection insurance as well.

19.2 Management Roles in Practice

Moving into a management role can provide an opportunity to develop business and leadership skills and utilise an RVN's unique insight into veterinary practice. Some RVNs may choose to move to a management only role and some may prefer to take on a role which combines management duties with clinical work.

Head Nurse

A head nurse leads the nursing team and, depending on the practice and the individual, may split time between management duties and clinical work, or focus solely on managing the team and the administration required. The responsibilities of a head nurse will vary between practices, but some common duties include:

- Creating and updating the rota for the nursing team to ensure adequate cover for each department and shift.
- Allocating duties to members of the nursing team.
- Recruitment – advertising, selecting candidates and interviewing.
- Arranging and recording annual leave, days off in lieu, other types of leave and sickness. Ensuring these are accounted for and providing adequate nursing cover for the practice.
- Recruiting locum nurses if required.
- Performance management – carrying out appraisals and regular evaluation of competency.

- Maintaining team morale and encouraging strong teamwork by holding regular nurses' meetings, utilising team building exercises and creating open, honest discussions with a no-blame culture.
- Training and mentoring members of the nursing team and ensuring that junior team members are supported effectively by senior nurses. Identifying training needs and creating and implementing plans to meet those needs.
- Create two-way communication between the nursing team and management.
- Ensure compliance with practice policies.

A head nurse may also take responsibility for areas such as stock control, infection control, preparing for RCVS inspections, promotions and initiatives.

This role can be demanding but also very rewarding. Strong people skills and excellent communication are essential qualities of a good head nurse. Creating a bonded and committed team is the ultimate goal.

Clinical Nursing Manager

The role of clinical nursing manager is similar to that of a head nurse and many duties may overlap. However, there are some key differences. It is not necessary for a clinical nursing manager to be an RVN although, it is important that the person has a strong understanding of veterinary practice and the role of the RVN. Therefore, the role could be filled by a veterinary surgeon for example. The duties of a clinical nursing manager are, as the title suggests, more focussed on management. The nursing manager is responsible for the performance management of the nursing team, and they may implement this in some or all of the following ways:

- Assessing competency and evaluating performance.
- Identifying training requirements and implementing that training.
- Recruiting new members of the team.
- Induction of new staff and ensuring their integration into the team (for example, allocating a mentor).
- Assessing the standard of patient care and the client experience and implementing measures to improve these.
- Facilitate effective, two-way communication between the nursing team and management.
- Facilitate effective communication and foster collaboration between the nursing team and other teams within the practice.

As these descriptions show, there are many similarities between the role of clinical nursing manager and head nurse. In practices where both roles exist, some of the duties may be interchangeable between the two positions, depending on the practice structure and the preferences, strengths and the relevant experience of the people fulfilling these roles.

Practice Manager

While practice management is very different to veterinary nursing, the knowledge and understanding of veterinary practice gained through a career in veterinary nursing is very useful in this role. The practice manager is responsible for the entire practice team, ensuring not only that the team performs to expectations, but also overseeing the wellbeing of the individual people involved and ensuring their needs are met. A practice manager is also expected to ensure that the practice meets its obligations to clients and patients and complies with any relevant legislative requirements. The practice manager ensures that the veterinary practice runs as a profitable, efficient business that provides a good service to clients and patients.

Practice manager duties may include:

- Staff recruitment.
- Staff performance management.
- Budgetary management.
- Creating and updating documents such as job descriptions, policies, procedures, consent forms and an employee handbook.
- Liaising with clients for feedback on their experience with the practice and implementing changes based on that feedback.
- Resolving client and staff grievances.
- Arranging collection of outstanding debts to the practice.
- Advertising the practice and utilising social media.

Moving from a nursing role to practice management may be a daunting transition but the knowledge RVNs have of how a veterinary practice runs and what all of the roles within that practice entails can be invaluable. RVNs driven to move into practice management may benefit from working in a head nurse or clinical nursing manager role first to develop strong leadership and management skills, while leading a smaller team of people in nursing roles, before moving on to managing a larger team with multiple departments. There are also many excellent courses available for learning and improving management skills which may be beneficial, and some veterinary corporate groups offer management training courses free for employees wishing to move from a clinical role into management.

Clinical Director

The role of clinical director is one with a high level of responsibility for the whole practice. The clinical director reports directly to the practice owner(s) and is expected to ensure the practice runs as a successful business. Typically, this role has been undertaken by veterinary surgeons however, an increasing number of RVNs are now taking up these positions. As well as taking responsibility for the performance of the team and clinical outcomes, the clinical director oversees the financial performance of the practice too. Some responsibilities which may be assigned to a clinical director include:

- Quality improvement practices such as clinical auditing, critical event analysis and running morbidity and mortality meetings.
- Managing staff performance.
- Managing the practice budget.
- Setting fees and pricing structures.
- Setting and monitoring key performance indicators (KPIs).

For an RVN at the beginning of their career, the prospect of becoming a clinical director may seem unrealistic or impossible. However, there is no reason that an experienced RVN cannot develop their management skills and progress to this level, if business and leadership are something they are passionate about.

Practice Owner

Opportunities for RVNs to become practice owners are scarce; however, that does not mean it is not possible for an RVN to follow this path. In small animal practice, it is becoming more common for RVNs to invest in practice ownership and some veterinary corporate groups run schemes to allow both RVNs and vets to achieve this. There are obviously financial benefits to practice ownership; however, this is balanced with the stress and risk of investment and so should not be entered into without careful consideration. As it is most likely that an RVN in this position would jointly own the practice with others, it is also important to ensure before entering a partnership that all involved parties are in agreement on the fundamental way in which you wish to run your practice. Becoming a practice owner will mean the freedom to run your practice exactly as you wish and provide a service that is in line with your personal values and in the way you believe a veterinary practice should run. Being able to select the premises and equipment, decide which services to offer and select a team who share the same ethos are all benefits of owning a practice. However, these benefits are balanced with the level of responsibility. Problems with the premises, licensing and legislation requirements, equipment malfunction and breakdown, staff shortages and ultimately the success or failure of the business are all the responsibility of the practice owner.

Roles in Sales and Technical Support

An RVN's knowledge and understanding from clinical practice can be transferred to a role within a company which provides medication, equipment or services to the veterinary industry. The applicable and practical understanding obtained from working in a clinical role in combination with an approachable manner and strong technical knowledge can allow an RVN to excel in these roles.

Pharmaceutical Sales

A scientific understanding of disease processes and medications in combination with the practical experiences of nursing patients and administering medications, make RVNs great candidates for a role in pharmaceutical sales. Being a representative (rep) for a pharmaceutical company usually involves visiting practices and establishing connections within the veterinary industry, to advise customers on suitable products and increase sales and revenue for the company. Typically, sales reps cover a designated area of the country and are expected to travel to the practices within that area. Comprehensive knowledge of all the products being sold is essential to be able to answer any questions the purchasers may have. A good understanding of the conditions the product is licensed to treat is also important so that a rep can provide informative presentations and explain why the product is required and how it works. As with any role in sales, it is very useful to develop relationships with the purchasers, as it is likely when choosing between two products of similar quality, the decision may be made based on who the purchaser would prefer to interact with. A role in this field can allow an RVN to utilise their existing knowledge while developing new skills in sales.

Equipment Sales and Technical Support

Companies that manufacture and sell veterinary equipment such as diagnostic imaging equipment, laboratory equipment or surgical instruments also employ sales reps. Much like pharmaceutical sales, this role involves visiting practices to demonstrate and explain the use of the products and answer any questions. Often equipment sales reps cover a larger territory than the pharmaceutical reps due to the specificity of their products and the lower number of reps. These companies may also employ RVNs as technical advisors, perhaps working remotely answering queries and arranging repairs and replacements by phone and email, or perhaps travelling to practices to do this. With some technical training on the specific products, RVNs are well placed to carry out these roles and have a unique insight having utilised them in practice, which gives an understanding of the practicalities of their use.

Insurance Assessor

Equine insurance companies employ claims assessors who review insurance claims and assess validity or query anomalies. A sound knowledge of conditions affecting horses and how those conditions are treated is essential and therefore RVNs are ideally suited to this role.

19.3 Roles in Education

Moving from clinical practice into education can be a very rewarding pathway for RVNs. Passing on knowledge and clinical skills developed over a nursing career to the next generation of veterinary nurses can provide a sense of giving back to the profession.

Lecturer

RVNs may wish to pass on their knowledge and teach the next generation. As well as opportunities to teach student veterinary nurses and in some instances veterinary students, RVNs are desirable candidates for animal care teaching positions and might also diversify into teaching other science subjects. Some lecturer positions require candidates to have a Bachelor's degree or higher and a postgraduate certificate in education can then be undertaken while teaching. Opportunities to teach part time alongside clinical practice are sometimes available as well as opportunities to teach full time.

Course Leader

A course leader is responsible for the delivery and administration of a veterinary nursing course. A course leader is usually an experienced lecturer who knows the course content well, has delivered it previously and understands the student experience of the course. This role is an excellent opportunity for an RVN in a lecturing position to take on more responsibility within the college or university.

Head of Centre

The head of centre oversees both lecturers and course leaders and takes responsibility for the entire department. This is primarily a management role and requires strong leadership skills. Responsibilities of the head of centre may include:

- Managing teaching and support staff.
- Budget management and allocation of resources.

- Development of courses and the curriculum.
- Dealing with complaints and feedback from students and staff.

An RVN with a combination of management experience and teaching experience may find this role an ideal prospect. For example, an RVN who has worked in a head nurse or practice manager position before moving to education, working as a lecturer and then course leader and wishes to progress to a more challenging role.

Examiner

To become a veterinary nursing examiner for the objective structured clinical examinations (OSCEs), RVNs must complete a training course run by the awarding body they wish to examine for [4]. To be become an examiner, an RVN must have a minimum of four years post-qualification experience. Once the RVN has attended the required training, they will be eligible to examine student veterinary nurses undertaking OSCEs as part of their end point assessment. RVN OSCE examiners are required to attend yearly standardisation sessions run by the awarding body that employs them.

Internal Quality Assurance (IQA)

Veterinary nursing colleges employ IQAs to support students and clinical supervisors in practice. The role primarily involves visiting training practices to meet with students and their clinical supervisors and provide support and guidance as well as assessing progress. The IQA also visits practices for training practice approval and renewal inspections. This role may also include some student support within the college classroom and taking responsibility for provision of clinical supervisor training and standardisation. To become an IQA, a Level 4 qualification in quality assurance will need to be completed.

Exam Question Writer

Veterinary nursing awarding bodies employ writers to create questions for veterinary nursing examinations. Writers provide multiple choice questions with a correct answer and false 'distracter' answers and these are added to a question bank. Questions are continually added to the bank to ensure that the same questions are not used repeatedly, and all learning outcomes are covered. Most question writers are RVNs, and they may be employed by the awarding body or provide content in a self-employed capacity. This is a role which can easily fit around a full-time job in clinical practice and is a good way to develop non-clinical skills and utilise knowledge.

Practice Standards Assessor

The RCVS run a practice standards scheme (PSS) which veterinary practices can join voluntarily and, depending on which criteria they meet, receive a level of accreditation [5]. To join the scheme, an inspection of the practice must be carried out and this is the job of practice standards assessors. The role consists of visiting veterinary practices and assessing all the elements detailed in the scheme requirements, advising on areas which do not meet standards or suggesting ways to achieve a higher level of accreditation. All PSS assessors are veterinary surgeons or RVNs and must have been registered with the RCVS for a minimum of five years, not have left clinical practice more than three years ago and have approval from the RCVS for suitability to carry out inspections.

19.4 Opportunities to Undertake Further Education

Obtaining a veterinary nursing qualification is never the end of learning for an RVN. If academic achievement and the challenge of progressing through higher levels of education are appealing, then there are many opportunities to undertake further education throughout your career either alongside clinical practice or as a standalone endeavour.

RCVS Diploma in Advanced Veterinary Nursing

Previously, equine RVNs working in clinical practice with at least one year of post-qualification experience could undertake the RCVS Diploma in Advanced Veterinary Nursing. This modular course involved studying core subjects and selecting some subjects of interest. Assessment took the form of assignments, written exams, practical exams, a literature review and an oral exam about the literature review. Unfortunately, at the time of writing, this is no longer available in the equine context.

Batchelor's Degree

Several Bachelor's degree courses for ns are available and the veterinary nursing qualification can fulfil the entry requirements for degrees in related subjects such as animal welfare or behaviour. It may also be possible to utilise the veterinary nursing qualification to meet entry requirements for other non-animal related science degrees.

Post Graduate Certificate/Post Graduate Diploma

Following on from a Bachelor's degree, there are some postgraduate courses available. The postgraduate certificate can

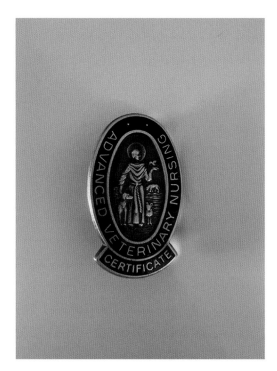

Figure 19.4 The Advanced Veterinary Nursing Certificate badge awarded by the RCVS for completion of an accredited post graduate certificate course. *Source:* Sarah Baillie.

be studied over one to three years if part time and the post graduate diploma in two years. These qualifications can be undertaken as the first year or two years of a master's degree, or as qualifications in their own right. Two equine specific postgraduate certificates are currently offered, one in critical care and one in diagnostic imaging and rehabilitation. A certificate and a badge are awarded after successful completion of these courses (Figure 19.4). Several universities in the United Kingdom offer these courses in general veterinary nursing related to One Health subjects, and many of the units are broadly applicable to all species of veterinary patients and/or veterinary nursing specialisations.

Master's Degree

There are a few Master's degrees open to RVNs in subjects such as advanced practice, veterinary education and One Health. Courses may involve full or part-time study, some are taught in person and some online. To obtain a master's degree, core and optional modules must be completed before undertaking a research study. It is possible to complete a master's degree while working full time in practice however, it does require a commitment of around 15 hours per week to study and complete assignments. The financial cost of a master's degree is significant but options for financial support are available. It may be possible to utilise your practice CPD allowance towards tuition fees, there are also several veterinary bursaries which may be applied for, a student loan may be helpful, and universities allow fees to be paid in instalments to spread the cost over the year.

Doctorate Degree

RVNs who have completed a master's degree may choose to continue their studies and obtain a doctorate degree. Doctor of Philosophy (PhD) opportunities are competitively sought and obtaining funding can be challenging. However, these obstacles are not insurmountable and if an RVN is driven to follow this academic path, it is entirely possible. Part-time PhD opportunities are available in some instances and would allow an RVN to continue practicing at least part time. Some RVNs choose to leave their clinical role and study full time in order to complete their doctorate degree more quickly.

19.5   Roles in Research

Veterinary nursing research may still be in its infancy compared to our human nursing counterparts, but it is rapidly growing thanks to increasing opportunities brought by the increasing numbers of further education pathways available. The development of awareness and understanding of One Health and increasing awareness of the links between public health and animal health, provide even more scope for RVNs to get involved in research.

Research Assistant

Some RVNs may find that in carrying out research during further education, they develop an interest or passion for generating new veterinary nursing research. It is possible to move from veterinary nursing to a full-time research position or to combine clinical work with a research role. One way to do this is to become a research assistant, usually at a university.

A research assistant plays an active role in carrying out studies and contributes directly to the research they are assigned. Some of the ways they may do this include:

- Recruiting and managing study participants.
- Carrying out literature reviews.
- Collecting data and data analysis.
- Obtaining equipment and supplies required for the study.
- Creating and distributing questionnaires for data collection.
- Conducting and recording interviews for data collection.
- Managing the allocated budget for the study.

- Sourcing funding.
- Providing progress reports throughout the research process.
- Maintaining data protection.

Research Compliance Officer

A research compliance officer is responsible for ensuring all legislative and ethical requirements for veterinary research are met. This role requires an excellent understanding of the research process, the legal requirements for producing research, the ethics review process, publishing process, funding application process and data protection requirements. Some duties of a research compliance officer may include:

- Reviewing and advising on research proposals.
- Reviewing and advising on publishing completed research.
- Assisting with obtaining ethical approval for a study.
- Assisting with funding applications for research.
- Advising researchers on data protection.

19.6   Charitable Volunteering of Time and Skills

Animal charities around the world welcome RVNs and offer volunteering opportunities. Volunteering abroad is a great way to visit regions that are not typically seen by tourists, and it allows you to experience different cultures and meet local people in an authentic situation. Some charities provide accommodation and meals for volunteers and some long-term positions even offer a small wage. Volunteering opportunities are also available within the United Kingdom at various equine and animal charities, and these are a great option if oversees travel is not possible, or for more regular, or occasional days volunteering. Volunteering presents many challenges and an opportunity to solve unconventional problems, which can be very rewarding (Figure 19.5).

19.7   Career Sustainability

As with any career, veterinary nursing comes with challenges and drawbacks in contrast to the rewarding elements and job satisfaction. Equine veterinary nursing is a vocation that most enter with a passion for improving their patients' lives and advocating for equids in need of care. The sense of satisfaction that comes from utilising clinical skills, knowledge and experience to nurse animals is motivation to go to work each day. But what happens when that motivation is no longer enough?

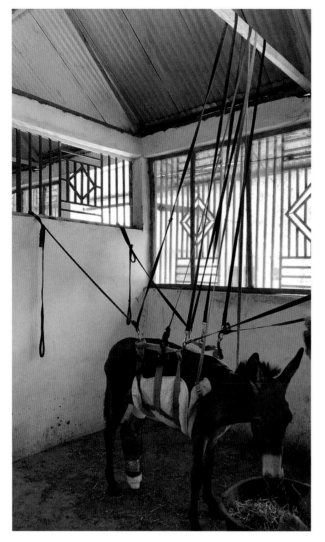

Figure 19.5 A donkey with a fractured leg and injuries from a road traffic accident in The Gambia, Africa. This patient required a sling which was created out of lunge lines, girths and transport straps. *Source:* Sarah Baillie.

For some, finding the area of practice which interests them the most and staying within that area to grow and develop as an RVN is the best pathway. For others they may wish to move between the many options available to an RVN in a way that allows them to find new challenges, and refresh their passion for the industry. What is best for one RVN may be the worst approach for another, and taking time to self-reflect regularly can ensure that you understand your personal preferences and motivations, to allow you to continue to thrive in equine veterinary nursing.

As this chapter shows there are a large number of options for career progression and this list is not exhaustive. The clinical and non-clinical skills of an RVN are largely transferable and the options to utilise them are vast.

References

1 College of Animal Welfare (2022). Veterinary physiotherapist career profile. www.caw.ac.uk/careers/veterinary-physiotherapist (accessed 13 February 2022).

2 VetSkill (2022). Becoming a suitably qualified person (SQP). www.vetskill.com/sqp/become-an-sqp (accessed 13 February 2022).

3 Jankovic, S. (2018). Could you offer a veterinary pharmacy service? *The Pharmaceutical Journal* https://doi.org/10.1211/PJ.2018.20205345.

4 Royal College of Veterinary Surgeons (2007). New VN examiner dates announced. https://www.rcvs.org.uk/news-and-views/news/new-vn-examiner-course-date-announced (accessed 13 February 2022).

5 Royal College of Veterinary Surgeons (2022). Practice standards scheme. https://www.rcvs.org.uk/setting-standards/practice-standards-scheme (accessed 13 February 2022).

Further Reading

www.rcvs.org.uk/veterinary-careeers/
www.bvna/careers/
www.beva.org.uk/nurses
www.baedt.com

Index

Textbook of Equine Veterinary Nursing, First Edition. Edited by Rosina Lillywhite and Marie Rippingale.
© 2025 John Wiley & Sons Ltd. Published 2025 by John Wiley & Sons Ltd.
Companion website: www.wiley.com/go/equineveterinarynursing